TEXTBOOK OF Laboratory and Diagnostic Testing

Practical Application at the Bedside

TEXTBOOK OF Laboratory and Diagnostic Testing

Practical Application at the Bedside

Anne M. Van Leeuwen, MA, BS, MT (ASCP)
Medical Laboratory Scientist & Independent Author
Greater Seattle Area, Washington

Mickey Bladh, RN, BSN, MSN
PIH Health Hospital
Nurse Educator, Training Center Coordinator
Los Angeles, California

F. A. DAVIS COMPANY • Philadelphia

F. A. Davis Company
1915 Arch Street
Philadelphia, PA 19103
www.fadavis.com

Printed in the United States of America

Last digit indicates print number: 10 9 8 7 6 5 4 3 2 1

Publisher, Nursing: Lisa B. Houck
Content Project Manager I: Julia L. Curcio
Design & Illustrations Manager: Carolyn O'Brien

As new scientific information becomes available through basic and clinical research, recommended
treatments and drug therapies undergo changes. The author(s) and publisher have done everything possible
to make this book accurate, up to date, and in accord with accepted standards at the time of publication.
The author(s), editors, and publisher are not responsible for errors or omissions or for consequences from
application of the book, and make no warranty, expressed or implied, in regard to the contents of the
book. Any practice described in this book should be applied by the reader in accordance with professional
standards of care used in regard to the unique circumstances that may apply in each situation. The reader is
advised always to check product information (package inserts) for changes and new information regarding
dose and contraindications before administering any drug. Caution is especially urged when using new or
infrequently ordered drugs.

Library of Congress Cataloging-in-Publication Data

Van Leeuwen, Anne M., author.
  Textbook of laboratory and diagnostic testing : practical application at
the bedside / Anne M. Van Leeuwen, Mickey Bladh.
    p. ; cm.
  Includes bibliographical references and index.
  ISBN 978-0-8036-2315-6—ISBN 0-8036-2315-1
  I. Bladh, Mickey Lynn, author. II. Title.
  [DNLM: 1. Clinical Laboratory Techniques—Case Reports. 2. Nursing
Diagnosis—methods—Case Reports. 3. Point-of-Care Systems—Case Reports.
QY 25]
  RT48.5
  616.07'5—dc23
                                                      2015015982

The connection between mind and body is sought by many people probing for answers on multiple levels.

My contribution to this distinctive text is dedicated to all the wonderful individuals whose passion is to be a nurse, especially those who have touched my life in so many ways. Mom, Lynda, Adele, and Mickey, you exemplify those heroes who demonstrate with perfect clarity how the Art of Nursing is a conduit into an amazing connection. Thank you to all my family, friends, and canine fans for supporting my efforts in coauthoring this book. My heartfelt thanks and appreciation to Lisa Houck, Rob Allen, Victoria White, and Julie Scardiglia—without your confidence, patience, and great skill, this book would not have been possible.

Anne M. Van Leeuwen, MA, BS, MT (ASCP)
Medical Laboratory Scientist and Independent Author
Greater Seattle Area, Washington

I am the proud mother of five wonderful children and am lucky to be married to the love of my life. They are the fire that keeps me going. My nursing career began as a volunteer at the age of 17, followed by working as a Certified Nursing Assistant, and then as a Registered Nurse. I have not just seen but experienced all aspects of clinical care. I would like to thank all of those nurses in my past who assisted in growing my clinical mind. Their kind contributions have allowed me to share the nursing wisdom I have gained with all of you. My work on this book is dedicated to every person with the dream of "becoming" a nurse. My desire is to help you to be successful. Your success is my success. Thanks to Julie, Victoria, and especially Anne for believing in the dream, and for all of the hard work of those at F.A. Davis. Last, I would like to thank my parents Buddy and Kay Harms who told me that I could achieve anything in this life with hard work. Thanks for believing in me, Mom and Dad—I miss you every day.

Mickey Bladh, RN, BSN, MSN
PIH Health Hospital
Nurse Educator, Training Center Coordinator
Los Angeles, California

Preface

Nursing is not for the faint of heart. This book was written for the love of the profession and the hope that the information provided can help you, our up-and-coming nursing generation, find your clinical feet. We believe the very best way to do this is to take diverse content and combine it for the best possible mix of unique nursing knowledge. We, the authors of this book, take that responsibility very seriously. Our goal in the development and presentation of the material within these pages is to take you on a journey of exploration that we call safe, effective nursing care (SENC). Each chapter was purposely designed to help you to figure out how to best care for your patients. Our goal is to help you provide the very best care possible to every single patient in various clinical settings. It is our sincere hope that by designing this book to be a practical text, you will find it useful during your years as a student and beyond into practice.

In considering feedback from experienced and novice nurses regarding "information overload," we decided to take a very different approach in the design of this textbook. This book is not intended to be used as a comprehensive reference for data, as it pertains to the interpretation of laboratory and diagnostic findings. We have already accomplished that in the publication, *Davis's Comprehensive Handbook of Laboratory and Diagnostic Testing with Nursing Implications.* We decided this book should focus on teaching ways to identify key aspects of ancillary testing and incorporate them into the application of nursing practice. Our Section I chapters provide a good mix of technical study-specific information, nursing implications, and a number of Learning Outcomes from which students should develop awareness of elements required to provide safe, effective nursing care (SENC). By providing examples of each type of ancillary testing, our goal is to help the student could see how all the data types they are required to learn about can be managed by consistent incorporation into the familiar framework of the nursing process. SENC includes mastery of core competencies and standards of care; it is based on a judicious application of nursing knowledge in combination with scientific principles. Our strong belief is that the Art of Nursing lies in blending knowledge with the ability to effectively apply that knowledge in a compassionate manner. For this reason, these thoughts about SENC are used to introduce the concepts of core competencies (Thinking, Doing, Caring) to the Learning Outcomes in each chapter. Thinking, Doing, Caring are also known, in other models, as KSAs (knowledge, skills, and attitude). We prepared case studies for the student to test his or her own ability to develop a successful frame of reference for day-to-day practice. The Clinical Reasoning Tool provides a framework for providing SENC in each patient encounter you experience as a nurse—it is up to you to learn how to best apply the Art of Nursing in your chosen profession.

About this Book

As authors, we recognize that some truths about writing on the topic of nursing practice are self-evident. First, we consider this book to be a living document and welcome any suggestions that will assist us to better help you reach your clinical goals. Second, as seasoned health-care professionals, we recognize that the reality of modern-day nursing includes a diverse population of speakers of English as a second language and older adults who choose nursing as a second or late-in-life career. Third, as students ourselves, we recognize the desire of the adult learner to be provided with information that is relevant and efficient. Last, we acknowledge that varied approaches in providing information help to match learning styles and make it easier to learn. It is for these reasons that we have included tables, photos, and illustrations to facilitate understanding of the content. The language used within the text itself was styled to be informal and inviting. We also acknowledge that time is a valuable commodity. Our success with this book is measured by its ability to save you time while assisting you to understand laboratory and diagnostic studies associated with patient care.

This book is divided into two sections. Each section can be used as a stand-alone, commonsense resource for the learner or in combination as an integrative approach to patient care. We organized the book with the goal of making information available "at your fingertips":

- *Section I, Understanding Laboratory and Diagnostic Testing,* presents commonly used laboratory and diagnostic studies in a simple-to-understand format. The format was specifically selected to walk you through the *Hows* and *Whys* of laboratory and diagnostic tools that are used in clinical situations. This approach individualizes learning and fosters clinical reasoning in patient care.
- *Section II, Clinical Reasoning Tool Case Studies: Applying Laboratory and Diagnostic Testing Clinically,* provides case studies designed to provide a step-by-step approach to the use of nursing process in a meaningful way. Cases have been developed to mimic real-life clinical situations and outcomes. Although presented most often as a linear concept, nursing process is really a dynamic, in-the-moment interactive investigative tool to develop an action plan for care. Nursing process helps us to see the why, what, when, where, and how of any clinical situation. People

learn through a combination of reading, seeing, and doing. To enhance the *"knowing how"* piece of nursing, we have updated the traditional linear nursing process and refashioned it into a visual format called the *Clinical Reasoning Tool*. This format allows you to see how the nursing process works and to learn to integrate nursing activities with clinical reasoning within the context of patient care, essentially not just learning but *seeing* how to think like a nurse.

Section I—Understanding Laboratory and Diagnostic Testing

Understanding how to integrate diagnostic and laboratory studies into a clinical experience in a meaningful way can be a challenge. Our goal is to make this easier for you. Coordination of patient care in relation to laboratory and diagnostic studies requires a clear understanding of three key concepts: (1) what the laboratory or diagnostic study is used for, (2) what the patient needs to know, and (3) any special preparation required for a procedure or to collect a specimen. This section of the book is a rich blend of scientific and commonsense information to assist in doing just that.

The Section I chapters are organized alphabetically by test category to allow for easy access of information; for example, the blood studies are listed in five distinct chapters beginning with <u>B</u>lood Studies: Clinical Chemistry through Blood Studies: Immunology, followed by <u>C</u>omputed Tomography Studies, and so on.

Each chapter includes an overview specific to the test category, a selection of related learning outcomes, an alphabetically arranged study listing followed by the detailed studies with nursing implications, a review of the learning outcomes, a thought-provoking section named Words of Wisdom, and the Bibliography.

Overview

Understanding why a laboratory or diagnostic study is being performed, how it is performed, and what it can tell you in relation to your patient is essential to providing good nursing care. Each study is presented in a commonsense way to answer those questions for you by breaking the information into chunks. We deliberately framed study information in nursing format to help you connect the dots between doing a task and understanding the meaning of that task in relation to patient care. Each laboratory and diagnostic procedure begins with the study name, what the study is most commonly used for, how the study is applied, and what the normal results would be. From there, the clinical significance of the laboratory or diagnostic study is reviewed in a nursing process format:

- **Assessment** links medical diagnoses and nursing problems to better understand their relationship and make it easier for you to connect the clinical dots.
- **Diagnosis** helps you to consider the abnormal findings and the clinical significance of the study results.
- **Planning** reviews what you should do and say in preparing your patient for the study to be performed.
- **Implementation** helps you to understand what you need to do for the performance of each study.
- **Evaluation** provides direction on what to do after the study has been completed.
- Communicating **critical findings** to the physician and assisting the patient and family in dealing with the study outcome is discussed.
- Because you may have questions about what other studies might be done for a similar situation, we have provided you with that information also. Each study has its own unique set of **expected outcomes** framed in goals for the study itself and, just as importantly, in goals for the patient who is experiencing the study. *Safety Tips* are built in throughout the discussions to prompt you to double-check specific points before proceeding.
- The *Overview* section provides general information about the type of laboratory or diagnostic studies that will be discussed.
- Information is organized in a way to help nursing students see how the five basic components of the nursing process can be applied to each phase of laboratory and diagnostic testing. The goal is to use nursing process to understand the integration of care (laboratory, diagnostic, nursing care) toward achieving a positive expected outcome. The basic tenants of nursing process—assessment, diagnosis, planning, implementation, and evaluation—are interwoven into each individual study and supported by Universal Pearls that focus on specific aspects of laboratory and diagnostic inquiry such as pretest (planning), intratest (implementation), and post-test (evaluation).
- *Universal Pretest Pearls (Planning).* Pretest pearls contain universal planning reminders to
  - Obtain pertinent clinical, laboratory, dietary, and therapeutic history of the patient, especially as it pertains to comparison of previous test results, and preparation for the test.
  - Provide a simple explanation that presents the patient with the requirements and restrictions related to the procedure as well as what to expect during the procedure.
  - Anticipate and allay patient and family concerns or anxieties with consideration for social and cultural issues during interactions.
- *Universal Intratest Pearls (Implementation).* Intratest pearls contain a number of universal implementation reminders to
  - Follow institutional policies for patient safety, especially as it pertains to providing positive patient identification using at least two person-specific identifiers.
  - Ensure the patient has complied with pretest requirements.
- *Universal Post-Test Pearls (Evaluation).* Post-test pearls contain various universal evaluation reminders to
  - Communicate critical findings to the requesting health-care provider (HCP).
  - Provide study-specific information and education to the patient and family.

Learning Outcomes

Each chapter's learning outcomes are offered as suggestions of valuable information to be obtained during the chapter review. These student learning objectives can act as a self-assessment tool that reflects how well you understand the content; they can help you discover areas you may need to review. Answers to each learning objective are given at the end of the chapter as a way to validate understanding.

Detailed Studies

The detailed studies are presented in alphabetical order for ease of access to the desired information. The goal of integrating nursing process with the studies presented is to help you understand how to link and integrate laboratory and diagnostic information with patient care. Understanding why a laboratory or diagnostic study is being performed, how it is performed, and what it can tell you in relation to your patient is essential to providing good nursing care. Each study is presented in a commonsense way to answer those questions for you by breaking the information into chunks:

- FEATURES: Discussion points, contraindications, general complications, safety tips, notes, and special considerations are identified for individual studies and groups of studies to highlight key points necessary for safe and effective practice. The detailed studies utilize a consistent format that includes these features.
- QUICK SUMMARY: Each laboratory and diagnostic procedure begins with a Quick Summary that provides the study name, what the study is most

commonly used for, how the study is applied, and what the normal results would be. From there the clinical significance of the laboratory or diagnostic study is reviewed in a nursing process format. Additional information is provided in each Quick Summary:

- *Synonyms* and *Acronyms* are listed where appropriate.
- *Common Use* is included to assist you to identify the most typical use of any specific laboratory or diagnostic study in the clinical setting. This information can be used as an educational tool for the patient and family as well as for yourself.

- **SPECIMEN:** In the case of laboratory studies, a *Specimen* section includes the type of specimen usually collected and, where appropriate, the type of collection tube or container commonly recommended. Specimen requirements vary by laboratory. The amount of specimen collected is usually more than what is minimally required so that additional specimen is available, if needed, for repeat testing (e.g., quality-control failure, dilutions, or confirmation of unexpected results).

- **AREA OF APPLICATION:** In the case of diagnostic studies, the *area of application* is given.

- **NORMAL FINDINGS:** *Normal findings* for each study include variations, when indicated, for age, gender, and ethnicity. For laboratory studies, it is important to consider the normal variation of values over the life span and across cultures; that sometimes what might be considered an abnormal value in one circumstance is actually what is expected in another; and that laboratory values can vary by method, and therefore, laboratory normal ranges are listed along with the associated methodology. Normal findings for laboratory tests are given in conventional and standard international (SI) units. The factor used to convert conventional to SI units is also given.

- **TEST EXPLANATION:** The *Test Explanation* section includes detailed information pertaining to the study's purpose and insight into how and why the test results can affect health. Some test descriptions also provide insight into how test results influence the development of national health guidelines.

- **ASSESSMENT:** The *Assessment* section lists the main indications for the study and some of the associated potential nursing problems. Assessment links medical diagnoses and nursing problems to better understand their relationship and make it easier for you to connect the clinical dots.

- **DIAGNOSIS:** The *Diagnosis* section presents a list of conditions in which findings may be abnormal, increased, or decreased, and in some cases, an explanation of variations that may be encountered. Diagnosis helps you to consider the abnormal

findings and the clinical significance of the study results.

- **PLANNING:** The *Planning* section reviews what you should do and say in preparing your patient for the study to be performed. Other study-specific information to consider in the care plan are contraindications and interfering factors:
  - *Contraindications* or circumstances that might put the patient at risk if the procedure is performed should be known prior to performance of the study.
  - *Interfering factors* are substances or circumstances that may influence the results of the test, rendering the results invalid or unreliable. Knowledge of interfering factors is an important aspect of quality assurance and includes pharmaceuticals, foods, natural and additive therapies, timing of the study in relation to other studies or procedures, specimen collection site, specimen handling, and underlying patient conditions.

- **IMPLEMENTATION:** The *Implementation* section helps you to understand what you need to do for the performance of each study.

- **EVALUATION:** The *Evaluation* section provides direction on what to do after the study has been completed. Examples might include
  - Specific monitoring and therapeutic measures that should be performed after the procedure (e.g., maintaining bedrest, obtaining vital signs to compare with baseline values, and observing signs and symptoms of complications)
  - Specific instructions for the patient and family, such as when to resume usual diet, medications, and activity
  - General nutritional guidelines related to excess or deficit as well as common food sources for dietary replacement
  - Indications for interventions from public health representatives or for special counseling related to test outcomes
  - Indications for follow-up testing that may be required within specific time frames

- **CRITICAL FINDINGS:** Communicating results that may be life-threatening or for which particular concern may be indicated is addressed in the *Critical Findings* section. Laboratory findings are given in conventional and SI units, along with age-span considerations where applicable. This section also includes signs and symptoms associated with a critical finding as well as possible nursing interventions and the nurse's role in communication of critical findings to the appropriate HCP.

- **STUDY-SPECIFIC COMPLICATIONS:** Health status can be complicated by the existence of multiple conditions or circumstances that lead to postprocedural complications. The *Study-Specific Complications* section lists the associated problems a patient may encounter after completing a laboratory or diagnostic study.

- **RELATED TESTS:** Because you may have questions about what other studies might be done for a similar situation, we have provided you with that information also. The alphabetical listing of related laboratory and/or diagnostic tests is intended to provoke a deeper and broader investigation of multiple pieces of information; the tests provide data that, when combined, can form a more complete picture of health or illness.

- **EXPECTED OUTCOMES:** The additional information included in the *Expected Outcomes* section is another opportunity to "drill" further down into the nursing implications. It is provided as a reminder of the nurse's role as educator and advocate for additional SENC teaching moments.

Review of Chapter Learning Outcomes

The review of learning objectives at the end of each chapter can be used as a self-assessment for understanding the concepts just discussed. All objectives are meant to be thought-provoking and meaningful.

Words of Wisdom

The contents of this section were created to instigate opportunities for self-reflection; it is provided to stimulate consideration of the intended and unintended impact that our attitudes and actions may have on a patient's experience.

Section II: Clinical Reasoning Tool Case Studies: Applying Laboratory and Diagnostic Testing Clinically

One of the greatest challenges of becoming a nurse is in understanding how to use nursing process in a practical way rather than as an abstract concept. We recognize that clinical learning occurs best within the context of patient care. Section II uses case studies to take you by the hand and walk you through how to think like a nurse. Two case studies are provided for each body system, one common and one uncommon. One full set of cases is found in Section II, and the second set is found on the F.A. Davis website (www.davisplus.com).

Cases are purposely written to reflect actual practice, including possible errors, uncooperative patients, family issues that can obstruct care, and imperfections in critical thinking. Case studies are presented as if you are the nurse in the room caring for the patient. You will be challenged to discover where those issues lie, identify them, and address them within the nursing role. The goal is to engage you in not just thinking about what you should do but in thinking about what might happen with the choices made.

Each case is presented in 10 steps. Cases are identified by body system and are linked with the laboratory and diagnostic studies presented in Section I. An added bonus to Section II is the Clinical Reasoning Tool. This tool has been designed by us to move nursing process away from an abstract concept to one in which you can actually see it in action. This is an invaluable tool for visual learners and learners of English as a second language. Each of the 10 steps is represented within this tool.

Step 1, Data Collection, begins each case with data collection, discussing pathophysiology, signs and symptoms, laboratory studies, diagnostic studies, and general medical management. This is meant to be an overview of how to manage a patient with a specific type of diagnosis. The Clinical Reasoning Tool allows you to see yourself walking the Nursing Pathway as data are collected, bringing a concrete feeling to an abstract process.

Step 2, Potential Problem/Diagnoses, encourages you to think about what potential nursing problems could arise based on the information gathered during data collection. You are encouraged to ask yourselves, "based upon your review of the content presented in Step 1, what potential problems would you expect for a patient with this diagnosis?" We want you to mentally walk into the Diagnoses corridor of the Clinical Reasoning Tool and create a working list of potential nursing problems.

Step 3, Potential Interventions and Expected Outcome, asks you to now select potential interventions for the potential problems you have just identified and describe what the expected outcome would be. A question is posed: "based upon the identification of patient problems, what possible interventions would you recommend for these diagnoses, and what would you expect to happen?" This would be considered your "grocery list" of the possible actions you could use to assist your patient. Visually, this is represented as the Interventions corridor on the Clinical Reasoning Tool. Picture yourself walking into this corridor and, just like a grocery store, place your interventions into the mental checkout cart to be taken out and used later.

Putting It All Together is where you are going to be challenged to blend the art and science of nursing to provide the best patient outcomes. We will ask you to take the possible problems and interventions and place them into the context of a patient situation.

To accomplish this, you will be directed to use Nursing Diagnosis, Nursing Interventions, Nursing Outcomes, and Nursing Theory to provide the palate for nursing care. Visually see yourself within the Clinical Reasoning Tool moving from the abstract concept of thinking about the care to the concrete act of doing the care. Patients, who are the point of it all, are located at the center of the hub of the wheel.

Step 4, Assessment, **introduces your patient with demographics of age, gender, and ethnicity. The chief complaint is provided along with history of present illness, past medical history, and family history.** Patient assessment information is provided by a chart review and shift report, combined with both a subjective and an objective assessment. The discussions with the patient are interactive, as if you were standing in the room with the patient and having the discussion described.

Step 5, Reality Check, **is where we take a moment and ask you to consider what may be happening in the patient's life that can have an impact on your plan.** Each case presents information about the patient that will have a positive or negative impact on that plan. The Clinical Reasoning Tool visually represents this step as the Reality Check corridor that links the patient at the hub of the tool to the nursing pathway at the outer rim. Mentally you have to walk into this corridor to discover what the "wrenches" are that create challenging situations in patient care. This is to act as a reminder that if the plan is not congruent with the patient's needs, then it does not work. **A *Critical Thinking Moment* reminds you that you have just completed your assessment and you need to make a decision on the patient's actual problems and nursing diagnoses based on the data you have collected and the potential problems you identified.** Outcomes must be realistic and measurable.

Step 6, Actual Problems/Diagnoses, **takes you one step further in problem identification and asks you to use the Clinical Reasoning Tool and revisit the list of potential diagnoses and choose actual diagnoses based on your interaction with patient, family, or others, as well as the assessment of the case study information provided.**

Step 7, Planning: Actual Interventions, **focuses on development of a plan and asks you to go back to your "grocery list" of potential interventions and now choose actual interventions that will fit with the actual diagnoses you just selected.** They should blend with the patient's reality and meet expected outcomes. Interventions are discussed in three categories: (1) assessment (what you need to look for), (2) therapeutic (what you need to do), and (3) education (what you need to tell the patient or family). Expected outcomes must be identified. You never implement an intervention without knowing what you expect to see happen.

Step 8, Implementation, **is the application of the plan. Here you are asked to consider your resources, and what or whom you need to help you implement the plan.** Nursing theorists have a lot of great ideas on how best to approach doing the job. We emphasize using multiple theorists for different aspects of care. We have created a table for the Practical Application of Nursing Theory, placed at the end of the book, to help you understand how to do this. No one eats the same food every day. Our food selections will vary depending on the situation. The nursing theories we use will also vary with the situation. The Clinical Reasoning Tool asks you to consider how to apply nursing theory in a commonsense way. Ancillary support is discussed as part of the equation of who can help you. Judicious use of resources, such as respiratory therapy, physical therapy, social services, case management, and more, is a nursing role.

Step 9, Plan of Care, **acknowledges the importance of creating a Plan of Care as a road map for patient care and a communication tool between disciplines.** Review of expected entries on the plan of care is discussed within each case.

Step 10, Evaluation, **is the end of the case.** Here you will be asked to evaluate the success of your plan. Were your goals met, partially met, or not met? If your goals were met, you can continue with the plan as outlined; if your goals were partially met, you need to revise the parts of the plan that did not work; if the goals were not met, you have to start all over with a new plan. Each case provides you with an end-of-shift narrative report that allows you to experience case closure in real time. Once this has been done, you will finish the case by answering the question that should be on your mind every time you do patient care: is my patient getting better, getting worse, or is there no change?

A valuable tool for nursing thought and action is the body of knowledge known as *Nursing Theory.* Each theorist provides her or his own unique perspective on the hows and whys of patient care. No one theorist has all of the answers, but each one provides direction for some aspect of doing the job. The table is designed to simplify theory into usable nuggets of information that you can use every day when interacting with patients and family. As nurses, we need to use all of our available resources. Please consider using the wisdom of those who have come before you to be successful in your chosen career.

DavisPlus

The following online materials can be found on the Davis*Plus* website (www.davisplus.com):

Appendices

A. Patient Preparation and Specimen Collection
- A summary of guidelines for preparing a patient to undergo laboratory and diagnostic studies, with considerations for special patient populations.
- The guidelines describe the types of specimen collection procedures and materials used in specimen collection.

B. Guidelines for Age-Specific Communication
- Age-specific nursing care guidelines with suggested approaches to persons at various developmental stages to assist the provider in facilitating cooperation and understanding

C. Introduction to CLIA
- Introduction to CLIA (Clinical Laboratory Improvement Amendments) with an explanation of the different levels of laboratory testing complexity and requirements for CLIA certification at each level

D. Transfusion Reactions: Laboratory Findings and Potential Nursing Interventions
- Transfusion reactions, their signs and symptoms, associated laboratory findings, and potential nursing interventions

E. Effects of Natural Products
- Herbs and nutraceuticals associated with adverse clinical reactions or drug interactions listed by body system

Interactive Case Studies

- Interactive Case Studies for students are formatted to help the novice learn how to clinically reason by using the nursing process to solve problems. Cases are purposefully designed to promote a discussion of situations that may occur in the clinical setting. Situations may be medical, ethical, family related, patient related, nurse related, or any combination.

Fast Find: Lab & Dx

- A searchable library of all Laboratory and Diagnostic Tests included within this textbook, along with monographs of additional related studies, is available online.

Audio Glossary

- Audio pronunciations of over 150 laboratory and diagnostic terms with written definitions.

Assumptions

- The authors recognize that preferences for the use of specific medical terminology may vary by institution. Much of the terminology used in this textbook is sourced from *Taber's Cyclopedic Medical Dictionary*, 22nd ed.
- The definition, implementation, and interpretation of national guidelines for the treatment of various medical conditions changes as new information and new technology emerge. The publication of updated information may at times be contentious among the professional institutions that offer either support or dissent for the proposed changes. This can cause confusion when a patient asks questions about how his or her condition will be identified and managed. The authors believe that the most important discussion about health care occurs between the patient and his or her health-care provider(s). While the individual studies may point out various screening tests used to identify a disease, the authors often refer the reader to websites maintained by nationally recognized authorities on a specific topic that reflect the most current information and recommendations for screening, diagnosis, and treatment.
- Most institutions have established policies, protocols, and interdisciplinary teams that provide for efficient and effective patient care within the appropriate scope of practice. While it is not our intention that the actual duties a nurse may perform be misunderstood due to misinterpreted inferences in writing style, the information prepared by the authors considers that specific limitations are understood by the licensed professionals and other team members involved in patient care activities, and that the desired outcomes are achieved by order of the appropriate health-care provider.

Reviewers

Marianne Adam, PhD, RN, CRNP
Assistant Professor
Moravian College
Bethlehem, Pennsylvania

Jocelyn Anderson, RN, MN
Skills Lab Instructor
Bellevue College
Bellevue, Washington

Ramona Anest, MSN, RNC-TNP, CNE
Associate Professor
Bob Jones University
Greenville, South Carolina

Candyce F. Antley, RN, MN
Instructor
Midlands Technical College
Columbia, South Carolina

Lisa Aymong, MS, MPA, BS, RN, APRN
Associate Professor
Suffolk County Community College
Selden, New York

Kathy Batton, PhD, RN-BC
Nursing Instructor
Hinds Community College
Jackson, Mississippi

Julia Behr, RN, DNP, APRN-BC
Assistant Dean for CONAT
Georgia Health Sciences University
Athens, Georgia

Susan J. Brillhart, DNS(c), RN, PNP-BC
Assistant Professor, Nursing
City University of New York
Assistant Professor, Nursing
Borough of Manhattan Community College
New York, New York

Ruth Chaplen, RN, DNP, APRN-BC, AOCN
Assistant Professor, Clinical
College of Nursing
Wayne State University
Oncology Nurse Practitioner
Adult Health Nursing
Karmanos Cancer Institute
Detroit, Michigan

Jennifer Chapman-Bullock, MSN, BSN, RN
Nursing Lab Director
Trident Technical College
Charleston, South Carolina

Kelly Coffin, RN, MSN, CCRN
Assistant Professor of Nursing
Colorado Mesa University
Grand Junction, Colorado

Theresa Cooper, RN, MSN, MBA
Clinical Educator
Wichita State University
Wichita, Kansas

Tina Cormio, RN, MSN, ANP
Professor of Nursing
Middlesex Community College
Lowell, Massachusetts

Denise Davidson, RN, MSN, CNE
Assistant Professor of Nursing
Montgomery County Community College
Blue Bell, Pennsylvania

Karen de la Cruz, MSN, AACNP/FNP
Assistant Teaching Professor
College of Nursing
Brigham Young University
Provo, Utah

Doreen DeAngelis, MSN, RN
Instructor
Penn State University, Fayette Campus
LaMont Furnace, Pennsylvania

Laurie DeGroot, RN, MSN, GCNS-BC
Associate Degree Nursing Instructor and Program Leader
North Iowa Area Community College
Mason City, Iowa

Debbie Dollmeyer, RN, MSN, ANP-C
Professor of Nursing
Scottsdale Community College
Scottsdale, Arizona

Rowena W. Elliott, PhD, RN, CNN, BC, CNE
Associate Professor
University of Southern Mississippi
Hattiesburg, Mississippi

Deborah Ellis, RN, MSN, NP-C

Associate Professor of Nursing
Missouri Western State University
St. Joseph, Missouri

Sally Erdel, MS, RN, CNE

Associate Professor of Nursing, Coordinator of
    Pre-Licensure Programs at Bethel Campus
Bethel College
Mishawaka, Indiana

Maria C. Farber, MSN, RN, BC, OCN

Instructor, Nursing Education
Middlesex County College
Edison, New Jersey

Sandra G. Fleischmann, MSN, RN-BC

Nurse Faculty
Southern Vermont College
Bennington, Vermont

Stephanie Franks, RN, MSN

Nursing Professor
St. Louis Community College, Meramec
St. Louis, Missouri

Margaret Fried, RN, MA, CNE

Adjunct Faculty
Pima Community College
Tucson, Arizona

Jason T. Garbarino, RN, MSN

Clinical Educator
University of Vermont
Burlington, Vermont

Pamela Gwin, MSN, RN-BC, CNE

Assistant Professor
College of the Mainland
Texas City, Texas

Rose Hasenmiller, RNC, MSN, CNM

Assistant Professor, Nursing Faculty
St. Ambrose University
Davenport, Iowa

Jayme G. Haynes, MSN, RN

Nursing Instructor
Pikes Peak Community College
Colorado Springs, Colorado

Amy Zlomek Hedden, RN, MS, NP

Associate Professor, Department of Nursing
California State University, Bakersfield
Bakersfield, California

Theresa Hoadley, PhD, RN, TNS

Associate Professor
Saint Francis Medical Center College of Nursing
Peoria, Illinois

Theresa M. Holsan, RN, DNP, FNP-C

Instructor
Regis University
Denver, Colorado

Charlene C. Hopkins, MSN, RN, CNE

Nursing Instructor
Western Technical College
La Crosse, Wisconsin

Karla Huntsman, RN, BSN, MSN/Ed

Faculty Member, Nursing Program
AmeriTech College
Draper, Utah

Mary Ann Johnston, RN, MSN

Lecturer in Nursing
California State University, Stanislaus
Turlock, California

Ellen Ketcherside, RN, CCRN, MA

Nursing Professor
Mineral Area College
Park Hills, Missouri

Norma Krumwiede, EdD, RN

Professor of Nursing
Minnesota State University
Mankato, Minnesota

Dawn Kuerschner, MSN, APN-BC, CNE

Associate Professor of Nursing
Oakton Community College
Des Plaines, Illinois

Laurel R. Lalicker, MSN, RN, CNN, CNE

Professor, Nursing
Aims Community College
Greeley, Colorado

Camella Marcom, RN, MSN, CNE

ADN Instructor
Vance-Granville Community College
Henderson, North Carolina

Lolita A. McCarthy, MSN, MBA-HCM, RN

Instructor of Nursing
Barry University
Miami Shores, Florida

Barbara McGraw, MSN, RN, CNE

Nursing Faculty
Central Community College
Grand Island, Nebraska

Kathleen A. Miller, MS, RN, FNP

Assistant Professor of Nursing
Morrisville State College
Morrisville, New York

Carrie O'Reilly, PhD, MSN, RN

Undergraduate Programs Coordinator/Assistant Professor
Touro University Nevada
Henderson, Nevada

Rosalynde Peterson, DNP, RN

Instructor
Shelton State Community College
Tuscaloosa, Alabama

Kimberly Porter, MNSc, RN, BA

Assistant Professor of Nursing
University of Arkansas at Little Rock
Little Rock, Arkansas

Colleen M. Quinn, RN, MSN, EdD

Assistant Professor of Nursing
Broward College
Pembroke Pines, Florida

Janice Ramirez, MSN, RN BC, CRRN, CNE

Nursing Instructor
North Idaho College
Coeur d' Alene, Idaho

Kevin R. Reilly, MSN, RN

Assistant Professor
Samuel Merritt University
Oakland, California

Nancy Jo Ross, PHDC, RN, CNE

Director, Nursing Program
Central Main Medical Center College of Nursing and
   Health Professions
Lewiston, Maine

Lynette Scianna-DeBellis, RN, MA

Assistant Professor of Nursing; Curriculum Chairperson
Westchester Community College
Valhalla, New York

Kathy Sheppard, PhD, MA, RN

Associate Dean and Professor School of Nursing
University of Mobile
Mobile, Alabama

Beryl Stetson, RNBC, MSN, CNE, LCCE, CLC

Associate Professor, Nursing
Raritan Valley Community College
Somerville, New Jersey

Debbie Strickert, MN, APRN-CNS

Associate Professor of Nursing
Newman University
Wichita, Kansas

Marie Huffmaster Thomas, RN, PhD, CNE

Lead Instructor
Forsyth Technical Community College
Winston Salem, North Carolina

Robin Benson Thompson, RN, MSN-Ed

ADN Nursing Instructor
Hinds Community College
Jackson, Mississippi

Diane Vangsness, MA (Nursing), RN

Nursing Instructor; Associate of Science Degree
Minnesota West Community and Technical College
Worthington, Minnesota

Mary Anne Vincent, PhD, RN, ACNS-BC

Assistant Professor
Sam Houston State University
Huntsville, Texas

Bonnie L. Welniak, MSN, RN

Assistant Professor of Nursing
   Monroe County Community College
Monroe, Michigan

Nancy Whetzel, RN, MS, CNS

Visiting Assistant Professor of Nursing
Colorado State University–Pueblo
Pueblo, Colorado

Barbara Wilder, DSN, CRNP

Professor
Auburn School of Nursing
Auburn, Alabama

Irish Patrick Williams, PhD, RN, MSN, CRRN

Instructor
Hinds Community College
Jackson, Mississippi

Wendy Woolston, MSN, RN

Nursing Instructor
Benedictine College
Atchison, Kansas

Tara Zacharzuk-Marciano, RN, MA

Nursing Instructor
Ulster County Community College (SUNY Ulster)
Stone Ridge, New York

Acknowledgments

Mickey and I are so grateful to all the people who have helped us make this book possible. We thank our readers for allowing us this important opportunity to touch their lives. We are also thankful for our association with the F.A. Davis Company. We value and appreciate the efforts of all the people associated with F.A. Davis, because without their hard work this publication could not succeed. We recognize all the wonderful people in leadership, the editors, freelance consultants, designers, IT gurus, and digital applications developers, as well as those in sales and marketing, distribution, and finance. We have a deep appreciation for the Davis Educational Consultants. They are tasked with being our voice. Their exceptional ability to communicate is what actually brings our book to the market. We would like to give special acknowledgment to the outstanding publishing professionals who were our core support team throughout the development of this edition:

Lisa Houck, Publisher
Robert Allen, Content Applications Developer
Victoria White, Content Project Manager II
Julia Curcio, Content Project Manager I
Julie Scardiglia, Freelance Development Editor
Cynthia Naughton, Production Manager, Digital Solutions
Sandra Glennie, Project Manager, Digital Solutions
Carolyn O'Brien, Art & Design Manager
Jaclyn Lux, Marketing Manager
Dan Clipner, Production Manager

Contents in Brief

Contents

Section I Studies

Understanding Laboratory and Diagnostic Testing

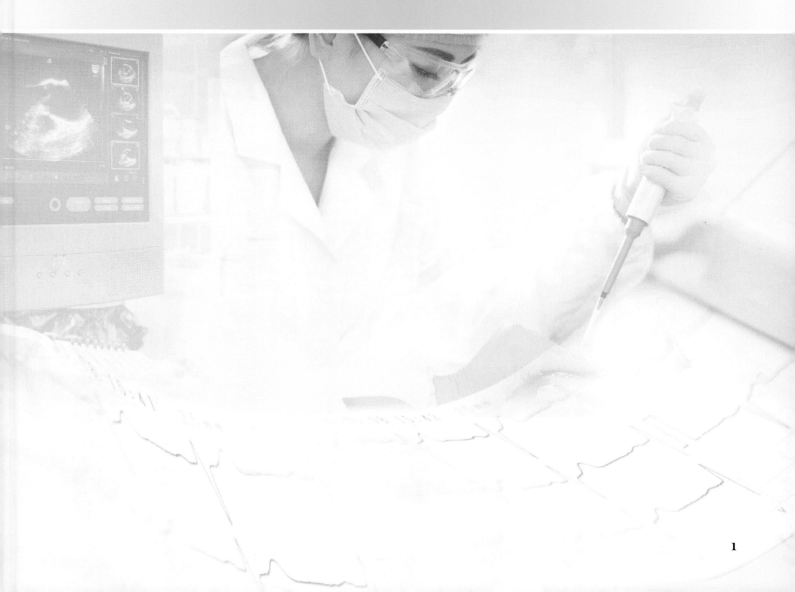

Blood Studies: Clinical Chemistry

OVERVIEW

Years of studying the physiology of humans have provided a lengthy list of measurable substances transported in blood and other body fluids. Blood chemistry studies are used to measure balance (normal findings) or imbalance (increased or decreased findings) in either the level of constituents used to drive cellular function or those generated as waste products of cellular metabolism. There are millions of cells in the body. During the various stages of human development, specialized cells are grouped to form organs, bones, tissue, and all the other anatomical structures of the body. The cells carry out both simple and complex life-sustaining biochemical reactions.

Blood chemistry studies can be classified into any number of specialized categories that cover a wide range of physiological functions in the body. Categories may group tests by chemical composition, organ-specific function, or a combination of composition and function because some of the commonly measured substances can impact multiple organ systems. Classical categories include carbohydrates, water and electrolytes, proteins, protein metabolites, enzymes, lipids and fatty acids, bilirubin, hormones, vitamins and minerals, as well as drugs and toxic substances. Studies in these categories can reveal evidence of normal physiology or the development of pathological conditions of the cardiovascular, endocrine, gastrointestinal, genitourinary, hematopoietic, hepatobiliary, immune, musculoskeletal, reproductive, and respiratory systems. This introduction will briefly describe basic clinical chemistry topics in terms of chemical composition.

Carbohydrates

Carbohydrate metabolism is the mechanism by which cellular processes in the body can quickly acquire energy. Dietary glucose is the main carbohydrate source for the body. It is a simple six-carbon sugar derived from the disaccharides sucrose, lactose, or maltose, and the polysaccharide starch (see Fig. 1.1). The body is capable of synthesizing glucose from other sources if needed. Amino acids, glycerol, and fatty acids can also be used to generate glucose in a process called *gluconeogenesis*. Glucose can be metabolized immediately into carbon dioxide, water, and ATP (energy), or it can be stored in muscle and liver cells as glycogen. There are a number of feedback loops in the body, regulated by hormones, which directly or indirectly influence glucose levels. The two organs that play a crucial role in the distribution and storage of glucose are the liver and pancreas.

Water and Electrolytes

Water and electrolyte balance are often discussed together because both are found in every type of intracellular and extracellular fluid. Most of the body is composed of water. In fact, water is much more crucial to survival than food. It has been demonstrated that a human can live up to a month without food but will perish in a matter of days without water. Water serves numerous macro- and microfunctions in the body that include contributing to the physical shape of blood cells, tissues, and organs; serving as a vehicle for the exchange of gases, electrolytes, and other small molecules into and out of cells; transporting substances to tissues and organs for absorption; transporting substances for excretion from the body; maintaining blood volume and pressure; and maintaining body temperature (see Fig. 1.2). It also serves a protective function as a basic component of the lubricant in joint fluids. Water is both created and consumed in numerous metabolic processes in the body. Water can carry materials to the intended targets via larger transport proteins, or it can

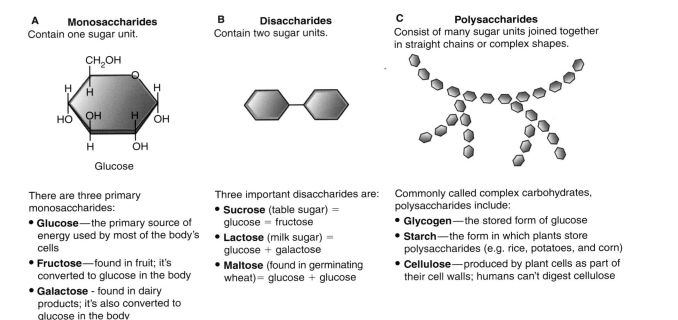

A   Monosaccharides
Contain one sugar unit.

Glucose

B   Disaccharides
Contain two sugar units.

C   Polysaccharides
Consist of many sugar units joined together in straight chains or complex shapes.

There are three primary monosaccharides:

- **Glucose**—the primary source of energy used by most of the body's cells
- **Fructose**—found in fruit; it's converted to glucose in the body
- **Galactose** - found in dairy products; it's also converted to glucose in the body

Three important disaccharides are:

- **Sucrose** (table sugar) = glucose = fructose
- **Lactose** (milk sugar) = glucose + galactose
- **Maltose** (found in germinating wheat)= glucose + glucose

Commonly called complex carbohydrates, polysaccharides include:

- **Glycogen**—the stored form of glucose
- **Starch**—the form in which plants store polysaccharides (e.g. rice, potatoes, and corn)
- **Cellulose**—produced by plant cells as part of their cell walls; humans can't digest cellulose

FIGURE 1.1 Diagram of the types of carbohydrates. (A) Monosaccharides. (B) Disaccharides. (C) Polysaccharides. *Used with permission, from Thompson, G. (2013). Understanding anatomy & physiology. FA Davis Company.*

provide direct transport as a solvent for some vitamins, minerals, and other smaller water-soluble substances such as glucose (see Fig. 1.3).

Body fluids normally contain an equal number of positive and negative charges. Proteins, minerals, and salts carry an electrical charge, but not all will dissolve in water and dissociate into electrically charged cations and anions as do electrolytes. Electrolytes are essential for the completion of many biological functions. They help maintain acid-base balance in the metabolic and respiratory compensatory systems, control the process of osmosis (the movement of water), and conduct significant and essential electrical currents in the neurological, musculoskeletal, and cardiovascular systems (see Fig. 1.4). The most significant body fluid electrolytes are sodium, potassium, chloride, and bicarbonate. Other electrolytes of interest are calcium, magnesium,

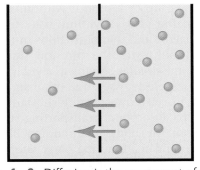

FIGURE 1.2 Diffusion is the movement of dissolved particles across a semipermeable membrane from higher to lower concentrations. *Used with permission, from Burton, M. (2011). Fundamentals of nursing care: Concepts, connections, & skills. FA Davis Company.*

and phosphorus. The balance of intracellular and extracellular electrolytes, as well electrolyte balance between various body fluid compartments, is controlled by the exchange of oxygen and carbon dioxide in the process of respiration; by various aspects of renal function (excretion, secretion, and absorption); and by complementary hormonal interaction and regulation from the endocrine system.

Proteins and Enzymes

Protein content is second only to water in the human body. While more than 500 proteins have been identified, 20 common amino acids are the building blocks for most of the protein that supports the body's structure, including muscle, cartilage, tendons, tissues, and organs, as well as hair, teeth, and bones (see Fig. 1.5). Proteins direct cellular functions such as growth, maintenance, regulation, and protection. Some examples of specialized proteins are enzymes, hormones, immunoglobulins, nucleoproteins (DNA and RNA), and transport proteins. Proteins can also be used as an energy source for the body's needs. Changes in protein intake, cellular synthesis or destruction, fluid balance, liver function (metabolism), and kidney function (excretion) create a situation of balance or imbalance in protein levels.

Enzymes are protein catalysts that enhance reactions without directly participating or being consumed in them. Enzymes are very specific, each having its own substrate and end product, and are involved in virtually all metabolic functions of the body. Some enzyme-mediated reactions occur in all cell types, and the related enzymes are found in cells throughout the body. Other enzymes participate in organ-specific biochemical

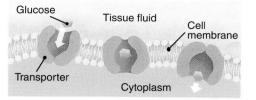

FIGURE 1.3 Facilitated diffusion of glucose across the cell membrane by a specific carrier protein. *Used with permission, from Hale, A. & Hovey, M. (2013). Fluid and electrolyte notes. FA Davis Company.*

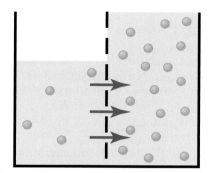

FIGURE 1.4 Osmosis is the movement of water across a semipermeable membrane from a less concentrated solution to a more concentrated solution. *Used with permission, from Burton, M. (2011). Fundamentals of nursing care: Concepts, connections, & skills. FA Davis Company.*

processes and are found only in those cell types. Enzymes are normally intracellular molecules. However, during the normal cycle of cell production and death, enzymes are released into the circulating blood at a consistent or "normal" level. Increased or "abnormal" levels of enzymes occur due to an abnormal increase in cellular enzyme production, an abnormal increase in the number of cells producing the enzyme, or the increased release of cellular contents related to trauma (e.g., poor specimen collection technique) or cell death (e.g., disease or exposure to toxins).

Cellular Waste Products

Cellular metabolism creates waste, and not all waste products are recycled by the body. The two most prevalent nitrogen-containing end products of protein metabolism are ammonia and urea. The main route for nitrogen excretion from the body is through the deamination of ammonia by the liver. Ammonia is converted into urea, a nonprotein nitrogenous waste product, in an enzymatic process known as the urea cycle. Creatinine is nonprotein nitrogenous waste generated by the chemical production of energy from phosphocreatine in skeletal muscles and some organs (notably the heart and brain). Urea and creatinine are transported to the kidneys and excreted in the urine. As such, both

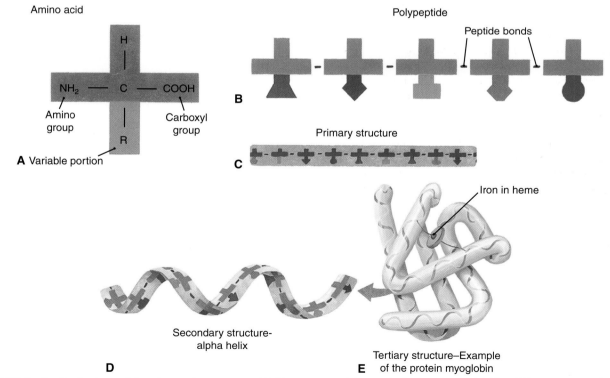

FIGURE 1.5 Amino acid and protein structure. (A) The structural formual of an amino acid. The "R" represents the variable portion of the molecule. (B) A polypeptide. Several Amino acides represented by different shapes, are linked by peptide bonds. (C) The primary structure of a protein. (D) The secondary structure of a protein. (E) The tertiary structure example of the protein myoglobin. *Used with permission, from Scanlon, V., & Sanders, T. (2010). Essentials of anatomy and physiology (6th Ed.). FA Davis Company.*

substances are important indicators of renal function. Uric acid is a nonprotein nitrogen-containing waste product synthesized by the liver and excreted by the kidneys. Uric acid is generated from the metabolism of two purine nucleic acid bases, adenine and guanine, during the normal process of cell turnover. Uric acid is also absorbed by the body from dietary sources. Another important waste product is bilirubin, an orange-yellow bile pigment formed from the breakdown of heme in red blood cells. A small amount of bilirubin circulates in the blood as a reflection of normal red blood cell turnover; the rest of the bilirubin is transported in the blood to the liver where it is changed into a soluble form in a process called *conjugation*, and then secreted into the bile. Most of the secreted bile is reabsorbed by the intestines and is converted by intestinal bacteria into a colorless pigment called *urobilinogen*. Half of the urobilinogen is recirculated to the liver, reabsorbed, and resecreted in the bile where it circulates as part of the hepatic portal circulatory system. The other half of the urobilinogen is converted into a brown pigment called stercobilin which is excreted in the feces. A very small amount of urobilinogen is converted into urobilin and excreted by the kidneys into the urine. The bilirubin level is considered a good indicator of liver health and function (see Fig. 1.6).

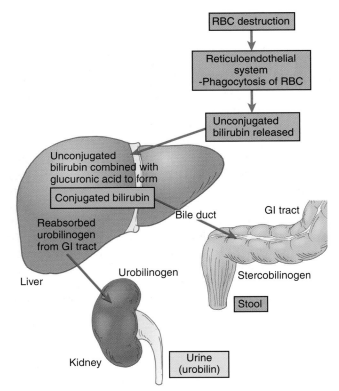

FIGURE 1.6 Pathway for the excretion of bilirubin. *Used with permission, from Ward, S. (2009). Maternal-child nursing care: Optimizing outcomes for mothers, children, and families. FA Davis Company.*

Lipids

Lipids and fatty acids are composed of the same three basic elements as carbohydrates: hydrogen, carbon, and oxygen. There are three basic categories of required lipids provided by dietary sources and internal synthesis:

1. Neutral fats (e.g., triglycerides)
2. Conjugated lipids (e.g., phospholipids)
3. Sterols (e.g., cholesterol)

Lipids and fatty acids have many essential functions that include providing:

1. A major fuel source and energy reserve for most body tissues
2. A means of transport for fat-soluble constituents, such as the cholesterols and vitamins D, A, E, and K
3. A subcutaneous layer of insulation that protects the body from extremes of heat or cold
4. Support and protection to vital organs from mechanical shock and trauma
5. A unique composition in cell membranes essential for the transport of substances into and out of cells
6. Lubrication of body tissues by oils secreted from the sebaceous glands

Cholesterol is a very important lipid that plays a crucial role in other specific functions in the body, including serving as a precursor molecule in the formation of vitamin D and sterol hormones such as corticosteroids and sex hormones, serving as a component in bile salts that aid in the emulsification and digestion of fats, and serving as a component in the myelin sheath to protect nerves and enhance the conduction of nerve impulses (see Fig. 1.7).

Hormones

Hormones are chemicals that participate in a wide range of essential functions. In the simplest grouping they comprise three chemical classes: peptide hormones (e.g., insulin, growth hormone), smaller amino hormones (e.g., thyroid hormones), and steroid hormones (e.g., cortisol, testosterone). Some exert their effects in the vicinity of their release, and others are transported in the extracellular fluid to distant tissues and organs. Like enzymes, some hormones affect numerous cells in the body while others affect specific targets. Hormones can exert their effects directly on the specific target by altering cell membrane permeability or indirectly by affecting the rates of the production and secretion of other hormones and enzymes. They act as sensors, messengers, regulators, and neuroprotectors with the ability to support and provide numerous functions. Hormones stimulate hunger pangs and regulate metabolism, stimulate or inhibit growth, influence emotions, prepare the body for survival responses such as

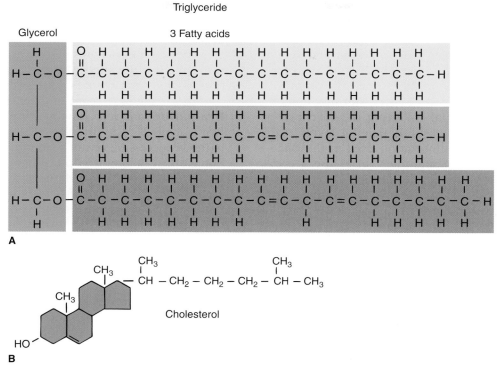

FIGURE 1.7 Structure of triglyceride and cholesterol. *Modified from Scanlon, V., & Sanders, T. (2010). Essentials of anatomy and physiology (6th Ed.). FA Davis Company.*

fight or flight, prepare the body for major changes (e.g., puberty, reproduction, and menopause), as well as provide anti-inflammatory and immunizing effects.

Hormone levels are mostly controlled by negative feedback loops in which hormones instigate mediated compensation to oppose or reverse a situation. An example of a common negative feedback loop relates to the endocrine system control of blood glucose levels by the hormone insulin. When blood glucose levels are high, the pancreas secretes insulin. Insulin acts on the liver and skeletal muscles to remove glucose from circulation and store it as glycogen. As the concentration of circulating glucose decreases, insulin levels also decrease until its effects have diminished to the point that glucose levels once again stimulate the secretion of insulin. There are also some positive feedback loops that exist in human physiology. Regulation by positive feedback is one in which the hormone causes a change to be amplified instead of reversed. An example is ovulation, which is regulated by hormones that affect the reproductive system. During the late follicular phase of the menstrual cycle, an unchallenged secretion of estradiol stimulates the increased secretion of luteinizing hormone, which increases further production of estradiol. The positive feedback encourages the continued hormonal secretion of both estradiol and luteinizing hormone until the follicle erupts, releasing the ovum.

Vitamins and Minerals

There are 13 biologically important vitamins to humans that are classified as water soluble or fat soluble. The water-soluble group includes vitamin C and the B vitamins: thiamine (B1), riboflavin (B2), niacin (B3), pantothenic acid (B5), pyridoxine (B6), biotin, folic acid (B9), and cobalamin (B12). The fat-soluble vitamins include A, D, E, and K. Vitamins are required in small amounts yet are essential for normal cellular metabolism, growth, and maintenance. The major minerals required by the body have already been listed and discussed as electrolytes. Trace minerals of clinical significance include iron (Fe), copper (Cu), and zinc (Zn). As with the vitamins, minerals are required in relatively small amounts. They may have a specific function, as with iron's ability to carry oxygen when incorporated in the hemoglobin molecule. They may also have important roles as cofactors, coenzymes, or regulators in critical cellular functions.

Drug Levels

The measurement of drug concentration is used to ensure that the prescribed medication has reached a level in which the desired effects will occur. Measurements are also taken to monitor the sustainability of therapeutic levels, to monitor patient compliance to the prescribed regimen, to avoid accidental excess dosing, to document workplace drug use, or to identify and treat suspected deliberate overdose. IMPORTANT NOTE: Information regarding peak and trough collection times must be clearly and accurately communicated to avoid misunderstanding of the dose time in relation to the collection time. Miscommunication between the individual administering the medication and the individual collecting the specimen is the most frequent cause of subtherapeutic levels, toxic levels, and misleading information used in the calculation of future doses. Some pharmacies use a computerized pharmacokinetics approach to dosing that eliminates the need to be concerned about peak and trough collections; random specimens are adequate. If the administration of the drug is delayed, notify the appropriate department(s) to reschedule the blood draw and notify the requesting health-care provider (HCP) if the delay has caused any real or perceived therapeutic harm.

The information in the Part I studies is organized in a manner to help the student see how the five basic components of the nursing process (assessment, diagnosis, planning, implementation, and evaluation) can be applied to each phase of laboratory and diagnostic testing. The goal is to use the nursing process to understand the integration of care (laboratory, diagnostic, nursing care) toward achieving a positive expected outcome.

- **Assessment** is the collection of information for the purpose of answering the question, "is there a problem?" Knowledge of the patient's health history, medications, complaints, and allergies as well as synonyms or alternate test names, common use for the procedure, specimen requirements, and normal ranges or interpretive comments provide the foundation for diagnosis.
- **Diagnosis** is the process of looking at the information gathered during assessment and answering the questions, "what is the problem?" and "what do I need to do about it?" Test indications tell us why the study has been requested, and potential diagnoses tell us the value or importance of the study relative to its clinical utility.
- **Planning** is a blueprint of the nursing care before the procedure. It is the process of determining how the nurse is going to partner with the patient to fix the problem (e.g., "The patient has a study ordered and this is what I should know before I successfully carry out the plan to have the study completed"). Knowledge of interfering factors, social and cultural issues, preprocedural restrictions, the need for written and informed consent, anxiety about the procedure, and concerns regarding pain are some considerations for planning a successful partnership.

- **Implementation** is putting the plan into action with an idea of what the expected outcome should be. Collaboration with the departments where the laboratory test or diagnostic study is to be performed is essential to the success of the plan. Implementation is where the work is done within each health-care team member's scope of practice.
- **Evaluation** answers the question, "did the plan work or not?" Was the plan completely successful, partially successful, or not successful? If the plan did not work, evaluation is the process used to determine what needs to be changed to make the plan work better. This includes a review of all expected outcomes. Nursing care after the procedure is where information is gathered to evaluate the plan. Review of results, including critical findings in relation to patient symptoms and other tests performed, provides data that form a more complete picture of health or illness.
- **Expected outcomes** are positive outcomes related to the test. They are the outcomes the nurse should expect if all goes well.

A number of pretest, intratest, and post-test universal points are presented in this overview section because the information applies to clinical chemistry blood studies in general.

Universal Pretest Pearls (Planning)

- Obtain a history of the patient's complaints, including a list of known allergens, especially allergies or sensitivities to medications or latex so their use can be avoided or their effects mitigated if an allergy is present. Carefully evaluate all medications currently being taken by the patient. A list of the patient's current medications, prescribed and over the counter (including anticoagulants, aspirin and other salicylates, herbs, nutritional supplements, and neutraceuticals), should also be obtained. Such products may be discontinued by medical direction for the appropriate number of days prior to the procedure. Ensure that all allergies are clearly noted in the medical record, and ensure that the patient is wearing an allergy and medical record armband. Report information that could interfere with, or delay proceeding with, the study to the HCP and laboratory.
- Obtain a history of the patient's affected body system, symptoms, and results of previously performed laboratory tests and diagnostic and surgical procedures. Previous test results will provide a basis of comparison between old and new data.
- An important aspect of planning is understanding the factors that may alter study findings or cause

abnormal results. Interdepartmental communication is a key factor in the planning process. The inability of a patient to cooperate or remain still during the procedure because of age, significant pain, or mental status should be among the anticipated factors. Recent or past procedures, medications, or existing medical conditions that could complicate or interfere with test results should be noted.

- Review the steps of the study with the patient or caregiver. Expect patients to be nervous about the procedure and the pending results. Educating the patient on his or her role during the procedure and what to expect can facilitate this. The patient's role during the procedure is to remain still. The actual time required to complete each study will depend on a number of conditions, including the type of equipment being used and how well a patient will cooperate.

- Explain that specimen collection by venipuncture takes approximately 5 to 10 minutes. Bleeding or bruising can be prevented, once the needle has been removed, by applying direct pressure to the venipuncture site with dry gauze for a minute or two. The site should be observed/assessed for bleeding or hematoma formation, and then covered with a gauze and adhesive bandage.

- Address any concerns about pain and explain or describe, as appropriate, the level and type of discomfort that may be expected. Advise the patient that some discomfort may be experienced during the venipuncture.

- Provide additional instructions and patient preparation regarding medication, diet, fluid intake, or activity, if appropriate. Unless specified in the individual study, there are no special instructions or restrictions.

- Always be sensitive to any cultural or psychosocial issues, including a concern for modesty before, during, and after the procedure.

Reminder

Ensure that a written and informed consent has been documented in the medical record prior to the study, if required. The consent must be obtained before medication is administered.

Universal Intratest Pearls (Implementation)

- Correct patient identification is crucial prior to any procedure. Positively identify the patient using two unique identifiers such as patient name, date of birth, Social Security number, or medical record number.

- Standard Precautions must be followed.

- Children and infants may be accompanied by a parent to calm them. Keep neonates and infants covered and in a warm room and provide a pacifier or gentle touch. The testing environment should be quiet, and the patient should be instructed, as appropriate, to remain still during the test as extraneous movements can affect results.

- Ensure that the patient has complied with pretesting instructions, including dietary, fluid, medication, and activity restrictions as given for the procedure.

- Before leaving the patient's side, appropriate specimen containers should always be labeled with the corresponding patient demographics, initials of the person collecting the sample, collection date, time of collection, applicable special notes, especially site location and laterality if appropriate, and then promptly transported to the laboratory for processing and analysis.

Universal Post Test Pearls (Evaluation)

- Note that completed test results are made available to the requesting HCP, who will discuss them with the patient.

- Answer questions and address concerns voiced by the patient or family, and reinforce information given by the patient's HCP regarding further testing, treatment, or referral to another HCP. Recognize that patients will have anxiety related to test results. Provide teaching and information regarding the clinical implications of the test results on the patient's lifestyle, as appropriate.

- Note that test results should be evaluated in context with the patient's signs, symptoms, and diagnosis. Depending on the results of the procedure, additional testing may be performed to evaluate or monitor progression of the disease process and determine the need for a change in therapy.

- Be aware that when a person goes through a traumatic event such as an illness or is being given information that will impact his or her lifestyle, there are universal human reactions that occur. These include knowledge deficit, fear, anxiety, and coping; in some situations, grieving may occur. HCPs should always be aware of the human response and how it may affect the plan of care and expected outcomes.

DISCUSSION POINT

Regarding Post-Test Critical Findings: Timely notification of a critical finding for lab or diagnostic studies is a role expectation of the professional nurse. Notification

processes will vary among facilities. Upon receipt of the critical finding, the information should be read back to the caller to verify accuracy. Most policies require immediate notification of the primary HCP, Hospitalist, or on-call HCP. Reported information includes the patient's name, unique identifiers, critical finding, name of the person giving the report, and name of the person receiving the report. Documentation of notification should be made in the medical record with the name of the HCP notified, time and date of notification, and any orders received. Any delay in a timely report of a critical finding may require completion of a notification form with review by Risk Management.

STUDIES

- Alanine Aminotransferase
- Albumin and Albumin/Globulin Ratio
- Alkaline Phosphatase and Isoenzymes
- Amylase
- Anticonvulsant Drugs: Carbamazepine, Ethosuximide, Lamotrigine, Phenobarbital, Phenytoin, Primidone, Valproic Acid
- Antidepressant Drugs (Cyclic): Amitriptyline, Nortriptyline, Protriptyline, Doxepin, Imipramine
- Antimicrobial Drugs-Aminoglycosides: Amikacin, Gentamicin, Tobramycin; Tricyclic Glycopeptide: Vancomycin
- Aspartate Aminotransferase
- Bilirubin and Bilirubin Fractions
- Calcium, Blood
- Carbon Dioxide
- Chloride, Blood
- Cholesterol, HDL and LDL
- Cholesterol, Total
- C-Reactive Protein
- Creatine Kinase and Isoenzymes
- Creatinine, Blood
- Glucose
- Glycated Hemoglobin
- Human Chorionic Gonadotropin
- Immunosuppressants: Cyclosporine, Methotrexate, Everolimus, Sirolimus, and Tacrolimus
- Lipase
- Magnesium, Blood
- Myoglobin
- Newborn Screening
- Parathyroid Hormone
- Potassium, Blood
- Prealbumin
- Protein, Blood, Total and Fractions
- Sodium, Blood
- Testosterone, Total

- Thyroid-Stimulating Hormone
- Thyroxine, Free
- Triglycerides
- Troponins I and T
- Urea Nitrogen, Blood
- Vitamin D

LEARNING OUTCOMES

Providing safe, effective nursing care (SENC) includes mastery of core competencies and standards of care. SENC is based on a judicious application of nursing knowledge in combination with scientific principles. The Art of Nursing lies in blending what you know with the ability to effectively apply your knowledge in a compassionate manner.

After reading/studying this chapter you will be able to:

Thinking

1. List the seven categories of studies included in clinical chemistry and the main cellular functions they fulfill.
2. List the two most common tests used to diagnose and manage diabetes.
3. List two studies commonly used to evaluate kidney function.

Doing

1. Name three complications of venipuncture the nurse should anticipate.
2. Discuss the main safety risk the nurse should anticipate prior to venipuncture.
3. Examine how the evaluation of a root cause analysis after a sentinel event can change practice.

Caring

1. Recognize the importance of the quality assurance process and evidenced-based practice in the provision of care.

Alanine Aminotransferase

Quick Summary

SYNONYM ACRONYM: ALT (previously known as serum glutamic pyruvic transaminase [SGPT]).

COMMON USE: To assess liver function related to liver disease and/or damage.

SPECIMEN: Serum collected in a gold-, red-, or red/gray-top tube. Plasma collected in a green-top (heparin) tube is also acceptable.

NORMAL FINDINGS: (Method: Spectrophotometry)

Age	Conventional & SI Units
Newborn–12 mo	13–45 units/L
13 mo–60 yr	
Male	10–40 units/L
Female	7–35 units/L
61–90 yr	
Male	13–40 units/L
Female	10–28 units/L
Greater than 90 yr	
Male	6–38 units/L
Female	5–24 units/L

Values may be slightly elevated in older adults due to the effects of medications and the presence of multiple chronic or acute diseases with or without muted symptoms.

Test Explanation

Alanine aminotransferase (ALT), formerly known as serum glutamic pyruvic transaminase (SGPT), is an enzyme produced by the liver. The highest concentration of ALT is found in liver cells; moderate amounts are found in kidney cells; and smaller amounts are found in heart, pancreas, spleen, skeletal muscle, and red blood cells. When liver damage occurs, serum levels of ALT may increase as much as 50 times normal, making this a sensitive test for evaluating liver function. ALT is part of a group of tests known as LFTs or liver function tests used to evaluate liver function: ALT, Albumin, Alkaline phosphatase, Aspartate aminotransferase (AST), Bilirubin, direct, Bilirubin, total, and Protein, total

Nursing Implications
Assessment

Indications	Potential Nursing Problems
Compare serially with aspartate aminotransferase (AST) levels to track the course of liver disease Monitor liver damage resulting from hepatotoxic drugs Monitor response to treatment of liver disease, with tissue repair indicated by gradually declining levels	• Activity • Breathing *(related to pressure from ascites on the diaphragm)* • Body Image • Confusion *(related to an accumulation of ammonia)* • Fear • Fluid Volume • Gas Exchange • Grief • Human Response • Infection • Nutrition • Pain • Self-image • Skin • Socialization

Diagnosis: Clinical Significance of Test Results
INCREASED IN
Release of ALT from damaged liver, kidney, heart, pancreas, red blood cells, or skeletal muscle cells.

- Acute pancreatitis
- AIDS (related to hepatitis B co-infection)
- Biliary tract obstruction
- Burns (severe)
- Chronic alcohol misuse
- Cirrhosis
- Fatty liver
- HELLP Syndrome
- Hepatic carcinoma
- Hepatitis
- Infectious mononucleosis
- Muscle injury from intramuscular injections, trauma, infection, and seizures (recent)
- Muscular dystrophy
- Myocardial infarction
- Myositis
- Pancreatitis
- Pre-eclampsia
- Shock (severe)

DECREASED IN
- Pyridoxal phosphate deficiency *(related to a deficiency of pyridoxal phosphate that results in decreased production of ALT)*

Planning
Considerations for planning a successful partnership should include clear communication of what to expect during the test to decrease anxiety and improve cooperation. Before the procedure is performed, plan to review the steps with the patient. Address concerns about pain and explain that there may be some discomfort during the venipuncture.

SPECIAL CONSIDERATIONS
An important aspect of planning is understanding the factors that may alter the study findings or cause abnormal results. Interdepartmental communication is a key factor in the planning process.

It is also important to understand which medications or substances the patient may be exposed to in the health-care setting that can interfere with accurate testing:

- Drugs that may increase ALT levels by causing cholestasis include anabolic steroids, dapsone, estrogens, ethionamide, icterogenin, mepazine, methandriol, oral contraceptives, oxymetholone, propoxyphene, sulfonylureas, and zidovudine. Drugs that may increase ALT levels by causing hepatocellular damage include acetaminophen (toxic), acetylsalicylic acid, anticonvulsants, asparaginase, carbutamide, cephalosporins, chloramphenicol, clofibrate, cytarabine,

danazol, dinitrophenol, enflurane, erythromycin, ethambutol, ethionamide, ethotoin, florantyrone, foscarnet, gentamicin, gold salts, halothane, ibufenac, indomethacin, interleukin-2, isoniazid, lincomycin, low-molecular-weight heparin, metahexamide, metaxalone, methoxsalen, methyldopa, methylthiouracil, naproxen, nitrofurans, oral contraceptives, probenecid, procainamide, and tetracyclines.
* Drugs that may decrease ALT levels include cyclosporine, interferons, metronidazole (affects enzymatic test methods), and ursodiol.

Implementation
Patient education is key to obtaining the patient's cooperation in following directions, and providing an explanation for the purpose of the procedure is an important part of this process. Inform the patient that this study can assist with the evaluation of liver function and the identification of disease. Perform the venipuncture.

Evaluation
Recognize anxiety related to test results and carefully observe the cirrhotic patient for the development of ascites, in which case fluid and electrolyte balance requires strict attention. Dietary and fluid restrictions may be required; diuretics may be ordered. The patient should be frequently monitored for weight gain, intake and output, and abdominal girth. The alcoholic patient should be encouraged to avoid alcohol and also to seek appropriate counseling for substance abuse.

NUTRITIONAL CONSIDERATIONS: Increased ALT levels may be associated with liver disease. Dietary recommendations may be indicated and vary depending on the severity of the condition. A low-protein diet may be in order if the patient's liver has lost the ability to process the end products of protein metabolism. A diet of soft foods may be required if esophageal varices have developed. Ammonia levels may be used to determine whether protein should be added to or reduced from the diet. Patients should be encouraged to eat simple carbohydrates and emulsified fats (e.g., homogenized milk or eggs) rather than complex carbohydrates (e.g., starch, fiber, and glycogen [animal carbohydrates]) and complex fats, which require additional bile to emulsify them so that they can be used. The cirrhotic patient should be carefully observed for the development of ascites, in which case fluid and electrolyte balance requires strict attention.

⊘ Critical Findings
N/A

⊘ Study Specific Complications
There are a number of complications associated with performing a venipuncture. **Pain** is commonly associated with needles, and although the pain experienced during venipuncture is usually mild, on a rare occasion the needle may strike a nerve causing permanent pain. Some patients experience a **vasovagal reaction** during the venipuncture procedure, evidenced by sweating, low blood pressure, fainting, or near fainting. The potential for a **fall injury** is a significant concern related to vasovagal reactions. Prolonged **bleeding** is a complication that occurs with patients who are taking blood thinners or who have coagulopathies such as hemophilia. A **hematoma** results when blood leaks into the tissue during or after a venipuncture, as evidenced by pain, bruising, and/or swelling at the venipuncture site. The swelling can cause injury by compression to surrounding nerves, which can be temporary or permanent. Health-care providers (HCPs) should watch for minor complications such as bruising and hematoma at the venipuncture site, which are fairly common. Hematomas occur more often in older adult or frail patients, or those with veins that are difficult to access. Bleeding or bruising can be prevented once the needle has been removed by applying direct pressure to the site with dry gauze for a minute or two. Some other more unusual complications of venipuncture include **cellulitis, phlebitis, inadvertent arterial puncture,** and **sepsis.** Sepsis can be caused by introduction of bacteria from the surface of the skin into the blood as the result of improper cleansing of the venipuncture site. Immunocompromised patients are at higher risk for developing this complication.

⊘ Related Tests
* Related tests include acetaminophen, ammonia, AST, bilirubin, biopsy liver, cholangiography percutaneous transhepatic, electrolytes, GGT, hepatitis antigens and antibodies, LDH, liver and spleen scan, US abdomen, and US liver.
* See the Hepatobiliary System table at the end of the book for related tests by body system.

Expected Outcomes
Expected outcomes associated with ALT are:

* Minimizing fatigue by pacing activities throughout the day
* Regaining a healthy nutritional status as demonstrated by the attainment and maintenance of a healthy weight
* Verbalizing an understanding of the disease and its cause; the patient is prepared to address addiction issues related to the disease
* Verbalizing the components of a healthy, balanced diet and being compliant with preparing meals that meet the patient's nutritional requirements
* Complying with ordered medication and the therapeutic regimen as demonstrated by lack of complications such as bleeding tendencies and the development of ascites, infection, or neurological dysfunction

Albumin and Albumin/Globulin Ratio

Quick Summary

SYNONYM ACRONYM: Alb, A/G ratio.

COMMON USE: To assess liver or kidney function and nutritional status.

SPECIMEN: Serum collected in a gold-, red-, or red/gray-top tube. Plasma collected in a green-top (heparin) tube is also acceptable.

NORMAL FINDINGS: (Method: Spectrophotometry) Normally the albumin/globulin (A/G) ratio is greater than 1.

Age	Conventional Units	SI Units (Conventional Units × 10)
Cord	2.8–4.3 g/dL	28–43 g/L
Newborn–7 days	2.6–3.6 g/dL	26–36 g/L
8–30 days	2–4.5 g/dL	20–45 g/L
1–3 mo	2–4.8 g/dL	20–48 g/L
4–6 mo	2.1–4.9 g/dL	21–49 g/L
7–12 mo	2.1–4.7 g/dL	21–47 g/L
1–3 yr	3.4–4.2 g/dL	34–42 g/L
4–6 yr	3.5–5.2 g/dL	35–52 g/L
7–19 yr	3.7–5.6 g/dL	37–56 g/L
20–40 yr	3.7–5.1 g/dL	37–51 g/L
41–60 yr	3.4–4.8 g/dL	34–48 g/L
61–90 yr	3.2–4.6 g/dL	32–46 g/L
Greater than 90 yr	2.9–4.5 g/dL	29–45 g/L

Test Explanation

Most of the body's total protein is a combination of albumin and globulins. Albumin, the protein present in the highest concentrations, is the main transport protein in the body for hormones, therapeutic drugs, calcium, magnesium, heme, and waste products such as bilirubin. Albumin also significantly affects plasma oncotic pressure, which regulates the distribution of body fluid between blood vessels, tissues, and cells. Albumin is synthesized in the liver. Low levels of albumin may be the result of inadequate intake, inadequate production, or excessive loss. Albumin levels are more useful as an indicator of chronic deficiency than of short-term deficiency. Hypoalbuminemia or low serum albumin, a level less than 3.4 g/dL, can stem from many causes and may be a useful predictor of mortality. Normally albumin is not excreted in urine. However, in cases of kidney damage some albumin may be lost due to decreased kidney function as seen in nephrotic syndrome, and in pregnant women with pre-eclampsia and eclampsia.

Albumin levels are affected by posture. Results from specimens collected in an upright posture are higher than results from specimens collected in a supine position.

The albumin/globulin (A/G) ratio is useful in the evaluation of liver and kidney disease. The ratio is calculated using the following formula:

$$albumin/(total\ protein - albumin)$$

where globulin is the difference between the total protein value and the albumin value. For example, with a total protein of 7 g/dL and albumin of 4 g/dL, the A/G ratio is calculated as 4/(7 − 4) or 4/3 = 1.33. A reversal in the ratio, where globulin exceeds albumin (i.e., ratio less than 1), is clinically significant.

Nursing Implications

Assessment

Indications	Potential Nursing Problems
Assess nutritional status of hospitalized patients, especially older adult patients Evaluate chronic illness Evaluate liver disease	• Activity • Bleeding • Body image • Cardiac Output • Confusion • Gas Exchange • Fear • Fluid Volume • Human Response • Infection • Injury Risk • Jaundice • Nutrition • Pain

Diagnosis: Clinical Significance of Test Results

INCREASED IN

Any condition that results in a decrease of plasma water (e.g., dehydration); look for increase in hemoglobin and hematocrit. Decreases in the volume of intravascular liquid automatically result in concentration of the components present in the remaining liquid, as reflected by an elevated albumin level.

• Hyperinfusion of albumin

DECREASED IN

• *Insufficient intake:*
  • Malabsorption *(related to lack of amino acids available for protein synthesis)*
  • Malnutrition *(related to insufficient dietary source of amino acids required for protein synthesis)*

- *Decreased synthesis by the liver:*
  - Acute and chronic liver disease (e.g., alcoholism, cirrhosis, hepatitis) *(evidenced by a decrease in normal liver function; the liver is the body's site of protein synthesis)*
  - Genetic analbuminemia *(related to genetic inability of liver to synthesize albumin)*
- *Inflammation and chronic diseases result in production of acute-phase reactant and other globulin proteins; the increase in globulins causes a corresponding relative decrease in albumin:*
  - Amyloidosis
  - Bacterial infections
  - Monoclonal gammopathies (e.g., multiple myeloma, Waldenström macroglobulinemia)
  - Neoplasm
  - Parasitic infestations
  - Peptic ulcer
  - Prolonged immobilization
  - Rheumatic diseases
  - Severe skin disease
- *Increased loss over body surface:*
  - Burns *(evidenced by loss of interstitial fluid albumin)*
  - Enteropathies (e.g., gluten sensitivity, Crohn disease, ulcerative colitis, Whipple disease) *(evidenced by sensitivity to ingested substances or related to inadequate absorption from intestinal loss)*
  - Fistula (gastrointestinal or lymphatic) *(related to loss of sequestered albumin from general circulation)*
  - Hemorrhage *(related to fluid loss)*
  - Kidney disease *(related to loss from damaged renal tubules)*
  - Pre-eclampsia *(evidenced by excessive renal loss)*
  - Rapid hydration or overhydration *(evidenced by dilution effect)*
  - Repeated thoracentesis or paracentesis (related to removal of a*lbumin in accumulated third-space fluid)*
- *Increased catabolism:*
  - Cushing disease *(related to excessive cortisol-induced protein metabolism)*
  - Thyroid dysfunction *(related to overproduction of albumin binding thyroid hormones)*
- *Increased blood volume (hypervolemia):*
  - Heart failure *(evidenced by dilution effect)*
  - Pre-eclampsia *(related to fluid retention)*
  - Pregnancy *(evidenced by increased circulatory volume from placenta and fetus)*

Planning

Considerations for planning a successful partnership should include clear communication of what to expect during the test to decrease anxiety and improve cooperation. Before the procedure is performed, plan to review the steps with the patient. The patient should be assessed for signs of edema or ascites. Address concerns about pain and explain that there may be some discomfort during the venipuncture.

SPECIAL CONSIDERATIONS

An important aspect of planning is understanding the factors that may alter the study findings or cause abnormal results. Interdepartmental communication is a key factor in the planning process.

It is also important to understand which medications or substances the patient may be exposed to in the healthcare setting that can interfere with accurate testing:

- Drugs that may increase albumin levels include carbamazepine, furosemide, phenobarbital, and prednisolone.
- Drugs that may decrease albumin levels include acetaminophen (poisoning), amiodarone, asparaginase, dextran, estrogens, ibuprofen, interleukin-2, methotrexate, methyldopa, niacin, nitrofurantoin, oral contraceptives, phenytoin, prednisone, and valproic acid.

DISCUSSION POINT

The availability of administered drugs is affected by variations in albumin levels. Patients receiving therapeutic drug treatments should have their drug levels monitored when levels of the transport protein, albumin, are decreased in order to prevent the development of toxic drug concentrations.

Implementation

Patient education is key to obtaining the patient's cooperation in following directions, and providing an explanation for the purpose of the procedure is an important part of this process. Inform the patient that this study can assist with the evaluation of liver and kidney function, as well as the effects of chronic disease. Perform the venipuncture.

Evaluation

Recognize anxiety related to test results and answer any questions or address any concerns voiced by the patient or family.

NUTRITIONAL CONSIDERATIONS: Dietary recommendations may be indicated and will vary depending on the severity of the condition. IV albumin may be administered for hypoalbuminemia. Ammonia levels may be used to determine whether protein should be added to or reduced from the diet.

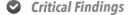 **Critical Findings**

N/A

 Study Specific Complications

There are a number of complications associated with performing a venipuncture. **Pain** is commonly associated with needles, and although the pain experienced during venipuncture is usually mild, on a rare occasion the needle may strike a nerve causing permanent pain. Some patients experience a **vasovagal reaction** during the venipuncture procedure, evidenced by sweating, low blood pressure, fainting, or near fainting. The potential for a **fall injury** is a significant concern related to vasovagal reactions. Prolonged **bleeding** is a complication that occurs with patients who are taking blood thinners or who have coagulopathies such as hemophilia. A **hematoma** results when blood leaks into the tissue during or after a venipuncture, as evidenced by pain, bruising, and/or swelling at the venipuncture site. The swelling can cause injury by compression to surrounding nerves, which can be temporary or permanent. Health-care providers should watch for minor complications such as bruising and hematoma at the venipuncture site, which are fairly common. Hematomas occur more often in older adult or frail patients, or those with veins that are difficult to access. Bleeding or bruising can be prevented once the needle has been removed by applying direct pressure to the site with dry gauze for a minute or two. Some other more unusual complications of venipuncture include **cellulitis, phlebitis, inadvertent arterial puncture,** and **sepsis.** Sepsis can be caused by introduction of bacteria from the surface of the skin into the blood as the result of improper cleansing of the venipuncture site. Immunocompromised patients are at higher risk for developing this complication.

✔ Related Tests

- Related tests include ALT, ALP, ammonia, antismooth muscle antibodies, AST, bilirubin, biopsy liver, CBC hematocrit, CBC hemoglobin, CT biliary tract and liver, GGT, hepatitis antibodies and antigens, KUB studies, laparoscopy abdominal, liver scan, MRI abdomen, osmolality, potassium, prealbumin, protein total and fractions, radiofrequency ablation liver, sodium, US abdomen, and US liver.
- See the Gastrointestinal, Genitourinary, and Hepatobiliary systems tables at the end of the book for related tests by body system.

Expected Outcomes

Expected outcomes associated with Albumin and Albumin/Globulin Ratio are:

- Agreeing to abstain from drinking alcohol with the assistance of a support group
- Decreasing extravascular fluid volume
- Making nutritional selections that support the maintenance of a healthy body weight
- Verbalizing an understanding of the patient's disease and possible treatment options, which may include treatment for alcoholism
- Describing an appropriately balanced meal plan that will restore the patient's albumin level and improve her or his health status

Alkaline Phosphatase and Isoenzymes

Quick Summary

SYNONYM ACRONYM: Alk Phos, ALP and fractionation, heat-stable ALP.

COMMON USE: To assist in the diagnosis of liver cancer and cirrhosis, or bone cancer and bone fracture.

SPECIMEN: Serum collected in a gold-, red-, or red/gray-top tube. Plasma collected in a green-top (heparin) tube is also acceptable.

NORMAL FINDINGS: (Method: Spectrophotometry for total alkaline phosphatase, inhibition/electrophoresis for fractionation)

Total ALP	Conventional & SI Units	Bone Fraction	Liver Fraction
0–30 days			
Male	75–375 units/L		
Female	65–350 units/L		
1–11 mo			
Male	70–350 units/L		
Female	80–330 units/L		
1–5 yr			
Male	56–350 units/L	39–308 units/L	Less than 8–101 units/L
Female	73–378 units/L	56–300 units/L	Less than 8–53 units/L
6–7 yr			
Male	70–364 units/L	50–319 units/L	Less than 8–76 units/L
Female	73–378 units/L	56–300 units/L	Less than 8–53 units/L
8 yr			
Male	70–364 units/L	50–258 units/L	Less than 8–62 units/L
Female	98–448 units/L	78–353 units/L	Less than 8–62 units/L
9–12 yr			
Male	112–476 units/L	78–339 units/L	Less than 8–81 units/L
Female	98–448 units/L	78–353 units/L	Less than 8–62 units/L
13 yr			
Male	112–476 units/L	78–389 units/L	Less than 8–48 units/L
Female	56–350 units/L	28–252 units/L	Less than 8–50 units/L

Continued

Table Continued

Total ALP	Conventional & SI Units	Bone Fraction	Liver Fraction
14 yr			
Male	112–476 units/L	78–389 units/L	Less than 8–48 units/L
Female	56–266 units/L	31–190 units/L	Less than 8–48 units/L
15 yr			
Male	70–378 units/L	48–311 units/L	Less than 8–39 units/L
Female	42–168 units/L	20–115 units/L	Less than 8–53 units/L
16 yr			
Male	70–378 units/L	48–311 units/L	Less than 8–39 units/L
Female	28–126 units/L	14–87 units/L	Less than 8–50 units/L
17 yr			
Male	56–238 units/L	34–190 units/L	Less than 8–39 units/L
Female	28–126 units/L	17–84 units/L	Less than 8–53 units/L
18 yr			
Male	56–182 units/L	34–146 units/L	Less than 8–39 units/L
Female	28–126 units/L	17–84 units/L	Less than 8–53 units/L
19 yr			
Male	42–154 units/L	25–123 units/L	Less than 8–39 units/L
Female	28–126 units/L	17–84 units/L	Less than 8–53 units/L
20 yr			
Male	45–138 units/L	25–73 units/L	Less than 8–48 units/L
Female	33–118 units/L	17–56 units/L	Less than 8–50 units/L
21 yr and older			
Male	35–142 units/L	11–73 units/L	0–93 units/L
Female	25–125 units/L	11–73 units/L	0–93 units/L

Values may be slightly elevated in older adults.

Test Explanation

Alkaline phosphatase (ALP) is an enzyme found in the liver; in Kupffer cells lining the biliary tract; and in bones, intestines, and placenta. Additional sources of ALP include the proximal tubules of the kidneys, pulmonary alveolar cells, germ cells, vascular bed, lactating mammary glands, and granulocytes of circulating blood. ALP is referred to as alkaline because it functions optimally at a pH of 9. This test is most useful for determining the presence of liver or bone disease.

Isoelectric focusing methods can identify 12 isoenzymes of ALP. Certain cancers produce small amounts of distinctive Regan and Nagao ALP isoenzymes. Elevations in three main ALP isoenzymes, however, are of clinical significance: ALP_1 of liver origin, ALP_2 of bone origin, and ALP_3 of intestinal origin (normal elevations are present in Lewis antibody positive individuals with blood types O and B). ALP levels vary by age and gender. Values in children are higher than in adults because of the level of bone growth and development. An immunoassay method is available for measuring bone-specific ALP as an indicator of increased bone turnover and estrogen deficiency in postmenopausal women.

Nursing Implications

Assessment

Indications	Potential Nursing Problems
Evaluate signs and symptoms of various disorders associated with elevated ALP levels, such as biliary obstruction, hepatobiliary disease, and bone disease, including malignant processes Differentiate obstructive hepatobiliary tract disorders from hepatocellular disease; greater elevations of ALP are seen in the former Determine effects of renal disease on bone metabolism Determine bone growth or destruction in children with abnormal growth patterns	• Anxiety • Dehydration • Fear • Fever • Grief • Human Response • Jaundice • Pain • Self-image • Skin

Diagnosis: Clinical Significance of Test Results
INCREASED IN
Release of alkaline phosphatase from damaged bone, biliary tract, and liver cells

- Liver disease:
  - Biliary atresia
  - Biliary obstruction (acute cholecystitis, cholelithiasis, intrahepatic cholestasis of pregnancy, primary biliary cirrhosis)
  - Cancer
  - Chronic active hepatitis
  - Cirrhosis
  - Diabetes (diabetic hepatic lipidosis)
  - Extrahepatic duct obstruction
  - Granulomatous or infiltrative liver diseases (sarcoidosis, amyloidosis, TB)
  - Infectious mononucleosis

- Intrahepatic biliary hypoplasia
- Toxic hepatitis
- Viral hepatitis
- Bone disease:
  - Healing fractures
  - Metabolic bone diseases (rickets, osteomalacia)
  - Metastatic tumors in bone
  - Osteogenic sarcoma
  - Osteoporosis
  - Paget disease (osteitis deformans)
- Other conditions:
  - Advanced pregnancy *(related to additional sources: placental tissue and new fetal bone growth; marked decline is seen with placental insufficiency and imminent fetal demise)*
  - Cancer of the breast, colon, gallbladder, lung, or pancreas
  - Familial hyperphosphatemia
  - Heart failure
  - HELLP syndrome
  - Hyperparathyroidism
  - Perforated bowel
  - Pneumonia
  - Pulmonary and myocardial infarctions
  - Pulmonary embolism
  - Ulcerative colitis

DECREASED IN
- Anemia (severe)
- Celiac disease
- Folic acid deficiency
- HIV-1 infection
- Hypervitaminosis D
- Hypophosphatasia *(related to insufficient phosphorus source for ALP production; congenital and rare)*
- Hypothyroidism (characteristic in infantile and juvenile cases)
- Nutritional deficiency of zinc or magnesium
- Pernicious anemia
- Scurvy *(related to vitamin C deficiency)*
- Whipple disease
- Zollinger-Ellison syndrome

Planning

Considerations for planning a successful partnership should include clear communication of what to expect during the test to decrease anxiety and improve cooperation. Before the procedure is performed, plan to review the steps with the patient. Address concerns about pain, and explain that there may be some discomfort during the venipuncture.

SPECIAL CONSIDERATIONS
An important aspect of planning is understanding the factors that may alter the study findings or cause abnormal results. Interdepartmental communication is a key factor in the planning process.

It is also important to understand which medications or substances the patient may be exposed to in the health-care setting that can interfere with accurate testing:

- Drugs that may increase ALP levels by causing cholestasis include anabolic steroids, erythromycin, ethionamide, gold salts, imipramine, interleukin-2, isocarboxazid, nitrofurans, oral contraceptives, phenothiazines, sulfonamides, and tolbutamide. Drugs that may increase ALP levels by causing hepatocellular damage include acetaminophen (toxic), amiodarone, anticonvulsants, arsenicals, asparaginase, bromocriptine, captopril, cephalosporins, chloramphenicol, enflurane, ethionamide, foscarnet, gentamicin, indomethacin, lincomycin, methyldopa, naproxen, nitrofurans, probenecid, procainamide, progesterone, ranitidine, tobramycin, tolcapone, and verapamil. Drugs that may cause an overall decrease in ALP levels include alendronate, azathioprine, calcitriol, clofibrate, estrogens with estrogen replacement therapy, and ursodiol.

Implementation

Patient education is key to obtaining the patient's cooperation in following directions, and providing an explanation for the purpose of the procedure is an important part of this process. Inform the patient that this study can assist with determining the presence of liver or bone disease. Perform the venipuncture.

NUTRITIONAL CONSIDERATIONS: Increased ALP levels may be associated with liver disease. Dietary recommendations may be indicated and may vary depending on the severity of the condition. A low-protein diet may be in order if the patient's liver has lost the ability to process the end products of protein metabolism. A diet of soft foods may be required if esophageal varices have developed. Ammonia levels may be used to determine whether protein should be added to or reduced from the diet. Patients should be encouraged to eat simple carbohydrates and emulsified fats (e.g., homogenized milk or eggs) rather than complex carbohydrates (e.g., starch, fiber, and glycogen [animal carbohydrates]) and complex fats, which require additional bile to emulsify them so that they can be used. The cirrhotic patient should be carefully observed for the development of ascites, in which case fluid and electrolyte balance requires strict attention.

Evaluation

Recognize anxiety related to test results and answer any questions or address any concerns voiced by the patient or family.

⊘ *Critical Findings*

N/A

Study Specific Complications

There are a number of complications associated with performing a venipuncture. **Pain** is commonly associated with needles, and although the pain experienced during venipuncture is usually mild, on a rare occasion the needle may strike a nerve causing permanent pain. Some patients experience a **vasovagal reaction** during the venipuncture procedure, evidenced by sweating, low blood pressure, fainting, or near fainting. The potential for a **fall injury** is a significant concern related to vasovagal reactions. Prolonged **bleeding** is a complication that occurs with patients who are taking blood thinners or who have coagulopathies such as hemophilia. A **hematoma** results when blood leaks into the tissue during or after a venipuncture, as evidenced by pain, bruising, and/or swelling at the venipuncture site. The swelling can cause injury by compression to surrounding nerves, which can be temporary or permanent. Health-care providers (HCPs) should watch for minor complications such as bruising and hematoma at the venipuncture site, which are fairly common. Hematomas occur more often in older adult or frail patients, or those with veins that are difficult to access. Bleeding or bruising can be prevented once the needle has been removed by applying direct pressure to the site with dry gauze for a minute or two. Some other more unusual complications of venipuncture include **cellulitis, phlebitis, inadvertent arterial puncture,** and **sepsis.** Sepsis can be caused by introduction of bacteria from the surface of the skin into the blood as the result of improper cleansing of the venipuncture site. Immunocompromised patients are at higher risk for developing this complication.

Related Tests

- Related tests include acetaminophen, ALT, albumin, ammonia, anti-DNA antibodies, AMA/ASMA, ANA, α_1-antitrypsin, α_1-antitrypsin phenotyping, AST, bilirubin, biopsy bone, biopsy liver, bone scan, BMD, calcium, ceruloplasmin, collagen cross-linked telopeptides, C3 and C4, complements, copper, ERCP, GGT, hepatitis antigens and antibodies, hepatobiliary scan, KUB studies, magnesium, MRI abdomen, MRI venography, osteocalcin, PTH, phosphorus, potassium, protein, protein electrophoresis, PT/INR, salicylate, sodium, US abdomen, US liver, vitamin D, and zinc.
- See the Hepatobiliary and Musculoskeletal systems tables at the end of the book for related tests by body system.

Expected Outcomes

Expected outcomes associated with Alkaline Phosphatase and Isoenzymes are:

- Demonstrating an understanding of the disease and potential treatment options

- Recognizing that body image changes may occur related to therapeutic treatment
- Receiving family support in relation to treatment option decisions

Amylase

Quick Summary

COMMON USE: To assist in diagnosis and evaluation of the treatment modalities used for pancreatitis.

SPECIMEN: Serum collected in a gold-, red-, or red/gray-top tube. Plasma collected in a green-top (heparin) tube is also acceptable.

NORMAL FINDINGS: (Method: Enzymatic)

Age	Conventional & SI Units
3–90 days	0–30 units/L
3–6 mo	6–40 units/L
7–11 mo	6–70 units/L
1–3 yr	11–80 units/L
4–9 yr	16–91 units/L
10–18 yr	19–76 units/L
Adult–older adult	30–110 units/L

Values may be slightly elevated in older adults due to the effects of medications and the presence of multiple chronic or acute diseases with or without muted symptoms.

Test Explanation

Amylase is a digestive enzyme mainly secreted by the acinar cells of the pancreas and by the parotid glands. Pancreatic amylase is secreted into the pancreatic common bile ducts and then into the duodenum where it assists in the digestion of carbohydrates by splitting starch into disaccharides. Amylase is a sensitive indicator of pancreatic acinar cell damage and pancreatic obstruction. Newborns and children up to 2 years old have little measurable serum amylase. In the early years of life, most of this enzyme is produced by the salivary glands. Amylase can be separated into pancreatic (P_1, P_2, P_3) and salivary (S_1, S_2, S_3) isoenzymes. Isoenzyme patterns are useful in identifying the organ source. Requests for amylase isoenzymes are rare because of the expense of the procedure and limited clinical utility of the result. Isoenzyme analysis is primarily used to assess decreasing pancreatic function in children 5 years and older who have been diagnosed with cystic fibrosis and who may be candidates for enzyme replacement. Cyst fluid amylase levels with isoenzyme analysis is useful in differentiating pancreatic neoplasms (low enzyme concentration) and pseudocysts (high enzyme concentration). Lipase is usually ordered in conjunction with amylase because lipase is more sensitive and specific to conditions affecting pancreatic function.

Nursing Implications

Assessment

Indications	Potential Nursing Problems
Assist in the diagnosis of early acute pancreatitis; serum amylase begins to rise within 6 to 24 hr after onset and returns to normal in 2 to 7 days Assist in the diagnosis of macroamylasemia, a disorder seen in alcoholism, malabsorption syndrome, and other digestive problems Assist in the diagnosis of pancreatic duct obstruction, which causes serum amylase levels to remain elevated Detect blunt trauma or inadvertent surgical trauma to the pancreas Differentiate between acute pancreatitis and other causes of abdominal pain that require surgery	• Activity • Fluid Volume **(related to vomiting or movement to another space)** • Gas Exchange • Human Response • Infection • Nutrition **(related to vomiting and a loss of appetite)** • Pain **(related to the release of digestive enzymes into the pertitoneum)**

Diagnosis: Clinical Significance of Test Results

INCREASED IN

Amylase is released from any damaged cell in which it is stored, so conditions that affect the pancreas and parotid glands and cause cellular destruction demonstrate elevated amylase levels.

- Acute appendicitis *(related to enzyme release from damaged pancreatic tissue)*
- Administration of some drugs (e.g., morphine) is known to increase amylase levels *(related to increased biliary tract pressure as evidenced by effect of narcotic analgesic drugs)*
- Afferent loop syndrome *(related to impaired pancreatic duct flow)*
- Aortic aneurysm *(elevated amylase levels following rupture are associated with a poor prognosis; both S and P subtypes have been identified following rupture. The causes for elevation are mixed and difficult to state as a generalization)*
- Abdominal trauma *(related to release of enzyme from damaged pancreatic tissue)*
- Alcoholism *(related to increased secretion; salivary origin most likely)*
- Biliary tract disease *(related to impaired pancreatic duct flow)*
- Burns and traumatic shock
- Carcinoma of the head of the pancreas (advanced) *(related to enzyme release from damaged pancreatic tissue)*
- Common bile duct obstruction, common bile duct stones *(related to impaired pancreatic duct flow)*
- Diabetic ketoacidosis *(related to increased secretion; salivary origin most likely)*
- Duodenal obstruction *(accumulation in the blood as evidenced by leakage from the gut)*
- Ectopic pregnancy *(related to ectopic enzyme production by the fallopian tubes)*
- Extrapancreatic tumors (especially esophagus, lung, ovary)
- Gastric resection *(accumulation in the blood as evidenced by leakage from the gut)*
- Hyperlipidemias (etiology is unclear, but there is a distinct association with amylasemia)
- Hyperparathyroidism (etiology is unclear, but there is a distinct association with amylasemia)
- Intestinal infarction *(related to impaired pancreatic duct flow)*
- Intestinal obstruction *(related to impaired pancreatic duct flow)*
- Macroamylasemia *(related to decreased ability of renal glomeruli to filter large molecules as evidenced by accumulation in the blood)*
- Mumps *(related to increased secretion from inflamed tissue; salivary origin most likely)*
- Pancreatic ascites *(related to release of pancreatic fluid into the abdomen and subsequent absorption into the circulation)*
- Pancreatic cyst and pseudocyst *(related to release of pancreatic fluid into the abdomen and subsequent absorption into the circulation)*
- Pancreatitis *(related to enzyme release from damaged pancreatic tissue)*
- Parotitis *(related to increased secretion from inflamed tissue; salivary origin most likely)*
- Perforated peptic ulcer whether or not the pancreas is involved *(related to enzyme release from damaged pancreatic tissue; involvement of the pancreas may be unnoticed upon gross examination yet be present as indicated by elevated enzyme levels)*
- Peritonitis *(accumulation in the blood as evidenced by leakage from the gut)*
- Postoperative period *(related to complications of the surgical procedure)*
- Pregnancy *(related to increased secretion; salivary origin most likely related to hyperemesis or hyperlipidemia-induced pancreatitis related to increased estrogen levels)*
- Renal disease *(related to decreased renal excretion as evidenced by accumulation in blood)*
- Some tumors of the lung and ovaries *(related to ectopic enzyme production)*
- Tumor of the pancreas or adjacent area *(related to release of enzyme from damaged pancreatic tissue)*

DECREASED IN

- Hepatic disease (severe) *(may be due to lack of amino acid production necessary for enzyme manufacture)*

- Pancreatectomy
- Pancreatic insufficiency
- Toxemia of pregnancy

Planning

Considerations for planning a successful partnership should include clear communication of what to expect during the test to decrease anxiety and improve cooperation. Before the procedure is performed, plan to review the steps with the patient. Address concerns about pain and explain that there may be some discomfort during the venipuncture.

SPECIAL CONSIDERATIONS

An important aspect of planning is understanding the factors that may alter the study findings or cause abnormal results. Elevated amylase levels frequently occur (75% of the time) after endoscopic retrograde cholangiopancreatography. Interdepartmental communication is a key factor in the planning process.

It is also important to understand which medications or substances the patient may be exposed to in the health-care setting that can interfere with accurate testing:

- Drugs that may increase amylase levels include acetaminophen, aminosalicylic acid, amoxapine, asparaginase, aspirin, azathioprine, bethanechol, calcitriol, chlorthalidone, cholinergics, clozapine, codeine, corticosteroids, corticotropin, desipramine, dexamethasone, diazoxide, ethyl alcohol, felbamate, fentanyl, fluvastatin, glucocorticoids, hydantoin derivatives, hydrochlorothiazide, hydroflumethiazide, meperidine, mercaptopurine, methacholine, methyclothiazide, methyldopa, metolazone, minocycline, morphine, nitrofurantoin, opium alkaloids, pegaspargase, pentazocine, potassium iodide, prednisone, procyclidine, tetracycline, thiazide diuretics, valproic acid, zalcitabine, and zidovudine.
- Drugs that may decrease amylase levels include anabolic steroids, citrates, fluorides, and glucose.

Implementation

Patient education is key to obtaining the patient's cooperation in following directions, and providing an explanation for the purpose of the procedure is an important part of this process. Inform the patient that this study can assist in evaluating pancreatic health and/or the effectiveness of medical treatment for pancreatitis. Perform the venipuncture.

Evaluation

Recognize anxiety related to test results and answer any questions or address any concerns voiced by the patient or family.

NUTRITIONAL CONSIDERATIONS:

Increased amylase levels may be associated with gastrointestinal disease or alcoholism. Small, frequent meals work best for patients with gastrointestinal disorders. Consideration should be given to dietary alterations in the case of gastrointestinal disorders. Usually after acute symptoms subside and bowel sounds return, patients are given a clear liquid diet, progressing to a low-fat, high-carbohydrate diet. Vitamin B_{12} may be ordered for parenteral administration to patients with decreased levels, especially if their disease prevents adequate absorption of the vitamin. The patients who are alcoholics should be encouraged to avoid alcohol and to seek appropriate counseling for substance abuse.

Critical Findings

N/A

Study Specific Complications

There are a number of complications associated with performing a venipuncture. **Pain** is commonly associated with needles, and although the pain experienced during venipuncture is usually mild, on a rare occasion the needle may strike a nerve causing permanent pain. Some patients experience a **vasovagal reaction** during the venipuncture procedure, evidenced by sweating, low blood pressure, fainting, or near fainting. The potential for a **fall injury** is a significant concern related to vasovagal reactions. Prolonged **bleeding** is a complication that occurs with patients who are taking blood thinners or who have coagulopathies such as hemophilia. A **hematoma** results when blood leaks into the tissue during or after a venipuncture, as evidenced by pain, bruising, and/or swelling at the venipuncture site. The swelling can cause injury by compression to surrounding nerves, which can be temporary or permanent. Health-care providers (HCPs) should watch for minor complications such as bruising and hematoma at the venipuncture site, which are fairly common. Hematomas occur more often in older adult or frail patients, or those with veins that are difficult to access. Bleeding or bruising can be prevented once the needle has been removed by applying direct pressure to the site with dry gauze for a minute or two. Some other more unusual complications of venipuncture include **cellulitis, phlebitis, inadvertent arterial puncture,** and **sepsis.** Sepsis can be caused by introduction of bacteria from the surface of the skin into the blood as the result of improper cleansing of the venipuncture site. Immunocompromised patients are at higher risk for developing this complication.

Related Tests

- Related tests include ALT, ALP, AST, bilirubin, cancer antigens, calcium, C-peptide, CBC, WBC count and differential, CT pancreas, ERCP, fecal fat, GGT, lipase, magnesium, MRI pancreas, mumps serology, peritoneal fluid analysis, triglycerides, US abdomen, and US pancreas.
- See the Gastrointestinal and Hepatobiliary systems tables at the end of the book for related tests by body system.

Expected Outcomes

Expected outcomes associated with Amylase are:

- Remaining normovolemic, evidenced by stable vital signs; successfully tolerating increasing levels of activity
- Collaborating with the HCP to select medications that will control the pain at a level acceptable to the patient
- Demonstrating an understanding of the disease and an ability to list the triggers and interventions for the disease
- Correctly describing well-balanced meals and successfully attaining a healthy weight
- Pain control at a level acceptable to the patient through compliance with the medication regimen
- Successfully tolerating increasing levels of activity

Antimicrobial Drugs—Aminoglycosides: Amikacin, Gentamicin, Tobramycin; Tricyclic Glycopeptide: Vancomycin

Quick Summary

SYNONYM ACRONYM: *Amikacin* (Amikin); *gentamicin* (Garamycin, Genoptic, Gentacidin, Gentafair, Gentak, Gentamar, Gentrasul, G-myticin, Oco-Mycin, Spectro-Genta); *tobramycin* (Nebcin, Tobrex); *vancomycin* (Lyphocin, Vancocin, Vancoled).

COMMON USE: To evaluate specific drugs for subtherapeutic, therapeutic, or toxic levels in the treatment of infection.

SPECIMEN: Serum collected in a red-top tube.

Drug	Route of Administration	Recommended Collection Time*
Amikacin	IV, IM	Trough: immediately before next dose
		Peak: 30 min after the end of a 30-min IV infusion
Gentamicin	IV, IM	Trough: immediately before next dose
		Peak: 30 min after the end of a 30-min IV infusion
Tobramycin	IV, IM	Trough: immediately before next dose
		Peak: 30 min after the end of a 30-min IV infusion
Tricyclic glycopeptide and vancomycin	IV, PO	Trough: immediately before next dose
		Peak: 30–60 min after the end of a 60-min IV infusion

*Usually after fifth dose if given every 8 hr or third dose if given every 12 hr.
IM = intramuscular; IV = intravenous; PO = by mouth.

NORMAL FINDINGS: (Method: Immunoassay)

Drug	Therapeutic Range Conventional Units	Conversion to SI Units	SI Units	Half-Life (hr)	Distribution (L/kg)	Volume of Binding (%)	Excretion
Amikacin							
Peak	15–30 mcg/mL	SI units = Conventional Units × 1.71	26–51 micromol/L	4–8	0.4–1.3	50	1° renal
Trough	4–8 mcg/mL	SI units = Conventional Units × 1.71	7–14 micromol/L				1° renal
Gentamicin (Standard dosing)							
Peak	5–10 mcg/mL	SI units = Conventional Units × 2.09	10–21 micromol/L	4–8	0.4–1.3	50	1° renal
Trough	Less than 2 mcg/mL	SI units = Conventional Units × 2.09	Less than 4 micromol/L				1° renal
Tobramycin (Standard dosing)							
Peak	4–8 mcg/mL	SI units = Conventional Units × 2.09	8.4–16.7 micromol/L	4–8	0.4–1.3	50	1° renal
Trough	Less than 1 mcg/mL	SI units = Conventional Units × 2.09	Less than 2.1 micromol/L				1° renal
Tobramycin (Once daily dosing)							
Peak	8–12 mcg/mL	SI units = Conventional Units × 2.09	16.7–25.1 micromol/L	4–8	0.4–1.3	50	1° renal
Trough	Less than 0.5 mcg/mL	SI units = Conventional Units × 2.09	Less than 1 micromol/L				1° renal
Vancomycin							
Trough (general) values vary with indication	5–15 mcg/mL	SI units = Conventional Units × 0.69	3.4–10.4 micromol/L	6–12	0.4–1	10–15	1° renal

Test Explanation

The aminoglycoside antibiotics amikacin, gentamicin, and tobramycin are used against many gram-negative (*Acinetobacter, Citrobacter, Enterobacter, Escherichia coli, Klebsiella, Proteus, Providencia, Pseudomonas, Raoultella, Salmonella, Serratia, Shigella,* and *Stenotrophomonas*) and some gram-positive (*Staphylococcus aureus*) pathogenic microorganisms. Aminoglycosides are poorly absorbed through the gastrointestinal tract and are most frequently administered IV.

Vancomycin is a tricyclic glycopeptide antibiotic used against many gram-positive microorganisms, such as staphylococci, *Streptococcus pneumoniae,* group A β-hemolytic streptococci, enterococci, *Corynebacterium,* and *Clostridium.* Vancomycin has also been used in an oral form for the treatment of pseudomembranous colitis resulting from *Clostridium difficile* infection. This approach is less frequently used because of the emergence of vancomycin-resistant enterococci (VRE).

Many factors must be considered in effective dosing and monitoring of therapeutic drugs, including patient age, patient weight, interacting medications, electrolyte balance, protein levels, water balance, conditions that affect absorption and excretion, and ingestion of substances (e.g., foods, herbals, vitamins, and minerals) that can either potentiate or inhibit the intended target concentration. The most serious side effects of the aminoglycosides and vancomycin are nephrotoxicity and irreversible ototoxicity (uncommon). Peak and trough collection times should be documented carefully in relation to the time of medication administration. Creatinine levels should be monitored every 2 to 3 days to detect renal impairment due to toxic drug levels.

Nursing Implications

Assessment

Indications	Potential Nursing Problems
Assist in the diagnosis and prevention of toxicity Monitor renal dialysis patients or patients with rapidly changing renal function Monitor therapeutic regimen	• Health Management *(related to potential subtherapeutic or toxic levels)* • Human Response • Infection • Noncompliance • Sensory Perception • Urination

Diagnosis: Clinical Significance of Test Results

Level	Response
Normal levels	Therapeutic effect
Subtherapeutic levels	Adjust dose as indicated
Toxic levels	Adjust dose as indicated
Amikacin	Renal, hearing impairment
Gentamicin	Renal, hearing impairment
Tobramycin	Renal, hearing impairment
Vancomycin	Renal, hearing impairment

Planning

Considerations for planning a successful partnership should include clear communication of what to expect during the test to decrease anxiety and improve cooperation. Nephrotoxicity and ototoxicity are risks associated with the administration of aminoglycosides. Obtain a complete history of the time and amount of the drug ingested by the patient. Obtain a history of the patient's known or suspected hearing loss, including the type and cause; ear conditions with treatment regimens; ear surgery; and other tests and procedures to assess and diagnose an auditory deficit. Before the procedure is performed, plan to review the steps with the patient. Address concerns about pain and explain that there may be some discomfort during the venipuncture.

Aminoglycosides are metabolized and excreted by the kidneys and are therefore contraindicated in patients with renal disease or impairment.

SPECIAL CONSIDERATIONS

An important aspect of planning is understanding the factors that may alter the study findings or cause abnormal results. Interdepartmental communication is a key factor in the planning process. The following should be noted when planning for this study:

• Obtain a culture before and after the first dose of aminoglycosides.
• The risks of ototoxicity and nephrotoxicity are increased by the concomitant administration of aminoglycosides.
• Blood drawn in serum separator tubes (gel tubes) will be rejected for analysis.

It is also important to understand which medications or substances the patient may be exposed to in the healthcare setting that can interfere with accurate testing:

• Drugs that may decrease aminoglycoside efficacy include penicillins (e.g., carbenicillin, piperacillin).

Implementation

Patient education is key to obtaining the patient's cooperation in following directions, and providing an explanation for the purpose of the procedure is an important part of this process. Inform the patient that this study can assist in monitoring for subtherapeutic, therapeutic, or toxic drug levels used in the treatment of infection. Consider the recommended collection time in relation to the dosing schedule. Perform the venipuncture.

Evaluation

Recognize anxiety related to test results and instruct the patient receiving aminoglycosides to immediately report any unusual symptoms (e.g., hearing loss, decreased urinary output) to his or her health-care provider (HCP). Administer antibiotic therapy if ordered and provide instructions regarding food and drug interactions. Remind the patient of the importance of completing the entire course of antibiotic therapy, even if signs and symptoms disappear before the completion of therapy. Instruct the patient to be prepared to provide the pharmacist with a list of other medications he or she is already taking in the event that the requesting HCP prescribes a medication.

NUTRITIONAL CONSIDERATIONS: Discuss avoiding alcohol consumption while taking these medications.

☑ Critical Findings

The adverse effects of subtherapeutic levels are important. Care should be taken to investigate signs and symptoms of too little and too much medication.

Note and immediately report to the requesting HCP any critical findings and related symptoms. A listing of these findings varies among facilities.

Signs and symptoms of toxic levels of these antibiotics are similar and include loss of hearing and decreased renal function. Suspected hearing loss can be evaluated by audiometry testing. Impaired renal function may be identified by monitoring blood urea nitrogen (BUN) and creatinine levels as well as intake and output. The most important intervention is accurate therapeutic drug monitoring so the medication can be discontinued before irreversible damage is done.

Drug Name	Toxic Levels Conventional Units	Toxic Levels SI Units
Amikacin	Greater than 10 mcg/mL	Greater than 17.1 micromol/L
Gentamicin	Peak greater than 12 mcg/mL, trough greater than 2 mcg/mL	Peak greater than 25.1 micromol/L, trough greater than 4.2 micromol/L
Tobramycin	Peak greater than 12 mcg/mL, trough greater than 2 mcg/mL	Peak greater than 25.1 micromol/L, trough greater than 4.2 micromol/L
Vancomycin	Trough greater than 30 mcg/mL	Trough greater than 20.7 micromol/L

☑ Study Specific Complications

Lack of consideration for the proper collection time relative to the dosing schedule can provide misleading information that may result in an erroneous interpretation of levels, creating the potential for a medication error–related injury to the patient.

There are a number of complications associated with performing a venipuncture. **Pain** is commonly associated with needles, and although the pain experienced during venipuncture is usually mild, on a rare occasion the needle may strike a nerve causing permanent pain. Some patients experience a **vasovagal reaction** during the venipuncture procedure, evidenced by sweating, low blood pressure, fainting, or near fainting. The potential for a **fall injury** is a significant concern related to vasovagal reactions. Prolonged **bleeding** is a complication that occurs with patients who are taking blood thinners or who have coagulopathies such as hemophilia. A **hematoma** results when blood leaks into the tissue during or after a venipuncture, as evidenced by pain, bruising, and/or swelling at the venipuncture site. The swelling can cause injury by compression to surrounding nerves, which can be temporary or permanent. HCPs should watch for minor complications such as bruising and hematoma at the venipuncture site, which are fairly common. Hematomas occur more often in older adult or frail patients, or those with veins that are difficult to access. Bleeding or bruising can be prevented once the needle has been removed by applying direct pressure to the site with dry gauze for a minute or two. Some other more unusual complications of venipuncture include **cellulitis, phlebitis, inadvertent arterial puncture,** and **sepsis.** Sepsis can be caused by introduction of bacteria from the surface of the skin into the blood as the result of improper cleansing of the venipuncture site. Immunocompromised patients are at higher risk for developing this complication.

☑ Related Tests

- Related tests include albumin, audiometry hearing loss, BUN, CBC WBC and differential, creatinine, creatinine clearance, cultures bacterial (ear, eye, skin, wound, blood, stool, sputum, urine), otoscopy, potassium, spondee speech recognition test, tuning fork tests, and UA.
- See the Auditory, Genitourinary, and Immune systems tables at the end of the book for related tests by body system.

Expected Outcomes

Expected outcomes associated with Antimicrobial (antibiotic) Drugs are:

- Medication is administered appropriately to assure therapeutic drug levels using peak and trough evaluation.
- Dosage is individualized to the appropriate renal clearance assessment.

- Hearing is not adversely affected by drug administration.
- Renal perfusion is not adversely affected by drug administration.
- Adherence to the recommended therapeutic drug regimen is obtained.
- An understanding of the proper use of the medication to maximize health benefits is verbalized.

Anticonvulsant Drugs: Carbamazepine, Ethosuximide, Lamotrigine, Phenobarbital, Phenytoin, Primidone, Valproic Acid

Quick Summary

SYNONYM ACRONYM: *Carbamazepine* (Carbamazepinum, Carbategretal, Carbatrol, Carbazep, CBZ, Epitol, Tegretol, Tegretol XR); *ethosuximide* (Suxinutin, Zarontin, Zartalin); *lamotrigine* (Lamictal); *phenobarbital* (Barbita, Comizial, Fenilcal, Gardenal, Phenemal, Phenemalum, Phenobarb, Phenobarbitone, Phenylethylmalonylurea, Solfoton, Stental Extentabs); *phenytoin* (Antisacer, Dilantin, Dintoina, Diphenylan Sodium, Diphenylhydantoin, Ditan, Epanutin, Epinat, Fenitoina, Fenytoin, Fosphenytoin); *primidone* (Desoxyphenobarbital, Hexamidinum, Majsolin, Mylepsin, Mysoline, Primaclone, Prysolin); *valproic acid* (Depacon, Depakene, Depakote, Depakote XR, Depamide, Dipropylacetic

Acid, Divalproex Sodium, Epilim, Ergenyl, Leptilan, 2–Propylpentanoic Acid, 2–Propylvaleric Acid, Valkote, Valproate Semisodium, Valproate Sodium).

COMMON USE: To monitor specific drugs for subtherapeutic, therapeutic, or toxic levels in the evaluation of treatment.

SPECIMEN: Serum collected in a red-top tube.

Drug*	Route of Administration
Carbamazepine	Oral
Ethosuximide	Oral
Lamotrigine	Oral
Phenobarbital	Oral
Phenytoin	Oral
Primidone	Oral
Valproic acid	Oral

*Recommended collection time = trough: immediately before next dose (at steady state) or at a consistent sampling time.

NORMAL FINDINGS: (Method: Immunoassay for all except lamotrigine; liquid chromatography/tandem mass spectrometry for lamotrigine)

Drug	Therapeutic Range Conventional Units	Conversion to SI Units	Therapeutic Range SI Units	Half-Life (hr)	Volume of Distribution (L/kg)	Protein Binding (%)	Excretion
Carbamazepine	4–12 mcg/mL	SI units = Conventional Units × 4.23	17–51 micromol/L	15–40	0.8–1.8	60–80	Hepatic
Ethosuximide	40–100 mcg/mL	SI units = Conventional Units × 7.08	283–708 micromol/L	25–70	0.7	0–5	Renal
Lamotrigine	1–4 mcg/mL	SI units = Conventional Units × 3.9	4–16 micromol/L	25–33	0.9–1.3	50–5	Hepatic
Phenobarbital	*Adult:* 15–40 mcg/mL	SI units = Conventional Units × 4.31	*Adult:* 65–172 micromol/L	*Adult:* 50–140	0.5–1	40–50	80% Hepatic and 20% renal
	Child: 15–30 mcg/mL	SI units = Conventional Units × 4.31	*Child:* 65–129 micromol/L	*Child:* 40–70			80% Hepatic and 20% renal
Phenytoin	10–20 mcg/mL	SI units = Conventional Units × 3.96	40–79 micromol/L	20–40	0.6–0.7	85–95	Hepatic
Primidone	*Adult:* 5–12 mcg/mL	SI units = Conventional Units × 4.58	*Adult:* 23–55 micromol/L	4–12	0.5–1	0–20	Hepatic
	Child: 7–10 mcg/mL	SI units = Conventional Units × 4.58	*Child:* 32–46 micromol/L				
Valproic acid	50–125 mcg/mL	SI units = Conventional Units × 6.93	347–866 micromol/L	8–15	0.1–0.5	85–95	Hepatic

Test Explanation

Anticonvulsants are used to reduce the frequency and severity of seizures for patients with epilepsy. Carbamazepine is also used for controlling neurogenic pain in trigeminal neuralgia and diabetic neuropathy and for treating bipolar disease and other neurological and psychiatric conditions. Valproic acid is also used for some psychiatric conditions like bipolar disease and for prevention of migraine headache.

Many factors must be considered in effective dosing and monitoring of therapeutic drugs, including patient age, patient weight, interacting medications, electrolyte balance, protein levels, water balance, conditions that affect absorption and excretion, and the ingestion of substances (e.g., foods, herbals, vitamins, and minerals) that can either potentiate or inhibit the intended target concentration. Peak and trough collection times should be documented carefully in relation to the time of medication administration.

The metabolism of many commonly prescribed medications is driven by the cytochrome P450 (CYP450) family of enzymes. Genetic variants can alter enzymatic activity that results in a spectrum of effects ranging from the total absence of drug metabolism to ultrafast metabolism. Impaired drug metabolism can prevent the intended therapeutic effect or even lead to serious adverse drug reactions. Poor metabolizers (PM) are at increased risk for drug-induced side effects due to accumulation of drug in the blood, while ultra-rapid metabolizers (UM) require a higher than normal dosage because the drug is metabolized over a shorter duration than intended. In the case of prodrugs, which require activation prior to metabolism, the opposite occurs: PM may require a higher dose because the activated drug becomes available more slowly than intended, and UM requires less because the activated drug becomes available sooner than intended. Other genetic phenotypes used to report CYP450 results are intermediate metabolizer (IM) and extensive metabolizer (EM). Genetic testing can be performed on blood samples submitted to a laboratory. The test method commonly used is polymerase chain reaction. Counseling and informed written consent are generally required for genetic testing. CYP2C9 is a gene in the CYP450 family that metabolizes phenytoin as well as other drugs like the antihypertensive drug, losartin and the anticoagulant drug warfarin. Testing for the most common genetic variants of CYP2C9 is used to predict altered enzyme activity and anticipate the most effective therapeutic plan.

Nursing Implications

Assessment

Indications	Potential Nursing Problems
Assist in the diagnosis of and prevention of toxicity	• Emotional Distress
	• Fear
Evaluate overdose, especially in combination with ethanol	• Health Maintenance **(related to potential toxic or subtherapeutic levels)**
Monitor compliance with therapeutic regimen	• Human Response
	• Noncompliance
	• Spirituality

Diagnosis: Clinical Significance of Test Results

Level	Response
Normal levels	Therapeutic effect
Subtherapeutic levels	Adjust dose as indicated
Toxic levels	Adjust dose as indicated
Carbamazepine	Hepatic impairment
Ethosuximide	Renal impairment
Lamotrigine	Hepatic impairment
Phenobarbital	Hepatic or renal impairment
Phenytoin	Hepatic impairment
Primidone	Hepatic impairment
Valproic acid	Hepatic impairment

Planning

Considerations for planning a successful partnership should include clear communication of what to expect during the test to decrease anxiety and improve cooperation. Obtain a complete history of the time and amount of drug ingested by the patient. Before the procedure is performed, plan to review the steps with the patient. Address concerns about pain and explain that there may be some discomfort during the venipuncture.

CONTRAINDICATIONS

These medications are metabolized and excreted by the liver and kidneys and are therefore contraindicated in patients with hepatic or renal disease. Caution is advised for patients with renal impairment.

SPECIAL CONSIDERATIONS

An important aspect of planning is understanding the factors that may alter the study findings or cause abnormal results. Interdepartmental communication is a key factor in the planning process. It should be noted when planning for this study that blood drawn in serum separator tubes (gel tubes) will be rejected for analysis.

It is also important to understand which medications or substances the patient may be exposed to in the healthcare setting that can interfere with accurate testing:

CARBAMAZEPINE

- Drugs that may increase carbamazepine levels or that increase the risk of toxicity include acetazolamide, azithromycin, bepridil, cimetidine, danazol, diltiazem, erythromycin, felodipine, fluoxetine, flurithromycin, fluvoxamine, gemfibrozil, isoniazid, itraconazole, josamycin, ketoconazole, loratadine, macrolides, niacinamide, nicardipine, nifedipine, nimodipine, nisoldipine, propoxyphene, ritonavir, terfenadine, troleandomycin, valproic acid, verapamil, and viloxazine.
- Drugs that may decrease carbamazepine levels include phenobarbital, phenytoin, and primidone. Carbamazepine may affect other body chemistries as seen by a decrease in calcium, sodium, T_3, T_4 levels, and white blood cell (WBC) count and an increase in alanine aminotransferase (ALT), alkaline phosphatase, ammonia, aspartate aminotransferase (AST), and bilirubin levels.

ETHOSUXIMIDE

- Drugs that may increase ethosuximide levels include isoniazid, ritonavir, and valproic acid.
- Drugs that may decrease ethosuximide levels include phenobarbital, phenytoin, and primidone.

LAMOTRIGINE

- Drugs that may increase lamotrigine levels include valproic acid.
- Drugs that may decrease lamotrigine levels include acetaminophen, carbamazepine, hydantoins (e.g., phenytoin), oral contraceptives, orlistat, oxcarbazepine, phenobarbital, primidone, protease inhibitors (e.g., ritonavir), rifamycins (e.g., rifampin), and succinimides (e.g., ethosuximide).

PHENOBARBITAL

- Drugs that may increase phenobarbital levels or that increase the risk of toxicity include barbital drugs, furosemide, primidone, salicylates, and valproic acid.
- Phenobarbital may affect the metabolism of other drugs, increasing their effectiveness, such as β-blockers, chloramphenicol, corticosteroids, doxycycline, griseofulvin, haloperidol, methylphenidate, phenothiazines, phenylbutazone, propoxyphene, quinidine, theophylline, tricyclic antidepressants, and valproic acid.
- Phenobarbital may affect the metabolism of other drugs, decreasing their effectiveness, such as

chloramphenicol, cyclosporine, ethosuximide, oral anticoagulants, oral contraceptives, phenytoin, theophylline, vitamin D, and vitamin K.
- Phenobarbital is an active metabolite of primidone, and both drug levels should be monitored while the patient is receiving primidone to avoid either toxic or subtherapeutic levels of both medications.
- Phenobarbital may affect other body chemistries as seen by a decrease in bilirubin and calcium levels, and an increase in alkaline phosphatase, ammonia, and gamma glutamyl transferase levels.

PHENYTOIN

- Drugs that may increase phenytoin levels or that increase the risk of phenytoin toxicity include amiodarone, azapropazone, carbamazepine, chloramphenicol, cimetidine, disulfiram, ethanol, fluconazole, halothane, ibuprofen, imipramine, levodopa, metronidazole, miconazole, nifedipine, phenylbutazone, sulfonamides, trazodone, tricyclic antidepressants, and trimethoprim.
- Small changes in formulation (i.e., changes in brand) also may increase phenytoin levels or increase the risk of phenytoin toxicity.
- Drugs that may decrease phenytoin levels include bleomycin, carbamazepine, cisplatin, disulfiram, folic acid, intravenous fluids containing glucose, nitrofurantoin, oxacillin, rifampin, salicylates, and vinblastine.

PRIMIDONE

- Primidone decreases the effectiveness of carbamazepine, ethosuximide, felbamate, lamotrigine, oral anticoagulants, oxcarbazepine, topiramate, and valproate.
- Primidone may affect other body chemistries as seen by a decrease in calcium levels and an increase in alkaline phosphatase levels.

VALPROIC ACID

- Drugs that may increase valproic acid levels or that increase the risk of toxicity include dicumarol, phenylbutazone, and high doses of salicylate.
- Drugs that may decrease valproic acid levels include carbamazepine, phenobarbital, phenytoin, and primidone.

Implementation

Patient education is key to obtaining the patient's cooperation in following directions, and providing an explanation for the purpose of the procedure is an important part of this process. Inform the patient this study can assist with monitoring for subtherapeutic, therapeutic, or toxic drug levels. Consider the recommended collection time in relation to the dosing schedule. Perform the venipuncture.

Evaluation

Recognize anxiety related to test results and explain to the patient the importance of following the medication regimen; provide instructions regarding drug interactions. Instruct the patient to immediately report any unusual sensations (e.g., ataxia, dizziness, dyspnea, lethargy, rash, tremors, mental changes, weakness, or visual disturbances) to his or her health-care provider (HCP). Instruct the patient to be prepared to provide the pharmacist with a list of other medications he or she is already taking in the event that the requesting HCP prescribes a medication.

NUTRITIONAL CONSIDERATIONS: Antiepileptic drugs antagonize folic acid, and there is a corresponding slight increase in the incidence of fetal malformations in children of epileptic mothers. Women of childbearing age who are taking carbamazepine, phenobarbital, phenytoin, primadone, and/or valproic acid should also be prescribed supplemental folic acid to reduce the incidence of neural tube defects. Neonates born to epileptic mothers taking antiseizure medications during pregnancy may experience a temporary drug-induced deficiency of vitamin K–dependent coagulation factors. This can be avoided by the administration of vitamin K to the mother in the last few weeks of pregnancy and to the infant at birth.

☑ Critical Findings

It is important to note the adverse effects of toxic and subtherapeutic levels. Care must be taken to investigate signs and symptoms of not enough medication and too much medication.

Note and immediately report to the requesting HCP any critical findings and related symptoms. A listing of these findings varies among facilities.

Carbamazepine: Greater Than 20 mcg/mL
(SI: Greater Than 85 micromol/L)
Signs and symptoms of carbamazepine toxicity include respiratory depression, seizures, leukopenia, hyponatremia, hypotension, stupor, and possible coma. Possible interventions include gastric lavage (contraindicated if ileus is present); airway protection; administration of fluids and vasopressors for hypotension; treatment of seizures with diazepam, phenobarbital, or phenytoin; cardiac monitoring; monitoring of vital signs; and discontinuing the medication. Emetics are contraindicated.

Ethosuximide: Greater Than 200 mcg/mL
(SI: Greater Than 1,416 micromol/L)
Signs and symptoms of ethosuximide toxicity include nausea, vomiting, and lethargy. Possible interventions include administration of activated charcoal, administration of saline cathartic and gastric lavage (contraindicated if ileus is present), airway protection, hourly assessment of neurologic function, and discontinuing the medication.

Lamotrigine: Greater Than 20 mcg/mL
(SI: Greater Than 78 micromol/L)
Signs and symptoms of lamotrigine toxicity include severe skin rash, nausea, vomiting, ataxia, decreased levels of consciousness, coma, increased seizures, and nystagmus. Possible interventions include administration of activated charcoal, administration of saline cathartic and gastric lavage (contraindicated if ileus is present), airway protection, hourly assessment of neurologic function, and discontinuing the medication.

Phenobarbital: Greater Than 60 mcg/mL
(SI: Greater Than 259 micromol/L)
Signs and symptoms of phenobarbital toxicity include cold, clammy skin; ataxia; central nervous system (CNS) depression; hypothermia; hypotension; cyanosis; Cheyne-Stokes respiration; tachycardia; possible coma; and possible renal impairment. Possible interventions include gastric lavage, administration of activated charcoal with cathartic, airway protection, possible intubation and mechanical ventilation (especially during gastric lavage if there is no gag reflex), monitoring for hypotension, and discontinuing the medication.

Phenytoin (Adults): Greater Than 40 mcg/mL
(SI: Greater Than 158 micromol/L)
Signs and symptoms of phenytoin toxicity include double vision, nystagmus, lethargy, CNS depression, and possible coma. Possible interventions include airway support, electrocardiographic monitoring, administration of activated charcoal, gastric lavage with warm saline or tap water, administration of saline or sorbitol cathartic, and discontinuing the medication.

Primidone: Greater Than 15 mcg/mL
(SI: Greater Than 69 micromol/L)
Signs and symptoms of primidone toxicity include ataxia, anemia, CNS depression, lethargy, somnolence, vertigo, and visual disturbances. Possible interventions include airway protection, treatment of anemia with vitamin B_{12} and folate, and discontinuing the medication.

Valproic Acid: Greater Than 200 mcg/mL
(SI: Greater Than 1,386 micromol/L)
Signs and symptoms of valproic acid toxicity include loss of appetite, mental changes, numbness, tingling, and weakness. Possible interventions include administration of activated charcoal and naloxone and discontinuing the medication.

☑ Study Specific Complications

Lack of consideration for the proper collection time relative to the dosing schedule can provide misleading information that may result in erroneous interpretation of levels, creating the potential for a medication error–related injury to the patient.

There are a number of complications associated with performing a venipuncture. **Pain** is commonly associated with needles, and although the pain experienced during venipuncture is usually mild, on a rare occasion the needle may strike a nerve causing permanent pain. Some patients experience a **vasovagal reaction** during the venipuncture procedure, evidenced by sweating, low blood pressure, fainting, or near fainting. The potential for a **fall injury** is a significant concern related to vasovagal reactions. Prolonged **bleeding** is a complication that occurs with patients who are taking blood thinners or who have coagulopathies such as hemophilia. A **hematoma** results when blood leaks into the tissue during or after a venipuncture, as evidenced by pain, bruising, and/or swelling at the venipuncture site. The swelling can cause injury by compression to surrounding nerves, which can be temporary or permanent. HCPs should watch for minor complications such as bruising and hematoma at the venipuncture site, which are fairly common. Hematomas occur more often in older adult or frail patients, or those with veins that are difficult to access. Bleeding or bruising can be prevented once the needle has been removed by applying direct pressure to the site with dry gauze for a minute or two. Some other more unusual complications of venipuncture include **cellulitis, phlebitis, inadvertent arterial puncture,** and **sepsis.** Sepsis can be caused by introduction of bacteria from the surface of the skin into the blood as the result of improper cleansing of the venipuncture site. Immunocompromised patients are at higher risk for developing this complication.

✔ Related Tests

- Related tests include ALT, albumin, AST, bilirubin, BUN, creatinine, electrolytes, GGT, and protein blood total and fractions.
- See the Genitourinary and Hepatobiliary systems tables at the end of the book for related tests by body system.

Expected Outcomes

Expected outcomes associated with Anticonvulsant Drugs are:

- Verification of the therapeutic drug level for treatment parameters
- Immediate notification of the HCP for toxic or subtherapeutic levels
- Demonstration of an understanding of taking the prescribed medication toward overall health

- Absence of convulsions while on the medication at a therapeutic level

Antidepressant Drugs (Cyclic): Amitriptyline, Nortriptyline, Protriptyline, Doxepin, Imipramine

Quick Summary

SYNONYM ACRONYM: *Cyclic antidepressants: amitriptyline* (Elavil, Endep, Etrafon, Limbitrol, Triavil); *nortriptyline* (Allegron, Aventyl HCL, Nortrilen, Norval, Pamelor); *protriptyline* (Aventyl, Sinequan, Surmontil, Tofranil, Vivactil); *doxepin* (Adapin, Co-Dax, Novoxapin, Sinequan, Triadapin); *imipramine* (Berkomine, Dimipressin, Iprogen, Janimine, Pentofrane, Presamine, SK-Pramine, Tofranil PM).

COMMON USE: To monitor subtherapeutic, therapeutic, or toxic drug levels in the evaluation of effective treatment modalities.

SPECIMEN: Serum collected in a red-top tube.

Drug	Route of Administration	Recommended Collection Time
Amitriptyline	Oral	Trough: immediately before next dose (at steady state)
Nortriptyline	Oral	Trough: immediately before next dose (at steady state)
Protriptyline	Oral	Trough: immediately before next dose (at steady state)
Doxepin	Oral	Trough: immediately before next dose (at steady state)
Imipramine	Oral	Trough: immediately before next dose (at steady state)

NORMAL FINDINGS: (Method: Chromatography for amitriptyline, nortriptyline, protriptyline, and doxepin; immunoassay for imipramine)

Drug	Therapeutic Range Conventional Units	Conversion to SI Units	Therapeutic Range SI Units	Half-Life (h)	Volume of Distribution (L/kg)	Protein Binding (%)	Excretion
Amitriptyline	125–250 ng/mL	SI units = Conventional Units × 3.6	450–900 nmol/L	20–40	10–36	85–95	Hepatic
Nortriptyline	50–150 ng/mL	SI units = Conventional Units × 3.8	190–570 nmol/L	20–60	15–23	90–95	Hepatic
Protriptyline	70–250 ng/mL	SI units = Conventional Units × 3.8	266–950 nmol/L	60–90	15–31	91–93	Hepatic
Doxepin	110–250 ng/mL	SI units = Conventional Units × 3.58	394–895 nmol/L	10–25	10–30	75–85	Hepatic
Imipramine	180–240 ng/mL	SI units = Conventional Units × 3.57	643–857 nmol/L	6–18	9–23	60–95	Hepatic

Test Explanation

Cyclic antidepressants are used in the treatment of major depression. They have also been used effectively to treat bipolar disorder, panic disorder, attention deficit-hyperactivity disorder (ADHD), obsessive-compulsive disorder (OCD), enuresis, eating disorders (bulimia nervosa, in particular), nicotine dependence (tobacco), and cocaine dependence. Numerous drug interactions occur with the cyclic antidepressants.

Many factors must be considered in effective dosing and monitoring of therapeutic drugs, including patient age, patient ethnicity, patient weight, interacting medications, electrolyte balance, protein levels, water balance, conditions that affect absorption and excretion, and the ingestion of substances (e.g., foods, herbals, vitamins, and minerals) that can either potentiate or inhibit the intended target concentration. Trough collection times should be documented carefully in relation to the time of medication administration.

The metabolism of many commonly prescribed medications is driven by the cytochrome P450 (CYP450) family of enzymes. Genetic variants can alter enzymatic activity that results in a spectrum of effects ranging from the total absence of drug metabolism to ultrafast metabolism. Impaired drug metabolism can prevent the intended therapeutic effect or even lead to serious adverse drug reactions. Poor metabolizers (PM) are at increased risk for drug-induced side effects due to accumulation of drug in the blood, while ultra-rapid metabolizers (UM) require a higher than normal dosage because the drug is metabolized over a shorter duration than intended. Other genetic phenotypes used to report CYP450 results are intermediate metabolizer (IM) and extensive metabolizer (EM). Genetic testing can be performed on blood samples submitted to a laboratory. The test method commonly used is polymerase chain reaction. Counseling and informed written consent are generally required for genetic testing. CYP2D6 is a gene in the CYP450 family that metabolizes drugs such as tricyclic antidepressants like nortriptyline, antipsychotics like haloperidol, and beta blockers. Testing for the most common genetic variants of CYP2D6 is used to predict altered enzyme activity and anticipate the most effective therapeutic plan.

Nursing Implications

Assessment

Indications	Potential Nursing Problems
Assist in the diagnosis and prevention of toxicity	• Emotional Distress
	• Grief
Evaluate overdose, especially in combination with ethanol (*Note:* Doxepin abuse is unusual.)	• Health Management (*related to potential toxic or subtherapeutic levels*)
	• Human Response
Monitor compliance with therapeutic regimen	• Noncompliance
	• Spirituality

Diagnosis: Clinical Significance of Test Results

Level	Response
Normal levels	Therapeutic effect
Subtherapeutic levels	Adjust dose as indicated
Toxic levels	Adjust dose as indicated
Amitriptyline	Hepatic impairment
Nortriptyline	Hepatic impairment
Protriptyline	Hepatic impairment
Doxepin	Hepatic impairment
Imipramine	Hepatic impairment

Planning

Considerations for planning a successful partnership should include clear communication of what to expect during the test to decrease anxiety and improve cooperation. Obtain a complete history of the time and amount of drug ingested by the patient. Before the procedure is performed, plan to review the steps with the patient. Address concerns about pain and explain that there may be some discomfort during the venipuncture.

CONTRAINDICATIONS

These medications are metabolized and excreted by the liver and are therefore contraindicated in patients with hepatic disease. Caution is advised in patients with renal impairment.

SPECIAL CONSIDERATIONS

An important aspect of planning is understanding the factors that may alter the study findings or cause abnormal results. Interdepartmental communication is a key factor in the planning process. It should be noted when planning for this study that blood drawn in serum separator tubes (gel tubes) will be rejected for analysis.

It is also important to understand which medications or substances the patient may be exposed to in the healthcare setting that can interfere with accurate testing:

• Cyclic antidepressants may potentiate the effects of oral anticoagulants.

Implementation

Patient education is key to obtaining the patient's cooperation in following directions, and providing an explanation for the purpose of the procedure is an important part of this process. Inform the patient that this study can assist in monitoring subtherapeutic, therapeutic, or toxic drug levels. Consider the recommended collection time in relation to the dosing schedule. Perform the venipuncture.

Evaluation

Recognize anxiety related to test results and explain to the patient the importance of following the medication regimen; provide instructions regarding drug interactions. Instruct the patient to immediately report any unusual sensations (e.g., severe headache, vomiting, sweating, visual disturbances) to his or her health-care provider (HCP). Blood pressure should be monitored regularly. Instruct the patient to be prepared to provide the pharmacist with a list of other medications he or she is already taking in the event that the requesting HCP prescribes a medication.

NUTRITIONAL CONSIDERATIONS: Discuss avoiding alcohol consumption while taking these medications.

✅ *Critical Findings*

It is important to note the adverse effects of toxic and subtherapeutic levels of antidepressants. Care must be taken to investigate signs and symptoms of too little and too much medication.

Note and immediately report to the requesting HCP any critical findings and related symptoms. A listing of these findings varies among facilities.

Cyclic Antidepressants

- Amitriptyline: Greater Than 500 ng/mL (SI: Greater Than 1,800 nmol/L)
- Nortriptyline: Greater Than 500 ng/mL (SI: Greater Than 1,900 nmol/L)
- Protriptyline: Greater Than 500 ng/mL (SI: Greater Than 1,900 nmol/L)
- Doxepin: Greater Than 500 ng/mL (SI: Greater Than 1,790 nmol/L)
- Imipramine: Greater Than 500 ng/mL (SI: Greater Than 1,785 nmol/L)

Signs and symptoms of cyclic antidepressant toxicity include agitation, drowsiness, hallucinations, confusion, seizures, dysrhythmias, hyperthermia, flushing, dilation of the pupils, and possible coma. Possible interventions include administration of activated charcoal; emesis; gastric lavage with saline; administration of physostigmine to counteract seizures, hypertension, or respiratory depression; administration of bicarbonate, propranolol, lidocaine, or phenytoin to counteract dysrhythmias; and electrocardiographic monitoring.

✅ *Study Specific Complications*

Lack of consideration for the proper collection time relative to the dosing schedule can provide misleading information that may result in erroneous interpretation of levels, creating the potential for a medication error–related injury to the patient.

There are a number of complications associated with performing a venipuncture. **Pain** is commonly associated with needles, and although the pain experienced during venipuncture is usually mild, on a rare occasion the needle may strike a nerve causing permanent pain. Some patients experience a **vasovagal reaction** during the venipuncture procedure, evidenced by sweating, low blood pressure, fainting, or near fainting. The potential for a **fall injury** is a significant concern related to vasovagal reactions. Prolonged **bleeding** is a complication that occurs with patients who are taking blood thinners or who have coagulopathies such as hemophilia. A **hematoma** results when blood leaks into the tissue during or after a venipuncture, as evidenced by pain, bruising, and/or swelling at the venipuncture site. The swelling can cause injury by compression to surrounding nerves, which can be temporary or permanent. HCPs should watch for minor complications such as bruising and hematoma at the venipuncture site, which are fairly common. Hematomas occur more often in older adult or frail patients, or those with veins that are difficult to access. Bleeding or bruising can be prevented once the needle has been removed by applying direct pressure to the site with dry gauze for a minute or two. Some other more unusual complications of venipuncture include **cellulitis, phlebitis, inadvertent arterial puncture,** and **sepsis.** Sepsis can be caused by introduction of bacteria from the surface of the skin into the blood as the result of improper cleansing of the venipuncture site. Immunocompromised patients are at higher risk for developing this complication.

✅ *Related Tests*

Related tests include ALT, albumin, AST, bilirubin, BUN, creatinine, CBC, electrolytes, GGT, and protein blood total and fractions.

See the Genitourinary and Hepatobiliary systems tables at the end of the book for related tests by body system.

Expected Outcomes

Expected outcomes associated with Antidepressant Drugs are:

- Demonstrating an understanding of the proper use of the medication and obtaining the maximum benefit from the medication regimen
- Demonstrating an ability to cope with stressful situations
- Agreeing to seek the assistance of a support group to manage emotional health

Aspartate Aminotransferase

Quick Summary

SYNONYM ACRONYM: Serum glutamic-oxaloacetic transaminase, AST, SGOT.

COMMON USE: Considered an indicator of cellular damage in liver disease, such as hepatitis or cirrhosis; and in heart disease, such as myocardial infarction.

SPECIMEN: Serum collected in a gold-, red-, or red/gray-top tube.

NORMAL FINDINGS: (Method: Spectrophotometry, enzymatic at 37°C)

Age	Conventional Units	SI Units (Conventional Units × 0.017)
Newborn	25–75 units/L	0.43–1.28 micro kat/L
10 days–23 mo	15–60 units/L	0.26–1.02 micro kat/L
2–3 yr	10–56 units/L	0.17–0.95 micro kat/L
4–6 yr	20–39 units/L	0.34–0.66 micro kat/L
7–19 yr	12–32 units/L	0.2–0.54 micro kat/L
20–49 yr		
Male	20–40 units/L	0.34–0.68 micro kat/L
Female	15–30 units/L	0.26–0.51 micro kat/L
Greater than 50 yr (older adult)		
Male	10–35 units/L	0.17–0.6 micro kat/L
Greater than 45 yr (older adult)		
Female	10–35 units/L	0.17–0.6 micro kat/L

Values may be slightly elevated in older adults due to the effects of medications and the presence of multiple chronic or acute diseases with or without muted symptoms.

Test Explanation

Aspartate aminotransferase (AST) is an enzyme that catalyzes the reversible transfer of an amino group between aspartate and α-ketoglutaric acid in the citric acid or Krebs cycle, a powerful and essential biochemical pathway for releasing stored energy. It was formerly known as serum glutamic-oxaloacetic transaminase (SGOT). AST exists in large amounts in liver and myocardial cells and in smaller but significant amounts in skeletal muscle, kidneys, pancreas, red blood cells, and the brain. Serum AST rises when there is damage to the tissues and cells where the enzyme is found and levels directly reflect the extent of damage. AST values greater than 500 units/L are usually associated with hepatitis and other hepatocellular diseases in an acute phase. AST levels are very elevated at birth, decrease with age to adulthood, and increase slightly in older adults. *Note:* Measurement of AST in evaluation of myocardial infarction has been replaced by more sensitive tests, such as creatine kinase–MB fraction (CK-MB) and troponin.

Nursing Implications

Assessment

Indications	Potential Nursing Problems
Assist in the diagnosis of disorders or injuries involving the tissues where AST is normally found	• Breathing **(related to pressure from ascites on the diaphragm)**
Assist (formerly) in the diagnosis of myocardial infarction (*Note:* AST rises within 6 to 8 hr, peaks at 24 to 48 hr, and declines to normal within 72 to 96 hr of a myocardial infarction if no further cardiac damage occurs) Compare serially with alanine aminotransferase levels to track the course of hepatitis Monitor response to therapy with potentially hepatotoxic or nephrotoxic drugs Monitor response to treatment for various disorders in which AST may be elevated, with tissue repair indicated by declining levels	• Confusion and Disturbed Thoughts **(related to an accumulation of ammonia)** • Human Response • Nutrition

Diagnosis: Clinical Significance of Test Results
INCREASED IN
AST is released from any damaged cell in which it is stored, so conditions that affect the liver, kidneys, heart, pancreas, red blood cells, or skeletal muscle, and cause cellular destruction demonstrate elevated AST levels.

SIGNIFICANTLY INCREASED IN (GREATER THAN FIVE TIMES NORMAL LEVELS)

- Acute hepatitis **(AST is very elevated in acute viral hepatitis)**
- Acute hepatocellular disease **(especially related to chemical toxicity or drug overdose; moderate doses of acetaminophen have initiated severe hepatocellular disease in patients who are alcoholics)**
- Acute pancreatitis
- Shock

MODERATELY INCREASED IN (THREE TO FIVE TIMES NORMAL LEVELS)

- Alcohol misuse (chronic)
- Biliary tract obstruction
- Cardiac dysrhythmias
- Cardiac catheterization, angioplasty, or surgery
- Chronic hepatitis
- Cirrhosis
- Heart failure
- HELLP Syndrome
- Infectious mononucleosis
- Liver tumors
- Muscle diseases (e.g., dermatomyositis, dystrophy, gangrene, polymyositis, trichinosis)
- Myocardial infarct
- Reye syndrome
- Trauma **(related to injury or surgery of liver, head, and other sites where AST is found)**

SLIGHTLY INCREASED IN (TWO TO THREE TIMES NORMAL)

- Cerebrovascular accident
- Cirrhosis, fatty liver *(related to obesity, diabetes, jejunoileal bypass, administration of total parenteral nutrition)*
- Delirium tremens
- Hemolytic anemia
- Pericarditis
- Pulmonary infarction

DECREASED IN

- Hemodialysis *(presumed to be related to a corresponding deficiency of vitamin B$_6$ observed in hemodialysis patients)*
- Uremia *(related to a buildup of toxins that modify the activity of coenzymes required for transaminase activity)*
- Vitamin B$_6$ deficiency *(related to the lack of vitamin B$_6$, a required cofactor for the transaminases)*

Planning

Considerations for planning a successful partnership should include clear communication of what to expect during the test to decrease anxiety and improve cooperation. Before the procedure is performed, plan to review the steps with the patient. Address concerns about pain, and explain that there may be some discomfort during the venipuncture.

SPECIAL CONSIDERATIONS

An important aspect of planning is understanding the factors that may alter the study findings or cause abnormal results. Interdepartmental communication is a key factor in the planning process. The following should be noted when planning for this study:

- With the specimen collection technique, note that intracellular concentration of the enzyme is much higher than in the circulating plasma; therefore, hemolysis falsely increases AST values.
- Hemodialysis falsely decreases AST values.

It is also important to understand which medications or substances the patient may be exposed to in the health-care setting that can interfere with accurate testing:

- Drugs that may increase AST levels by causing cholestasis include amitriptyline, anabolic steroids, androgens, benzodiazepines, chlorothiazide, chlorpropamide, dapsone, erythromycin, estrogens, ethionamide, gold salts, imipramine, mercaptopurine, nitrofurans, oral contraceptives, penicillins, phenothiazines, progesterone, propoxyphene, sulfonamides, tamoxifen, and tolbutamide. Drugs that may increase AST levels by causing hepatocellular damage include acetaminophen, acetylsalicylic acid, allopurinol, amiodarone, anabolic steroids, anticonvulsants, asparaginase, azithromycin, bromocriptine, captopril, cephalosporins, chloramphenicol, clindamycin, clofibrate, danazol, enflurane, ethambutol, ethionamide, fenofibrate, fluconazole, fluoroquinolones, foscarnet, gentamicin, indomethacin, interferon, interleukin-2, levamisole, levodopa, lincomycin, low-molecular-weight heparin, methyldopa, monoamine oxidase inhibitors, naproxen, nifedipine, nitrofurans, oral contraceptives, probenecid, procainamide, quinine, ranitidine, retinol, ritodrine, sulfonylureas, tetracyclines, tobramycin, and verapamil.
- Drugs that may decrease AST levels include allopurinol, cyclosporine, interferon alpha, naltrexone, progesterone, trifluoperazine, and ursodiol.

Implementation

Patient education is key to obtaining the patient's cooperation in following directions, and providing an explanation for the purpose of the procedure is an important part of this process. Inform the patient that this study can assist in assessing liver function. Perform the venipuncture.

Evaluation

Recognize anxiety related to test results and be supportive of fear of a shortened life expectancy. Instruct the patient to immediately report chest pain or changes in breathing pattern to the health-care provider (HCP). Carefully observe the cirrhotic patient for the development of ascites, in which case fluid and electrolyte balance requires strict attention. Dietary and fluid restrictions may be required; diuretics may be ordered. The patient should be frequently monitored for weight gain, intake and output, and abdominal girth. The alcoholic patient should be encouraged to avoid alcohol and also to seek appropriate counseling for substance abuse. Discuss the implications of abnormal test results on the patient's lifestyle. Provide teaching and information regarding the clinical implications of the test results as appropriate. Provide contact information, if desired, for the American Heart Association (www.americanheart.org) or the National Heart, Lung, and Blood Institute (NHLBI) (www.nhlbi.nih.gov).

SPECIAL CONSIDERATIONS

Numerous studies point to the prevalence of excess body weight in American children and adolescents. Experts estimate that obesity is present in 25% of the population ages 6 to 11 years. The medical, social, and emotional consequences of excess body weight are significant. Special attention should be given to instructing the child and caregiver regarding health risks and weight-control education.

NUTRITIONAL CONSIDERATIONS FOR THE CARDIAC PATIENT: Increases in AST levels may be associated with coronary artery disease (CAD). Nutritional therapy is recommended for the patient identified to be at risk for developing CAD or for individuals who have specific risk factors and/or existing medical conditions (e.g., elevated LDL cholesterol levels, other lipid disorders, insulin-dependent diabetes, insulin resistance, or metabolic syndrome). Other changeable risk factors warranting patient education include strategies to encourage patients, especially those who are overweight and with high blood pressure, to safely decrease sodium intake, achieve a normal weight, ensure regular participation of moderate aerobic physical activity three to four times per week, eliminate tobacco use, and adhere to a heart-healthy diet. If triglycerides also are elevated, the patient should be advised to eliminate or reduce alcohol. The Guideline on Lifestyle Management to Reduce Cardiovascular Risk published by the American College of Cardiology (ACC) and the American Heart Association (AHA) in conjunction with the NHLBI recommends a "Mediterranean"-style diet rather than a low-fat diet. The guideline emphasizes inclusion of vegetables, whole grains, fruits, low-fat dairy, nuts, legumes, and nontropical vegetable oils (e.g., olive, canola, peanut, sunflower, flaxseed) along with fish and lean poultry. A similar dietary pattern known as the Dietary Approaches to Stop Hypertension (DASH) diet makes additional recommendations for the reduction of dietary sodium. Both dietary styles emphasize a reduction in consumption of red meats, which are high in saturated fats and cholesterol, and other foods containing sugar, saturated fats, trans fats, and sodium.

⚫ *Critical Findings*

N/A

⚫ *Study Specific Complications*

There are a number of complications associated with performing a venipuncture. **Pain** is commonly associated with needles, and although the pain experienced during venipuncture is usually mild, on a rare occasion the needle may strike a nerve causing permanent pain. Some patients experience a **vasovagal reaction** during the venipuncture procedure, evidenced by sweating, low blood pressure, fainting, or near fainting. The potential for a **fall injury** is a significant concern related to vasovagal reactions. Prolonged **bleeding** is a complication that occurs with patients who are taking blood thinners or who have coagulopathies such as hemophilia. A **hematoma** results when blood leaks into the tissue during or after a venipuncture, as evidenced by pain, bruising, and/or swelling at the venipuncture site. The swelling can cause injury by compression to surrounding nerves, which can be temporary or permanent. HCPs should watch for minor complications such as bruising and hematoma at the venipuncture site, which are fairly common. Hematomas occur more often in older adult or frail patients, or those with veins that are difficult to access. Bleeding or bruising can be prevented once the needle has been removed by applying direct pressure to the site with dry gauze for a minute or two. Some other more unusual complications of venipuncture include **cellulitis, phlebitis, inadvertent arterial puncture,** and **sepsis.** Sepsis can be caused by introduction of bacteria from the surface of the skin into the blood as the result of improper cleansing of the venipuncture site. Immunocompromised patients are at higher risk for developing this complication.

⚫ *Related Tests*

Related tests include acetaminophen, ALT, albumin, ALP, ammonia, AMA/ASMA, α_1-antitrypsin/phenotyping, bilirubin and fractions, biopsy liver, cholangiography percutaneous transhepatic, cholangiography post-op, CT biliary tract and liver, ERCP, ethanol, ferritin, GGT, hepatitis antigens and antibodies, hepatobiliary scan, iron/total iron-binding capacity, liver and spleen scan, protein and fractions, PT/INR, US abdomen, and US liver if liver disease is suspected; and antidysrhythmic drugs, apolipoprotein A and B, ANP, BNP, blood gases, CRP, calcium/ionized calcium, CT scoring, cholesterol (total, HDL, and LDL), CK, echocardiography, Holter monitor, homocysteine, LDH, MRI chest, myocardial infarct scan, myocardial perfusion heart scan, myoglobin, PET heart, potassium, triglycerides, and troponin if myocardial infarction is suspected.

See the Cardiovascular and Hepatobiliary systems tables at the end of the book for related tests by body system.

Expected Outcomes

Expected outcomes associated with Aspartate Aminotransferase (AST) are:

- Displaying respiratory effort that is normally evidenced by absence of the use of accessory muscles with ventilatory effort
- Verbalizing an understanding of the disease and possible treatment options
- Listing and discussing lifestyle adjustments required to promote healing and reduce risk factors
- Verbalizing an understanding of the disease and its cause; the patient is prepared to address addiction issues related to the disease
- Describing components of a healthy, balanced diet and being compliant with preparing meals that meet nutritional requirements demonstrated by attainment of a healthy weight
- Complying with ordered medication and the therapeutic regimen as demonstrated by the lack of complications such as bleeding tendencies, the development of ascites, infection, or neurological dysfunction

Bilirubin and Bilirubin Fractions

Quick Summary

SYNONYM ACRONYM: Conjugated/direct bilirubin, unconjugated/indirect bilirubin, delta bilirubin, TBil.

COMMON USE: A multipurpose lab test that acts as an indicator for various diseases of the liver or for disease that affects the liver, or conditions associated with RBC hemolysis.

SPECIMEN: Serum collected in gold-, red-, or red/gray-top tube. Plasma collected in green-top (heparin) tube or in a heparinized microtainer is also acceptable. Protect sample from direct light.

NORMAL FINDINGS: (Method: Spectrophotometry) Total bilirubin levels in infants should decrease to adult levels by day 10 as the development of the hepatic circulatory system matures. Values in breastfed infants may take longer to reach normal adult levels. Values in premature infants may initially be higher than in full-term infants and also take longer to decrease to normal levels.

Age	Conventional Units	SI Units (Conventional Units × 17.1)
Total bilirubin		
Newborn–1 day	Less than 5.8 mg/dL	Less than 99 micromol/L
1–2 days	Less than 8.2 mg/dL	Less than 140 micromol/L
3–5 days	Less than 11.7 mg/dL	Less than 200 micromol/L
6–7 days	Less than 8.4 mg/dL	Less than 144 micromol/L
8–9 days	Less than 6.5 mg/dL	Less than 111 micromol/L
10–11 days	Less than 4.6 mg/dL	Less than 79 micromol/L
12–13 days	Less than 2.7 mg/dL	Less than 46 micromol/L
14–30 days	Less than 0.8 mg/dL	Less than 14 micromol/L
1 mo–older adult	Less than 1.2 mg/dL	Less than 21 micromol/L
Unconjugated bilirubin	Less than 1.1 mg/dL	Less than 19 micromol/L
Conjugated bilirubin		
Neonate	Less than 0.6 mg/dL	Less than 10 micromol/L
29 days–older adult	Less than 0.3 mg/dL	Less than 5 micromol/L
Delta bilirubin	Less than 0.2 mg/dL	Less than 3 micromol/L

Test Explanation

Bilirubin is a by-product of heme catabolism from aged red blood cells (RBCs). Bilirubin is primarily produced in the liver, spleen, and bone marrow. Total bilirubin is the sum of unconjugated or indirect bilirubin, monoglucuronide and diglucuronide, conjugated or direct bilirubin, and albumin-bound delta bilirubin. Unconjugated bilirubin is carried to the liver by albumin, where it becomes conjugated. In the small intestine, conjugated bilirubin converts to urobilinogen and then to stercobilin and urobilin. Stercobilin is then excreted in the feces and urobilin is excreted in the urine. Defects in bilirubin excretion can be identified in a routine urinalysis. Increases in bilirubin levels can result from prehepatic, hepatic, and/or posthepatic conditions, making fractionation useful in determining the cause of the increase in total bilirubin levels. Delta bilirubin has a longer half-life than the other bilirubin fractions and therefore remains elevated during convalescence after the other fractions have decreased to normal levels. Delta bilirubin can be calculated using the formula:

$$\text{Delta bilirubin} = \text{Total bilirubin} - (\text{Indirect bilirubin} + \text{Direct bilirubin})$$

When bilirubin concentration increases, the yellowish pigment deposits in skin and sclera. This increase in yellow pigmentation is termed *jaundice* or *icterus*. Bilirubin levels can also be checked using noninvasive methods. Hyperbilirubinemia in neonates can be reliably evaluated using transcutaneous measurement devices (see Fig. 1.8).

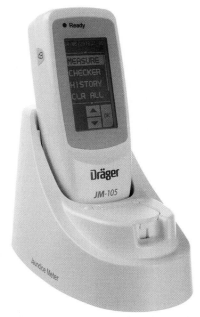

FIGURE 1.8 Transcutaneous bilirubinometer.

Nursing Implications

Assessment

Indications	Potential Nursing Problems
Assist in the differential diagnosis of obstructive jaundice Assist in the evaluation of liver and biliary disease Monitor the effects of drug reactions on liver function Monitor the effects of phototherapy on jaundiced newborns Monitor jaundice in newborn patients	• Body Image • Confusion • Dehydration *(related to insufficient fluids or phototherapy in the case of a neonate)* • Emotional Distress • Gas Exchange • Hyperthermia *(related to phototherapy in the case of a neonate)* • Human Response • Jaundice *(related to deposition of the bilirubin pigment in skin tissue or sclera)* • Nutrition • Skin *(related to dehydration in the case of a neonate)*

Diagnosis: Clinical Significance of Test Results

INCREASED IN

- Prehepatic (hemolytic) jaundice *(related to excessive amounts of heme released from RBC destruction. Heme is catabolized to bilirubin in concentrations that exceed the liver's conjugation capacity, and indirect bilirubin accumulates)*
  - Erythroblastosis fetalis
  - Hematoma
  - Hemolytic anemia
  - Pernicious anemia
  - Physiological jaundice of the newborn
  - The post blood transfusion period, when a number of units are rapidly infused or in the case of a delayed transfusion reaction
  - RBC enzyme abnormalities (i.e., glucose-6-phosphate dehydrogenase, pyruvate kinase, spherocytosis)
- Hepatic jaundice *(related to bilirubin conjugation failure)*
  - Crigler-Najjar syndrome
- Hepatic jaundice *(related to disturbance in bilirubin transport)*
  - Dubin-Johnson syndrome *(related to preconjugation transport failure)*
  - Gilbert syndrome *(related to postconjugation transport failure)*
- Hepatic jaundice *(evidenced by liver damage or necrosis that interferes with excretion into bile ducts either by physical obstruction or drug inhibition and bilirubin accumulates)*
  - Alcoholism
  - Cholangitis

  - Cholecystitis
  - Cholestatic drug reactions
  - Cirrhosis
  - Hepatitis
  - Hepatocellular damage
  - Infectious mononucleosis
- Posthepatic jaundice *(evidenced by blockage that interferes with excretion into bile ducts, resulting in accumulated bilirubin)*
  - Advanced tumors of the liver
  - Biliary obstruction
- Other conditions
  - Anorexia or starvation *(related to liver damage)*
  - HELLP Syndrome *(related to hemolysis)*
  - Hypothyroidism *(related to effect on the liver whereby hepatic enzyme activity for formation of conjugated or direct bilirubin is enhanced in combination with decreased flow of bile and secretion of bile acids; results in accumulation of direct bilirubin)*
  - Premature or breastfed infants *(evidenced by diminished hepatic function of the liver in premature infants; related to inability of neonate to feed in sufficient quantity. Insufficient breast milk intake results in weight loss, decreased stool formation, and decreased elimination of bilirubin)*

DECREASED IN
N/A

Planning

Considerations for planning a successful partnership should include clear communication of what to expect during the test to decrease anxiety and improve cooperation. Before the procedure is performed, plan to review the steps with the patient. Address concerns about pain and explain that there may be some discomfort during the venipuncture.

SPECIAL CONSIDERATIONS

An important aspect of planning is understanding the factors that may alter the study findings or cause abnormal results. Interdepartmental communication is a key factor in the planning process. The following should be noted when planning for this study: Bilirubin is light-sensitive. Therefore, the collection container should be suitably covered to protect the specimen from light between the time of collection and analysis.

It is also important to understand which medications or substances the patient may be exposed to in the health-care setting that can interfere with accurate testing:

- Drugs that may increase bilirubin levels by causing cholestasis include anabolic steroids, androgens, butaperazine, chlorothiazide, chlorpromazine, chlorpropamide, cinchophen, dapsone, dienoestrol, erythromycin, estrogens, ethionamide, gold salts, hydrochlorothiazide, icterogenin, imipramine, iproniazid, isocarboxazid, isoniazid, meprobamate, mercaptopurine, meropenem, methandriol, nitrofurans, norethandrolone, nortriptyline, oleandomycin, oral contraceptives, penicillins, phenothiazines, prochlorperazine, progesterone, promazine, promethazine, propoxyphene, protriptyline, sulfonamides, tacrolimus, thiouracil, tolazamide, tolbutamide, thiacetazone, trifluoperazine, and trimeprazine.

- Drugs that may increase bilirubin levels by causing hepatocellular damage include acetaminophen (toxic), acetylsalicylic acid, allopurinol, aminothiazole, anabolic steroids, asparaginase, azathioprine, azithromycin, carbamazepine, carbutamide, chloramphenicol, clindamycin, clofibrate, chlorambucil, chloramphenicol, chlordane, chloroform, chlorzoxazone, clonidine, colchicine, coumarin, cyclophosphamide, cyclopropane, cycloserine, cyclosporine, dactinomycin, danazol, desipramine, dexfenfluramine, diazepam, diethylstilbestrol, dinitrophenol, enflurane, ethambutol, ethionamide, ethoxazene, factor IX complex, felbamate, flavaspidic acid, flucytosine, fusidic acid, gentamicin, glycopyrrolate, guanoxan, haloperidol, halothane, hycanthone, hydroxyacetamide, ibuprofen, interferon, interleukin-2, isoniazid, kanamycin, labetalol, levamisole, lincomycin, melphalan, mesoridazine, metahexamide, metaxalone, methotrexate, methoxsalen, methyldopa, nitrofurans, oral contraceptives, oxamniquine, oxyphenisatin, pemoline, penicillin, perphenazine, phenazopyridine, phenelzine, phenindione, pheniprazine, phenothiazines, piroxicam, probenecid, procainamide, pyrazinamide, quinine, sulfonylureas, thiothixene, timolol, tobramycin, tolcapone, tretinoin, trimethadione, urethan, and verapamil.
- Drugs that may increase bilirubin levels by causing hemolysis include aminopyrine, amphotericin B, carbamazepine, cephaloridine, cephalothin, chloroquine, dimercaprol, dipyrone, furadaltone, furazolidone, mefenamic acid, melphalan, mephenytoin, methylene blue, nitrofurans, nitrofurazone, pamaquine, penicillins, pentaquine, phenylhydrazine, piperazine, pipobroman, primaquine, procainamide, quinacrine, quinidine, quinine, stibophen, streptomycin, sulfonamides, triethylenemelamine, tyrothricin, and vitamin K.
- Drugs that may decrease bilirubin levels include anticonvulsants, barbiturates (newborns), chlorophenothane, cyclosporine, flumecinolone (newborns), and salicylates.

Implementation
Patient education is key to obtaining the patient's cooperation in following directions, and providing an explanation for the purpose of the procedure is an important part of this process. Inform the patient that this study can assist in assessing liver function. Perform the venipuncture or heel stick.

Evaluation
Recognize anxiety related to test results and answer any questions or address any concerns voiced by the patient or family. Educate the patient regarding the cause of the hyperbilirubinemia. Explain the importance of adequate fluid intake and teach the patient skin care for the neonate.

Complications: There are several types of jaundice that may occur in the neonate, and it is important to quickly determine the cause so that effective treatment can be initiated.

1. Physiologic jaundice occurs as a normal response to the neonate's limited ability to excrete bilirubin in the first days of life. Intervention may include early, frequent feeding to stimulate gastrointestinal motility and phototherapy. This type of jaundice usually lasts 10 to 14 days, premature neonates may take up to a month, and it resolves in reverse to the pattern of development with the legs looking normal first and the face remaining yellowish longer (see Fig. 1.9).
2. Breastfeeding jaundice is seen in breastfed neonates during the first week of life, peaking during the second or third week. It occurs due to dehydration in neonates who do not nurse well or if the mother's milk is slow to come in; the bilirubin levels are elevated relative to the decreased total fluid volume. The goal is to provide adequate fluid and nutrition to the breastfeeding neonate by providing water or formula between feedings until the mother's milk supply is adequate. Phototherapy may also be ordered in order to accelerate the breakdown of bilirubin and to prevent accumulation to dangerous levels. Skin turgor, input and output, vital signs, and the

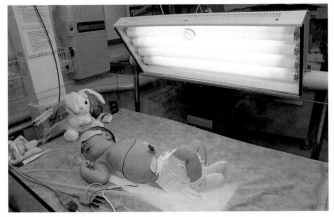

F I G U R E 1 . 9 Phototherapy for jaundice. *Used with permission, from Ward, S. (2009). Maternal-child nursing care: Optimizing outcomes for mothers, children, and families. FA Davis Company.*

number and quality of stools should be frequently monitored. Total bilirubin and fractions should be monitored regularly until levels decrease to normal neonatal values.

3. Breast milk jaundice is different than breastfeeding jaundice, occurs in about 2% of breastfed neonates after the first week of life, takes up to 12 weeks to resolve, and is believed to have a familial relationship; assessment of the family history is very helpful. Hyperbilirubinemia occurs due to substances in the mother's milk that interfere with the development of enzymes required to break down bilirubin. The main goals are to increase fluids by more frequent feeding, or additional fluids given orally or by IV and through the use of phototherapy. Fiberoptic blankets and special beds that shine light up from the mattresses are available.

4. Severe jaundice may occur as the result of an ABO or Rh incompatibility between the mother and baby. The jaundice occurs as the result of hemolysis or red blood cell (RBC) breakdown due to the incompatibility.

NUTRITIONAL CONSIDERATIONS: Increased bilirubin levels may be associated with liver disease. Dietary recommendations may be indicated depending on the condition and severity of the condition. For example, there are currently no specific medications that can be given to cure hepatitis, but the elimination of alcohol consumption and a diet optimized for convalescence are commonly included in the treatment plan. A high-calorie, high-protein, moderate-fat diet with a high fluid intake is often recommended for the patient with hepatitis. Treatment of cirrhosis is different because a low-protein diet may be in order if the patient's liver has lost the ability to process the end products of protein metabolism. A diet of soft foods may also be required if esophageal varices have developed. Ammonia levels may be used to determine whether protein should be added to or reduced from the diet. Patients should be encouraged to eat simple carbohydrates and emulsified fats (e.g., homogenized milk or eggs) rather than complex carbohydrates (e.g., starch, fiber, and glycogen [animal carbohydrates]) and complex fats, which require additional bile to emulsify them so that they can be used. The cirrhotic patient should be carefully observed for the development of ascites, in which case fluid and electrolyte balance requires strict attention. The alcoholic patient should be encouraged to avoid alcohol and also to seek appropriate counseling for substance abuse.

✅ Critical Findings
Adults and children
● Greater than 15 mg/dL (SI: Greater than 257 micromol/L)

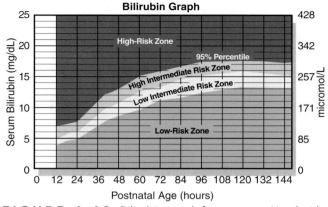

FIGURE 1.10 Bilirubin graph for neonate. *Used with permission, from Ward, S. (2009). Maternal-child nursing care: Optimizing outcomes for mothers, children, and families. FA Davis Company.*

Newborns
● Greater than 13 mg/dL (SI: Greater than 222 micromol/L)

Note and immediately report to the requesting healthcare provider (HCP) any critical findings and related symptoms. A listing of these findings varies among facilities.

Sustained hyperbilirubinemia can result in brain damage. Kernicterus refers to the deposition of bilirubin in the basal ganglia and brainstem nuclei. There is no exact level of bilirubin that puts infants at risk for developing kernicterus. Symptoms of kernicterus in infants include lethargy, poor feeding, upward deviation of the eyes, and seizures. Intervention for infants may include early frequent feedings to stimulate gastrointestinal motility, phototherapy, and exchange transfusion (see Fig. 1.10).

✅ Study Specific Complications
There are a number of complications associated with performing a venipuncture. **Pain** is commonly associated with needles, and although the pain experienced during venipuncture is usually mild, on a rare occasion the needle may strike a nerve causing permanent pain. Some patients experience a **vasovagal reaction** during the venipuncture procedure, evidenced by sweating, low blood pressure, fainting, or near fainting. The potential for a **fall injury** is a significant concern related to vasovagal reactions. Prolonged **bleeding** is a complication that occurs with patients who are taking blood thinners or who have coagulopathies such as hemophilia. A **hematoma** results when blood leaks into the tissue during or after a venipuncture, as evidenced by pain, bruising, and/or swelling at the venipuncture site. The swelling can cause injury by compression to surrounding nerves, which can be temporary or permanent. Health-care providers (HCPs) should watch for minor complications such as bruising and hematoma at the venipuncture site,

which are fairly common. Hematomas occur more often in older adult or frail patients, or those with veins that are difficult to access. Bleeding or bruising can be prevented once the needle has been removed by applying direct pressure to the site with dry gauze for a minute or two. Some other more unusual complications of venipuncture include **cellulitis, phlebitis, inadvertent arterial puncture,** and **sepsis.** Sepsis can be caused by introduction of bacteria from the surface of the skin into the blood as the result of improper cleansing of the venipuncture site. Immunocompromised patients are at higher risk for developing this complication.

✅ *Related Tests*

Related tests include ALT, albumin, ALP, ammonia, amylase, AMA/ASMA, α_1-antitrypsin/phenotyping, AST, biopsy liver, cholesterol, coagulation factor assays, CBC, cholangiography percutaneous transhepatic, cholangiography post-op, CT biliary tract and liver, copper, ERCP, GGT, hepatobiliary scan, hepatitis serologies, infectious mononucleosis screen, lipase, liver and spleen scan, protein total and fractions, PT/INR, US abdomen, US liver, and UA.

See the Hepatobiliary System table at the end of the book for related tests by body system.

Expected Outcomes

Expected outcomes associated with Bilirubin and Bilirubin Fractions are:

- Decreasing neonatal values to normal in response to appropriate treatments
- Demonstrating emotional stability in relation to worry over the newborn's jaundice
- Adapting to body image changes associated with ongoing jaundice
- Verbalizing an understanding of the disease, available treatment options, and lifestyle changes that are required to achieve an improvement in health status
- Describing symptoms that should be immediately communicated to the HCP
- Complying with the ordered therapy and the jaundice resolves
- Verbalizing an understanding of the disease and its cause; the patient is prepared to address addiction issues related to the disease
- Verbalizing components of a healthy, balanced diet and being compliant with preparing meals that meet their nutritional requirements evidenced by the attainment and maintenance of a healthy weight
- Complying with ordered medication and the therapeutic regimen as demonstrated by the lack of complications such as bleeding tendencies, the development of ascites, infection, or neurological dysfunction
- Accepting body image changes related to ongoing disease pathology

Calcium, Blood

Quick Summary

SYNONYM ACRONYM: Total calcium, Ca.

COMMON USE: To investigate various conditions related to abnormally increased or decreased calcium levels.

SPECIMEN: Serum collected in a red- or red/gray-top tube. Plasma collected in a green-top (heparin) tube is also acceptable.

NORMAL FINDINGS: (Method: Spectrophotometry)

Age	Conventional Units	SI Units (Conventional Units × 0.25)
Cord	8.2–11.2 mg/dL	2.1–2.8 mmol/L
0–10 days	7.6–10.4 mg/dL	1.9–2.6 mmol/L
11 days–2 yr	9–11 mg/dL	2.2–2.8 mmol/L
3–12 yr	8.8–10.8 mg/dL	2.2–2.7 mmol/L
13–18 yr	8.4–10.2 mg/dL	2.1–2.6 mmol/L
Adult	8.2–10.2 mg/dL	2.1–2.6 mmol/L
Adult older than 90 yr	8.2–9.6 mg/dL	2.1–2.4 mmol/L

Test Explanation

Calcium, the most abundant cation in the body, participates in almost all of the body's vital processes. Calcium concentration is largely regulated by the parathyroid glands and by the action of vitamin D. Of the body's calcium reserves, 98% to 99% is stored in the teeth and skeleton. Calcium values are higher in children because of growth and active bone formation. About 45% of the total amount of blood calcium circulates as free ions that participate in numerous regulatory functions to include bone development and maintenance, blood coagulation, transmission of nerve impulses, activation of enzymes, stimulating the glandular secretion of hormones, and control of skeletal and cardiac muscle contractility. The remaining calcium is bound to circulating proteins (40% bound mostly to albumin) and anions (15% bound to anions such as bicarbonate, citrate, phosphate, and lactate) and plays no physiological role. Calcium values can be adjusted up or down by 0.8 mg/dL for every 1 g/dL that albumin is greater than or less than 4 g/dL. Calcium and phosphorus levels are inversely proportional.

Fluid and electrolyte imbalances are often seen in patients with serious illness or injury; in these clinical situations, the normal homeostatic balance of the body is altered. During surgery or in the case of a critical illness, bicarbonate, phosphate, and lactate concentrations can change dramatically. Therapeutic treatments may also cause or contribute to electrolyte imbalance. This is why total calcium values can sometimes be misleading. Abnormal calcium levels are used to indicate general malfunctions in various body systems. Ionized calcium is used in more specific conditions.

Calcium values should be interpreted in conjunction with results of other tests. Normal calcium with an abnormal phosphorus value indicates impaired calcium absorption (possibly because of altered parathyroid hormone level or activity). Normal calcium with an elevated urea nitrogen value indicates possible hyperparathyroidism (primary or secondary). Normal calcium with decreased albumin value is an indication of hypercalcemia (high calcium levels). The most common cause of hypocalcemia (low calcium levels) is hypoalbuminemia. The most common causes of hypercalcemia are hyperparathyroidism and cancer (with or without bone metastases).

Nursing Implications

Assessment

Indications	Potential Nursing Problems
Detect parathyroid gland loss after thyroid or other neck surgery, as indicated by decreased levels	• Airway
	• Body Image
	• Cardiac Output **(related to hyper- or hypocalcemia)**
Evaluate cardiac dysrhythmias and coagulation disorders to determine if altered serum calcium level is contributing to the problem	• Emotional Distress
	• Fall Risk **(related to hyper- or hypocalcemia)**
Evaluate the effects of various disorders on calcium metabolism, especially diseases involving bone	• Health Management
	• Human Response
	• Injury Risk **(related to seizures secondary to hypocalcemia)**
Monitor the effectiveness of therapy being administered to correct abnormal calcium levels, especially calcium deficiencies	• Mobility
	• Nutrition **(related to hypocalcemia due to insufficient intake or hypoalbuminemia)**
Monitor the effects of renal failure and various drugs on calcium levels	• Sensory Perception

Diagnosis: Clinical Significance of Test Results

INCREASED IN

- Acidosis *(related to imbalance in electrolytes; longstanding acidosis can result in osteoporosis and release of calcium into circulation)*
- Acromegaly *(related to alteration in vitamin D metabolism, resulting in increased calcium)*
- Addison disease *(related to adrenal gland dysfunction; decreased blood volume and dehydration occur in the absence of aldosterone)*
- Cancers (bone, Burkitt lymphoma, Hodgkin lymphoma, leukemia, myeloma, and metastases from other organs)
- Dehydration *(related to a decrease in the fluid portion of blood, causing an overall increase in the concentration of most plasma constituents)*
- Hyperparathyroidism *(related to increased parathyroid hormone [PTH] and vitamin D levels, which increase circulating calcium levels)*
- Idiopathic hypercalcemia of infancy
- Lung disease (tuberculosis, histoplasmosis, coccidioidomycosis, berylliosis) *(related to activity by macrophages in the epithelium that interfere with vitamin D regulation by converting it to its active form; vitamin D increases circulating calcium levels)*
- Malignant disease without bone involvement *(some cancers [e.g., squamous cell carcinoma of the lung and kidney cancer] produce PTH-related peptide that increases calcium levels)*
- Milk-alkali syndrome (Burnett syndrome) *(related to excessive intake of calcium-containing milk or antacids, which can increase calcium levels)*
- Paget disease *(related to calcium released from bone)*
- Pheochromocytoma *(hyperparathyroidism related to multiple endocrine neoplasia type 2A [MEN2A] syndrome associated with some pheochromocytomas; PTH increases calcium levels)*
- Polycythemia vera *(related to dehydration; decreased blood volume due to excessive production of red blood cells)*
- Renal transplant *(related to imbalances in electrolytes; a common post-transplant issue)*
- Sarcoidosis *(related to activity by macrophages in the granulomas that interfere with vitamin D regulation by converting it to its active form; vitamin D increases circulating calcium levels)*
- Thyrotoxicosis *(related to increased bone turnover and release of calcium into the blood)*
- Vitamin D toxicity *(vitamin D increases circulating calcium levels)*

DECREASED IN

- Acute pancreatitis *(complication of pancreatitis related to hypoalbuminemia and calcium binding by excessive fats)*
- Alcoholism *(related to insufficient nutrition)*
- Alkalosis *(increased blood pH causes intracellular uptake of calcium to increase)*
- Chronic renal failure *(related to decreased synthesis of vitamin D)*
- Cystinosis *(hereditary disorder of the renal tubules that results in excessive calcium loss)*
- Hepatic cirrhosis *(related to impaired metabolism of vitamin D and calcium)*
- Hyperphosphatemia *(phosphorus and calcium have an inverse relationship)*

- Hypoalbuminemia *(related to insufficient levels of albumin, an important carrier protein)*
- Hypomagnesemia *(lack of magnesium inhibits PTH and thereby decreases calcium levels)*
- Hypoparathyroidism (congenital, idiopathic, surgical) *(related to lack of PTH)*
- Inadequate nutrition
- Leprosy *(related to increased bone retention)*
- Long-term anticonvulsant therapy *(these medications block calcium channels and interfere with calcium transport)*
- Malabsorption (celiac disease, tropical sprue, pancreatic insufficiency) *(related to insufficient absorption)*
- Massive blood transfusion *(related to the presence of citrate preservative in blood product that chelates or binds calcium and removes it from circulation)*
- Neonatal prematurity
- Osteomalacia (advanced) *(bone loss is so advanced there is little calcium remaining to be released into circulation)*
- Renal tubular disease *(related to decreased synthesis of vitamin D)*
- Vitamin D deficiency (rickets) *(related to insufficient amounts of vitamin D, resulting in decreased calcium metabolism)*

Planning

Considerations for planning a successful partnership should include clear communication of what to expect during the test to decrease anxiety and improve cooperation. Before the procedure is performed, plan to review the steps with the patient. Address concerns about pain, and explain that there may be some discomfort during the venipuncture.

SPECIAL CONSIDERATIONS

An important aspect of planning is understanding the factors that may alter the study findings or cause abnormal results. Interdepartmental communication is a key factor in the planning process. The following should be noted when planning for this study:

- Calcium exhibits diurnal variation; serial samples should be collected at the same time of day for comparison.
- Patients on ethylenediaminetetraacetic acid (EDTA) therapy (chelation) may show falsely decreased calcium values.
- Patients receiving massive blood transfusions may experience decreased ionized calcium values related to chelation of the free calcium by the anticoagulant in the blood products.
- Patients with very low albumin levels (e.g., in cases of malnutrition or dilutional effect of IV fluid overload) will have low total calcium levels.
- Patients who ingest large amounts of milk, calcium or Vitamin D supplements, or antacid tablets shortly before specimen collection will have increased calcium values.

- Patients with chronic kidney disease, especially those on hemodialysis, may have low calcium levels. The inability of the kidneys to filter excess phosphorus from the blood into urine stimulates abnormal excretion of calcium resulting in lower circulating calcium levels. If the calcium concentration in the dialysate fluid is not adjusted to correct the blood levels, the parathyroid glands secrete PTH, which causes calcium to be lost from the bones. Over time, bone loss results in deformities and loss of function.
- Hemolysis and icterus cause false-positive results because of interference from biological pigments.
- Specimens should never be collected above an IV line because of the potential for dilution when the specimen and the IV solution combine in the collection container, falsely decreasing the result. There is also the potential of contaminating the sample with the substance of interest if it is present in the IV solution, falsely increasing the result.

It is also important to understand which medications or substances the patient may be exposed to in the healthcare setting that can interfere with accurate testing:

- Drugs that may increase calcium levels include anabolic steroids, some antacids, calcitriol, calcium salts, danazol, diuretics (long-term), ergocalciferol, hydralazine, isotretinoin, lithium, oral contraceptives, parathyroid extract, parathyroid hormone, prednisone, progesterone, tamoxifen, vitamin A, and vitamin D.
- Drugs that may decrease calcium levels include acetazolamide, albuterol, alprostadil, aminoglycosides, anticonvulsants, asparaginase, aspirin, calcitonin, cisplatin, diuretics (initially), estrogens, gastrin, glucagon, glucocorticoids, glucose, heparin, insulin, laxatives (excessive use), magnesium salts, methicillin, phosphates, plicamycin, sodium sulfate (given IV), tetracycline (in pregnancy), trazodone, and viomycin.

Implementation

Patient education is key to obtaining the patient's cooperation in following directions, and providing an explanation for the purpose of the procedure is an important part of this process. Inform the patient that this study can assist as a general indicator in diagnosing health concerns. Perform the venipuncture.

Evaluation

Recognize anxiety related to test results, and assess the patient for signs and symptoms of calcium imbalance. Teach the patient the signs and symptoms associated with a calcium imbalance. Assess associated studies such as electrocardiogram (ECG), phosphorus, and albumin so the correct therapeutic measures can be taken. Hypoalbuminemia may initiate symptoms of hypocalcemia in the presence of near normal calcium levels. Educate the patient regarding access to nutritional counseling services. Provide contact information, if desired, for the Institute of Medicine of the National Academies (www.iom.edu) and the U.S. Department of Agriculture (www.choosemyplate.gov).

NUTRITIONAL CONSIDERATIONS: Patients with abnormal calcium values should be informed that a daily intake of calcium is important even though body stores in the bones can be called on to supplement circulating levels. Dietary calcium can be obtained from animal or plant sources. Milk and milk products, sardines, clams, oysters, salmon, refried beans, rhubarb, spinach, beet greens, broccoli, kale, tofu, legumes, and fortified orange juice are high in calcium. Milk and milk products also contain vitamin D and lactose, which assist calcium absorption. Cooked vegetables yield more absorbable calcium than raw vegetables. Patients should be informed of the substances that can inhibit calcium absorption by irreversibly binding to some of the calcium, making it unavailable for absorption, such as oxalates, which naturally occur in some vegetables (e.g., beet greens, collards, leeks, okra, parsley, quinoa, spinach, Swiss chard) and are found in tea; phytic acid, found in some cereals (e.g., wheat bran, wheat germ); phosphoric acid, found in dark cola; and insoluble dietary fiber (in excessive amounts). Excessive protein intake can also negatively affect calcium absorption, especially if it is combined with foods high in phosphorus and in the presence of a reduced dietary calcium intake (see Fig. 1.11).

✅ Critical Findings

- Less than 7 mg/dL (SI: Less than 1.8 mmol/L)
- Greater than 12 mg/dL (SI: Greater than 3 mmol/L) (some patients can tolerate higher concentrations)

Note and immediately report to the requesting health-care provider (HCP) any critical findings and related symptoms. A listing of these findings varies among facilities.

Consideration may be given to verify the critical findings before action is taken. Policies vary among facilities and may include requesting immediate recollection and retesting by the laboratory or retesting using a rapid Point of Care instrument at the bedside, if available.

Observe the patient for symptoms of critically decreased or elevated calcium levels. Hypocalcemia is evidenced by convulsions, nervousness, dysrhythmias, changes in ECG in the form of prolonged ST segment and Q-T interval, facial spasms (positive Chvostek sign), tetany, lethargy, muscle cramps, tetany, numbness in extremities, tingling, and muscle twitching (positive Trousseau sign). Possible interventions include seizure precautions, increased frequency of ECG monitoring, and administration of calcium or magnesium (see Figs. 1.12 through 1.14).

Severe hypercalcemia is manifested by excessive thirst, polyuria, constipation, changes in ECG (shortened QT interval due to shortening of the ST segment and prolonged PR interval), lethargy, confusion, muscle weakness, joint aches, apathy, anorexia, headache,

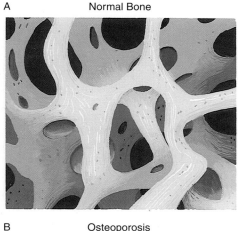

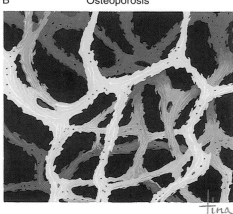

FIGURE 1.11 (A) Normal bone and (B) bone showing osteoporosis. *Used with permission, from Scanlon, V., & Sanders, T. (2010). Essentials of anatomy and physiology (6th Ed.). FA Davis Company.*

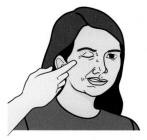

FIGURE 1.12 A positive Chvostek sign. *Used with permission, from Hale, A., & Hovey, M. (2013). Fluid and electrolyte notes. FA Davis Company.*

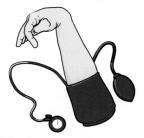

FIGURE 1.13 A positive Trousseau sign. *Used with permission, from Hale, A., & Hovey, M. (2013). Fluid and electrolyte notes. FA Davis Company.*

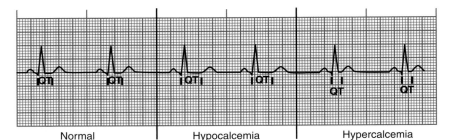

FIGURE 1.14 ECG lead II changes comparing normal calcium to calcium imbalances. *Used with permission, from Hale, A., & Hovey, M. (2013). Fluid and electrolyte notes. FA Davis Company.*

nausea, vomiting, and ultimately may result in coma. Possible interventions include the administration of normal saline and diuretics to speed up dilution and excretion or administration of calcitonin or steroids to force the circulating calcium into the cells.

● *Study Specific Complications*

There are a number of complications associated with performing a venipuncture. **Pain** is commonly associated with needles, and although the pain experienced during venipuncture is usually mild, on a rare occasion the needle may strike a nerve causing permanent pain. Some patients experience a **vasovagal reaction** during the venipuncture procedure, evidenced by sweating, low blood pressure, fainting, or near fainting. The potential for a **fall injury** is a significant concern related to vasovagal reactions. Prolonged **bleeding** is a complication that occurs with patients who are taking blood thinners or who have coagulopathies such as hemophilia. A **hematoma** results when blood leaks into the tissue during or after a venipuncture, as evidenced by pain, bruising, and/or swelling at the venipuncture site. The swelling can cause injury by compression to surrounding nerves, which can be temporary or permanent. HCPs should watch for minor complications such as bruising and hematoma at the venipuncture site, which are fairly common. Hematomas occur more often in older adult or frail patients, or those with veins that are difficult to access. Bleeding or bruising can be prevented once the needle has been removed by applying direct pressure to the site with dry gauze for a minute or two. Some other more unusual complications of venipuncture include **cellulitis, phlebitis, inadvertent arterial puncture, and sepsis.** Sepsis can be caused by introduction of bacteria from the surface of the skin into the blood as the result of improper cleansing of the venipuncture site. Immunocompromised patients are at higher risk for developing this complication.

● *Related Tests*

- Related tests include ACTH, albumin, aldosterone, ALP, biopsy bone marrow, BMD, bone scan, calcitonin, calcium ionized, urine calcium, calculus kidney stone analysis, catecholamines, chloride, collagen cross-linked telopeptides, CBC, CT pelvis, CT spine, cortisol, CK and isoenzymes, DHEA, fecal fat, glucose, HVA, magnesium, metanephrines, osteocalcin, PTH, phosphorus, potassium, protein total, radiography bone, renin, sodium, thyroid scan, thyroxine, US abdomen, US thyroid and parathyroid, UA, and vitamin D.
- Refer to the Cardiovascular, Gastrointestinal, Genitourinary, Hematopoietic, Hepatobiliary, and Musculoskeletal systems tables at the end of the book for related tests by body system.

Expected Outcomes

Expected outcomes associated with Calcium, Blood are:

- Absence of any evidence of dementia, and remaining oriented to person, place, time, and purpose
- Calcium levels that reach the normal range and the patient's verbalizing the absence of symptoms associated with calcium imbalance
- Correct identification of signs and symptoms that should prompt immediate notification of the HCP
- Compliance with dietary and fluid intake recommendations; chloride intake meets the minimum daily requirements to help correct calcium levels
- Acknowledgment of lifestyle changes required to avoid injury and bone fractures
- Demonstration of the ability to manage symptoms related to calcium imbalance (thirst, cramps, nausea, vomiting, constipation) and verbalization of a reduction or an absence of symptoms
- Verbalization of an understanding of medications that contain calcium, as well as their proper use and adverse effects

Carbon Dioxide

Quick Summary

SYNONYM ACRONYM: CO_2 combining power, CO_2, Tco_2.

COMMON USE: To assess the effect of total carbon dioxide levels on respiratory and metabolic acid-base balance.

SPECIMEN: Serum collected in a gold-, red-, or red/gray-top tube, plasma collected in a green-top (lithium or sodium heparin) tube; or whole blood collected in a green-top (lithium or sodium heparin) tube or heparinized syringe.

NORMAL FINDINGS: (Method: Colorimetry, enzyme assay, or Pco_2 electrode)

Carbon Dioxide	Conventional & SI Units
Plasma or serum (venous)	
Infant–2 yr	13–29 mEq/L or mmol/L
2 yr–older adult	23–29 mEq/L or mmol/L
Whole blood (venous)	
Infant–2 yr	18–28 mEq/L or mmol/L
2 yr–older adult	22–26 mEq/L or mmol/L

Test Explanation

Serum or plasma carbon dioxide (CO_2) measurement is usually done as part of an electrolyte panel. Total CO_2 (Tco_2) is an important component of the body's buffering capability, and measurements are used mainly in the evaluation of acid-base balance. It is important to understand the differences between Tco_2 (CO_2 content) and CO_2 gas (Pco_2). Total CO_2 reflects the majority of CO_2 in the body, mainly in the form of bicarbonate (HCO_3^-); is present as a base; and is regulated by the kidneys. CO_2 gas contributes little to the Tco_2 level, is acidic, and is regulated by the lungs (see study titled "Blood Gases").

CO_2 provides the basis for the principal buffering system of the extracellular fluid system, which is the bicarbonate–carbonic acid buffer system. CO_2 circulates in the body either bound to protein or physically dissolved. Constituents in the blood that contribute to Tco_2 levels are bicarbonate, carbamino compounds, and carbonic acid (carbonic acid includes undissociated carbonic acid and dissolved CO_2). Bicarbonate is the second-largest group of anions in the extracellular fluid (chloride is the largest). Tco_2 levels closely reflect bicarbonate levels in the blood, because 90% to 95% of CO_2 circulates as HCO_3^-.

Nursing Implications
Assessment

Indications	Potential Nursing Problems
Evaluate decreased venous CO_2 in the case of compensated metabolic acidosis	• Breathing
	• Confusion
	• Emotional Distress
Evaluate increased venous CO_2 in the case of compensated metabolic alkalosis	• Fatigue
	• Fluid Volume
Monitor decreased venous CO_2 as a result of compensated respiratory alkalosis	• Gas Exchange **(related to the retention of carbon dioxide)**
Monitor increased venous CO_2 as a result of compensation for respiratory acidosis secondary to significant respiratory system infection or cancer; decreased respiratory rate	• Human Response
	• Injury Risk
	• Sensory Perception
	• Spirituality

Diagnosis: Clinical Significance of Test Results
INCREASED IN
Interpretation requires clinical information and evaluation of other electrolytes.

- Acute intermittent porphyria *(related to severe vomiting associated with acute attacks)*
- Airway obstruction *(related to impaired elimination from weak breathing responses)*
- Asthmatic shock *(related to impaired elimination from abnormal breathing responses)*
- Brain tumor *(related to abnormal blood circulation)*
- Bronchitis (chronic) *(related to impaired elimination from weak breathing responses)*
- Cardiac disorders *(related to lack of blood circulation)*
- Chronic obstructive pulmonary disease *(related to impaired elimination from weak breathing responses)*
- Depression of respiratory center *(related to impaired elimination from weak breathing responses)*
- Electrolyte disturbance (severe) *(response to maintain acid-base balance)*
- Hypothyroidism *(related to impaired elimination from weak breathing responses)*
- Hypoventilation *(related to impaired elimination from weak breathing responses)*
- Metabolic alkalosis *(various causes; excessive vomiting)*
- Myopathy *(related to impaired ventilation)*
- Pneumonia *(related to impaired elimination from weak breathing responses)*
- Poliomyelitis *(related to impaired elimination from weak breathing responses)*
- Respiratory acidosis *(related to impaired elimination)*
- Tuberculosis (pulmonary) *(related to impaired elimination from weak breathing responses)*

DECREASED IN
Interpretation requires clinical information and evaluation of other electrolytes.

- Acute renal failure *(response to buildup of ketoacids)*
- Anxiety *(related to hyperventilation; too much CO_2 is exhaled)*
- Dehydration *(response to metabolic acidosis that develops)*
- Diabetic ketoacidosis *(response to buildup of ketoacids)*
- Diarrhea (severe) *(acidosis related to loss of base ions like HCO_3; most of CO_2 content is in this form)*
- High fever *(response to neutralize acidosis present during fever)*
- Metabolic acidosis *(response to neutralize acidosis)*
- Respiratory alkalosis *(hyperventilation; too much CO_2 is exhaled)*
- Salicylate intoxication *(response to neutralize related metabolic acidosis)*
- Starvation *(CO_2 buffer system used to neutralize buildup of ketoacids)*

Planning

Considerations for planning a successful partnership should include clear communication of what to expect during the test to decrease anxiety and improve cooperation. Before the procedure is performed, plan to review the steps with the patient. Address concerns about pain, and explain that there may be some discomfort during the venipuncture.

SPECIAL CONSIDERATIONS

An important aspect of planning is understanding the factors that may alter the study findings or cause abnormal results. Interdepartmental communication is a key factor in the planning process.

It is also important to understand which medications or substances the patient may be exposed to in the health-care setting that can interfere with accurate testing:

- Drugs that may cause an increase in TCO_2 levels include acetylsalicylic acid, aldosterone, bicarbonate, carbenicillin, carbenoxolone, corticosteroids, dexamethasone, ethacrynic acid, laxatives (chronic abuse), and x-ray contrast agents.
- Drugs that may cause a decrease in TCO_2 levels include acetazolamide, acetylsalicylic acid (initially), amiloride, ammonium chloride, fluorides, metformin, methicillin, nitrofurantoin, paraldehyde, tetracycline, triamterene, and xylitol.

The specimen should be stored under anaerobic conditions after collection to prevent the diffusion of CO_2 gas from the specimen. Falsely decreased values result from uncovered specimens. It is estimated that CO_2 diffuses from the sample at the rate of 6 mEq/hr or mmol/hr.

Implementation

Patient education is key to obtaining the patient's cooperation in following directions, and providing an explanation for the purpose of the procedure is an important part of this process. Inform the patient that this study can assist in measuring the amount of carbon dioxide in the body. Perform the venipuncture.

Evaluation

Recognize anxiety related to test results, and answer any questions or address any concerns voiced by the patient or family. Assist the patient with the administration of oxygen as ordered. Teach and assist the patient with deep breathing exercises. Monitor respiratory rate and depth.

NUTRITIONAL CONSIDERATIONS:

Abnormal CO_2 values may be associated with diseases of the respiratory system. Malnutrition is commonly seen in patients with severe respiratory disease for reasons including fatigue, lack of appetite, and gastrointestinal distress. Research has estimated that the daily caloric intake required for respiration in patients with chronic obstructive pulmonary disease is 10 times higher than that of normal individuals. Adequate intake of vitamins A and C is also important to prevent pulmonary infection and to decrease the extent of lung tissue damage. The importance of following the prescribed diet should be stressed to the patient and/or caregiver.

✔ Critical Findings

- Less than 15 mEq/L or mmol/L (SI: Less than 15 mmol/L)
- Greater than 40 mEq/L or mmol/L (SI: Greater than 40 mmol/L)

Note and immediately report to the requesting health-care provider (HCP) any critical findings and related symptoms. A listing of these findings varies among facilities.

Consideration may be given to verification of critical findings before action is taken. Policies vary among facilities and may include requesting immediate recollection and retesting by the laboratory or retesting using a rapid Point of Care testing instrument at the bedside, if available.

Observe the patient for signs and symptoms of excessive or insufficient CO_2 levels, and report these findings to the HCP. If the patient has been vomiting for several days and is breathing shallowly, or if the patient has had gastric suctioning and is breathing shallowly, this may indicate elevated CO_2 levels. Decreased CO_2 levels are evidenced by deep, vigorous breathing and flushed skin.

✔ Study Specific Complications

There are a number of complications associated with performing a venipuncture. **Pain** is commonly associated with needles, and although the pain experienced during venipuncture is usually mild, on a rare occasion the needle may strike a nerve causing permanent pain. Some patients experience a **vasovagal reaction** during the venipuncture procedure, evidenced by sweating, low blood pressure, fainting, or near fainting. The potential for a **fall injury** is a significant concern related to vasovagal reactions. Prolonged **bleeding** is a complication that occurs with patients who are taking blood thinners or who have coagulopathies such as hemophilia. A **hematoma** results when blood leaks into the tissue during or after a venipuncture, as evidenced by pain, bruising, and/or swelling at the venipuncture site. The swelling can cause injury by compression to surrounding nerves, which can be temporary or permanent. HCPs should watch for minor complications such as bruising and hematoma at the venipuncture site, which are fairly common. Hematomas occur more often in older adult or frail patients, or those with veins that are difficult to access. Bleeding or bruising can be prevented once the needle has been removed by applying direct pressure to the site with dry gauze for a minute or two. Some other more unusual complications of venipuncture include **cellulitis, phlebitis, inadvertent arterial puncture,** and **sepsis.** Sepsis can be caused by introduction of bacteria from the surface of the skin into the blood as the result of improper cleansing of the venipuncture site. Immunocompromised patients are at higher risk for developing this complication.

⊘ *Related Tests*

Related tests include anion gap, arterial/alveolar oxygen ratio, biopsy lung, blood gases, chest x-ray, chloride, cold agglutinin titer, CBC white blood cell count and differential, culture bacterial blood, culture bacterial sputum, culture mycobacterium, culture viral, cytology sputum, eosinophil count, ESR, gallium scan, Gram stain, IgE, ketones, lung perfusion scan, osmolality, phosphorus, plethysmography, pleural fluid analysis, potassium, PFT, pulse oximetry, salicylate, and US abdomen.

Refer to the Cardiovascular, Genitourinary, and Respiratory systems tables at the end of the book for related tests by body system.

Expected Outcomes

Expected outcomes associated with Carbon Dioxide are:

- Maintaining an oxygen saturation greater than 93%
- Maintaining a fluid volume to support blood pressure and prevent postural hypotension
- Demonstrating a cognitive status that remains within normal limits
- Having an absence of suicidal ideation
- Demonstrating improved breathing and carbon dioxide levels within the normal range after the appropriate interventions were taken

Chloride, Blood

Quick Summary

SYNONYM ACRONYM: Cl^-.

COMMON USE: To evaluate electrolytes, acid-base balance, and hydration level.

SPECIMEN: Serum collected in a gold-, red-, or red/gray-top tube. Plasma collected in a green-top (heparin) tube is also acceptable.

NORMAL FINDINGS: (Method: Ion-selective electrode)

Age	Conventional & SI Units
Premature	95–110 mEq/L or mmol/L
0–1 mo	98–113 mEq/L or mmol/L
2 mo–older	adult 97–107 mEq/L or mmol/L

Test Explanation

Chloride is the most abundant anion in the extracellular fluid. Its most important function is in the maintenance of acid-base balance, in which it competes with bicarbonate for sodium. Chloride levels generally increase and decrease proportionally to sodium levels and inversely proportional to bicarbonate levels. Chloride also participates with sodium in the maintenance of water balance and aids in the regulation of osmotic pressure. Chloride contributes to gastric acid (hydrochloric acid) for digestion and activation of enzymes. The chloride content of venous blood is slightly higher than that of arterial blood because chloride ions enter red blood cells in response to absorption of carbon dioxide into the cell. As carbon dioxide enters the blood cell, bicarbonate leaves, and chloride is absorbed in exchange to maintain electrical neutrality within the cell.

Chloride is provided by dietary intake, mostly in the form of sodium chloride. It is absorbed by the gastrointestinal system, filtered out by the glomeruli, and reabsorbed by the renal tubules. Excess chloride is excreted in the urine. Serum values normally remain fairly stable. A slight decrease may be detectable after meals because chloride is used to produce hydrochloric acid as part of the digestive process. Measurement of chloride levels is not as essential as measurement of other electrolytes such as sodium or potassium. Chloride is usually included in standard electrolyte panels to detect the presence of unmeasured anions via calculation of the anion gap. Chloride levels are usually not interpreted apart from sodium, potassium, carbon dioxide, and anion gap.

The patient's clinical picture needs to be considered in the evaluation of electrolytes. Fluid and electrolyte imbalances are often seen in patients with serious illness or injury, because in these cases the clinical situation has affected the normal homeostatic balance of the body. It is also possible that therapeutic treatments being administered are causing or contributing to the electrolyte imbalance. Children and older adults are at high risk for fluid and electrolyte imbalances when chloride levels are depleted. Children are considered to be at high risk during chloride imbalance because a positive serum chloride balance is important for expansion of the extracellular fluid compartment. Anemia, the result of decreased hemoglobin levels, is a frequent issue for older adult patients. Because hemoglobin participates in a major buffer system in the body, depleted hemoglobin levels affect the efficiency of chloride ion exchange for bicarbonate in red blood cells, which in turn affects acid-base balance. Older adult patients are also at high risk because their renal response to change in pH is slower, resulting in a more rapid development of electrolyte imbalance.

Nursing Implications

Assessment

Indications	Potential Nursing Problems
Assist in confirming a diagnosis of disorders associated with abnormal chloride values, as seen in acid-base and fluid imbalances Differentiate between types of acidosis (hyperchloremic versus anion gap) Monitor effectiveness of drug therapy to increase or decrease serum chloride levels	• Activity **(lethargy, related to hyperchloremia)** • Confusion • Diarrhea • Electrolytes **(edema, related to electrolyte imbalance)** • Fall Risk **(tremors, twitching, related to hyper- or hypochloremia)** • Fluid Volume • Human Response • Injury Risk **(Dysrhythmias, related to hyperchloremia)** • Nutrition

Diagnosis: Clinical Significance of Test Results
INCREASED IN
- Acute kidney injury *(related to decreased renal excretion)*
- Cushing disease *(related to sodium retention as a result of increased levels of aldosterone; typically, chloride levels follow sodium levels)*
- Dehydration *(related to hemoconcentration)*
- Diabetes insipidus *(hemoconcentration related to excessive urine production)*
- Excessive infusion of normal saline *(related to excessive intake)*
- Head trauma with hypothalamic stimulation or damage
- Hyperparathyroidism (primary) *(high chloride-to-phosphate ratio is used to assist in diagnosis)*
- Metabolic acidosis *(associated with prolonged diarrhea)*
- Renal tubular acidosis *(acidosis related to net retention of chloride ions)*
- Respiratory alkalosis (e.g., hyperventilation) *(related to metabolic exchange of intracellular chloride replaced by bicarbonate; chloride levels increase)*
- Salicylate intoxication *(related to acid-base imbalance resulting in a hyperchloremic acidosis)*

DECREASED IN
- Addison disease *(related to insufficient production of aldosterone; potassium is retained while sodium and chloride are lost)*
- Burns *(dilutional effect related to sequestration of extracellular fluid)*
- Diabetic ketoacidosis *(related to acid-base imbalance with accumulation of ketone bodies and increased chloride)*
- Excessive sweating *(related to excessive loss of chloride without replacement)*
- Gastrointestinal loss from vomiting (severe), diarrhea, nasogastric suction, or fistula
- Heart failure *(related to dilutional effect of fluid buildup)*
- Metabolic alkalosis *(related to homeostatic response in which intracellular chloride increases to reduce alkalinity of extracellular fluid)*
- Overhydration *(related to dilutional effect)*
- Respiratory acidosis (chronic)
- Salt-losing nephritis *(related to excessive loss)*
- Syndrome of inappropriate antidiuretic hormone secretion *(related to dilutional effect)*
- Water intoxication *(related to dilutional effect)*

Planning
Considerations for planning a successful partnership should include clear communication of what to expect during the test to decrease anxiety and improve cooperation. Before the procedure is performed, plan to review the steps with the patient. Address concerns about pain, and explain that there may be some discomfort during the venipuncture.

SPECIAL CONSIDERATIONS
An important aspect of planning is understanding the factors that may alter the study findings or cause abnormal results. Interdepartmental communication is a key factor in the planning process. The following should be noted when planning for this study:

- Specimens should not be collected during hemodialysis.
- Elevated triglyceride or protein levels may cause a volume displacement error in the specimen, reflecting falsely decreased chloride values when chloride measurement methods employing predilution specimens are used (e.g., indirect ion-selective electrode).
- Specimens should never be collected above an IV line because of the potential for dilution when the specimen and the IV solution combine in the collection container, falsely decreasing the result. There is also the potential of contaminating the sample with the normal saline contained in the IV solution, falsely increasing the result.
- Use of triamterene, which has nephrotoxic and azotemic effects, and when organ damage has occurred result in increased serum chloride levels.
- Potassium chloride (found in salt substitutes) can lower blood chloride levels and raise urine chloride levels.

It is also important to understand which medications or substances the patient may be exposed to in the healthcare setting that can interfere with accurate testing:

- Drugs that may cause an increase in chloride levels include acetazolamide, acetylsalicylic acid, ammonium

chloride, androgens, bromide, chlorothiazide, cholestyramine, cyclosporine, estrogens, guanethidine, hydrochlorothiazide, lithium, methyldopa, NSAIDs, oxyphenbutazone, phenylbutazone, and triamterene.
- Drugs that may cause a decrease in chloride levels include aldosterone, bicarbonate, corticosteroids, corticotropin, cortisone, diuretics, ethacrynic acid, furosemide, hydroflumethiazide, laxatives (if chronic abuse occurs), mannitol, meralluride, mersalyl, methyclothiazide, metolazone, and triamterene. Many of these drugs can cause a diuretic action that inhibits the tubular reabsorption of chloride.

Implementation
Patient education is key to obtaining the patient's cooperation in following directions, and providing an explanation for the purpose of the procedure is an important part of this process. Inform the patient that this study can assist in evaluating the amount of chloride in the blood. Perform the venipuncture.

Evaluation
Recognize anxiety related to test results and observe the patient on saline IV fluid replacement therapy for signs of overhydration, especially in cases in which there is a history of cardiac or renal disease. Signs of overhydration include constant, irritable cough; chest rales; dyspnea; or engorgement of neck and hand veins. Evaluate the patient for signs and symptoms of dehydration. Check the patient's skin turgor, mucous membrane moisture, and ability to produce tears. Dehydration is a significant and common finding in older adult patients and other patients in whom renal function has deteriorated. Monitor daily weights as well as intake and output to determine whether fluid retention is occurring because of sodium and chloride excess. Patients at risk for or with a history of fluid imbalance are also at risk for electrolyte imbalance. Educate the patient regarding access to nutritional counseling services. Provide contact information, if desired, for the Institute of Medicine of the National Academies (www.iom.edu) and U.S. Department of Agriculture (www.choosemyplate.gov).

NUTRITIONAL CONSIDERATIONS: Careful observation of the patient on IV fluid replacement therapy is important. A patient receiving a continuous 5% dextrose solution (D5W) may not be taking in an adequate amount of chloride to meet the body's needs. The patient, if allowed, should be encouraged to drink fluids such as broths, tomato juice, or colas, and to eat foods such as meats, seafood, or eggs, which contain sodium and chloride. The use of table salt may also be appropriate.

Instruct patients with elevated chloride levels to avoid eating or drinking anything containing sodium chloride salt. The patient or caregiver should also be encouraged to read food labels to determine which products are suitable for a low-sodium diet.

Instruct patients with low chloride levels that a decrease in iron absorption may occur as a result of less chloride available to form gastric acid, which is essential for iron absorption. In prolonged periods of chloride deficit, iron-deficiency anemia could develop.

⊘ Critical Findings
- Less than 80 mEq/L or mmol/L (SI: Less than 80 mmol/L)
- Greater than 115 mEq/L or mmol/L (SI: Greater than 115 mEq/L or mmol/L)

Note and immediately report to the requesting healthcare provider (HCP) any critical findings and related symptoms. A listing of these findings varies among facilities. Consideration may be given to verification of critical findings before action is taken. Policies vary among facilities and may include requesting immediate recollection and retesting by the laboratory or retesting using a rapid Point of Care testing instrument at the bedside, if available.

The following may be seen in hypochloremia: twitching or tremors, which may indicate excitability of the nervous system; slow and shallow breathing; and decreased blood pressure as a result of fluid loss. Possible interventions relate to treatment of the underlying cause.

Signs and symptoms associated with hyperchloremia are weakness; lethargy; and deep, rapid breathing. Proper interventions include treatments that correct the underlying cause.

⊘ Study Specific Complications
There are a number of complications associated with performing a venipuncture. **Pain** is commonly associated with needles, and although the pain experienced during venipuncture is usually mild, on a rare occasion the needle may strike a nerve causing permanent pain. Some patients experience a **vasovagal reaction** during the venipuncture procedure, evidenced by sweating, low blood pressure, fainting, or near fainting. The potential for a **fall injury** is a significant concern related to vasovagal reactions. Prolonged **bleeding** is a complication that occurs with patients who are taking blood thinners or who have coagulopathies such as hemophilia. A **hematoma** results when blood leaks into the tissue during or after a venipuncture, as evidenced by pain, bruising, and/or swelling at the venipuncture site. The swelling can cause injury by compression to surrounding nerves, which can be temporary or permanent. Health-care providers (HCPs) should watch for minor complications such as bruising and hematoma at the venipuncture site, which are fairly common. Hematomas occur more often in older adult or frail patients, or those with veins that are difficult to access. Bleeding or bruising can be prevented once the needle has been removed by

applying direct pressure to the site with dry gauze for a minute or two. Some other more unusual complications of venipuncture include **cellulitis, phlebitis, inadvertent arterial puncture,** and **sepsis.** Sepsis can be caused by introduction of bacteria from the surface of the skin into the blood as the result of improper cleansing of the venipuncture site. Immunocompromised patients are at higher risk for developing this complication.

✔ Related Tests

- Related tests include ACTH, anion gap, blood gases, carbon dioxide, CBC hematocrit, CBC hemoglobin, osmolality, potassium, protein total and fractions, sodium, and US abdomen.
- Refer to the Cardiovascular, Endocrine, Gastrointestinal, Genitourinary, and Respiratory systems tables at the end of the book for related test by body system.

Expected Outcomes

Expected outcomes associated with Chloride, Blood are:

- Maintenance of normovolemic status
- Nutritional intake of chloride that meets the minimum daily requirements and supports maintaining electrolyte balance
- Absence of vomiting or diarrhea
- Verbalization of signs and symptoms related to the disease process secondary to an altered chloride level
- Compliance with the ordered medication regimen

Cholesterol, HDL and LDL

Quick Summary

SYNONYM ACRONYM: α_1-Lipoprotein cholesterol, high-density cholesterol, HDLC, and β-lipoprotein cholesterol, low-density cholesterol, LDLC.

COMMON USE: To assess risk and monitor for coronary artery disease.

SPECIMEN: Serum collected in a gold-, red-, or red/gray-top tube.

NORMAL FINDINGS: (Method: Spectrophotometry)

HDLC	Conventional Units	SI Units (Conventional Units × 0.0259)
Birth	6–56 mg/dL	0.16–1.45 mmol/L
Children, adults, and older adults		
Desirable	Greater than 60 mg/dL	Greater than 1.55 mmol/L
Acceptable	40–60 mg/dL	1–1.55 mmol/L
Low	Less than 40 mg/dL	Less than 1 mmol/L

LDLC	Conventional Units	SI Units (Conventional Units × 0.0259)
Optimal	Less than 100 mg/dL	Less than 2.59 mmol/L
Near optimal	100–129 mg/dL	2.59–3.34 mmol/L
Borderline high	130–159 mg/dL	3.37–4.11 mmol/L
High	160–189 mg/dL	4.14–4.9 mmol/L
Very high	Greater than 190 mg/dL	Greater than 4.92 mmol/L

	NMR LDLC Particle Number	NMR LDLC Small Particle Size
High-risk CAD	Less than 1,000 nmol/L	Less than 528 nmol/L
Moderately high-risk CAD	Less than 1,300 nmol/L	Less than 528 nmol/L

CAD, coronary artery disease; NMR, nuclear magnetic resonance.

Test Explanation

High-density lipoprotein cholesterol (HDLC) and low-density lipoprotein cholesterol (LDLC) are the major transport proteins for cholesterol in the body. It is believed that HDLC may have protective properties in that its role includes transporting cholesterol from the arteries to the liver. LDLC is the major transport protein for cholesterol to the arteries from the liver. LDLC can be calculated using total cholesterol, total triglycerides, and HDLC levels. Beyond the total cholesterol, HDL and LDL cholesterol values, other important risk factors must be considered. Guidelines for the prevention of cardiovascular disease (CVD) have been developed by the American College of Cardiology (ACC) and the American Heart Association (AHA) in conjunction with members of the National Heart, Lung, and Blood Institute's (NHLBI) ATP IV Expert Panel. The updated, evidence-based guidelines redefine the condition of concern as atherosclerotic cardiovascular disease (ASCVD) and expand ASCVD to include CVD, stroke, and peripheral artery disease. Some of the important highlights include the following:

- Movement away from the use of LDL cholesterol targets in determining treatment with statins. Recommendations focus on selecting (a) the patients that fall into four groups most likely to benefit from statin therapy, and (b) the level of statin intensity most likely to affect or reduce development of ASCVD.
- Development of a new 10-year risk assessment tool based on findings from a large, diverse population. Evidence-based risk factors include age, sex, ethnicity, total cholesterol, HDLC, blood pressure,

blood-pressure treatment status, diabetes, and current use of tobacco products.

- Recommendations for aspects of lifestyle that would encourage prevention of ASCVD to include adherence to a Mediterranean-style or DASH (Dietary Approaches to Stop Hypertension)–style diet; dietary restriction of saturated fats, trans fats, sugar, and sodium; and regular participation in aerobic exercise. The guidelines contain reductions in body mass index (BMI) cutoffs for men and women designed to promote discussions between health-care providers (HCPs) and their patients regarding the benefits of maintaining a healthy weight.
- Recognition that additional biological markers, such as family history, high-sensitivity C-reactive protein, ankle-brachial index (ABI), and coronary artery calcium (CAC) score, may be selectively used with the assessment tool to assist in predicting and evaluating risk.
- Recognition that other biomarkers such as apolipoprotein B, eGFR, creatinine, lipoprotein (a) or Lp(a), and microalbumin warrant further study and may be considered for inclusion in future guidelines.

Studies have shown that CAD is inversely related to LDLC particle number and size. The NMR lipid profile uses NMR imaging spectroscopy to determine LDLC particle number and size in addition to measurement of the traditional lipid markers.

HDLC levels less than 40 mg/dL in men and women represent a coronary risk factor. There is an inverse relationship between HDLC and risk of CAD (i.e., lower HDLC levels represent a higher risk of CAD). Levels of LDLC in terms of risk for CAD are directly proportional to risk and vary by age group. The LDLC can be estimated using the Friedewald formula:

$$LDLC = (Total\ Cholesterol) - (HDLC) - (VLDLC)$$

Very-low-density lipoprotein cholesterol (VLDLC) is estimated by dividing the triglycerides (conventional units) by 5. Triglycerides in SI units would be divided by 2.18 to estimate VLDLC. It is important to note that the formula is valid only if the triglycerides are less than 400 mg/dL or 4.52 mmol/L.

Nursing Implications

Assessment

Indications	Potential Nursing Problems
Determine the risk of cardiovascular disease Evaluate the response to dietary and drug therapy for hypercholesterolemia	• Activity • Cardiac Output *(related to blocked vessels)* • Fatigue *(related to poor physical condition as a result of the disease process)*

Indications	Potential Nursing Problems
Investigate hypercholesterolemia in light of family history of cardiovascular disease	• Gas Exchange • Health Maintenance • Human Response • Mobility *(related to poor physical condition as a result of the disease process)* • Nutrition *(related to a lack of knowledge or financial limitations)* • Pain *(related to reduced blood flow and oxygen to the heart)*

Diagnosis: Clinical Significance of Test Results

Although the exact pathophysiology is unknown, cholesterol is required for many functions at the cellular and organ levels. Elevations of cholesterol are associated with conditions caused by an inherited defect in lipoprotein metabolism, liver disease, kidney disease, or a disorder of the endocrine system. Decreases in cholesterol levels are associated with conditions caused by enzyme deficiencies, malnutrition, malabsorption, liver disease, and sudden increased utilization.

HDLC INCREASED IN
- Alcoholism
- Biliary cirrhosis
- Chronic hepatitis
- Exercise
- Familial hyper-α-lipoproteinemia

HDLC DECREASED IN
- Abetalipoproteinemia
- Cholestasis
- Chronic kidney disease
- Fish-eye disease
- Genetic predisposition or enzyme/cofactor deficiency
- Hepatocellular disorders
- Hypertriglyceridemia
- Nephrotic syndrome
- Obesity
- Premature CAD
- Sedentary lifestyle
- Smoking
- Tangier disease
- Syndrome X (metabolic syndrome)
- Uncontrolled diabetes

LDLC INCREASED IN
- Anorexia nervosa
- Chronic kidney disease
- Corneal arcus
- Cushing syndrome
- Diabetes
- Diet high in cholesterol and saturated fat

- Dysglobulinemias
- Hepatic disease
- Hepatic obstruction
- Hyperlipoproteinemia types IIA and IIB
- Hypothyroidism
- Nephrotic syndrome
- Porphyria
- Pregnancy
- Premature CAD
- Syndrome X (metabolic syndrome)
- Tendon and tuberous xanthomas

LDLC DECREASED IN

- Acute stress (severe burns, illness)
- Chronic anemias
- Chronic pulmonary disease
- Genetic predisposition or enzyme/cofactor deficiency
- Hyperthyroidism
- Hypolipoproteinemia and abetalipoproteinemia
- Inflammatory joint disease
- Myeloma
- Reye syndrome
- Severe hepatocellular destruction or disease
- Tangier disease

Planning

Considerations for planning a successful partnership should include clear communication of what to expect during the test to decrease anxiety and improve cooperation. The presence of other risk factors, such as a family history of heart disease, smoking, obesity, diet, lack of physical activity, hypertension, diabetes, previous myocardial infarction, and previous vascular disease, should be investigated. Before the procedure is performed, plan to review the steps with the patient. Address concerns about pain, and explain that there may be some discomfort during the venipuncture.

SPECIAL CONSIDERATIONS

An important aspect of planning is understanding the factors that may alter the study findings or cause abnormal results. Interdepartmental communication is a key factor in the planning process. The following should be noted when planning for this study:

- Ideally, the patient should be on a stable diet for 3 weeks and should fast for 12 hours before specimen collection. Failure to follow dietary restrictions before the procedure may cause the procedure to be canceled or repeated. Protocols may vary among facilities.
- Confirm with the requesting HCP that the patient should withhold medications known to influence test results, and instruct the patient accordingly.

It is also important to understand which medications or substances the patient may be exposed to in the health-care setting that can interfere with accurate testing:

HDLC

- Drugs that may increase HDLC levels include albuterol, anticonvulsants, cholestyramine, cimetidine, clofibrate and other fibric acid derivatives, estrogens, ethanol (moderate use), lovastatin, niacin, oral contraceptives, pindolol, pravastatin, prazosin, and simvastatin.
- Drugs that may decrease HDLC levels include acebutolol, atenolol, danazol, diuretics, etretinate, interferon, isotretinoin, linseed oil, metoprolol, neomycin, nonselective β-adrenergic blocking agents, probucol, progesterone, steroids, and thiazides.

LDLC

- Drugs that may increase LDLC levels include androgens, catecholamines, chenodiol, cyclosporine, danazol, diuretics, etretinate, glucogenic corticosteroids, and progestins.
- Drugs that may decrease LDLC levels include aminosalicylic acid, cholestyramine, colestipol, estrogens, fibric acid derivatives, interferon, lovastatin, neomycin, niacin, pravastatin, prazosin, probucol, simvastatin, terazosin, and thyroxine.

Some of the drugs used to lower total cholesterol and LDLC or increase HDLC may cause liver damage.

Grossly elevated triglyceride levels invalidate the Friedewald formula for mathematical estimation of LDLC; if the triglyceride level is greater than 400 mg/dL (SI = 4.52 mmol/L), the formula should not be used.

Implementation

Patient education is key to obtaining the patient's cooperation in following directions, and providing an explanation for the purpose of the procedure is an important part of this process. Inform the patient that this study can assist with evaluation of the cholesterol level. Ensure that the patient has complied with dietary and medication restrictions as well as other pretesting preparations; ensure that food has been restricted for at least 12 hours prior to the procedure. Perform the venipuncture.

Evaluation

Recognize anxiety related to test results, and be supportive of the fear of a shortened life expectancy. Discuss the implications of abnormal test results on the patient's lifestyle. Provide teaching and information regarding the clinical implications of the test results as appropriate. Educate the patient regarding access to counseling services. Provide contact information, if desired, for the American Heart Association (AHA) (www.american-heart.org) or the NHLBI (www.nhlbi.nih.gov).

SPECIAL CONSIDERATIONS

Numerous studies point to the prevalence of excess body weight in American children and adolescents. Experts estimate that obesity is present in 25% of the population ages 6 to 11 years. The medical, social, and emotional consequences of excess body weight are significant. Special attention should be given to instructing the child and caregiver regarding health risks and weight-control education.

NUTRITIONAL CONSIDERATIONS FOR THE CARDIAC PATIENT: Increases in LDLC and decreases in HDLC levels may be associated with CAD. Nutritional therapy is recommended for the patient identified to be at risk for developing CAD or for individuals who have specific risk factors and/or existing medical conditions (e.g., elevated LDL cholesterol levels, other lipid disorders, insulin-dependent diabetes, insulin resistance, or metabolic syndrome). Other changeable risk factors warranting patient education include strategies to encourage patients, especially those who are overweight and with high blood pressure, to safely decrease sodium intake, achieve a normal weight, ensure regular participation of moderate aerobic physical activity three to four times per week, eliminate tobacco use, and adhere to a heart-healthy diet. If triglycerides also are elevated, the patient should be advised to eliminate or reduce alcohol. The Guideline on Lifestyle Management to Reduce Cardiovascular Risk published by the American College of Cardiology (ACC) and AHA in conjunction with the NHLBI recommends a "Mediterranean"-style diet rather than a low-fat diet. The guideline emphasizes inclusion of vegetables, whole grains, fruits, low-fat dairy, nuts, legumes, and nontropical vegetable oils (e.g., olive, canola, peanut, sunflower, flaxseed) along with fish and lean poultry. A similar dietary pattern known as the Dietary Approaches to Stop Hypertension (DASH) diet makes additional recommendations for the reduction of dietary sodium. Both dietary styles emphasize a reduction in consumption of red meats, which are high in saturated fats and cholesterol, and other foods containing sugar, saturated fats, trans fats, and sodium.

✓ Critical Findings

N/A

✓ Study Specific Complications

There are a number of complications associated with performing a venipuncture. **Pain** is commonly associated with needles, and although the pain experienced during venipuncture is usually mild, on a rare occasion the needle may strike a nerve causing permanent pain. Some patients experience a **vasovagal reaction** during the venipuncture procedure, evidenced by sweating, low blood pressure, fainting, or near fainting. The potential for a **fall injury** is a significant concern related to vasovagal reactions. Prolonged **bleeding** is a complication that occurs with patients who are taking blood thinners or who have coagulopathies such as hemophilia. A **hematoma** results when blood leaks into the tissue during or after a venipuncture, as evidenced by pain, bruising, and/or swelling at the venipuncture site. The swelling can cause injury by compression to surrounding nerves, which can be temporary or permanent. HCPs should watch for minor complications such as bruising and hematoma at the venipuncture site, which are fairly common. Hematomas occur more often in older adult or frail patients, or those with veins that are difficult to access. Bleeding or bruising can be prevented once the needle has been removed by applying direct pressure to the site with dry gauze for a minute or two. Some other more unusual complications of venipuncture include **cellulitis, phlebitis, inadvertent arterial puncture,** and **sepsis.** Sepsis can be caused by introduction of bacteria from the surface of the skin into the blood as the result of improper cleansing of the venipuncture site. Immunocompromised patients are at higher risk for developing this complication.

✓ Related Tests

- Related tests include antidysrhythmic drugs, apolipoprotein A and B, AST, ANP, blood gases, BNP, calcium (total and ionized), cholesterol total, CT cardiac scoring, CRP, CK and isoenzymes, echocardiography, glucose, glycated hemoglobin, Holter monitor, homocysteine, ketones, LDH and isoenzymes, lipoprotein electrophoresis, magnesium, MRI chest, MI scan, myocardial perfusion heart scan, myoglobin, PET heart, potassium, triglycerides, and troponin.
- Refer to the Cardiovascular System table at the end of the book for related tests by body system.

Expected Outcomes

Expected outcomes associated with HDL and LDL Cholesterol are:

- Identifying healthy food choices and creating a strategy to adapt to better eating habits
- Achieving a heart rate that is within normal limits in relation to the baseline value
- Verbalizing an understanding of the disease process and causative factors; the patient commits to alterations in lifestyle that will decrease risk factors
- Participating in desired activities at the desired level of activity without dyspnea

Cholesterol, Total

Quick Summary

COMMON USE: To assess and monitor risk for coronary artery disease (CAD).

SPECIMEN: Serum collected in a gold-, red-, or red/gray-top tube. Plasma collected in a green-top (heparin) tube is also acceptable. It is important to use the same tube type when serial specimen collections are anticipated for consistency in testing.

NORMAL FINDINGS: (Method: Spectrophotometry)

Risk	Conventional Units	SI Units (Conventional Units × 0.0259)
Children and Adolescents (Less Than 20 yr)		
Desirable	Less than 170 mg/dL	Less than 4.4 mmol/L
Borderline	170–199 mg/dL	4.4–5.2 mmol/L
High	Greater than 200 mg/dL	Greater than 5.2 mmol/L
Adults and Older Adults		
Desirable	Less than 200 mg/dL	Less than 5.2 mmol/L
Borderline	200–239 mg/dL	5.2–6.2 mmol/L
High	Greater than 240 mg/dL	Greater than 6.2 mmol/L

Plasma values may be 10% lower than serum values.

Test Explanation

Cholesterol is a lipid needed to form cell membranes, bile salts, adrenal corticosteroid hormones, and other hormones such as estrogen and the androgens. Cholesterol is obtained from the diet and also synthesized in the body, mainly by the liver and intestinal mucosa. Very low cholesterol values, as are sometimes seen in critically ill patients, can be as life-threatening as very high levels. According to the National Cholesterol Education Program, maintaining cholesterol levels less than 200 mg/dL (SI: Less than 5.2 mmol/L) significantly reduces the risk of coronary heart disease. Beyond the total cholesterol and high-density lipoprotein cholesterol (HDLC) values, other important risk factors must be considered. Many myocardial infarctions occur even in patients whose cholesterol levels are considered to be within acceptable limits or who are in a moderate-risk category. The combination of risk factors and lipid values helps identify individuals at risk so that appropriate interventions can be taken. If the cholesterol level is greater than 200 mg/dL (SI: Greater than 5.2 mmol/L), repeat testing after a 12- to 24-hour fast is recommended.

Guidelines for the prevention of cardiovascular disease (CVD) have been developed by the American College of Cardiology (ACC) and the American Heart Association (AHA) in conjunction with members of the National Heart, Lung, and Blood Institute's (NHLBI) ATP IV Expert Panel. The updated, evidence-based guidelines redefine the condition of concern as atherosclerotic cardiovascular disease (ASCVD) and expand ASCVD to include CVD, stroke, and peripheral artery disease. Some of the important highlights include the following:

- Movement away from the use of LDL cholesterol targets in determining treatment with statins. Recommendations that focus on selecting (a) the patients who fall into four groups most likely to benefit from statin therapy, and (b) the level of statin intensity most likely to affect or reduce development of ASCVD.
- Development of a new 10-year risk assessment tool is based on findings from a large, diverse population. Evidence-based risk factors include age, sex, ethnicity, total cholesterol, HDLC, blood pressure, blood-pressure treatment status, diabetes, and current use of tobacco products.
- Development of recommendations for aspects of lifestyle that would encourage prevention of ASCVD include adherence to a Mediterranean- or DASH (Dietary Approaches to Stop Hypertension)-style diet; dietary restriction of saturated fats, trans fats, sugar, and sodium; and regular participation in aerobic exercise. The guidelines contain reductions in body mass index (BMI) cutoffs for men and women designed to promote discussions between healthcare providers (HCPs) and their patients regarding the benefits of maintaining a healthy weight.
- Recognition that additional biological markers, such as family history, high-sensitivity C-reactive protein, ankle-brachial index (ABI), and coronary artery calcium (CAC) score, may be selectively used with the assessment tool to assist in predicting and evaluating risk.
- Recognition that other biomarkers such as apolipoprotein B, eGFR, creatinine, lipoprotein (a) or Lp(a), and microalbumin warrant further study and may be considered for inclusion in future guidelines.

Nursing Implications

Assessment

Indications	Potential Nursing Problems
Assist in determining risk of cardiovascular disease	• Activity
	• Cardiac Output (*related to blocked vessels*)
Assist in the diagnosis of nephrotic syndrome, hepatic disease, pancreatitis, and thyroid disorders	• Fatigue (*related to poor physical condition as a result of the disease process*)
	• Gas Exchange
Evaluate the response to dietary and drug therapy for hypercholesterolemia	• Health Maintenance
	• Human Response
	• Mobility (*related to poor physical condition as a result of the disease process*)
Investigate hypercholesterolemia in light of family history of cardiovascular disease	• Nutrition (*related to a lack of knowledge or financial limitations*)
	• Pain (*related to reduced blood flow and oxygen to the heart*)
	• Tissue Perfusion

Diagnosis: Clinical Significance of Test Results

INCREASED IN

Although the exact pathophysiology is unknown, cholesterol is required for many functions at the cellular and organ levels. Elevations of cholesterol are associated with conditions caused by an inherited defect in lipoprotein metabolism, liver disease, kidney disease, or a disorder of the endocrine system.

- Acute intermittent porphyria
- Alcoholism
- Anorexia nervosa
- Cholestasis
- Chronic kidney disease
- Diabetes (with poor control)
- Diets high in cholesterol and fats
- Familial hyperlipoproteinemia
- Glomerulonephritis
- Glycogen storage disease (von Gierke disease)
- Gout
- Hypothyroidism (primary)
- Ischemic heart disease
- Nephrotic syndrome
- Obesity
- Pancreatic and prostatic malignancy
- Pregnancy
- Syndrome X (metabolic syndrome)
- Werner syndrome

DECREASED IN

Although the exact pathophysiology is unknown, cholesterol is required for many functions at the cellular and organ levels. Decreases in cholesterol levels are associated with conditions caused by malnutrition, malabsorption, liver disease, and sudden increased utilization.

- Burns
- Chronic myelocytic leukemia
- Chronic obstructive pulmonary disease
- Hyperthyroidism
- Liver disease (severe)
- Malabsorption and malnutrition syndromes
- Myeloma
- Pernicious anemia
- Polycythemia vera
- Severe illness
- Sideroblastic anemias
- Tangier disease
- Thalassemia
- Waldenström macroglobulinemia

Planning

Considerations for planning a successful partnership should include clear communication of what to expect during the test to decrease anxiety and improve cooperation. Assess the patient for the presence of other risk factors, such as a family history of heart disease, smoking, obesity, diet, lack of physical activity, hypertension, diabetes, previous myocardial infarction, and previous vascular disease. Before the procedure is performed, plan to review the steps with the patient. Address concerns about pain, and explain that there may be some discomfort during the venipuncture.

SPECIAL CONSIDERATIONS

An important aspect of planning is understanding the factors that may alter the study findings or cause abnormal results. Interdepartmental communication is a key factor in the planning process. The following should be noted when planning for this study:

- Fasting 6 to 12 hours before specimen collection is required if triglyceride measurements are included; it is recommended if cholesterol levels alone are measured for screening. Failure to follow dietary restrictions before the procedure may cause the procedure to be canceled or repeated. Protocols may vary among facilities.
- Instruct the patient to withhold alcohol 12 to 24 hours before the test as alcohol consumption can falsely elevate results.
- At the direction of the HCP, instruct the patient to withhold drugs known to alter cholesterol levels for 12 to 24 hours before specimen collection.
- Positioning can affect results; lower levels are obtained if the specimen is from a patient who has been supine for 20 minutes.

It is also important to understand which medications or substances the patient may be exposed to in the healthcare setting that can interfere with accurate testing:

- Drugs that may increase cholesterol levels include amiodarone, androgens, β-blockers, calcitriol, cortisone, cyclosporine, danazol, diclofenac, disulfiram, fluoxymesterone, glucogenic corticosteroids, ibuprofen, isotretinoin, levodopa, mepazine, methyclothiazide, miconazole (owing to castor oil vehicle, not the drug), nafarelin, nandrolone, some oral contraceptives, oxymetholone, phenobarbital, phenothiazine, prochlorperazine, sotalol, thiabendazole, thiouracil, tretinoin, and trifluoperazine.
- Drugs that may decrease cholesterol levels include acebutolol, amiloride, aminosalicylic acid, androsterone, ascorbic acid, asparaginase, atenolol, atorvastatin, beclobrate, bezafibrate, carbutamide, cerivastatin, cholestyramine, ciprofibrate, clofibrate, clonidine, colestipol, dextrothyroxine, doxazosin, enalapril, estrogens, fenfluramine, fenofibrate, fluvastatin, gemfibrozil, haloperidol, hormone replacement therapy, hydralazine, hydrochlorothiazide, interferon, isoniazid, kanamycin, ketoconazole, lincomycin, lisinopril, lovastatin, metformin, nafenopin, nandrolone, neomycin, niacin, nicotinic acid, nifedipine, oxandrolone, paromomycin, pravastatin, probucol, simvastatin, tamoxifen, terazosin, thyroxine, trazodone, triiodothyronine, ursodiol, valproic acid, and verapamil.

Implementation

Patient education is key to obtaining the patient's cooperation in following directions, and providing an explanation for the purpose of the procedure is an important part of this process. Inform the patient that this study can assist with evaluation of cholesterol level.

DISCUSSION POINT

Ensure that the patient has complied with dietary restrictions and pretesting preparations; ensure that food has been restricted for at least 6 to 12 hours prior to the procedure if triglycerides are to be measured. Perform the venipuncture.

Evaluation

Recognize anxiety related to test results and be supportive of fear of a shortened life expectancy. Discuss the implications of abnormal test results on the patient's lifestyle. Provide teaching and information regarding the clinical implications of the test results as appropriate. Educate the patient regarding access to counseling services. Provide contact information, if desired, for the AHA (www.americanheart.org) or the NHLBI (www.nhlbi.nih.gov).

SPECIAL CONSIDERATIONS

Numerous studies point to the prevalence of excess body weight in American children and adolescents. Experts estimate that obesity is present in 25% of the population ages 6 to 11 years. The medical, social, and emotional consequences of excess body weight are significant. Special attention should be given to instructing the child and caregiver regarding health risks and weight-control education.

NUTRITIONAL CONSIDERATIONS FOR THE CARDIAC PATIENT: Increases in total cholesterol levels may be associated with coronary artery disease (CAD) (see Fig. 1.15). Nutritional therapy is recommended for the patient identified to be at risk for developing CAD or for individuals who have specific risk factors and/or existing medical conditions (e.g., elevated LDL cholesterol levels, other lipid disorders, insulin-dependent diabetes, insulin resistance, or metabolic syndrome). Other changeable risk factors warranting patient education include strategies to encourage patients, especially those who are overweight and with high blood pressure, to safely decrease sodium intake, achieve a normal weight, ensure regular participation of moderate aerobic physical activity three to four times per week, eliminate tobacco use, and adhere to a heart-healthy diet. If triglycerides also are elevated, the patient should be advised to eliminate or reduce alcohol. The Guideline on Lifestyle Management to Reduce Cardiovascular Risk published by the American College of Cardiology (ACC) and AHA in conjunction with the NHLBI recommends a "Mediterranean"-style diet rather than a low-fat diet. The guideline emphasizes inclusion of vegetables, whole grains, fruits, low-fat dairy, nuts, legumes, and nontropical vegetable oils (e.g., olive, canola, peanut, sunflower, flaxseed) along with fish and lean poultry. A similar dietary pattern known as the Dietary Approaches to Stop Hypertension (DASH) diet makes additional recommendations for the reduction of dietary sodium. Both dietary styles emphasize a reduction in consumption of red meats, which are high in saturated fats and cholesterol, and other foods containing sugar, saturated fats, trans fats, and sodium.

✓ *Critical Findings*

N/A

✓ *Study Specific Complications*

There are a number of complications associated with performing a venipuncture. **Pain** is commonly associated with needles, and although the pain experienced during venipuncture is usually mild, on a rare occasion the needle may strike a nerve causing permanent pain. Some patients experience a **vasovagal reaction** during the venipuncture procedure, evidenced by sweating, low blood pressure, fainting, or near fainting. The potential for a **fall injury** is a significant concern related to vasovagal reactions. Prolonged **bleeding** is a complication that occurs with patients who are taking blood thinners or who have coagulopathies such as hemophilia. A **hematoma** results when blood leaks into the tissue during or after a venipuncture, as evidenced

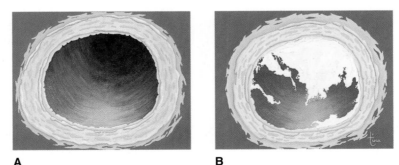

A　　　　　**B**

FIGURE 1.15 Normal and diseased coronary artery. *Used with permission from Venes, D. (Ed.). (2009). Taber's cyclopedic medical dictionary (21st Ed.). FA Davis Company.*

by pain, bruising, and/or swelling at the venipuncture site. The swelling can cause injury by compression to surrounding nerves, which can be temporary or permanent. Health-care providers should watch for minor complications such as bruising and hematoma at the venipuncture site, which are fairly common. Hematomas occur more often in older adult or frail patients, or those with veins that are difficult to access. Bleeding or bruising can be prevented once the needle has been removed by applying direct pressure to the site with dry gauze for a minute or two. Some other more unusual complications of venipuncture include **cellulitis, phlebitis, inadvertent arterial puncture,** and **sepsis.** Sepsis can be caused by introduction of bacteria from the surface of the skin into the blood as the result of improper cleansing of the venipuncture site. Immunocompromised patients are at higher risk for developing this complication.

✓ Related Tests

- Related tests include antidysrhythmic drugs, apolipoprotein A and B, AST, ANP, blood gases, BNP, calcium, cholesterol (HDL and LDL), CT cardiac scoring, CRP, CK and isoenzymes, echocardiography, glucose, glycated hemoglobin, Holter monitor, homocysteine, ketones, LDH and isoenzymes, lipoprotein electrophoresis, MRI chest, magnesium, MI scan, myocardial perfusion heart scan, myoglobin, PET heart, potassium, triglycerides, and troponin.
- Refer to the Cardiovascular, Gastrointestinal, and Hepatobiliary systems tables at the end of the book for related tests by body system.

Expected Outcomes

Expected outcomes associated with total Cholesterol are:

- Displaying no evidence of peripheral edema with capillary refill less than 3 seconds
- Verbalizing the importance of taking cholesterol to decrease disease risk
- Verbalizing an understanding of the disease process and causative factors; the patient commits to alterations in lifestyle that will decrease risk factors
- Participating in activities of daily living without evidence of dyspnea

C-Reactive Protein

Quick Summary

SYNONYM ACRONYM: CRP.

COMMON USE: Indicates a nonspecific inflammatory response; this highly sensitive test is used to assess risk for cardiovascular and peripheral artery disease.

SPECIMEN: Serum collected in a gold-, red-, or red/gray-top tube.

NORMAL FINDINGS: (Method: Nephelometry)

High-Sensitivity Immunoassay (Cardiac Applications)	Conventional & SI Units
Low risk	Less than 1 mg/L
Average risk	1–3 mg/L
High risk	Greater than 10 mg/L (after repeat testing)

Conventional Assay	Conventional & SI Units
Adult	Less than 8 mg/L

Test Explanation

C-reactive protein (CRP) is a glycoprotein produced by the liver in response to acute inflammation. The CRP assay is a nonspecific test that determines the presence (not the cause) of inflammation; it is often ordered in conjunction with erythrocyte sedimentation rate (ESR). CRP assay is a more sensitive and rapid indicator of the presence of an inflammatory process than ESR. CRP disappears from the serum rapidly when inflammation has subsided. The inflammatory process and its association with atherosclerosis make the presence of CRP, as detected by highly sensitive CRP assays, a potential marker for coronary artery disease. It is believed that the inflammatory process may instigate the conversion of a stable plaque to a weaker one that can rupture and occlude an artery.

Nursing Implications

Assessment

Indications	Potential Nursing Problems
Assist in the differential diagnosis of appendicitis and acute pelvic inflammatory disease	• Activity
	• Cardiac Output
Assist in the differential diagnosis of Crohn disease and ulcerative colitis	• Death
	• Fatigue
Assist in the differential diagnosis of rheumatoid arthritis and uncomplicated systemic lupus erythematosus (SLE)	• Fear
	• Human Response
	• Infection
Assist in the evaluation of coronary artery disease	• Mobility **(related to decreased strength, decreased coordination, or physical deformity)**
Detect the presence or exacerbation of inflammatory processes	
Monitor response to therapy for autoimmune disorders such as rheumatoid arthritis	• Pain **(related to inflammation)**
	• Skin
	• Tissue Perfusion

Diagnosis: Clinical Significance of Test Results
INCREASED IN
Conditions associated with an inflammatory response stimulate production of CRP.

- Acute bacterial infections
- Crohn disease
- Inflammatory bowel disease
- Myocardial infarction *(inflammation of the coronary vessels is associated with increased CRP levels and increased risk for coronary vessel injury, which may result in distal vessel plaque occlusions)*
- Pregnancy (second half)
- Rheumatic fever
- Rheumatoid arthritis
- SLE
- Syndrome X (metabolic syndrome) *(inflammation of the coronary vessels is associated with increased CRP levels and increased risk for coronary vessel injury, which may result in distal vessel plaque occlusions)*

DECREASED IN
N/A

Planning
Considerations for planning a successful partnership should include clear communication of what to expect during the test to decrease anxiety and improve cooperation. Assess the patient for pain related to the inflammatory process in connective or other tissues. Before the procedure is performed, plan to review the steps with the patient. Address concerns about pain, and explain that there may be some discomfort during the venipuncture.

SPECIAL CONSIDERATIONS
An important aspect of planning is understanding the factors that may alter the study findings or cause abnormal results. Interdepartmental communication is a key factor in the planning process. The following should be noted when planning for this study:

- NSAIDs, salicylates, and steroids, which may cause false-negative results because of suppression of inflammation
- Falsely elevated levels, which may occur with the presence of an intrauterine device
- Lipemic samples that are turbid in appearance, which may be rejected for analysis when nephelometry is the test method

It is also important to understand which medications or substances the patient may be exposed to in the health-care setting that can interfere with accurate testing:

- Drugs that may increase CRP levels include chemotherapy, interleukin-2, oral contraceptives, and pamidronate.
- Drugs that may decrease CRP levels include aurothiomalate, dexamethasone, gemfibrozil, leflunomide, methotrexate, NSAIDs, oral contraceptives (progestogen effect), penicillamine, pentopril, prednisolone, prinomide, and sulfasalazine.

Implementation
Patient education is key to obtaining the patient's cooperation in following directions, and providing an explanation for the purpose of the procedure is an important part of this process. Inform the patient that this study can assist in assessing for inflammation. Perform the venipuncture.

Evaluation
Recognize anxiety related to test results, and assist with pain management as ordered. Ensure the patient receives a referral for physical therapy as appropriate. Explain the importance of maintaining an upright position when standing, sitting, and walking to maximize joint function and mobility. Discuss the proper mix of rest and activity and the importance of taking regular rest periods throughout the day to prevent exhaustion. Teach the patient to use pillows to properly position him- or herself and to provide relief to stressed joints.

✓ Critical Findings
N/A

✓ Study Specific Complications
There are a number of complications associated with performing a venipuncture. **Pain** is commonly associated with needles, and although the pain experienced during venipuncture is usually mild, on a rare occasion the needle may strike a nerve causing permanent pain. Some patients experience a **vasovagal reaction** during the venipuncture procedure, evidenced by sweating, low blood pressure, fainting, or near fainting. The potential for a **fall injury** is a significant concern related to vasovagal reactions. Prolonged **bleeding** is a complication that occurs with patients who are taking blood thinners or who have coagulopathies such as hemophilia. A **hematoma** results when blood leaks into the tissue during or after a venipuncture, as evidenced by pain, bruising, and/or swelling at the venipuncture site. The swelling can cause injury by compression to surrounding nerves, which can be temporary or permanent. Health-care providers (HCPs) should watch for minor complications such as bruising and hematoma at the venipuncture site, which are fairly common. Hematomas occur more often in older adult or frail patients, or those with veins that are difficult to access. Bleeding or bruising can be prevented once the needle has been removed by applying direct pressure to the site with dry gauze for a minute or two. Some other more unusual complications of venipuncture include **cellulitis, phlebitis, inadvertent arterial puncture,** and **sepsis.** Sepsis can be caused by introduction of bacteria from the surface of the skin into the blood

as the result of improper cleansing of the venipuncture site. Immunocompromised patients are at higher risk for developing this complication.

⊘ Related Tests

- Related tests include antidysrhythmic drugs, antibodies anticyclic citrullinated peptide, ANA, apolipoprotein A and B, AST, arthroscopy, ANP, blood gases, BMD, bone scan, BNP, calcium (blood and ionized), cholesterol (total, HDL, and LDL), CBC, CBC WBC count and differential, CT, cardiac scoring, CK and isoenzymes, echocardiography, ESR, glucose, glycated hemoglobin, Holter monitor, homocysteine, ketones, LDH and isoenzymes, MRI chest, MRI musculoskeletal, MI scan, myocardial perfusion scan, myoglobin, PET heart, potassium, procalcitonin, radiography bone, RF, synovial fluid analysis, triglycerides, and troponin.
- Refer to the Cardiovascular and Immune systems tables at the end of the book for related tests by body system.

Expected Outcomes

Expected outcomes associated with CRP are:

- Able to attain adequate tissue perfusion demonstrated by capillary refill of less than 3 seconds
- Able to remain nomothermic for 48 hours
- Compliant with physical therapy and able to demonstrate improved strength, endurance, and mobility
- Able to verbalize that pain is relieved at an acceptable level

Creatine Kinase and Isoenzymes

Quick Summary

SYNONYM ACRONYM: CK and isoenzymes.

COMMON USE: To monitor myocardial infarction and some disorders of the musculoskeletal system such as Duchenne muscular dystrophy.

SPECIMEN: Serum collected in a red- or red/gray-top tube. Serial specimens are highly recommended. Care must be taken to use the same type of collection container if serial measurements are to be taken.

NORMAL FINDINGS: (Method: Enzymatic for CK, electrophoresis for isoenzymes; enzyme immunoassay techniques are in common use for CK-MB)

	Conventional & SI Units
Total CK	
Newborn–1 yr	Up to 2 × adult values
Male (children and adults)	50–204 units/L
Female (children and adults)	36–160 units/L

	Conventional & SI Units
CK Isoenzymes by Electrophoresis	
CK-BB	Absent
CK-MB	0–4%
CK-MM	96–100%
CK-MB by Immunoassay	0–3 ng/mL
CK-MB Index	0–2.5

CK = creatine kinase; CK-BB = CK isoenzyme in brain; CK-MB = CK isoenzyme in heart; CK-MM = CK isoenzyme in skeletal muscle.

The CK-MB index is the CK-MB (by immunoassay) divided by the total CK and then multiplied by 100. For example, a CK-MB by immunoassay of 25 ng/mL with a total CK of 250 units/L would have a CK-MB index of 10.

Elevations in total CK occur after exercise. Values in older adults may decline slightly related to loss of muscle mass.

Test Explanation

Creatine kinase (CK) is an enzyme that exists almost exclusively in skeletal muscle, heart muscle, and, in smaller amounts, in the brain and lungs. This enzyme is important for intracellular storage and release of energy. Three isoenzymes, based on primary location, have been identified by electrophoresis: brain and lungs CK-BB, cardiac CK-MB, and skeletal muscle CK-MM. When injury to these tissues occurs, the enzymes are released into the bloodstream. Levels increase and decrease in a predictable time frame. Measuring the serum levels can help determine the extent and timing of the damage. Noting the presence of the specific isoenzyme helps determine the location of the tissue damage. Atypical forms of CK can be identified. Macro-CK, an immunoglobulin complex of normal CK isoenzymes, has no clinical significance. Mitochondrial-CK is sometimes identified in the sera of seriously ill patients, especially those with metastatic carcinoma.

Acute myocardial infarction (MI) releases CK into the serum within the first 48 hours; values return to normal in about 3 days. The isoenzyme CK-MB appears in the first 4 to 6 hours, peaks in 24 hours, and usually returns to normal in 72 hours. Recurrent elevation of CK suggests reinfarction or extension of ischemic damage. Significant elevations of CK are expected in early phases of muscular dystrophy, even before the clinical signs and symptoms appear. CK elevation diminishes as the disease progresses and muscle mass decreases. Differences in total CK with age and gender relate to the fact that the predominant isoenzyme is muscular in origin. Body builders have higher values, whereas older individuals have lower values because of deterioration of muscle mass.

Serial use of the mass assay for CK-MB with serial cardiac troponin I, myoglobin, and serial electrocardiograms in the assessment of MI have largely replaced the use of CK isoenzyme assay by electrophoresis. CK-MB mass assays are more sensitive and rapid than electrophoresis. Studies have demonstrated a high positive predictive value for acute MI when the CK-MB (by immunoassay) is greater than 10 ng/mL with a relative CK-MB index greater than 3.

Timing for Appearance and Resolution of Serum/Plasma Cardiac Markers in Acute MI

Cardiac Marker	Appearance (hr)	Peak (hr)	Resolution (days)
AST	6–8	24–48	3–4
CK (total)	4–6	24	2–3
CK-MB	4–6	15–20	2–3
LDH	12	24–48	10–14
Myoglobin	1–3	4–12	1
Troponin I	2–6	15–20	5–7

Nursing Implications

Assessment

Indications	Potential Nursing Problems
Assist in the diagnosis of acute MI and evaluate cardiac ischemia (CK-MB) Detect musculoskeletal disorders that do not have a neurological basis, such as dermatomyositis or Duchenne muscular dystrophy (CK-MM) Determine the success of coronary artery reperfusion after streptokinase infusion or percutaneous transluminal angioplasty, as evidenced by a decrease in CK-MB	• Activity **(related to the deprivation of oxygen to heart muscle)** • Cardiac Output • Constipation • Family • Fear • Human Response • Nausea • Pain **(related to the deprivation of oxygen and nutrients to heart muscle)** • Self-concept • Sleep • Tissue Perfusion **(related to ineffective circulation to the heart)**

Diagnosis: Clinical Significance of Test Results
INCREASED IN
CK is released from any damaged cell in which it is stored, so conditions that affect the brain, heart, or skeletal muscle and cause cellular destruction demonstrate elevated CK levels and correlating isoenzyme source CK-BB, CK-MB, CK-MM.

- Alcoholism *(CK-MM)*
- Brain infarction (extensive) *(CK-BB)*
- Congestive heart failure *(CK-MB)*
- Delirium tremens *(CK-MM)*
- Dermatomyositis *(CK-MM)*
- Gastrointestinal (GI) tract infarction *(CK-MM)*

- Head injury *(CK-BB)*
- Hypothyroidism *(CK-MM related to metabolic effect on and damage to skeletal muscle tissue)*
- Hypoxic shock *(CK-MM related to muscle damage from lack of oxygen)*
- Loss of blood supply to any muscle *(CK-MM)*
- Malignant hyperthermia *(CK-MM related to skeletal muscle injury)*
- MI *(CK-MB)*
- Muscular dystrophies *(CK-MM)*
- Myocarditis *(CK-MB)*
- Neoplasms of the prostate, bladder, and GI tract *(CK-MM)*
- Polymyositis *(CK-MM)*
- Pregnancy; during labor *(CK-MM)*
- Prolonged hypothermia *(CK-MM)*
- Pulmonary edema *(CK-MM)*
- Pulmonary embolism *(CK-MM)*
- Reye syndrome *(CK-BB)*
- Rhabdomyolysis *(CK-MM)*
- Surgery *(CK-MM)*
- Tachycardia *(CK-MB)*
- Tetanus *(CK-MM related to muscle injury from injection)*
- Trauma *(CK-MM)*

DECREASED IN
- Small stature *(related to lower muscle mass than average stature)*
- Sedentary lifestyle *(related to decreased muscle mass)*

Planning
Considerations for planning a successful partnership should include clear communication of what to expect during the test to decrease anxiety and improve cooperation. The patient should be assessed for a personal and family history of heart disease as well as risk factors associated with heart disease. Before the procedure is performed, plan to review the steps with the patient. Inform the patient that a series of samples will be required. (Samples at the time of admission and 2 to 4 hours, 6 to 8 hours, and 12 hours after admission are the minimal recommendations. Protocols may vary among facilities. Additional samples may be requested.) Address concerns about pain, and explain that there may be some discomfort during the venipuncture.

SPECIAL CONSIDERATIONS
An important aspect of planning is understanding the factors that may alter the study findings or cause abnormal results. Any intramuscularly injected preparations will increase CK levels because of tissue trauma caused by the injection. Interdepartmental communication is a key factor in the planning process.

It is also important to understand which medications or substances the patient may be exposed to in the health-care setting that can interfere with accurate testing:

- Drugs that may increase total CK levels include aspirin, captopril, clofibrate, ethyl alcohol, propranolol, statins, and any intramuscularly injected preparations because of tissue damage caused by the injection.
- Drugs that may decrease total CK levels include dantrolene.

Implementation

Patient education is key to obtaining the patient's cooperation in following directions, and providing an explanation for the purpose of the procedure is an important part of this process. Inform the patient that this study can assist in assessing for heart or skeletal muscle cell damage. Perform the venipuncture.

Evaluation

Recognize anxiety related to test results and be supportive of the fear of a shortened life expectancy. Discuss the implications of abnormal test results on the patient's lifestyle. Provide teaching and information regarding the clinical implications of the test results as appropriate. Educate the patient regarding access to counseling services. Provide contact information, if desired, for the American Heart Association (AHA) (www.americanheart.org) or the National Heart, Lung, and Blood Institute (NHLBI) (www.nhlbi.nih.gov).

SPECIAL CONSIDERATIONS

Numerous studies point to the prevalence of excess body weight in American children and adolescents. Experts estimate that obesity is present in 25% of the population ages 6 to 11 years. The medical, social, and emotional consequences of excess body weight are significant. Special attention should be given to instructing the child and caregiver regarding health risks and weight-control education.

NUTRITIONAL CONSIDERATIONS FOR THE CARDIAC PATIENT: Increases in CPK levels may be associated with coronary artery disease (CAD). Nutritional therapy is recommended for the patient identified to be at risk for developing CAD or for individuals who have specific risk factors and/or existing medical conditions (e.g., elevated LDL cholesterol levels, other lipid disorders, insulin-dependent diabetes, insulin resistance, or metabolic syndrome). Other changeable risk factors warranting patient education include strategies to encourage patients, especially those who are overweight and with high blood pressure, to safely decrease sodium intake, achieve a normal weight, ensure regular participation of moderate aerobic physical activity three to four times per week, eliminate tobacco use, and adhere to a heart-healthy diet. If triglycerides also are elevated, the patient should be advised to eliminate or reduce alcohol. The Guideline on Lifestyle Management to Reduce Cardiovascular Risk published by the American College

of Cardiology (ACC) and the AHA in conjunction with the NHLBI recommends a "Mediterranean"-style diet rather than a low-fat diet. The guideline emphasizes inclusion of vegetables, whole grains, fruits, low-fat dairy, nuts, legumes, and nontropical vegetable oils (e.g., olive, canola, peanut, sunflower, flaxseed) along with fish and lean poultry. A similar dietary pattern known as the Dietary Approaches to Stop Hypertension (DASH) diet makes additional recommendations for the reduction of dietary sodium. Both dietary styles emphasize a reduction in consumption of red meats, which are high in saturated fats and cholesterol, and other foods containing sugar, saturated fats, trans fats, and sodium.

✓ Critical Findings

N/A

✓ Study Specific Complications

There are a number of complications associated with performing a venipuncture. **Pain** is commonly associated with needles, and although the pain experienced during venipuncture is usually mild, on a rare occasion the needle may strike a nerve causing permanent pain. Some patients experience a **vasovagal reaction** during the venipuncture procedure, evidenced by sweating, low blood pressure, fainting, or near fainting. The potential for a **fall injury** is a significant concern related to vasovagal reactions. Prolonged **bleeding** is a complication that occurs with patients who are taking blood thinners or who have coagulopathies such as hemophilia. A **hematoma** results when blood leaks into the tissue during or after a venipuncture, as evidenced by pain, bruising, and/or swelling at the venipuncture site. The swelling can cause injury by compression to surrounding nerves, which can be temporary or permanent. HCPs should watch for minor complications such as bruising and hematoma at the venipuncture site, which are fairly common. Hematomas occur more often in older adult or frail patients, or those with veins that are difficult to access. Bleeding or bruising can be prevented once the needle has been removed by applying direct pressure to the site with dry gauze for a minute or two. Some other more unusual complications of venipuncture include **cellulitis, phlebitis, inadvertent arterial puncture,** and **sepsis.** Sepsis can be caused by introduction of bacteria from the surface of the skin into the blood as the result of improper cleansing of the venipuncture site. Immunocompromised patients are at higher risk for developing this complication.

✓ Related Tests

- Related tests include antidysrhythmic drugs, apolipoprotein A and B, AST, ANP, blood gases, BNP, calcium (blood and ionized), cholesterol (total, HDL, and LDL), CRP, CT cardiac scoring, echocardiography, glucose, glycated hemoglobin, Holter monitor, homocysteine, ketones, LDH and isoenzymes, lipoprotein electrophoresis, magnesium, MRI chest, MRI venography, MI scan, myocardial perfusion scan, myoglobin, pericardial fluid, PET heart, potassium, triglycerides, and troponin.

- Refer to the Cardiovascular and Musculoskeletal systems tables at the end of the book for related tests by body system.

Expected Outcomes

Expected outcomes associated with Creatinine Kinase (CK) and Isoenzymes are:

- Verbalized relief of chest pain with treatment
- Maintenance of normal sinus rhythm with adequate cardiac output
- Absence of nausea or vomiting
- Verbalized understanding of the disease and compliance with lifestyle changes that will reduce risk factors
- Compliance with the medication regimen

Creatinine, Blood

Quick Summary

COMMON USE: To assess kidney function found in acute and chronic renal failure, related to drug reaction and disease such as diabetes.

SPECIMEN: Serum collected in a red- or red/gray-top tube. Plasma collected in a green-top (heparin) tube is also acceptable.

NORMAL FINDINGS: (Method: Spectrophotometry)

Age	Conventional Units	SI Units (Conventional Units × 88.4)
Newborn	0.31–1.21 mg/dL	27–107 micromol/L
Infant	0.31–0.71 mg/dL	27–63 micromol/L
1–5 yr	0.31–0.51 mg/dL	27–45 micromol/L
6–10 yr	0.51–0.81 mg/dL	45–72 micromol/L
Adult male	0.61–1.21 mg/dL	54–107 micromol/L
Adult female	0.51–1.11 mg/dL	45–98 micromol/L

Values in older adults remain relatively stable after a period of decline related to loss of muscle mass during the transition from adult to older adult.

The National Kidney Foundation recommends the use of two decimal places in reporting serum creatinine for use in calculating estimated glomerular filtration rate.

Test Explanation

Creatine resides almost exclusively in skeletal muscle, where it participates in energy-requiring metabolic reactions. A small amount of creatine is irreversibly converted to creatinine by the liver, which then circulates to the kidneys and is excreted. The amount of creatinine generated in an individual is proportional to the mass of skeletal muscle present and remains fairly constant throughout the life span; its consistency in production and clearance is the reason that creatinine is used as an indicator of renal function. Creatinine values normally decrease with age owing to diminishing muscle mass. Conditions involving degenerative muscle wasting or massive muscle trauma from a crushing injury will also result in decreased creatinine levels. Blood urea nitrogen (BUN) is often ordered with creatinine for comparison. The BUN/creatinine ratio is also a useful indicator of kidney disease. The ratio should be between 10:1 and 20:1. The creatinine clearance test measures a blood sample and a urine sample to determine the rate at which the kidneys are clearing creatinine from the blood; this reflects the glomerular filtration rate, or GFR (see study titled "Creatinine, Urine, and Creatinine Clearance, Urine").

Chronic kidney disease (CKD) is a significant health concern worldwide. An international effort to standardize methods to identify and monitor CKD has been undertaken by the National Kidney Disease Education Program (NKDEP), the International Confederation of Clinical Chemistry and Laboratory Medicine, and the European Communities Confederation of Clinical Chemistry. International efforts have resulted in development of an isotope dilution mass spectrometry (IDMS) reference method for standardized measurement of creatinine. The National Kidney Foundation (NKF) has recommended use of an equation to estimate glomerular filtration rate (eGFR). The equation is based on factors identified in the NKF Modification of Diet in Renal Disease (MDRD) study. The equation includes four factors: serum or plasma creatinine value, age (in years), gender, and ethnicity. The equation is valid only for patients between the ages of 18 and 70. A correction factor is incorporated in the equation if the patient is African American because CKD is more prevalent in African Americans; results are approximately 20% higher. An IDMS-traceable equation using serum creatinine results from a method that has a calibration traceable to the IDMS and referred to as the "bedside" Schwartz equation is recommended for estimating GFR for children less 18 years of age. The formula uses the patient's height in centimeters and the serum creatinine value where the GFR (mL/min/1.73 m^2) = (0.41 × height cm)/serum creatinine mg/dL (SI Units: GFR (mL/min/1.73 m^2) = (36.2 × height cm)/serum creatinine micromol/L. It is very important to know whether the creatinine has been measured using an IDMS traceable test method because the values will differ; results are lower. The equations have not been validated for pregnant women (GFR is significantly increased in pregnancy); patients older than 70; patients with serious comorbidities; or patients with extremes in body size, muscle mass, or nutritional status. eGFR calculators can be found at the National Kidney Disease Education Program (www.nkdep.nih.gov/professionals/gfr_calculators/index.htm).

Cystatin C, also known as cystatin 3 and CST3, is now recognized as a useful marker for kidney damage and monitor of function in transplanted kidneys. It is a low-molecular-weight molecule belonging in the family of proteinase inhibitors. Cystatin C is produced by all nucleated cells in the body and is freely filtered by the glomerular membrane in the kidney. It is not secreted by the kidney tubules, and although a small amount is reabsorbed by the kidney tubules, it is metabolized in the tubules and does not reenter circulation. Therefore, its serum concentration is directly proportional to kidney function. It is believed to be a better marker of kidney function than creatinine because levels are independent of weight and height, diet, muscle mass, age, and sex. Normal values for individuals ages 1 to 50 years are 0.56 to 0.9 mg/L (SI: 2.3–3.7 micromol/L) and 0.58 to 1.08 mg/L (SI: 2.4–4.47 micromol/L) for age 50 years and older.

Nursing Implications

Assessment

Indications	Potential Nursing Problems
Assess a known or suspected disorder involving muscles in the absence of renal disease Evaluate known or suspected impairment of renal function	• Confusion • Constipation **(related to dehydration or fluid restriction)** • Fatigue • Fluid Volume • Human Response • Infection • Injury Risk **(related to fatigue and anemia due to the insufficient renal production of erythropoietin)** • Nutrition **(related to possible restrictions in protein and some electrolytes)** • Protection • Skin **(related to skin breakdown due to uremia)** • Urination

Diagnosis: Clinical Significance of Test Results

INCREASED IN

- Acromegaly *(related to increased muscle mass)*
- Dehydration *(related to hemoconcentration)*
- Gigantism *(related to increased muscle mass)*
- Heart failure *(related to decreased renal blood flow)*
- Poliomyelitis *(related to increased release from damaged muscle)*
- Pregnancy-induced hypertension *(related to reduced GFR and decreased urinary excretion)*
- Renal calculi *(related to decreased renal excretion due to obstruction)*
- Renal disease, acute kidney injury and chronic kidney disease *(related to decreased urinary excretion)*
- Rhabdomyolysis *(related to increased release from damaged muscle)*
- Shock *(related to increased release from damaged muscle)*

DECREASED IN

- Decreased muscle mass *(related to debilitating disease or increasing age)*
- Hyperthyroidism *(related to increased GFR)*
- Inadequate protein intake *(related to decreased muscle mass)*
- Liver disease (severe) *(related to fluid retention)*
- Muscular dystrophy *(related to decreased muscle mass)*
- Pregnancy *(related to increased GFR and renal clearance)*
- Small stature *(related to decreased muscle mass)*

Planning

Considerations for planning a successful partnership should include clear communication of what to expect during the test to decrease anxiety and improve cooperation. Before the procedure is performed, plan to review the steps with the patient. Address concerns about pain, and explain that there may be some discomfort during the venipuncture.

SPECIAL CONSIDERATIONS

An important aspect of planning is understanding the factors that may alter the study findings or cause abnormal results. Interdepartmental communication is a key factor in the planning process. The following should be noted when planning for this study:

- The patient must be instructed to refrain from excessive exercise for 8 hours before the test as it may cause a transient increase in the creatinine level.
- High blood levels of bilirubin and glucose can cause false decreases in creatinine.
- A diet high in meat can cause increased creatinine levels.
- Ketosis can cause a significant increase in creatinine.
- Hemolyzed specimens are unsuitable for analysis.

It is also important to understand which medications or substances the patient may be exposed to in the healthcare setting that can interfere with accurate testing:

- Drugs and substances that may increase creatinine levels include acebutolol, acetaminophen (overdose), acetylsalicylic acid, aldatense, amikacin, amiodarone, amphotericin B, arginine, arsenicals, ascorbic acid, asparaginase, barbiturates, capreomycin, captopril, carbutamide, carvedilol, cephalothin, chlorthalidone, cimetidine, cisplatin, clofibrate, colistin, corn oil (Lipomul), cyclosporine, dextran, doxycycline, enalapril, ethylene glycol, gentamicin, indomethacin, ipodate, kanamycin, levodopa, mannitol, methicillin, methoxyflurane, mitomycin, neomycin, netilmicin, nitrofurantoin, NSAIDs, oxyphenbutazone, paromomycin, penicillin, pentamidine, phosphorus, plicamycin, radiographic agents, semustine, streptokinase, streptozocin, tetracycline, thiazides, tobramycin, triamterene, vancomycin, vasopressin, viomycin, and vitamin D.

- Drugs that may decrease creatinine levels include citrates, dopamine, ibuprofen, and lisinopril.

Implementation

Patient education is key to obtaining the patient's cooperation in following directions, and providing an explanation for the purpose of the procedure is an important part of this process. Inform the patient that this study can assist in assessing kidney function. Ensure that the patient has complied with activity restrictions; assure that activity has been restricted for at least 8 hours prior to the procedure. Perform the venipuncture.

Evaluation

Recognize anxiety related to test results and be supportive of impaired activity related to fear of a shortened life expectancy. Discuss the implications of abnormal test results on the patient's lifestyle. Provide teaching and information regarding the clinical implications of the test results as appropriate. Patients with elevated creatinine levels may require adjustments in medications and dosages, especially regarding drugs excreted by the kidneys. There is a potential for prolonged effects or overdose in cases of compromised renal function with administration of some commonly prescribed medications such as digoxin, phenothiazines, meperidine, and some antibiotics. Educate the patient regarding access to counseling services. Help the patient to cope with long-term implications. Recognize that anticipatory anxiety and grief related to potential lifestyle changes may be expressed when someone is faced with a chronic disorder. Provide contact information, if desired, for the National Kidney Foundation (www.kidney.org) or the National Kidney Disease Education Program (www.nkdep.nih.gov).

NUTRITIONAL CONSIDERATIONS: Increased creatinine levels may be associated with kidney disease. The nutritional needs of patients with kidney disease vary widely and are in constant flux. Anorexia, nausea, and vomiting commonly occur, prompting the need for continuous monitoring for malnutrition, especially among patients receiving long-term hemodialysis therapy.

Critical Findings

Adults. Potential critical finding is greater than 7.4 mg/dL (SI: 654.2 micromol/L) (nondialysis patient).

Children. Potential critical finding is greater than 3.8 mg/dL (SI: 336 micromol/L) (nondialysis patient).

Note and immediately report to the requesting health-care provider (HCP) any critical findings and related symptoms. A listing of these findings varies among facilities.

Chronic renal insufficiency is identified by creatinine levels between 1.5 and 3 mg/dL (SI: 132.6 and 265.2 micromol/L); chronic kidney disease is present at levels greater than 3 mg/dL (SI: 265.2 micromol/L).

Possible interventions may include renal or peritoneal dialysis and organ transplant, but early discovery of the cause of elevated creatinine levels might avoid such drastic interventions.

Study Specific Complications

There are a number of complications associated with performing a venipuncture. **Pain** is commonly associated with needles, and although the pain experienced during venipuncture is usually mild, on a rare occasion the needle may strike a nerve causing permanent pain. Some patients experience a **vasovagal reaction** during the venipuncture procedure, evidenced by sweating, low blood pressure, fainting, or near fainting. The potential for a **fall injury** is a significant concern related to vasovagal reactions. Prolonged **bleeding** is a complication that occurs with patients who are taking blood thinners or who have coagulopathies such as hemophilia. A **hematoma** results when blood leaks into the tissue during or after a venipuncture, as evidenced by pain, bruising, and/or swelling at the venipuncture site. The swelling can cause injury by compression to surrounding nerves, which can be temporary or permanent. Health-care providers should watch for minor complications such as bruising and hematoma at the venipuncture site, which are fairly common. Hematomas occur more often in older adult or frail patients, or those with veins that are difficult to access. Bleeding or bruising can be prevented once the needle has been removed by applying direct pressure to the site with dry gauze for a minute or two. Some other more unusual complications of venipuncture include **cellulitis, phlebitis, inadvertent arterial puncture,** and **sepsis.** Sepsis can be caused by introduction of bacteria from the surface of the skin into the blood as the result of improper cleansing of the venipuncture site. Immunocompromised patients are at higher risk for developing this complication.

Related Tests

- Related tests include anion gap, antimicrobial drugs, ANF, BNP, biopsy muscle, blood gases, BUN, calcium, calculus kidney stone panel, CT abdomen, CT renal, CK and isoenzymes, creatinine clearance, cystoscopy, echocardiography, echocardiography transesophageal, electrolytes, EMG, ENG, glucagon, glucose, glycolated hemoglobin, insulin, IVP, KUB studies, lung perfusion scan, MRI venography, microalbumin, osmolality, phosphorus, renogram, retrograde ureteropyelography, TSH, thyroxine, US abdomen, uric acid, and UA.
- Refer to the Genitourinary and Musculoskeletal systems tables at the end of the book for related tests by body system.

Expected Outcomes

Expected outcomes associated with Creatinine, Blood are:

- Caloric intake is sufficient to meet nutritional needs.
- Urinary output is in excess of 30 mL per hour.
- Injury risk associated with uremia is recognized.
- An understanding of the disease is verbalized, and there is compliance with fluid and dietary restrictions as ordered.
- The importance of taking stool softeners to help prevent constipation is verbalized.
- Collaboration with the requesting HCP takes place in selecting treatment options related to end-of-life care, including the use of dialysis.
- Positive coping is demonstrated in relation to the chronic nature of the disease.

Glucose

Quick Summary

SYNONYM ACRONYM: Blood sugar, fasting blood sugar (FBS), postprandial glucose, 2-hr PC (post cibum).

COMMON USE: To assist in the diagnosis of diabetes and to evaluate disorders of carbohydrate metabolism such as malabsorption syndrome.

SPECIMEN: Serum collected in a gold-, red-, or red/gray-top tube. Plasma is recommended for diagnosis of diabetes. Plasma collected in a gray-top (sodium fluoride) or a green-top (heparin) tube.

NORMAL FINDINGS: (Method: Spectrophotometry)

Age	Conventional Units	SI Units (Conventional Units × 0.0555)
Fasting		
Cord blood	45–96 mg/dL	2.5–5.3 mmol/L
Premature infant	20–80 mg/dL	1.1–4.4 mmol/L
Newborn 2 days–2 yr	30–100 mg/dL	1.7–5.6 mmol/L
Child	60–100 mg/dL	3.3–5.6 mmol/L
Adult–older adult	Less than 100 mg/dL	Less than 5.6 mmol/L
Other		
Prediabetes or impaired fasting glucose	100–125 mg/dL	5.6–6.9 mmol/L
2-hr postprandial (PC)	65–139 mg/dL	3.6–7.7 mmol/L
Prediabetes or impaired 2-hr sample	140–199 mg/dL	7.8–11 mmol/L
Random	Less than 200 mg/dL	Less than 11.1 mmol/L

The American Diabetes Association and National Institute of Diabetes and Digestive and Kidney Diseases consider a confirmed fasting blood glucose greater than 126 mg/dL to be consistent with a diagnosis of diabetes. Fasting means no caloric intake for 8 or more hours. Values tend to increase in older adults.

Test Explanation

Glucose, a simple six-carbon sugar (monosaccharide), enters the diet as part of the sugars sucrose, lactose, and maltose and from the complex polysaccharide, dietary starch. The body acquires most of its energy from the oxidative metabolism of glucose. Excess glucose is stored in the liver or in muscle tissue as glycogen. Glucose levels in plasma (one of the components of blood) are generally 10%–15% higher than glucose measurements in whole blood (and even more after eating). This is important because home blood glucose meters measure the glucose in whole blood while most laboratory tests measure the glucose in either plasma or serum.

Diabetes is a group of diseases characterized by hyperglycemia, or elevated glucose levels. Hyperglycemia results from a defect in insulin secretion due to destruction of the beta cells of the pancreas (type 1 diabetes), a defect in insulin action, or a combination of defects in secretion and action (type 2 diabetes). The chronic hyperglycemia of diabetes may result over time in damage, dysfunction, and eventually failure of the eyes (retinopathy), kidneys (nephropathy), nerves (neuropathy), heart (cardiovascular disease), and blood vessels (micro- and macrovascular conditions). The American Diabetes Association and National Institute of Diabetes and Digestive and Kidney Disease have established criteria for diagnosing diabetes to include any combination of the following findings or confirmation of any of the individual findings by repetition of the same test on a subsequent day:

- Symptoms of diabetes (e.g., polyuria, polydipsia, unexplained weight loss) in addition to a random glucose level greater than 200 mg/dL (SI: 11.1 mmol/L)
- Fasting blood glucose greater than 126 mg/dL (SI: 7 mmol/L) after fasting for a minimum of 8 hours
- A1C equal to or greater 6.5% in adults
- Glucose level greater than 200 mg/dL (SI: 11.1 mmol/L) 2 hours after glucose challenge with standardized 75-mg load

Glucose measurements have been used for many years as an indicator of short-term glycemic control to identify diabetes and assist in management of the disease. Glycated hemoglobin, or hemoglobin A_{1c}, is used to indicate long-term glycemic control over a period of several months. The estimated average glucose (eAG) is a mathematical relationship between hemoglobin A_{1c} and glucose levels expressed by the formula

$$eAG = (mg/dL) = [(A_{1c} \times 28.7) - 46.7]$$

For example, eAG for a patient with an A_{1c} of 6% would be calculated as $[(6 \times 28.7) - 46.7] = 125.5$ mg/dL. Studies have documented the need for markers that reflect intermediate glycemic control, or the period of time between 2 to 4 weeks as opposed to hours or months. Many patients who appear to be well controlled according to glucose and A_{1c} values actually have significant postprandial hyperglycemia. Management of postprandial hyperglycemia is considered to be of high importance in preventing or delaying the development of diabetes related complications. The GlycoMark assay measures serum 1,5-anhydroglucitol, is a validated marker of short-term glycemic control, and can be used in combination with glucose and hemoglobin A1C measurements to provide a more complete picture of glucose levels over time. GlycoMark values greater than 8 mcg/mL are considered normal for adults. Serum 1,5-anhydroglucitol is a naturally occurring monosaccharide found in most foods. It is not normally metabolized by the body and is excreted by the kidneys. During periods of normal glucose levels, there is an equilibrium between glucose and 1,5-anhydroglucitol concentrations. When blood glucose concentration rises above 180 mg/dL, the renal threshold for glucose, levels of circulating serum 1,5-anhydroglucitol decrease due to competitive inhibition of renal tubular absorption favouring glucose over serum 1,5-anhydroglucitol. As glucose is retained in the circulating blood and levels of glucose increase, correspondingly higher amounts of 1,5-anhydroglucitol are excreted in the urine resulting in lower serum concentrations. The change in serum 1,5-anhydroglucitol levels is directly proportional to the severity and frequency of hyperglycemic episodes. Serum 1,5-anhydroglucitol concentration returns to normal after 2 wk with no recurrence of hyperglycemia. Reports from the medical community indicate that over half of the U.S. population will have diabetes or prediabetes by 2020. The combined use of available markers of glycemic control will greatly improve the ability to achieve tighter, more timely glycemic control.

Comparison of Markers of Glycemic Control to Approximate Blood Glucose Concentration

1,5-Anhydroglucitol Measured Using the GlycoMark Assay	Hemo-globin A_{1c}	Estimated Blood Glucose (mg/dL)	Degree of Diabetic Control
14 mcg/mL or greater	4–5%	68–97 mg/dL	Normal/nondiabetic
10–12 mcg/mL	4–6%	68–126 mg/dL	Well controlled
5–10 mcg/mL	6–8%	126–183 mg/dL	Moderately well controlled
2–5 mcg/mL	8–10%	183–240 mg/dL	Poorly controlled
Less than 2 mcg/mL	Greater than 10% (11–14%)	269–355 mg/dL	Very poorly controlled

Assessment of medications used to manage diabetes is an important facet of controlling the disease and its health-related complications. Drug response is an active area of study to ensure that the medications prescribed are meeting the needs of the patients who are taking them. Insulin and metformin are two commonly prescribed medications for the treatment of diabetes. See the "Insulin Antibodies" study for more detailed information. The AccuType Metformin Assay is a genetic test that identifies individuals who may not respond appropriately or have a suboptimal response to metformin related to a genetic mutation in the proteins responsible for transporting metformin.

Nursing Implications
Assessment

Indications	Potential Nursing Problems
Assist in the diagnosis of insulinoma Determine insulin requirements Evaluate disorders of carbohydrate metabolism Identify hypoglycemia Screen for diabetes	• Blood Glucose (*related to hypoglycemia or hyperglycemia*) • Confusion • Fatigue (*related to insufficient nutrition*) • Fluid Loss (*diaphoresis related to hypoglycemia or more rarely to autonomic neuropathy*) • Human Response • Infection (*related to neuropathy and the inability to feel injury and poor circulation*) • Noncompliance (*related to denial of the disease process*) • Nutrition • Pain (*headache related to altered blood glucose*) • Sensory Perception (*blurred vision and diminished hearing related to altered glucose over time*) • Urination (*related to overworked renal filtering at the cellular level*)

Diagnosis: Clinical Significance of Test Results
INCREASED IN
- Acromegaly, gigantism (*growth hormone [GH] stimulates the release of glucagon, which in turn increases glucose levels*)
- Acute stress reaction (*hyperglycemia is stimulated by the release of catecholamines and glucagon*)
- Cerebrovascular accident (*possibly related to stress*)
- Cushing syndrome (*related to elevated cortisol*)
- Diabetes (*glucose intolerance and elevated glucose levels define diabetes*)
- Glucagonoma (*glucagon releases stored glucose; glucagon-secreting tumors will increase glucose levels*)

- Hemochromatosis *(related to iron deposition in the pancreas; subsequent damage to pancreatic tissue releases cell contents, including glucagon, resulting in hyperglycemia)*
- Liver disease (severe) *(damaged liver tissue releases cell contents, including stored glucose, into circulation)*
- Myocardial infarction *(related to stress and/or preexisting diabetes)*
- Pancreatic adenoma *(damage to pancreatic tissue releases cell contents, including glucagon, resulting in hyperglycemia)*
- Pancreatitis (acute and chronic) *(damage to pancreatic tissue releases cell contents, including glucagon, resulting in hyperglycemia)*
- Pancreatitis due to mumps *(damage to pancreatic tissue releases cell contents, including glucagon, resulting in hyperglycemia)*
- Pheochromocytoma *(related to increased catecholamines, which increase glucagon; glucagon increases glucose levels)*
- Renal disease (severe) *(glucagon is degraded by the kidneys; when damaged kidneys cannot metabolize glucagon, glucagon levels in blood rise and result in hyperglycemia)*
- Shock, trauma *(hyperglycemia is stimulated by the release of catecholamines and glucagon)*
- Somatostatinoma *(somatostatin-producing tumor of pancreatic delta cells, associated with diabetes)*
- Strenuous exercise *(hyperglycemia is stimulated by the release of catecholamines and glucagon)*
- Syndrome X (metabolic syndrome) *(related to the development of diabetes)*
- Thyrotoxicosis *(related to loss of kidney function)*
- Vitamin B$_1$ deficiency *(thiamine is involved in the metabolism of glucose; deficiency results in accumulation of glucose)*

DECREASED IN
- Acute alcohol ingestion *(most glucose metabolism occurs in the liver; alcohol inhibits the liver from making glucose)*
- Addison disease *(cortisol affects glucose levels; insufficient levels of cortisol result in diminished glucose levels)*
- Ectopic insulin production from tumors (adrenal carcinoma, carcinoma of the stomach, fibrosarcoma)
- Excess insulin by injection
- Galactosemia *(inherited enzyme disorder that results in accumulation of galactose in excessive proportion to glucose levels)*
- Glucagon deficiency *(glucagon controls glucose levels; hypoglycemia occurs in the absence of glucagon)*
- Glycogen storage diseases *(deficiencies in enzymes involved in conversion of glycogen to glucose)*
- Hereditary fructose intolerance *(inherited disorder of fructose metabolism; phosphates needed for intermediate steps in gluconeogenesis are trapped from further action by the enzyme deficiency responsible for fructose metabolism)*
- Hypopituitarism *(decreased levels of hormones such as adrenocorticotropin hormone [ACTH] and GH result in decreased glucose levels)*
- Hypothyroidism *(thyroid hormones affect glucose levels; decreased thyroid hormone levels result in decreased glucose levels)*
- Insulinoma *(the function of insulin is to decrease glucose levels)*
- Malabsorption syndromes *(insufficient absorption of carbohydrates)*
- Maple syrup urine disease *(inborn error of amino acid metabolism; accumulation of leucine is believed to inhibit the rate of gluconeogenesis, independently of insulin, and thereby diminish release of hepatic glucose stores)*
- Poisoning resulting in severe liver disease *(decreased liver function correlates with decreased glucose metabolism)*
- Postgastrectomy *(insufficient intake of carbohydrates)*
- Starvation *(insufficient intake of carbohydrates)*
- von Gierke disease *(most common glycogen storage disease; G6PD deficiency)*

Planning
Other considerations for planning a successful partnership should include clear communication of what to expect during the test to decrease anxiety and improve cooperation. Obtain a list of medications the patient is taking, including herbs, nutritional supplements, nutraceuticals, insulin, and any other substances used to regulate glucose levels. Before the procedure is performed, plan to review the steps with the patient. Address concerns about pain, and explain that there may be some discomfort during the venipuncture.

SPECIAL CONSIDERATIONS
An important aspect of planning is understanding the factors that may alter the study findings or cause abnormal results. Interdepartmental communication is a key factor in the planning process. The following should be noted when planning for this study:

- For the fasting glucose test, the patient should fast for at least 8 hours before specimen collection and not consume any caffeinated products or chew any type of gum before specimen collection for the fasting glucose test; these factors are known to elevate glucose levels. Protocols may vary among facilities. The patient should follow the instructions given by the HCP for a 2-hour postprandial glucose test. Some HCPs may order the administration of a standard glucose solution, whereas others may instruct the patient to eat a meal with a known carbohydrate composition.

- Elevated urea levels and uremia, which can lead to falsely elevated glucose levels *(related to dehydration)*
- Extremely elevated white blood cell counts, which can lead to falsely decreased glucose values *(related to stress and increased metabolism that increases the demand for glucose)*
- Failure to follow dietary restrictions before the fasting test, which can lead to falsely elevated glucose values
- Administration of insulin or oral hypoglycemic drugs within 8 hours of a fasting blood glucose, which can lead to falsely decreased values
- Specimens collected above an IV line, which should never be done due to the potential for dilution when the specimen and the IV solution combine in the collection container, falsely decreasing the result

It is also important to understand which medications or substances the patient may be exposed to in the healthcare setting that can interfere with accurate testing:

- Drugs that may increase glucose levels include acetazolamide, alanine, albuterol, anesthetic agents, antipyrine, atenolol, betamethasone, cefotaxime, chlorpromazine, chlorprothixene, clonidine, clorexolone, corticotropin, cortisone, cyclic AMP, cyclopropane, dexamethasone, dextroamphetamine, diapamide, epinephrine, enflurane, ethacrynic acid, ether, fludrocortisone, fluoxymesterone, furosemide, glucagon, glucocorticoids, homoharringtonine, hydrochlorothiazide, hydroxydione, isoniazid, maltose, meperidine, meprednisone, methyclothiazide, metolazone, niacin, nifedipine, nortriptyline, octreotide, oral contraceptives, oxyphenbutazone, pancreozymin, phenelzine, phenylbutazone, piperacetazine, polythiazide, prednisone, quinethazone, reserpine, rifampin, ritodrine, salbutamol, secretin, somatostatin, thiazides, thyroid hormone, and triamcinolone.
- Drugs that may decrease glucose levels include acarbose, acetylsalicylic acid, acipimox, alanine, allopurinol, antimony compounds, arsenicals, ascorbic acid, benzene, buformin, cannabis, captopril, carbutamide, chloroform, clofibrate, dexfenfluramine, enalapril, enprostil, erythromycin, fenfluramine, gemfibrozil, glibornuride, glyburide, guanethidine, niceritrol, nitrazepam, oral contraceptives, oxandrolone, oxymetholone, phentolamine, phosphorus, promethazine, ramipril, rotenone, sulfonylureas, thiocarlide, tolbutamide, tromethamine, and verapamil.

Implementation

Patient education is key to obtaining the patient's cooperation in following directions, and providing an explanation for the purpose of the procedure is an important part of this process. Inform the patient that this study can assist in evaluating blood sugar levels. Ensure that the patient has complied with dietary restrictions and other pretesting preparations; assure that food has been restricted for at least 8 hours prior to the fasting procedure. Perform the venipuncture.

Evaluation

Recognize anxiety related to test results, and be supportive of a perceived loss of independence and fear of a shortened life expectancy. Discuss the implications of abnormal test results on the patient's lifestyle. Provide teaching and information regarding the clinical implications of the test results as appropriate. Instruct the patient and caregiver to report signs and symptoms of hypoglycemia (e.g., weakness, confusion, diaphoresis, rapid pulse) or hyperglycemia (e.g., polydipsia, polyuria, polyphagia, lethargy). Emphasize, if indicated, that good glycemic control delays the onset and slows the progression of diabetic retinopathy, nephropathy, and neuropathy. Provide teaching on foot care. Instruct the patient in the use of home testing strips or meters approved for glucose, ketones, or A_{1c} by the U.S. Food and Drug Administration, if prescribed (see Fig. 1.16). Answer any questions or address any concerns voiced by the patient or family. Educate the patient regarding access to counseling services as appropriate. Provide contact information, if desired, for the American Diabetes Association (ADA) (www.diabetes.org) or the American Heart Association (AHA) (www.americanheart.org). The ADA recommends A_{1c} testing four times a year when glycemic targets are not being met or whose therapy has changed and twice a year when treatment goals are being met. The ADA also recommends that testing for diabetes commence at age 45 for asymptomatic individuals, be considered for adults of any age who are overweight and have additional risk factors, and continue every 3 years in the absence of symptoms.

SPECIAL CONSIDERATIONS
NUTRITIONAL CONSIDERATIONS FOR THE DIABETIC PATIENT

Abnormal glucose levels may be associated with conditions resulting from poor glucose control. There is

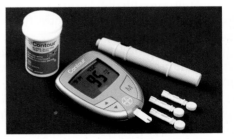

FIGURE 1.16 Materials for fingerstick glucose measurement. *Used with permission, from Wilkinson, J., & Treas, L. (2010). Fundamentals of nursing (2nd Ed.). FA Davis Company.*

no "diabetic diet"; however, many meal-planning approaches with nutritional goals are endorsed by the American Diabetes Association. Patients who adhere to dietary recommendations report a better general feeling of health, better weight management, greater control of glucose and lipid values, and improved use of insulin. Instruct the patient, as appropriate, in nutritional management of diabetes. The nutritional needs of each diabetic patient need to be determined individually (especially during pregnancy) with the appropriate HCPs, particularly professionals educated in nutrition.

⊘ Critical Findings

Glucose
ADULTS & CHILDREN
- Less than 40 mg/dL (SI: Less than 2.22 mmol/L)
- Greater than 400 mg/dL (SI: Greater than 22.2 mmol/L)

NEWBORNS
- Less than 32 mg/dL (SI: Less than 1.8 mmol/L)
- Greater than 328 mg/dL (SI: Greater than 18.2 mmol/L)

Consideration may be given to verify the critical findings before action is taken. Policies vary among facilities and may include requesting immediate recollection and retesting by the laboratory or retesting using a rapid Point of Care instrument at the bedside, if available.

Note and immediately report to the requesting HCP any critical findings and related symptoms. A listing of these findings varies among facilities.

Glucose monitoring is an important measure in achieving tight glycemic control. The enzymatic GDH-PQQ test method may produce falsely elevated results in patients who are receiving products that contain other sugars (e.g., oral xylose, parenterals containing maltose or galactose, and peritoneal dialysis solutions that contain icodextrin). The GDH-NAD, glucose oxidase, and glucose hexokinase methods can distinguish between glucose and other sugars.

Symptoms of decreased glucose levels include headache, confusion, polyphagia, irritability, nervousness, restlessness, diaphoresis, and weakness. Possible interventions include oral or intravenous (IV) administration of glucose, IV or intramuscular injection of glucagon, and continuous glucose monitoring.

Symptoms of elevated glucose levels include abdominal pain, fatigue, muscle cramps, nausea, vomiting, polyuria, polyphagia, and polydipsia. Possible interventions include fluid replacement in addition to subcutaneous or IV injection of insulin with continuous glucose monitoring.

⊘ Study Specific Complications

There are a number of complications associated with performing a venipuncture. **Pain** is commonly associated with needles, and although the pain experienced during venipuncture is usually mild, on a rare occasion the needle may strike a nerve causing permanent pain. Some patients experience a **vasovagal reaction** during the venipuncture procedure, evidenced by sweating, low blood pressure, fainting, or near fainting. The potential for a **fall injury** is a significant concern related to vasovagal reactions. Prolonged **bleeding** is a complication that occurs with patients who are taking blood thinners or who have coagulopathies such as hemophilia. A **hematoma** results when blood leaks into the tissue during or after a venipuncture, as evidenced by pain, bruising, and/or swelling at the venipuncture site. The swelling can cause injury by compression to surrounding nerves, which can be temporary or permanent. HCPs should watch for minor complications such as bruising and hematoma at the venipuncture site, which are fairly common. Hematomas occur more often in older adult or frail patients, or those with veins that are difficult to access. Bleeding or bruising can be prevented once the needle has been removed by applying direct pressure to the site with dry gauze for a minute or two. Some other more unusual complications of venipuncture include **cellulitis, phlebitis, inadvertent arterial puncture,** and **sepsis.** Sepsis can be caused by introduction of bacteria from the surface of the skin into the blood as the result of improper cleansing of the venipuncture site. Immunocompromised patients are at higher risk for developing this complication.

⊘ Related Tests

- Related tests include ACTH, angiography adrenal, BUN, calcium, catecholamines, cholesterol (HDL, LDL, total), cortisol, C-peptide, CT cardiac scoring, CRP, CK and isoenzymes, creatinine, DHEA, echocardiography, fecal analysis, fecal fat, fluorescein angiography, fructosamine, fundus photography, gastric emptying scan, glucagon, GTT, glycated hemoglobin gonioscopy, Holter monitor, HVA, insulin, insulin antibodies, ketones, LDH and isoenzymes, lactic acid, lipoprotein electrophoresis, MRI chest, metanephrines, microalbumin, myoglobin, MI infarct scan, myocardial perfusion heart scan, plethysmography, PET heart, renin, sodium, troponin, and visual fields test.
- Refer to the Endocrine System table at the end of the book for related tests by body system.

Expected Outcomes
Expected outcomes associated with Glucose are:

- Demonstrating blood glucose that remains within normal limits

- Being compliant with a diet that supports glucose control through demonstrating an understanding of what constitutes well-balanced, healthy meals
- Describing symptoms of hypoglycemia and how to effectively reverse a hypoglycemic event
- Being compliant with and reliably performing daily blood glucose monitoring as ordered
- Being compliant with the medication regimen as ordered
- Successfully maintaining a healthy weight and activity level
- Describing proper foot care and what to look for each day when the feet are inspected

Glycated Hemoglobin

Quick Summary

SYNONYM ACRONYM: Hemoglobin A_{1c}, A_{1c}.

COMMON USE: To monitor treatment in individuals with diabetes by evaluating their long-term glycemic control.

SPECIMEN: Whole blood collected in a lavender-top (EDTA) tube.

NORMAL FINDINGS: (Method: Chromatography)

Non-diabetic	4–5.5%
Prediabetes	5.7–6.4%
Diabetes	6.5% or less

Values vary widely by method. The treatment goal assumes the use of a standardized test as referenced to the National Glycohemoglobin Standardization Program-Diabetes Control and Complications Trial and the absence of clinical conditions such as hemoglobinopathies, anemias, renal and hepatic diseases known to affect the accuracy of the test results.

American Diabetes Association (ADA).

Test Explanation

Glycosylated or *glycated hemoglobin* is the combination of glucose and hemoglobin into a ketamine; the rate at which this occurs is proportional to glucose concentration. The average life span of a red blood cell (RBC) is approximately 120 days; measurement of glycated hemoglobin is a way to monitor long-term diabetic management. A change of 1% in the A_{1c} is roughly equivalent to a change in glucose concentration of 29 mg/dL or 1.6 mmol/L. The average plasma glucose can be estimated using the formula:

Average plasma glucose

$$(mg/dL) = [(A1c \times 28.7) - 46.7]$$

The same formula can be used to convert the eAG to glucose in SI units (after multiplying the eAG by 0.555 to convert from mg/dL to mmol/L). For example, an A_{1c} value of 6% would reflect an average plasma glucose

of 125.5 mg/dL or $[(6 \times 28.7) - 46.7]$. Expressed in SI units $[(6 \times 28.7) - 46.7] = 125.5 \times 0.555 = 7$ mmol/L.

Diabetes is a group of diseases characterized by hyperglycemia or elevated glucose levels. Hyperglycemia results from a defect in insulin secretion (type 1 diabetes), a defect in insulin action, or a combination of dysfunctional secretion and action (type 2 diabetes). The chronic hyperglycemia of diabetes over time results in damage, dysfunction, and eventually failure of the eyes, kidneys, nerves, heart, and blood vessels. Hemoglobin A_{1c} levels are not age dependent and are not affected by exercise, diabetic medications, or nonfasting state before specimen collection. The hemoglobin A_{1c} assay would not be useful for patients with hemolytic anemia or abnormal hemoglobins (e.g., hemoglobin S) accompanied by abnormal RBC turnover. These patients would be screened, diagnosed, and managed using symptoms, clinical risk factors, short-term glycemic indicators (glucose), and intermediate glycemic indicators (1,5-anhydroglucitol or glycated albumin).

Nursing Implications

Assessment

Indications	Potential Nursing Problems
Assess long-term glucose control in individuals with diabetes	• Blood Glucose • Confusion • Fatigue *(related to insufficient nutrition)* • Fluid Loss *(related to diaphoresis)* • Infection • Health Management • Human Response • Noncompliance • Pain *(headache related to altered glucose)* • Sensory Perception *(blurred vision and hearing loss related to altered glucose over time)*

Diagnosis: Clinical Significance of Test Results

INCREASED IN

- Diabetes (poorly controlled or uncontrolled) *(related to and evidenced by elevated glucose levels)*
- Pregnancy *(evidenced by gestational diabetes)*
- Splenectomy *(related to prolonged RBC survival, which extends the amount of time hemoglobin is available for glycosylation)*

DECREASED IN

- Chronic blood loss *(related to decreased concentration of RBC-bound glycated hemoglobin due to blood loss)*
- Chronic kidney disease *(low RBC count associated with this condition reflects corresponding decrease in RBC-bound glycated hemoglobin)*

- Conditions that decrease RBC life span *(evidenced by anemia and low RBC count, reflecting a corresponding decrease in RBC-bound glycated hemoglobin)*
- Hemolytic anemia *(evidenced by low RBC count due to hemolysis, reflecting a corresponding decrease in RBC-bound glycated hemoglobin)*
- Pregnancy *(evidenced by anemia and low RBC count, reflecting a corresponding decrease in RBC-bound glycated hemoglobin)*

Planning

Considerations for planning a successful partnership should include clear communication of what to expect during the test to decrease anxiety and improve cooperation. Before the procedure is performed, plan to review the steps with the patient. Address concerns about pain, and explain that there may be some discomfort during the venipuncture.

SPECIAL CONSIDERATIONS

An important aspect of planning is understanding the factors that alter the study findings or cause abnormal results. Interdepartmental communication is a key factor in the planning process.

It is also important to understand which medications or substances the patient may be exposed to in the health-care setting that can interfere with accurate testing:

- Drugs that may increase glycated hemoglobin values include aspirin (large doses), atenolol, chronic use of opiates, drugs that increase glucose levels, propranolol, and sulfonylureas.
- Drugs that may decrease glycated hemoglobin values include antiretroviral drugs, aspirin (small doses), cholestyramine, drugs that cause RBC hemolysis (e.g., dapsone), drugs that decrease glucose levels (e.g., metformin), vitamin C, and vitamin E.

Conditions involving abnormal hemoglobins (hemoglobinopathies) affect the reliability of glycated hemoglobin values, causing (1) falsely increased values, (2) falsely decreased values, or (3) discrepancies in either direction depending on the method.

Implementation

Patient education is key to obtaining the patient's cooperation in following directions, and providing an explanation for the purpose of the procedure is an important part of this process. Inform the patient that this study can assist in evaluating blood sugar control over approximately the past 3 months. Perform the venipuncture.

Evaluation

Recognize anxiety related to test results, and be supportive of a perceived loss of independence and fear of a shortened life expectancy. Discuss the implications of abnormal test results on the patient's lifestyle. Provide teaching and information regarding the clinical implications of the test results as appropriate. Instruct the

patient and caregiver to report signs and symptoms of hypoglycemia (e.g., weakness, confusion, diaphoresis, rapid pulse) or hyperglycemia (e.g., polydipsia, polyuria, polyphagia, lethargy). Emphasize, if indicated, that good glycemic control delays the onset and slows the progression of diabetic retinopathy, nephropathy, neuropathy, cardiovascular disease, and micro- and macrovascular conditions. Provide teaching on foot care. Instruct the patient in the use of home test kits approved by the U.S. Food and Drug Administration, if prescribed. The ADA recommends A_{1c} testing four times a year for type 1 or type 2 diabetes when glycemic targets are not being met or whose therapy has changed, and twice a year when treatment goals are being met for type 2 diabetes. The ADA also recommends that testing for diabetes commence at age 45 for asymptomatic individuals, be considered for adults of any age who are overweight and have additional risk factors, and continue every 3 yr in the absence of symptoms. Educate the patient regarding access to counseling services, as appropriate. Provide contact information, if desired, for the American Diabetes Association (ADA) (www.diabetes.org) or the American Heart Association (AHA) (www.americanheart.org).

SPECIAL CONSIDERATIONS
NUTRITIONAL CONSIDERATIONS FOR THE DIABETIC PATIENT

Abnormal glucose levels may be associated with conditions resulting from poor glucose control. There is no "diabetic diet"; however, many meal-planning approaches with nutritional goals are endorsed by the American Dietetic Association. Patients who adhere to dietary recommendations report a better general feeling of health, better weight management, greater control of glucose and lipid values, and improved use of insulin. Instruct the patient, as appropriate, in nutritional management of diabetes. The nutritional needs of each diabetic patient need to be determined individually (especially during pregnancy) with the appropriate HCPs, particularly professionals educated in nutrition.

Critical Findings

N/A

Study Specific Complications

There are a number of complications associated with performing a venipuncture. **Pain** is commonly associated with needles, and although the pain experienced during venipuncture is usually mild, on a rare occasion the needle may strike a nerve causing permanent pain. Some patients experience a **vasovagal reaction** during the venipuncture procedure, evidenced by sweating, low blood pressure, fainting, or near fainting. The potential for a **fall injury** is a significant concern related to vasovagal reactions. Prolonged **bleeding** is a complication that occurs with patients who are taking blood thinners or who have coagulopathies such as hemophilia. A **hematoma** results when blood leaks into the tissue during or after a venipuncture, as evidenced by pain, bruising, and/or swelling at the venipuncture site. The swelling can cause injury by compression to surrounding nerves, which can be temporary or permanent. Health-care providers (HCPs) should watch for minor complications such as bruising and hematoma at the venipuncture site, which are fairly common. Hematomas occur more often in older adult or frail patients, or those with veins that are difficult to access. Bleeding or bruising can be prevented once the needle has been removed by applying direct pressure to the site with dry gauze for a minute or two. Some other more unusual complications of venipuncture include **cellulitis, phlebitis, inadvertent arterial puncture,** and **sepsis.** Sepsis can be caused by introduction of bacteria from the surface of the skin into the blood as the result of improper cleansing of the venipuncture site. Immunocompromised patients are at higher risk for developing this complication.

✔ Related Tests

- Related tests include C-peptide, cholesterol (total and HDL), CT cardiac scoring, creatinine/eGFR, EMG, ENG, fluorescein angiography, fructosamine, fundus photography, gastric emptying scan, glucagon, glucose, glucose tolerance tests, insulin, insulin antibodies, ketones, microalbumin, plethysmography, slit-lamp biomicroscopy, triglycerides, and visual fields test.
- Refer to the Endocrine System table at the end of the book for related tests by body system.

Expected Outcomes

Expected outcomes associated with Glycated Hemoglobin are:

- Accepting the diagnosis of diabetes
- Recognizing the need for a change in diet to support health
- Collaborating with the medical team to design an effective treatment plan that fits with lifestyle choices
- Identifying symptoms of hypoglycemia and how to effectively reverse a hypoglycemic event
- Complying with and reliably performing daily blood glucose monitoring as ordered
- Maintaining a healthy weight and activity level
- Describing proper foot care and what to look for each day when the feet are inspected

Human Chorionic Gonadotropin

Quick Summary

SYNONYM ACRONYM: Chorionic gonadotropin, pregnancy test, HCG, hCG, α-HCG, β-subunit HCG.

COMMON USE: To assist in verification of pregnancy, screen for neural tube defects, and evaluate human chorionic gonadotropin (HCG)–secreting tumors.

SPECIMEN: Serum collected in a gold-, red-, or red/gray-top tube. Plasma collected in a green-top (heparin) tube is also acceptable.

NORMAL FINDINGS: (Method: Immunoassay)

Patient	Conventional Units	SI Units (Conventional Units × 1)
Males and nonpregnant females	Less than 5 milli international units/mL	Less than 5 international units/L
Pregnant females by week of gestation:		
Less than 1 wk	5–50 milli international units/mL	5–50 international units/L
2 wk	5–100 milli international units/mL	5–100 international units/L
3 wk	200–3,000 milli international units/mL	200–3,000 international units/L
4 wk	10,000–80,000 milli international units/mL	10,000–80,000 international units/L
5–12 wk	10,000–200,000 milli international units/mL	10,000–200,000 international units/L
13–24 wk	5,000–80,000 milli international units/mL	5,000–80,000 international units/L
26–28 wk	3,000–15,000 milli international units/mL	3,000–15,000 international units/L

Test Explanation

Human chorionic gonadotropin (HCG) is a hormone secreted by the placenta beginning 8 to 10 days after conception, which coincides with implantation of the fertilized ovum. It stimulates secretion of progesterone by the corpus luteum. HCG levels peak at 8 to 12 weeks of gestation and then fall to less than 10% of first trimester levels by the end of pregnancy. By postpartum week 2, levels are undetectable. HCG levels increase at a slower rate in ectopic pregnancy and spontaneous abortion than in normal pregnancy; a low rate of change between serial specimens is predictive of a nonviable fetus. As assays improve in sensitivity over time, ectopic pregnancies are increasingly being identified before rupture. HCG is used along with α-fetoprotein, dimeric inhibin-A, and estriol in prenatal screening for neural tube defects. These prenatal measurements are also known as *triple* or *quad markers,* depending on which tests are included. Serial measurements are needed for an accurate estimate of gestational stage and determination of fetal viability.

Triple- and quad-marker testing has also been used to screen for trisomy 21 (Down syndrome). (To compare HCG to other tests in the triple- and quad-marker screening procedure, see study titled "α_1-Fetoprotein.") HCG is also produced by some germ cell tumors. Most assays measure both the intact and free β-HCG subunit, but if HCG is to be used as a tumor marker, the assay must be capable of detecting both intact and free β-HCG. Pregnancy testing is performed in many settings: at home using over-the-counter test kits, in the HCP's office using CLIA approved test kits or point of care instruments, and in full-service laboratories. HCG can be reliably measured using urine or blood specimens. Blood specimens are preferred because blood levels of HCG are detectable earlier than in urine specimens; urine specimens are susceptible to false-negative results if the specific gravity is too low, which is not a factor for blood specimens.

Nursing Implications

Assessment

Indications	Potential Nursing Problems
Assist in the diagnosis of suspected HCG-producing tumors, such as choriocarcinoma, germ cell tumors of the ovary and testes, or hydatidiform moles	• Fear *(related to the ability to carry a potential child to full term, and congenital deformity)*
Confirm pregnancy, assist in the diagnosis of suspected ectopic pregnancy, or determine threatened or incomplete abortion	• Grief *(related to the viability of pregnancy, and an altered perception of a child's future potential)*
Determine adequacy of hormonal levels to maintain pregnancy	• Human Response
Monitor effects of surgery or chemotherapy	• Spirituality *(related to acceptance and peace with the pregnancy outcome)*
Monitor ovulation induction treatment	• Powerlessness *(related to the possible loss of a potential child)*
Prenatally detect neural tube defects and trisomy 21 (Down syndrome)	

Diagnosis: Clinical Significance of Test Results
INCREASED IN
- Choriocarcinoma *(related to HCG-producing tumor)*
- Ectopic HCG-producing tumors (stomach, lung, colon, pancreas, liver, breast) *(related to HCG-producing tumor)*
- Erythroblastosis fetalis *(hemolytic anemia as a result of fetal sensitization by incompatible maternal blood group antigens such as Rh, Kell, Kidd, and Duffy is associated with increased HCG levels)*
- Germ cell tumors (ovary and testes) *(related to HCG-producing tumors)*

- Hydatidiform mole *(related to HCG-secreting mole)*
- Islet cell tumors *(related to HCG-producing tumors)*
- Multiple gestation pregnancy *(related to increased levels produced by the presence of multiple fetuses)*
- Pregnancy *(related to increased production by placenta)*

DECREASED IN
Any condition associated with diminished viability of the placenta will reflect decreased levels.

- Ectopic pregnancy *(HCG levels increase slower than in viable intrauterine pregnancies, plateau, and then decrease prior to rupture)*
- Incomplete abortion
- Intrauterine fetal demise
- Spontaneous abortion
- Threatened abortion

Planning
Considerations for planning a successful partnership should include clear communication of what to expect during the test to decrease anxiety and improve cooperation. Record the date of the last menstrual period and determine the possibility of pregnancy in perimenopausal women. Before the procedure is performed, plan to review the steps with the patient. Address concerns about pain, and explain that there may be some discomfort during the venipuncture.

SPECIAL CONSIDERATIONS
An important aspect of planning is understanding the factors that may alter the study findings or cause abnormal results. Interdepartmental communication is a key factor in the planning process. The following should be noted when planning for this study:

- Results may vary widely depending on the sensitivity of the assay. Performance of the test too early in pregnancy may cause false-negative results.
- Results may vary widely depending on the specificity of the assay. HCG is composed of an α and a β subunit. The structure of the α subunit is essentially identical to the α-subunit of follicle-stimulating hormone, luteinizing hormone, and thyroid-stimulating hormone. The structure of the β-subunit differentiates HCG from the other hormones. Therefore, false-positive results can be obtained if the HCG assay does not detect β-subunit.

It is also important to understand which medications or substances the patient may be exposed to in the healthcare setting that can interfere with accurate testing:

- Drugs that may decrease HCG levels include epostane and mifepristone.

Implementation
Patient education is key to obtaining the patient's cooperation in following directions, and providing an explanation for the purpose of the procedure is an important

part of this process. Inform the patient that this study can assist in screening for pregnancy, identifying tumors, and evaluating fetal health. Perform the venipuncture.

Evaluation

Recognize anxiety related to test results, and encourage the family to seek counseling if concerned with pregnancy termination or to seek genetic counseling if a chromosomal abnormality is determined. Provide teaching and information regarding the clinical implications of the test results as appropriate. Decisions regarding elective abortion should take place in the presence of both parents. Provide a nonjudgmental, nonthreatening atmosphere for discussing the risks and difficulties of delivering and raising a developmentally challenged infant, as well as exploring other options (e.g., termination of pregnancy or adoption). It is also important to discuss feelings the mother and father may experience (e.g., guilt, depression, anger) if fetal abnormalities are detected. Instruct the patient in the use of home test kits for pregnancy approved by the U.S. Food and Drug Administration as appropriate.

Offer support, as appropriate, to patients who may be the victims of rape or sexual assault. Educate the patient regarding access to counseling services. Provide a nonjudgmental, nonthreatening atmosphere for a discussion during which risks of sexually transmitted diseases are explained. It is also important to discuss problems the victim of sexual assault may experience (e.g., guilt, depression, anger) if there is possibility of pregnancy related to the assault.

In patients with carcinoma, recognize anxiety related to abnormal test results and offer support. Provide teaching and information regarding the clinical implications of abnormal test results, as appropriate. Educate the patient regarding access to counseling services as appropriate.

⊘ Critical Findings

N/A

⊘ Study Specific Complications

There are a number of complications associated with performing a venipuncture. **Pain** is commonly associated with needles, and although the pain experienced during venipuncture is usually mild, on a rare occasion the needle may strike a nerve causing permanent pain. Some patients experience a **vasovagal reaction** during the venipuncture procedure, evidenced by sweating, low blood pressure, fainting, or near fainting. The potential for a **fall injury** is a significant concern related to vasovagal reactions. Prolonged **bleeding** is a complication that occurs with patients who are taking blood thinners or who have coagulopathies such as hemophilia. A **hematoma** results when blood leaks into the tissue during or after a venipuncture, as evidenced by pain, bruising, and/or swelling at the venipuncture

site. The swelling can cause injury by compression to surrounding nerves, which can be temporary or permanent. Health-care providers should watch for minor complications such as bruising and hematoma at the venipuncture site, which are fairly common. Hematomas occur more often in older adult or frail patients, or those with veins that are difficult to access. Bleeding or bruising can be prevented once the needle has been removed by applying direct pressure to the site with dry gauze for a minute or two. Some other more unusual complications of venipuncture include **cellulitis, phlebitis, inadvertent arterial puncture, and sepsis.** Sepsis can be caused by introduction of bacteria from the surface of the skin into the blood as the result of improper cleansing of the venipuncture site. Immunocompromised patients are at higher risk for developing this complication.

⊘ Related Tests

- Related tests include biopsy chorionic villus, *Chlamydia* group antibody, chromosome analysis, CMV, estradiol, fetal fibronectin, α_1-fetoprotein, CBC, hematocrit, CBC hemoglobin, CBC WBC count and differential, progesterone, rubella antibody, rubeola antibody, syphilis serology, toxoplasma antibody, US abdomen, and US biophysical profile obstetric.
- Refer to the Endocrine, Immune, and Reproductive systems tables at the end of the book for related tests by body system.

Expected Outcomes

Expected outcomes associated with Human Chorionic Gonadotropin (HCG) are:

- Accepting the possibility of fetal birth defects
- Seeking emotional support for adaptation to a potential child
- Recognizing fear related to congenital deformity and seeking constructive ways to allay fear

Immunosuppressants: Cyclosporine, Methotrexate, Everolimus, Sirolimus, and Tacrolimus

Quick Summary

SYNONYM ACRONYM: *Cyclosporine* (Sandimmune), *methotrexate* (MTX, amethopterin, Folex, Rheumatrex), methotrexate sodium (Mexate), *everolimus* (Afinitor, Certican, Zortress), *sirolimus* (Rapamycin), *tacrolimus* (Prograf).

COMMON USE: To monitor appropriate drug dosage of immunosuppressant related to organ transplant maintenance.

SPECIMEN: Whole blood collected in lavender-top tube for cyclosporine, everolimus; sirolimus; tacrolimus. Serum collected in a red-top tube for methotrexate; specimen must be protected from light.

Immunosuppressant	Route of Administration	Recommended Collection Time
Cyclosporine	Oral or intravenous	12 hr after dose or immediately prior to next dose
Methotrexate	Oral	Varies according to dosing protocol
	Intramuscular	Varies according to dosing protocol
Everolimus	Oral	Immediately prior to next dose
Sirolimus	Oral	Immediately prior to next dose
Tacrolimus	Oral	Immediately prior to next dose

Leucovorin therapy, also called leucovorin rescue, is used in conjunction with administration of methotrexate. Leucovorin, a fast-acting form of folic acid, protects healthy cells from the toxic effects of methotrexate

NORMAL FINDINGS: (Method: Immunoassay for cyclosporine and methotrexate; liquid chromatography with tandem mass spectrometry for everolimus, sirolimus, and tacrolimus)

Test Explanation

Cyclosporine is an immunosuppressive drug used in the management of organ rejection, especially rejection of heart, liver, pancreas, and kidney transplants. Its most serious side effect is renal impairment or renal failure. Cyclosporine is often administered in conjunction with corticosteroids (e.g., prednisone) for its anti-inflammatory or immune-suppressing properties and with other drugs (e.g., everolimus, sirolimus, tacrolimus) to reduce graft-versus-host disease. Methotrexate is a highly toxic drug that causes cell death by disrupting DNA synthesis. Methotrexate is also used in the treatment of rheumatoid arthritis, psoriasis, polymyositis, and Reiter syndrome. Cyclosporine, sirolimus, and tacrolimus are metabolized by the cytochrome enzyme, CYP3A4 and CYP3A5, which is essential to achieve the desired therapeutic effect. Testing for specific CYP450 genotype defects can be performed in some laboratories on blood and buccal specimens. Counseling and informed written consent are generally required for genetic testing. Test results can

	Therapeutic Dose		Half-Life (hr)	Volume of Distribution (L/kg)	Protein Binding (%)	Excretion
	Conventional Units	SI Units (Conventional Units × 0.832)				
Cyclosporine	100–300 ng/mL renal transplant	83–250 nmol/L	8–24	4–6	90	Renal
	200–350 ng/mL cardiac, hepatic, pancreatic transplant	166–291 nmol/L	8–24	4–6	90	Renal
	100–300 ng/mL bone marrow transplant	83–250 nmol/L	8–24	4–6	90	Renal
Methotrexate		SI Units (Conventional Units × 1)	5–9	0.4–1	50–70	Renal
	Low dose: 0.5–1 micromol/L	Low dose: 0.5–1 micromol/L				
	High dose: Less than 5 micromol/L at 24 hr; less than 0.5 micromol/L at 48 hr; less than 0.1 micromol/L at 72 hr	High dose: Less than 5 micromol/L at 24 hr; less than 0.5 micromol/L at 48 hr; less than 0.1 micromol/L at 72 hr				
		SI Units (Conventional Units × 1.04)				
Everolimus	Transplant: 3–8 ng/mL	3–8 nmol/L	18–35 (kidney); 30–35 (liver)	128–589	75	Biliary
	Oncology: 5–10 ng/mL	5–10 nmol/L	18–35	128–589	75	Biliary
		SI Units (Conventional Units × 1.1)				
Sirolimus	Maintenance phase: renal transplant: 4–12 ng/mL; liver transplant: 12–20 ng/mL	Renal transplant: 4–12 nmol/L; liver transplant: 12–20 nmol/L	46–78	4–20	92	Biliary
		SI Units (Conventional Units × 1.24)				
Tacrolimus	Maintenance phase: renal transplant: 6–12 ng/mL; liver transplant: 4–10 ng/mL; pancreas transplant: 10–18 ng/mL; bone marrow transplant: 10–20 ng/mL	Renal transplant: 7–15 nmol/L; liver transplant: 5–12 nmol/L; pancreas transplant: 12–22 nmol/L; bone marrow transplant: 12–25 nmol/L	10–14	1.5	99	Biliary

Therapeutic targets are highly dependent on the therapeutic approach. The testing laboratory should be consulted for their specific guidelines. Therapeutic targets for the initial phase post-transplantation are slightly higher than during the maintenance phase and are influenced by the specific therapy chosen for each patient with respect to coordination of treatment for other conditions and corresponding therapies. Therapeutic ranges for everolimus, sirolimus, and tacrolimus assume concomitant administration of cyclosporine and steroids.

identify poor and ultrasensitive drug metabolizers. This allows for the possibility of personalized adjustments to their medication regimen or decisions to seek alternative drugs which in turn results in safer, more effective treatment.

Many factors must be considered in effective dosing and monitoring of therapeutic drugs, including patient age; weight; interacting medications; electrolyte balance; protein levels; water balance; conditions that affect absorption and excretion; as well as foods, herbals, vitamins, and minerals that can either potentiate or inhibit the intended target concentration.

Nursing Implications

Assessment

Indications	Potential Nursing Problems
Cyclosporine, Sirolimus, Tacrolimus Assist in the management of treatments to prevent organ rejection Monitor for toxicity Everolimus Assist in the management of treatments to prevent organ rejection Assist in the management of treatments for subependymal giant cell astrocytoma Monitor effectiveness of treatment of renal cell carcinoma Monitor for toxicity Methotrexate Monitor effectiveness of treatment of cancer and some autoimmune disorders Monitor for toxicity	• Body Image • Health Maintenance • Human Response • Infection • Noncompliance **(related to subtherapeutic drug levels)** • Protection • Skin • Tissue Integrity • Toxic Levels

Diagnosis: Clinical Significance of Test Results

Level	Response
Normal levels	Therapeutic effect
Toxic levels	Adjust dose as indicated
Cyclosporine	Renal impairment
Methotrexate	Renal impairment
Everolimus, sirolimus, tacrolimus	Hepatic impairment

Planning

Considerations for planning a successful partnership should include clear communication of what to expect during the test to decrease anxiety and improve cooperation. Before the procedure is performed, plan to review the steps with the patient. Obtain a complete history of the time and amount of drug ingested by the patient. Address concerns about pain, and explain that there may be some discomfort during the venipuncture.

CONTRAINDICATIONS

These medications are metabolized and excreted by the liver and kidneys and are therefore contraindicated in patients with hepatic and renal disease. Caution is advised in patients with renal impairment.

SPECIAL CONSIDERATIONS

An important aspect of planning is understanding the factors that may alter the study findings or cause abnormal results. Interdepartmental communication is a key factor in the planning process. It should be noted when planning for this study that blood drawn in serum separator tubes (gel tubes) will be rejected for analysis.

It is also important to understand which medications or substances the patient may be exposed to in the healthcare setting that can interfere with accurate testing:

CYCLOSPORINE

• Numerous drugs interact with cyclosporine and either increase cyclosporine levels or increase the risk of toxicity. These drugs include acyclovir, aminoglycosides, amiodarone, amphotericin B, anabolic steroids, cephalosporins, cimetidine, danazol, erythromycin, furosemide, ketoconazole, melphalan, methylprednisolone, miconazole, NSAIDs, oral contraceptives, and trimethoprimsulfamethoxazole.
• Drugs that may decrease cyclosporine levels include carbamazepine, ethotoin, mephenytoin, phenobarbital, phenytoin, primidone, and rifampin.

METHOTREXATE

• Drugs that may increase methotrexate levels or increase the risk of toxicity include NSAIDs, probenecid, salicylate, and sulfonamides.
• Antibiotics may decrease the absorption of methotrexate.

EVEROLIMUS

• Drugs and foods that may increase everolimus levels include ketoconazole, amprenavir, aprepitant, atazanavir, clarithromycin, delavirdine, diltiazem, erythromycin, fluconazole, fosamprenavir, grapefruit juice, indinavir, itraconazole, nefazodone, nelfinavir, ritonavir, saquinavir, telithromycin, verapamil, and voriconazole.
• Drugs and herbs that may decrease everolimus levels include carbamazepine, dexamethasone, phenobarbital, phenytoin, rifabutin, rifampin, and St. John's Wort.

SIROLIMUS

• Drugs and foods that may increase sirolimus levels include bromocriptine, cimetidine, cisapride, clotrimazole, danazol, diltiazem, fluconazole, indinavir, metoclopramide, nicardipine, ritonavir, troleandomycin, and verapamil.

- Drugs and herbs that may increase sirolimus levels include carbamazepine, phenobarbital, phenytoin, rifapentine, and St. John's Wort.

TACROLIMUS

- Drugs and foods that may increase tacrolimus levels include bromocriptine, chloramphenicol, cimetidine, cisapride, clarithromycin, clotrimazole, cyclosporine, danazol, diltiazem, erythromycin, fluconazole, grapefruit juice, itraconazole, ketoconazole, methylprednisolone, metoclopramide, nelfinavir, nicardipine, nifedipine, torinavir, troleandomycin, verapamil, and voriconazole.
- Drugs and herbs that may decrease tacrolimus levels include carbamazepine, ethotoin, mephenytoin, octreotide, phenobarbital, primidone, rifabutin, rifampin, sirolimus, and St. John's Wort.

Implementation

Patient education is key to obtaining the patient's cooperation in following directions, and providing an explanation for the purpose of the procedure is an important part of this process. Inform the patient that this study can assist with monitoring subtherapeutic, therapeutic, or toxic drug levels. Consider the recommended collection time in relation to the dosing schedule. Perform the venipuncture.

Evaluation

Recognize anxiety related to test results, and explain to the patient the importance of following the medication regimen; provide instructions regarding drug interactions. Instruct the patient to be prepared to provide the pharmacist with a list of other medications he or she is already taking in the event that the requesting health-care provider (HCP) prescribes a medication.

NUTRITIONAL CONSIDERATIONS: Discuss avoidance of alcohol consumption while taking these medications.

Critical Findings

It is important to note the adverse effects of toxic and subtherapeutic levels. Care must be taken to investigate signs and symptoms of too little and too much medication.

Note and immediately report to the requesting health-care provider HCP any critical findings and related symptoms. A listing of these findings varies among facilities.

Cyclosporine: Greater Than 500 ng/mL (SI: Greater Than 416 nmol/L)

Signs and symptoms of cyclosporine toxicity include increased severity of expected side effects, which include nausea, stomatitis, vomiting, anorexia, hypertension, infection, fluid retention, hypercalcemic metabolic

acidosis, tremor, seizures, headache, and flushing. Possible interventions include close monitoring of blood levels to make dosing adjustments, inducing emesis (if orally ingested), performing gastric lavage (if orally ingested), withholding the drug, and initiating alternative therapy for a short time until the patient is stabilized.

Methotrexate: Greater Than 1 micromol/L After 48 Hr With High-Dose Therapy; Greater Than 0.02 micromol/L After 48 Hr With Low-Dose Therapy

Signs and symptoms of methotrexate toxicity include increased severity of expected side effects, which include nausea, stomatitis, vomiting, anorexia, bleeding, infection, bone marrow depression, and, over a prolonged period of use, hepatotoxicity. The effect of methotrexate on normal cells can be reversed by administration of 5-formyltetrahydrofolate (citrovorum or leucovorin). 5-Formyltetrahydrofolate allows higher doses of methotrexate to be given.

Everolimus: Greater Than 15 ng/mL (SI: Greater Than 15 mcg/L)

Signs and symptoms of everolimus pulmonary toxicity include hypoxia, pleural effusion, cough, and dyspnea. Possible interventions include dosing adjustments, administration of corticosteroids, and monitoring of pulmonary function with chest x-ray. Use of everolimus is contraindicated in patients with severe hepatic impairment. Concomitant administration of strong CYP3A4 inhibitors may significantly increase everolimus levels.

Sirolimus: Greater Than 25 ng/mL (SI: Greater Than 25 mcg/L)

Signs and symptoms of sirolimus pulmonary toxicity include cough, shortness of breath, chest pain, and rapid heart rate. Possible interventions include dosing adjustments, administration of corticosteroids, and monitoring of pulmonary function with chest x-ray.

Tacrolimus: Greater Than 25 ng/mL (SI: Greater Than 25 mcg/L)

Signs and symptoms of tacrolimus toxicity include tremors, seizures, headache, high blood pressure, hyperkalemia, tinnitus, nausea, and vomiting. Possible interventions include treatment of hypertension, administration of antiemetics for nausea and vomiting, and dosing adjustments.

Study Specific Complications

Lack of consideration for the proper collection time relative to the dosing schedule can provide misleading information that may result in an erroneous interpretation of levels, creating the potential for a medication-error-related injury to the patient.

There are a number of complications associated with performing a venipuncture. **Pain** is commonly associated with needles, and although the pain experienced during venipuncture is usually mild, on a rare occasion the needle may strike a nerve causing permanent pain. Some patients experience a **vasovagal reaction** during the venipuncture procedure, evidenced by sweating, low blood pressure, fainting, or near fainting. The potential for a **fall injury** is a significant concern related to vasovagal reactions. Prolonged **bleeding** is a complication that occurs with patients who are taking blood thinners or who have coagulopathies such as hemophilia. A **hematoma** results when blood leaks into the tissue during or after a venipuncture, as evidenced by pain, bruising, and/or swelling at the venipuncture site. The swelling can cause injury by compression to surrounding nerves, which can be temporary or permanent. HCPs should watch for minor complications such as bruising and hematoma at the venipuncture site, which are fairly common. Hematomas occur more often in older adult or frail patients, or those with veins that are difficult to access. Bleeding or bruising can be prevented once the needle has been removed by applying direct pressure to the site with dry gauze for a minute or two. Some other more unusual complications of venipuncture include **cellulitis, phlebitis, inadvertent arterial puncture,** and **sepsis.** Sepsis can be caused by introduction of bacteria from the surface of the skin into the blood as the result of improper cleansing of the venipuncture site. Immunocompromised patients are at higher risk for developing this complication.

⊘ Related Tests

- Related tests include ALT, AST, bilirubin, BUN, CBC platelet count, CBC WBC count and differential, and creatinine.
- Refer to the Genitourinary and Immune systems tables at the end of the book for related tests by body system.

Expected Outcomes

Expected outcomes associated with Immunosuppressant Drugs are:

- Adhering to a medication plan to support the viability of organ transplant
- Taking appropriate self-care measures to prevent infection
- Adapting to the physical changes associated with transplant

Lipase

Quick Summary

SYNONYM ACRONYM: Triacylglycerol acylhydrolase.

COMMON USE: To assess for pancreatic disease related to inflammation, tumor, or cyst, specific to the diagnosis of pancreatitis.

SPECIMEN: Serum collected in a gold-, red-, or red/gray-top tube. Plasma collected in a green-top (heparin) tube is also acceptable.

NORMAL FINDINGS: (Method: Enzymatic spectrophotometry)

Age	Conventional & SI Units
Newborn–older adult	0–60 units/L

Test Explanation

Lipases are digestive enzymes secreted by the pancreas into the duodenum. There are different lipolytic enzymes with specific substrates, but they are collectively described as lipase. Lipase participates in fat digestion by breaking down triglycerides into fatty acids and glycerol so the fatty acids can be absorbed and either used for energy or stored for later use. Lipase is released into the bloodstream when damage occurs to the pancreatic acinar cells. Its presence in the blood indicates pancreatic disease because the pancreas is the only organ that secretes this enzyme.

Nursing Implications

Assessment

Indications	Potential Nursing Problems
Assist in the diagnosis of acute and chronic pancreatitis Assist in the diagnosis of pancreatic carcinoma	• Breathing • Fear • Fluid Volume (*deficient, related to loss from vomiting*) • Gas Exchange • Human Response • Nutrition (*inadequate, related to loss of appetite due to nausea and other GI symptoms from altered fat digestion*) • Pain

Diagnosis: Clinical Significance of Test Results
INCREASED IN
Lipase is contained in pancreatic tissue and is released into the serum when cell damage or necrosis occurs.

- Acute cholecystitis
- End stage renal disease or chronic kidney disease (*related to decreased renal excretion*)
- Obstruction of the pancreatic duct
- Pancreatic carcinoma (early)
- Pancreatic cyst or pseudocyst
- Pancreatic inflammation
- Pancreatitis (acute and chronic)

DECREASED IN
N/A

Planning

Considerations for planning a successful partnership should include clear communication of what to expect during the test to decrease anxiety and improve cooperation. Before the procedure is performed, plan to review the steps with the patient. Address concerns about pain, and explain that there may be some discomfort during the venipuncture.

SPECIAL CONSIDERATIONS

An important aspect of planning is understanding the factors that may alter the study findings or cause abnormal results. Interdepartmental communication is a key factor in the planning process. The following should be noted when planning for this study:

- Endoscopic retrograde cholangiopancreatography may increase lipase levels.
- Serum lipase levels increase with hemodialysis; therefore, predialysis specimens should be collected for lipase analysis.

It is also important to understand which medications or substances the patient may be exposed to in the health-care setting that can interfere with accurate testing:

- Drugs that may increase lipase levels include acetaminophen, asparaginase, azathioprine, calcitriol, cholinergics, codeine, deoxycholate, diazoxide, didanosine, felbamate, glycocholate, hydrocortisone, indomethacin, meperidine, methacholine, methylprednisolone, metolazone, morphine, narcotics, nitrofurantoin, pancreozymin, pegaspargase, pentazocine, and taurocholate.
- Drugs that may decrease lipase levels include protamine and saline (IV infusions).

Implementation

Patient education is key to obtaining the patient's cooperation in following directions, and providing an explanation for the purpose of the procedure is an important part of this process. Inform the patient that this study can assist in diagnosing pancreatitis. Perform the venipuncture.

Evaluation

Recognize anxiety related to test results and answer any questions or address any concerns voiced by the patient or family. Administer vitamin B$_{12}$, as ordered, to the patient with decreased lipase levels, especially if his or her disease prevents adequate absorption of the vitamin. Encourage the alcoholic patient to avoid alcohol and to seek appropriate counseling for substance abuse.

NUTRITIONAL CONSIDERATIONS: Instruct the patient to ingest small, frequent meals if he or she has a gastrointestinal disorder; advise the patient to consider other dietary alterations as well. After acute symptoms subside and bowel sounds return, patients are usually prescribed a clear liquid diet, progressing to a low-fat, high-carbohydrate diet.

Critical Findings

N/A

Specific Complications

There are a number of complications associated with performing a venipuncture. **Pain** is commonly associated with needles, and although the pain experienced during venipuncture is usually mild, on a rare occasion the needle may strike a nerve causing permanent pain. Some patients experience a **vasovagal reaction** during the venipuncture procedure, evidenced by sweating, low blood pressure, fainting, or near fainting. The potential for a **fall injury** is a significant concern related to vasovagal reactions. Prolonged **bleeding** is a complication that occurs with patients who are taking blood thinners or who have coagulopathies such as hemophilia. A **hematoma** results when blood leaks into the tissue during or after a venipuncture, as evidenced by pain, bruising, and/or swelling at the venipuncture site. The swelling can cause injury by compression to surrounding nerves, which can be temporary or permanent. Health-care providers (HCPs) should watch for minor complications such as bruising and hematoma at the venipuncture site, which are fairly common. Hematomas occur more often in older adult or frail patients, or those with veins that are difficult to access. Bleeding or bruising can be prevented once the needle has been removed by applying direct pressure to the site with dry gauze for a minute or two. Some other more unusual complications of venipuncture include **cellulitis, phlebitis, inadvertent arterial puncture,** and **sepsis.** Sepsis can be caused by introduction of bacteria from the surface of the skin into the blood as the result of improper cleansing of the venipuncture site. Immunocompromised patients are at higher risk for developing this complication.

Related Tests

- Related tests include ALT, ALP, amylase, AST, bilirubin, calcitonin stimulation, calcium, cancer antigens, cholangiography percutaneous transhepatic, cholesterol, CBC, CBC WCB count and diff, ERCP, fecal fat, GGT, hepatobiliary scan, magnesium, MRI pancreas, mumps serology, pleural fluid analysis, peritoneal fluid analysis, triglycerides, US abdomen, and US pancreas.
- Refer to the Gastrointestinal and Hepatobiliary systems tables at the end of the book for related tests by body system.

Expected Outcomes

Expected outcomes associated with Lipase are:

- Pain that is relieved at a manageable level acceptable to the patient
- Respiratory rate that remains within baseline normal
- Adequate fluid intake with urinary output at a minimum of 30 mL/hr

Magnesium, Blood

Quick Summary

SYNONYM ACRONYM: Mg^{2+}.

COMMON USE: To assess electrolyte balance related to magnesium levels to assist in diagnosis, monitoring diseases, and therapeutic interventions such as hemodialysis.

SPECIMEN: Serum collected in a gold-, red-, or red/gray-top tube.

NORMAL FINDINGS: (Method: Spectrophotometry)

Age	Conventional Units	SI Units (Conventional Units × 0.4114)
Newborn	1.7–2.5 mg/dL	0.7–1 mmol/L
Child	1.7–2.3 mg/dL	0.7–0.95 mmol/L
Adult	1.6–2.2 mg/dL	0.66–0.91 mmol/L

Test Explanation

Magnesium is required as a cofactor in numerous crucial enzymatic processes, such as protein synthesis, nucleic acid synthesis, and muscle contraction. Magnesium is also required for the use of adenosine diphosphate as a source of energy. It is the fourth most abundant cation and the second most abundant intracellular ion. Magnesium is needed for the transmission of nerve impulses and muscle relaxation. It controls absorption of sodium, potassium, calcium, and phosphorus; utilization of carbohydrate, lipid, and protein; and activation of enzyme systems that enable the B vitamins to function. Magnesium is also essential for oxidative phosphorylation, nucleic acid synthesis, and blood clotting. Urine magnesium levels reflect magnesium deficiency before serum levels. Magnesium deficiency severe enough to cause hypocalcemia and cardiac dysrhythmias can exist despite normal serum magnesium levels.

Nursing Implications

Assessment

Indications	Potential Nursing Problems
Determine electrolyte balance in renal failure and chronic alcoholism	• Activity
Evaluate cardiac dysrhythmias (decreased magnesium levels can lead to excessive ventricular irritability)	• Cardiac Output
Evaluate known or suspected disorders associated with altered magnesium levels	• Electrolytes
Monitor the effects of various drugs on magnesium levels	• Fluid Volume
	• Human Response
	• Nutrition

Diagnosis: Clinical Significance of Test Results

INCREASED IN

- Addison disease *(related to insufficient production of aldosterone; decreased renal excretion)*
- Adrenocortical insufficiency *(related to decreased renal excretion)*
- Dehydration *(related to hemoconcentration)*
- Diabetic acidosis (severe) *(related to acid-base imbalance)*
- Hypothyroidism *(pathophyiology is unclear)*
- Massive hemolysis *(related to release of intracellular magnesium; intracellular concentration is three times higher than normal plasma levels)*
- Overuse of antacids *(related to excessive intake of magnesium-containing antacids)*
- Renal insufficiency *(related to decreased urinary excretion)*
- Tissue trauma

DECREASED IN

- Alcoholism *(related to increased renal excretion and possible insufficient dietary intake)*
- Diabetic acidosis *(insulin treatment lowers blood glucose and appears to increase intracellular transport of magnesium)*
- Glomerulonephritis (chronic) *(related to diminished renal function; magnesium is reabsorbed in the renal tubules)*
- Hemodialysis *(related to loss of magnesium due to dialysis treatment)*
- Hyperaldosteronism *(related to increased excretion)*
- Hypocalcemia *(decreased magnesium is associated with decreased calcium and vitamin D levels)*
- Hypoparathyroidism *(related to decreased calcium)*
- Inadequate intake
- Inappropriate secretion of antidiuretic hormone *(related to fluid overload)*
- Long-term hyperalimentation
- Malabsorption *(related to impaired absorption of calcium and vitamin D)*
- Pancreatitis *(secondary to alcoholism)*
- Pregnancy
- Severe loss of body fluids *(diarrhea, lactation, sweating, laxative abuse)*

Planning

Considerations for planning a successful partnership should include clear communication of what to expect during the test to decrease anxiety and improve cooperation. Before the procedure is performed, plan to review the steps with the patient. Address concerns about pain, and explain that there may be some discomfort during the venipuncture.

SPECIAL CONSIDERATIONS

An important aspect of planning is understanding the factors that may alter the study findings or cause abnormal results. Interdepartmental communication is a key factor in the planning process. The following should be noted when planning for this study:

- Magnesium is present in higher intracellular concentrations. Therefore, hemolysis will result in a false elevation in values; such specimens should be rejected for analysis.
- Specimens should never be collected above an IV line because of the potential for dilution when the specimen and the IV solution combine in the collection container, falsely decreasing the result. There is also the potential of contaminating the sample with the substance of interest, if it is present in the IV solution, falsely increasing the result.

It is also important to understand which medications or substances the patient may be exposed to in the healthcare setting that can interfere with accurate testing:

- Drugs that may increase magnesium levels include acetylsalicylic acid and progesterone.
- Drugs that may decrease magnesium levels include albuterol, aminoglycosides, amphotericin B, bendroflumethiazide, chlorthalidone, cisplatin, citrates, cyclosporine, digoxin, gentamicin, glucagon, and oral contraceptives.

Implementation

Patient education is key to obtaining the patient's cooperation in following directions, and providing an explanation for the purpose of the procedure is an important part of this process. Inform the patient that this study can assist in the evaluation of electrolyte balance. Perform the venipuncture.

Evaluation

Recognize anxiety related to test results, and instruct the patient to report any signs or symptoms of electrolyte imbalance, such as dehydration, diarrhea, vomiting, or prolonged anorexia. Educate the patient regarding access to nutritional counseling services. Provide contact information, if desired, for the Institute of Medicine of the National Academies (www.iom.edu) and the U.S. Department of Agriculture (www.choosemyplate.gov).

NUTRITIONAL CONSIDERATIONS: Educate the magnesium-deficient patient regarding good dietary sources of magnesium, such as green vegetables, seeds, legumes, shrimp, and some bran cereals. Advise the patient that a high intake of substances such as phosphorus, calcium, fat, and protein interferes with the absorption of magnesium.

Critical Findings

Adults
- Less than 1.2 mg/dL (SI: Less than 0.5 mmol/L)
- Greater than 4.9 mg/dL (SI: Greater than 2 mmol/L)

Children
- Less than 1.2 mg/dL (SI: Less than 0.5 mmol/L)
- Greater than 4.3 mg/dL (SI: Greater than 1.8 mmol/L)

Note and immediately report to the requesting healthcare provider (HCP) any critical findings and related symptoms. A listing of these findings varies among facilities.

Symptoms such as tetany, weakness, dizziness, tremors, hyperactivity, nausea, vomiting, and convulsions occur at decreased (less than 1.2 mg/dL ; SI: Less than 0.5 mmol/L) concentrations. Electrocardiographic (ECG) changes (prolonged P-R and Q-T intervals; broad, flat T waves; and ventricular tachycardia) may also occur. Treatment may include IV or oral administration of magnesium salts, monitoring for respiratory depression and areflexia (IV administration of magnesium salts), and monitoring for diarrhea and metabolic alkalosis (oral administration to replace magnesium).

Respiratory paralysis, decreased reflexes, and cardiac arrest occur at grossly elevated (greater than 15 mg/dL; SI: greater than 6.2 mmol/L) levels. ECG changes, such as prolonged P-R and Q-T intervals, and bradycardia may be seen. Toxic levels of magnesium may be reversed with the administration of calcium, dialysis treatments, and removal of the source of excessive intake.

Study Specific Complications

There are a number of complications associated with performing a venipuncture. **Pain** is commonly associated with needles, and although the pain experienced during venipuncture is usually mild, on a rare occasion the needle may strike a nerve causing permanent pain. Some patients experience a **vasovagal reaction** during the venipuncture procedure, evidenced by sweating, low blood pressure, fainting, or near fainting. The potential for a **fall injury** is a significant concern related to vasovagal reactions. Prolonged **bleeding** is a complication that occurs with patients who are taking blood thinners or who have coagulopathies such as hemophilia. A **hematoma** results when blood leaks into the tissue during or after a venipuncture, as evidenced by pain, bruising, and/or swelling at the venipuncture site. The swelling can cause injury by compression to surrounding nerves, which can be temporary or permanent. HCPs should watch for minor complications such as bruising and hematoma at the venipuncture site, which are fairly common. Hematomas occur more often in older adult or frail patients, or those with veins that are difficult to access. Bleeding or bruising can be prevented once the needle has been removed by applying direct pressure to the site with dry gauze for a minute or two. Some other more unusual complications of venipuncture include **cellulitis, phlebitis, inadvertent arterial puncture,** and **sepsis.** Sepsis can be caused by introduction of bacteria from the surface of the skin into the blood as the result of improper cleansing of the venipuncture site. Immunocompromised patients are at higher risk for developing this complication.

Related Tests

- Related tests include ACTH, aldosterone, anion gap, antidysrhythmic drugs, AST, BUN, calcium, calculus kidney stone panel, CBC WBC count and differential, cortisol, CRP, CK and isoenzymes, creatinine, glucose, homocysteine, LDH and isoenzymes, magnesium urine, myoglobin, osmolality, PTH, phosphorus, potassium, renin, sodium, troponin, US abdomen, and vitamin D.
- Refer to the Cardiovascular, Endocrine, Gastrointestinal, Genitourinary, and Reproductive systems tables at the end of the book for related tests by body system.

Expected Outcomes

Expected outcomes associated with Magnesium, Blood are:

- Heart remains in normal sinus rhythm
- Report that muscle weakness is resolved
- Serum magnesium levels return to normal

Myoglobin

Quick Summary

SYNONYM ACRONYM: MB.

COMMON USE: A general assessment of damage to skeletal or cardiac muscle from trauma or inflammation.

SPECIMEN: Serum collected in a red- or red/gray-top tube.

NORMAL FINDINGS: (Method: Electrochemiluminescent immunoassay)

	Conventional Units	SI Units (Conventional Units × 0.0571)
Male	28–72 ng/mL	1.6–4.1 nmol/L
Female	25–58 ng/mL	1.4–3.3 nmol/L

Values are higher in males.

Test Explanation

Myoglobin is an oxygen-binding muscle protein normally found in skeletal and cardiac muscle. It is released into the bloodstream after muscle damage from ischemia, trauma, or inflammation. Although myoglobin testing is more sensitive than creatinine kinase and isoenzymes, it does not indicate the specific site involved.

Timing for Appearance and Resolution of Serum/Plasma *Cardiac Markers* in *Acute Myocardial Infarction*

Cardiac Marker	Appearance (Hours)	Peak (Hours)	Resolution (Days)
AST	6–8	24–48	3–4
CK (total)	4–6	24	2–3
CK-MB	4–6	15–20	2–3
LDH	12	24–48	10–14
Myoglobin	1–3	4–12	1
Troponin I	2–6	15–20	5–7

Nursing Implications

Assessment

Indications	Potential Nursing Problems
Assist in predicting a flare-up of polymyositis Estimate damage from skeletal muscle injury or myocardial infarction (MI)	• Activity *(related to the deprivation of oxygen to heart muscle)* • Breathing • Cardiac Output • Communication • Fatigue • Gas Exchange • Human Response • Pain *(related to the deprivation of oxygen and nutrients to heart muscle)* • Swallowing • Tissue Perfusion *(related to ineffective circulation to the heart)*

Diagnosis: Clinical Significance of Test Results

INCREASED IN
Conditions that cause muscle damage; damaged muscle cells release myoglobin into circulation.

- Cardiac surgery
- Cocaine use *(rhabdomyolysis is a complication of cocaine use or overdose)*
- Exercise
- Malignant hyperthermia
- MI
- Progressive muscular dystrophy
- Renal failure
- Rhabdomyolysis
- Shock
- Thrombolytic therapy

DECREASED IN
- Myasthenia gravis
- Presence of antibodies to myoglobin, as seen in patients with polymyositis
- Rheumatoid arthritis

Planning

Considerations for planning a successful partnership should include clear communication of what to expect during the test to decrease anxiety and improve cooperation. Before the procedure is performed, plan to review the steps with the patient. Address concerns about pain, and explain that there may be some discomfort during the venipuncture.

SPECIAL CONSIDERATIONS
An important aspect of planning is understanding the factors that may alter the study findings or cause abnormal results. Interdepartmental communication is a key factor in the planning process.

Implementation

Patient education is key to obtaining the patient's cooperation in following directions, and providing an explanation for the purpose of the procedure is an important part of this process. Inform the patient that this study can assist in diagnosing cardiac or skeletal muscle damage. Perform the venipuncture.

Evaluation

Recognize anxiety related to test results, and be supportive of the fear of a shortened life expectancy. Discuss the implications of abnormal test results on the patient's lifestyle. Provide teaching and information regarding the clinical implications of the test results as appropriate. Educate the patient regarding access to counseling services. Provide contact information, if desired, for the American Heart Association (AHA) (www.americanheart.org) or the National Heart, Lung, and Blood Institute (NHLBI) (www.nhlbi.nih.gov).

SPECIAL CONSIDERATIONS

Numerous studies point to the prevalence of excess body weight in American children and adolescents. Experts estimate that obesity is present in 25% of the population ages 6 to 11 years. The medical, social, and emotional consequences of excess body weight are significant. Special attention should be given to instructing the child and caregiver regarding health risks and weight-control education.

NUTRITIONAL CONSIDERATIONS FOR THE CARDIAC PATIENT:

Increases in myoglobin levels may be associated with coronary artery disease (CAD). Nutritional therapy is recommended for the patient identified to be at risk for developing CAD or for individuals who have specific risk factors and/or existing medical conditions (e.g., elevated LDL cholesterol levels, other lipid disorders, insulin-dependent diabetes, insulin resistance, or metabolic syndrome). Other changeable risk factors warranting patient education include strategies to encourage patients, especially those who are overweight and with high blood pressure, to safely decrease sodium intake, achieve a normal weight, ensure regular participation of moderate aerobic physical activity three to four times per week, eliminate tobacco use, and adhere to a heart-healthy diet. If triglycerides also are elevated, the patient should be advised to eliminate or reduce alcohol. The Guideline on Lifestyle Management to Reduce Cardiovascular Risk published by the American College of Cardiology (ACC) and AHA in conjunction with the NHLBI recommends a "Mediterranean"-style diet rather than a low-fat diet. The guideline emphasizes inclusion of vegetables, whole grains, fruits, low-fat dairy, nuts, legumes, and nontropical vegetable oils (e.g., olive, canola, peanut, sunflower, flaxseed) along with fish and lean poultry. A similar dietary pattern known as the Dietary Approaches to Stop Hypertension (DASH) diet makes additional recommendations for the reduction of dietary sodium. Both dietary styles emphasize a reduction in consumption of red meats, which are high in saturated fats and cholesterol, and other foods containing sugar, saturated fats, trans fats, and sodium.

✅ Critical Findings

N/A

✅ Specific Complications

There are a number of complications associated with performing a venipuncture. **Pain** is commonly associated with needles, and although the pain experienced during venipuncture is usually mild, on a rare occasion the needle may strike a nerve causing permanent pain. Some patients experience a **vasovagal reaction** during the venipuncture procedure, evidenced by sweating, low blood pressure, fainting, or near fainting. The potential for a **fall injury** is a significant concern related to vasovagal reactions. Prolonged **bleeding** is a complication that occurs with patients who are taking blood thinners or who have coagulopathies such as hemophilia. A **hematoma** results when blood leaks into the tissue during or after a venipuncture, as evidenced by pain, bruising, and/or swelling at the venipuncture site. The swelling can cause injury by compression to surrounding nerves, which can be temporary or permanent. Health-care providers (HCPs) should watch for minor complications such as bruising and hematoma at the venipuncture site, which are fairly common. Hematomas occur more often in older adult or frail patients, or those with veins that are difficult to access. Bleeding or bruising can be prevented once the needle has been removed by applying direct pressure to the site with dry gauze for a minute or two. Some other more unusual complications of venipuncture include **cellulitis, phlebitis, inadvertent arterial puncture,** and **sepsis.** Sepsis can be caused by introduction of bacteria from the surface of the skin into the blood as the result of improper cleansing of the venipuncture site. Immunocompromised patients are at higher risk for developing this complication.

✅ Related Tests

- Related tests include antidysrhythmic drugs, apolipoprotein A and B, AST, ANP, blood gases, BNP, calcium, cholesterol (total, HDL, and LDL), CRP, CK and isoenzymes, CT cardiac scoring, echocardiography, echocardiography transesophageal, ECG, exercise stress test, glucose, glycated hemoglobin, Holter monitor, homocysteine, ketones, LDH and isoenzymes, lipoprotein electrophoresis, magnesium, MRI chest, MI infarct scan, myoglobin, pericardial fluid analysis, PET heart, potassium, triglycerides, and troponin.
- Refer to the Cardiovascular and Musculoskeletal systems tables at the end of the book for related tests by body system.

Expected Outcomes

Expected outcomes associated with Myoglobin are:

- Successfully swallowing food without aspiration
- Collaborating with the dietician to select foods that are easy to swallow
- Agreeing to use assistive devices to support activity and prevent falls
- Verbalizing an understanding of the disease and being compliant with lifestyle changes that will reduce risk factors
- Verbalizing an absence of pain and being compliant with the medication regimen

Newborn Screening

Quick Summary

SYNONYM ACRONYM: NBS, newborn metabolic screening, tests for inborn errors of metabolism.

COMMON USE: To evaluate newborns for congenital abnormalities, which may include hearing loss; identification of hemoglobin variants such as thalassemias and sickle cell anemia; presence of antibodies that would indicate a HIV infection; or metabolic disorders such as homocystinuria, maple syrup urine disease (MSUD), phenylketonuria (PKU), tyrosinuria, and unexplained intellectual disabilities. Ears for hearing tests.

SPECIMEN: Whole blood for metabolic tests.

NORMAL FINDINGS: (Method: Thyroxine, TSH, and HIV—immunoassay; amino acids—tandem mass spectrometry; hemoglobin variants—electrophoresis)

Hearing Test	
Age	**Normal Findings**
Neonates–3 days	Normal pure tone average of −10 to 15 dB

Thyroid-Stimulating Hormone (TSH)		
Age	**Conventional Units**	**SI Units (Conventional Units × 1)**
Neonates–3 days	Less than 40 micro-international units/mL	Less than 40 milli-international units/L

Thyroxine, Total		
Age	**Conventional Units**	**SI Units (Conventional Units × 17.1)**
Neonates–30 days	5.4–22.6 mcg/dL	92–386 nmol/L

Hemoglobinopathies	Normal Hemoglobin Pattern
Blood spot amino acid analysis	Normal findings. Numerous amino acids are evaluated by blood spot testing, and values vary by method and laboratory. The testing laboratory should be consulted for corresponding reference ranges.
HIV antibodies	Negative

Test Explanation

Newborn screening is a process used to evaluate infants for disorders that are treatable but difficult to identify by direct observation of diagnosable symptoms. The testing is conducted shortly after birth and is mandated in all 50 states and U.S. territories through a collaborative effort between government agencies, local public health departments, hospitals, and parents. Testing is categorized as core tests and second-tier tests. The testing included in mandatory newborn screening programs varies among states and territories; testing of interest that is not included in the mandatory list can be requested by a health-care provider (HCP), as appropriate. Confirmatory testing is performed if abnormal findings are produced by screening methods. Properly collected blood spot cards contain sufficient sample to perform both screening and confirmatory testing. Confirmatory testing varies depending on the initial screen and can include fatty acid oxidation probe tests on skin samples, enzyme uptake testing of skin or muscle tissue samples, enzyme assays of blood samples, DNA testing, gas chromatography/mass spectrometry, and tandem mass spectrometry. Testing for common genetically transferred conditions can be performed on either or both prospective parents by blood tests, skin tests, or DNA testing. DNA testing can also be performed on the fetus, in utero, through the collection of fetal cells by amniocentesis or chorionic villus sampling. Counseling and written, informed consent are recommended and sometimes required before genetic testing.

Every state and U.S. territory has a newborn screening program that includes early hearing loss detection and intervention (EHDI). The goal of EHDI is to assure that permanent hearing loss is identified before 3 months of age, appropriate and timely intervention services are provided before 6 months of age, families of infants with hearing loss receive culturally competent support, and tracking and data management systems for newborn hearing screens are linked with other relevant public health information systems. For more detailed information refer to the study titled "Audiometry Hearing Loss."

The adrenal glands are responsible for production of the hormones cortisol, aldosterone, and male sex androgens. Most infants born with congenital adrenal hyperplasia (CAH) make too much of the androgen hormones and not enough cortisol or aldosterone. The complex feedback loops in the body call for the adrenal glands to increase production of cortisol and aldosterone, and as the adrenal glands work harder to increase production, they increase in size, resulting in hyperplasia. CAH is a group of conditions. Most frequently, lack of or dysfunction of an enzyme called 21-hydroxylase results in one of two types of CAH. The first is a salt-wasting condition in which insufficient levels of aldosterone cause too much salt and water to be lost in the urine. Newborns with this condition are poor feeders and appear lethargic or sleepy. Other symptoms include vomiting, diarrhea, and dehydration, which can lead to weight loss, low blood pressure, and decreased electrolytes. If untreated, these symptoms can result in metabolic acidosis and shock, which in CAH infants is called an *adrenal crisis.* Signs of an adrenal crisis include confusion, irritability, tachycardia, and coma. The second most common type of CAH is a condition in which having too much of the androgen hormones in the blood causes female babies to develop masculinized or virilized genitals. High levels of androgens lead to precocious sexual development, well before the normal age of puberty, in both boys and girls.

Inadequate production of the thyroid hormone thyroxine can result in congenital hypothyroidism, which when untreated manifests in severely delayed physical and intellectual development. Inadequate production may be due to a defect such as a missing, misplaced, or malfunctioning thyroid gland. Inadequate production may also be due to the mother's thyroid condition or treatment during pregnancy or, less commonly encountered in developed nations, a maternal deficiency of iodine. Most newborns do not exhibit signs and symptoms of thyroxine deficiency during the first few weeks of life while they function on the hormone provided by their mother. As the maternal thyroxine is metabolized, some of the symptoms that ensue include coarse, swollen facial features; wide, short hands; respiratory problems; a hoarse-sounding cry; poor weight gain and small stature; delayed occurrence of developmental milestones such as sitting up, crawling, walking, and talking; goiter; anemia; bradycardia; myxedema (accumulation of fluid under the skin); and hearing loss. Children who remain untreated usually demonstrate intellectual and physical disabilities; they may have an unsteady gait and lack coordination. Most demonstrate delays in development of speech, and some have behavioral problems.

Hemoglobin (Hgb) A is the main form of Hgb in the healthy adult. Hgb F is the main form of Hgb in the fetus, the remainder being composed of Hgb A_1 and A_2. Hgb S and C result from abnormal amino acid substitutions during the formation of Hgb and are inherited hemoglobinopathies. Hgb S results from an amino acid substitution during Hgb synthesis whereby valine replaces glutamic acid. Hemoglobin C Harlem results from the substitution of lysine for glutamic acid. Hgb electrophoresis is a separation process used to identify normal and abnormal forms of Hgb. Electrophoresis and high-performance liquid chromatography as well as molecular genetics testing for mutations can also be used to identify abnormal forms of Hgb. Individuals with sickle cell disease have chronic anemia because the abnormal Hgb is unable to carry oxygen. The red blood cells of affected individuals are also abnormal in shape, resembling a crescent or sickle rather than the normal disk shape. This abnormality, combined with cell-wall rigidity, prevents the cells from passing through smaller blood vessels. Blockages in blood vessels result in hypoxia, damage, and pain. Individuals with the sickle cell trait do not have the clinical manifestations of the disease but may pass the disease on to children if the other parent has the trait (or the disease) as well.

Amino acids are required for the production of proteins, enzymes, coenzymes, hormones, nucleic acids used to form DNA, pigments such as hemoglobin, and neurotransmitters. Testing for specific aminoacidopathies is generally performed on infants after an initial screening test with abnormal results. Certain congenital enzyme deficiencies interfere with normal amino acid metabolism and cause excessive accumulation of or deficiencies in amino acid levels. The major genetic disorders include phenylketonuria (PKU), maple syrup urine disease (MSUD), and tyrosinuria. Enzyme disorders can also result in conditions of dysfunctional fatty acid or organic acid metabolism in which toxic substances accumulate in the body and, if untreated, can result in death. Infants with these conditions often appear normal and healthy at birth. Symptoms can appear soon after feeding begins or not until the first months of life, depending on the specific condition. Most of the signs and symptoms of amino acid disorders in infants include poor feeding, lethargy, vomiting, and irritability. Newborns with MSUD produce urine that smells like maple syrup or burned sugar. Accumulation of ammonia, a by-product of protein metabolism, and the corresponding amino acids, results in progressive liver damage, hepatomegaly, jaundice, and tendency to bruise and bleed. If untreated, there may be delays in growth, lack of coordination, and permanent learning and intellectual disabilities. Early diagnosis and treatment of certain aminoacidopathies can prevent intellectual disabilities, reduced growth rates, and various unexplained symptoms.

Cystic fibrosis (CF) is a genetic disease that affects normal functioning of the exocrine glands, causing them to excrete large amounts of electrolytes. CF is characterized by abnormal exocrine secretions within the lungs, pancreas, small intestine, bile ducts, and skin. Some of the signs and symptoms that may be demonstrated by the newborn with CF include failure to thrive, salty sweat, chronic respiratory problems (constant coughing or wheezing, thick mucus, recurrent lung and sinus infections, nasal polyps), and chronic gastrointestinal problems (diarrhea, constipation, pain, gas, and greasy, malodorous stools that are bulky and pale colored). Patients with CF have sweat electrolyte levels two to five times normal. Sweat test values, with family history and signs and symptoms, are required to establish a diagnosis of CF. Clinical presentation may include chronic problems of the gastrointestinal and/or respiratory system. CF is more common in Caucasians than in other populations. Testing of stool samples for decreased trypsin activity has been used as a screen for CF in infants and children, but this is a much less reliable method than the sweat test. Sweat conductivity is a screening method that estimates chloride levels. Sweat conductivity values greater than or equal to 50 mEq/L should be referred for quantitative analysis of sweat chloride. The sweat electrolyte test is still considered the gold standard diagnostic for CF.

Biotin is an important water-soluble vitamin/cofactor that aids in the metabolism of fats, carbohydrates, and proteins. A congenital enzyme deficiency of biotinidase prevents biotin released during normal cellular turnover or via digested dietary proteins from being properly recycled and absorbed, resulting in biotin deficiency. Signs and symptoms of biotin deficiency appear within the first few months and can result in hypotonia, poor coordination, respiratory problems, delays in development, seizures, behavioral disorders, and learning disabilities. Untreated, the deficiency can lead to loss of vision and hearing, ataxia, skin rashes, and hair loss.

Lactose, the main sugar in milk and milk products, is composed of galactose and glucose. Galactosemia occurs when there is a deficiency of the enzyme galactose-1-phosphate uridyl transferase, which is responsible for the conversion of galactose into glucose. The inability of dietary galactose and lactose to be metabolized results in the accumulation of galactose-1-phosphate, which causes damage to the liver, central nervous system, and other body systems. Newborns with galactosemia usually have diarrhea and vomiting within a few days of drinking milk or formula containing lactose. Other early symptoms include poor suckling and feeding, failure to gain weight or grow in length, lethargy, and irritability. The accumulation of galactose-1-phosphate and ammonia is damaging to the liver, and symptoms likely to follow if untreated include hypoglycemia, seizures, coma, hepatomegaly, jaundice, bleeding, shock, and life-threatening bacteremia or septicemia. Early cataracts can occur in about 10% of children with galactosemia. Most untreated children eventually die of liver failure.

HIV is the etiological agent of AIDS and is transmitted through bodily secretions, especially by blood or sexual contact. The virus preferentially binds to the T4 helper lymphocytes and replicates within the cells. Current assays detect several viral proteins. Positive results should be confirmed by Western blot assay. This test is routinely recommended as part of a prenatal work-up and is required for evaluating donated blood units before release for transfusion. The Centers for Disease Control and Prevention (CDC) has structured its recommendations to increase identification of HIV-infected patients as early as possible; early identification increases treatment options, increases frequency of successful treatment, and can decrease further spread of disease.

Core Conditions Evaluated in Many States

Condition	Affected Component	Marker for Disease	Incidence	Potential Therapeutic Interventions	Outcomes of Therapeutic Interventions
Hearing loss	Damage to or malformations of the inner ear	Abnormal audiogram	1 in 3,000 births	Surgery, medications for infections, removal of substances blocking the ear canal, hearing aids	A shorter period of auditory deprivation has a positive impact on normal development.
Congenital adrenal hyperplasia (CAH) (classical)	Multiple types of CAH; majority have a deficiency of or nonfunctioning enzyme: 21-hydroxylase	17-hydroxy-progesterone (17-OHP)	1 in 15,000 births (75% have salt-wasting type; 25% have virilization type)	Oral cortisone administration, surgery for females with virilization	Patients who begin treatment soon after birth usually have normal growth and development.
Congenital hypothyroidism	Missing, misplaced, or malfunctioning thyroid gland resulting in insufficient thyroxine; insufficient thyroxine due to maternal thyroid condition or treatment with anti-thyroid medications during pregnancy	Thyroxine (total), thyroid-stimulating hormone	1 in 3,000–4,000 births	Administration of L-thyroxine	Patients who begin treatment soon after birth usually have normal growth and development.

Core Conditions Evaluated in Many States

Condition	Affected Component	Marker for Disease	Incidence	Potential Therapeutic Interventions	Outcomes of Therapeutic Interventions
Sickle cell disease (SCD) and thalassemia	Variant hemoglobin	Hgb S: amino acid substitution of valine for glutamic acid in the beta-globin chain; Hgb C: amino acid substitution of lysine for glutamic acid in the beta-globin chain; thalassemia: loss of two amino acids in the alpha-globin chain or decreased production of the beta-globin chain	Hgb S: 1 in 3,700 births; Hgb S/C: 1 in 7,400 births; Hgb S/beta-thalassemia 1 in 50,000 births (found more often in people of African, Mediterranean, Middle Eastern, and Asian ancestry and in parts of the world where malaria is endemic).	Care of patients with Hgb S is complex, and the main goal is to prevent complications from infection, blindness from damaged blood vessels in the eye, anemia, dehydration, and fatigue. Some thalassemias may require iron supplementation.	The goal with treatment is to lessen symptoms. Treatment cannot cure the condition. Symptoms may occur in spite of good treatment.

Inborn Errors of Amino Acid Metabolism

Condition	Affected Component	Marker for Disease	Incidence	Potential Therapeutic Interventions	Outcomes of Therapeutic Interventions
Arginosuccinic aciduria (ASA)	Deficiency of or non-functioning enzyme: arginosuccinic acid lysase	Arginosuccinic acid lysase	Less than 1 in 70,000 births	Consultation with a dietician; low-protein diet supplemented by special medical foods and formula	Patients who begin treatment soon after birth and continue treatment throughout life usually have normal growth and development. Early treatment can help prevent high ammonia levels. Accumulation of ammonia can cause brain damage, resulting in lifelong learning problems, intellectual disabilities, or lack of coordination.
Citrullinemia type I	Deficiency of or non-functioning enzyme: argininosuccinate synthetase	Citrulline	1 in 57,000 births	Consultation with a dietician; low-protein diet supplemented by special medical foods and formula	Patients who begin treatment soon after birth and continue treatment throughout life usually have normal growth and development. Early treatment can help prevent high ammonia levels. Accumulation of ammonia can cause brain damage, resulting in lifelong learning problems, intellectual disabilities, or lack of coordination.

Continued

Table Continued

Core Conditions Evaluated in Many States

Condition	Affected Component	Marker for Disease	Incidence	Potential Therapeutic Interventions	Outcomes of Therapeutic Interventions
Homocystin-uria	Deficiency of or non-functioning enzyme: cystathionine beta-synthase	Methionine	Less than 1 in 50,000 births (found more often in white people from the New England region of the United States and in people of Irish ancestry)	Consultation with dietician; diet low in methionine supplemented by special medical foods; administration of vitamin B_6, vitamin B_{12}, folic acid, betaine, and L-cystine	Patients who begin treatment soon after birth and continue treatment throughout life usually have normal growth and development. Treatment may lower the chance for blood clots, heart disease, and stroke. Treatment also lessens the chance of eye problems such as cataract or lens dislocation, which can often be corrected by surgery.
Maple syrup urine disease (MSUD)	Deficiency of or non-functioning enzyme group: branched-chain ketoacid dehydrogenase	Leucine and isoleucine	Less than 1 in 100,000 births (found more often in Mennonite people: about 1 in 380 babies of Mennonite background is born with MSUD; also found more often in people of French-Canadian ancestry)	Consultation with a dietician; diet low in branched-chain amino acids supplemented by special medical foods and formula, administration of thiamine; liver transplant	Patients who begin treatment soon after birth and continue treatment throughout life usually have normal growth and development. Untreated or delayed treatment results in brain damage and mental retardation.
Phenylketon-uria	Deficiency of or non-functioning enzyme: phenylalanine hydroxylase (PAH)	Phenylalanine	1 in 10,000 births; found more often in people of Irish, Northern European, Turkish, or Native American ancestry	Consultation with a dietician; diet low in phenylalanine supplemented by special medical foods and formula; administration of BH4 (tetrahydrobiopterin), which helps the PAH enzyme convert phenylalanine into tyrosine. Patients with this condition should avoid foods and vitamins containing the sugar substitute aspartame, which increases blood levels of phenylalanine	Patients who begin treatment soon after birth and continue treatment throughout life usually have normal growth and development. Some patients may experience delays in learning even after treatment, but without treatment or if treatment is delayed until after 6 mo of age, intellectual disabilities usually result.

Core Conditions Evaluated in Many States

Condition	Affected Component	Marker for Disease	Incidence	Potential Therapeutic Interventions	Outcomes of Therapeutic Interventions
Tyrosinemia type 1	Deficiency of or non-functioning enzyme: fumarylace-toacetase	Tyrosine	Less than 1 in 100,000 births (found more often in people of French-Canadian ancestry)	Consultation with a dietician; diet low in tyrosine and phenylalanine supplemented by special medical foods and formula; administration of nitisinone to prevent liver and kidney damage; liver transplant	Patients who begin treatment soon after birth and continue treatment throughout life usually have normal growth and development. Without treatment, liver and kidney damage will occur.

Inborn Errors of Fatty Acid Metabolism

Condition	Affected Component	Marker for Disease	Incidence	Potential Therapeutic Interventions	Outcomes of Therapeutic Interventions
Carnitine up-take disorder	Deficiency of or non-functioning enzyme: carnitine transporter	Free and total carnitine	Less than 1 in 50,000 births	Consultation with a dietician; diet low in tyrosine and phenylalanine supplemented by special medical foods and formula	Patients who begin treatment soon after birth and continue treatment throughout life usually have normal growth and development. Without treatment, infants may incur brain damage resulting in permanent learning or intellectual disabilities.
Long-chain L-3-hydroxy-acyl-CoA dehydrogenase deficiency	Deficiency of or nonfunctioning enzyme: long-chain L-3-hydroxyacyl-CoA dehydrogenase	Acylcarnitines	Very rare; actual incidence is unknown (found more often in people of Finnish ancestry)	Consultation with a dietician; low-fat, high-carbohydrate diet supplemented by special medical foods and formula consumed in small, frequent meals to avoid hypoglycemia; infants may need to be woken up to eat if they do not wake up on their own; administration of medium-chain triglyceride oil (MCT oil), L-carnitine and DHA (docosahexa-noic acid) which may help prevent loss of eyesight	Patients who begin treatment soon after birth and continue treatment throughout life usually have normal growth and development. Continued episodes of hypoglycemia can lead to learning or intellectual disabilities. With treatment, some people still develop vision, muscle, liver, or heart problems.
Medium-chain acyl-CoA dehydrogenase deficiency	Deficiency of or non-functioning enzyme: medium-chain acyl-CoA dehydrogenase	Octanoyl carnitine and acyl carnitine	1 in 15,000 births (found more often in white people from Northern Europe and the United States)	Consultation with a dietician; low-fat, high-carbohydrate diet supplemented by special medical foods and formula consumed in small, frequent meals to avoid hypoglycemia; infants may need to be woken up to eat if they do not wake up on their own; administration of MCT oil and L-carnitine	Patients who begin treatment soon after birth and continue treatment throughout life usually have normal growth and development. Continued episodes of hypoglycemia can lead to lack of coordination, chronic muscle weakness, learning or intellectual disabilities.

Continued

Table Continued

Core Conditions Evaluated in Many States

Condition	Affected Component	Marker for Disease	Incidence	Potential Therapeutic Interventions	Outcomes of Therapeutic Interventions
Trifunctional protein (TFP) deficiency	Deficiency of or non-functioning enzyme group: mitochondrial trifunctional protein	3-Hydroxy-hexadec-anoylcarnitine	Very rare; actual incidence is unknown	Consultation with a dietician; low-fat, high-carbohydrate diet supplemented by special medical foods and formula consumed in small, frequent meals to avoid hypoglycemia; infants may need to be woken up to eat if they do not wake up on their own; administration of MCT oil and L-carnitine	Most newborns with early TFP deficiency die of cardiac or respiratory problems, even when treated. Patients with childhood TFP deficiency who begin treatment soon after birth and continue treatment throughout life usually have normal growth and development. Continued episodes of hypoglycemia can lead to lack of coordination, chronic muscle weakness, learning or intellectual disabilities. Patients with mild/muscle TFP deficiency who begin treatment soon after birth and continue treatment throughout life usually have normal growth and development. This form does not affect intelligence.
Very-long-chain acyl-CoA de-hydrogenase deficiency	Deficiency of or non-functioning enzyme: very-long-chain acyl-CoA dehydrogenase	Tetradecenoyl-carnitine	Greater than 1 in 30,000 to 100,000 births worldwide; incidence is not higher in any geographic area or ethnic group than in another	Consultation with a dietician; low-fat, high-carbohydrate diet supplemented by special medical foods and formula consumed in small, frequent meals to avoid hypoglycemia; infants may need to be woken up to eat if they do not wake up on their own; administration of MCT oil and L-carnitine	Patients who begin treatment soon after birth and continue treatment throughout life usually have normal growth and development.

Inborn Errors of Organic Acid Metabolism

Condition	Affected Component	Marker for Disease	Incidence	Potential Therapeutic Interventions	Outcomes of Therapeutic Interventions
Glutaric acide-mia Type 1	Deficiency of or non-functioning enzyme: glutaryl-CoA dehydrogenase	Glutarylcarni-tine	1 in 40,000 births (found more often in people of Amish background in the United States, the Ojibway Indian population in Canada, and people of Swedish ancestry)	Consultation with a dietician; diet high in carbohydrates, low in protein, especially lysine and tryptophan, supplemented by special medical foods and formula consumed in small, frequent meals; administration of riboflavin, carnitine	Patients who begin treatment soon after birth and continue treatment throughout life usually have normal growth and development.

Core Conditions Evaluated in Many States

Condition	Affected Component	Marker for Disease	Incidence	Potential Therapeutic Interventions	Outcomes of Therapeutic Interventions
3-Hydroxy, 3-methylglutaric aciduria	Deficiency of or non-functioning enzyme: HMG CoA lyase	Acylcarnitines	Very rare; actual incidence is unknown (found more often in people of Saudi Arabian, Portuguese, and Spanish ancestry)	Consultation with a dietician; diet high in carbohydrates, low in protein, especially leucine, supplemented by special medical foods and formula consumed in small, frequent meals; administration of carnitine	Patients who begin treatment soon after birth and continue treatment throughout life usually have normal growth and development.
Isovaleric acidemia	Deficiency of or non-functioning enzyme: isovaleryl-CoA dehydrogenase	Isovaleryl carnitine	1 in 230,000 births	Consultation with a dietician; diet high in carbohydrates, low in protein, especially leucine, supplemented by special medical foods and formula consumed in small, frequent meals; administration of glycine, carnitine	Patients who begin treatment soon after birth and continue treatment throughout life usually have normal growth and development.
Methyl malonic acidemias (vitamin B_{12} disorders)	Deficiency of or non-functioning enzyme: methylmalonyl-CoA mutase combined with mutations causing defects in vitamin B_{12} metabolism	Propionylcarnitine	Less than 1 in 80,000 births	Consultation with a dietician; diet high in carbohydrates, low in protein, especially leucine, valine, methionine, and threonine, supplemented by special medical foods and formula consumed in small, frequent meals; administration of betaine, carnitine, vitamin B_{12}	Treatment may help some patients but not others. Some infants die even with treatment. Patients who begin treatment soon after birth and continue treatment throughout life may have permanent learning or intellectual disabilities, psychiatric disorders.
Beta ketothiolase	Deficiency of or non-functioning enzyme: mitochondrial aceto-acetyl-CoA thiolase	3-Methylcrotonyl carnitine	Very rare; actual incidence is unknown	Consultation with a dietician; diet high in carbohydrates, low in protein, supplemented by special medical foods and formula consumed in small, frequent meals; administration of carnitine	Patients who begin treatment soon after birth and continue treatment throughout life usually have normal growth and development.

Continued

Table Continued

Core Conditions Evaluated in Many States

Condition	Affected Component	Marker for Disease	Incidence	Potential Therapeutic Interventions	Outcomes of Therapeutic Interventions
Proprionic acidemia	Deficiency of or non-functioning enzyme: propionyl-CoA car-boxylase	Acylcarnitines	Greater than 1 in 100,000 births (found more often in people of Saudi Arabian ancestry and the Inuit Indian population of Greenland)	Consultation with a dietician; diet high in carbohydrates, low in protein, especially leucine, valine, methionine, and threonine, supplemented by special medical foods and formula consumed in small, frequent meals; administration of biotin, carnitine	Patients who begin treatment soon after birth and continue treatment through-out life usually have normal growth and development. Some patients, even with treatment, may have seizures, involuntary movement disorders, chronic infections, permanent learning or intellectual disabilities.
Multiple carboxylase (holocarbox-ylase)	Deficiency of or non-functioning enzyme: 3-methylcrotonyl-CoA carboxylase, 2-methylbutyryl-CoA dehydrogenase	3-Hydroxy-isovaleryl carnitine	Less than 1 in 100,000 births	Consultation with a dietician; diet high in carbohydrates, low in protein, supplemented by special medical foods and formula consumed in small, frequent meals; administration of carnitine	Patients who begin treatment soon after birth and continue treatment throughout life usually have normal growth and development.

Other Multisystem Diseases

Condition	Affected Component	Marker for Disease	Incidence	Potential Therapeutic Interventions	Outcomes of Therapeutic Interventions
Biotinidase deficiency	Deficiency of or non-functioning enzyme: biotinidase	Biotinidase	Greater than 1 in 75,000 to 80,000 births	Consultation with a dietician; diet supplemented by special medical foods and formula; administration of biotin	Patients who begin treatment soon after birth and continue treatment throughout life usually have normal growth and development.
Cystic fibrosis	Deficiency of or nonfunctioning protein: cystic fibrosis transmembrane conductance regulator protein	CF mutation analysis or im-munoreactive trypsinogen	1 in 3,600–3,700 births	Consultation with a dietician; higher calorie diet supplemented by special medical foods and formula, additional hydration, administration of pancreatic enzymes and vitamins; bronchodilators, antibiotics, mucus thinners; percussive therapy, ThAIRapy vest; gene therapy, lung transplant	Patients who begin treatment soon after birth and continue treatment throughout life usually have normal growth and development. The goal with treatment is to lessen symptoms. Treatment cannot cure the condition. Symptoms may occur in spite of good treatment.

Core Conditions Evaluated in Many States

Condition	Affected Component	Marker for Disease	Incidence	Potential Therapeutic Interventions	Outcomes of Therapeutic Interventions
Core Conditions Evaluated in Many States					
Galactosemia (classical)	Deficiency of or nonfunctioning enzyme: galactose-1-phosphate uridyl transferase	Galactose-1-phosphate	Greater than 1 in 50,000 births	Consultation with a dietician; diet free of lactose and galactose supplemented by special medical foods and formula; administration of calcium, vitamin D, and vitamin K	Patients who begin treatment soon after birth and continue treatment throughout life usually have normal growth and development. Some patients may experience delays in learning even after treatment, but without treatment or if treatment is delayed until after 10 days of age, developmental delays and learning disabilities usually result.

Nursing Implications

Assessment

Indications	Potential Nursing Problems
Hearing Tests Screen for hearing loss in infants to determine the need for a referral to an audiologist Blood Spot Testing Assist in the diagnosis of CAH Assist in the diagnosis of congenital hypothyroidism Assist in the diagnosis of abnormal hemoglobins as with Hgb C disease, sickle cell trait or sickle cell disease, and thalassemias, especially in patients with a family history positive for any the disorders Assist in identifying the cause of hemolytic anemia resulting from G-6-PD enzyme deficiency Detect congenital errors of amino acid, fatty acid, or organic acid metabolism Detect congenital errors responsible for urea cycle disorders Screen for multisystem disorders such as CF, biotinidase deficiency, or galactosemia Test for HIV antibodies in infants who have documented and significant exposure to other infected individuals	• Communication • Family • Fear **(related to the possibility of a congenital anomaly)** • Human Response • Spirituality **(related to the loss of an expected potential child)** • Sensory Perception **(related to hearing loss)**

Diagnosis: Clinical Significance of Test Results
ABNORMAL FINDINGS RELATED TO HEARING TEST:
- Abnormal audiogram *(related to congenital damage or malformations of the inner ear, infections, residual amniotic fluid or vernix in the ear canal)*

ENDOCRINE DISORDERS
INCREASED IN
- Congenital hypothyroidism (TSH) *(related to decrease in total thyroxine hormone levels, which activates the feedback loop to increase production of TSH)*
- CAH (adrenocorticotropic hormone [ACTH] and androgens) *(related to an autosomal recessive inherited disorder that results in missing or malfunctioning enzymes responsible for the production of cortisol and which may result in a salt-wasting condition or virilization of female genitalia)*

DECREASED IN
- Congenital hypothyroidism (total T4) *(related to missing or malfunctioning thyroid gland resulting in absence or decrease in total thyroxine hormone levels)*
- CAH (21-hydroxylase) *(related to an autosomal recessive inherited disorder that results in missing or malfunctioning enzymes responsible for the production of cortisol and which may result in one of several conditions, including a salt-wasting condition or virilization of female genitalia)*
- CAH (cortisol) *(related to an autosomal recessive inherited disorder that results in missing or*

malfunctioning enzymes responsible for the production of cortisol and which may result in a salt-wasting condition or virilization of female genitalia)

- CAH (aldosterone) *(related to an autosomal recessive inherited disorder that results in missing or malfunctioning enzymes responsible for the production of cortisol and which may result in a salt-wasting condition)*

ABNORMAL FINDINGS RELATED TO HEMOGLOBINOPATHIES

- Hgb S: sickle cell trait or sickle cell anemia (most common variant in the United States; occurs with a frequency of about 8% among African Americans) *(related to an autosomal recessive inherited disorder that results in a genetic variation in the β-chain of hemoglobin, causing a conformational change in the hemoglobin molecule and affecting the oxygen-binding properties of hemoglobin, which results in sickle-shaped red blood cells)*
- Hgb SC disease *(related to an autosomal recessive inherited disorder that results in the presence of an abnormal combination of Hgb S with Hgb C and presents a milder form of sickle cell anemia)*
- Hgb S/β-thalassemias *(related to an autosomal recessive inherited disorder that results in the presence of abnormal hemoglobin S/β-thalassemia, which combines the effects of thalassemia, a genetic disorder that results in decreased production of hemoglobin and sickle cell anemia, where sickled red blood cells lack the ability to combine effectively with oxygen)*

RBC ENZYME DEFECT
DECREASED IN

- G6PD deficiency *(usually related to an X-linked recessive inherited disorder that results in a deficiency of glucose-6-phosphate dehydrogenase, which causes a hemolytic anemia)*

INBORN ERRORS OF AMINO ACID METABOLISM/ DISORDERS OF THE UREA CYCLE

- Aminoacidopathies *(usually related to an autosomal recessive inherited disorder that results in insufficient or nonfunctional enzyme levels; specific amino acids are implicated)*
- Disorders of the urea cycle; specifically argininemia, argininosuccinic acidemia, citrullinemia, and hyperammonemia/hyperornithinemia/homocitrullinemia *(usually related to an autosomal recessive inherited disorder that results in insufficient or nonfunctional enzyme levels; specific amino acids are implicated)*

INBORN ERRORS OF ORGANIC ACID METABOLISM

- Organic acid disorders *(usually related to an autosomal recessive inherited disorder that results in insufficient or nonfunctional enzyme levels; specific organic acids are implicated)*

INBORN ERRORS OF FATTY ACID METABOLISM

- Fatty acid oxidation disorders *(usually related to an autosomal recessive inherited disorder that results in insufficient or nonfunctional enzyme levels; specific fatty acids are implicated)*

OTHER MULTISYSTEM DISEASES

- Biotinidase deficiency *(related to an autosomal recessive inherited disorder that results in deficiency of the enzyme biotinidase, which prevents absorption or recycling of the essential vitamin biotin)*
- Cystic fibrosis *(related to an autosomal recessive inherited disorder that results in insufficient or nonfunctional CF transmembrane conductance regulator protein, which results in poor transport of salts, especially sodium and chloride, and significantly impairs pulmonary and gastrointestinal function)*
- Galactosemia (classical) *(usually related to an autosomal recessive inherited disorder that results in insufficient or nonfunctional galactose-1-phosphate uridyl transferase enzyme levels)*

INFECTIOUS DISEASES
Positive finding in

- HIV-1 or HIV-2 infection

Planning
Considerations for planning a successful partnership should include clear communication of what to expect during the test to decrease anxiety and improve cooperation. Before the procedure is performed, plan to review the steps with the patient's parents or caregivers. Address concerns about pain, and explain that there may be some discomfort during the venipuncture.

NEONATAL BLOOD SCREEN
Explain that blood specimens from neonates are collected by heel stick and applied to filter paper spots on the birth state's specific screening program card. Most state regulations require screening specimens to be collected between 24 and 48 hours after birth to allow sufficient time after protein intake for abnormal metabolites to be detected, and preferably before blood product transfusion or physical transfer to another facility (see Figs. 1.17 and 1.18).

HEARING TEST
Review the procedure with the patient's parents or caregivers. Address concerns about pain, and explain that no discomfort will be experienced during the test. Inform the parents or caregiver that an audiologist or HCP trained in this procedure performs the test in a quiet room and that the test can take up 20 minutes to evaluate both ears. Explain that each ear is tested separately by using earphones and/or a device placed behind the ear to deliver sounds of varying intensities.

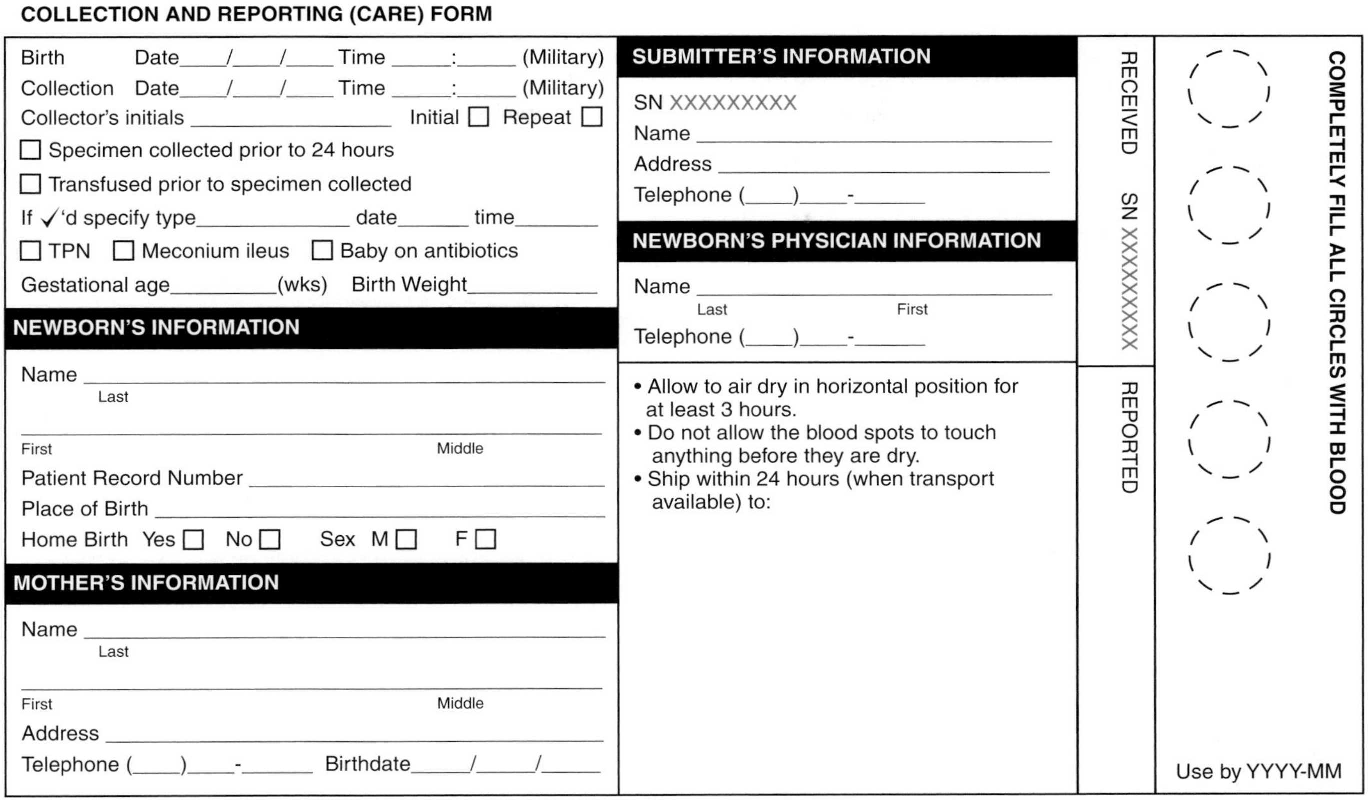

COLLECTION AND REPORTING (CARE) FORM

Birth Date____/____/____ Time _____:_____ (Military)
Collection Date____/____/____ Time _____:_____ (Military)
Collector's initials _____ Initial ☐ Repeat ☐
☐ Specimen collected prior to 24 hours
☐ Transfused prior to specimen collected
If ✓'d specify type_____ date_____ time_____
☐ TPN ☐ Meconium ileus ☐ Baby on antibiotics
Gestational age_____(wks) Birth Weight_____

NEWBORN'S INFORMATION

Name _____
      Last

_____
First   Middle
Patient Record Number _____
Place of Birth _____
Home Birth Yes ☐ No ☐ Sex M ☐ F ☐

MOTHER'S INFORMATION

Name _____
      Last

_____
First   Middle
Address _____
Telephone (____)____-_____ Birthdate____/____/____

SUBMITTER'S INFORMATION

SN XXXXXXXXX
Name _____
Address _____
Telephone (____)____-_____

NEWBORN'S PHYSICIAN INFORMATION

Name _____
      Last   First
Telephone (____)____-_____

• Allow to air dry in horizontal position for at least 3 hours.
• Do not allow the blood spots to touch anything before they are dry.
• Ship within 24 hours (when transport available) to:

RECEIVED   SN XXXXXXXX   REPORTED

COMPLETELY FILL ALL CIRCLES WITH BLOOD

Use by YYYY-MM

FIGURE 1.17 Blank neonatal screening card

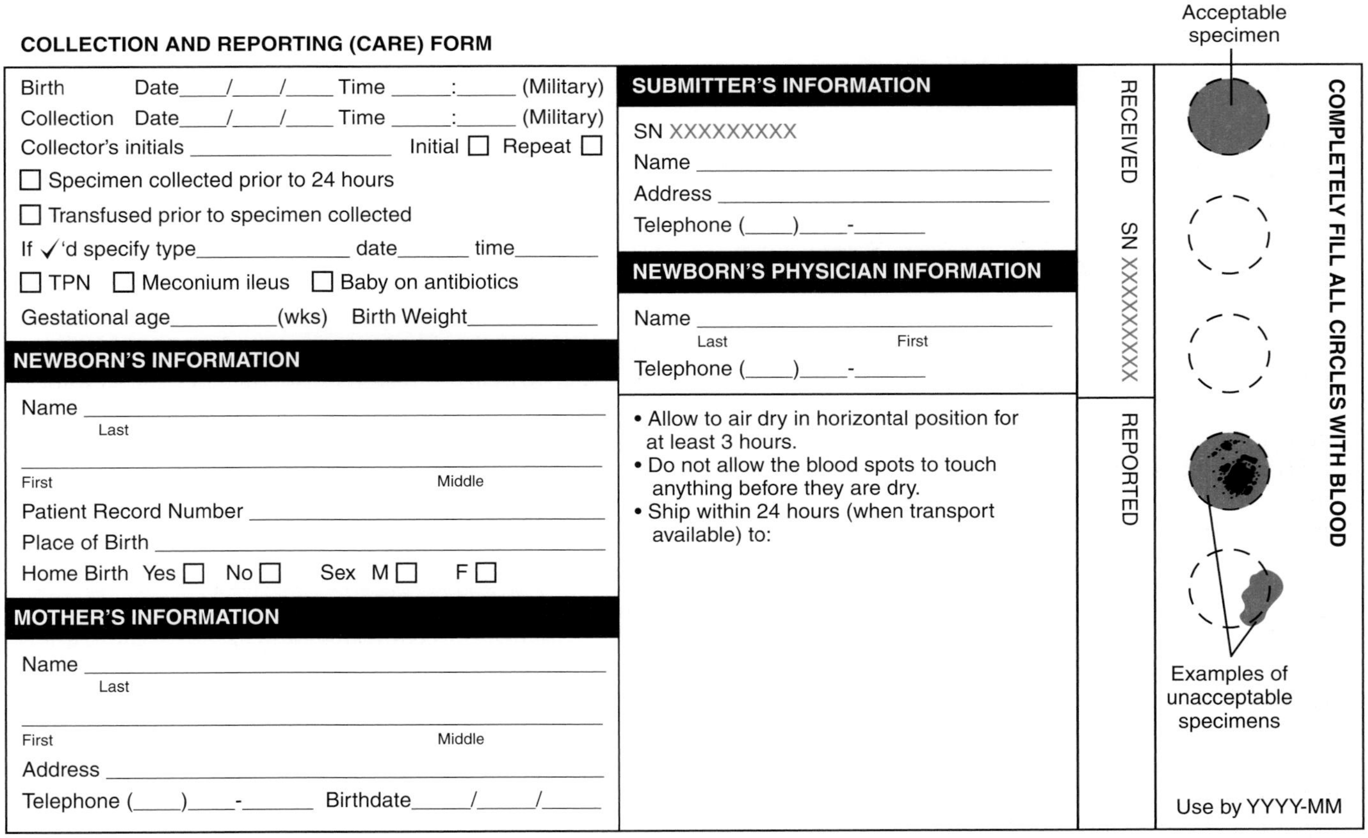

COLLECTION AND REPORTING (CARE) FORM

Birth Date____/____/____ Time _____:_____ (Military)
Collection Date____/____/____ Time _____:_____ (Military)
Collector's initials _____ Initial ☐ Repeat ☐
☐ Specimen collected prior to 24 hours
☐ Transfused prior to specimen collected
If ✓'d specify type_____ date_____ time_____
☐ TPN ☐ Meconium ileus ☐ Baby on antibiotics
Gestational age_____(wks) Birth Weight_____

NEWBORN'S INFORMATION

Name _____
      Last

_____
First   Middle
Patient Record Number _____
Place of Birth _____
Home Birth Yes ☐ No ☐ Sex M ☐ F ☐

MOTHER'S INFORMATION

Name _____
      Last

_____
First   Middle
Address _____
Telephone (____)____-_____ Birthdate____/____/____

SUBMITTER'S INFORMATION

SN XXXXXXXXX
Name _____
Address _____
Telephone (____)____-_____

NEWBORN'S PHYSICIAN INFORMATION

Name _____
      Last   First
Telephone (____)____-_____

• Allow to air dry in horizontal position for at least 3 hours.
• Do not allow the blood spots to touch anything before they are dry.
• Ship within 24 hours (when transport available) to:

RECEIVED   SN XXXXXXXX   REPORTED

COMPLETELY FILL ALL CIRCLES WITH BLOOD

Acceptable specimen

Examples of unacceptable specimens

Use by YYYY-MM

FIGURE 1.18 Completed neonatal screening card with acceptable and unacceptable specimens

DISCUSSION POINT

Education regarding newborn screening should begin during the prenatal period and should be reinforced at the time of preadmission testing. Many birthing facilities and hospitals provide educational brochures to the parents. Physicians and physician delegates are responsible to inform parents of the newborn screening process before discharge. Inform the patient that these procedures can assist in evaluating a number of congenital conditions, including hearing loss, thyroid function, adrenal gland function, and other metabolic enzyme disorders. Evaluation may also include HIV antibody testing if not performed prenatally or if otherwise clinically indicated.

SPECIAL CONSIDERATIONS

An important aspect of planning is understanding the factors that may alter the study findings or cause abnormal results. Interdepartmental communication is a key factor in the planning process. The following should be noted when planning for this study:

- Specimens for newborn screening collected earlier than 24 hours after the first feeding or collected from neonates receiving total parenteral nutrition may produce invalid results.
- Specimens for newborn screening that are improperly applied to the filter paper circles may produce invalid results.
- Touching blood spots on the filter paper card after collection may contaminate the sample and produce invalid results.
- Failure to let the filter paper sample dry may affect test results.
- Specimens for newborn screening collected after transfusion may produce invalid results.
- Nonreactive HIV test results occur during the acute stage of the disease, when the virus is present but antibodies have not sufficiently developed to be detected. Explain that it may take up to 6 months for the test to become positive. During this stage, the test for HIV antigen may not confirm an HIV infection.

Implementation

Patient education is key to obtaining the patient's cooperation in following directions, and providing an explanation for the purpose of the procedure is an important part of this process. Inform the patient that this study can assist in identifying conditions that are not apparent at birth and that may be treatable with early intervention. Perform the venipuncture.

HEARING TEST

First perform an otoscopy examination to ensure that the external ear canal is free from any obstruction (see the study titled "Otoscopy"). Also test for closure of the canal from the pressure of the earphones by compressing the tragus. There is a tendency for the canal to close in children. This can be corrected by the careful insertion of a small, stiff plastic tube into the anterior canal. The test starts by providing a trial tone of 15 to 20 dB above the expected threshold to the ear for 1 to 2 seconds to familiarize the patient with the sounds. If no response is indicated, the level is increased until a response is obtained, and then it is raised in 10-dB increments or until the audiometer's limit is reached for the test frequency. The test results are plotted on a graph called an audiogram using symbols that indicate the ear tested and responses using earphones (air conduction) or oscillator (bone conduction).

In the air conduction test, the tone is delivered to an infant through insert earphones or ear muffins, and the auditory response is measured through electrodes placed on the infant's scalp. Air conduction is tested first by starting at 1,000 Hz and gradually decreasing the intensity 10 dB at a time until there is no response, indicating that the tone is no longer heard. The intensity is then increased 5 dB at a time until the tone is heard again. This is repeated until the same response is achieved at a 50% response rate at the same hertz level. The threshold is derived from the lowest decibel level at which the patient correctly responds to three out of six trials to a tone at that hertz level. The test is continued for each ear with tones delivered at 1,000 Hz, 2,000 Hz, 4,000 Hz, and 8,000 Hz, and then again at 1,000 Hz, 500 Hz, and 250 Hz to determine a second threshold. Results are recorded on an audiogram. Averaging the air conduction thresholds at the 500-Hz, 1,000-Hz, and 2,000-Hz levels reveals the degree of hearing loss and is called the pure tone average (PTA). Bone conduction testing is performed in a similar manner to air conduction testing; a vibrator placed on the skull is used to deliver tones to an infant instead of earphones as in the air conduction test. The raised and lowered tones are delivered as in air conduction using 250 Hz, 500 Hz, 1,000 Hz, 2,000 Hz, and 4,000 Hz to determine the thresholds. An analysis of thresholds for air and bone conduction tones is done to determine the type of hearing loss (conductive, sensorineural, or mixed).

In otoacoustic testing, microphones are placed in the infant's ears. Nearby sounds should echo in the ear canal and be detected by the microphones if the infant's hearing is normal.

FILTER PAPER TEST

Obtain a kit and cleanse the heel with antiseptic. Observe standard precautions, and follow the general guidelines in Appendix A. Use gauze to dry the stick area completely. Perform the heel stick, gently squeezing the infant's heel and touching the filter paper to the puncture site. When collecting samples for newborn screening, it is important to apply each blood drop to the correct side of the filter paper card and fill each circle with a single application of blood. Overfilling or underfilling the circles will cause the specimen card to be rejected by the testing facility. Additional information is required on newborn screening cards and may vary by state. Newborn screening cards should be allowed to air dry for several hours on a level, nonabsorbent, unenclosed area. If multiple patients are tested, do not stack cards. State regulations usually require the specimen cards to be submitted within 24 hours of collection. Observe/assess the puncture site for bleeding or hematoma formation, and secure the gauze with adhesive bandage.

Evaluation

Recognize anxiety related to test results, and answer any questions or address any concerns voiced by the patient or family. Be supportive of the parents' or caregivers' perceived loss of impaired activity or independence related to hearing loss or physical limitations, as well as their fear of a shortened life expectancy for the newborn. Inform the parents or caregivers that positive neonatal HIV findings must be reported to local health department officials. Discuss the implications of abnormal test results on the patient's lifestyle. Provide teaching and information regarding the clinical implications of the test results, as appropriate. Provide information regarding vaccine-preventable diseases where indicated. Provide contact information, if desired, for the Centers for Disease Control and Prevention (www.cdc.gov/vaccines/vpd-vac). Educate the parents or caregivers regarding access to genetic or other counseling services. Provide contact information, if desired, for the March of Dimes (www.marchofdimes.com), the National Library or Medicine (www.nlm.nih.gov/medlineplus/newbornscreening.html), general information (newbornscreening.info/Parents/facts.html), or the state department of health newborn screening program. There are numerous support groups and informational Web sites for specific conditions, including the National Center for Hearing Assessment and Management (www.infanthearing.org), the American Speech-Language-Hearing Association (www.asha.org), ABLEDATA (for assistive technology; sponsored by the National Institute on Disability and Rehabilitation Research [www.abledata.com]), the Sickle Cell Disease Association of America (www.sicklecelldisease.org), the Fatty Oxidation Disorders (FOD) Family Support Group (www.fodsupport.org), the Organic Acidemia Association (www.oaanews.org), the United Mitochondrial Disease Foundation (www.umdf.org), the Cystic Fibrosis Foundation (www.cff.org), and, for AIDS information, the National Institutes of Health (www.aidsinfo.nih.gov) and the CDC (www.cdc.gov).

SOCIAL AND CULTURAL CONSIDERATIONS: Offer support, as appropriate, to parents who may be the victims of rape or sexual assault. Educate the parents regarding access to counseling services. Provide a nonjudgmental, nonthreatening atmosphere for a discussion during which risks of sexually transmitted diseases to the newborn are explained. It is also important to discuss problems the parents may experience (e.g., guilt, depression, anger).

NUTRITIONAL CONSIDERATIONS: Instruct the parents or caregiver in special dietary modifications to treat deficiency, and refer parents or caregivers to a qualified nutritionist, as appropriate. Amino acids are classified as essential (i.e., must be present simultaneously in sufficient quantities), conditionally or acquired essential (i.e., under certain stressful conditions, they become essential), and nonessential (i.e., can be produced by the body, when needed, if the diet does not provide them). Essential amino acids include lysine, threonine, histidine, isoleucine, methionine, phenylalanine, tryptophan, and valine. Conditionally essential amino acids include cysteine, tyrosine, arginine, citrulline, taurine, and carnitine. Nonessential amino acids include alanine, glutamic acid, aspartic acid, glycine, serine, proline, glutamine, and asparagine. A high intake of specific amino acids can cause other amino acids to become essential.

✅ Critical Findings

N/A

✅ Study Specific Complications

There are a number of complications associated with performing a venipuncture. **Pain** is commonly associated with needles, and although the pain experienced during venipuncture is usually mild, on a rare occasion the needle may strike a nerve causing permanent pain. Prolonged **bleeding** is a complication that occurs with patients who are taking blood thinners or who have coagulopathies such as hemophilia. A **hematoma** results when blood leaks into the tissue during or after a venipuncture, as evidenced by pain, bruising, and/or swelling at the venipuncture site. The swelling can cause injury by compression to surrounding nerves, which can be temporary or permanent. HCPs should watch for minor complications such as bruising and hematoma at the venipuncture site, which are fairly common. Hematomas occur more often in those with veins that are difficult to access. Bleeding or bruising can be prevented once the needle has been removed by applying direct pressure to the site with dry gauze for a minute or two. Some other more unusual complications of venipuncture include **cellulitis, phlebitis, inadvertent arterial puncture,** and **sepsis.** Sepsis can be caused by introduction of bacteria from the surface of the skin into the blood as the result of improper cleansing of the venipuncture site. Immunocompromised patients are at higher risk for developing this complication.

Related Tests

- Related tests include amino acid screen, amniotic fluid analysis, audiometry hearing loss, biopsy chorionic villus, chloride sweat, chromosome analysis, CBC, evoked brain potential studies for hearing loss, glucose-6-phosphate dehydrogenase, hemoglobin electrophoresis, human immunodeficiency virus type 1 and type 2 antibodies, otoscopy, sickle cell screen, TSH, thyroxine total, and US thyroid.
- Refer to the Auditory, Endocrine, Genitourinary, Hematopoietic, Hepatobiliary, and Reproductive systems tables at the end of the book for related tests by body system.

Expected Outcomes

Expected outcomes associated with Newborn Screening are:

- Expressing appropriate concerns about the infant's birth disability
- Agreeing to attend a support group to better understand how to care for a disabled child
- Accepting the support of a spiritual leader to better cope with the infant's disability

Parathyroid Hormone

Quick Summary

SYNONYM ACRONYM: Parathormone, PTH, intact PTH, whole molecule PTH.

COMMON USE: To assist in the diagnosis of parathyroid disease and disorders of calcium balance. Also used to monitor patients receiving renal dialysis.

SPECIMEN: Serum collected in a gold-, red-, or red/gray-top tube. Specimen should be transported tightly capped and in an ice slurry.

NORMAL FINDINGS: (Method: Immunoassay)

Age	Conventional Units	SI Units (Conventional Units × 1)
Cord blood	Less than 3 pg/mL	Less than 3 ng/L
2–20 yr	9–52 pg/mL	9–52 ng/L
Adult	10–65 pg/mL	10–65 ng/L

Test Explanation

Parathyroid hormone (PTH) is secreted by the parathyroid glands in response to decreased levels of circulating calcium. PTH assists in raising serum calcium levels by:

- Stimulating the release of calcium from bone into the bloodstream

- Promoting renal tubular reabsorption of calcium and decreased reabsorption of phosphate
- Enhancing renal production of active vitamin D metabolites which increases calcium absorption in the small intestine (see Fig. 1.19). C-terminal and N-terminal assays were used prior to the development of reliable intact or whole molecule PTH assays. A rapid PTH assay has been developed specifically for intraoperative monitoring of PTH in the surgical treatment of primary hyperparathyroidism. Rapid PTH assays have proved valuable because the decision of whether the hyperparathyroidism involves one or multiple glands depends on measurement of circulating PTH levels. Surgical outcomes indicate that a 50% decrease or more in intraoperative PTH from baseline measurements can predict successful treatment with up to 97% accuracy. An intraoperative decrease of less than 50% indicates the need to identify and remove additional malfunctioning parathyroid tissue. In healthy individuals, intact PTH has a circulating half-life of about 5 min. N-terminal PTH has a circulating half-life of about 2 min and is found in very small quantities. Intact and N-terminal PTH are the only biologically active forms of the hormone. Ninety percent of circulating PTH is composed of inactive C-terminal and midregion fragments. PTH is cleared from the body by the kidneys.

Nursing Implications

Assessment

Indications	Potential Nursing Problems
Assist in the diagnosis of hyperparathyroidism Assist in the diagnosis of suspected secondary hyperparathyroidism due to chronic renal failure, malignant tumors that produce ectopic PTH, and malabsorption syndromes Detect incidental damage or inadvertent removal of the parathyroid glands during thyroid or neck surgery Differentiate parathyroid and nonparathyroid causes of hypercalcemia Evaluate autoimmune destruction of the parathyroid glands Evaluate parathyroid response to altered serum calcium levels, especially those that result from malignant processes, leading to decreased PTH production Evaluate source of altered calcium metabolism	• Airway Clearance • Body Image • Human Response • Injury Risk • Mobility • Nutrition • Pain • Renal • Sensory Perception • Urination

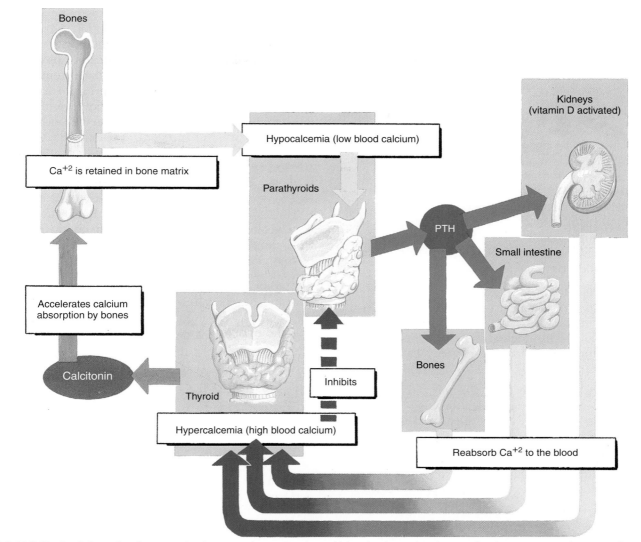

FIGURE 1.19 Role of PTH and calcitonin in maintenance of blood calcium levels. *Used with permission, from Scanlon, V., & Sanders, T. (2010). Essentials of anatomy and physiology (6th Ed.). FA Davis Company.*

Diagnosis: Clinical Significance of Test Results
INCREASED IN

- Fluorosis *(skeletal fluorosis can cause a condition resembling secondary hyperparathyroidism, disruption in calcium homeostasis, and excessive PTH production)*
- Hyperparathyroidism: primary, secondary, or tertiary *(all result in excess PTH production)*
- Hypocalcemia *(compensatory response to low calcium levels)*
- Pseudogout *(calcium is lost due to deposits in the joint; decrease in calcium stimulates PTH production)*
- Pseudohypoparathyroidism *(related to a congenital defect of the kidney that prevents a normal response to PTH in the presence of low calcium levels; signaling the parathyroid glands to secrete additional PTH)*

- Zollinger-Ellison syndrome *(related to poor intestinal absorption of calcium and vitamin D; decreased calcium stimulates PTH production)*

DECREASED IN

- Autoimmune destruction of the parathyroids *(related to decreased parathyroid function)*
- DiGeorge's syndrome *(related to hypoparathyroidism)*
- Hypercalcemia for any reason (e.g., tumors of the bone, breast, lung, kidney, pancreas, ovary) *(compensatory response to high calcium levels)*
- Hyperthyroidism *(related to increased calcium from bone loss; increased calcium levels inhibit PTH production)*
- Hypomagnesemia *(magnesium is a calcium channel blocker; low magnesium levels allow for increased calcium, which inhibits PTH production)*

- Nonparathyroid hypercalcemia (in the absence of renal failure) *(increased calcium levels inhibit PTH production)*
- Sarcoidosis *(related to increased calcium levels)*
- Secondary hypoparathyroidism due to surgery

Planning

Considerations for planning a successful partnership should include clear communication of what to expect during the test to decrease anxiety and improve co-operation. Before the procedure is performed, plan to review the steps with the patient. Inform the patient undergoing parathyroidectomy that multiple specimens may be collected intraoperatively. Address concerns about pain, and explain that there may be some discomfort during the routine venipuncture; there will be no discomfort experienced during intraoperative specimen collection.

SPECIAL CONSIDERATIONS

An important aspect of planning is understanding the factors that may alter the study findings or cause abnormal results. Interdepartmental communication is a key factor in the planning process. The following should be noted when planning for this study:

- PTH levels are subject to diurnal variation, with highest levels occurring in the morning.
- PTH levels should always be measured in conjunction with calcium for proper interpretation.

It is also important to understand which medications or substances the patient may be exposed to in the health-care setting that can interfere with accurate testing:

- Drugs that may increase PTH levels include anticonvulsants, clodronate, estrogen/progestin therapy, foscarnet, furosemide, hydrocortisone, isoniazid, lithium, nifedipine, octreotide, pamidronate, phosphates, prednisone, rifampin, steroids, tamoxifen, and verapamil.
- Drugs and vitamins that may decrease PTH levels include alfacalcidol, aluminum hydroxide, calcitriol, cimetidine, diltiazem, magnesium sulfate, parathyroid hormone, pindolol, prednisone, propranolol, and vitamin D.

Implementation

Patient education is key to obtaining the patient's cooperation in following directions, and providing an explanation for the purpose of the procedure is an important part of this process. Inform the patient that this study can assist in diagnosing parathyroid disease. Perform the venipuncture.

SPECIAL CONSIDERATIONS

In most patients with primary hyperparathyroidism, it is usually a single gland that is abnormal, rather than multiple of the four glands present. Removal of abnormal glands, combined with intraoperative PTH monitoring, has become the surgical treatment of choice.

Inform the surgical patient that a baseline PTH level will be collected prior to resection of the abnormal parathyroid glands. Explain that additional specimens will be collected during the procedure to indicate that all abnormal parathyroid tissue has been removed and the procedure can be concluded. The protocol may vary among health-care providers (HCPs) regarding when the baseline level should be drawn (i.e., prior to anesthesia or prior to incision). The amount of change between the baseline and the intraoperative values considered adequate for determining successful, complete resection of the abnormal tissue may also vary by HCP; a decrease of 50% is typically used as a cutoff.

The sample should be placed in an ice slurry immediately after collection. Information on the specimen label should be protected from water in the ice slurry by first placing the specimen in a protective plastic bag.

Evaluation

Recognize anxiety related to test results, and instruct the patient to report signs and symptoms of hypocalcemia and hypercalcemia to the HCP.

NUTRITIONAL CONSIDERATIONS: Patients with abnormal parathyroid levels are also likely to experience the effects of calcium-level imbalances.

✅ Critical Findings

N/A

✅ Study Specific Complications

There are a number of complications associated with performing a venipuncture. **Pain** is commonly associated with needles, and although the pain experienced during venipuncture is usually mild, on a rare occasion the needle may strike a nerve causing permanent pain. Some patients experience a **vasovagal reaction** during the venipuncture procedure, evidenced by sweating, low blood pressure, fainting, or near fainting. The potential for a **fall injury** is a significant concern related to vasovagal reactions. Prolonged **bleeding** is a complication that occurs with patients who are taking blood thinners or who have coagulopathies such as hemophilia. A **hematoma** results when blood leaks into the tissue during or after a venipuncture, as evidenced by pain, bruising, and/or swelling at the venipuncture site. The swelling can cause injury by compression to surrounding nerves, which can be temporary or permanent. HCPs should watch for minor complications such as bruising and hematoma at the venipuncture site, which are fairly common. Hematomas occur more often in older adult or frail patients, or those with veins that are difficult to access. Bleeding or bruising can be prevented once the needle has been removed by applying direct pressure to the site with dry gauze for a minute or two. Some other more unusual complications of venipuncture include **cellulitis, phlebitis, inadvertent**

arterial puncture, and **sepsis.** Sepsis can be caused by introduction of bacteria from the surface of the skin into the blood as the result of improper cleansing of the venipuncture site. Immunocompromised patients are at higher risk for developing this complication.

⊘ *Related Tests*

- Related tests include ALP, arthroscopy, calcitonin, calcium, collagen cross-linked telopeptides, evoked brain potentials, fecal fat, gastric emptying scan, gastric acid stimulation, gastrin stimulation test, parathyroid scan, phosphorus, RAIU, synovial fluid analysis, TSH, thyroxine, US thyroid and parathyroid, uric acid, UA, and vitamin D.
- Refer to the Endocrine System table at the end of the book for related tests by body system.

Expected Outcomes

Expected outcomes associated with Parathyroid Hormone (PTH) are:
- Managing oral secretions and maintaining an open airway
- Maintaining body equilibrium without injury
- Identifying coping strategies for emotional support associated with potential surgery

Potassium, Blood

Quick Summary

SYNONYM ACRONYM: Serum K+.

COMMON USE: To evaluate fluid and electrolyte balance related to potassium levels toward diagnosing disorders such as acidosis, renal failure, and dehydration, and to monitor the effectiveness of therapeutic interventions.

SPECIMEN: Serum collected in a gold-, red-, or red/gray-top tube. Plasma collected in green-top (heparin) tube is also acceptable.

NORMAL FINDINGS: (Method: Ion-selective electrode)

Serum	Conventional & SI Units
Birth–7 days	3.2–5.5 mEq/L or mmol/L
8 days–1 mo	3.4–6 mEq/L or mmol/L
1–5 mo	3.5–5.6 mEq/L or mmol/L
6 mo–1 yr	3.5–6.1 mEq/L or mmol/L
2–19 yr	3.8–5.1 mEq/L or mmol/L
Adult–older adult	3.5–5.3 mEq/L or mmol/L

Note: Serum values are 0.1 mmol/L higher than plasma values, and reference ranges should be adjusted accordingly. It is important that serial measurements be collected using the same type of collection container to reduce variability of results from collection to collection.

Older adults are at risk for hyperkalemia due to the decline in aldosterone levels, decline in renal function, and effects of commonly prescribed medications that inhibit the renin-angiotensin-aldosterone system.

Test Explanation

Electrolytes dissociate into electrically charged ions when dissolved. Cations, including potassium, carry a positive charge. Body fluids contain approximately equal numbers of anions and cations, although the nature of the ions and their mobility differs between the intracellular and extracellular compartments. Both types of ions affect the electrical and osmolar functions of the body. Electrolyte quantities and the balance among them are controlled by oxygen and carbon dioxide exchange in the lungs; absorption, secretion, and excretion of many substances by the kidneys; and secretion of regulatory hormones by the endocrine glands. Potassium is the most abundant intracellular cation with a number of essential functions to include transmission of electrical impulses in cardiac and skeletal muscle and participation in enzyme reactions that transform glucose into energy and amino acids into proteins. Potassium also helps maintain acid-base equilibrium, and it has a significant and inverse relationship to pH: A decrease in pH of 0.1 increases the potassium level by 0.6 mmol/L.

Abnormal potassium levels can be caused by a number of contributing factors, which can be categorized as follows:

- *Altered renal excretion:* Normally, 80% to 90% of the body's potassium is filtered out through the kidneys each day (the remainder is excreted in sweat and stool); renal disease can result in abnormally high potassium levels.
- *Altered dietary intake:* A severe potassium deficiency can be caused by an inadequate intake of dietary potassium.
- *Altered cellular metabolism:* Damaged red blood cells (RBCs) release potassium into the circulating fluid, resulting in increased potassium levels.

Nursing Implications

Assessment

Indications	Potential Nursing Problems
Assess a known or suspected disorder associated with renal disease, glucose metabolism, trauma, or burns	• Activity
	• Cardiac Output
	• Electrolytes
Assist in the evaluation of electrolyte imbalances; this test is especially indicated in older adult patients, patients receiving hyperalimentation supplements, patients on hemodialysis, and patients with hypertension	• Fluid Volume
	• Health Management
	• Human Response
	• Injury Risk

Continued

Table Continued

Indications	Potential Nursing Problems
Evaluate cardiac dysrhythmia to determine whether altered potassium levels are contributing to the problem, especially during digitalis therapy, which leads to ventricular irritability Evaluate the effects of drug therapy, especially diuretics Evaluate the response to treatment for abnormal potassium levels Monitor known or suspected acidosis, because potassium moves from RBCs into the extracellular fluid in acidotic states Routine screen of electrolytes in acute and chronic illness	• Renal • Urination

Diagnosis: Clinical Significance of Test Results
INCREASED IN

- Acidosis *(intracellular potassium ions are expelled in exchange for hydrogen ions in order to achieve electrical neutrality)*
- Acute kidney injury *(potassium excretion is diminished, and it accumulates in the blood)*
- Addison disease *(due to lack of aldosterone, potassium excretion is diminished, and it accumulates in the blood)*
- Asthma *(related to chronic inflammation and damage to lung tissue)*
- Burns *(related to tissue damage and release by damaged cells)*
- Chronic interstitial nephritis *(potassium excretion is diminished, and it accumulates in the blood)*
- Dehydration *(related to hemoconcentration)*
- Dialysis *(dialysis treatments simulate kidney function, but potassium builds up between treatments)*
- Diet *(related to excessive intake of salt substitutes or of potassium salts in medications)*
- Exercise *(related to tissue damage and release by damaged cells)*
- Hemolysis (massive) *(potassium is the major intracellular cation)*
- Hyperventilation *(in response to respiratory alkalosis, blood levels of potassium are increased in order to achieve electrical neutrality)*
- Hypoaldosteronism *(due to lack of aldosterone, potassium excretion is diminished, and it accumulates in the blood)*
- Insulin deficiency *(insulin deficiency results in movement of potassium from the cell into the extracellular fluid)*

- Ketoacidosis *(insulin deficiency results in movement of potassium from the cell into the extracellular fluid)*
- Leukocytosis
- Muscle necrosis *(related to tissue damage and release by damaged cells)*
- Near drowning
- Pregnancy
- Prolonged periods of standing
- Tissue trauma *(related to release by damaged cells)*
- Transfusion of old banked blood *(aged cells hemolyze and release intracellular potassium)*
- Tubular unresponsiveness to aldosterone
- Uremia

DECREASED IN

- Alcoholism *(related to insufficient dietary intake)*
- Alkalosis *(potassium uptake by cells is increased in response to release of hydrogen ions from cells)*
- Anorexia nervosa *(related to significant changes in renal function that result in hypokalemia)*
- Bradycardia *(hypokalemia can cause bradycardia)*
- Chronic, excessive licorice ingestion (from licorice root) *(Licorice inhibits short-chain dehydrogenase/reductase enzymes. These enzymes normally prevent cortisol from binding to aldosterone receptor sites in the kidney. In the absence of these enzymes, cortisol acts on the kidney and triggers the same effects as aldosterone, which include increased potassium excretion, sodium retention, and water retention.)*
- Crohn disease *(insufficient intestinal absorption)*
- Cushing syndrome *(aldosterone facilitates the excretion of potassium by the kidneys)*
- Diet deficient in meat and vegetables *(insufficient dietary intake)*
- Excess insulin *(insulin causes glucose and potassium to move into cells)*
- Familial periodic paralysis *(related to fluid retention)*
- Gastrointestinal (GI) loss due to vomiting, diarrhea, nasogastric suction, or intestinal fistula
- Heart failure *(related to fluid retention and hemodilution)*
- Hyperaldosteronism *(aldosterone facilitates the excretion of potassium by the kidneys)*
- Hypertension *(medications used to treat hypertension may result in loss of potassium; hypertension is often related to diabetes and renal disease, which affect cellular retention and renal excretion of potassium, respectively)*
- Hypomagnesemia *(magnesium levels tend to parallel potassium levels)*
- IV therapy with inadequate potassium supplementation
- Laxative abuse *(related to medications that cause potassium wasting)*
- Malabsorption *(related to insufficient intestinal absorption)*

- Pica (eating substances of no nutritional value, e.g., clay)
- Renal tubular acidosis *(condition results in excessive loss of potassium)*
- Sweating *(related to increased loss)*
- Theophylline administration, excessive *(theophylline drives potassium into cells, reducing circulating levels)*
- Thyrotoxicosis *(related to changes in renal function)*

Planning

Considerations for planning a successful partnership should include clear communication of what to expect during the test to decrease anxiety and improve cooperation. Especially note complaints of weakness and confusion. Before the procedure is performed, plan to review the steps with the patient. Address concerns about pain, and explain that there may be some discomfort during the venipuncture.

SPECIAL CONSIDERATIONS

An important aspect of planning is understanding the factors that may alter the study findings or cause abnormal results. Interdepartmental communication is a key factor in the planning process. The following should be noted when planning for this study:

- Leukocytosis, as seen in leukemia, causes elevated potassium levels.
- False elevations can occur with vigorous pumping of the hand during venipuncture.
- Hemolysis of the sample and high platelet counts also increase potassium levels, as follows: (1) Because potassium is an intracellular ion and concentrations are approximately 150 times extracellular concentrations, even a slight amount of hemolysis can cause a significant increase in levels. (2) Platelets release potassium during the clotting process, and therefore serum samples collected from patients with elevated platelet counts may produce spuriously high potassium levels. Plasma is the specimen of choice in patients known to have elevated platelet counts.
- False increases are seen in unprocessed samples left at room temperature because a significant amount of potassium leaks out of the cells within a few hours; plasma or serum should be separated from cells within 4 hours of collection.
- Specimens should never be collected above an IV line because of the potential for dilution when the specimen and the IV solution combine in the collection container, falsely decreasing the result. There is also the potential of contaminating the sample with the substance of interest, if it is present in the IV solution, falsely increasing the result.

It is also important to understand which medications or substances the patient may be exposed to in the health-care setting that can interfere with accurate testing:

- Drugs that can cause an increase in potassium levels include ACE inhibitors, atenolol, basiliximab, captopril, clofibrate in association with renal disease, cyclosporine, dexamethasone, enalapril, etretinate, lisinopril in association with heart failure or hypertension, NSAIDs, some drugs with potassium salts (e.g., antibiotics such as penicillin), spironolactone, succinylcholine, and tacrolimus.
- Drugs that can cause a decrease in potassium levels include acetazolamide, acetylsalicylic acid, aldosterone, ammonium chloride, amphotericin B, bendroflumethiazide, benzthiazide, bicarbonate, captopril, cathartics, chlorothiazide, chlorthalidone, cisplatin, clorexolone, corticosteroids, cyclothiazide, dichlorphenamide, digoxin, diuretics, enalapril, foscarnet, fosphenytoin, furosemide, insulin, laxatives, metolazone, moxalactam (common when coadministered with amikacin), large doses of any IV penicillin, phenolphthalein (with chronic laxative abuse), polythiazide, quinethazone, sodium bicarbonate, tacrolimus, IV theophylline, thiazides, triamterene, and trichlormethiazide. A number of these medications initially increase the serum potassium level, but they also have a diuretic effect, which promotes potassium loss in the urine except in cases of renal insufficiency.

Implementation

Patient education is key to obtaining the patient's cooperation in following directions, and providing an explanation for the purpose of the procedure is an important part of this process. Inform the patient that this study can assist in evaluating electrolyte balance. Instruct the patient not to clench and unclench the fist immediately before or during specimen collection. Perform the venipuncture.

Evaluation

Recognize anxiety related to test results, and monitor potassium levels carefully because cardiac dysrhythmias can occur. Observe the patient for signs and symptoms of hyperkalemia. Increased potassium levels may be associated with dehydration, a significant and common finding in older adult patients and other patients in whom renal function has deteriorated. Assess the patient for fluid volume excess related to excess potassium intake. The patient should also be observed for fluid volume deficit reflected by decreased potassium levels, which may occur in patients receiving digoxin or potassium-wasting diuretics. Instruct the patient in electrolyte replacement therapy and changes in dietary intake that affect electrolyte levels as ordered. Educate the patient regarding access to nutritional counseling services. Provide contact information, if desired, for the Institute of Medicine of the National Academies (www.iom.edu) and the U.S. Department of Agriculture (www.choosemyplate.com).

NUTRITIONAL CONSIDERATIONS: Potassium is present in all plant and animal cells, making dietary replacement simple to achieve in the potassium-deficient patient. Fruits, vegetables, and meats are rich in potassium (artichokes, avocados, bananas, cantaloupe, dried fruits, kiwi, mango, meats, milk, dried beans, nuts, oranges, peaches, pears, pomegranate, potatoes, prunes, pumpkin, spinach, sunflower seeds, swiss chard, tomatoes, and winter squash).

✔ *Critical Findings*

ADULTS & CHILDREN

- Less than 2.5 mEq/L or mmol/L (SI: Less than 2.5 mEq/L or mmol/L)
- Greater than 6.2 mEq/L or mmol/L (SI: Greater than 6.2 mEq/L or mmol/L)

NEWBORNS

- Less than 2.8 mEq/L or mmol/L (SI: Less than 2.8 mmol/L)
- Greater than 6.4 mEq/L or mmol/L (SI: Greater than 6.4 mmol/L)

Consideration may be given to verifying the critical findings before action is taken. Policies vary among facilities and may include requesting immediate recollection and retesting by the laboratory or retesting using a rapid Point of Care instrument at the bedside, if available.

Note and immediately report to the requesting HCP any critical findings and related symptoms. A listing of these findings varies among facilities.

Symptoms of hyperkalemia include irritability, diarrhea, cramps, oliguria, difficulty speaking, and cardiac dysrhythmias (peaked T waves and ventricular fibrillation). Continuous cardiac monitoring is indicated. Administration of sodium bicarbonate or calcium chloride may be requested. If the patient is receiving an IV supplement, verify that the patient is voiding (see Figs. 1.20 and 1.21).

Symptoms of hypokalemia include malaise, thirst, polyuria, anorexia, weak pulse, low blood pressure, vomiting, decreased reflexes, and electrocardiographic changes (depressed T waves and ventricular ectopy). Replacement therapy is indicated.

✔ *Study Specific Complications*

There are a number of complications associated with performing a venipuncture. **Pain** is commonly associated with needles, and although the pain experienced during venipuncture is usually mild, on a rare occasion the needle may strike a nerve causing permanent pain. Some patients experience a **vasovagal reaction** during the venipuncture procedure, evidenced

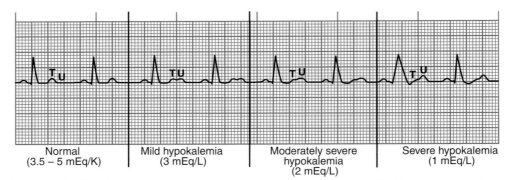

| Normal (3.5 – 5 mEq/K) | Mild hypokalemia (3 mEq/L) | Moderately severe hypokalemia (2 mEq/L) | Severe hypokalemia (1 mEq/L) |

FIGURE 1.20 ECG lead II changes comparing normal potassium to hypokalemia. *Used with permission, from Hale, A., & Hovey, M. (2013). Fluid and electrolyte notes. FA Davis Company.*

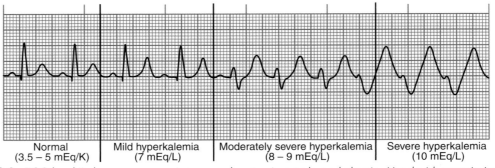

| Normal (3.5 – 5 mEq/K) | Mild hyperkalemia (7 mEq/L) | Moderately severe hyperkalemia (8 – 9 mEq/L) | Severe hyperkalemia (10 mEq/L) |

FIGURE 1.21 ECG lead II changes comparing normal potassium to hyperkalemia. *Used with permission, from Hale, A., & Hovey, M. (2013). Fluid and electrolyte notes. FA Davis Company.*

by sweating, low blood pressure, fainting, or near fainting. The potential for a **fall injury** is a significant concern related to vasovagal reactions. Prolonged **bleeding** is a complication that occurs with patients who are taking blood thinners or who have coagulopathies such as hemophilia. A **hematoma** results when blood leaks into the tissue during or after a venipuncture, as evidenced by pain, bruising, and/or swelling at the venipuncture site. The swelling can cause injury by compression to surrounding nerves, which can be temporary or permanent. HCPs should watch for minor complications such as bruising and hematoma at the venipuncture site, which are fairly common. Hematomas occur more often in older adult or frail patients, or those with veins that are difficult to access. Bleeding or bruising can be prevented once the needle has been removed by applying direct pressure to the site with dry gauze for a minute or two. Some other more unusual complications of venipuncture include **cellulitis, phlebitis, inadvertent arterial puncture,** and **sepsis.** Sepsis can be caused by introduction of bacteria from the surface of the skin into the blood as the result of improper cleansing of the venipuncture site. Immunocompromised patients are at higher risk for developing this complication.

⊙ *Related Tests*

Related tests include ACTH, aldosterone, anion gap, antidysrhythmic drugs, alveolar/arterial gradient, ANP, BNP, blood gases, BUN, calcium, carbon dioxide, chloride, complement, CBC hematocrit, CBC hemoglobin, CBC WBC count and differential, Coomb antiglobulin (direct and indirect), cortisol, CK and isoenzymes, creatinine, DHEAS, echocardiography, echocardiography transesophageal, fecal fat, glucose, G6PD, Ham test, haptoglobin, hemosiderin, insulin, ketones, lactic acid, lung perfusion scan, magnesium, osmolality, osmotic fragility, plethysmography, urine potassium, PFT, PK, renin, sickle cell screen, sodium, and US abdomen.

Refer to the Cardiovascular, Endocrine, Gastrointestinal, Genitourinary, Immune, and Respiratory systems tables at the end of the book for related tests by body system.

Expected Outcomes

Expected outcomes associated with Potassium, Blood are:

* Keeping consistent daily weight as verified by daily weigh-ins
* Having breath sounds that remain clear in the presence of elevated potassium levels that may cause fluid retention
* Maintaining blood pressure within normal limits
* Understanding that altered potassium can place the patient at risk for cardiac injury
* Identifying five favorite potassium-rich foods to include in the diet

Prealbumin

Quick Summary

SYNONYM ACRONYM: Transthyretin.

COMMON USE: To assess nutritional status and evaluate liver function toward diagnosing disorders such as malnutrition and chronic renal failure.

SPECIMEN: Serum collected in a gold-, red-, or red/gray-top tube.

NORMAL FINDINGS: (Method: Nephelometry)

Age	Conventional Units	SI Units (Conventional Units × 10)
Newborn–1 mo	7–39 mg/dL	70–390 mg/L
1–6 mo	8–34 mg/dL	80–340 mg/L
6 mo–4 yr	2–36 mg/dL	20–360 mg/L
5–6 yr	12–30 mg/dL	120–300 mg/L
7 yr–adult/older adult	12–42 mg/dL	120–420 mg/L

Test Explanation

Prealbumin is a protein primarily produced by the liver. It is the major transport protein for triiodothyronine and thyroxine. It is also important in the metabolism of retinol-binding protein, which is needed for transporting vitamin A (retinol). Prealbumin has a short biological half-life of 2 days. It is used as an indicator of protein status and a marker for malnutrition. Prealbumin is often measured simultaneously with transferrin and albumin. The role of prealbumin in nutritional management has come into question by some health-care providers (HCPs) because it is a negative acute phase protein. Prealbumin levels decrease during the acute phase of an inflammatory process such as in burns, infection, neoplasms, strenuous exercise, surgery, tissue infarction, and trauma, making the use of prealbumin less reliable as a predictor of malnutrition in certain clinical situations. Prealbumin may also be measured with C-reactive protein to assess for the coexistence of an inflammatory process and provide a more complete interpretation of the results.

Nursing Implications

Assessment

Indications	Potential Nursing Problems
Evaluate nutritional status	• Body Image
	• Fluid Volume
	• Human Response
	• Infection
	• Nutrition
	• Renal
	• Skin

Diagnosis: Clinical Significance of Test Results

INCREASED IN

- Alcoholism *(related to leakage of prealbumin from damaged hepatocytes and/or poor nutrition)*
- Chronic kidney disease *(related to rapid turnover of prealbumin, which reflects a perceived elevation in the presence of overall loss of other proteins that take longer to produce)*
- Patients receiving steroids *(these drugs stimulate production of prealbumin)*

DECREASED IN

- Acute-phase inflammatory response *(prealbumin is a negative acute-phase reactant protein; levels decrease in the presence of inflammation)*
- Diseases of the liver *(related to decreased ability of the damaged liver to synthesize protein)*
- Hepatic damage *(related to decreased ability of the damaged liver to synthesize protein)*
- Malnutrition *(synthesis is decreased due to lack of proper diet)*
- Tissue necrosis *(prealbumin is a negative acute-phase reactant protein; levels decrease in the presence of inflammation)*

Planning

Considerations for planning a successful partnership should include clear communication of what to expect during the test to decrease anxiety and improve cooperation. Before the procedure is performed, plan to review the steps with the patient. Address concerns about pain, and explain that there may be some discomfort during the venipuncture.

SPECIAL CONSIDERATIONS

An important aspect of planning is understanding the factors that may alter the study findings or cause abnormal results. Interdepartmental communication is a key factor in the planning process. The following should be noted when planning for this study:

- Fasting 8 hours before specimen collection may be required. Protocols may vary among institutions. Reference ranges are often based on fasting populations to provide some level of standardization for comparison.
- The presence of lipids in the blood may also interfere with the test method; fasting eliminates this potential source of error, especially if the patient has elevated lipid levels.

It is also important to understand which medications or substances the patient may be exposed to in the healthcare setting that can interfere with accurate testing:

- Drugs that may increase prealbumin levels include anabolic steroids, anticonvulsants, danazol, oral contraceptives, prednisolone, prednisone, and propranolol.
- Drugs that may decrease prealbumin levels include amiodarone and diethylstilbestrol.

Implementation

Patient education is key to obtaining the patient's cooperation in following directions, and providing an explanation for the purpose of the procedure is an important part of this process. Inform the patient that this study can assist in assessing nutritional status. Ensure that the patient has complied with dietary restrictions and that food has been restricted for at least 8 hours prior to the procedure, if required. Perform the venipuncture.

Evaluation

Recognize anxiety related to test results, and inform the patient that nutritional therapy may be indicated for significantly decreased prealbumin levels.

NUTRITIONAL CONSIDERATIONS: Educate the patient, as appropriate, that good dietary sources of complete protein (containing all eight essential amino acids) include meat, fish, eggs, and dairy products and that good sources of incomplete protein (lacking one or more of the eight essential amino acids) include grains, nuts, legumes, vegetables, and seeds.

✔ Critical Findings

N/A

✔ Specific Complications

There are a number of complications associated with performing a venipuncture. **Pain** is commonly associated with needles, and although the pain experienced during venipuncture is usually mild, on a rare occasion the needle may strike a nerve causing permanent pain. Some patients experience a **vasovagal reaction** during the venipuncture procedure, evidenced by sweating, low blood pressure, fainting, or near fainting. The potential for a **fall injury** is a significant concern related to vasovagal reactions. Prolonged **bleeding** is a complication that occurs with patients who are taking blood thinners or who have coagulopathies such as hemophilia. A **hematoma** results when blood leaks into the tissue during or after a venipuncture, as evidenced by pain, bruising, and/or swelling at the venipuncture site. The swelling can cause injury by compression to surrounding nerves, which can be temporary or permanent. HCPs should watch for minor complications such as bruising and hematoma at the venipuncture site, which are fairly common. Hematomas occur more often in older adult or frail patients, or those with veins that are difficult to access. Bleeding or bruising can be prevented once the needle has been removed by applying direct pressure to the site with dry gauze for a minute or two. Some other more unusual complications of venipuncture include **cellulitis, phlebitis, inadvertent arterial puncture,** and **sepsis.** Sepsis can be caused by introduction of bacteria from the surface of the skin into the blood as the result of improper cleansing of the venipuncture site. Immunocompromised patients are at higher risk for developing this complication.

Related Tests

- Related tests include albumin, chloride, ferritin, iron/TIBC, potassium, protein, sodium, T_4, T_3, transferrin, and vitamin A.
- Refer to the Endocrine, Gastrointestinal, and Hepatobiliary systems tables at the end of the book for related tests by body system.

Expected Outcomes

Expected outcomes associated with Prealbumin are:

- Verbalizing an understanding of body image alterations in relation to disease process
- Verbalizing the importance of reporting symptoms of infection timely to prevent injury
- Maintaining normal renal perfusion evidenced by laboratory values within normal limits
- Understanding the importance of and agreeing to fast as requested prior to specimen collection

Protein, Blood, Total and Fractions

Quick Summary

SYNONYM ACRONYM: TP, SPEP (fractions include albumin, α_1-globulin, α_2-globulin, β-globulin, and γ-globulin).

COMMON USE: To assess nutritional status related to various disease and conditions such as dehydration, burns, and malabsorption.

SPECIMEN: Serum collected in a gold-, red-, or red/gray-top tube.

NORMAL FINDINGS: (Method: Spectrophotometry for total protein, electrophoresis for protein fractions)

Total Protein

Age	Conventional Units	SI Units (Conventional Units × 10)
Newborn–5 days	3.8–6.2 g/dL	38–62 g/L
1–3 yr	5.9–7 g/dL	59–70 g/L
4–6 yr	5.9–7.8 g/dL	59–78 g/L
7–9 yr	6.2–8.1 g/dL	62–81 g/L
10–19 yr	6.3–8.6 g/dL	63–86 g/L
Adult	6–8 g/dL	60–80 g/L

Values may be slightly decreased in older adults due to insufficient intake or the effects of medications and the presence of multiple chronic or acute diseases with or without muted symptoms.

Protein Fractions

	Conventional Units	SI Units (Conventional Units × 10)
Albumin	3.4–4.8 g/dL	34–48 g/L
α_1-Globulin	0.2–0.4 g/dL	2–4 g/L
α_2-Globulin	0.4–0.8 g/dL	4–8 g/L

Protein Fractions

	Conventional Units	SI Units (Conventional Units × 10)
β-Globulin	0.5–1 g/dL	5–10 g/L
γ-Globulin	0.6–1.2 g/dL	6–12 g/L

Values may be slightly decreased in older adults due to insufficient intake or the effects of medications and the presence of multiple chronic or acute diseases with or without muted symptoms.

Test Explanation

Protein is essential to all physiological functions. Proteins consist of amino acids, the building blocks of blood and body tissues. Protein is also required for the regulation of metabolic processes, immunity, and proper water balance. Total protein includes albumin and globulins. Albumin, the protein present in the highest concentrations, is the main transport protein in the body. Albumin also significantly affects plasma oncotic pressure, which regulates the distribution of body fluid between blood vessels, tissues, and cells. α_1-Globulin includes α_1-antitrypsin, α_1-fetoprotein, α_1-acidglycoprotein, α_1-antichymotrypsin, inter-α_1-trypsin inhibitor, high-density lipoproteins, and group-specific component (vitamin D–binding protein). α_2-Globulin includes haptoglobin, ceruloplasmin, and α_2-macroglobulin. β-Globulin includes transferrin, hemopexin, very-low-density lipoproteins, low-density lipoproteins, β_2-microglobulin, fibrinogen, complement, and C-reactive protein. γ-Globulin includes immunoglobulin (Ig) G, IgA, IgM, IgD, and IgE. After an acute infection or trauma, levels of many of the liver-derived proteins increase, whereas albumin level decreases; these conditions may not reflect an abnormal total protein determination (see Fig. 1.22).

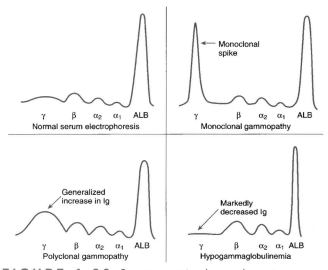

FIGURE 1.22 Serum protein electrophoresis patterns. *Used with permission, from Cavanaugh, B. (2003). Nurse's manual of laboratory and diagnostic tests. FA Davis Company.*

Nursing Implications
Assessment

Indications	Potential Nursing Problems
Evaluation of edema, as seen in patients with low total protein and low albumin levels Evaluation of nutritional status	• Breathing • Body Image • Fatigue • Fluid Volume • Human Response • Infection Risk • Jaundice • Nutrition • Powerlessness • Self-care • Self-image • Skin

Diagnosis: Clinical Significance of Test Results
INCREASED IN

- α_1-Globulin proteins in acute and chronic inflammatory diseases
- α_2-Globulin proteins occasionally in diabetes, pancreatitis, and hemolysis
- β-Globulin proteins in hyperlipoproteinemias and monoclonal gammopathies
- γ-Globulin proteins in chronic liver diseases, chronic infections, autoimmune disorders, hepatitis, cirrhosis, and lymphoproliferative disorders
- Total protein:
  - Dehydration *(related to hemoconcentration)*
  - Monoclonal and polyclonal gammopathies *(related to excessive γ-globulin protein synthesis)*
  - Myeloma *(related to excessive γ-globulin protein synthesis)*
  - Sarcoidosis *(related to excessive γ-globulin protein synthesis)*
  - Some types of chronic liver disease
  - Tropical diseases (e.g., leprosy) *(related to inflammatory reaction)*
  - Waldenström macroglobulinemia *(related to excessive γ-globulin protein synthesis)*

DECREASED IN

- α_1-Globulin proteins in hereditary deficiency
- α_2-Globulin proteins in nephrotic syndrome, malignancies, numerous subacute and chronic inflammatory disorders, and recovery stage of severe burns
- β-Globulin proteins in hypo-β-lipoproteinemias and IgA deficiency
- γ-Globulin proteins in immune deficiency or suppression

- Total protein:
  - Administration of IV fluids *(related to hemodilution)*
  - Burns *(related to fluid retention, loss of albumin from chronic open burns)*
  - Chronic alcoholism *(related to insufficient dietary intake; diminished protein synthesis by damaged liver)*
  - Chronic ulcerative colitis *(related to poor intestinal absorption)*
  - Cirrhosis *(related to damaged liver, which cannot synthesize adequate amount of protein)*
  - Crohn disease *(related to poor intestinal absorption)*
  - Glomerulonephritis *(related to alteration in permeability that results in excessive loss by kidneys)*
  - Heart failure *(related to fluid retention)*
  - Hyperthyroidism *(possibly related to increased metabolism and corresponding protein synthesis)*
  - Malabsorption *(related to insufficient intestinal absorption)*
  - Malnutrition *(related to insufficient intake)*
  - Neoplasms
  - Nephrotic syndrome *(related to alteration in permeability that results in excessive loss by kidneys)*
  - Pregnancy *(related to fluid retention, dietary insufficiency, increased demands of growing fetus)*
  - Prolonged immobilization *(related to fluid retention)*
  - Protein-losing enteropathies *(related to excessive loss)*
  - Severe skin disease
  - Starvation *(related to insufficient intake)*

Planning

Considerations for planning a successful partnership should include clear communication of what to expect during the test to decrease anxiety and improve cooperation. Before the procedure is performed, plan to review the steps with the patient. Address concerns about pain, and explain that there may be some discomfort during the venipuncture.

SPECIAL CONSIDERATIONS

An important aspect of planning is understanding the factors that may alter the study findings or cause abnormal results. Interdepartmental communication is a key factor in the planning process. The following should be noted when planning for this study:

- Recumbent patients have values that are significantly lower (5% to 10%).
- Hemolysis can falsely elevate results.
- Venous stasis can falsely elevate results; the tourniquet should not be left on the arm for longer than 60 seconds.

It is also important to understand which medications or substances the patient may be exposed to in the health-care setting that can interfere with accurate testing:

- Drugs that may increase protein levels include amino acids (if given IV), anabolic steroids, angiotensin, anticonvulsants, corticosteroids, corticotropin, furosemide, insulin, isotretinoin, levonorgestrel, oral contraceptives, progesterone, radiographic agents, and thyroid agents.
- Drugs and substances that may decrease protein levels include acetylsalicylic acid, arginine, benzene, carvedilol, citrates, floxuridine, laxatives, mercury compounds, oral contraceptives, pentastarch, phosgene, pyrazinamide, rifampin, trimethadione, and valproic acid.

Implementation

Patient education is key to obtaining the patient's cooperation in following directions, and providing an explanation for the purpose of the procedure is an important part of this process. Inform the patient that this study can assist in assessing nutritional status related to the disease process. Perform the venipuncture.

Evaluation

Recognize anxiety related to test results, and answer any questions or address any concerns voiced by the patient or family.

NUTRITIONAL CONSIDERATIONS: Educate the patient, as appropriate, that good dietary sources of complete protein (containing all eight essential amino acids) include meat, fish, eggs, and dairy products and that good sources of incomplete protein (lacking one or more of the eight essential amino acids) include grains, nuts, legumes, vegetables, and seeds.

Critical Findings

N/A

Study Specific Complications

There are a number of complications associated with performing a venipuncture. **Pain** is commonly associated with needles, and although the pain experienced during venipuncture is usually mild, on a rare occasion the needle may strike a nerve causing permanent pain. Some patients experience a **vasovagal reaction** during the venipuncture procedure, evidenced by sweating, low blood pressure, fainting, or near fainting. The potential for a **fall injury** is a significant concern related to vasovagal reactions. Prolonged **bleeding** is a complication that occurs with patients who are taking blood thinners or who have coagulopathies such as hemophilia. A **hematoma** results when blood leaks into the tissue during or after a venipuncture, as evidenced by pain, bruising, and/or swelling at the venipuncture site. The swelling can cause injury by compression to surrounding nerves, which can be temporary or permanent. HCPs should watch for minor complications such as bruising and hematoma at the venipuncture site, which are fairly common. Hematomas occur more often in older adult or frail patients, or those with veins that are difficult to access. Bleeding or bruising can be prevented once the needle has been removed by applying direct pressure to the site with dry gauze for a minute or two. Some other more unusual complications of venipuncture include **cellulitis, phlebitis, inadvertent arterial puncture,** and **sepsis.** Sepsis can be caused by introduction of bacteria from the surface of the skin into the blood as the result of improper cleansing of the venipuncture site. Immunocompromised patients are at higher risk for developing this complication.

Related Tests

- Related tests include albumin, ALP, ACE, anion gap, AST, biopsy liver, biopsy lung, calcium, carbon dioxide, chloride, CBC WBC count and differential, cryoglobulin, fecal analysis, fecal fat, gallium scan, GGT, IgA, IgG, IgM, IFE, liver and spleen scan, magnesium, mediastinoscopy, β_2-microglobulin, osmolality, protein urine total and fractions, PFT, radiography bone, RF, sodium, TSH, thyroxine, and UA.
- Refer to the Gastrointestinal, Hepatobiliary, and Immune systems tables at the end of the book for related tests by body system.

Expected Outcomes

Expected outcomes associated with Protein, Blood, Total and Fractions, are:

- Safely performing self-care activities
- Recognizing and verbalizing positive aspects of the self
- Beginning to gain control over personal health by accepting education to support better choices

Sodium, Blood

Quick Summary

SYNONYM ACRONYM: Serum Na$^+$.

COMMON USE: To assess electrolyte balance related to hydration levels and disorders such as diarrhea and vomiting and to monitor the effect of diuretic use.

SPECIMEN: Serum collected in a gold-, red-, or red/gray-top tube. Plasma collected in a green-top (heparin) tube is also acceptable.

NORMAL FINDINGS: (Method: Ion-selective electrode)

Age	Conventional & SI Units
Newborn	135–145 mEq/L or mmol/L
7 day–1 mo	134–144 mEq/L or mmol/L
2 mo–5 mo	134–142 mEq/L or mmol/L
6 mo–1 yr	133–142 mEq/L or mmol/L
Child-Adult–older adult	135–145 mEq/L or mmol/L

Note: Older adults are at increased risk for both hypernatremia and hyponatremia. Diminished thirst, illness, and lack of mobility are common causes for hypernatremia in older adults. There are multiple causes of hyponatremia in older adults, but the most common factor may be related to the use of thiazide diuretics.

Test Explanation

Electrolytes dissociate into electrically charged ions when dissolved. Cations, including sodium, carry a positive charge. Body fluids contain approximately equal numbers of anions and cations, although the nature of the ions and their mobility differs between the intracellular and extracellular compartments. Both types of ions affect the electrical and osmolar functions of the body. Electrolyte quantities and the balance among them are controlled by oxygen and carbon dioxide exchange in the lungs; absorption, secretion, and excretion of many substances by the kidneys; and secretion of regulatory hormones by the endocrine glands. Sodium is the most abundant extracellular cation that together with chloride and bicarbonate participate in a number of essential functions to include maintaining the osmotic pressure of extracellular fluid, regulating renal retention and excretion of water, maintaining acid-base balance, regulating potassium levels, stimulating neuromuscular reactions, and maintaining systemic blood pressure. *Hypernatremia* (elevated sodium level) occurs when there is excessive water loss or abnormal retention of sodium. *Hyponatremia* (low sodium level) occurs when there is inadequate sodium retention or inadequate intake.

Nursing Implications

Assessment

Indications	Potential Nursing Problems
Determine whole-body stores of sodium, because the ion is predominantly extracellular Monitor the effectiveness of drug therapy, especially diuretics, on serum sodium levels	• Confusion • Diarrhea • Electrolyte • Fluid Volume • Human Response • Sexuality • Vomiting

Diagnosis: Clinical Significance of Test Results

INCREASED IN

- Azotemia *(related to increased renal retention)*
- Burns *(hemoconcentration related to excessive loss of free water)*
- Cushing disease
- Dehydration
- Diabetes *(dehydration related to frequent urination)*
- Diarrhea *(related to water loss in excess of salt loss)*
- Excessive intake
- Excessive saline therapy *(related to administration of IV fluids)*
- Excessive sweating *(related to loss of free water, which can cause hemoconcentration)*
- Fever *(related to loss of free water through sweating)*
- Hyperaldosteronism *(related to excessive production of aldosterone, which increases renal absorption of sodium and increases blood levels)*
- Lactic acidosis *(related to diabetes)*
- Nasogastric feeding with inadequate fluid *(related to dehydration and hemoconcentration)*
- Vomiting *(related to dehydration)*

DECREASED IN

- Central nervous system disease
- Cystic fibrosis *(related to loss from chronic diarrhea; poor intestinal absorption)*
- Excessive antidiuretic hormone production *(related to excessive loss through renal excretion)*
- Excessive use of diuretics *(related to excessive loss through renal excretion; renal absorption is blocked)*
- Heart failure *(diminished renal blood flow due to reduced cardiac capacity decreases urinary excretion and increases blood sodium levels)*
- Hepatic failure *(hemodilution related to fluid retention)*
- Hypoproteinemia *(related to fluid retention)*
- Insufficient intake
- IV glucose infusion *(hypertonic glucose draws water into extracellular fluid and sodium is diluted)*
- Mineralocorticoid deficiency (Addison disease) *(related to inadequate production of aldosterone, which results in decreased absorption by the kidneys)*
- Nephrotic syndrome *(related to decreased ability of renal tubules to reabsorb sodium)*

Planning

Considerations for planning a successful partnership should include clear communication of what to expect during the test to decrease anxiety and improve cooperation. Before the procedure is performed, plan to review the steps with the patient. Address concerns about pain, and explain that there may be some discomfort during the venipuncture.

SPECIAL CONSIDERATIONS

An important aspect of planning is understanding the factors that may alter the study findings or cause abnormal results. Interdepartmental communication is a key factor in the planning process. The following should be noted when planning for this study:

- Specimens should never be collected above an IV line because of the potential for dilution when the specimen and the IV solution combine in the collection container, falsely decreasing the result. There is also the potential of contaminating the sample with the substance of interest, if it is present in the IV solution, falsely increasing the result.

It is also important to understand which medications or substances the patient may be exposed to in the health-care setting that can interfere with accurate testing:

- Drugs that may increase serum sodium levels include anabolic steroids, angiotensin, bicarbonate, carbenoxolone, cisplatin, corticotropin, cortisone, gamma globulin, and mannitol.
- Drugs that may decrease serum sodium levels include amphotericin B, bicarbonate, cathartics (excessive use), chlorpropamide, chlorthalidone, diuretics, ethacrynic acid, fluoxetine, furosemide, laxatives (excessive use), methyclothiazide, metolazone, nicardipine, quinethazone, theophylline (IV infusion), thiazides, and triamterene.

Implementation

Patient education is key to obtaining the patient's cooperation in following directions, and providing an explanation for the purpose of the procedure is an important part of this process. Inform the patient that this study can assist in evaluating electrolyte balance. Perform the venipuncture.

Evaluation

Recognize anxiety related to test results, and evaluate the patient for signs and symptoms of dehydration. Decreased skin turgor, dry mouth, and multiple longitudinal furrows in the tongue are symptoms of dehydration. Dehydration is a significant and common finding in older adult patients and other patients in whom renal function has deteriorated. Educate the patient regarding access to nutritional counseling services. Provide contact information, if desired, for the Institute of Medicine of the National Academies (www.iom.edu) and the United States Department of Agriculture (www.choosemyplate.com).

NUTRITIONAL CONSIDERATIONS: If appropriate, educate patients with low sodium levels that the major source of dietary sodium is found in table salt. Many foods, such as milk and other dairy products, are also good sources of dietary sodium. Most other dietary sodium is available through the consumption of processed foods; some examples are baking mixes (pancakes or muffins), sauces (barbecue), butter, canned soups and sauces, dry soup mixes, frozen or microwave meals,

ketchup, pickles, and snack foods (potato chips, pretzels). Patients on low-sodium diets should be advised to avoid beverages such as colas, ginger ale, sports drinks, lemon-lime sodas, and root beer. Many over-the-counter medications, including antacids, laxatives, analgesics, sedatives, and antitussives, contain significant amounts of sodium. The best advice is to emphasize the importance of reading all food, beverage, and medicine labels.

Critical Findings

- *Hyponatremia:* Less than 120 mEq/L or mmol/L (SI: Less than 120 mmol/L)
- *Hypernatremia:* Greater than 160 mEq/L or mmol/L (SI: Greater than 160 mmol/L)

Consideration may be given to verifying the critical findings before action is taken. Policies vary among facilities and may include requesting immediate recollection and retesting by the laboratory or retesting using a rapid Point of Care instrument at the bedside, if available.

Note and immediately report to the requesting health-care provider (HCP) any critical findings and related symptoms. A listing of these findings varies among facilities.

Signs and symptoms of hyponatremia include confusion, irritability, convulsions, tachycardia, nausea, vomiting, and loss of consciousness. Possible interventions include maintenance of airway, monitoring for convulsions, fluid restriction, and performance of hourly neurological checks. Administration of saline for replacement requires close attention to serum and urine osmolality.

Signs and symptoms of hypernatremia include restlessness, intense thirst, weakness, swollen tongue, seizures, and coma. Possible interventions include treatment of the underlying cause of water loss or sodium excess, which includes sodium restriction and administration of diuretics combined with IV solutions of 5% dextrose in water (D_5W).

Study Specific Complications

There are a number of complications associated with performing a venipuncture. **Pain** is commonly associated with needles, and although the pain experienced during venipuncture is usually mild, on a rare occasion the needle may strike a nerve causing permanent pain. Some patients experience a **vasovagal reaction** during the venipuncture procedure, evidenced by sweating, low blood pressure, fainting, or near fainting. The potential for a **fall injury** is a significant concern related to vasovagal reactions. Prolonged **bleeding** is a complication that occurs with patients who are taking blood thinners or who have coagulopathies such as hemophilia. A **hematoma** results when blood leaks into the tissue during or after a venipuncture, as evidenced by pain, bruising, and/or swelling at the venipuncture site. The swelling can cause injury by compression to surrounding nerves, which can be temporary or permanent. HCPs should watch for minor complications such as bruising and hematoma at the venipuncture site, which are fairly common. Hematomas occur more often in older adult or frail patients, or those with veins that are difficult to access. Bleeding or bruising can be prevented once the needle has been removed by applying direct pressure to the site with dry gauze for a minute or two. Some other more unusual complications of venipuncture include **cellulitis, phlebitis, inadvertent arterial puncture,** and **sepsis.** Sepsis can be caused by introduction of bacteria from the surface of the skin into the blood as the result of improper cleansing of the venipuncture site. Immunocompromised patients are at higher risk for developing this complication.

Related Tests

- Related tests include ACTH, aldosterone, anion gap, ANP, BNP, blood gases, BUN, calculus kidney stone panel, BUN, calcium, carbon dioxide, chloride, chloride sweat, cortisol, creatinine, DHEAS, echocardiography, glucose, insulin, ketones, lactic acid, lung perfusion scan, magnesium, osmolality, potassium, renin, US abdomen, urine sodium, and UA.
- Refer to the Cardiovascular, Endocrine, and Genitourinary systems tables at the end of the book for related tests by body system.

Expected Outcomes

Expected outcomes associated with Sodium, Blood are:

- Verbalizing the importance of maintaining a normal sodium level to overall health
- Adhering to a plan to decrease vomiting and diarrhea to prevent the depletion of sodium stores
- Recognizing the risk of altered sexual function associated with an altered sodium level

Testosterone, Total and Free

Quick Summary

COMMON USE: To evaluate testosterone to assist in identification of disorders related to early puberty, late puberty, and infertility while assessing gonadal and adrenal function.

SPECIMEN: Serum collected in a red- or red/gray-top tube. Plasma collected in green-top (heparin) tube is also acceptable.

NORMAL FINDINGS: (Method: HPLC/Tandem MS for total and Immunochemiluminometric assay [ICMA] for free testosterone)

Free Testosterone

Age	Conventional Units	SI Units (Conventional Units × 3.47)
1–12 yr		
Male and Female	Less than 2 pg/mL	Less than 6.94 pmol/L
12–14 yr		
Male	Less than 60 pg/mL	Less than 208 pmol/L
Female	Less than 2 pg/mL	Less than 6.94 pmol/L
14–18 yr		
Male	4–100 pg/mL	13.88–347 pmol/L
Female	Less than 4 pg/mL	Less than 13.88 pmol/L
Adult		
Male	50–224 pg/mL	173.5–777.28 pmol/L
Female	1–8.5 pg/mL	3.47–29.5 pmol/L
Older Adult		
Male	5–75 pg/mL	17.35–260.25 pmol/L
Female	1–8.5 pg/mL	3.47–29.5 pmol/L

Total Testosterone

Age	Conventional Units	SI Units (Conventional Units × 0.0347)
Newborn		
Male	17–61 ng/dL	0.59–2.12 nmol/L
Female	16–44 ng/dL	0.56–1.53 nmol/L
1–5 mo		
Male	Less than 300 ng/dL	Less than 10.41 nmol/L
Female	Less than 20 ng/dL	Less than 0.69 nmol/L
6–11 mo		
Male	Less than 40 ng/dL	Less than 1.39 nmol/L
Female	Less than 9 ng/dL	Less than 0.31 nmol/L
1–5 yr		
Male and female	Less than 10 ng/dL	Less than 0.35 nmol/L
6–7 yr		
Male	Less than 20 ng/dL	Less than 0.69 nmol/L
Female	Less than10 ng/dL	Less than 0.35 nmol/L
8–10 yr		
Male	2–25 ng/dL	0.07–0.87 nmol/L
Female	1–30 ng/dL	0.04–1 nmol/L
11–12 yr		
Male	Less than 350 ng/dL	Less than 12.1 nmol/L
Female	Less than 50 ng/dL	Less than 1.74 nmol/L

Total Testosterone

Age	Conventional Units	SI Units (Conventional Units × 0.0347)
13–15 yr		
Male	15–500 ng/dL	0.52–17.35 nmol/L
Female	Less than 50 ng/dL	Less than 1.74 nmol/L
Adult		
Male	241–827 ng/dL	8.36–28.7 nmol/L
Female	15–70 ng/dL	0.52–2.43 nmol/L
Older adult		
Male	300–720 ng/dL	10.41–24.98
Female	5-32 ng/dL	0.17–1.11

Post menopausal levels are about half the normal adult level for females; levels in pregnant women are 3–4 times the normal adult level for non-pregnant females.

Tanner Stage	Male	Female
I	2–15 ng/dL	2–10 ng/dL
II	5–170 ng/dL	5–30 ng/dL
III	15–280 ng/dL	10–30 ng/dL
IV	105–545 ng/dL	15–40 ng/dL
V	265–800 ng/dL	10–40 ng/dL

Test Explanation

Testosterone is the major androgen responsible for sexual differentiation. In males, testosterone is made by the Leydig cells in the testicles and is responsible for spermatogenesis and the development of secondary sex characteristics. In females, the ovary and adrenal gland secrete small amounts of this hormone; however, most of the testosterone in females comes from the metabolism of androstenedione. Testosterone levels have a slight diurnal variation, with the highest levels occurring around 8 a.m. and lowest levels around 8 p.m. Measurements of total testosterone levels are used most often in evaluating suspected hormone imbalances. Free testosterone is the active form of the hormone. It is used in conjunction with total testosterone to evaluate hormone levels in conditions known to alter the effectiveness of testosterone binding protein, also called sex hormone binding globulin (SHBG). Alterations in the affinity of SHBG to bind free testosterone are known to occur with obesity, liver disease, and hyperthyroidism. In males, a testicular, adrenal, or pituitary tumor can cause an overabundance of testosterone, triggering precocious puberty. In females, adrenal tumors, hyperplasia, and medications can cause an overabundance of this hormone, resulting in masculinization or hirsutism.

Nursing Implications

Assessment

Indications	Potential Nursing Problems
Assist in the diagnosis of hypergonadism	• Human Response
Assist in the diagnosis of male sexual precocity before age 10	• Role Performance
Distinguish between primary and secondary hypogonadism	• Self-esteem
Evaluate hirsutism	• Sexuality
Evaluate male infertility	

Diagnosis: Clinical Significance of Test Results

INCREASED IN

- Adrenal hyperplasia *(oversecretion of the androgen precursor dehydroepiandrosterone [DHEA])*
- Adrenocortical tumors *(oversecretion of the androgen precursor DHEA)*
- Hirsutism *(any condition that results in increased production of testosterone or its precursors)*
- Hyperthyroidism *(high thyroxine levels increase the production of sex hormone–binding protein, which increases measured levels of total testosterone)*
- Idiopathic sexual precocity *(related to stimulation of testosterone production by elevated levels of luteinizing hormone [LH])*
- Polycystic ovaries *(high estrogen levels increase the production of sex hormone–binding protein, which increases measured levels of total testosterone)*
- Syndrome of androgen resistance
- Testicular or extragonadal tumors *(related to excessive secretion of testosterone)*
- Trophoblastic tumors during pregnancy
- Virilizing ovarian tumors

DECREASED IN

- Anovulation
- Cryptorchidism *(related to dysfunctional testes)*
- Delayed puberty
- Down syndrome *(related to diminished or dysfunctional testes)*
- Excessive alcohol intake *(alcohol inhibits secretion of testosterone)*
- Hepatic insufficiency *(related to decreased binding protein and reflects decreased measured levels of total testosterone)*
- Impotence *(decreased testosterone levels can result in impotence)*

- Klinefelter syndrome *(chromosome abnormality XXY associated with testicular failure)*
- Malnutrition
- Myotonic dystrophy *(related to testicular atrophy)*
- Orchiectomy *(testosterone production occurs in the testes)*
- Primary and secondary hypogonadism
- Primary and secondary hypopituitarism
- Uremia

Planning
Considerations for planning a successful partnership should include clear communication of what to expect during the test to decrease anxiety and improve cooperation. Before the procedure is performed, plan to review the steps with the patient. Address concerns about pain, and explain that there may be some discomfort during the venipuncture.

SPECIAL CONSIDERATIONS
An important aspect of planning is understanding the factors that may alter the study findings or cause abnormal results. Interdepartmental communication is a key factor in the planning process.

It is also important to understand which medications or substances the patient may be exposed to in the health-care setting that can interfere with accurate testing:

- Drugs that may increase testosterone levels include barbiturates, bromocriptine, cimetidine, flutamide, gonadotropin, levonorgestrel, mifepristone, moclobemide, nafarelin (males), nilutamide, oral contraceptives, rifampin, and tamoxifen.
- Drugs that may decrease testosterone levels include cyclophosphamide, cyproterone, danazol, dexamethasone, diethylstilbestrol, digoxin, D-Trp-6-LHRH, fenoldopam, goserelin, ketoconazole, leuprolide, magnesium sulfate, medroxyprogesterone, methylprednisone, nandrolone, oral contraceptives, pravastatin, prednisone, pyridoglutethimide, spironolactone, stanozolol, tetracycline, and thioridazine.

Implementation
Patient education is key to obtaining the patient's cooperation in following directions, and providing an explanation for the purpose of the procedure is an important part of this process. Inform the patient that this study can assist with evaluating hormone levels. Perform the venipuncture.

Evaluation
Recognize anxiety related to test results, and offer support as appropriate. Discuss the implications of abnormal test results on the patient's lifestyle. Provide teaching and information regarding the clinical implications of the test results as appropriate. Educate the patient regarding access to counseling services.

✔ Critical Findings
N/A

✔ Study Specific Complications
There are a number of complications associated with performing a venipuncture. **Pain** is commonly associated with needles, and although the pain experienced during venipuncture is usually mild, on a rare occasion the needle may strike a nerve causing permanent pain. Some patients experience a **vasovagal reaction** during the venipuncture procedure, evidenced by sweating, low blood pressure, fainting, or near fainting. The potential for a **fall injury** is a significant concern related to vasovagal reactions. Prolonged **bleeding** is a complication that occurs with patients who are taking blood thinners or who have coagulopathies such as hemophilia. A **hematoma** results when blood leaks into the tissue during or after a venipuncture, as evidenced by pain, bruising, and/or swelling at the venipuncture site. The swelling can cause injury by compression to surrounding nerves, which can be temporary or permanent. Health-care providers (HCPs) should watch for minor complications such as bruising and hematoma at the venipuncture site, which are fairly common. Hematomas occur more often in older adult or frail patients, or those with veins that are difficult to access. Bleeding or bruising can be prevented once the needle has been removed by applying direct pressure to the site with dry gauze for a minute or two. Some other more unusual complications of venipuncture include **cellulitis, phlebitis, inadvertent arterial puncture,** and **sepsis.** Sepsis can be caused by introduction of bacteria from the surface of the skin into the blood as the result of improper cleansing of the venipuncture site. Immunocompromised patients are at higher risk for developing this complication.

✔ Related Tests
- Related tests include angiography adrenal gland scan, ACE, antibodies antisperm, biopsy thyroid, chromosome analysis, CT renal, DHEAS, estradiol, FSH, LH, PTH, RAIU, semen analysis, thyroid scan, TSH, thyroxine, and US scrotal.
- Refer to the Endocrine and Reproductive systems tables at the end of the book for related test by body system.

Expected Outcomes
Expected outcomes associated with total Testosterone are:

- Agreeing to explore the cause of infertility
- Expressing concerns over potential parenting ability
- Expressing willingness to attend an infertility support group

Thyroid-Stimulating Hormone

Quick Summary

SYNONYM ACRONYM: Thyrotropin, TSH.

COMMON USE: To evaluate thyroid gland function related to the primary cause of hypothyroidism and assess for congenital disorders, tumor, cancer, and inflammation.

SPECIMEN: Serum collected in a gold-, red-, or tiger-top tube; for a neonate, use filter paper.

NORMAL FINDINGS: (Method: Immunoassay)

Age	Conventional Units	SI Units (Conventional Units × 1)
Neonates–3 days	Less than 40 micro-international units/mL	Less than 40 milli-international units/L
2 wk–5 mo	1.7–9.1 micro-international units/mL	1.7–9.1 milli-international units/L
6 mo–1 yr	0.7–6.4 micro-international units/mL	0.7–6.4 milli-international units/L
2 yr–19 yr	0.5–4.5 micro-international units/mL	0.5–4.5 milli-international units/L
Greater than 20 yr	0.4–4.2 micro-international units/mL	0.4–4.2 milli-international units/L

Trimester	Conventional Units	SI Units (Conventional Units × 1)
First Trimester	0.3–2.7 micro-international units/mL	0.3–2.7 milli-international units/L
Second Trimester	0.5–2.7 micro-international units/mL	0.5–2.7 milli-international units/L
Third Trimester	0.4–2.9 micro-international units/mL	0.4–2.9 milli-international units/L

Test Explanation

Thyroid-stimulating hormone (TSH) is produced by the pituitary gland in response to stimulation by thyrotropin-releasing hormone (TRH), a hypothalamic-releasing factor. TRH regulates the release and circulating levels of thyroid hormones in response to variables such as cold, stress, and increased metabolic need. Thyroid and pituitary function can be evaluated by TSH measurement. TSH exhibits diurnal variation, peaking between midnight and 4 a.m. and troughing between 5 and 6 p.m. TSH values are high at birth but reach adult levels in the first year of life. Elevated TSH levels combined with decreased thyroxine (T_4) levels indicate hypothyroidism and thyroid gland dysfunction. In general, decreased TSH and T_4 levels indicate secondary congenital hypothyroidism and pituitary hypothalamic dysfunction. A normal TSH level and a depressed T_4 level may indicate (1) hypothyroidism owing to a congenital defect in T_4-binding globulin or (2) transient congenital hypothyroidism owing to hypoxia or prematurity. Early diagnosis and treatment in the neonate are crucial for the prevention of cretinism and intellectual disabilities.

Nursing Implications

Assessment

Indications	Potential Nursing Problems
Assist in the diagnosis of congenital hypothyroidism Assist in the diagnosis of hypothyroidism or hyperthyroidism or suspected pituitary or hypothalamic dysfunction Differentiate functional euthyroidism from true hypothyroidism in debilitated individuals	• Cardiac Output • Communication • Confusion • Human Response • Nutrition • Self-esteem • Sensory Perception

Diagnosis: Clinical Significance of Test Results

INCREASED IN

A decrease in thyroid hormone levels activates the feedback loop to increase production of TSH.

- Congenital hypothyroidism in the neonate (filter paper test)
- Ectopic TSH-producing tumors (lung, breast)
- Primary hypothyroidism *(related to a dysfunctional thyroid gland)*
- Secondary hyperthyroidism owing to pituitary hyperactivity
- Thyroid hormone resistance
- Thyroiditis (Hashimoto autoimmune disease)

DECREASED IN

An increase in thyroid hormone levels activates the feedback loop to decrease production of TSH.

- Excessive thyroid hormone replacement
- Graves disease
- Primary hyperthyroidism
- Secondary hypothyroidism *(related to pituitary involvement that decreases production of TSH)*
- Tertiary hypothyroidism *(related to hypothalamic involvement that decreases production of TRH)*

Planning

Considerations for planning a successful partnership should include clear communication of what to expect during the test to decrease anxiety and improve cooperation. Before the procedure is performed, plan to review the steps with the patient. Address concerns about pain, and explain that there may be some discomfort during the venipuncture.

SPECIAL CONSIDERATIONS

An important aspect of planning is understanding the factors that may alter the study findings or cause abnormal results. Interdepartmental communication is a key factor in the planning process. The following should be noted when planning for this study:

- Failure to let the filter paper sample dry may affect neonatal screening test results.

It is also important to understand which medications or substances the patient may be exposed to in the healthcare setting that can interfere with accurate testing:

- Drugs and hormones that may increase TSH levels include amiodarone, benserazide, erythrosine, flunarizine (males), iobenzamic acid, iodides, lithium, methimazole, metoclopramide, morphine, propranolol, radiographic agents, TRH, and valproic acid.
- Drugs and hormones that may decrease TSH levels include acetylsalicylic acid, amiodarone, anabolic steroids, carbamazepine, corticosteroids, glucocorticoids, hydrocortisone, interferon-alfa-2b, iodamide, levodopa (in hypothyroidism), levothyroxine, methergoline, nifedipine, T_4, and triiodothyronine (T_3).

Implementation

Patient education is key to obtaining the patient's cooperation in following directions, and providing an explanation for the purpose of the procedure is an important part of this process. Inform the patient that this study can assist in evaluating thyroid function. Perform the venipuncture.

FILTER PAPER TEST (NEONATE)

Obtain a neonatal collection kit and cleanse the infant's heel with an antiseptic. Observe standard precautions. Perform the heel stick, gently squeeze the infant's heel, and touch the filter paper to the puncture site. Use gauze to dry the stick area completely. When collecting samples for newborn screening, it is important to apply blood drop to the correct side of the filter paper card and fill each circle with a single application of blood. Overfilling or underfilling the circles will cause the specimen card to be rejected by the testing facility. Additional information is required on newborn screening cards and may vary by state. Newborn screening cards should be allowed to air dry for several hours on a level, nonabsorbent, unenclosed area. If multiple patients are tested, do not stack cards. State regulations usually require the specimen cards to be submitted within 24 hours of collection.

Evaluation

Recognize anxiety related to the test results and answer any questions or address any concerns voiced by the patient or family.

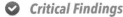 Critical Findings

N/A

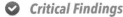 Study Specific Complications

There are a number of complications associated with performing a venipuncture. **Pain** is commonly associated with needles, and although the pain experienced during venipuncture is usually mild, on a rare occasion the needle may strike a nerve causing permanent pain. Some patients experience a **vasovagal reaction** during the venipuncture procedure, evidenced by sweating, low blood pressure, fainting, or near fainting. The potential for a **fall injury** is a significant concern related to vasovagal reactions. Prolonged **bleeding** is a complication that occurs with patients who are taking blood thinners or who have coagulopathies such as hemophilia. A **hematoma** results when blood leaks into the tissue during or after a venipuncture, as evidenced by pain, bruising, and/or swelling at the venipuncture site. The swelling can cause injury by compression to surrounding nerves, which can be temporary or permanent. Health-care providers (HCPs) should watch for minor complications such as bruising and hematoma at the venipuncture site, which are fairly common. Hematomas occur more often in older adult or frail patients, or those with veins that are difficult to access. Bleeding or bruising can be prevented once the needle has been removed by applying direct pressure to the site with dry gauze for a minute or two. Some other more unusual complications of venipuncture include **cellulitis, phlebitis, inadvertent arterial puncture,** and **sepsis.** Sepsis can be caused by introduction of bacteria from the surface of the skin into the blood as the result of improper cleansing of the venipuncture site. Immunocompromised patients are at higher risk for developing this complication.

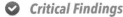 Related Tests

- Related tests include adrenocorticotropin hormone, albumin, antibodies antithyroglobulin, biopsy thyroid, copper, follicle-stimulating hormone, growth hormone, luteinizing hormone, newborn screening, PTH, protein total, RAIU, thyroglobulin, TSI, TBII, thyroid scan, T_4, free T_4, T_3, free T_3, and US thyroid.
- Refer to the Endocrine System table at the end of the book for related tests by body system.

Expected Outcomes

Expected outcomes associated with Thyroid-Stimulating Hormone (TSH) are:

- Maintaining a stable weight
- Agreeing to a weight reduction program as appropriate to achieve a healthy BMI
- Having an absence of bradycardia with a pulse greater than 60 beats per minute

Thyroxine, Free

Quick Summary

SYNONYM ACRONYM: Free T_4, Free$_4$.

COMMON USE: A reflex test for thyroid function related to deficiency or excess to assist in diagnosing hyperthyroidism and hypothyroidism in the presence of an abnormal TSH level.

SPECIMEN: Serum collected in a gold-, red-, or red/gray-top tube. Plasma collected in a green-top (heparin) tube is also acceptable.

NORMAL FINDINGS: (Method: Immunoassay)

Age	Conventional Units	SI Units (Conventional Units × 12.9)
Newborn	0.8–2.8 ng/dL	10–36 pmol/L
1–12 mo	0.8–2 ng/dL	10–26 pmol/L
1–18 yr	0.8–1.7 ng/dL	10–22 pmol/L
Adult–older adult	0.8–1.5 ng/dL	10–19 pmol/L
Pregnancy (first trimester)	0.9–1.4 ng/dL	12–18 pmol/L
Pregnancy (second trimester)	0.7–1.3 ng/dL	9–17 pmol/L

Test Explanation

Thyroxine (T_4) is a hormone produced and secreted by the thyroid gland (see Fig. 1.23). Most T_4 in the serum (99.97%) is bound to thyroxine-binding globulin (TBG), prealbumin, and albumin. The remainder (0.03%) circulates as unbound or free T_4, which is the physiologically active form. Levels of free T_4 are proportional to levels of total T_4. The advantage of measuring free T_4 instead of total T_4 is that, unlike total T_4 measurements, free T_4 levels are not affected by fluctuations in TBG levels; as a result, free T_4 levels are considered the most accurate indicator of T_4 and its thyrometabolic activity. Free T_4 measurements are useful in evaluating thyroid disease when thyroid-stimulating hormone (TSH) levels alone provide insufficient information. Free T_4 and TSH levels are inversely proportional. Measurement of free T_4 is also recommended during treatment for hyperthyroidism until symptoms have abated and levels have decreased into the normal range.

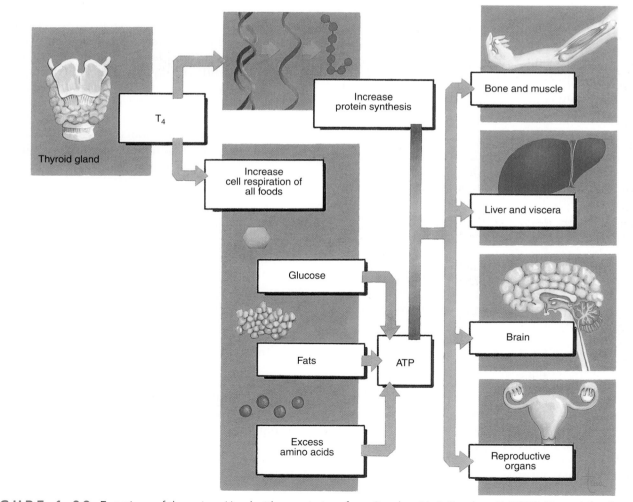

FIGURE 1.23 Functions of thyroxine. *Used with permission, from Scanlon, V., & Sanders, T. (2010). Essentials of anatomy and physiology (6th Ed.). FA Davis Company.*

Nursing Implications

Assessment

Indications	Potential Nursing Problems
Evaluate signs of hypothyroidism or hyperthyroidism Monitor response to therapy for hypothyroidism or hyperthyroidism	• Body Image • Cardiac Output • Communication • Confusion • Human Response • Nutrition • Self-esteem • Skin • Thermoregulation

Diagnosis: Clinical Significance of Test Results

INCREASED IN

- Hyperthyroidism *(thyroxine is produced independently of stimulation by TSH)*
- Hypothyroidism treated with T_4 *(laboratory tests do not distinguish between endogenous and exogenous sources)*

DECREASED IN

- Hypothyroidism *(thyroid hormones are not produced in sufficient quantities regardless of TSH levels)*
- Pregnancy (late)

Planning

Considerations for planning a successful partnership should include clear communication of what to expect during the test to decrease anxiety and improve cooperation. Before the procedure is performed, plan to review the steps with the patient. Address concerns about pain, and explain that there may be some discomfort during the venipuncture.

SPECIAL CONSIDERATIONS

An important aspect of planning is understanding the factors that may alter the study findings or cause abnormal results. Interdepartmental communication is a key factor in the planning process.

It is also important to understand which medications or substances the patient may be exposed to in the health-care setting that can interfere with accurate testing:

- Drugs that may increase free T_4 levels include acetylsalicylic acid, amiodarone, halofenate, heparin, iopanoic acid, levothyroxine, methimazole, and iodinated radiographic agents.
- Drugs that may decrease free T_4 levels include amiodarone, anabolic steroids, asparaginase, methadone, methimazole, oral contraceptives, and phenylbutazone.

Implementation

Patient education is key to obtaining the patient's cooperation in following directions, and providing an explanation for the purpose of the procedure is an important part of this process. Inform the patient that this study can assist in assessing thyroid gland function. Perform the venipuncture.

Evaluation

Recognize anxiety related to test results, and answer any questions or address any concerns voiced by the patient or family.

✓ Critical Findings

N/A

✓ Study Specific Complications

There are a number of complications associated with performing a venipuncture. **Pain** is commonly associated with needles, and although the pain experienced during venipuncture is usually mild, on a rare occasion the needle may strike a nerve causing permanent pain. Some patients experience a **vasovagal reaction** during the venipuncture procedure, evidenced by sweating, low blood pressure, fainting, or near fainting. The potential for a **fall injury** is a significant concern related to vasovagal reactions. Prolonged **bleeding** is a complication that occurs with patients who are taking blood thinners or who have coagulopathies such as hemophilia. A **hematoma** results when blood leaks into the tissue during or after a venipuncture, as evidenced by pain, bruising, and/or swelling at the venipuncture site. The swelling can cause injury by compression to surrounding nerves, which can be temporary or permanent. HCPs should watch for minor complications such as bruising and hematoma at the venipuncture site, which are fairly common. Hematomas occur more often in older adult or frail patients, or those with veins that are difficult to access. Bleeding or bruising can be prevented once the needle has been removed by applying direct pressure to the site with dry gauze for a minute or two. Some other more unusual complications of venipuncture include **cellulitis, phlebitis, inadvertent arterial puncture,** and **sepsis.** Sepsis can be caused by introduction of bacteria from the surface of the skin into the blood as the result of improper cleansing of the venipuncture site. Immunocompromised patients are at higher risk for developing this complication.

✓ Related Tests

- Related tests include albumin, antibodies antithyroglobulin, biopsy thyroid, copper, PTH, prealbumin, protein, RAIU, thyroglobulin, TBII, thyroid scan, TSH, TSI, T$_4$, T$_3$, free T$_3$, and US thyroid.

- Refer to the Endocrine System table at the end of the book for related tests by body system.

Expected Outcomes

Expected outcomes associated with Thyroxine, Free, (FT$_4$), are:

- No confusion or altered processing of thoughts
- Acceptance of the diagnosis and agreeing to the corrective therapeutic regime
- Skin that remains clear

Triglycerides

Quick Summary

SYNONYM ACRONYM: Trigs, TG.

COMMON USE: To evaluate triglyceride levels to assess cardiovascular disease risk and evaluate the effectiveness of therapeutic interventions.

SPECIMEN: Serum collected in a gold-, red-, or red/gray-top tube. Plasma collected in a green-top (heparin) tube is also acceptable.

NORMAL FINDINGS: (Method: Spectrophotometry)

ATP III Classification	Conventional Units	SI Units (Conventional Units × 0.0113)
Normal	Less than 150 mg/dL	Less than 1.7 mmol/L
Borderline high	150–199 mg/dL	1.7–2.2 mmol/L
High	200–499 mg/dL	2.3–5.6 mmol/L
Very high	Greater than 500 mg/dL	Greater than 5.6 mmol/L

Test Explanation

Fat or adipose is an important source of energy. Triglycerides (TGs) are a combination of three fatty acids and one glycerol molecule. Much of the fatty acids used in various metabolic processes come from dietary sources. However, the body also generates fatty acids, from available glucose and amino acids, that are converted into glycogen or stored energy by the liver. Beyond triglyceride, total cholesterol, high-density lipoprotein (HDL), and low-density lipoprotein (LDL) cholesterol values, other important risk factors must be considered. Guidelines for the prevention of cardiovascular disease (CVD) have been developed by the American College of Cardiology (ACC) and the American Heart Association (AHA) in conjunction with members of the National Heart, Lung, and Blood Institute's (NHLBI) ATP IV Expert Panel. The updated, evidence-based guidelines redefine the condition of concern as atherosclerotic cardiovascular disease (ASCVD) and expand ASCVD to include CVD, stroke, and peripheral artery disease. Some of the important highlights include:

- Movement away from the use of LDL cholesterol targets in determining treatment with statins. Recommendations that focus on selecting (a) the patients that fall into four groups most likely to benefit from statin therapy, and (b) the level of statin intensity most likely to affect or reduce development of ASCVD.
- Development of a new 10-year risk assessment tool based on findings from a large, diverse population. Evidence-based risk factors include age, sex, ethnicity, total cholesterol, HDL cholesterol, blood pressure, blood-pressure treatment status, diabetes, and current use of tobacco products.
- Recommendations for aspects of lifestyle that would encourage prevention of ASCVD to include adherence to a Mediterranean- or DASH (Dietary Approaches to Stop Hypertension)-style diet; dietary restriction of saturated fats, trans fats, sugar, and sodium; and regular participation in aerobic exercise. The guidelines contain reductions in BMI cutoffs for men and women designed to promote discussions between health-care providers (HCPs) and their patients regarding the benefits of maintaining a healthy weight.
- Recognition that additional biological markers, such as family history, high-sensitivity C-reactive protein, ankle-brachial index (ABI), and coronary artery calcium (CAC) score may be selectively used with the assessment tool to assist in predicting and evaluating risk.
- Recognition that other biomarkers such as apolipoprotein B, eGFR, creatinine, lipoprotein (a) or Lp (a), and microalbumin warrant further study and may be considered for inclusion in future guidelines.

Triglyceride levels vary by age, gender, weight, and ethnicity:

- Levels increase with age.
- Levels are higher in men than in women (among women, those who take oral contraceptives have levels that are 20 to 40 mg/dL higher than those who do not).
- Levels are higher in overweight and obese people than in those with normal weight.
- Levels in African Americans are approximately 10 to 20 mg/dL lower than in whites.

Nursing Implications

Assessment

Indications	Potential Nursing Problems
Evaluate known or suspected disorders associated with altered triglyceride levels Identify hyperlipoproteinemia (hyperlipidemia) in patients with a family history of the disorder Monitor the response to drugs known to alter triglyceride levels Screen adults who are either over 40 yr or obese to estimate the risk for atherosclerotic cardiovascular disease	• Activity **(related to shortness of breath associated with poor physical fitness, and fatigue with poor oxygenation)** • Cardiac Output **(related to blocked vessels)** • Fatigue **(related to poor physical condition as a result of the disease process)** • Fear **(related to potential death)** • Health Management **(related to insufficient health-seeking behaviors)** • Human Response • Mobility **(related to poor physical condition as a result of the disease process)** • Nutrition **(related to a lack of knowledge, financial limitations, and/or overeating)** • Pain **(related to reduced blood flow and oxygen to the heart)** • Tissue Perfusion

Diagnosis: Clinical Significance of Test Results

INCREASED IN

- Acute myocardial infarction *(elevated TG is identified as an independent risk factor in the development of CAD)*
- Alcoholism *(related to decreased breakdown of fats in the liver and increased blood levels)*
- Anorexia nervosa *(compensatory increase secondary to starvation)*
- Chronic ischemic heart disease *(elevated TG is identified as an independent risk factor in the development of CAD)*
- Cirrhosis *(increased TG blood levels related to decreased breakdown of fats in the liver)*
- Glycogen storage disease *(G6PD deficiency, e.g., von Gierke disease, results in hepatic overproduction of very-low-density lipoprotein [VLDL] cholesterol, the TG-rich lipoprotein)*
- Gout *(TG is frequently elevated in patients with gout, possibly related to alterations in apolipoprotein E genotypes)*
- Hyperlipoproteinemia *(related to increase in transport proteins)*

- Hypertension *(associated with elevated TG, which is identified as an independent risk factor in the development of CAD)*
- Hypothyroidism *(significant relationship between elevated TG and decreased metabolism)*
- Impaired glucose tolerance *(increase in insulin stimulates production of TG by liver)*
- Metabolic syndrome *(syndrome consisting of obesity, high blood pressure, and insulin resistance)*
- Nephrotic syndrome *(related to absence or insufficient levels of lipoprotein lipase to remove circulating TG and to decreased catabolism of TG-rich VLDL lipoproteins)*
- Obesity *(significant and complex relationship between obesity and elevated TG)*
- Pancreatitis *(acute and chronic; related to effects on insulin production)*
- Pregnancy *(increased demand for production of hormones related to pregnancy)*
- Renal failure *(related to diabetes; elevated insulin levels stimulate production of TG by liver)*
- Respiratory distress syndrome *(related to artificial lung surfactant used for therapy)*
- Stress *(related to poor diet; effect of hormones secreted under stressful situations that affect glucose levels)*
- Syndrome X *(metabolic syndrome consisting of obesity, high blood pressure, and insulin resistance)*
- Werner syndrome *(clinical features resemble syndrome X)*

DECREASED IN

- End-stage liver disease *(related to cessation of liver function that results in decreased production of TG and TG transport proteins)*
- Hyperthyroidism *(related to increased catabolism of VLDL transport proteins and general increase in metabolism)*
- Hypolipoproteinemia and abetalipoproteinemia *(related to decrease in transport proteins)*
- Intestinal lymphangiectasia
- Malabsorption disorders *(inadequate supply from dietary sources)*
- Malnutrition *(inadequate supply from dietary sources)*

Planning

Considerations for planning a successful partnership should include clear communication of what to expect during the test to decrease anxiety and improve cooperation. Assess the patient for the presence of other risk factors, such as smoking, obesity, diet, a lack of physical activity, hypertension, diabetes, previous myocardial infarction, previous vascular disease, and a family history of heart disease. Before the procedure is performed, plan to review the steps with the patient. Address concerns about pain, and explain that there may be some discomfort during the venipuncture.

SPECIAL CONSIDERATIONS

An important aspect of planning is understanding the factors that may alter the study findings or cause abnormal results. Interdepartmental communication is a key factor in the planning process. The following should be noted when planning for this study:

- Ideally, the patient should be on a stable diet for 3 weeks and should avoid alcohol consumption for 3 days before specimen collection. Protocols may vary among facilities. The patient should be instructed to fast for 12 hours before specimen collection. Failure to follow dietary restrictions before the procedure may cause the procedure to be canceled or repeated.

It is also important to understand which medications or substances the patient may be exposed to in the health-care setting that can interfere with accurate testing:

- Drugs that may increase triglyceride levels include acetylsalicylic acid, aldatense, atenolol, bisoprolol, β-blockers, bendroflumethiazide, cholestyramine, conjugated estrogens, cyclosporine, estrogen/progestin therapy, estropipate, ethynodiol, etretinate, furosemide, glucocorticoids, hydrochlorothiazide, isotretinoin, labetalol, levonorgestrel, medroxyprogesterone, mepindolol, methyclothiazide, metoprolol, miconazole, mirtazapine, nadolol, nafarelin, oral contraceptives, oxprenolol, pindolol, prazosin, propranolol, tamoxifen, thiazides, ticlopidine, timolol, and tretinoin.
- Drugs and substances that may decrease triglyceride levels include anabolic steroids, ascorbic acid, beclobrate, bezafibrate, captopril, carvedilol, celiprolol, celiprolol, chenodiol, cholestyramine, cilazapril, ciprofibrate, clofibrate, colestipol, danazol, dextrothyroxine, doxazosin, enalapril, eptastatin (type IIb only), fenofibrate, flaxseed oil, fluvastatin, gemfibrozil, halofenate, insulin, levonorgestrel, levothyroxine, lifibrol, lovastatin, medroxyprogesterone, metformin, nafenopin, niacin, niceritrol, Norplant, pentoxifylline, pinacidil, pindolol, pravastatin, prazosin, probucol, simvastatin, and verapamil.

Implementation

Patient education is key to obtaining the patient's cooperation in following directions, and providing an explanation for the purpose of the procedure is an important part of this process. Inform the patient that this study can assist in monitoring and evaluating lipid levels. Ensure that the patient has complied with dietary restrictions and other pretesting preparations; assure that food has been restricted for at least 12 hours prior to the procedure. Perform the venipuncture.

Evaluation

Recognize anxiety related to test results, and be supportive of fear of a shortened life expectancy. Discuss the implications of abnormal test results on the patient's lifestyle. Provide teaching and information regarding the clinical implications of the test results as appropriate. Educate the patient regarding access to counseling services. Provide contact information, if desired, for the American Heart Association (AHA) (www.americanheart.org) or the National Heart, Lung, and Blood Institute (NHLBI) (www.nhlbi.nih.gov).

SPECIAL CONSIDERATIONS

Numerous studies point to the prevalence of excess body weight in American children and adolescents. Experts estimate that obesity is present in 25% of the population ages 6 to 11 years. The medical, social, and emotional consequences of excess body weight are significant. Special attention should be given to instructing the child and caregiver regarding health risks and weight-control education.

NUTRITIONAL CONSIDERATIONS FOR THE CARDIAC PATIENT: Increases in triglyceride levels may be associated with coronary artery disease (CAD). Nutritional therapy is recommended for the patient identified to be at risk for developing CAD or for individuals who have specific risk factors and/or existing medical conditions (e.g., elevated LDL cholesterol levels, other lipid disorders, insulin-dependent diabetes, insulin resistance, or metabolic syndrome). Other changeable risk factors warranting patient education include strategies to encourage patients, especially those who are overweight and with high blood pressure, to safely decrease sodium intake, achieve a normal weight, ensure regular participation of moderate aerobic physical activity three to four times per week, eliminate tobacco use, and adhere to a heart-healthy diet. If triglycerides also are elevated, the patient should be advised to eliminate or reduce alcohol. The Guideline on Lifestyle Management to Reduce Cardiovascular Risk published by the American College of Cardiology (ACC) and AHA in conjunction with the NHLBI recommends a "Mediterranean"-style diet rather than a low-fat diet. The guideline emphasizes inclusion of vegetables, whole grains, fruits, low-fat dairy, nuts, legumes, and nontropical vegetable oils (e.g., olive, canola, peanut, sunflower, flaxseed) along with fish and lean poultry. A similar dietary pattern known as the Dietary Approaches to Stop Hypertension (DASH) diet makes additional recommendations for the reduction of dietary sodium. Both dietary styles emphasize a reduction in consumption of red meats, which are high in saturated fats and cholesterol, and other foods containing sugar, saturated fats, trans fats, and sodium.

✓ Critical Findings

N/A

✓ Study Specific Complications

There are a number of complications associated with performing a venipuncture. **Pain** is commonly associated with needles, and although the pain experienced during venipuncture is usually mild, on a rare occasion the needle may strike a nerve causing permanent pain. Some patients experience a **vasovagal reaction** during the venipuncture procedure, evidenced by sweating, low blood pressure, fainting, or near fainting. The potential for a **fall injury** is a significant concern related to vasovagal reactions. Prolonged **bleeding** is a complication that occurs with patients who are taking blood thinners or who have coagulopathies such as hemophilia. A **hematoma** results when blood leaks into the tissue during or after a venipuncture, as evidenced by pain, bruising, and/or swelling at the venipuncture site. The swelling can cause injury by compression to surrounding nerves, which can be temporary or permanent. HCPs should watch for minor complications such as bruising and hematoma at the venipuncture site, which are fairly common. Hematomas occur more often in older adult or frail patients, or those with veins that are difficult to access. Bleeding or bruising can be prevented once the needle has been removed by applying direct pressure to the site with dry gauze for a minute or two. Some other more unusual complications of venipuncture include **cellulitis, phlebitis, inadvertent arterial puncture,** and **sepsis.** Sepsis can be caused by introduction of bacteria from the surface of the skin into the blood as the result of improper cleansing of the venipuncture site. Immunocompromised patients are at higher risk for developing this complication.

✓ Related Tests

• Related tests include antidysrhythmic drugs, apolipoprotein A and B, AST, atrial natriuretic peptide, blood gases, BNP, calcium (total and ionized), cholesterol (total, HDL, and LDL), CT cardiac scoring, C-reactive protein, CK and isoenzymes, echocardiography, glucose, glycated hemoglobin, Holter monitor, homocysteine, ketones, LDH and isoenzymes, lipoprotein electrophoresis, magnesium, MRI chest, myocardial infarct scan, myocardial perfusion heart scan, myoglobin, PET heart, potassium, and troponin.
• Refer to the Cardiovascular System table at the end of the book for related tests by body system.

Expected Outcomes

Expected outcomes associated with Triglycerides are:

• Creating a diet that incorporates heart-healthy foods to improve health

• Recognizing that failure to comply with the therapeutic regime places the patient's life at risk
• Managing activity to one's best capacity
• Adhering to instructions regarding dietary and alcohol consumption prior to the laboratory draw
• Demonstrating an understanding of the disease process and causative factors; the patient commits to alterations in lifestyle that will decrease risk factors

Troponins I and T

Quick Summary

SYNONYM ACRONYM: Cardiac troponin, cardiac troponin I (cTnI), cardiac troponin T (cTnT).

COMMON USE: To assist in evaluating myocardial muscle damage related to disorders such as myocardial infarction.

SPECIMEN: Serum collected in a gold-, red-, or red/gray-top tube. Plasma collected in a green-top (heparin) tube is also acceptable. Serial sampling is highly recommended. Care must be taken to use the same type of collection container if serial measurements are to be taken.

NORMAL FINDINGS: (Method: Enzyme immunoassay)

Age	Conventional & SI Units
Troponin I	Less than 4.8 ng/mL
0–30 days	Less than 4.8 ng/mL
1–3 mo	Less than 0.4 ng/mL
3–6 mo	Less than 0.3 ng/mL
7–12 mo	Less than 0.2 ng/mL
1–18 yr	Less than 0.1 ng/mL
Adult	Less than 0.05 ng/mL
Troponin T	Less than 0.2 ng/mL

Normal values can vary significantly due to differences in test kit reagents and instrumentation. The testing laboratory should be consulted for comparison of results to the corresponding reference range.

Test Explanation

Troponin is a complex of three contractile proteins that regulate the interaction of actin and myosin. Troponin C is the calcium-binding subunit; it does not have a cardiac muscle–specific subunit. Troponin I and troponin T, however, do have cardiac muscle–specific subunits. They are detectable a few hours to 7 days after the onset of symptoms of myocardial damage. Troponin I is thought to be a more specific marker of cardiac damage than troponin T. Cardiac troponin I begins to rise 2 to 6 hours after myocardial infarction (MI). It has a biphasic peak: It initially peaks at 15 to 24 hours after MI and then exhibits a lower peak after 60 to 80 hours. Cardiac troponin T levels rise 2 to 6 hours after MI and

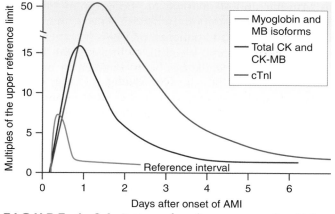

FIGURE 1.24 Pattern of cardiac enzymes after AMI

remain elevated. Both proteins return to the reference range 7 days after MI (see Fig. 1.24).

Timing for Appearance and Resolution of Serum/Plasma Cardiac Markers in Acute MI

Cardiac Marker	Appearance (hr)	Peak (hr)	Resolution (days)
AST	6–8	24–48	3–4
CK (total)	4–6	24	2–3
CK-MB	4–6	15–20	2–3
LDH	12	24–48	10–14
Myoglobin	1–3	4–12	1
Troponin I	2–6	15–20	5–7

AST = aspartate aminotransferase; CK = creatine kinase; CK-MB = creatine kinase MB fraction; LDH = lactate dehydrogenase.

Nursing Implications

Assessment

Indications	Potential Nursing Problems
Assist in establishing a diagnosis of MI Evaluate myocardial cell damage	• Activity *(related to the derivation of oxygen to heart muscle)* • Fear *(related to a potential loss of life)* • Health Management *(related to failure to actively participate in positive health choices)* • Human Response • Pain *(related to the deprivation of oxygen and nutrients to heart muscle)* • Tissue Perfusion *(related to ineffective circulation to the heart)*

Diagnosis: Clinical Significance of Test Results
INCREASED IN
Conditions that result in cardiac tissue damage; troponin is released from damaged tissue into the circulation.

- Acute MI
- Minor myocardial damage
- Myocardial damage after coronary artery bypass graft surgery or percutaneous transluminal coronary angioplasty
- Unstable angina pectoris

DECREASED IN
N/A

Planning
Considerations for planning a successful partnership should include clear communication of what to expect during the test to decrease anxiety and improve cooperation. Before the procedure is performed, plan to review the steps with the patient. Inform the patient that a number of samples will be collected. Collection at time of admission, 2 to 4 hours, 6 to 8 hours, and 12 hours after admission are the minimal recommendations. Additional samples may be requested. Address concerns about pain, and explain that there may be some discomfort during the venipuncture.

SPECIAL CONSIDERATIONS
An important aspect of planning is understanding the factors that may alter the study findings or cause abnormal results. Interdepartmental communication is a key factor in the planning process.

Implementation
Patient education is key to obtaining the patient's cooperation in following directions, and providing an explanation for the purpose of the procedure is an important part of this process. Inform the patient that this study can assist in evaluating heart damage. Perform the venipuncture.

Evaluation
Recognize anxiety related to test results, and be supportive of fear of a shortened life expectancy. Discuss the implications of abnormal test results on the patient's lifestyle. Provide teaching and information regarding the clinical implications of the test results as appropriate. Educate the patient regarding access to counseling services. Provide contact information, if desired, for the American Heart Association (AHA) (www.americanheart.org) or the National Heart, Lung, and Blood Institute (NHLBI) (www.nhlbi.nih.gov).

SPECIAL CONSIDERATIONS
Numerous studies point to the prevalence of excess body weight in American children and adolescents. Experts estimate that obesity is present in 25% of the population ages 6 to 11 years. The medical, social, and emotional consequences of excess body weight are significant. Special attention should be given to instructing the child and caregiver regarding health risks and weight-control education.

NUTRITIONAL CONSIDERATIONS FOR THE CARDIAC PATIENT: Increases in troponin levels may be associated with coronary artery disease (CAD). Nutritional therapy is recommended for the patient identified to be at risk for developing CAD or for individuals who have specific risk factors and/or existing medical conditions (e.g., elevated LDL cholesterol levels, other lipid disorders, insulin-dependent diabetes, insulin resistance, or metabolic syndrome). Other changeable risk factors warranting patient education include strategies to encourage patients, especially those who are overweight and with high blood pressure, to safely decrease sodium intake, achieve a normal weight, ensure regular participation of moderate aerobic physical activity three to four times per week, eliminate tobacco use, and adhere to a heart-healthy diet. If triglycerides also are elevated, the patient should be advised to eliminate or reduce alcohol. The Guideline on Lifestyle Management to Reduce Cardiovascular Risk published by the American College of Cardiology (ACC) and AHA in conjunction with the NHLBI recommends a "Mediterranean"-style diet rather than a low-fat diet. The guideline emphasizes inclusion of vegetables, whole grains, fruits, low-fat dairy, nuts, legumes, and nontropical vegetable oils (e.g., olive, canola, peanut, sunflower, flaxseed) along with fish and lean poultry. A similar dietary pattern known as the Dietary Approaches to Stop Hypertension (DASH) diet makes additional recommendations for the reduction of dietary sodium. Both dietary styles emphasize a reduction in consumption of red meats, which are high in saturated fats and cholesterol, and other foods containing sugar, saturated fats, trans fats, and sodium.

⊘ Critical Findings

N/A

⊘ Study Specific Complications

There are a number of complications associated with performing a venipuncture. **Pain** is commonly associated with needles, and although the pain experienced during venipuncture is usually mild, on a rare occasion the needle may strike a nerve causing permanent pain. Some patients experience a **vasovagal reaction** during the venipuncture procedure, evidenced by sweating, low blood pressure, fainting, or near fainting. The potential for a **fall injury** is a significant concern related to vasovagal reactions. Prolonged **bleeding** is a complication that occurs with patients who are taking blood thinners or who have coagulopathies such as hemophilia. A **hematoma** results when blood leaks into the tissue during or after a venipuncture, as evidenced by pain, bruising, and/or swelling at the venipuncture site. The swelling can cause injury by compression to surrounding nerves, which can be temporary or permanent. HCPs should watch for minor complications such

as bruising and hematoma at the venipuncture site, which are fairly common. Hematomas occur more often in older adult or frail patients, or those with veins that are difficult to access. Bleeding or bruising can be prevented once the needle has been removed by applying direct pressure to the site with dry gauze for a minute or two. Some other more unusual complications of venipuncture include **cellulitis, phlebitis, inadvertent arterial puncture,** and **sepsis.** Sepsis can be caused by introduction of bacteria from the surface of the skin into the blood as the result of improper cleansing of the venipuncture site. Immunocompromised patients are at higher risk for developing this complication.

⊘ Related Tests

- Related tests include antidysrhythmic drugs, apolipoprotein A and B, AST, ANP, blood gases, blood pool imaging, BNP, calcium, ionized calcium, cholesterol (total, HDL, and LDL), CRP, CT cardiac scoring, CK and isoenzymes, culture viral, echocardiography, echocardiography transesophageal, ECG, exercise stress test, glucose, glycated hemoglobin, Holter monitor, homocysteine, ketones, LDH and isoenzymes, lipoprotein electrophoresis, magnesium, MRI chest, MI infarct scan, myocardial perfusion heart scan, myoglobin, pericardial fluid analysis, PET heart, potassium, and triglycerides.
- Refer to the Cardiovascular System table at the end of the book for related tests by body system.

Expected Outcomes

Expected outcomes associated with Troponin are:

- Having heart rate and blood pressure return to normal limits as defined by the baseline assessment
- Ambulating in the room without shortness of breath or chest pain
- Expressing a desire to participate in education associated with changing personal choices to better protect overall health
- Demonstrating an understanding of the disease and being compliant with lifestyle changes that reduce risk factors
- Verbalizing an absence of pain and being compliant with the medication regimen

Urea Nitrogen, Blood

Quick Summary

SYNONYM ACRONYM: BUN.

COMMON USE: To assist in assessing for renal function toward diagnosing disorders such as kidney failure and dehydration. Also used in monitoring the effectiveness of therapeutic interventions such as hemodialysis.

SPECIMEN: Serum collected in a gold-, red-, or red/gray-top tube. Plasma collected in a green-top (heparin) tube is also acceptable.

NORMAL FINDINGS: (Method: Spectrophotometry)

Age	Conventional Units	SI Units (Conventional Units × 0.357)
Newborn–3 yr	5–17 mg/dL	1.8–6.1 mmol/L
4–13 yr	7–17 mg/dL	2.5–6.1 mmol/L
14 yr–adult	8–21 mg/dL	2.9–7.5 mmol/L
Adult older than 90 yr	10–31 mg/dL	3.6–11.1 mmol/L

Test Explanation

Unlike fats and carbohydrates, protein cannot be stored by the body. The amino acids and nitrogen used to make proteins are either obtained from dietary sources or from the normal turnover of aging cells in the body. Urea is a nonprotein nitrogen (NPN) compound formed in the liver from ammonia and excreted by the kidneys as an end product of protein metabolism. Other NPN compounds excreted by the kidneys include uric acid and creatinine. Blood urea nitrogen (BUN) levels reflect the balance between the amount of nitrogen ingested and excreted which is a representation of overall protein metabolism. BUN and creatinine values are commonly evaluated together. The normal BUN/creatinine ratio is 15:1 to 24:1. (e.g., if a patient has a BUN of 15 mg/dL, the creatinine should be approximately 0.6 to 1 mg/dL). BUN is used in the following calculation to estimate serum osmolality: $(2 \times Na^+) + (glucose/18) + (BUN/2.8)$.

Nursing Implications

Assessment

Indications	Potential Nursing Problems
Assess nutritional support Evaluate hemodialysis therapy Evaluate hydration Evaluate liver function Evaluate patients with lymphoma after chemotherapy (tumor lysis) Evaluate renal function Monitor the effects of drugs known to be nephrotoxic or hepatotoxic	• Cardiac Output • Electrolytes *(alterations associated with renal and liver function degradation)* • Fluid Volume • Gas Exchange • Gastrointestinal *(related to constipation due to dehydration or fluid restriction)* • Human Response • Injury Risk *(related to fatigue and anemia due to the insufficient renal production of erythropoietin)* • Liver *(functional degradation related to the toxic effects of drugs)* • Nutrition *(related to possible restrictions in protein and some electrolytes)*

Indications	Potential Nursing Problems
	• Protection • Skin *(related to skin breakdown due to uremia)* • Urination *(functional degradation of the kidneys related to the toxic effects of drugs)*

Diagnosis: Clinical Significance of Test Results
INCREASED IN
- Acute kidney injury *(related to decreased renal excretion)*
- Chronic glomerulonephritis *(related to decreased renal excretion)*
- Decreased renal perfusion *(reflects decreased renal excretion and increased blood levels)*
- Diabetes *(related to decreased renal excretion)*
- Excessive protein ingestion *(related to increased protein metabolism)*
- Gastrointestinal (GI) bleeding *(excessive blood protein in the GI tract and increased protein metabolism)*
- Heart failure *(related to decreased blood flow to the kidneys, decreased renal excretion, and accumulation in circulating blood)*
- Hyperalimentation *(related to increased protein metabolism)*
- Hypovolemia *(related to decreased blood flow to the kidneys, decreased renal excretion, and accumulation in circulating blood)*
- Ketoacidosis *(dehydration from ketoacidosis correlates with decreased renal excretion of urea nitrogen)*
- Muscle wasting from starvation *(related to increased protein metabolism)*
- Neoplasms *(related to increased protein metabolism or to decreased renal excretion)*
- Nephrotoxic agents *(related to decreased renal excretion and accumulation in circulating blood)*
- Pyelonephritis *(related to decreased renal excretion)*
- Shock *(related to decreased blood flow to the kidneys, decreased renal excretion, and accumulation in circulating blood)*
- Urinary tract obstruction *(related to decreased renal excretion and accumulation in circulating blood)*

DECREASED IN
- Inadequate dietary protein *(urea nitrogen is a by-product of protein metabolism; less available protein is reflected in decreased BUN levels)*
- Low-protein/high-carbohydrate diet *(urea nitrogen is a by-product of protein metabolism; less available protein is reflected in decreased BUN levels)*
- Malabsorption syndromes *(urea nitrogen is a by-product of protein metabolism; less available protein is reflected in decreased BUN levels)*

- Pregnancy
- Severe liver disease *(BUN is synthesized in the liver, so liver damage results in decreased levels)*

Planning

Considerations for planning a successful partnership should include clear communication of what to expect during the test to decrease anxiety and improve cooperation. Before the procedure is performed, plan to review the steps with the patient. Address concerns about pain, and explain that there may be some discomfort during the venipuncture.

SPECIAL CONSIDERATIONS

An important aspect of planning is understanding the factors that may alter the study findings or cause abnormal results. Interdepartmental communication is a key factor in the planning process.

It is also important to understand which medications or substances the patient may be exposed to in the health-care setting that can interfere with accurate testing:

- Drugs, substances, and vitamins that may increase BUN levels include acetaminophen, alanine, aldatense, alkaline antacids, amphotericin B, antimony compounds, arsenicals, bacitracin, bismuth subsalicylate, capreomycin, carbenoxolone, carbutamide, cephalosporins, chloral hydrate, chloramphenicol, chlorthalidone, colistimethate, colistin, cotrimoxazole, dexamethasone, dextran, diclofenac, doxycycline, ethylene glycol, gentamicin, guanethidine, guanoxan, ibuprofen, ifosfamide, ipodate, kanamycin, mephenesin, metolazone, mitomycin, neomycin, phosphorus, plicamycin, tertatolol, tetracycline, triamterene, triethylenemelamine, viomycin, and vitamin D.
- Drugs that may decrease BUN levels include acetohydroxamic acid, chloramphenicol, fluorides, paramethasone, phenothiazine, and streptomycin.

Implementation

Patient education is key to obtaining the patient's cooperation in following directions, and providing an explanation for the purpose of the procedure is an important part of this process. Inform the patient this study can assist in assessing kidney function. Perform the venipuncture.

Evaluation

Recognize anxiety related to test results and be supportive of impaired activity related to fear of a shortened life expectancy. Discuss the implications of abnormal test results on the patient's lifestyle. Provide teaching and information regarding the clinical implications of the test results as appropriate. Educate the patient regarding access to counseling services. Help the patient cope with long-term implications. Recognize that anticipatory anxiety and grief related to potential lifestyle changes may be expressed when someone is faced with a chronic disorder. Provide contact information, if desired, for the National Kidney Foundation (www.kidney.org) or the National Kidney Disease Education Program (www.nkdep.nih.gov).

NUTRITIONAL CONSIDERATIONS: Increased BUN levels may be associated with kidney disease. The nutritional needs of patients with kidney disease vary widely and are in constant flux. Anorexia, nausea, and vomiting commonly occur, prompting the need for continuous monitoring for malnutrition, especially among patients receiving long-term hemodialysis therapy.

Critical Findings

Adults

- Greater than 100 mg/dL (SI: Greater than 35.7 mmol/L) (nondialysis patients)

Children

- Greater than 55 mg/dL (SI: Greater than 19.6 mmol/L) (nondialysis patients)

Consideration may be given to verification of critical findings before action is taken. Policies vary among facilities and may include requesting immediate recollection and retesting by the laboratory or retesting using a rapid Point of Care testing instrument at the bedside, if available.

Note and immediately report to the requesting health-care provider (HCP) any critical findings and related symptoms. A listing of these findings varies among facilities.

A patient with a grossly elevated BUN may have signs and symptoms including acidemia, agitation, confusion, fatigue, nausea, vomiting, and coma. Possible interventions include treatment of the cause, administration of IV bicarbonate, a low-protein diet, hemodialysis, and caution with respect to prescribing and continuing nephrotoxic medications.

Study Specific Complications

There are a number of complications associated with performing a venipuncture. **Pain** is commonly associated with needles, and although the pain experienced during venipuncture is usually mild, on a rare occasion the needle may strike a nerve causing permanent pain. Some patients experience a **vasovagal reaction** during the venipuncture procedure, evidenced by sweating, low blood pressure, fainting, or near fainting. The potential for a **fall injury** is a significant concern related to vasovagal reactions. Prolonged **bleeding** is a complication that occurs with patients who are taking blood thinners or who have coagulopathies such as hemophilia. A **hematoma** results when blood leaks into the tissue during or after a venipuncture, as evidenced by pain, bruising, and/or swelling at the venipuncture site. The swelling can cause injury by compression to surrounding nerves, which can be temporary or permanent. HCPs should watch for minor complications such as bruising and hematoma at the venipuncture site, which are fairly common. Hematomas occur more often in older adult or frail patients, or those with veins that are difficult to access. Bleeding or bruising can be prevented once the needle has been removed by applying direct pressure to the site with dry gauze for a minute or two. Some other more unusual complications of venipuncture include **cellulitis, phlebitis, inadvertent arterial puncture,** and **sepsis.** Sepsis can be caused by introduction of bacteria from the surface of the skin into the blood as the result of improper cleansing of the venipuncture site. Immunocompromised patients are at higher risk for developing this complication.

✓ *Related Tests*

- Related tests include anion gap, antimicrobial drugs, biopsy kidney, calcium, calculus kidney stone panel, CT spleen, creatinine, creatinine clearance, cytology urine, cystoscopy, electrolytes, gallium scan, glucose, glycated hemoglobin, 5–HIAA, IVP, ketones, magnesium, MRI venography, microalbumin, osmolality, oxalate, phosphorus, protein total and fractions, renogram, US abdomen, US kidney, UA, urea nitrogen urine, and uric acid.
- Refer to the Genitourinary and Hepatobiliary systems tables at the end of the book for related tests by body system.

Expected Outcomes

Expected outcomes associated with Urea Nitrogen are:

- Having kidney function studies return to normal, with urinary elimination no less than 30 mL per hour
- Being compliant with dietary and fluid restrictions that will prevent further liver or kidney damage
- Verbalizing an understanding of the diagnosed renal or liver disease and being compliant with the recommended therapeutic regime
- Verbalizing an understanding of the need for stool softeners to assist with relief from constipation
- Participating in an active discussion of the available treatment options, and verbalizing an understanding of the impact to him- or herself as well as the patient's family if dialysis is chosen as an option to extend his or her life span
- Identifying coping strategies that can successfully assist in adjusting to the chronic nature of the patient's disease

Vitamin D

Quick Summary

SYNONYM ACRONYM: Cholecalciferol, vitamin D 1,25-dihydroxy.

COMMON USE: To assess vitamin D levels toward diagnosing disorders such as vitamin toxicity, malabsorption, and vitamin deficiency.

SPECIMEN: Serum collected in a red-top tube. Plasma collected in a green-top (heparin) tube is also acceptable.

NORMAL FINDINGS: (Method: High-performance liquid chromatography)

Form	Conventional Units	SI Units (Conventional Units × 2.496)
Vitamin D 25-hydroxy		
Deficient	Less than 20 ng/mL	Less than 49.9 nmol/L
Insufficient	20–30 ng/mL	49.9–74.9 nmol/L
Optimal	30–100 ng/mL	74.9–249.6 nmol/L
Possible toxicity	Greater than 150 ng/mL	Greater than 374.4 nmol/L
	Conventional Units	SI Units (Conventional Units × 2.496)
Vitamin D 1,25-dihydroxy	18–72 pg/mL	45–180 pmol/L

Test Explanation

Vitamin D is a group of interrelated sterols that have hormonal activity in multiple organs and tissues of the body, including the kidneys, liver, skin, and bones. There are two metabolically active forms of vitamin D: vitamin D 25-hydroxy and vitamin D 1,25-dihydroxy. Ergocalciferol (vitamin D_2) is formed when ergosterol in plants is exposed to sunlight. Ergocalciferol is absorbed by the stomach and intestine when orally ingested. Cholecalciferol (vitamin D_3) is formed when the skin is exposed to sunlight or ultraviolet light. Vitamins D_2 and D_3 enter the bloodstream after absorption. Vitamin D_3 is converted to vitamin D 25-hydroxy by the liver and is the major circulating form of the vitamin. Vitamin D_2 is converted to vitamin D 1,25-dihydroxy (calcitriol) by the kidneys and is the more biologically active form. Vitamin D acts with parathyroid hormone and calcitonin to regulate calcium metabolism and osteoblast function. The effects of vitamin D deficiency have been studied for many years, and continued research indicates a link between vitamin D deficiency and the development of diseases such as heart failure, stroke, hypertension, cancer, autism, multiple sclerosis, type 2 diabetes, systemic lupus erythematosus, depression, and immune function. The amount of vitamin D_3 produced by exposure of the skin to ultraviolet (UV) radiation depends on the intensity of the radiation as well as the duration of exposure. The use of lotions containing sun block significantly decreases production of vitamin D_3.

Nursing Implications

Assessment

Indications	Potential Nursing Problems
Consider differential diagnosis of disorders of calcium and phosphorus metabolism Evaluate deficiency or suspected toxicity Investigate bone diseases Investigate malabsorption	• Diarrhea • Fluid Volume • Health Maintenance • Human Response • Mobility • Nutrition • Pain

Diagnosis: Clinical Significance of Test Results

INCREASED IN
- Endogenous vitamin D intoxication *(in conditions such as sarcoidosis, cat scratch disease, and some lymphomas, extrarenal conversion of 25-hydroxy to 1,25-dihydroxy vitamin D occurs with a corresponding abnormal elevation of calcium)*
- Exogenous vitamin D intoxication

DECREASED IN
- Bowel resection *(related to lack of absorption)*
- Celiac disease *(related to lack of absorption)*
- Inflammatory bowel disease *(related to lack of absorption)*
- Malabsorption *(related to lack of absorption)*
- Osteomalacia *(related to dietary insufficiency)*
- Pancreatic insufficiency *(lack of digestive enzymes to metabolize fat-soluble vitamin D; malabsorption)*
- Rickets *(related to dietary insufficiency)*
- Thyrotoxicosis *(possibly related to increased calcium loss through sweat, urine, or feces with corresponding decrease in vitamin D levels)*

Planning

Considerations for planning a successful partnership should include clear communication of what to expect during the test to decrease anxiety and improve cooperation. Before the procedure is performed, plan to review the steps with the patient. Address concerns about pain, and explain that there may be some discomfort during the venipuncture.

SPECIAL CONSIDERATIONS

An important aspect of planning is understanding the factors that may alter the study findings or cause abnormal results. Interdepartmental communication is a key factor in the planning process.

It is also important to understand which medications or substances the patient may be exposed to in the health-care setting that can interfere with accurate testing:

- Drugs that may decrease vitamin D levels include cholestyramine, orlistat (a medication for weight loss), and phenytoin.

Implementation

Patient education is key to obtaining the patient's cooperation in following directions, and providing an explanation for the purpose of the procedure is an important part of this process. Inform the patient that this study can assist in diagnosing vitamin toxicity or deficiency. Perform the venipuncture.

Evaluation

Recognize anxiety related to test results, and educate the patient regarding access to nutritional counseling services. Provide contact information, if desired, for the Institute of Medicine of the National Academies (www.iom.edu).

NUTRITIONAL CONSIDERATIONS: Educate the patient with vitamin D deficiency, as appropriate, that the main dietary sources of vitamin D are fortified dairy foods and cod liver oil. Explain to the patient that vitamin D is also synthesized by the body and in the skin, and is activated by sunlight.

✓ Critical Findings

Note and immediately report to the requesting health-care provider (HCP) any critical findings and related symptoms. A listing of these findings varies among facilities.

Vitamin toxicity can be as significant as problems brought about by vitamin deficiencies. The potential for toxicity is especially important to consider with respect to fat-soluble vitamins, which are not eliminated from the body as quickly as water-soluble vitamins and can accumulate in the body. Most cases of toxicity are brought about by oversupplementing and can be avoided by consulting a qualified nutritionist for recommended daily dietary and supplemental allowances. Signs and symptoms of vitamin D toxicity include nausea, loss of appetite, vomiting, polyuria, muscle weakness, and constipation.

✓ Study Specific Complications

There are a number of complications associated with performing a venipuncture. **Pain** is commonly associated with needles, and although the pain experienced during venipuncture is usually mild, on a rare occasion the needle may strike a nerve causing permanent pain. Some patients experience a **vasovagal reaction** during the venipuncture procedure, evidenced by sweating, low blood pressure, fainting, or near fainting. The potential for a **fall injury** is a significant concern related to vasovagal reactions. Prolonged **bleeding** is a complication that occurs with patients who are taking blood thinners or who have coagulopathies such as hemophilia. A **hematoma** results when blood leaks into the tissue during or after a venipuncture, as evidenced by pain, bruising, and/or swelling at the venipuncture site. The swelling can cause injury by compression to surrounding nerves, which can be temporary or permanent. HCPs should watch for minor complications such as bruising and hematoma at the venipuncture site, which are fairly common. Hematomas occur more often in older adult or frail patients, or those with veins that are difficult to access. Bleeding or bruising can be prevented once the needle has been removed by applying direct pressure to the site with dry gauze for a minute or two. Some other more unusual complications of venipuncture include **cellulitis, phlebitis, inadvertent arterial puncture,** and **sepsis.** Sepsis can be caused by introduction of bacteria from the surface of the skin into the blood as the result of improper cleansing of the venipuncture site. Immunocompromised patients are at higher risk for developing this complication.

Related Tests

- Related tests include amylase, ANCA, biopsy intestinal, calcium, capsule endoscopy, colonoscopy, fecal analysis, fecal fat, antibodies gliadin antibodies, kidney stone panel, laparoscopy abdominal, lipase, osteocalcin, oxalate, phosphorus, and proctosigmoidoscopy.
- Refer to the Gastrointestinal and Musculoskeletal systems tables at the end of the book for related tests by body system.

Expected Outcomes

Expected outcomes associated with Vitamin D are:

- Being compliant with taking the vitamin D supplement
- Not having diarrhea
- Exploring health management strategies to identify contributors to the disease process, such as taking more supplement than is required for healthy living
- Understanding the importance of managing an adequate fluid intake with episodes of diarrhea to prevent dehydration

REVIEW OF LEARNING OUTCOMES

Thinking

1. The area of clinical chemistry covers many different types of studies. List seven categories of studies included in clinical chemistry and the main cellular functions they fulfill. Answer: Carbohydrates (energy), water and electrolytes (transportation and electrical conductivity), proteins and enzymes (structure and metabolic functions), cellular waste products (indicate a breakdown in health status when increased), lipids (energy and transportation), hormones (regulation), and vitamins and minerals (many are cofactors required for normal cellular production, maturation, and metabolism).
2. Diabetes is the most common endocrine disorder in the United States. List the two most common tests used in diagnosis and management. Answer: Glucose testing is used to identify diabetes. Glucose reflects short-term levels and glycated hemoglobin reflects glucose levels over the past 3 months; both

are used in the management of diabetes. Other tests are being developed to reflect glucose levels over shorter, intermediate time frames.
3. List two studies commonly used to evaluate kidney function. Answer: Blood urea nitrogen (BUN) and creatinine.

Doing

1. Name three complications of venipuncture the nurse should anticipate. Answer: Pain is commonly associated with needles, and although the pain experienced during venipuncture is usually mild, on a rare occasion the needle may strike a nerve, causing permanent pain. Some patients experience a vasovagal reaction during the venipuncture procedure, evidenced by sweating, low blood pressure, fainting, or near fainting. Prolonged bleeding is a complication that occurs with patients who are taking blood thinners or who have coagulopathies such as hemophilia. A hematoma results when blood leaks into the tissue during or after a venipuncture, as evidenced by pain, and bruising and/or swelling at the venipuncture site. The swelling can cause injury by compression to the surrounding nerves, which can be temporary or permanent. Some other more unusual complications of venipuncture include cellulitis, phlebitis, inadvertent arterial puncture, and sepsis. Sepsis can be caused by the introduction of bacteria from the surface of the skin into the blood as the result of improper cleansing of the venipuncture site.
2. Discuss the main safety risk the nurse should anticipate prior to venipuncture. Answer: The potential for a fall injury is a significant concern related to vasovagal reactions. This potential can be anticipated by obtaining a history of fainting or near-fainting prior to venipuncture.
3. Examine how the evaluation of a root cause analysis after a sentinel event can change practice. Answer: Sometimes it is the attention to details that makes an event safe or unsafe. When shortcuts are taken, the outcome can be devastating for the patient and the nurse. A root cause analysis is designed to look at the details of a sentinel event to discover causal factors. Causal factors can be process errors, human errors, or both. Taking the opportunity to be involved in this type of review can strengthen the sense of accountability and clarify the concept of do no harm.

Caring

1. Recognize the importance of the quality assurance process and evidence-based practice in the provision of care. Answer: Constant change is the new normal in nursing. Advancing technology in disease management is and will continue to

change how we use laboratory studies in conjunction with patient care. It is each individual nurse's responsibility to remain current with the changes in patient management as pertains to the use of laboratory studies. Examples are updated management for congestive heart failure and diabetes.

Words OF Wisdom: Blood studies are a common part of patient care used to diagnose multiple medical problems. As nurses, we use blood study results in patient care to correlate what we see (objective), what our patient says (subjective), and what is going on internally (laboratory results). This correlation provides direction to design care and factual evidence to determine the success of that plan. A simple analogy is infection. A septic patient will have an elevated white blood count. Collaborating with the healthcare provider (HCP) and administering antibiotics will help to resolve the sepsis. One piece of evidence that the sepsis is resolving is repeated white blood count study showing the level is decreasing. Conversely, continued elevated white blood count levels are evidence that the plan is not working. Trending the results over time can provide insight as to how quickly the infection is resolving or not. Remember that the blood study results are not just a number to be reported to the HCP but an indicator of patient progress and the success of the overall plan of care.

BIBLIOGRAPHY

Bilirubin. (n.d.). Retrieved from www.rnceus.com/lf/lfbili.html.

Cavanaugh, B. (2003). Nurse's manual of laboratory and diagnostic tests. (4th ed.). Philadelphia, PA: F.A. Davis Company.

Darlington, D., & Dallman, M. (Dec 19, 2011). Chapter 5: Feedback control in endocrine systems. Retrieved from www.medtextfree.wordpress.com/2011/12/19/chapter-5-feedback-control-in-endocrine-systems/.

Eckel, R., Jakicic, J., Ard, J., Hubbard, V., de Jesus, J., Lee, I., Lichtenstein, A., Loria, C., Millen, B., Houston Miller, N., Nonas, C., Sacks, F., Smith, S., Svetkey, L., Wadden, T., & Yanovski, S. (2013). 2013 AHA/ACC Guideline on Lifestyle Management to Reduce Cardiovascular Risk: A Report of the American College of Cardiology/American Heart Association Task Force on Practice Guidelines. Retrieved from whttp://circ.ahajournals.org/content/early/2013/11/01.cir.0000437740.48606.d1.full.pdf.

Electrolytes. (n.d.). Retrieved from www.medicinenet.com/electrolytes/article.htm.

Goff, D., Lloyd-Jones, D., Bennett, G., Coady, S., D'Agostino, R., Gibbons, R., Greenland, P., Lackland, D., Levy, D., O'Donnell, C., Robinson, J., Schwartz, J., Shero, S., Smith, S., Sorlie, P., Stone, N., & Wilson, P. (2013). 2013 ACC/AHA Guideline on the Assessment of Cardiovascular Risk: A Report of the American College of Cardiology/American Heart Association Task Force on Practice Guidelines. Retrieved from http://circ.ahajournals.org/content/early/2013/11/01.cir.0000437741.48606.98.full.pdf.

Gutiérrez-Preciado, A., Romero, H., & Peimbert, M. (2010). An evolutionary perspective on amino acids. Retrieved from www.nature.com/scitable/topicpage/an-evolutionary-perspective-on-amino-acids-14568445.

Hermann, J. (n.d.). Minerals and the body. Retrieved from www.fcs.okstate.edu/documents/nutrition/T-3164%20Minerals.pdf.

Introduction to human physiology. (n.d.). Retrieved from www.highered.mcgraw-hill.com/sites/dl/free/0073403490/578766/sample_chapter01.pdf.

Jensen, M., Ryan, D., Apovian, C., Ard, J., Comuzzie, A., Donato, K., Hu, F., Hubbard, V., Jakicic, J., Kushner, R., Loria, C., Millen, B., Nonas, C., Pi-Sunyer, F., Stevens, J., Stevens,V., Wadden, T., Wolfe, B., & Yanovski, S. (2013). 2013 AHA/ACC/TOS Guideline for the Management of Overweight and Obesity in Adults: A Report of the American College of Cardiology/American Heart Association Task Force on Practice Guidelines and The Obesity Society. Retrieved from http://circ.ahajournals.org/content/early/2013/11/11/01.cir.0000437739.71477.ee.

Lutz, C., & Przytulski, K. (2011). Nutrition and diet therapy. (5th ed.). Philadelphia, PA: F.A. Davis Company.

Mandal, A. Cholesterol physiology. (n.d.). Retrieved from www.news-medical.net/health/Cholesterol-Physiology.aspx.

Mayo Clinic staff. (October 13, 2012). Bilirubin. Retrieved from www.mayoclinic.com/health/bilirubin/MY00094.

Minerals. (n.d.). Retrieved from www.nlm.nih.gov/medlineplus/minerals.html.

Nutrition Care Systems. (n.d.). Hypoalbuminemia: Malnutrition versus inflammatory response. Retrieved from www.nutritioncaresystems.com/hypoalbuminemia-malnutrition-versus-inflammatory-response.

Ophardt, C. (2003). Fluid and electrolyte balance. Retrieved from http://elmhcx9.elmhurst.edu/~chm/vchembook/250fluidbal.html.

Popat, V. (2011). Gonadotropin-releasing hormone deficiency in adults. Retrieved from emedicine.medscape.com/article/255152-overview.

Sterols. (n.d.). Retrieved from www.encyclopedia2.thefreedictionary.com/Sterol.

Stone, N., Robinson, J., Lichtenstein, A., Bairey Merz, C., Blum, C., Eckel, R., Goldberg, A., Gordon, D., Levy, D., Lloyd-Jones, D., McBride, P., Schwartz, S., Shero, S., Smith, S., Watson, K., & Wilson, P. (2013). 2013 ACC/AHA Guideline on the Treatment of Blood Cholesterol to Reduce Atherosclerotic Cardiovascular Risk in Adults: A report of the American College of Cardiology/American Heart Association Task Force on Practice Guidelines. Retrieved from http://circ.ahajournals.org/content/early/2013/11/11/01.cir.0000437738.63853.7a.

Understanding the 2013 AHA Lipid guidelines. (2013). Retrieved from http://cardiologydoc.wordpress.com/2013/11/24/understanding-the-2013-aha-lipid-guidelines/.

Van Leeuwen, A., and Bladh, M. (2015). Davis's comprehensive handbook of laboratory and diagnostic tests with nursing implications. (6th ed.). Philadelphia, PA: F.A. Davis Company.

Vincent, J., Dubois, M., Navickis, R., & Wilkes, M. (2003). Hypoalbuminemia in acute illness: Is there a rationale for intervention? Retrieved from www.ncbi.nlm.nih.gov/pmc/articles/PMC1514323/.

Go to Section II of this book and http://www.davisplus.com for the Clinical Reasoning Tool and its case studies to provide you with a safe place to explore patient care situations. There are a total of 26 different case studies; 2 cases are presented for each of 13 body systems: One set of 13 cases are found in the Section II chapters, and a second set of 13 cases are available online at http://www.davisplus.com. Each case is designed with the specific goal of helping you to connect the dots of clinical reasoning. Cases are designed to reflect possible clinical scenarios; the outcomes may or may not be positive—you decide.

Blood Studies: Hematology

OVERVIEW

Hematology studies are in the area of medical science that examines the cellular components of blood, the organs that produce blood, and diseases of the blood, bone marrow, and lymphatic system. A number of studies from the other subsections found in this chapter will be mentioned to emphasize the interrelationships that exist between various types of blood studies. Blood volume as a percent of total body weight varies with a number of factors to include height, weight, degree of hydration, sex, and age. Circulating plasma and red blood cell (RBC) volumes can be estimated by injecting an artery with a dye, a radioisotope, or carbon dioxide gas in a procedure called *blood volume testing*. Knowing the circulating blood volume may be useful in situations in which the patient has experienced a traumatic acute loss of blood, would benefit from monitoring during extensive surgical procedures, or can be diagnosed with treatable conditions such as hypovolemia (low plasma volume), hypervolemia (high plasma volume), anemia (low RBC volume), or polycythemia (high RBC volume). RBC volume can also be used to evaluate therapies such as hemodialysis or precision volume blood product transfusion. Blood constitutes 6% to 8% of total body weight and is composed of a liquid portion (plasma) and a solid cellular portion (RBCs, white blood cells [WBCs], and platelets are the major circulating cell types). Males generally have a higher volume of blood than females at 6 L (12 pints) for males and 4.5 L (9 pints) for females. The average total blood volume is estimated at 70 mL/kg body weight (see Fig. 2.1). Plasma volume starts out lower in the newborn at about 40 to 46 mL/kg of body weight, increases rapidly during the first week of life to 52 mL/kg, levels out after the first year to 50 mL/kg, and after age 18 years reaches the adult range of 40 to 45 mL/kg. The

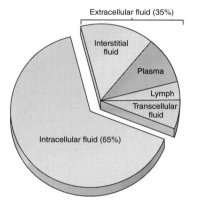

FIGURE 2.1 Plasma as a fraction of fluid volume. *Used with permission, from Thompson, G. (2013). Understanding anatomy & physiology. FA Davis Company.*

proportion of blood represented by the RBC fraction begins around 43 to 50 mL/kg at birth as reflected by a hematocrit (Hct) of 45% to 70% seen in normal newborns and infants during the first month of life. The Hct and corresponding RBC volume then decrease to much lower values in the range of 30% to 50% based on age and sex.

Blood has a number of different functions in the body:

- Its main role is the **transportation** of substances required for critical processes to their intended targets. Examples include the transport of oxygen to the lungs for respiration, and of enzymes, coenzymes, vitamins, minerals, other nutrients, and hormones to cells as required for metabolism. The transportation role also involves the movement of waste products for excretion, such as the carbon dioxide produced from respiration and the numerous by-products of cellular metabolism (see Fig. 2.2).

- A second role is **regulation**. The hypothalamus is a part of the brain that helps maintain homeostatic

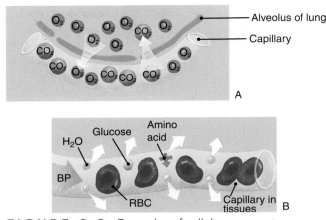

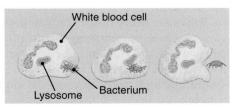

FIGURE 2.2 Examples of cellular transport mechanisms. (A) diffusion; (B) filtration. *Used with permission, from Scanlon, V. (2010). Essentials of anatomy and physiology (6th Ed.). FA Davis Company.*

control over a number of bodily functions that include a constant core body temperature of 37°C. Feedback from temperature sensors in the skin, mucous membranes, and internal structures results in regulatory responses. Blood participates in the regulation of body temperature. When the body is cold, one mechanism it uses to decrease heat loss is preventing the blood vessels from coming in close proximity to the skin's surface (vasoconstriction). The opposite occurs when the body is hot and vasodilation occurs: The blood vessels widen and come close to the skin surface. This allows heat from the warm blood to be lost through the skin by radiation. Blood also serves as an important buffer system to regulate pH or acid-base balance in the various body fluid compartments with which it comes into direct contact.

- A third role of blood is **protection**. Blood provides a defensive function by transporting antibodies and components of the body's cell-mediated defense system to the site of infection or inflammation, or to fight invasion by foreign elements (e.g., bacteria, viruses, parasites, toxins) (see Fig. 2.3). The ability of blood to form clots assists in the healing of wounds and prevents the loss of blood and fluids from the body.

Hematopoiesis is the process of blood cell formation that takes place in the liver, spleen, and bone marrow.

FIGURE 2.3 Phagocytosis. *Used with permission, from Scanlon, V. (2010). Essentials of anatomy and physiology (6th Ed.). FA Davis Company.*

The extramedullary formation of blood begins in the yolk sac, then continues in the liver and spleen of the developing embryo. In the newborn and in children, hematopoiesis occurs in the red marrow of all bones. In adults, hematopoiesis normally occurs in the red marrow of bones such as the sternum, ribs, vertebral bodies, pelvis, and proximal portions of the humerus and femur; the long bones contain relatively little red marrow. There are two types of bone marrow, red and yellow (see Fig. 2.4). Gradually, with age, red marrow is converted to yellow, and by adulthood the bones contain 5 to 6 pounds of marrow in approximately equal amounts of red and yellow. Yellow marrow can revert to the production of blood cells during times of severe stress on the hematopoietic system. Bone marrow is also an important part of the lymphatic system. There are two types of cells found in bone marrow: hematopoietic, which mainly produces blood cells, and stromal, which produces macrophages, plasma cells, reticular cells, and cells that form fat, cartilage, and bone. The pleuripotent hematopoietic stem cell is believed to be an undifferentiated stem cell from which

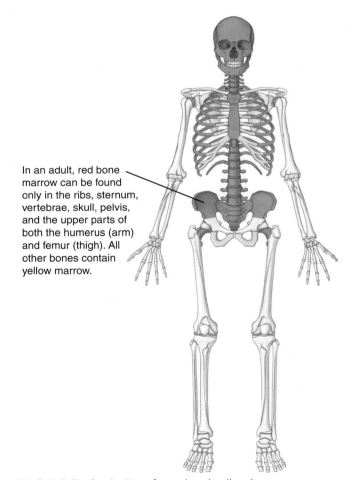

In an adult, red bone marrow can be found only in the ribs, sternum, vertebrae, skull, pelvis, and the upper parts of both the humerus (arm) and femur (thigh). All other bones contain yellow marrow.

FIGURE 2.4 Sites for red and yellow bone marrow formation *Used with permission, from Thompson, G. (2013). Understanding anatomy & physiology. FA Davis Company.*

all the different blood cell types are derived. Each cell line goes through a developmental process beginning with the most immature or "blast" stage in which hematopoietic stem cells form a specific clone or type of blood cells. Mature red blood cells and platelets do not have a nucleus; mature white blood cells are nucleated but none of the blood cell types are able to replicate on their own, so hematopoiesis is an ongoing process to replace old or damaged blood cells.

A complete blood count (CBC) includes automated (1) enumeration of the cellular elements of the blood; (2) assessment of cellular indices (RBC, WBC, and platelet) that provide information regarding cell age, size, and hemoglobin content; and (3) determination of cellular morphology regarding descriptions of RBC size, shape, color, or the presence of inclusions. Automated instruments have software that alerts the operator of suspicious results, which can be confirmed manually

Blood Cell Line	Least Mature Cell Type	→	→	→	→	Circulating Cell Type
RBC	Pronormoblast	Basophilic normoblast	Polychromatic normoblast	Orthochromic normoblast	Reticulocyte	Erythrocyte
Platelet	Megakaryoblast	Promegakaryocyte	Megakaryocyte	Metamegakaryocyte		Thrombocyte
Polysegmented WBC	Myeloblast	Promyelocyte	Eosinophilic Myelocyte	Eosinophilic Metamyelocyte		Eosinophil
Polysegmented WBC	Myeloblast	Promyelocyte	Neutrophilic Myelocyte	Neutrophilic Metamyelocyte	Band Neutrophil	Band Segmented Neutrophil
Polysegmented WBC	Myeloblast	Promyelocyte	Basophilic Myelocyte	Basophilic Metamyelocyte		Basophil
Monocytic WBC	Monoblast	Promonocyte				Monocyte
Lymphocytic WBC	Lymphoblast	Prolymphocyte				Lymphocyte
Plasma Cell	Plasmoblast	Proplasmocyte			Plasmocyte	

by review of a stained smear (see Fig. 2.5). Reference values for the elements in a CBC vary across the age continuum and by sex. For example, the developing neonate has a very high demand for oxygen. Therefore, the RBC count is also high. Also, in females, hemoglobin and hematocrit decrease when puberty begins, while the same measurements increase at puberty in males. The difference between females and males can be partially explained by menstrual blood loss in females and the effects of androgens in males.

RBCs contain hemoglobin (Hgb), which transports oxygen from the lungs for distribution to all cells in the body. Hgb is able to reversibly bind both oxygen and carbon dioxide. Carbon dioxide is a waste product of cellular metabolism, and while some of it is removed by hemoglobin, the majority of it is transported as dissolved bicarbonate in the RBCs and blood plasma. (For additional information about the relationship between the respiratory and renal components of the hemoglobin buffer system, see the chapter 14 pulmonary function study titled Blood Gases. Each Hgb molecule is made of two polypeptide alpha chains and two polypeptide beta chains. Each chain has an iron and a porphyrin-containing heme group in which oxygen binding

occurs and gives blood its characteristic red color. The chains of the Hgb tetramer are bound together by the forces of several types of chemical bonds, resulting in an almost spherically shaped molecule, many of which are contained in a single erythrocyte. After childhood, hematopoiesis normally occurs in the red marrow of the sternum, ribs, vertebral bodies, pelvis, and proximal portions of the humerus and femur. Marrow concentration in the posterior iliac crest, a common site for bone marrow biopsy, is about half red and half yellow marrow by age 50 years and declines by approximately 10% every 10 years after, such that the sternum, ribs, and vertebral bodies are the main sites for erythropoiesis, the production of RBCs, in older adults. Erythropoiesis normally occurs at a rate of about 2 million cells per second or 1.7 trillion cells per day. Copper, vitamin B_{12}, folate, iron, and vitamin E are essential to normal RBC formation, development, and the maintenance of membrane integrity. The mature RBC is a biconcave disk with an average life span of 120 days. The biconcave shape allows for an increased surface area upon which gas exchange will occur and allows the RBC membrane to be very flexible in adapting to the size and contours of the various blood vessel lumens through which it

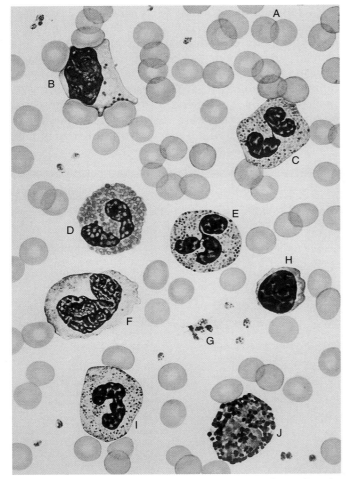

FIGURE 2.5 Cell types found in smears of peripheral blood from normal individuals. (A) Red blood cells (RBCs), (B) large lymphocyte, (C) segmented neutrophil, (D) eosinophil, (E) segmented neutrophil, (F) monocyte, (G) platelets, (H) small lymphocyte, (I) neutrophilic band, and (J) basophil. *Used with permission, from Harmening, D. (2008). Clinical hematology and fundamentals of hemostasis (5th Ed.). FA Davis Company.*

of the conjugated bilirubin is excreted into the stool and urine. Stercobilin gives stool its brown color and urobilin gives urine its yellow color. RBC production is related to the rate of RBC turnover and can also be stimulated in response to erythropoietin, a hormone produced and secreted by the kidneys when the level of renal tissue oxygenation decreases below an acceptable set point. There are numerous factors and conditions that affect normal erythropoiesis, such as blood loss, malnutrition, disorders of other organs (e.g., kidney disease or injury that results in deficient production of erythropoietin), acquired or inherited RBC enzyme defects that disturb metabolic function or cell membrane integrity, hemoglobinopathies (e.g., thalassemias, sickle cell), inflammatory conditions that affect the manner in which the cells are attracted to or repelled by each other, malignancies, bone marrow failure, and the effects of drugs, toxic chemicals, or ionizing radiation (see Fig. 2.6).

Leukopoiesis is the production of WBCs that occurs mainly in the hematopoietic or red bone marrow. The main types of WBCs in descending order of normal circulating levels are neutrophils (band and segmented neutrophils), lymphocytes, monocytes, eosinophils, and basophils. There are two types of lymphocytes: B-cell lymphocytes, which remain in the bone marrow to mature, and T-cell lymphocytes, which migrate to and mature in the thymus. WBCs are also classified as granular (neutrophils, eosinophils, and basophils) and agranular (monocytes and lymphocytes). Granular WBCs are also referred to as polymorphonuclear cells because their nucleus is lobed in segments. The main function of WBCs is to protect the body against foreign organisms, tissues, and other substances; as such the WBC count can change rapidly and significantly in response to various stimuli. Each WBC cell has a unique and specific method for defending the body. WBC production varies diurnally with counts being lowest in the morning and highest in the late afternoon; thus, the time of collection should be taken into consideration when reviewing or comparing WBC counts. Counts also vary with age and are influenced by nonpathological factors such as stress and high levels of physical activity (e.g., a woman in childbirth or an actively crying infant). The life span of a normal WBC is 13 to 20 days. Old WBCs are destroyed by the lymphatic system and excreted in the feces.

Leukocytosis reflects an increase in the WBC count; leukopenia reflects a decrease in the WBC count. An increase in the WBC count usually occurs in a single cell type rather than by a proportional increase in all WBC types. Bandemia is defined by the presence of greater than 10% band neutrophils in the total WBC population. Neutrophils are the body's first line of defense through the process of phagocytosis or engulfment of the foreign element. Granules in the cytoplasm of neutrophils contain enzymes and pyogens

must travel. The spleen removes old or damaged RBCs from circulation. When the RBCs are destroyed, the cellular contents, mainly iron, are recycled.

The human body contains between 4 and 5 grams of iron, about 65% of which is present in hemoglobin and 3% of which is present in myoglobin, the oxygen storage protein found in skeletal and cardiac muscle. During the process of RBC turnover, iron is carried by its specific transport protein, transferrin, back to the red marrow to be used by developing RBCs. Excess iron is stored in the liver and spleen as ferritin and hemosiderin. The breakdown of heme results in the production of bilirubin, which is carried to the liver, is conjugated with glucuronic acid to make it water soluble, is excreted in bile, and is stored in the gallbladder. A portion

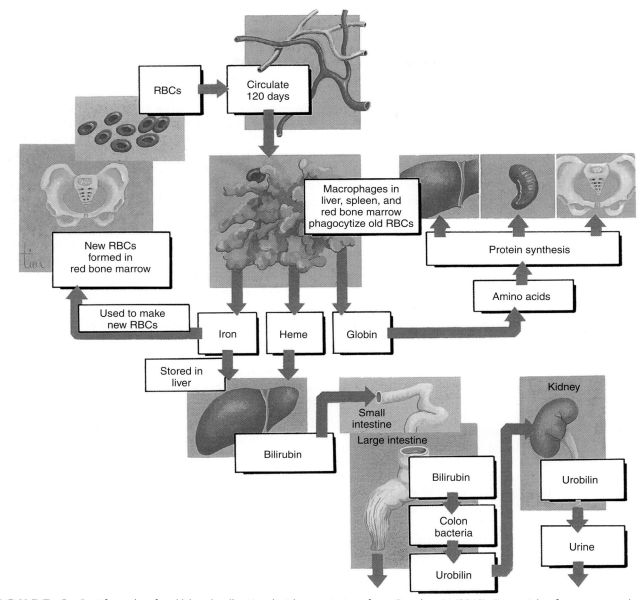

FIGURE 2.6 Life cycle of red blood cells. *Used with permission, from Scanlon, V. (2010). Essentials of anatomy and physiology (6th Ed.). FA Davis Company.*

that destroy invading microorganisms. The life span of neutrophils is relatively short and averages 5 to 6 days in the circulating blood. Lymphocytes are smaller than granulocytes and also play a major role in the body's natural defense system. The B-lymphocytes differentiate into immunoglobulin-synthesizing plasma cells.

There are five classes of immunoglobulins: G, M, A, D, and E. Some immunoglobulin classes have a number of subclasses. All types of immunoglobulins have specificity for their targets and carry out their protective functions by binding to the targets in a manner that fatally disables the toxin's chemical action or prevents an organism from causing infection. The T-lymphocytes function as cellular mediators of immunity and

include helper/inducer (CD4) lymphocytes, delayed hypersensitivity lymphocytes, cytotoxic (CD8 or CD4) lymphocytes, and suppressor (CD8) lymphocytes. The T-lymphocyte cells interact directly with the invading element. The major function of monocytes is phagocytosis. Monocytes provide protection as they circulate in the peripheral blood for about 1 to 5 days, after which they migrate into the tissues and develop into macrophages, a type of phagocytic tissue cell. Eosinophils are another type of specialized cell of the immune system normally found in small numbers in the circulating blood, with the majority normally residing in the tissues of the lungs and gastrointestinal tract. They have a variety of functions that are known and some that have not yet been well established. Eosinophils move to areas of established inflammation, responding to allergic and parasitic diseases. They have granules that contain histamine, which is used to kill foreign cells in the body, and proteolytic enzymes that damage parasitic worms. The granules break open when the cells are activated and sometimes do damage to the body as the contents of the granules do not distinguish between foreign proteins and a person's own cells. Once the cells are activated, they circulate for 8 to 12 hours before arriving at the target location, where they then remain for 1 to 2 weeks. Basophils are the least understood of the WBC types. They are found in small numbers in the circulating blood for 10 to 15 days after which they migrate into the tissue and develop into mast cells. They have a phagocytic function and, similar to eosinophils, contain numerous specific granules that contain heparin, which prevents blood from clotting too quickly, histamines that dilate blood vessels and blood flow to tissues, and proteolytic enzymes that damage the proteins of invaders.

Thrombopoiesis is the production of thrombocytes or platelets. Mature platelets are nonnucleated, round- or oval-shaped disks, formed by budding off larger multinucleated cells called megakaryocytes in the bone marrow. Approximately 70% of the platelets produced by the bone marrow circulate in the blood, surviving 8 to 10 days once released from the bone marrow. The spleen removes old or damaged platelets from circulation and holds in reserve the remaining 30% of mature platelets. Generally, platelet production is stimulated by an increased need for platelets either through hemostasis or bone marrow stimulation. Decreased platelet counts occur whenever a condition results in decreased production or increased consumption or destruction. The main function of platelets is to prevent bleeding when there has been trauma to a blood vessel wall. A more detailed discussion of platelet function is available in the hemostasis subsection.

Many disorders of the hematopoietic system do not present with obvious signs and symptoms. Correct diagnosis often requires laboratory testing to provide scientific data that correlate with a clinical condition. Therefore, it is important to listen carefully to the patient's complaints and to ask questions that may provide more information regarding symptoms and a more thorough assessment. Some common questions to obtain information regarding the patient's current and past history might include

- Have you ever had any problems with your blood—like anemia or cancers such as leukemia? *The patient's ability to recall past medical issues relating to the hematopoietic system can be a very helpful baseline in determining which studies should be used to provide further information.*

- Do you feel fatigued? *One of the hallmarks of anemia is fatigue due to a decreased RBC count and the ensuing ramifications that occur when there is an insufficient number of RBCs to support the normal functions of the body.*
- Have you been getting sick or having fevers more often than usual? *Conditions such as leukemia or chronic infections may be implicated by general symptoms reflected by compromised immune function.*
- Have you had your spleen removed? Have you had any surgeries of your gastrointestinal system? *Surgical manipulation of the components of the hematopoietic system can affect their normal function for a period of time. There are many examples of how other conditions can affect the hematopoietic system. Some examples include the effect of kidney disease on erythropoietin levels and the effect of gastrointestinal disease or surgery on the absorption of iron and vitamins that are essential to RBC formation and maturation.*
- Have any of your family members been diagnosed with any type of anemia (iron deficient, thalessemia, or sickle cell) or other blood disease? *A number of hematologic disorders can be inherited, so obtaining a family history of disease is an important area of discussion.*

Traditional risk factors such as smoking, poor diet, excessive alcohol consumption, and a lack of physical exercise have a very negative effect on the hematopoietic system, and health issues with other organs can have a negative impact on the hematopietic system.

DISCUSSION POINT
Hematology tests have some common factors that may impair the procedure or cause abnormal results:

- Review the results from other studies to help identify potentially confounding information. For example, a hematocrit level greater than 55% may affect results because of anticoagulant excess relative to plasma volume. Having this information in advance provides the opportunity, using established guidelines, to adjust the volume of anticoagulant in the tube prior to specimen collection, thus avoiding a potentially erroneous finding.
- Be aware that specimen collection technique has a significant impact on the validity of test results. Placement of the tourniquet for longer than 1 minute can result in venous stasis and changes in the results. Hgb and Hct levels can be falsely increased by 2% to 5%. RBC and WBC counts are also falsely increased due to venous stasis. Vascular injury caused during the venipuncture procedure can cause erroneous results (e.g., Hgb, Hct, RBC, and erythrocyte sedimentation rate [ESR] levels may be falsely decreased). Evidence of this type of interference is

evident in hemolyzed specimens, which must be rejected for analysis.

- Note that specimen collection above an IV infusion could result in falsely decreased values due to hemodilution.
- Reject specimens for analysis if there are incompletely filled collection tubes, inadequately mixed specimens, or clotted specimens.
- For CBC studies, obtain an EDTA Microtainer sample from infants, children, and adults for whom venipuncture may not be feasible. The specimen should be mixed gently by inverting the tube 10 times. The specimen should be analyzed within 24 hours when stored at room temperature or within 48 hours if stored at refrigerated temperature. If it is anticipated the specimen will not be analyzed within 24 hours, two blood smears should be made immediately after the venipuncture and submitted with the blood sample. Smears made from specimens older than 24 hours will contain an unacceptable number of misleading artifactual abnormalities of the RBCs, such as echinocytes and spherocytes, as well as necrobiotic WBCs.

The information in the Part I studies is organized in a manner to help the student see how the five basic components of the nursing process (assessment, diagnosis, planning, implementation, and evaluation) can be applied to each phase of laboratory and diagnostic testing. The goal is to use nursing process to understand the integration of care (laboratory, diagnostic, nursing care) toward achieving a positive expected outcome.

- **Assessment** is the collection of information for the purpose of answering the question, "is there a problem?" Knowledge of the patient's health history, medications, complaints, and allergies, as well as synonyms or alternate test names, common use for the procedure, specimen requirements, and normal ranges or interpretive comments provide the foundation for diagnosis.
- **Diagnosis** is the process of looking at the information gathered during assessment and answering the questions, "what is the problem?" and "what do I need to do about it?" Test indications tell us why the study has been requested, and potential diagnoses tell us the value or importance of the study relative to its clinical utility.
- **Planning** is a blueprint of the nursing care before the procedure. It is the process of determining how the nurse is going to partner with the patient to fix the problem (e.g., "The patient has a study ordered and this is what I should know before I successfully carry out the plan to have the study completed"). Knowledge of interfering factors, social and cultural issues,

preprocedural restrictions, the need for written and informed consent, anxiety about the procedure, and concerns regarding pain are some considerations for planning a successful partnership.

- **Implementation** is putting the plan into action with an idea of what the expected outcome should be. Collaboration with the departments where the laboratory test or diagnostic study is to be performed is essential to the success of the plan. Implementation is where the work is done within each health-care team member's scope of practice.
- **Evaluation** answers the question, "did the plan work or not?" Was the plan completely successful, partially successful, or not successful? If the plan did not work, evaluation is the process used to determine what needs to be changed to make the plan work better. This includes a review of all expected outcomes. Nursing care after the procedure is where information is gathered to evaluate the plan. Review of results, including critical findings, in relation to patient symptoms and other tests performed, provides data that form a more complete picture of health or illness.
- **Expected outcomes** are positive outcomes related to the test. They are the outcomes the nurse should expect if all goes well.

A number of pretest, intratest, and post-test universal points are presented in this overview section because the information applies to hematologic blood studies in general.

Universal Pretest Pearls (Planning)

- Obtain a history of the patient's complaints, including a list of known allergens, especially allergies or sensitivities to medications or latex so their use can be avoided or their effects mitigated if an allergy is present. Carefully evaluate all medications currently being taken by the patient. A list of the patient's current medications, prescribed and over the counter (including anticoagulants, aspirin and other salicylates, and dietary supplements), should also be obtained. Such products may be discontinued by medical direction for the appropriate number of days prior to the procedure. Ensure that all allergies are clearly noted in the medical record, and ensure that the patient is wearing an allergy and medical record armband. Report information that could interfere with, or delay proceeding with, the study to the health-care provider (HCP) and laboratory.
- Obtain a history of the patient's affected body system, symptoms, and results of previously performed laboratory tests and diagnostic and surgical

procedures. Previous test results will provide a basis of comparison between old and new data.

- An important aspect of planning is understanding the factors that may alter study findings or cause abnormal results. Interdepartmental communication is a key factor in the planning process. The inability of a patient to cooperate or remain still during the procedure because of age, significant pain, or mental status should be among the anticipated factors. Recent or past procedures, medications, or existing medical conditions that could complicate or interfere with test results should be noted.
- Review the steps of the study with the patient or caregiver. Expect patients to be nervous about the procedure and the pending results. Educating the patient about his or her role during the procedure and what to expect can facilitate this. The patient's role during the procedure is to remain still. The actual time required to complete each study will depend on a number of conditions, including the type of equipment being used and how well a patient will cooperate.
- Explain that specimen collection by venipuncture takes approximately 5 to 10 minutes. Bleeding or bruising can be prevented, once the needle has been removed, by applying direct pressure to the venipuncture site with dry gauze for a minute or two. The site should be observed/assessed for bleeding or hematoma formation, and then covered with a gauze and an adhesive bandage.
- Address any concerns about pain, and explain or describe, as appropriate, the level and type of discomfort that may be expected. Advise the patient that some discomfort may be experienced during the venipuncture.
- Provide additional instructions and patient preparation regarding medication, diet, fluid intake, or activity, if appropriate. Unless specified in the individual study, there are no special instructions or restrictions.
- Always be sensitive to any cultural or psychosocial issues, including a concern for modesty before, during, and after the procedure.

Reminder

Ensure that a written and informed consent has been documented in the medical record prior to the study, if required. The consent must be obtained before medication is administered.

Universal Intratest Pearls (Implementation)

- Correct patient identification is crucial prior to any procedure. Positively identify the patient using two unique identifiers such as patient name, date

of birth, Social Security number, or medical record number.

- Standard Precautions must be followed.
- Children and infants may be accompanied by a parent to calm them. Keep neonates and infants covered and in a warm room and provide a pacifier or gentle touch. The testing environment should be quiet, and the patient should be instructed, as appropriate, to remain still during the test as extraneous movements can affect results.
- Ensure that the patient has complied with pretesting instructions, including dietary, fluid, medication, and activity restrictions as given for the procedure.
- Before leaving the patient's side, appropriate specimen containers should always be labeled with the corresponding patient demographics, initials of the person collecting the sample, collection date, time of collection, and applicable special notes, especially site location and laterality if appropriate and then promptly transported to the laboratory for processing and analysis.

Universal Post Test Pearls (Evaluation)

- Note that completed test results are made available to the requesting HCP who will discuss them with the patient.
- Answer questions and address concerns voiced by the patient or family, and reinforce information given by the patient's HCP regarding further testing, treatment, or referral to another HCP. Recognize that patients will have anxiety related to test results. Provide teaching and information regarding the clinical implications of the test results on the patient's lifestyle as appropriate.
- Note that test results should be evaluated in context with the patient's signs, symptoms, and diagnosis. Depending on the results of the procedure, additional testing may be performed to evaluate or monitor progression of the disease process and determine the need for a change in therapy.
- Be aware that when a person goes through a traumatic event such as an illness or being given information that will impact his or her lifestyle, there are universal human reactions that occur. These include knowledge deficit, fear, anxiety, and coping; in some situations, grieving may occur. HCPs should always be aware of the human response and how it may affect the plan of care and expected outcomes.

DISCUSSION POINT

Regarding Post-Test Critical Findings: Timely notification of a critical finding for lab or diagnostic studies is a role expectation of the professional nurse. Notification

processes will vary among facilities. Upon receipt of the critical finding, the information should be read back to the caller to verify accuracy. Most policies require immediate notification of the primary HCP, hospitalist, or on-call HCP. Reported information includes the patient's name, unique identifiers, critical finding, name of the person giving the report, and name of the person receiving the report. Documentation of notification should be made in the medical record with the name of the HCP notified, time and date of notification, and any orders received. Any delay in a timely report of a critical finding may require completion of a notification form with review by risk management.

STUDIES

- Complete Blood Count, Hematocrit
- Complete Blood Count, Hemoglobin
- Complete Blood Count, RBC Count
- Complete Blood Count, RBC Indices
- Complete Blood Count, RBC Morphology and Inclusions
- Complete Blood Count, WBC Count and Differential
- Erythrocyte Sedimentation Rate
- Hemoglobin Electrophoresis
- Reticulocyte Count
- Sickle Cell Screen

LEARNING OUTCOMES

Providing safe, effective nursing care (SENC) includes mastery of core competencies and standards of care. SENC is based on a judicious application of nursing knowledge in combination with scientific principles. The Art of Nursing lies in blending what you know with the ability to effectively apply your knowledge in a compassionate manner.

After reading/studying this chapter you will be able to:

Thinking

1. Define hematopoiesis.
2. Name the three basic elements incorporated in hematology studies.
3. Name the seven different types of blood cells and associate each of them with one of three main functions: transportation, regulation, or protection.
4. Give two common examples for when an abnormal WBC count is "normal."

Doing

1. Discuss a few of the reasons why variables such as collection time, age, race, and gender must be considered when reviewing results of a CBC.
2. Accept the leadership role required to meet specific clinical situations.

3. Describe appropriate nursing assessment/responsibilities related to the hematologic system.

Caring

1. Recognize the value of differing clinical points of view and associated responsibilities.

Complete Blood Count, Hematocrit

Quick Summary

SYNONYM ACRONYM: Packed cell volume (PCV), Hct.

COMMON USE: To evaluate anemia, polycythemia, and hydration status and to monitor therapy.

SPECIMEN: Whole blood from one full lavender-top (EDTA) tube, Microtainer, or capillary. Whole blood from a green-top (lithium or sodium heparin) tube may also be submitted.

NORMAL FINDINGS: (Method: Automated, computerized, multichannel analyzers)

Age	Conventional Units (%)	SI Units (Conventional Units × 0.01) (Volume fraction)
Cord blood	42–62	0.42–0.62
0–1 wk	46–68	0.46–0.68
2–3 wk	41–56	0.41–0.56
1–2 mo	39–59	0.39–0.59
3–6 mo	35–49	0.35–0.49
7 mo–1 yr	31–43	0.31–0.43
2–6 yr	30–40	0.3–0.4
7–15 yr	32–42	0.32–0.42
16–18 yr	33–45	0.33–0.45
Adult		
Male	42–52	0.42–0.52
Female	36–48	0.36–0.48
Pregnant Female		
1st Trimester	35–42	0.35–0.42
2nd and 3rd Trimester	28–33	0.28–0.33

Values are slightly lower in older adults

Test Explanation

Blood consists of a liquid plasma portion and a solid cellular portion. The solid portion is composed of red blood cells (RBCs), white blood cells (WBCs), and platelets.

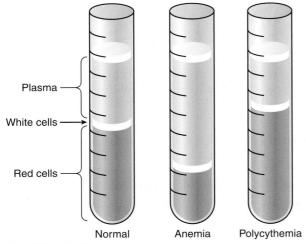

Plasma

White cells

Red cells

Normal   Anemia   Polycythemia

F I G U R E   2 . 7 Diagram depicting normal and abnormal packed cell volume (hematocrit)

It is important to be able to assess whether there is a sufficient number of circulating RBCs to transport the required amount of oxygen throughout the body. The hematocrit (Hct) is a mathematical expression of the number of RBCs, or packed cell volume, expressed as a percentage of whole blood. For example, a packed cell volume, or Hct of 45% means that a 100-mL sample of blood contains 45 mL of packed RBCs, which would reflect an acceptable level of RBCs for a patient of any given age (see Fig. 2.7). The Hct depends primarily on the number of RBCs; however, the average size of the RBCs influences Hct. Conditions that cause RBC size to be increased (e.g., swelling of the RBC due to change in osmotic pressure related to elevated sodium levels) may increase the Hct, while conditions that result in smaller than normal RBCs (e.g., microcytosis related to iron-deficiency anemia) may decrease the Hct. Hematocrit can be estimated directly by centrifuging a sample of whole blood for a specific time period. As the blood spins, it is separated into fractions. The RBC fraction is read against a scale. Most often the Hct is measured indirectly, by multiplying the RBC count and mean cell volume (MCV), using an automated cell counter. Hct can also be estimated by multiplying the hemoglobin by three.

The Hct level is part of the complete blood count (CBC). It is also frequently requested together with hemoglobin (Hgb) as an H&H (Hgb and Hct). Hgb and Hct levels parallel each other and are the best determinant of the degree of anemia or polycythemia. *Polycythemia* is a term used in conjunction with conditions resulting from an abnormal increase in Hgb, Hct, and RBC counts. *Anemia* is a term associated with conditions resulting from an abnormal decrease in Hgb, Hct, and RBC counts. Results of the Hgb, Hct, and RBC counts should be evaluated simultaneously, because

the same underlying conditions affect this triad of tests similarly. The RBC count multiplied by three should approximate the Hgb concentration. The Hct should be within three times the Hgb if the RBC population is normal in size and shape. The Hct plus six should approximate the first two figures of the RBC count within three (e.g., Hct is 40%; therefore 40 + 6 = 46, and the RBC count should be 4.6 or in the range of 4.3 to 4.9). There are some cultural variations in H&H values. After the first decade of life, the mean Hgb in African Americans is 0.5 to 1 g lower than in whites. Mexican Americans and Asian Americans have higher H&H values than whites.

Nursing Implications

Assessment

Indications	Potential Nursing Problems
Detect hematological disorder, neoplasm, or immunological abnormality	• Activity **(related to insufficient energy stores associated with anemia)**
Determine the presence of hereditary hematological abnormality	• Bleeding
Evaluate known or suspected anemia and related treatment, in combination with Hgb	• Breathing **(related to an inadequate number of RBCs to provide the required oxygen levels)**
Monitor blood loss and response to blood replacement, in combination with Hgb	• Confusion **(related to inadequate oxygenation)**
Monitor the effects of physical or emotional stress on the patient	• Fatigue **(related to insufficient energy stores associated with anemia)**
Monitor fluid imbalances or their treatment	• Gas Exchange **(related to an inadequate number of oxygen-carrying red cells)**
Monitor hematological status during pregnancy, in combination with Hgb	• Human Response
Monitor the progression of nonhematological disorders such as chronic obstructive pulmonary disease, malabsorption syndromes, cancer, and kidney disease	• Infection **(related to decreased effectiveness of the immune system as a result of a nutritional deficit related to anemia)**
Monitor response to drugs or chemotherapy, and evaluate undesired reactions to drugs that may cause blood dyscrasias	• Injury **(related to weakness or fatigue associated with anemia)**
	• Nutrition
Provide screening as part of a CBC in a general physical examination, especially upon admission to a health-care facility or before surgery	• Palpitations **(related to an inadequate number of RBCs to provide nutrients and the required oxygen levels to heart tissue)**
	• Tissue Perfusion **(related to an inadequate number of RBCs to provide the required oxygen levels)**

Diagnosis: Clinical Significance of Test Results
INCREASED IN

- Burns *(related to dehydration; total blood volume is decreased, but RBC count remains the same)*
- Chronic obstructive pulmonary disease *(related to chronic hypoxia that stimulates production of RBC and a corresponding increase in Hct)*
- Dehydration *(total blood volume is decreased, but RBC count remains the same)*
- Erythrocytosis *(total blood volume remains the same, but RBC count is increased)*
- Heart failure *(when the underlying cause is anemia, the body responds by increasing production of RBCs with a corresponding increase in Hct)*
- Hemoconcentration *(same effect as seen in dehydration)*
- High altitudes *(related to hypoxia that stimulates production of RBC and therefore increases Hct)*
- Polycythemia *(abnormal bone marrow response resulting in overproduction of RBC)*
- Shock

DECREASED IN

- Anemia *(overall decrease in RBC and corresponding decrease in Hct)*
- Blood loss (acute and chronic) *(overall decrease in RBC and corresponding decrease in Hct)*
- Bone marrow hyperplasia *(bone marrow failure that results in decreased RBC production)*
- Carcinoma *(anemia is often associated with chronic disease)*
- Cirrhosis *(related to accumulation of fluid)*
- Chronic disease *(anemia is often associated with chronic disease)*
- Fluid retention *(dilutional effect of increased blood volume while RBC count remains stable)*
- Hemoglobinopathies *(reduced RBC survival with corresponding decrease in Hgb)*
- Hemolytic disorders (e.g., hemolytic anemias, prosthetic valves) *(reduced RBC survival with corresponding decrease in Hct)*
- Hemorrhage (acute and chronic) *(related to loss of RBC that exceeds rate of production)*
- Hodgkin disease *(bone marrow failure that results in decreased RBC production)*
- Incompatible blood transfusion *(reduced RBC survival with corresponding decrease in Hgb)*
- Intravenous overload *(dilutional effect)*
- Fluid retention *(dilutional effect of increased blood volume while RBC count remains stable)*
- Kidney disease *(related to decreased levels of erythropoietin, which stimulates production of RBCs)*
- Leukemia *(bone marrow failure that results in decreased RBC production)*
- Lymphomas *(bone marrow failure that results in decreased RBC production)*

- Nutritional deficit *(anemia related to dietary deficiency in iron, vitamins, folate needed to produce sufficient RBC; decreased RBC count with corresponding decrease in Hct)*
- Pregnancy *(related to anemia)*
- Splenomegaly *(total blood volume remains the same, but spleen retains RBCs and Hct reflects decreased RBC count)*

Planning

Considerations for planning a successful partnership should include clear communication of what to expect during the test to decrease anxiety and improve cooperation. Before the procedure is performed, plan to review the steps with the patient. Address concerns about pain, and explain that there may be some discomfort during the venipuncture or fingerstick (if the microhematocrit collection will be used).

SPECIAL CONSIDERATIONS

An important aspect of planning is understanding the factors that may alter study findings or cause abnormal results. Interdepartmental communication is a key factor in the planning process. The following should be noted when planning for this study:

- The patient's age. *Newborns normally have increased values due to hemoconcentration. Older adults may also have slightly increased values due to hemoconcentration. Dehydration is a significant and common finding in older adult patients with decreased fluid intake and/or decreased kidney function.*
- The patient's position. *Hct can decrease when the patient is recumbent as a result of hemodilution and can increase when the patient rises as a result of hemoconcentration.*
- Acute blood loss or transfusion. *Care should be taken in evaluating the Hct during transfusion or acute blood loss because the value may appear to be normal and may not be a reliable indicator of anemia or therapeutic response to treatment.*
- Elevated blood glucose or serum sodium levels may produce elevated Hct levels *related to swelling of the erythrocytes.*
- Diseases and conditions including sickle cell anemia, hereditary spherocytosis, and iron deficiency *related to abnormalities in the RBC size (macrocytes, microcytes) or shape (spherocytes, sickle cells) that may alter Hct values.*

It is also important to understand which medications or substances the patient may be exposed to in the health-care setting that can interfere with accurate testing:

- Some drugs may also affect Hct values by increasing the RBC count (see the "Complete Blood Count, RBC Count" study).

● **Safety Tip**

The results of a CBC should be carefully evaluated during transfusion or acute blood loss because the body is not in a state of homeostasis and values may be misleading. Considerations for draw times after transfusion include the type of product, the amount of product transfused, and the patient's clinical situation. Generally, specimens collected an hour after transfusion will provide an acceptable reflection of the effects of the transfused product. Measurements taken during a massive transfusion are an exception, providing essential guidance for therapeutic decisions during critical care.

Implementation

Patient education is key to obtaining the patient's cooperation in following directions, and providing an explanation for the purpose of the procedure is an important part of this process. Inform the patient that this study can assist in evaluating the body's blood cell volume status during an acute or chronic illness. Perform the venipuncture.

Evaluation

Recognize anxiety related to test results, and assess the color of the patient's skin as pallor is an indication of poor tissue perfusion. Inform the patient, as appropriate, that oxygen or a blood product transfusion may be necessary to alleviate some of the symptoms the patient is experiencing due to the effects of the anemia. Frequently assess vital signs, and explain to the patient that elevating the head of the bed may reduce difficulty in breathing. Educate the patient regarding access to nutritional counseling services. Provide contact information, if desired, for the Institute of Medicine of the National Academies (www.iom.edu) and the U.S. Department of Agriculture (www.choosemyplate.com).

NUTRITIONAL CONSIDERATIONS: Nutritional therapy may be indicated for patients with increased Hct if iron levels are also elevated. Educate the patient with abnormally elevated iron values, as appropriate, on the importance of reading food labels. Patients with hemochromatosis or acute pernicious anemia should be educated to avoid foods rich in iron. Iron absorption is affected by numerous factors that may enhance or decrease absorption regardless of the original content of the iron-containing dietary source. The iron levels in foods can be increased if foods are cooked in cookware that contain iron. The consumption of large amounts of alcohol damages the intestine and allows an increased absorption of iron. A high intake of calcium and ascorbic acid also increases iron absorption. Iron absorption after a meal is also increased by factors in meat, fish, and poultry.

NUTRITIONAL CONSIDERATIONS: Nutritional therapy may be indicated for patients with decreased Hct. Iron deficiency is the most common nutrient deficiency in the United States. Patients at risk (e.g., children,

pregnant women, women of childbearing age, and low-income populations) should be instructed to include in their diet foods that are high in iron, such as meats (especially liver), eggs, grains, green leafy vegetables, and multivitamins with iron. Educate the patient with abnormally elevated iron values, as appropriate, about the importance of reading food labels. Iron absorption is affected by numerous factors, enhancing or decreasing absorption regardless of the original content of the iron-containing dietary source. Iron absorption is decreased by the absence (gastric resection) or diminished presence (use of antacids) of gastric acid. Phytic acids from cereals, tannins from tea and coffee, oxalic acid from vegetables, and minerals such as copper, zinc, and manganese interfere with iron absorption.

✓ Critical Findings

Adults & Children
Less than 19.8% (SI: Less than 0.2 Volume fraction)
Greater than 60% (SI: Greater than 0.6 Volume fraction)

Newborns
Less than 28.5% (SI: Less than 0.28 Volume fraction)
Greater than 66.9% (SI: Greater than 0.67 Volume fraction)

Consideration may be given to verification of critical findings before action is taken. Policies vary among facilities and may include requesting immediate recollection and retesting by the laboratory or retesting using a rapid Point of Care testing instrument at the bedside, if available.

Note and immediately report to the requesting health-care provider (HCP) any critical findings and related symptoms. A listing of these findings varies among facilities.

Low Hct leads to anemia. Anemia can be caused by blood loss, decreased blood cell production, increased blood cell destruction, and hemodilution. Causes of blood loss include menstrual excess or frequency, gastrointestinal bleeding, inflammatory bowel disease, and hematuria. Decreased blood cell production can be caused by folic acid deficiency, vitamin B_{12} deficiency, iron deficiency, and chronic disease. Increased blood cell destruction can be caused by a hemolytic reaction, chemical reaction, medication reaction, and sickle cell disease. Hemodilution can be caused by heart failure, kidney disease or injury, polydipsia, and overhydration. Symptoms of anemia (due to these causes) include anxiety, dyspnea, edema, hypertension, hypotension, hypoxia, jugular venous distention, fatigue, pallor, rales, restlessness, and weakness. Treatment of anemia depends on the cause.

High Hct leads to polycythemia. Polycythemia can be caused by dehydration, decreased oxygen levels in the body, and an overproduction of RBCs by the bone marrow. Dehydration from diuretic use, vomiting, diarrhea, excessive sweating, severe burns, or decreased fluid intake decreases the plasma component of whole blood, thereby increasing the ratio of RBCs to plasma, and leads to a higher than normal Hct. Causes of decreased oxygen include smoking, exposure to carbon monoxide, high altitude, and chronic lung disease, which leads to a mild hemoconcentration of blood in the body to carry more oxygen to the body's tissues. An overproduction of RBCs by the bone marrow leads to polycythemia vera, which is a rare chronic myeloproliferative disorder that leads to a severe hemoconcentration of blood. Severe hemoconcentration can lead to thrombosis (spontaneous blood clotting). Symptoms of hemoconcentration include decreased pulse pressure and volume, loss of skin turgor, dry mucous membranes, headaches, hepatomegaly, low central venous pressure, orthostatic hypotension, pruritus (especially after a hot bath), splenomegaly, tachycardia, thirst, tinnitus, vertigo, and weakness. Treatment of polycythemia depends on the cause. Possible interventions for hemoconcentration due to dehydration include intravenous fluids and discontinuance of diuretics if they are believed to be contributing to critically elevated Hct. Polycythemia due to decreased oxygen states can be treated by removal of the offending substance, such as smoke or carbon monoxide. Treatment includes oxygen therapy in cases of smoke inhalation, carbon monoxide poisoning, and desaturating chronic lung disease. Symptoms of polycythemic overload crisis include signs of thrombosis, pain and redness in the extremities, facial flushing, and irritability. Possible interventions for hemoconcentration due to polycythemia include therapeutic phlebotomy and intravenous fluids.

● *Study Specific Complications*

There are a number of complications associated with performing a venipuncture. **Pain** is commonly associated with needles, and although the pain experienced during venipuncture is usually mild, on a rare occasion the needle may strike a nerve causing permanent pain. Some patients experience a **vasovagal reaction** during the venipuncture procedure, evidenced by sweating, low blood pressure, fainting, or near fainting. The potential for a **fall injury** is a significant concern related to vasovagal reactions. Prolonged **bleeding** is a complication that occurs with patients who are taking blood thinners or who have coagulopathies such as hemophilia. A **hematoma** results when blood leaks into the tissue during or after a venipuncture, as evidenced by pain, bruising, and/or swelling at the venipuncture site. The swelling can cause injury by compression to surrounding nerves, which can be temporary or permanent. HCPs should watch for minor complications such as bruising and hematoma at the venipuncture site, which are fairly common. Hematomas occur more often in older adult or frail patients, or those with veins that are difficult to access. Bleeding or bruising can be prevented once the needle has been removed by applying direct pressure to the site with dry gauze for a minute or two. Some other more unusual complications of venipuncture include **cellulitis, phlebitis, inadvertent arterial puncture,** and **sepsis.** Sepsis can be caused by introduction of bacteria from the surface of the skin into the blood as the result of improper cleansing of the venipuncture site. Immunocompromised patients are at higher risk for developing this complication.

● *Related Tests*

Related tests include biopsy bone marrow, CBC, CBC hemoglobin, CBC RBC indices, CBC RBC morphology, erythropoietin, ferritin, iron/TIBC, reticulocyte count, and US abdomen.

Refer to the Cardiovascular, Gastrointestinal, Hematopoietic, Hepatobiliary, Immune, and Respiratory systems tables at the end of the book for related tests by body system.

Expected Outcomes

Expected outcomes associated with Complete Blood Count, Hematocrit, are:

* Understanding that the purpose of a preoperative evaluation is to prevent injury from an inadequate number of red cells during surgery
* Verbalizing the importance of eating iron-rich foods to maintain adequate cellular iron stores
* Managing the fatigue associated with inadequate red cells by pacing activities to current functional status
* Understanding the importance of reporting any alterations in breathing to the HCP

Complete Blood Count, Hemoglobin

Quick Summary

SYNONYM ACRONYM: Hgb.

COMMON USE: To evaluate anemia, polycythemia, and hydration status, and monitor therapy such as transfusion.

SPECIMEN: Whole blood from one full lavender-top (EDTA) tube, Microtainer, or capillary. Whole blood from a green-top (lithium or sodium heparin) tube may also be submitted.

NORMAL FINDINGS: (Method: Spectrophotometry)

Age	Conventional Units	SI Units (Conventional Units × 10)
Cord blood	13.5–20.7 g/dL	135–207 g/L
0–1 wk	15.2–23.6 g/dL	152–236 g/L
2–3 wk	13.3–18.7 g/dL	133–187 g/L
1–2 mo	10.7–18 g/dL	107–180 g/L

Continued

Table Continued

Age	Conventional Units	SI Units (Conventional Units × 10)
3–6 mo	11.7–16.3 g/dL	117–163 g/L
7 mo–1 yr	10.3–14.3	103–143
2–6 yr	10–13.3	100–133
7–15 yr	10.7–14 g/dL	107–144 g/L
16–18 yr	11–15 g/dL	110–150 g/L
Adult		
Male	14–17.3 g/dL	140–173 g/L
Female	11.7–15.5 g/dL	117–155 g/L
Pregnant Female		
1st Trimester	11.6–13.9 g/dL	116–139 g/L
2nd and 3rd Trimester	9.5–11 g/dL	95–110 g/L

Values are slightly lower in older adults

Test Explanation

Hemoglobin (Hgb) is the main intracellular protein of erythrocytes. It carries oxygen (O_2) to and removes carbon dioxide (CO_2) from red blood cells (RBCs). It also serves as a buffer to maintain acid-base balance in the extracellular fluid. Each Hgb molecule consists of heme and globulin. Copper is a cofactor necessary for the enzymatic incorporation of iron molecules into heme. Heme contains iron and porphyrin molecules that have a high affinity for O_2. The affinity of Hgb molecules for O_2 is influenced by 2,3-diphosphoglyc-erate (2,3-DPG), a substance produced by anaerobic glycolysis to generate energy for the RBCs. When Hgb binds with 2,3-DPG, O_2 affinity decreases. The ability of Hgb to bind and release O_2 can be graphically represented by an oxyhemoglobin dissociation curve. The term *shift to the left* describes an increase in the affinity of Hgb for O_2. Conditions that can cause this leftward shift include decreased body temperature, decreased 2,3-DPG, decreased CO_2 concentration, and increased pH. Conversely, a *shift to the right* represents a decrease in the affinity of Hgb for O_2. Conditions that can cause a rightward shift include increased body temperature, increased 2,3-DPG levels, increased CO_2 concentration, and decreased pH.

Hgb levels are a direct reflection of the O_2-combining capacity of the blood. It is the combination of heme and O_2 that gives blood its characteristic red color. RBC counts parallel the O_2-combining capacity of Hgb, but because some RBCs contain more Hgb than others, the relationship is not directly proportional. As CO_2 diffuses into RBCs, an enzyme called carbonic anhydrase converts the CO_2 into bicarbonate and hydrogen ions. Hgb that is not bound to O_2 combines with the free hydrogen ions, increasing pH. As this binding is occurring, bicarbonate is leaving the RBC in exchange for chloride ions. (For additional information about the relationship between the respiratory and renal components of this buffer system, see study titled "Blood Gases.")

Hgb is included in the complete blood count (CBC). It is also frequently requested together with hemoglobin (Hgb) as an H&H. Hgb and Hct levels parallel each other and are frequently used to evaluate anemia. *Polycythemia* is a condition resulting from an abnormal increase in Hgb, Hct, and RBC count. *Anemia* is a condition resulting from an abnormal decrease in Hgb, Hct, and RBC count. Results of the Hgb, Hct, and RBC count should be evaluated simultaneously because the same underlying conditions affect this triad of tests similarly. The RBC count multiplied by three should approximate the Hgb concentration. The Hct should be within three times the Hgb if the RBC population is normal in size and shape. The Hct plus six should approximate the first two figures of the RBC count within three (e.g., Hct is 40%; therefore 40 + 6 = 46, and the RBC count should be 4.6 or in the range of 4.3 to 4.9). There are some cultural variations in Hgb and Hct (H&H) values. After the first decade of life, the mean Hgb in African Americans is 0.5 to 1 g lower than in whites. Mexican Americans and Asian Americans have higher Hgb and H&H values than whites.

Nursing Implications

Assessment

Indications	Potential Nursing Problems
Detect hematological disorder, neoplasm, or immunological abnormality Determine the presence of hereditary hematological abnormality Evaluate known or suspected anemia and related treatment, in combination with Hct Monitor blood loss and response to blood replacement, in combination with Hct Monitor the effects of physical or emotional stress on the patient Monitor fluid imbalances or the patient's treatment Monitor hematological status during pregnancy, in combination with Hct	• Activity • Bleeding • Breathing (*related to an inadequate number of RBCs to provide the required oxygen levels*) • Confusion (*related to inadequate oxygenation to support cerebral perfusion*) • Fatigue (*related to inadequate oxygen stores to support energy use*) • Gas Exchange (*related to adequate red cells to support oxygen demand*) • Health Management • Human Response

Indications	Potential Nursing Problems
Monitor the progression of nonhematological disorders, such as chronic obstructive pulmonary disease (COPD), malabsorption syndromes, cancer, and kidney disease Monitor response to drugs or chemotherapy and evaluate undesired reactions to drugs that may cause blood dyscrasias Provide screening as part of a CBC in a general physical examination, especially upon admission to a health-care facility or before surgery	• Infection *(related to the decreased effectiveness of the immune system as a result of a nutritional deficit related to anemia)* • Injury *(related to weakness or fatigue associated with anemia)* • Palpitations *(related to an inadequate number of RBCs to provide nutrients and the required oxygen levels to the heart tissue)* • Tissue Perfusion *(related to an inadequate number of RBCs to provide the required oxygen levels)*

Diagnosis: Clinical Significance of Test Results

INCREASED IN

- Burns *(related to dehydration; total blood volume is decreased, but RBC count remains the same)*
- COPD *(related to chronic hypoxia that stimulates production of RBCs and a corresponding increase in Hgb)*
- Dehydration *(total blood volume is decreased, but RBC count remains the same)*
- Erythrocytosis *(total blood volume remains the same, but RBC count is increased)*
- Heart failure *(when the underlying cause is anemia, the body will respond by increasing production of RBCs; with a responding increase in Hct)*
- Hemoconcentration *(same effect as seen in dehydration)*
- High altitudes *(related to hypoxia that stimulates production of RBCs and therefore increases Hgb)*
- Polycythemia vera *(abnormal bone marrow response resulting in overproduction of RBCs)*
- Shock

DECREASED IN

- Anemias *(overall decrease in RBCs and corresponding decrease in Hgb)*
- Blood loss (acute and chronic) *(overall decrease in RBC and corresponding decrease in Hct)*
- Bone marrow hyperplasia *(bone marrow failure that results in decreased RBC production)*
- Carcinoma *(anemia is often associated with chronic disease)*
- Cirrhosis *(related to accumulation of fluid)*
- Chronic disease *(anemia is often associated with chronic disease)*
- Fluid retention *(dilutional effect of increased blood volume while RBC count remains stable)*
- Hemoglobinopathies *(reduced RBC survival with corresponding decrease in Hgb)*
- Hemolytic disorders (e.g., hemolytic anemias, prosthetic valves) *(reduced RBC survival with corresponding decrease in Hct)*
- Hemorrhage (acute and chronic) *(overall decrease in RBCs and corresponding decrease in Hgb)*
- Hodgkin disease *(bone marrow failure that results in decreased RBC production)*
- Incompatible blood transfusion *(reduced RBC survival with corresponding decrease in Hgb)*
- Intravenous overload *(dilutional effect)*
- Kidney disease *(related to decreased levels of erythropoietin, which stimulates production of RBCs)*
- Leukemia *(bone marrow failure that results in decreased RBC production)*
- Lymphomas *(bone marrow failure that results in decreased RBC production)*
- Nutritional deficit *(anemia related to dietary deficiency in iron, vitamins, folate needed to produce sufficient RBCs; decreased RBC count with corresponding decrease in Hgb)*
- Pregnancy *(related to anemia)*
- Splenomegaly *(total blood volume remains the same, but spleen retains RBCs and Hgb reflects decreased RBC count)*

Planning

Considerations for planning a successful partnership should include clear communication of what to expect during the test to decrease anxiety and improve cooperation. Before the procedure is performed, plan to review the steps with the patient. Address concerns about pain, and explain that there may be some discomfort during the venipuncture or fingerstick (if the microhematocrit collection will be used).

SPECIAL CONSIDERATIONS

An important aspect of planning is understanding the factors that may alter study findings or cause abnormal results. Interdepartmental communication is a key factor in the planning process. The following should be noted when planning for this study:

- The patient's age. *Newborns normally have increased values due to hemoconcentration. Older adults may also have slightly increased values due to hemoconcentration. Dehydration is a significant and common finding in older adult patients with decreased fluid intake and/or decreased kidney function.*
- The patient's position. *Hgb can decrease when the patient is recumbent as a result of hemodilution and can increase when the patient rises as a result of hemoconcentration.*
- Acute blood loss or transfusion. *Care should be taken in evaluating the Hgb during transfusion or acute*

blood loss because the value may appear to be normal and may not be a reliable indicator of anemia or a therapeutic response to treatment.

- Lipemia will falsely increase the Hgb measurement because the turbidity in the sample caused by excessive levels of lipids is measured as Hgb by the instrument, also affecting the MCH and MCHC. This can be corrected by replacing the plasma with saline, repeating the measurement, and manually correcting the Hgb, MCH, and MCHC using specific mathematical formulas.
- Diseases and conditions including sickle cell anemia, hereditary spherocytosis, and iron deficiency *related to abnormalities in the RBC size (macrocytes, microcytes) or shape (spherocytes, sickle cells) that may alter Hgb values.*
- A severe copper deficiency may also result in decreased Hgb levels.
- Use of the nutraceutical liver extract is strongly contraindicated in iron-storage disorders, such as hemochromatosis, because it is rich in heme (the iron-containing pigment in Hgb).

It is also important to understand which medications or substances the patient may be exposed to in the healthcare setting that can interfere with accurate testing:

- Drugs and substances that may cause a decrease in Hgb include those that induce hemolysis due to drug sensitivity or enzyme deficiency and those that result in anemia (see the "Complete Blood Count, RBC Count" study within this chapter).
- Some drugs may also affect Hgb values by increasing the RBC count (see the "Complete Blood Count, RBC Count" study) or Hgb level.

● Safety Tip

The results of a CBC should be carefully evaluated during transfusion or acute blood loss because the body is not in a state of homeostasis and values may be misleading. Considerations for draw times after transfusion include the type of product, the amount of product transfused, and the patient's clinical situation. Generally, specimens collected an hour after transfusion will provide an acceptable reflection of the effects of the transfused product. Measurements taken during a massive transfusion are an exception, providing essential guidance for therapeutic decisions during critical care.

Implementation

Patient education is key to obtaining the patient's cooperation in following directions, and providing an explanation for the purpose of the procedure is an important part of this process. Inform the patient that this study can assist in evaluating the amount of hemoglobin in the blood to assist in diagnosis and monitor therapy. Perform the venipuncture.

Evaluation

Recognize anxiety related to test results, and assess the color of the patient's skin as pallor is an indication of poor tissue perfusion. Inform the patient, as appropriate, that oxygen or blood product transfusion may be necessary to alleviate some of the symptoms the patient is experiencing due to the effects of the anemia. Frequently assess vital signs and explain to the patient that elevating the head of the bed may reduce difficulty in breathing. Educate the patient regarding access to nutritional counseling services. Provide contact information, if desired, for the Institute of Medicine of the National Academies (www.iom.edu) or the U.S. Department of Agriculture (www.choosemyplate.com).

NUTRITIONAL CONSIDERATIONS: Nutritional therapy may be indicated for patients with increased Hgb if iron levels are also elevated. Educate the patient with abnormally elevated iron values, as appropriate, about the importance of reading food labels. Patients with hemochromatosis or acute pernicious anemia should be educated to avoid foods rich in iron. Iron absorption is affected by numerous factors that may enhance or decrease absorption regardless of the original content of the iron-containing dietary source. Iron levels in foods can be increased if foods are cooked in cookware that contain iron. The consumption of large amounts of alcohol damages the intestine and allows increased absorption of iron. A high intake of calcium and ascorbic acid also increases iron absorption. Iron absorption after a meal is also increased by factors in meat, fish, and poultry.

Nutritional therapy may be indicated for patients with decreased Hgb because this may indicate corresponding iron deficiency. Iron deficiency is the most common nutrient deficiency in the United States. Patients at risk (e.g., children, pregnant women, women of childbearing age, and low-income populations) should be instructed to include in their diet foods that are high in iron, such as meats (especially liver), eggs, grains, green leafy vegetables, and multivitamins with iron. Instruct these patients in the in the administration of iron supplements, including side effects, as appropriate. The Hgb level should increase by about 1 g/dL (SI: 10 g/L) after 3–4 weeks of oral iron supplementation. Educate the patient with abnormally decreased Hgb values, as appropriate, about the importance of reading food labels and of dietary inclusion of iron-rich foods. Iron absorption is affected by numerous factors, enhancing or decreasing absorption regardless of the original content of the iron-containing dietary source. Iron absorption is decreased by the absence (gastric resection) or diminished presence (use of antacids) of gastric acid. Phytic acids from cereals, tannins from tea and coffee, oxalic acid from vegetables, and minerals such as copper, zinc, and manganese interfere with iron absorption.

✓ Critical Findings

Adults & Children

Less than 6.6 g/dL (SI: Less than 66 g/L)
Greater than 20 g/dL (SI: Greater than 200 g/L)

Newborns

Less than 9.5 g/dL (SI: Less than 95 g/L)
Greater than 22.3 g/dL (SI: Greater than 223 g/L)

Consideration may be given to verification of critical findings before action is taken. Policies vary among facilities and may include requesting immediate recollection and retesting by the laboratory or retesting using a rapid Point of Care testing instrument at the bedside, if available.

Note and immediately report to the requesting HCP any critical findings and related symptoms. A listing of these findings varies among facilities.

Low Hgb leads to anemia. Anemia can be caused by blood loss, decreased blood cell production, increased blood cell destruction, and hemodilution. Causes of blood loss include menstrual excess or frequency, gastrointestinal bleeding, inflammatory bowel disease, and hematuria. Decreased blood cell production can be caused by folic acid deficiency, vitamin B_{12} deficiency, iron deficiency, and chronic disease. Increased blood cell destruction can be caused by a hemolytic reaction, chemical reaction, medication reaction, and sickle cell disease. Hemodilution can be caused by heart failure, kidney disease or injury, polydipsia, and overhydration. Symptoms of anemia (due to these causes) include anxiety, dyspnea, edema, fatigue, hypertension, hypotension, hypoxia, jugular venous distention, pallor, rales, restlessness, and weakness. Treatment of anemia depends on the cause.

High Hgb leads to polycythemia. Polycythemia can be caused by dehydration, decreased oxygen levels in the body, and an overproduction of RBCs by the bone marrow. Dehydration from diuretic use, vomiting, diarrhea, excessive sweating, severe burns, or decreased fluid intake decreases the plasma component of whole blood, thereby increasing the ratio of RBCs to plasma, and leads to a higher than normal Hgb. Causes of decreased oxygen include smoking, exposure to carbon monoxide, high altitude, and chronic lung disease, which leads to a mild hemoconcentration of blood in the body to carry more oxygen to the body's tissues. An overproduction of RBCs by the bone marrow leads to polycythemia vera, which is a rare chronic myeloproliferative disorder that leads to a severe hemoconcentration of blood. Severe hemoconcentration can lead to thrombosis (spontaneous blood clotting). Symptoms of hemoconcentration include decreased pulse pressure and volume, loss of skin turgor, dry mucous membranes, headaches, hepatomegaly, low central venous pressure, orthostatic hypotension, pruritus (especially after a hot bath), splenomegaly, tachycardia, thirst, tinnitus, vertigo, and weakness. Treatment of polycythemia depends on the cause. Possible interventions for hemoconcentration due to dehydration include intravenous fluids and discontinuance of diuretics if they are believed to be contributing to critically elevated Hgb. Polycythemia due to decreased oxygen states can be treated by removal of the offending substance, such as smoke or carbon monoxide. Treatment includes oxygen therapy in cases of smoke inhalation, carbon monoxide poisoning, and desaturating chronic lung disease. Symptoms of polycythemic overload crisis include signs of thrombosis, pain and redness in extremities, facial flushing, and irritability. Possible interventions for hemoconcentration due to polycythemia include therapeutic phlebotomy and intravenous fluids.

✓ Study Specific Complications

There are a number of complications associated with performing a venipuncture. **Pain** is commonly associated with needles, and although the pain experienced during venipuncture is usually mild, on a rare occasion the needle may strike a nerve causing permanent pain. Some patients experience a **vasovagal reaction** during the venipuncture procedure, evidenced by sweating, low blood pressure, fainting, or near fainting. The potential for a **fall injury** is a significant concern related to vasovagal reactions. Prolonged **bleeding** is a complication that occurs with patients who are taking blood thinners or who have coagulopathies such as hemophilia. A **hematoma** results when blood leaks into the tissue during or after a venipuncture, as evidenced by pain, bruising, and/or swelling at the venipuncture site. The swelling can cause injury by compression to surrounding nerves, which can be temporary or permanent. HCPs should watch for minor complications such as bruising and hematoma at the venipuncture site, which are fairly common. Hematomas occur more often in older adult or frail patients, or those with veins that are difficult to access. Bleeding or bruising can be prevented once the needle has been removed by applying direct pressure to the site with dry gauze for a minute or two. Some other more unusual complications of venipuncture include **cellulitis, phlebitis, inadvertent arterial puncture,** and **sepsis.** Sepsis can be caused by introduction of bacteria from the surface of the skin into the blood as the result of improper cleansing of the venipuncture site. Immunocompromised patients are at higher risk for developing this complication.

✓ Related Tests

Related tests include biopsy bone marrow, biopsy lymph node, biopsy kidney, blood groups and antibodies, CBC, CBC hematocrit, Coombs antiglobulin, CT thoracic, erythropoietin, fecal analysis (occult blood), ferritin, gallium scan, haptoglobin, hemoglobin electrophoresis, iron/TIBC, lymphangiogram, Meckel diverticulum scan, reticulocyte count, sickle cell screen, and US abdomen.

Refer to the Cardiovascular, Gastrointestinal, Hematopoietic, Hepatobiliary, Immune, and Respiratory systems tables at the end of the book for related tests by body system.

Expected Outcomes

Expected outcomes associated with Complete Blood Count, Hemoglobin, are:

- Maintaining normal hemoglobin and hematocrit levels by adhering to the therapeutic regime recommended by the HCP
- Reporting fatigue as manageable while preforming daily activities
- Collaborating with the HCP to identify the cause of blood loss
- Identifying and incorporating iron-rich foods into the daily diet

Complete Blood Count, RBC Count

Quick Summary

SYNONYM ACRONYM: RBC.

COMMON USE: To evaluate the number of circulating red cells in the blood toward diagnosing disease and monitoring therapeutic treatment. Variations in the number of cells is most often seen in anemias, cancer, and hemorrhage.

SPECIMEN: Whole blood collected in a lavender-top (EDTA) tube.

NORMAL FINDINGS: (Method: Automated, computerized, multichannel analyzers)

Age	Conventional Units (10⁶ cells/microL)	SI Units (10¹² cells/L) (Conventional Units × 1)
Cord blood	3.61–5.81	3.61–5.81
0–1 wk	4.51–6.01	4.51–6.01
2–3 wk	3.99–6.11	3.99–6.11
1–2 mo	3.71–6.11	3.71–6.11
3–6 mo	3.81–5.61	3.81–5.61
7 mo–1 yr	3.81–5.21	3.81–5.21
2–6 yr	3.91–5.31	3.91–5.31
7–15 yr	3.99–5.21	3.99–5.21
16–18 yr	4.21–5.41	4.21–5.41
Adult		
Male	4.21–5.81	4.21–5.81
Female	3.61–5.11	3.61–5.11

Values are decreased in pregnancy related to the dilutional effects of increased fluid volume and potential nutritional deficiency related to decreased intake, nausea, and/or vomiting. Values are slightly lower in older adults associated with potential nutritional deficiency.

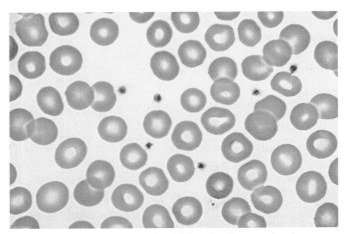

FIGURE 2.8 Normal red blood cells. *Used with permission, from Harmening, D. (2008). Clinical hematology and fundamentals of hemostasis (5th Ed.). FA Davis Company.*

Test Explanation

The red blood cell (RBC) count is a component of the CBC (see Fig. 2.8). It determines the number of RBCs per cubic millimeter of whole blood. The main role of RBCs, which contain the pigmented protein hemoglobin (Hgb), is the transport and exchange of oxygen to the tissues. Some carbon dioxide is returned from the tissues to the lungs by RBCs. RBC production in healthy adults takes place in the bone marrow of the vertebrae, pelvis, ribs, sternum, skull, and proximal ends of the femur and humerus. Production of RBCs is regulated by a hormone called erythropoietin which is produced and secreted by the kidneys. Normal RBC development and function are dependent on adequate levels of vitamin B_{12}, folic acid, vitamin E, and iron. The average life span of normal RBCs is 120 days. Old or damaged RBCs are removed from circulation by the spleen. The liver is responsible for the breakdown of hemoglobin and other cellular contents released from destroyed RBCs. *Polycythemia* is a condition resulting from an abnormal increase in Hgb, hematocrit (Hct), and RBC count. *Anemia* is a condition resulting from an abnormal decrease in Hgb, Hct, and RBC count. Results of the Hgb, Hct, and RBC count should be evaluated simultaneously because the same underlying conditions affect this triad of tests similarly. The RBC count multiplied by three should approximate the Hgb concentration. The Hct should be within three times the Hgb if the RBC population is normal in size and shape. The Hct plus six should approximate the first two figures of the RBC count within three (e.g., Hct is 40%; therefore 40 + 6 = 46, and the RBC count should be 4.6 or in the range 4.3 to 4.9). (See "Complete Blood Count, Hematocrit," "Complete Blood Count, Hemoglobin," and "Complete Blood Count, RBC Indices.")

Nursing Implications

Assessment

Indications	Potential Nursing Problems
Detect a hematological disorder involving RBC destruction (e.g., hemolytic anemia) Determine the presence of hereditary hematological abnormality Monitor the effects of acute or chronic blood loss Monitor the effects of physical or emotional stress on the patient Monitor patients with disorders associated with elevated erythrocyte counts (e.g., polycythemia vera, chronic obstructive pulmonary disease [COPD]) Monitor the progression of nonhematological disorders associated with elevated erythrocyte counts, such as COPD, liver disease, hypothyroidism, adrenal dysfunction, bone marrow failure, malabsorption syndromes, cancer, and kidney disease Monitor the response to drugs or chemotherapy and evaluate undesired reactions to drugs that may cause blood dyscrasias Provide screening as part of a CBC in a general physical examination, especially upon admission to a health-care facility or before surgery	• Bleeding • Cardiac Output • Confusion *(related to inadequate oxygenation to support cerebral perfusion)* • Fatigue *(related to inadequate oxygen stores to support energy use)* • Fear • Gas Exchange *(related to adequate red cells to support oxygen demand)* • Human Response • Pain • Role Performance • Tissue Perfusion *(related to an inadequate number of RBCs to provide the required oxygen levels)*

Diagnosis: Clinical Significance of Test Results

INCREASED IN

- Anxiety or stress *(related to physiological response)*
- Bone marrow failure *(initial response is stimulation of RBC production)*
- COPD with hypoxia and secondary polycythemia *(related to chronic hypoxia that stimulates production of RBCs and a corresponding increase in RBCs)*
- Dehydration with hemoconcentration *(related to decrease in total blood volume relative to unchanged RBC count)*
- Erythremic erythrocytosis *(related to unchanged total blood volume relative to increase in RBC count)*

- High altitude *(related to hypoxia that stimulates production of RBCs)*
- Polycythemia vera *(related to abnormal bone marrow response resulting in overproduction of RBCs)*

DECREASED IN

- Chemotherapy *(related to reduced RBC survival)*
- Chronic inflammatory diseases *(related to anemia of chronic disease)*
- Hemoglobinopathy *(related to reduced RBC survival)*
- Hemolytic anemia *(related to reduced RBC survival)*
- Hemorrhage *(related to overall decrease in RBC count)*
- Hodgkin disease *(evidenced by bone marrow failure that results in decreased RBC production)*
- Kidney disease *(related to decreased production of erythropoietin)*
- Leukemia *(evidenced by bone marrow failure that results in decreased RBC production)*
- Multiple myeloma *(evidenced by bone marrow failure that results in decreased RBC production)*
- Nutritional deficit *(related to deficiency of iron or vitamins required for RBC production and/or maturation)*
- Overhydration *(related to increase in blood volume relative to unchanged RBC count)*
- Pregnancy *(related to anemia; normal dilutional effect)*
- Subacute endocarditis

Planning

Considerations for planning a successful partnership should include clear communication of what to expect during the test to decrease anxiety and improve cooperation. Before the procedure is performed, plan to review the steps with the patient. Address concerns about pain, and explain that there may be some discomfort during the venipuncture or fingerstick (if the microhematocrit collection will be used).

SPECIAL CONSIDERATIONS

An important aspect of planning is understanding the factors that may alter study findings or cause abnormal results. Interdepartmental communication is a key factor in the planning process. The following should be noted when planning for this study:

- The patient's position. *RBC count can decrease when the patient is recumbent as a result of hemodilution and can increase when the patient rises as a result of hemoconcentration.*
- Acute blood loss or transfusion. *Care should be taken in evaluating the Hgb during transfusion or acute blood loss because the value may appear to be normal and may not be a reliable indicator of anemia or a therapeutic response to treatment.*
- Hemodilution (e.g., excessive administration of intravenous fluids, normal pregnancy) in the presence

of a normal number of RBCs may lead to false decreases in the RBC count.

- Excessive exercise, anxiety, pain, and dehydration may cause false elevations in RBC count.
- Cold agglutinins may falsely increase the mean corpuscular volume (MCV) and decrease the RBC count. This can be corrected by warming the blood or diluting the sample with warmed saline and repeating the analysis.

It is also important to understand which medications or substances the patient may be exposed to in the health-care setting that can interfere with accurate testing:

- Drugs and vitamins that may increase the RBC count include erythropoietin, glucocorticosteroids, pilocarpine, and vitamin B_{12}. The use of the nutraceutical liver extract is strongly contraindicated in patients with iron-storage disorders such as hemochromatosis because it is rich in heme (the iron-containing pigment in Hgb).
- Drugs and substances that may decrease RBC count by causing hemolysis that results from drug sensitivity or enzyme deficiency include acetaminophen, aminopyrine, aminosalicylic acid, amphetamine, anticonvulsants, antipyrine, arsenicals, benzene, busulfan, carbenicillin, cephalothin, chemotherapy drugs, chlorate, chloroquine, chlorothiazide, chlorpromazine, colchicine, diphenhydramine, dipyrone, glucosulfone, gold, hydroflumethiazide, indomethacin, mephenytoin, nalidixic acid, neomycin, nitrofurantoin, penicillin, phenacemide, phenazopyridine, and phenothiazine.
- Drugs that may decrease RBC count by causing anemia include miconazole, penicillamine, phenylhydrazine, primaquine, probenecid, pyrazolones, pyrimethamine, quinines, streptomycin, sulfamethizole, sulfamethoxypyridazine, sulfisoxazole, suramin, thioridazine, tolbutamide, trimethadione, and tripelennamine.
- Drugs that may decrease RBC count by causing bone marrow suppression include amphotericin B, floxuridine, and phenylbutazone.

● Safety Tip

The results of a CBC should be carefully evaluated during transfusion or acute blood loss because the body is not in a state of homeostasis and values may be misleading. Considerations for draw times after transfusion include the type of product, the amount of product transfused, and the patient's clinical situation. Generally, specimens collected an hour after transfusion will provide an acceptable reflection of the effects of the transfused product. Measurements taken during a massive transfusion are an exception, providing essential guidance for therapeutic decisions during critical care.

Implementation

Patient education is key to obtaining the patient's cooperation in following directions, and providing an explanation for the purpose of the procedure is an important part of this process. Inform the patient that this study can assist in assessing for anemia and disorders that affect the number of circulating RBCs. Perform the venipuncture.

Evaluation

Recognize anxiety related to test results, and talk to the patient about access to nutritional counseling services. Provide contact information, if desired, for the Institute of Medicine of the National Academies (www.iom.edu) or the U.S. Department of Agriculture (www.choosemyplate.com).

Nutritional therapy may be indicated for patients with a decreased RBC count. Iron deficiency is the most common nutrient deficiency in the United States. Patients at risk (e.g., children, pregnant women, women of childbearing age, and low-income populations) should be instructed to include foods that are high in iron in their diet, such as meats (especially liver), eggs, grains, green leafy vegetables, and multivitamins with iron. Iron absorption is affected by numerous factors.

Patients at risk for vitamin B_{12} or folate deficiency include those with the following conditions: malnourishment (inadequate intake), pregnancy (increased need), infancy, malabsorption syndromes (inadequate absorption/increased metabolic rate), infections, cancer, hyperthyroidism, serious burns, excessive blood loss, and gastrointestinal damage. Instruct the patient with vitamin B_{12} deficiency, as appropriate, in the use of vitamin supplements. Inform the patient, as appropriate, that the best dietary sources of vitamin B_{12} are meats, milk, cheese, eggs, and fortified soy milk products. Instruct the folate-deficient patient (especially pregnant women), as appropriate, to eat foods rich in folate, such as meats (especially liver), salmon, eggs, beets, asparagus, green leafy vegetables such as spinach, cabbage, oranges, broccoli, sweet potatoes, kidney beans, and whole wheat.

A diet deficient in vitamin E puts the patient at risk for increased RBC destruction, which could lead to anemia. Nutritional therapy may be indicated for these patients. Educate the patient with a vitamin E deficiency, if appropriate, that the main dietary sources of vitamin E are vegetable oils (including olive oil), whole grains, wheat germ, nuts, milk, eggs, meats, fish, and green leafy vegetables. Vitamin E is fairly stable at most cooking temperatures (except frying) and when exposed to acidic foods. Supplemental vitamin E may also be taken, but the danger of toxicity should be explained to the patient. Very large supplemental doses, in excess of 600 mg of vitamin E over a period of 1 year, may result in excess bleeding. Vitamin E is heat stable but is very negatively affected by light.

Critical Findings

The presence of abnormal cells, other morphological characteristics, or cellular inclusions may signify a potentially life-threatening or serious health condition and should be investigated. Examples are the presence of sickle cells, moderate numbers of spherocytes, marked schistocytosis, oval macrocytes, basophilic stippling, nucleated RBCs (if the patient is not an infant), or malarial organisms.

Consideration may be given to verification of critical findings before action is taken. Policies vary among facilities and may include requesting immediate recollection and retesting by the laboratory.

Note and immediately report to the requesting health-care provider (HCP) any critical findings and related symptoms. A listing of these findings varies among facilities.

Low RBC count leads to anemia. Anemia can be caused by blood loss, decreased blood cell production, increased blood cell destruction, or hemodilution. Causes of blood loss include menstrual excess or frequency, gastrointestinal bleeding, inflammatory bowel disease, or hematuria. Decreased blood cell production can be caused by folic acid deficiency, vitamin B_{12} deficiency, iron deficiency, or chronic disease. Increased blood cell destruction can be caused by a hemolytic reaction, chemical reaction, medication reaction, or sickle cell disease. Hemodilution can be caused by heart failure, kidney disease or injury, polydipsia, or overhydration. Symptoms of anemia (due to these causes) include anxiety, dyspnea, edema, hypertension, hypotension, hypoxia, jugular venous distention, fatigue, pallor, rales, restlessness, and weakness. Treatment of anemia depends on the cause.

High RBC count leads to polycythemia. Polycythemia can be caused by dehydration, decreased oxygen levels in the body, and an overproduction of RBCs by the bone marrow. Dehydration by diuretic use, vomiting, diarrhea, excessive sweating, severe burns, or decreased fluid intake decreases the plasma component of whole blood, thereby increasing the ratio of RBCs to plasma, and leads to a higher than normal Hct. Causes of decreased oxygen include smoking, exposure to carbon monoxide, high altitude, and chronic lung disease, which leads to a mild hemoconcentration of blood in the body to carry more oxygen to the body's tissues. An overproduction of RBCs by the bone marrow leads to polycythemia vera, which is a rare chronic myeloproliferative disorder that leads to a severe hemoconcentration of blood. Severe hemoconcentration can lead to thrombosis (spontaneous blood clotting). Symptoms of hemoconcentration include decreased pulse pressure and volume, loss of skin turgor, dry mucous membranes, headaches, hepatomegaly, low central venous pressure, orthostatic hypotension, pruritus (especially after a hot bath), splenomegaly, tachycardia, thirst, tinnitus, vertigo, and weakness. Treatment of polycythemia depends on the cause. Possible interventions for hemoconcentration due to dehydration include intravenous fluids and discontinuance of diuretics if they are believed to be contributing to critically elevated Hct. Polycythemia due to decreased oxygen states can be treated by removal of the offending substance, such as smoke or carbon monoxide. Treatment includes oxygen therapy in cases of smoke inhalation, carbon monoxide poisoning, and desaturating chronic lung disease. Symptoms of polycythemic overload crisis include signs of thrombosis, pain and redness in extremities, facial flushing, and irritability. Possible interventions for hemoconcentration due to polycythemia include therapeutic phlebotomy and intravenous fluids.

Study Specific Complications

There are a number of complications associated with performing a venipuncture. **Pain** is commonly associated with needles, and although the pain experienced during venipuncture is usually mild, on a rare occasion the needle may strike a nerve causing permanent pain. Some patients experience a **vasovagal reaction** during the venipuncture procedure, evidenced by sweating, low blood pressure, fainting, or near fainting. The potential for a **fall injury** is a significant concern related to vasovagal reactions. Prolonged **bleeding** is a complication that occurs with patients who are taking blood thinners or who have coagulopathies such as hemophilia. A **hematoma** results when blood leaks into the tissue during or after a venipuncture, as evidenced by pain, bruising, and/or swelling at the venipuncture site. The swelling can cause injury by compression to surrounding nerves, which can be temporary or permanent. HCPs should watch for minor complications such as bruising and hematoma at the venipuncture site, which are fairly common. Hematomas occur more often in older adult or frail patients, or those with veins that are difficult to access. Bleeding or bruising can be prevented once the needle has been removed by applying direct pressure to the site with dry gauze for a minute or two. Some other more unusual complications of venipuncture include **cellulitis, phlebitis, inadvertent arterial puncture,** and **sepsis.** Sepsis can be caused by introduction of bacteria from the surface of the skin into the blood as the result of improper cleansing of the venipuncture site. Immunocompromised patients are at higher risk for developing this complication.

Related Tests

Related tests include biopsy bone marrow, biopsy kidney, blood groups and antibodies, CBC, CBC hematocrit, CBC hemoglobin, CBC RBC morphology and inclusions, Coombs antiglobulin, erythropoietin, fecal analysis, ferritin, folate, gallium scan, haptoglobin, iron/TIBC, lymphangiogram, Meckel diverticulum scan, reticulocyte count, and vitamin B$_{12}$.

Refer to the Cardiovascular, Gastrointestinal, Genitourinary, Hematopoietic, Hepatobiliary, Immune, and Respiratory systems tables at the end of the book for related tests by body system.

Expected Outcomes

Expected outcomes associated with Complete Blood Count, RBC Count, are:

- Verbalizing an understanding of how low RBC can place one's life at risk
- Altering activities to decrease fatigue and still meet role performance needs
- Expressing anxiety about a decrease in health and working with the HCP to effect positive improvement

Complete Blood Count, RBC Indices

Quick Summary

SYNONYM ACRONYM: Mean corpuscular hemoglobin (MCH), mean corpuscular volume (MCV), mean corpuscular hemoglobin concentration (MCHC), red blood cell distribution width (RDW).

COMMON USE: To evaluate cell size, shape, weight, and hemoglobin concentration. Used to diagnose and monitor therapy for diagnoses such as iron-deficiency anemia.

SPECIMEN: Whole blood collected in a lavender-top (EDTA) tube.

NORMAL FINDINGS: (Method: Automated, computerized, multichannel analyzers)

Age	MCV (fL)	MCH (pg/cell)	MCHC (g/dL)	RDWCV	RDWSD
Cord blood	107–119	35–39	31–35	14.9–18.7	51–66
0–1 wk	104–116	29–45	24–36	14.9–18.7	51–66
2–3 wk	95–117	26–38	26–34	14.9–18.7	51–66
1–2 mo	81–125	25–37	26–34	14.9–18.7	44–55
3–11 mo	78–110	22–34	26–34	14.9–18.7	35–46
1–5 yr	74–94	24–32	30–34	11.6–14.8	35–42
6–8 yr	73–93	24–32	32–36	11.6–14.8	35–42
9–14 yr	74–94	25–33	32–36	11.6–14.8	37–44
15 yr–adult					
Male	77–97	26–34	32–36	11.6–14.8	38–48
Female	78–98	26–34	32–36	11.6–14.8	38–48
Older adult					
Male	79–103	27–35	32–36	11.6–14.8	38–48
Female	78–102	27–35	32–36	11.6–14.8	38–48

MCV = mean corpuscular volume; MCH = mean corpuscular hemoglobin; MCHC = mean corpuscular hemoglobin concentration; RDWCV = coefficient of variation in red blood cell distribution width; RDWSD = standard deviation in RBC distribution width index.

Test Explanation

Red blood cell (RBC) indices provide information about RBC size and hemoglobin content. The indices are derived from mathematical relationships between the RBC count, Hgb level, and Hct. RBC indices are frequently used to assist in the classification of anemias. The MCV reflects the average size of circulating RBCs and classifies size as normocytic, microcytic (smaller than normal), and macrocytic (larger than normal). MCV is determined by dividing the Hct by the total RBC. The RDW is a measurement of cell size distribution. Many of the commonly used automated cell counters report the more sophisticated statistical indices, RDWCV and RDWSD, instead of RDW. The RDWCV is an indication of variation in cell size over the circulating RBC population. The RDWSD is also an indicator of variation in RBC size, is not affected by the MCV as with the RDWCV index, and is a more accurate measurement of the degree of variation in cell size. Review of peripheral smears is used to corroborate findings from automated instruments. Excessive variations in cell size are graded from 1+ to 4+, with 4+ indicating the most severe degree of anisocytosis, or variation in cell size. MCH (or average amount of Hgb in RBCs) and MCHC (or average amount of Hgb per volume of RBCs) are used to measure hemoglobin content. Microscopic review of the peripheral smear can also be used to visually confirm automated values. Terms used to describe the hemoglobin content of RBCs are normochromic, hypochromic, and hyperchromic. The findings are also visually graded from 1+ to 4+. The MCH is determined by dividing the total hemoglobin by the RBC count. MCHC is determined by dividing total hemoglobin by hematocrit. (See "Complete Blood Count, Hemoglobin," "Complete Blood Count, Hematocrit," "Complete Blood Count, RBC Count," and "Complete Blood Count, RBC Morphology and Inclusions.")

Nursing Implications

Assessment

Indications	Potential Nursing Problems
Assist in the diagnosis of anemia Detect a hematological disorder, neoplasm, or immunological abnormality Determine the presence of a hereditary hematological abnormality Monitor the effects of physical or emotional stress Monitor the progression of nonhematological disorders such as chronic obstructive pulmonary disease, malabsorption syndromes, cancer, and kidney disease Monitor the response to drugs or chemotherapy, and evaluate undesired reactions to drugs that may cause blood dyscrasias Provide screening as part of a complete blood count (CBC) in a general physical examination, especially upon admission to a health-care facility or before surgery	• Cardiac Output • Confusion • Fatigue • Gas Exchange • Health Management • Human Response • Tissue Perfusion

Diagnosis: Clinical Significance of Test Results
INCREASED IN
MCV

- Alcoholism *(vitamin deficiency related to malnutrition)*
- Antimetabolite therapy *(the therapy inhibits vitamin B$_{12}$ and folate)*

- Liver disease *(complex effect on RBCs that includes malnutrition, alterations in RBC shape and size, effects of chronic disease)*
- Pernicious anemia (vitamin B$_{12}$/folate anemia)

MCH

- Macrocytic anemias *(related to increased hemoglobin or cell size)*

MCHC

- Spherocytosis *(artifact in measurement caused by abnormal cell shape)*

RDW

- Anemias with heterogeneous cell size as a result of hemoglobinopathy, hemolytic anemia, anemia following acute blood loss, iron-deficiency anemia, vitamin- and folate-deficiency anemia *(related to a mixture of cell sizes as the bone marrow responds to the anemia and/or to a mixture of cell shapes due to cell fragmentation as a result of the disease)*

DECREASED IN
MCV

- Iron-deficiency anemia *(related to low hemoglobin)*
- Thalassemias *(related to low hemoglobin)*

MCH

- Hypochromic anemias *(related to low hemoglobin)*
- Microcytic anemias *(related to low hemoglobin)*

MCHC

- Iron-deficiency anemia *(the amount of hemoglobin in the RBC is small relative to RBC size)*

RDW

- N/A

Planning
Considerations for planning a successful partnership should include clear communication of what to expect during the test to decrease anxiety and improve cooperation. Before the procedure is performed, plan to review the steps with the patient. Address concerns about pain, and explain that there may be some discomfort during the venipuncture.

SPECIAL CONSIDERATIONS
An important aspect of planning is understanding the factors that may alter study findings or cause abnormal results. Interdepartmental communication is a key factor in the planning process. The following should be noted when planning for this study:

- The patient's position. *RBC count and RBC indices can decrease when the patient is recumbent as a result of hemodilution and can increase when the patient rises as a result of hemoconcentration.*

- Acute blood loss or transfusion. *Care should be taken in evaluating the RBC count and indices during transfusion or acute blood loss because the values may appear to be normal and may not be a reliable indicator of anemia.*
- Cold agglutinins may falsely increase the MCH, MCHC, and decrease the RBC count. This can be corrected by warming the blood or diluting the sample with warmed saline and then correcting the RBC count mathematically.
- Lipemia may falsely increase the MCHC and MCH by falsely increasing Hgb.
- Diseases and conditions related to abnormalities in the RBC size (macrocytes, microcytes) or RBC shape (spherocytes, sickle cells), or that cause RBC agglutination may alter the values of RBC indices.

It is also important to understand which medications or substances the patient may be exposed to in the health-care setting that can interfere with accurate testing:

- Drugs that may increase the MCV include colchicine, pentamidine, pyrimethamine, and triamterene.
- Drugs that may increase the MCH and MCHC include oral contraceptives (long-term use).
- Drugs and substances that may decrease the MCHC include styrene (occupational exposure).
- Drugs that may decrease the MCV include nitrofurantoin.

● Safety Tip

The results of a CBC should be carefully evaluated during transfusion or acute blood loss because the body is not in a state of homeostasis, and values may be misleading. Considerations for draw times after transfusion include the type of product, the amount of product transfused, and the patient's clinical situation. Generally, specimens collected an hour after transfusion will provide an acceptable reflection of the effects of the transfused product. Measurements taken during a massive transfusion are an exception, providing essential guidance for therapeutic decisions during critical care.

Implementation

Patient education is key to obtaining the patient's cooperation in following directions, and providing an explanation for the purpose of the procedure is an important part of this process. Inform the patient that this study can assist in assessing RBC shape and size. Perform the venipuncture.

Evaluation

◉ Critical Findings

N/A

◉ Study Specific Complications

There are a number of complications associated with performing a venipuncture. **Pain** is commonly associated with needles, and although the pain experienced during venipuncture is usually mild, on a rare occasion the needle may strike a nerve causing permanent pain. Some patients experience a **vasovagal reaction** during the venipuncture procedure, evidenced by sweating, low blood pressure, fainting, or near fainting. The potential for a **fall injury** is a significant concern related to vasovagal reactions. Prolonged **bleeding** is a complication that occurs with patients who are taking blood thinners or who have coagulopathies such as hemophilia. A **hematoma** results when blood leaks into the tissue during or after a venipuncture, as evidenced by pain, bruising, and/or swelling at the venipuncture site. The swelling can cause injury by compression to surrounding nerves, which can be temporary or permanent. Health-care providers should watch for minor complications such as bruising and hematoma at the venipuncture site, which are fairly common. Hematomas occur more often in older adult or frail patients, or those with veins that are difficult to access. Bleeding or bruising can be prevented once the needle has been removed by applying direct pressure to the site with dry gauze for a minute or two. Some other more unusual complications of venipuncture include **cellulitis, phlebitis, inadvertent arterial puncture,** and **sepsis.** Sepsis can be caused by introduction of bacteria from the surface of the skin into the blood as the result of improper cleansing of the venipuncture site. Immunocompromised patients are at higher risk for developing this complication.

◉ Related Tests

Related tests include biopsy bone marrow, CBC, CBC hematocrit, CBC hemoglobin, CBC RBC count, CBC RBC morphology and inclusions, CBC WBC count and differential, erythropoietin, ferritin, folate, Hgb electrophoresis, iron/TIBC, lead, reticulocyte count, sickle cell screen, and vitamin B_{12}.

Refer to the Gastrointestinal, Hematopoietic, Immune, and Respiratory systems tables at the end of the book for related tests by body system.

Expected Outcomes

Expected outcomes associated with Complete Blood Count, RBC Indices, are:

- Identifying iron-rich foods and integrates them into the diet.
- Complying with iron replacement therapy as recommended by the HCP.
- Understanding that the purpose of a post-transfusion draw is to evaluate the transfusions effectiveness in improving red cell levels
- Verbalizing symptoms that should be reported that may indicate a transfusion reaction

Complete Blood Count, RBC Morphology and Inclusions

Quick Summary

COMMON USE: To make a visual evaluation of the red cell shape and/or size as a confirmation in assisting to diagnose and monitor disease progression.

SPECIMEN: Whole blood from one full lavender-top (EDTA) tube or Wright-stained, thin-film peripheral blood smear. The laboratory should be consulted as to the necessity of thick-film smears for the evaluation of malarial inclusions.

NORMAL FINDINGS: (Method: Microscopic, manual review of stained blood smear)

Red Blood Cell Morphology	Within Normal Limits	1+	2+	3+	4+
Size					
Anisocytosis	0–5	5–10	10–20	20–50	Greater than 50
Macrocytes	0–5	5–10	10–20	20–50	Greater than 50
Microcytes	0–5	5–10	10–20	20–50	Greater than 50
Shape					
Poikilocytes	0–2	3–10	10–20	20–50	Greater than 50
Burr cells	0–2	3–10	10–20	20–50	Greater than 50
Acanthocytes	Less than 1	2–5	5–10	10–20	Greater than 20
Schistocytes	Less than 1	2–5	5–10	10–20	Greater than 20
Dacryocytes (teardrop cells)	0–2	2–5	5–10	10–20	Greater than 20
Codocytes (target cells)	0–2	2–10	10–20	20–50	Greater than 50
Spherocytes	0–2	2–10	10–20	20–50	Greater than 50
Ovalocytes	0–2	2–10	10–20	20–50	Greater than 50
Stomatocytes	0–2	2–10	10–20	20–50	Greater than 50
Drepanocytes (sickle cells)	Absent	Reported as present or absent			
Helmet cells	Absent	Reported as present or absent			
Agglutination	Absent	Reported as present or absent			
Rouleaux	Absent	Reported as present or absent			
Hemoglobin (Hgb) Content					
Hypochromia	0–2	3–10	10–50	50–75	Greater than 75
Polychromasia					
Adult	Less than 1	2–5	5–10	10–20	Greater than 20
Newborn	1–6	7–15	15–20	20–50	Greater than 50
Inclusions					
Cabot rings	Absent	Reported as present or absent			
Basophilic stippling	0–1	1–5	5–10	10–20	Greater than 20
Howell-Jolly bodies	Absent	1–2	3–5	5–10	Greater than 10
Heinz bodies	Absent	Reported as present or absent			
Hgb C crystals	Absent	Reported as present or absent			
Pappenheimer bodies	Absent	Reported as present or absent			
Intracellular parasites (e.g., Plasmodium, Babesia, Trypanosoma)	Absent	Reported as present or absent			

Test Explanation

The decision to manually review a peripheral blood smear for abnormalities in red blood cell (RBC) shape or size is made on the basis of criteria established by the reporting laboratory. Cues in the results of the complete blood count (CBC) will point to specific abnormalities that can be confirmed visually by microscopic review of the sample on a stained blood smear (see Fig. 2.9).

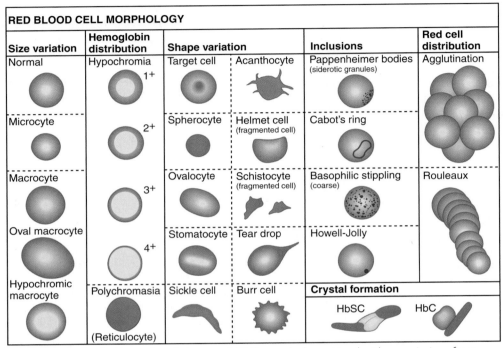

FIGURE 2.9 Normal and abnormal RBC morphology. *Used with permission, from Harmening, D. (2008). Clinical hematology and fundamentals of hemostasis (5th Ed.). FA Davis Company.*

Nursing Implications

Assessment

Indications	Potential Nursing Problems
Assist in the diagnosis of anemia	• Confusion
Detect a hematological disorder, neoplasm, or immunological abnormality	• Fear
Determine the presence of a hereditary hematological abnormality	• Gas Exchange
Monitor the effects of physical or emotional stress on the patient	• Human Response
Monitor the progression of nonhematological disorders, such as chronic obstructive pulmonary disease, malabsorption syndromes, cancer, and kidney disease	• Powerlessness
Monitor the response to drugs or chemotherapy, and evaluate undesired reactions to drugs that may cause blood dyscrasias	• Tissue Perfusion
Provide screening as part of a CBC in a general physical examination, especially upon admission to a health-care facility or before surgery	

Diagnosis: Clinical Significance of Test Results

RED BLOOD CELL SIZE INCREASED IN

- Alcoholism
- Aplastic anemia
- Chemotherapy
- Chronic hemolytic anemia
- Grossly elevated glucose (hyperosmotic)
- Hemolytic disease of the newborn
- Hypothyroidism
- Leukemia
- Lymphoma
- Metastatic carcinoma
- Myelofibrosis
- Myeloma
- Refractory anemia
- Sideroblastic anemia
- Vitamin B_{12}/folate deficiency *(related to impaired DNA synthesis and delayed cell division, which permits the cells to grow for a longer period than normal)*

RED BLOOD CELL SIZE DECREASED IN

- Hemoglobin C disease
- Hemolytic anemias
- Hereditary spherocytosis
- Inflammation
- Iron-deficiency anemia
- Thalassemias

RED BLOOD CELL SHAPE

Variations in cell shape are the result of hereditary conditions such as elliptocytosis, sickle cell anemia, spherocytosis, thalassemias, or hemoglobinopathies (e.g., hemoglobin C disease). Irregularities in cell shape can also result from acquired conditions, such as physical/mechanical cellular trauma, exposure to chemicals, or reactions to medications.

- Acquired spherocytosis can result from Heinz body hemolytic anemia, microangiopathic hemolytic anemia, secondary isoimmunohemolytic anemia, and transfusion of old banked blood.
- Acanthocytes are associated with acquired conditions such as alcoholic cirrhosis with hemolytic anemia, disorders of lipid metabolism, hepatitis of newborns, malabsorptive diseases, metastatic liver disease, the postsplenectomy period, and pyruvate kinase deficiency.
- Burr cells are commonly seen in acquired renal insufficiency, burns, cardiac valve disease, disseminated intravascular coagulation (DIC), hypertension, intravenous fibrin deposition, metastatic malignancy, normal neonatal period, and uremia.
- Codocytes are seen in hemoglobinopathies, iron-deficiency anemia, obstructive liver disease, and the postsplenectomy period.
- Dacryocytes are most commonly associated with metastases to the bone marrow, myelofibrosis, myeloid metaplasia, pernicious anemia, and tuberculosis.
- Schistocytes are seen in burns, cardiac valve disease, DIC, glomerulonephritis, hemolytic anemia, microangiopathic hemolytic anemia, renal graft rejection, thrombotic thrombocytopenic purpura, uremia, and vasculitis.

RED BLOOD CELL HEMOGLOBIN CONTENT

- RBCs with a normal hemoglobin (Hgb) level have a clear central pallor and are referred to as *normochromic.*
- Cells with low Hgb and lacking in central pallor are referred to as *hypochromic.* Hypochromia is associated with iron-deficiency anemia, thalassemias, and sideroblastic anemia.
- Cells with excessive Hgb levels are referred to as *hyperchromic* even though they technically lack a central pallor. Hyperchromia is usually associated with an elevated mean corpuscular Hgb concentration as well as hemolytic anemias.

- Cells referred to as *polychromic* are young erythrocytes that still contain ribonucleic acid (RNA). The RNA is picked up by the Wright stain. Polychromasia is indicative of premature release of RBCs from bone marrow secondary to increased erythropoietin stimulation.

RED BLOOD CELL INCLUSIONS

RBC inclusions can result from certain types of anemia, abnormal Hgb precipitation, or parasitic infection.

- Cabot rings may be seen in megaloblastic and other anemias, lead poisoning, and conditions in which RBCs are destroyed before they are released from bone marrow.
- Basophilic stippling is seen whenever there is altered Hgb synthesis, as in thalassemias, megaloblastic anemias, alcoholism, and lead or arsenic intoxication.
- Howell-Jolly bodies are seen in sickle cell anemia, other hemolytic anemias, megaloblastic anemia, congenital absence of the spleen, and the postsplenectomy period.
- Pappenheimer bodies may be seen in cases of sideroblastic anemia, thalassemias, refractory anemia, dyserythropoietic anemias, hemosiderosis, and hemochromatosis.
- Heinz bodies are most often seen in the blood of patients who have ingested drugs known to induce the formation of these inclusion bodies. They are also seen in patients with hereditary glucose-6-phosphate dehydrogenase (G6PD) deficiency.
- Hgb C crystals can often be identified in stained peripheral smears of patients with hereditary hemoglobin C disease.
- Parasites such as Plasmodium (transmitted by mosquitoes and causing malaria) and Babesia (transmitted by ticks), known to invade human RBCs, can be visualized with Wright stain and other special stains of the peripheral blood.

Planning

Considerations for planning a successful partnership should include clear communication of what to expect during the test to decrease anxiety and improve cooperation. Before the procedure is performed, plan to review the steps with the patient. Address concerns about pain and explain that there may be some discomfort during the venipuncture or fingerstick (if the microhematocrit collection will be used).

SPECIAL CONSIDERATIONS

An important aspect of planning is understanding the factors that may alter study findings or cause abnormal results. Interdepartmental communication is a key factor in the planning process.

It is also important to understand which medications or substances the patient may be exposed to in the health-care setting that can interfere with accurate testing:

- Drugs and substances that may increase Heinz body formation as an initial precursor to significant hemolysis include acetanilid, acetylsalicylic acid, aminopyrine, antimalarials, antipyretics, furaltadone, furazolidone, methylene blue, naphthalene, and nitrofurans.

Morphology can be evaluated to some extent via indices.

Implementation
Patient education is key to obtaining the patient's cooperation in following directions, and providing an explanation for the purpose of the procedure is an important part of this process. Inform the patient that this study can assist in assessing red cell appearance. Perform the venipuncture.

Evaluation
Recognize anxiety related to test results, and educate the patient about proper diet.

NUTRITIONAL CONSIDERATIONS: Instruct patients to consume a variety of foods within the basic food groups, maintain a healthy weight, be physically active, limit salt intake, limit alcohol intake, and avoid the use of tobacco.

✅ Critical Findings
The presence of sickle cells or parasitic inclusions should be brought to the immediate attention of the requesting health-care provider (HCP).

Note and immediately report to the requesting HCP any critical findings and related symptoms. A listing of these findings varies among facilities.

✅ Study Specific Complications
There are a number of complications associated with performing a venipuncture. **Pain** is commonly associated with needles, and although the pain experienced during venipuncture is usually mild, on a rare occasion the needle may strike a nerve causing permanent pain. Some patients experience a **vasovagal reaction** during the venipuncture procedure, evidenced by sweating, low blood pressure, fainting, or near fainting. The potential for a **fall injury** is a significant concern related to vasovagal reactions. Prolonged **bleeding** is a complication that occurs with patients who are taking blood thinners or who have coagulopathies such as hemophilia. A **hematoma** results when blood leaks into the tissue during or after a venipuncture, as evidenced by pain, bruising, and/or swelling at the venipuncture site. The swelling can cause injury by compression to surrounding nerves, which can be temporary or permanent. HCPs should watch for minor complications such as bruising and hematoma at the venipuncture site, which are fairly common. Hematomas occur more often in older adult or frail patients, or those with veins that are difficult to access. Bleeding or bruising can be prevented once the needle has been removed

by applying direct pressure to the site with dry gauze for a minute or two. Some other more unusual complications of venipuncture include **cellulitis, phlebitis, inadvertent arterial puncture,** and **sepsis.** Sepsis can be caused by introduction of bacteria from the surface of the skin into the blood as the result of improper cleansing of the venipuncture site. Immunocompromised patients are at higher risk for developing this complication.

✅ Related Tests
Related tests include biopsy bone marrow, CBC, CBC hematocrit, CBC hemoglobin, CBC platelet count, CBC RBC count, CBC RBC indices, CBC WBC count with differential, δ-aminolevulinic acid, erythropoietin, ferritin, G6PD, hemoglobin electrophoresis, iron/TIBC, lead, and reticulocyte count.

Refer to the Gastrointestinal, Hematopoietic, Hepatobiliary, Immune, and Respiratory systems tables at the end of the book for related tests by body system.

Expected Outcomes
Expected outcomes associated with Complete Blood Count, RBC Morphology and Inclusions, are:

- Correctly classifying anemia with the corresponding care plan, resulting in improved health and well-being of the patient
- Agreeing to have genetic counseling prior to pregnancy related to the potential for inherited disease
- Understanding health-care options, which increases one's sense of control
- Being emotionally stable in expressing fear related to a disquieting diagnosis

Complete Blood Count, WBC Count and Differential

Quick Summary
SYNONYM ACRONYM: WBC with diff, leukocyte count, white cell count.

COMMON USE: To evaluate viral and bacterial infections and to assist in diagnosing and monitoring leukemic disorders.

SPECIMEN: Whole blood from one full lavender-top (EDTA) tube.

NORMAL FINDINGS: (Method: Automated, computerized, multichannel analyzers. Many analyzers can determine a five- or six-part WBC differential. The six-part automated WBC differential identifies and enumerates neutrophils, lymphocytes, monocytes, eosinophils, basophils, and immature granulocytes (IG), where IG represents the combined enumeration of promyelocytes, metamyelocytes, and myelocytes as both an absolute number and a percentage. The five-part WBC differential includes all but the immature granulocyte parameters.)

White Blood Cell Count and Differential

Age	Conventional Units WBC × 10³/microL	Neutrophils	Lymphocytes	Monocytes	Eosinophils	Basophils
		(Absolute) and %	(Absolute) and %	(Absolute) and %	(Absolute) and %	(Absolute) and %
Birth	9.1–30.1	(5.5–18.3) 24%–58%	(2.8–9.3) 26%–56%	(0.5–1.7) 7%–13%	(0.02–0.7) 0%–8%	(0.1–0.2) 0%–2.5%
1–23 mo	6.1–17.5	(1.9–5.4) 21%–67%	(3.7–10.7) 20%–64%	(0.3–0.8) 4%–11%	(0.2–0.5) 0%–3.3%	(0–0.1) 0%–1%
2–10 yr	4.5–13.5	(2.4–7.3) 30%–77%	(1.7–5.1) 14%–50%	(0.2–0.6) 4%–9%	(0.1–0.3) 0%–5.8%	(0–0.1) 0%–1%
11 yr–older adult	4.5–11.1	(2.7–6.5) 40%–75%	(1.5–3.7) 12%–44%	(0.2–0.4) 4%–9%	(0.05–0.5) 0%–5.5%	(0–0.1) 0%–1%

*SI Units (Conventional Units × 1 or WBC count x 10^9/L).

White Blood Cell Count and Differential

Age	Immature Granulocytes (Absolute) (10³/microL)	Immature Granulocyte Fraction (IGF) (%)
Birth–9 yr	0–0.03	0%–0.4%
10 yr–older adult	0–0.09	0%–0.9%

Test Explanation

White blood cells (WBCs) constitute the body's primary defense system against foreign organisms, tissues, and other substances. The life span of a normal WBC is 13 to 20 days. Old WBCs are destroyed by the lymphatic system and excreted in the feces. Reference values for WBC counts vary significantly with age. WBC counts vary diurnally, with counts being lowest in the morning and highest in the late afternoon. Other variables such as stress and high levels of activity or physical exercise can trigger transient increases of $2–5 \times 10^3$/microL. The main WBC types are neutrophils (band and segmented neutrophils), eosinophils, basophils, monocytes, and lymphocytes. WBCs are produced in the bone marrow. B-cell lymphocytes remain in the bone marrow to mature. T-cell lymphocytes migrate to and mature in the thymus. The WBC count can be performed alone with the differential cell count or as part of the complete blood count (CBC). The WBC differential can be performed by an automated instrument or manually on a slide prepared from a stained peripheral blood sample. Automated instruments provide excellent, reliable information, but the accuracy of the WBC count can be affected by the presence of circulating nucleated red blood cells (RBCs), clumped platelets, fibrin strands, cold agglutinins, cryoglobulins, intracellular parasitic organisms, or other significant blood cell inclusions and may not be identified in the interpretation of an automated blood count. The decision to report a manual or automated differential is based on specific criteria established by the laboratory. The criteria are designed to identify findings that warrant further investigation or confirmation by manual review. An increased WBC count is termed *leukocytosis,* and a decreased WBC count is termed *leukopenia.* A total WBC count indicates the degree of response to a pathological process, but a more complete evaluation for specific diagnoses for any one disorder is provided by the differential count. The WBCs in the count and differential are reported as an *absolute value* and as a percentage. The relative percentages of cell types are arrived at by basing the enumeration of each cell type on a 100-cell count. The absolute value is obtained by multiplying the relative percentage value of each cell type by the total WBC count. For example, on a CBC report, with a total WBC of 9×10^3/microL and WBC differential with 92% segmented neutrophils, 1% band neutrophils, 5% lymphocytes, and 1% monocytes, the absolute values are calculated as follows: $92/100 \times 9 = 8.3$ segs, $1/100 \times 9 = 0.01$ bands, $5/100 \times 9 = 0.45$ lymphs, $1/100 \times 9 = 0.1$ monos for a total of 9 WBC count. The absolute neutrophil count (ANC) for this patient would be $9 \times (0.92 + 0.01) = 8.4$.

The absolute neutrophil count (ANC) reflects the number of segmented and band type neutrophils in the total WBC count. It is used as an indicator of immune status because it reflects the type and number of WBC available to rapidly respond to an infection. Neutropenia is a decrease below normal in the number of neutrophils. ANC = Total WBC × ((Segs/100) + (Bands/100)) or total WBC × (% Segs + % Bands). The normal value varies with age but in general mild neutropenia is less than 1.5, moderate neutropenia is between 0.5 and 1, and severe neutropenia is less than 0.5. The ANC is helpful when managing patients receiving chemotherapy. It can drive decisions to place a hospitalized patient in isolation in order to protect them from exposure to infectious agents. When the patient is aware of his or her ANC, the patient can also make informed decisions in taking actions to avoid exposure to crowds, avoid touching things in public places that may carry germs, or avoiding friends and family who may be sick.

Acute leukocytosis is initially accompanied by changes in the WBC count population, followed by changes within the individual WBCs. Leukocytosis usually occurs by way of increase in a single WBC family rather than a proportional increase in all cell types. Toxic granulation and vacuolation are commonly seen in leukocytosis accompanied by a *shift to the left,* or increase in the percentage of immature neutrophils to mature segmented neutrophils. An increased number or percentage of immature granulocytes, reflected by a shift to the left, represents production of WBCs and is useful as an indicator of infection. Immature neutrophils are called bands and can represent 3% to 5% of total circulating neutrophils in healthy individuals. *Bandemia* is defined by the presence of greater than 6% to 10% band neutrophils in the total neutrophil cell population. These changes in the white cell population are most commonly associated with an infectious process, usually bacterial, but they can occur in healthy individuals who are under stress (in response to epinephrine production), such as women in childbirth and very young infants. The WBC count and differential of a woman in labor or of an actively crying infant may show an overall increase in WBCs with a shift to the left. Before initiating any kind of intervention, it is important to determine whether an increased WBC count is the result of a normal condition involving physiological stress or a pathological process. The use of multiple specimen types may confuse the interpretation of results in infants. Multiple samples from the same collection site (i.e., capillary versus venous) may be necessary to obtain an accurate assessment of the WBC picture in these young patients.

Neutrophils are normally found as the predominant WBC type in the circulating blood. Also called *polymorphonuclear cells,* they are the body's first line of defense through the process of phagocytosis. They also contain enzymes and pyogenes, which combat foreign invaders.

Lymphocytes are agranular, mononuclear blood cells that are smaller than granulocytes. They are found in the next highest percentage in normal circulation. Lymphocytes are classified as B cells and T cells. Both types are formed in the bone marrow, but B cells mature in the bone marrow and T cells mature in the thymus. Lymphocytes play a major role in the body's natural defense system. B cells differentiate into immunoglobulin-synthesizing plasma cells. T cells function as cellular mediators of immunity and compose helper/inducer (CD4) lymphocytes, delayed hypersensitivity lymphocytes, cytotoxic (CD8 or CD4) lymphocytes, and suppressor (CD8) lymphocytes.

Monocytes are mononuclear cells similar to lymphocytes, but they are related more closely to granulocytes in terms of their function. They are formed in the bone marrow from the same cells as those that produce neutrophils. The major function of monocytes is phagocytosis. Monocytes stay in the peripheral blood for about 70 hours, after which they migrate into the tissues and become macrophages.

The function of eosinophils is phagocytosis of antigen-antibody complexes. They become active in the later stages of inflammation. Eosinophils respond to allergic and parasitic diseases: They have granules that contain histamine used to kill foreign cells in the body and proteolytic enzymes that damage parasitic worms (see study titled "Eosinophil Count").

Basophils are found in small numbers in the circulating blood. They have a phagocytic function and, similar to eosinophils, contain numerous specific granules. Basophilic granules contain heparin, histamines, and serotonin. Basophils may also be found in tissue and as such are classified as mast cells. Basophilia is noted in conditions such as leukemia, Hodgkin disease, polycythemia vera, ulcerative colitis, nephrosis, and chronic hypersensitivity states.

Nursing Implications

Assessment

Indications	Potential Nursing Problems
Assist in confirming suspected bone marrow depression	• Confusion
Assist in determining the cause of an elevated WBC count (e.g., infection, inflammatory process)	• Fatigue (related to the expenditure of energy stores to fight infection)
Detect hematological disorder, neoplasm, or immunological abnormality	• Fever (related to infection)
Determine the presence of a hereditary hematological abnormality	• Fluid Volume (insufficiency related to insensible loss from fever, and inadequate intake)
Monitor the effects of physical or emotional stress	
Monitor the progression of nonhematological disorders, such as chronic obstructive pulmonary disease, malabsorption syndromes, cancer, and kidney disease	• Health Management
	• Human Response
Monitor the response to drugs or chemotherapy and evaluate undesired reactions to drugs that may cause blood dyscrasias	• Infection
Provide screening as part of a CBC in a general physical examination, especially on admission to a healthcare facility or before surgery	• Nutrition (related to inadequate caloric intake associated with the disease process, and emotional status)

Diagnosis: Clinical Significance of Test Results

WBC INCREASED (LEUKOCYTOSIS)

Normal physiological and environmental conditions:

- Early infancy *(increases are believed to be related to the physiological stress of birth and metabolic demands of rapid development)*
- Emotional stress *(related to secretion of epinephrine)*
- Exposure to extreme heat or cold *(related to physiological stress)*
- Pregnancy and labor *(WBC counts may be modestly elevated due to increased neutrophils into the third trimester and during labor, returning to normal within a week postpartum)*
- Strenuous exercise *(related to epinephrine secretion; increases are short in duration, minutes to hours)*
- Ultraviolet light *(related to physiological stress and possible inflammatory response)*

Pathological conditions:

- Acute hemolysis, especially due to splenectomy or transfusion reactions *(related to leukocyte response to remove lysed RBC fragments)*
- All types of infections *(related to an inflammatory or infectious response)*
- Anemias *(bone marrow disorders affecting RBC production may result in elevated WBC count)*
- Appendicitis
- Collagen disorders *(related to an inflammatory or infectious response)*
- Cushing disease *(related to overproduction of cortisol, a corticosteroid, which stimulates WBC production)*
- Inflammatory disorders *(related to an inflammatory or infectious response)*
- Leukemias and other malignancies *(related to bone marrow disorders that result in abnormal WBC production)*
- Parasitic infestations *(related to an inflammatory or infectious response)*
- Polycythemia vera *(myeloproliferative bone marrow disorder causing an increase in all cell lines)*

WBC DECREASED (LEUKOPENIA)

Normal physiological conditions

- Diurnal rhythms (lowest in the morning)

Pathological conditions

- Alcoholism *(related to WBC changes associated with nutritional deficiencies of vitamin B_{12} or folate)*
- Anemias *(related to WBC changes associated with nutritional deficiencies of vitamin B_{12} or folate, especially in megaloblastic anemias)*

- Bone marrow depression *(related to decreased production)*
- Malaria *(related to hypersplenism)*
- Malnutrition *(related to WBC changes associated with nutritional deficiencies of vitamin B_{12} or folate)*
- Radiation *(related to physical cell destruction due to toxic effects of radiation)*
- Rheumatoid arthritis *(related to side effect of medications used to treat the condition)*
- Systemic lupus erythematosus (SLE) and other autoimmune disorders *(related to side effect of medications used to treat the condition)*
- Toxic and antineoplastic drugs *(related to bone marrow suppression)*
- Very low birth weight neonates *(related to bone marrow activity being diverted to develop RBCs in response to hypoxia)*
- Viral infections *(leukopenia, lymphocytopenia, and abnormal lymphocytes may be present in the early stages of viral infections)*

NEUTROPHILS INCREASED (NEUTROPHILIA)

- Acute hemolysis
- Acute hemorrhage
- Extremes in temperature
- Infectious diseases
- Inflammatory conditions (rheumatic fever, gout, rheumatoid arthritis, vasculitis, myositis)
- Malignancies
- Metabolic disorders (uremia, eclampsia, diabetic ketoacidosis, thyroid storm, Cushing's syndrome)
- Myelocytic leukemia
- Physiological stress (e.g., allergies, asthma, exercise, childbirth, surgery)
- Tissue necrosis (burns, crushing injuries, abscesses, myocardial infarction)
- Tissue poisoning with toxins and venoms

NEUTROPHILS DECREASED (NEUTROPENIA)

- Acromegaly
- Addison disease
- Anaphylaxis
- Anorexia nervosa, starvation, malnutrition
- Bone marrow depression (viruses, toxic chemicals, overwhelming infection, radiation, Gaucher disease)
- Disseminated SLE
- Thyrotoxicosis
- Viral infection (mononucleosis, hepatitis, influenza)
- Vitamin B_{12} or folate deficiency

LYMPHOCYTES INCREASED (LYMPHOCYTOSIS)

- Addison disease
- Felty syndrome
- Infections (viral [e.g., CMV, hepatitis, HIV, infectious mononucleosis, rubella, varicella] or bacterial [e.g., tuberculosis, whooping cough])

- Lymphocytic leukemia
- Lymphomas
- Lymphosarcoma
- Myeloma
- Rickets
- Thyrotoxicosis
- Ulcerative colitis
- Waldenström macroglobulinemia

LYMPHOCYTES DECREASED (LYMPHOPENIA)

- Antineoplastic drugs
- Aplastic anemia
- Bone marrow failure
- Burns
- Gaucher disease
- Hemolytic disease of the newborn
- High doses of adrenocorticosteroids
- Hodgkin disease
- Hypersplenism
- Immunodeficiency diseases
- Infections
- Malnutrition
- Pernicious anemia
- Pneumonia
- Radiation
- Rheumatic fever
- Septicemia
- Thrombocytopenic purpura
- Toxic chemical exposure
- Transfusion reaction

MONOCYTES INCREASED (MONOCYTOSIS)

- Carcinomas
- Cirrhosis
- Collagen diseases
- Gaucher disease
- Hemolytic anemias
- Hodgkin disease
- Infections
- Lymphomas
- Monocytic leukemia
- Polycythemia vera
- Radiation
- Sarcoidosis
- SLE
- Thrombocytopenic purpura
- Ulcerative colitis

Planning

Considerations for planning a successful partnership should include clear communication of what to expect during the test to decrease anxiety and improve cooperation. Before the procedure is performed, plan to review the steps with the patient. Address concerns about pain and explain that there may be some discomfort during the venipuncture.

SPECIAL CONSIDERATIONS

An important aspect of planning is understanding the factors that may alter study findings or cause abnormal results. Interdepartmental communication is a key factor in the planning process. The following should be noted when planning for this study:

- The patient's age. *Newborns normally have increased values. Older adults may also have slightly increased values due to hemoconcentration. Dehydration is a significant and common finding in older adult patients with decreased fluid intake and/or decreased kidney function.*
- The patient's position. *WBC count can decrease when the patient is recumbent as a result of hemodilution and can increase when the patient rises as a result of hemoconcentration.*
- Drug allergies. They may have a significant effect on eosinophil count and may affect the overall WBC count. (See the Eosinophil study found at http://www.davisplus.com.)
- Presence of nucleated RBCs or giant or clumped platelets. They affect the automated WBC, requiring a manual correction of the WBC count.
- Patients with cold agglutinins or monoclonal gammopathies. *A falsely decreased WBC count can occur as a result of cell clumping due to high concentrations of protein.*

It is also important to understand which medications or substances the patient may be exposed to in the healthcare setting that can interfere with accurate testing:

- Drugs that may increase the overall WBC count include amphetamine, amphotericin B, chloramphenicol, chloroform (normal response to anesthesia), colchicine (leukocytosis follows leukopenia), corticotropin, erythromycin, ether (normal response to anesthesia), fluroxene (normal response to anesthesia), isoflurane (normal response to anesthesia), niacinamide, phenylbutazone, prednisone, and quinine.
- Drugs that may decrease the overall WBC count include acetyldigitoxin, acetylsalicylic acid, aminoglutethimide, aminopyrine, aminosalicylic acid, ampicillin, amsacrine, antazoline, anticonvulsants, antineoplastic agents (therapeutic intent), antipyrine, barbiturates, busulfan, carbutamide, carmustine, chlorambucil, chloramphenicol, chlordane, chlorophenothane, chlortetracycline, chlorthalidone, cisplatin, colchicine, colistimethate, cycloheximide, cyclophosphamide, cytarabine, dacarbazine, dactinomycin, diaprim, diazepam, diethylpropion, digitalis, dipyridamole, dipyrone, fumagillin, glaucarubin, glucosulfone, hexachlorobenzene, hydroflumethiazide, hydroxychloroquine, iothiouracil, iproniazid, lincomycin, local anesthetics, mefenamic acid, mepazine, meprobamate, mercaptopurine, methotrexate, methylpromazine, mitomycin, paramethadione,

parathion, penicillin, phenacemide, phenindione, phenothiazine, pipamazine, prednisone (by Coulter S method), primaquine, procainamide, procarbazine, prochlorperazine, promazine, promethazine, pyrazolones, quinacrine, quinines, radioactive compounds, razoxane, ristocetin, sulfa drugs, tamoxifen, tetracycline, thenalidine, thioridazine, tolazamide, tolazoline, tolbutamide, trimethadione, and urethane. A significant decrease in basophil count occurs rapidly after the intravenous injection of propanidid and thiopental. A significant decrease in lymphocyte count occurs rapidly after the administration of corticotropin, mechlorethamine, methysergide, and x-ray therapy; and after megadoses of niacin, pyridoxine, and thiamine.

Implementation

Patient education is key to obtaining the patient's cooperation in following directions, and providing an explanation for the purpose of the procedure is an important part of this process. Inform the patient this study can assist in assessing for infection or monitoring leukemia. Perform the venipuncture.

Evaluation

Recognize anxiety related to test results, and be supportive of a fear of a shortened life expectancy. Discuss the implications of abnormal test results on the patient's lifestyle. Provide teaching and information regarding the clinical implications of the test results as appropriate. Educate the patient about access to counseling services. Provide contact information, if desired, for the National Cancer Institute (www.nci.nih.org) and for the Institute of Medicine of the National Academies (www.iom.edu). Infection, fever, sepsis, and trauma can result in an impaired nutritional status. Malnutrition can occur for many reasons, including fatigue, lack of appetite, and gastrointestinal distress.

Adequate intake of vitamins A and C, and zinc are also important for regenerating body stores depleted by the effort exerted in fighting infections. Educate the patient or caregiver about the importance of following the prescribed diet. Educate the patient with a vitamin A deficiency, as appropriate, that the main dietary source of vitamin A comes from carotene, a yellow pigment noticeable in most fruits and vegetables, especially carrots, sweet potatoes, squash, apricots, and cantaloupe. It is also present in spinach, collards, broccoli, and cabbage. This vitamin is fairly stable at most cooking temperatures, but it is destroyed easily by light and oxidation. Educate the patient with vitamin C deficiency, as appropriate, that citrus fruits are excellent dietary sources of vitamin C. Other good sources are green and red peppers, tomatoes, white potatoes, cabbage, broccoli, chard, kale, turnip greens, asparagus, berries, melons, pineapple, and guava. Vitamin C is destroyed by exposure to air, light, heat, or alkalis. Boiling water before cooking eliminates dissolved oxygen that destroys vitamin C in the process of boiling. Vegetables should be crisp and cooked as quickly as possible. Topical or oral supplementation may be ordered for patients with zinc deficiency. Dietary sources high in zinc include shellfish, red meat, wheat germ, nuts, and processed foods such as canned pork and beans and canned chili. Patients should be informed that phytates (from whole grains, coffee, cocoa, or tea) bind zinc and prevent it from being absorbed. Decreases in zinc also can be induced by an increased intake of iron, copper, or manganese. Vitamin and mineral supplements with a greater than 3:1 iron-to-zinc ratio inhibit zinc absorption.

✔ Critical Findings

- Total WBC count of less than 2×10^3/microL (SI: Less than 2×10^9/L)
- ANC of less than 0.5×10^3/microL (SI: Less than 0.5×10^9/L)
- Total WBC count of greater than 30×10^3/microL (SI: Greater than 30×10^9/L)

Note and immediately report to the requesting healthcare provider (HCP) any critical findings and related symptoms. A listing of these findings varies among facilities.

The presence of abnormal cells, other morphological characteristics, or cellular inclusions may signify a potentially life-threatening or serious health condition and should be investigated. Examples are hypersegmented neutrophils, agranular neutrophils, blasts or other immature cells, Auer rods, Döhle bodies, marked toxic granulation, or plasma cells.

✔ Study Specific Complications

There are a number of complications associated with performing a venipuncture. **Pain** is commonly associated with needles, and although the pain experienced during venipuncture is usually mild, on a rare occasion the needle may strike a nerve causing permanent pain. Some patients experience a **vasovagal reaction** during the venipuncture procedure, evidenced by sweating, low blood pressure, fainting, or near fainting. The potential for a **fall injury** is a significant concern related to vasovagal reactions. Prolonged **bleeding** is a complication that occurs with patients who are taking blood thinners or who have coagulopathies such as hemophilia. A **hematoma** results when blood leaks into the tissue during or after a venipuncture, as evidenced by pain, bruising, and/or swelling at the venipuncture site. The swelling can cause injury by compression to surrounding nerves, which can be temporary or permanent. HCPs should watch for minor complications such as bruising and hematoma at the venipuncture site, which are fairly common. Hematomas occur more often in older adult or frail patients, or those with veins that are difficult to access. Bleeding or bruising can be prevented once the needle has been removed by applying direct pressure to the site with dry gauze for a minute or two. Some other more unusual complications of venipuncture include **cellulitis, phlebitis, inadvertent arterial puncture,** and **sepsis.** Sepsis can be caused by introduction of bacteria from the surface of the skin into the blood as the result of improper cleansing of the venipuncture site. Immunocompromised patients are at higher risk for developing this complication.

⊘ *Related Tests*

Related tests include albumin, antibody, antineutrophilic cytoplasmic biopsy bone marrow, biopsy lymph node, CBC, CBC RBC count, CBC RBC indices, CBC RBC morphology, culture bacterial (see individually listed culture studies), culture fungal, culture viral, eosinophil count, ESR, fecal analysis, Gram stain, infectious mononucleosis, LAP, procalcitonin, UA, US abdomen, and WBC scan.

Refer to the Hematopoietic, Immune, and Respiratory systems tables at the end of the book for related tests by body system.

Expected Outcomes

Expected outcomes associated with Complete Blood Count, WBC Count and Differential, are:

- Nurse collaboration with the HCP to correlate laboratory results with other diagnostic information and presenting symptoms toward making a diagnosis regarding the presence or absence of disease
- Nurse administration of the appropriate treatment for abnormally increased or decreased WBC count that results in improved health status, without relapse
- Patient demonstration of good handwashing technique to prevent further infection
- Patient maintaining a normal temperature, and an understanding that fever is a symptom of disease severity

Erythrocyte Sedimentation Rate

Quick Summary

SYNONYM ACRONYM: Sed rate, ESR.

COMMON USE: To assist in diagnosing acute infection in diseases such as tissue necrosis, chronic infection, and acute inflammation.

SPECIMEN: Whole blood collected in a completely filled lavender-top (EDTA) tube for the modified Westergren method or a completely filled gray-top (3.8% sodium citrate) tube for the original Westergren method.

NORMAL FINDINGS: (Method: Westergren or modified Westergren)

Age	Male	Female
Newborn	0–2 mm/hr	0–2 mm/hr
Less than 50 yr	0–15 mm/hr	0–25 mm/hr
50 yr and older	0–20 mm/hr	0–30 mm/hr

- Glucose-6-phosphate dehydrogenase deficiency
- Heart failure
- Hemoglobin C disease
- Hypofibrinogenemia
- Polycythemia
- Sickle cell anemia
- Spherocytosis

Test Explanation

The erythrocyte sedimentation rate (ESR) is a measure of the rate of sedimentation of red blood cells (RBCs) in an anticoagulated whole blood sample over a specified period of time. The basis of the ESR test is the alteration of blood proteins by inflammatory and necrotic processes that cause the RBCs to stick together, become heavier, and rapidly settle at the bottom of a vertically held, calibrated tube over time. The most common promoter of rouleaux is an increase in circulating fibrinogen levels. In general, relatively little settling occurs in normal blood because normal RBCs do not form rouleaux and would not stack together. The sedimentation rate is proportional to the size or mass of the falling RBCs and is inversely proportional to plasma viscosity. The test is a nonspecific indicator of disease but is fairly sensitive and is frequently the earliest indicator of widespread inflammatory reaction due to infection or autoimmune disorders. Prolonged elevations are also present in malignant disease. The ESR can also be used to monitor the course of a disease and the effectiveness of therapy. The most commonly used method to measure the ESR is the Westergren (or modified Westergren) method.

Nursing Implications

Assessment

Indications	Potential Nursing Problems
Assist in the diagnosis of acute infection, such as tuberculosis or tissue necrosis	• Activity
Assist in the diagnosis of acute inflammatory processes	• Health Management
Assist in the diagnosis of chronic infections	• Human Response
Assist in the diagnosis of rheumatoid or autoimmune disorders	• Infection
Assist in the diagnosis of temporal arthritis and polymyalgia rheumatica	• Mobility
Monitor inflammatory and malignant disease	• Nutrition
	• Pain
	• Skin
	• Tissue Integrity

Diagnosis: Clinical Significance of Test Results

INCREASED IN

- *Increased rouleaux formation is associated with increased levels of fibrinogen and/or production of cytokines and other acute-phase reactant proteins in response to inflammation. Anemia of chronic disease as well as acute anemia influence the ESR because the decreased number of RBCs falls faster with the relatively increased plasma volume.*
- Acute myocardial infarction
- Anemia *(RBCs fall faster with increased plasma volume)*
- Carcinoma
- Cat scratch fever (*Bartonella henselae*)
- Collagen diseases, including systemic lupus erythematosus (SLE)
- Crohn disease *(due to anemia or related to acute-phase reactant proteins)*
- Elevated blood glucose *(hyperglycemia in older patients can induce production of cytokines responsible for the inflammatory response; hyperglycemia related to insulin resistance can cause hepatocytes to shift protein synthesis from albumin to production of acute-phase reactant proteins)*
- Endocarditis
- Heavy metal poisoning *(related to anemia affecting size and shape of RBCs)*
- Increased plasma protein level *(RBCs fall faster with increased plasma viscosity)*
- Infections (e.g., pneumonia, syphilis)
- Inflammatory diseases
- Lymphoma
- Lymphosarcoma
- Multiple myeloma *(RBCs fall faster with increased plasma viscosity)*
- Nephritis
- Pregnancy *(related to anemia)*
- Pulmonary embolism
- Rheumatic fever
- Rheumatoid arthritis
- Subacute bacterial endocarditis
- Temporal arteritis
- Toxemia
- Tuberculosis
- Waldenström macroglobulinemia *(RBCs fall faster with increased plasma viscosity)*

DECREASED IN

- Conditions resulting in high hemoglobin and RBC count

Planning

Considerations for planning a successful partnership should include clear communication of what to expect during the test to decrease anxiety and improve cooperation. Before the procedure is performed, plan to review the steps with the patient. Address concerns about pain, and explain that there may be some discomfort during the venipuncture. Obtain a history of infectious, autoimmune, or neoplastic diseases.

SPECIAL CONSIDERATIONS

An important aspect of planning is understanding the factors that may alter study findings or cause abnormal results. Interdepartmental communication is a key factor in the planning process. The following should be noted when planning for this study:

- Normal circumstances, such as menstruation and pregnancy, may cause falsely increased test results.
- Specimen handling as well as procedural technique can affect test results. A false elevation in values may occur in overheparinized specimens. Other factors that affect results include introducing bubbles in the ESR measurement tube as the specimen is added, tilting the ESR measurement tube more than 3° from vertical, subjecting the ESR tube to any movement or vibration of the surface on which the test is being conducted, inaccurate timing of the test period, or a delay in performing the test once the specimen has been collected. The test should be performed within 4 hours of collection when the specimen has been stored at room temperature. If a delay in testing is anticipated, refrigerate the sample at 2°C to 4°C; a refrigerated temperature is reported to extend the stability of the sample from 4 to 12 hours. If refrigerated, the specimen should be normalized to room temperature prior to testing.

It is also important to understand which medications or substances the patient may be exposed to in the health-care setting that can interfere with accurate testing:

- Some drugs cause an SLE-like syndrome that results in a physiological increase in ESR. These include anticonvulsants, hydrazine derivatives, nitrofurantoin, procainamide, and quinidine. Other drugs that may cause an increased ESR include acetylsalicylic acid, cephalothin, cephapirin, cyclosporin A, dextran, and oral contraceptives.
- Drugs that may cause a decrease in ESR include aurothiomalate, corticotropin, cortisone, dexamethasone, methotrexate, minocycline, NSAIDs, penicillamine, prednisolone, prednisone, quinine, sulfasalazine, tamoxifen, and trimethoprim.

Implementation

Patient education is key to obtaining the patient's cooperation in following directions, and providing an explanation for the purpose of the procedure is an important part of this process. Inform the patient that this study can assist in identifying the presence of inflammation. Perform the venipuncture.

Evaluation

Recognize anxiety related to test results, and address any concerns voiced by the patient or family.

✓ Critical Findings

N/A

✓ Study Specific Complications

There are a number of complications associated with performing a venipuncture. **Pain** is commonly associated with needles, and although the pain experienced during venipuncture is usually mild, on a rare occasion the needle may strike a nerve causing permanent pain. Some patients experience a **vasovagal reaction** during the venipuncture procedure, evidenced by sweating, low blood pressure, fainting, or near fainting. The potential for a **fall injury** is a significant concern related to vasovagal reactions. Prolonged **bleeding** is a complication that occurs with patients who are taking blood thinners or who have coagulopathies such as hemophilia. A **hematoma** results when blood leaks into the tissue during or after a venipuncture, as evidenced by pain, bruising, and/or swelling at the venipuncture site. The swelling can cause injury by compression to surrounding nerves, which can be temporary or permanent. HCPs should watch for minor complications such as bruising and hematoma at the venipuncture site, which are fairly common. Hematomas occur more often in older adult or frail patients, or those with veins that are difficult to access. Bleeding or bruising can be prevented once the needle has been removed by applying direct pressure to the site with dry gauze for a minute or two. Some other more unusual complications of venipuncture include **cellulitis, phlebitis, inadvertent arterial puncture,** and **sepsis.** Sepsis can be caused by introduction of bacteria from the surface of the skin into the blood as the result of improper cleansing of the venipuncture site. Immunocompromised patients are at higher risk for developing this complication.

✓ Related Tests

Related tests include antibodies, anticyclic citrullinated peptide, ANA, arthroscopy, arthrogram, blood pool imaging, BMD, bone scan, CBC, CBC hematocrit, CBC hemoglobin, CBC RBC indices, CBC RBC morphology, CT cardiac scoring, copper, CRP, d-dimer, exercise stress test, fibrinogen, glucose, iron, lead, MRI musculoskeletal, MRI venography, microorganism-specific serologies and related cultures, myocardial perfusion heart scan, procalcitonin, radiography bone, RF, synovial fluid analysis, and troponin.

Refer to the Cardiovascular, Hematopoietic, Immune, and Respiratory systems tables at the end of the book for related tests by body system.

Expected Outcomes

Expected outcomes associated with Erythrocyte Sedimentation Rate are:

* Recognizing the importance of seeking early medical treatment to prevent worsening infection
* Being able to describe the signs and symptoms of infection that should be reported to HCP
* Adhering to the therapeutic regime designed by HCP to treat infection

Hemoglobin Electrophoresis

Quick Summary

COMMON USE: To assist in evaluating hemolytic anemias and identifying hemoglobin variants, diagnose thalassemias, and sickle cell anemia.

SPECIMEN: Whole blood collected in a lavender-top (EDTA) tube.

NORMAL FINDINGS: (Method: Electrophoresis)

Age	Hgb A
Adult	Greater than 95%
	Hgb A$_2$
Adult	1.5%–3.7%
	Hgb F
Newborns and infants	
1 day–3 wk	70%–77%
6–9 wk	42%–64%
3–4 mo	7%–39%
6 mo	3%–7%
8–11 mo	0.6%–2.6%
Adult–older adult	Less than 2%

Test Explanation

Hemoglobin (Hgb) electrophoresis is a separation process used to identify normal and abnormal forms of Hgb. Electrophoresis and high-performance liquid chromatography as well as molecular genetics testing for mutations can also be used to identify abnormal forms of Hgb. Hgb A is the main form of Hgb in the normal adult. Hgb F is the main form of Hgb in the fetus, the remainder being composed of Hgb A$_1$ and A$_2$. Small amounts of Hgb F are normal in the adult. Hgb D, E, S, and C result from abnormal amino acid substitutions

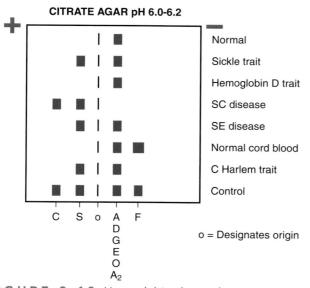

CITRATE AGAR pH 6.0-6.2

Normal
Sickle trait
Hemoglobin D trait
SC disease
SE disease
Normal cord blood
C Harlem trait
Control

C S o A F
         D
         G
         E
         O
         A₂

o = Designates origin

FIGURE 2.10 Hemoglobin electrophoresis.
Used with permission, from Harmening, D. (2008). Clinical hematology and fundamentals of hemostasis (5th Ed.). FA Davis Company.

during the formation of Hgb and are inherited hemoglobinopathies (see Fig. 2.10).

Nursing Implications
Assessment

Indications	Potential Nursing Problems
Assist in the diagnosis of Hgb C disease	• Activity
Assist in the diagnosis of thalassemia, especially in patients with a family history positive for the disorder	• Fear
	• Gas Exchange
	• Health Management
Differentiate among thalassemia types	• Human Response
Evaluate hemolytic anemia of unknown cause	• Pain
	• Tissue Perfusion
Evaluate a positive sickle cell screening test to differentiate sickle cell trait from sickle cell disease	

Diagnosis: Clinical Significance of Test Results
INCREASED IN
HGB A₂

- Hyperthyroidism
- Megaloblastic anemia
- β-Thalassemias
- Sickle trait

HGB F

- Anemia (aplastic, associated with chronic disease or due to blood loss)
- Erythropoietic porphyria
- Hereditary elliptocytosis or spherocytosis
- Hereditary persistence of fetal Hgb
- Hyperthyroidism
- Leakage of fetal blood into maternal circulation
- Leukemia (acute or chronic)
- Myeloproliferative disorders
- Paroxysmal nocturnal hemoglobinuria
- Pernicious anemia
- Sickle cell disease
- Thalassemias
- Unstable hemoglobins

HGB C

- Hgb C disease (second most common variant in the United States; has a higher prevalence among African Americans)

HGB D

- Hgb D (rare hemoglobinopathy that may also be found in combination with Hgb S or thalassemia)

HGB E

- Hgb E disease; thalassemia-like condition (second most common hemoglobinopathy in the world; occurs with the highest frequency in Southeast Asians and African Americans)

HGB S

- Sickle cell trait or disease (most common variant in the United States; occurs with a frequency of about 8% among African Americans)

HGB H

- α-Thalassemias
- Hgb Bart hydrops fetalis syndrome

DECREASED IN
HGB A₂

- Erythroleukemia
- Hgb H disease
- Iron-deficiency anemia (untreated)
- Sideroblastic anemia

Planning
Considerations for planning a successful partnership should include clear communication of what to expect during the test to decrease anxiety and improve cooperation. Before the procedure is performed, plan to review the steps with the patient. Address concerns

about pain, and explain that there may be some discomfort during the venipuncture.

SPECIAL CONSIDERATIONS
An important aspect of planning is understanding the factors that may alter study findings or cause abnormal results. Interdepartmental communication is a key factor in the planning process. The following should be noted when planning for this study:

- Red blood cell (RBC) transfusion within 4 months of the test can mask abnormal Hgb levels and can invalidate test findings.
- Some conditions that may increase values include high altitude exposure *related to a compensatory mechanism whereby RBC production is increased to increase availability of oxygen binding to Hgb* and dehydration *related to hemoconcentration*. Iron deficiency may decrease Hgb A$_2$, C, and S *related to decreased amounts of Hgb in smaller, iron-deficient RBCs*. In patients less than 3 months of age, false-negative results for Hgb S may occur due to the normal polycythemia of infancy *related to technical limitations of the procedure where increased total Hgb levels reflect a small, possibly undetectable percentage of Hgb S when compared to large amounts of Hgb F.*

Implementation
Patient education is key to obtaining the patient's cooperation in following directions, and providing an explanation for the purpose of the procedure is an important part of this process. Inform the patient that this study can assist in diagnosing various types of anemias. Perform the venipuncture.

Evaluation
Recognize anxiety related to test results, and answer any questions or address any concerns voiced by the patient or family.

✅ Critical Findings
N/A

✅ Study Specific Complications

There are a number of complications associated with performing a venipuncture. **Pain** is commonly associated with needles, and although the pain experienced during venipuncture is usually mild, on a rare occasion the needle may strike a nerve causing permanent pain. Some patients experience a **vasovagal reaction** during the venipuncture procedure, evidenced by sweating, low blood pressure, fainting, or near fainting. The potential for a **fall injury** is a significant concern related to vasovagal reactions. Prolonged **bleeding** is a complication that occurs with patients who are taking blood thinners or who have coagulopathies such as hemophilia. A **hematoma** results when

blood leaks into the tissue during or after a venipuncture, as evidenced by pain, bruising, and/or swelling at the venipuncture site. The swelling can cause injury by compression to surrounding nerves, which can be temporary or permanent. HCPs should watch for minor complications such as bruising and hematoma at the venipuncture site, which are fairly common. Hematomas occur more often in older adult or frail patients, or those with veins that are difficult to access. Bleeding or bruising can be prevented once the needle has been removed by applying direct pressure to the site with dry gauze for a minute or two. Some other more unusual complications of venipuncture include **cellulitis, phlebitis, inadvertent arterial puncture,** and **sepsis.** Sepsis can be caused by introduction of bacteria from the surface of the skin into the blood as the result of improper cleansing of the venipuncture site. Immunocompromised patients are at higher risk for developing this complication.

✅ Related Tests

Related tests include biopsy bone marrow, blood gases, CBC, CBC hematocrit, CBC hemoglobin, CBC RBC morphology, methemoglobin, newborn screening, osmotic fragility, and sickle cell screen.

Refer to the Hematopoietic System table at the end of the book for related tests by body system.

Expected Outcomes

Expected outcomes associated with Hemoglobin Electrophoresis are:

- Exhibiting strong peripheral pulses
- Activity level that increases with disease management
- Willingness to attend a support group for parents of children with disorders such as sickle cell disease or thalassemia
- Collaborating with the HCP to develop a management plan tailored to the child's needs

Reticulocyte Count

Quick Summary

SYNONYM ACRONYM: Retic count.

COMMON USE: To assess reticulocyte count in relation to bone marrow activity toward diagnosing anemias such as pernicious iron deficiency, and hemolytic; to monitor response of therapeutic interventions.

SPECIMEN: Whole blood collected in a lavender-top (EDTA) tube.

NORMAL FINDINGS: (Method: Automated analyzer or microscopic examination of specially stained peripheral blood smear)

Age	Reticulocyte Count %
Newborn	3%–6%
Infant	0.4%–2.8%
Child	0.8%–2.1%
Adult–older adult	0.5%–1.5%
	Reticulocyte Count (absolute number)
Birth–older adult	0.02–0.10 (10^6 cells/microL)
	Immature Reticulocyte Fraction %
Birth	2.5%–6.5%
Newborn–older adult	2.5%–17%
	Reticulocyte Hemoglobin
Birth	22–32 pg/cell
Newborn–18 yr	23–34 pg/cell
Adult–older adult	30–35 pg/cell

Test Explanation

Normally, as it matures, the red blood cell (RBC) loses its nucleus. The remaining ribonucleic acid (RNA) produces a characteristic color when special stains are used, making these cells easy to identify and enumerate. Some automated cell counters have the ability to provide a reticulocyte panel, which includes the enumeration of circulating reticulocytes as an absolute count and as a percentage of total RBCs; the immature reticulocyte fraction (IRF), which reflects the number of reticulocytes released into the circulation within the past 24 to 48 hours; and the reticulocyte hemoglobin (Ret-He) content, which reflects the amount of iron incorporated into the maturing RBCs. The presence of reticulocytes is an indication of the level of erythropoietic activity in the bone marrow. The information provided by the reticulocyte panel is useful in the evaluation of anemias, bone marrow response to therapy, degree of bone marrow engraftment following transplant, and the effectiveness of altitude training in high-performance athletes. In abnormal conditions, reticulocytes are prematurely released into circulation. (See studies titled "Complete Blood Count, RBC Count" and "Complete Blood Count, RBC Morphology and Inclusions.")

Nursing Implications

Assessment

Indications	Potential Nursing Problems
Evaluate erythropoietic activity Monitor response to therapy for anemias	• Activity • Confusion • Fatigue • Gas Exchange • Health Management • Human Response • Pain • Self-care

The reticulocyte production index (RPI) is a good estimate of RBC production. The calculation corrects the count for anemia and for the premature release of reticulocytes into the peripheral blood during periods of hemolysis or significant bleeding. The RPI also takes into consideration the maturation time of large polychromatophilic cells or nucleated RBCs seen on the peripheral smear:

$$\text{RPI} = \% \text{ reticulocytes} \times [\text{patient hematocrit (Hct)/normal Hct}] \times (1/\text{maturation time})$$

As the formula shows, the RPI is inversely proportional to Hct, as follows:

Hematocrit (%)	Maturation Time (days)
45	1
35	1.5
25	2
15	2.5

INCREASED IN

Conditions that result in excessive RBC loss or destruction stimulate a compensatory bone marrow response by increasing production of RBCs.

- Blood loss
- Hemolytic anemias
- Iron-deficiency anemia
- Malaria
- Megaloblastic anemia

Other

- Pregnancy
- Treatment for anemia

DECREASED IN

- Alcoholism *(decreased production related to nutritional deficit)*
- Anemia of chronic disease
- Aplastic anemia *(related to overall lack of RBC)*
- Bone marrow replacement *(new marrow fails to produce RBCs until it engrafts)*
- Endocrine disease *(hypometabolism related to hypothyroidism is reflected by decreased bone marrow activity)*
- Kidney disease *(diseased kidneys cannot produce erythropoietin, which stimulates the bone marrow to produce RBCs)*
- RBC aplasia *(related to overall lack of RBCs)*
- Sideroblastic anemia *(RBCs are produced but are abnormal in that they cannot incorporate iron into hemoglobin, resulting in anemia)*

Planning

Considerations for planning a successful partnership should include clear communication of what to expect during the test to decrease anxiety and improve cooperation. Before the procedure is performed, plan to review the steps with the patient. Address concerns about pain and explain that there may be some discomfort during the venipuncture.

SPECIAL CONSIDERATIONS

An important aspect of planning is understanding the factors that may alter study findings or cause abnormal results. Interdepartmental communication is a key factor in the planning process. The following should be noted when planning for this study:

- The presence of RBC inclusions (Howell-Jolly bodies, Heinz bodies, basophilic stippling, Pappenheimer bodies, and intracellular RBC parasites such as seen with malaria and babesiosis) may cause mature RBCs to be counted as reticulocytes, falsely increasing the results. Automated instruments will often flag the results, prompting a manual review of the blood smear in which the inclusions can be identified.
- The reticulocyte count may be falsely decreased as a result of the dilutional effect after a recent blood transfusion.

It is also important to understand which medications or substances the patient may be exposed to in the healthcare setting that can interfere with accurate testing:

- Drugs that may decrease reticulocyte counts include azathioprine, dactinomycin, hydroxyurea, methotrexate, and zidovudine.
- Drugs that may increase reticulocyte counts include acetanilid, acetylsalicylic acid, amyl nitrate, antimalarials, antipyretics, antipyrine, arsenicals, corticotropin, dimercaprol, etretinate, furaltadone, furazolidone, levodopa, methyldopa, nitrofurans, penicillin, procainamide, and sulfones.

Implementation

Patient education is key to obtaining the patient's cooperation in following directions, and providing an explanation for the purpose of the procedure is an important part of this process. Inform the patient that this study can assist in assessing for anemia. Perform the venipuncture.

Evaluation

Recognize anxiety related to test results, and answer any questions or concerns voiced by the patient or family.

✅ *Critical Findings*

N/A

✅ *Study Specific Complications*

There are a number of complications associated with performing a venipuncture. **Pain** is commonly associated with needles, and although the pain experienced during venipuncture is usually mild, on a rare occasion the needle may strike a nerve causing permanent pain. Some patients experience a **vasovagal reaction** during the venipuncture procedure, evidenced by sweating, low blood pressure, fainting, or near fainting. The potential for a **fall injury** is a significant concern related to vasovagal reactions. Prolonged **bleeding** is a complication that occurs with patients who are taking blood thinners or who have coagulopathies such as hemophilia. A **hematoma** results when blood leaks into the tissue during or after a venipuncture, as evidenced by pain, bruising, and/or swelling at the venipuncture site. The swelling can cause injury by compression to surrounding nerves, which can be temporary or permanent. Healthcare providers should watch for minor complications such as bruising and hematoma at the venipuncture site, which are fairly common. Hematomas occur more often in older adult or frail patients, or those with veins that are difficult to access. Bleeding or bruising can be prevented once the needle has been removed by applying direct pressure to the site with dry gauze for a minute or two. Some other more unusual complications of venipuncture include **cellulitis, phlebitis, inadvertent arterial puncture,** and **sepsis.** Sepsis can be caused by introduction of bacteria from the surface of the skin into the blood as the result of improper cleansing of the venipuncture site. Immunocompromised patients are at higher risk for developing this complication.

✅ *Related Tests*

Related tests include biopsy bone marrow, complement, CBC, CBC hematocrit, CBC hemoglobin, CBC RBC count, CBC RBC indices, CBC RBC morphology, Coomb antiglobulin direct and indirect, erythropoietin, iron/TIBC, ferritin, folate, G6PD, Ham test, Hgb electrophoresis, lead, osmotic fragility, PK, sickle cell screen, and vitamin B_{12}.

Refer to the Hematopoietic System table at the end of the book for related tests by body system.

Expected Outcomes

Expected outcomes associated with Reticulocyte Count are:

- Maintaining an optimal gas exchange with an oxygen saturation greater than 92%
- Appropriately interacting with others without evidence of confusion

Sickle Cell Screen

Quick Summary

SYNONYM ACRONYM: Sickle cell test.

COMMON USE: To assess for hemoglobin S to assist in diagnosing sickle cell anemia.

SPECIMEN: Whole blood collected in a lavender-top (EDTA) tube.

NORMAL FINDINGS: (Method: Hemoglobin high-salt solubility) Negative.

Test Explanation

The sickle cell screen is one of several screening tests for a group of hereditary hemoglobinopathies. The test is positive in the presence of rare sickling hemoglobin (Hgb) variants such as Hgb S and Hgb C Harlem. Electrophoresis and high-performance liquid chromatography as well as molecular genetics testing for beta-globin mutations can also be used to identify Hgb S. Hgb S results from an amino acid substitution during Hgb synthesis, whereby valine replaces glutamic acid. Hemoglobin C Harlem results from the substitution of lysine for glutamic acid. Individuals with sickle cell disease have chronic anemia because the abnormal Hgb is unable to carry oxygen. The red blood cells of affected individuals are also abnormal in shape, resembling a crescent or sickle rather than the normal disk shape (see Fig. 2.11). This abnormality, combined with cell-wall rigidity, prevents the cells from passing through smaller blood vessels. Blockages in blood vessels result in hypoxia, damage, and pain. Individuals with the sickle cell trait do not have the clinical manifestations of the disease but may pass the disease on to children if the other parent has the trait (or the disease) as well (see Fig. 2.12).

Nursing Implications

Assessment

Indications	Potential Nursing Problems
Detect sickled red blood cells Evaluate hemolytic anemias	• Activity • Fear • Gas Exchange • Health Management • Human Response • Pain • Stress

Diagnosis: Clinical Significance of Test Results
POSITIVE FINDINGS IN
Deoxygenated Hgb S is insoluble in the presence of a high-salt solution and will form a cloudy turbid suspension when present.

- Combination of Hgb S with other hemoglobinopathies
- Hgb C Harlem anemia
- Sickle cell anemia
- Sickle cell trait
- Thalassemias
- N/A

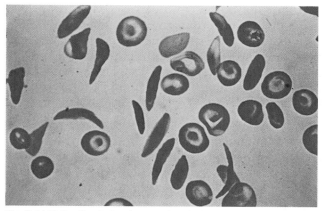

FIGURE 2.11 Shape of red blood cells as seen in sickle cell disease. *Used with permission, from Ward, S. (2009). Maternal-child nursing care: Optimizing outcomes for mothers, children, and families. FA Davis Company.*

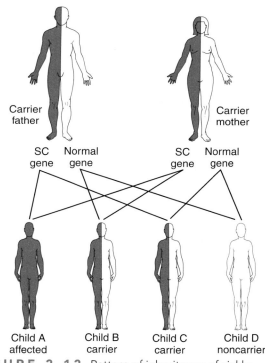

FIGURE 2.12 Pattern of inheritance of sickle cell disease. *Used with permission, from Ward, S. (2009). Maternal-child nursing care: Optimizing outcomes for mothers, children, and families. FA Davis Company.*

Planning

Considerations for planning a successful partnership should include clear communication of what to expect during the test to decrease anxiety and improve cooperation. Assess the patient for a family history of sickle cell trait or disease. Before the procedure is performed, plan to review the steps with the patient. Address concerns about pain and explain that there may be some discomfort during the venipuncture.

SPECIAL CONSIDERATIONS

An important aspect of planning is understanding the factors that may alter study findings or cause abnormal results. Interdepartmental communication is a key factor in the planning process. The following should be noted when planning for this study as false-negative results may occur:

- Children younger than 3 months of age *related to elevated levels of Hgb F*
- Patients who have received a recent blood transfusion before specimen collection *related to a dilutional effect of abnormal petient cells with normal transfused cells*

Implementation

Patient education is key to obtaining the patient's cooperation in following directions, and providing an explanation for the purpose of the procedure is an important part of this process. Inform the patient that this study can assist in diagnosing anemia. Perform the venipuncture.

Evaluation

Recognize anxiety related to test results, and offer support, as appropriate. Discuss the implications of abnormal test results on the patient's lifestyle. Explain that a positive screening test does not distinguish between the sickle trait and sickle cell anemia. To make this determination, follow-up testing by Hgb electrophoresis would be the next step in confirming the findings of the screening test. Provide teaching and information regarding the clinical implications of the test results as appropriate. Educate the patient about access to counseling services. Provide contact information, if desired, for the Sickle Cell Disease Association of America (www.sicklecelldisease.org).

SPECIAL CONSIDERATIONS

Advise the patient with sickle cell disease to avoid situations in which hypoxia may occur, such as strenuous exercise, staying at high altitudes, or traveling in an unpressurized aircraft. Obstetric and surgical patients with sickle cell anemia are at risk for hypoxia and therefore require close observation. Obstetric patients are at risk for hypoxia during the stress of labor and delivery, and surgical patients may become hypoxic while under general anesthesia.

✓ Critical Findings

N/A

✓ Study Specific Complications

There are a number of complications associated with performing a venipuncture. **Pain** is commonly associated with needles, and although the pain experienced during venipuncture is usually mild, on a rare occasion the needle may strike a nerve causing permanent pain.

Some patients experience a **vasovagal reaction** during the venipuncture procedure, evidenced by sweating, low blood pressure, fainting, or near fainting. The potential for a **fall injury** is a significant concern related to vasovagal reactions. Prolonged **bleeding** is a complication that occurs with patients who are taking blood thinners or who have coagulopathies such as hemophilia. A **hematoma** results when blood leaks into the tissue during or after a venipuncture, as evidenced by pain, bruising, and/or swelling at the venipuncture site. The swelling can cause injury by compression to surrounding nerves, which can be temporary or permanent. Health-care providers should watch for minor complications such as bruising and hematoma at the venipuncture site, which are fairly common. Hematomas occur more often in older adult or frail patients, or those with veins that are difficult to access. Bleeding or bruising can be prevented once the needle has been removed by applying direct pressure to the site with dry gauze for a minute or two. Some other more unusual complications of venipuncture include **cellulitis, phlebitis, inadvertent arterial puncture,** and **sepsis.** Sepsis can be caused by introduction of bacteria from the surface of the skin into the blood as the result of improper cleansing of the venipuncture site. Immunocompromised patients are at higher risk for developing this complication.

✓ Related Tests

Related tests include biopsy bone marrow, CBC, CBC RBC morphology, CBC RBC indices, ESR, Hgb electrophoresis, hemosiderin, LAP, MRI musculoskeletal, newborn screening, RBC cholinesterase, and US spleen.

Refer to the Hematopoietic System table at the end of the book for related tests by body system.

Expected Outcomes

Expected outcomes associated with Sickle Cell Screen are:

- Managing pain to an acceptable level
- Recognizing the importance of developing a lifestyle to prevent crises events
- Identifying activities that can create a flare-up and avoiding them

REVIEW OF LEARNING OUTCOMES

Thinking

1. Define hematopoiesis. Answer: Hematopoiesis is the process of blood cell formation that takes place in the liver, spleen, and bone marrow. Erythropoiesis refers to the generation of RBCs, leukopoiesis to the production of WBCs, and thrombopoiesis to the production of platelets.

2. Name the three basic elements incorporated in hematology studies. Answer: Hematology studies are in the area of medical science that examines the cellular components of blood, the organs that produce blood, and diseases of the blood, bone marrow, and lymphatic system.

3. Name seven different types of blood cells and associate each of them with one of three main functions. Answer: The main function of RBCs is transportation and an important secondary function is to assist in regulating some body functions such as body temperature and pH balance. Each WBC cell has a unique and specific method for defending the body: neutrophils, monocytes, eosinophils, and basophils are involved in defense or protection; lymphocytes and plasma cells are key to either cellular or humoral immunity or protection. As discussed in the next subsection on hemostasis, platelets perform a protective function to help prevent blood loss. The three main functions of blood components are transportation, regulation, and defense or protection.

4. Give two common examples for when an abnormal WBC count is "normal." Answer: WBC counts vary with age, so it is important to use the appropriate normal range when evaluating results. WBC counts are also influenced by nonpathological factors such as stress and high levels of physical activity (e.g., a woman in childbirth or an actively crying infant).

Doing

1. Discuss a few of the reasons why variables such as collection time, age, race, and gender must be considered when reviewing the results of a CBC. Answer: Reference values for the elements in a CBC vary across the age continuum and by sex. For example, the developing neonate has a very high demand for oxygen. Therefore, the RBC count is also high. Also, in females, hemoglobin and hematocrit decrease when puberty begins while the same measurements increase at puberty in males. The difference between females and males can be partially explained by menstrual blood loss in females and the effects of androgens in males. Care must also be taken when reviewing RBC counts after a blood transfusion—documentation should clearly reflect the time and date of the last transfusion with respect to the collection time of the study. WBC production varies diurnally with counts being lowest in the morning and highest in the late afternoon. Counts are also affected by high levels of physical activity or stress. Thus, the time of collection and the activity status of the patient should be taken into consideration when reviewing or comparing WBC counts.

2. Accept the leadership role required to meet specific clinical situations. Answer: Nurses have multiple roles in the care of their patients and need to understand when to use their roles to the best effect. For example, a nurse may act as a team leader when assessing laboratory results for indications of sepsis, but as a team member when collaborating with the HCP to design effective interventions to treat the infection.

3. Describe appropriate nursing assessment/responsibilities related to the hematologic system. Answer: Many disorders of the hematopoietic system do not present with obvious signs and symptoms. Correct diagnosis often requires laboratory testing to provide scientific data that correlate with a clinical condition. Therefore, it is important to listen carefully to the patient's complaints and to ask questions that may provide more information about symptoms as well as a past or family history that can result in a more thorough assessment. There are numerous factors and conditions that affect normal erythropoiesis, such as blood loss (e.g., acute or chronic loss via nose bleeds or blood in stool may be important clues); malnutrition or disorders of other organs (e.g., kidney disease or injury that results in a deficient production of erythropoietin or the effect of gastrointestinal disease or surgery on the absorption of iron and vitamins that are essential to RBC formation and maturation). Personal and family history taken during the patient interview may also reveal information regarding genetic RBC enzyme defects that disturb metabolic function or cell membrane integrity, inherited hemoglobinopathies (e.g., thalassemias, sickle cell disease) that have a significant effect on health as well as inflammatory conditions that affect the manner in which the cells are attracted to or repelled by each other, malignancies, or bone marrow failure. Finally, information about the patient's environment and lifestyle is important. The acquired effects of drugs, toxic chemicals, or ionizing radiation can definitely affect hemostasis. Traditional risk factors such as smoking, poor diet, excessive alcohol consumption, and a lack of physical exercise have a very negative effect on the hematopoietic system and create health issues with other organs, which can also have a negative impact on the hematopietic system.

Caring

1. Recognize the value of differing clinical points of view and associated responsibilities. Answer: Depending on the results of laboratory study, it may be necessary to ask for assistance from other health-care professionals to assist your patient to deal with the results. An example is parents who unknowingly passed a devastating inherited disease to their child, such as sickle cell anemia. Let the results of the laboratory studies guide whom you select to assist in coping with the outcomes.

◐ **Words OF Wisdom:** Many of the studies in this chapter are what nurses would consider to be "common" tests. And to us they are common in that it would be a rare day that one or more of our patients would not have one of them done for some reason or another. But stop and ask yourself if this is common for your patient. What is your patient's perception of you if you are the one who is explaining the test or are collecting the blood specimen? Does your patient perceive you as caring or uncaring? It's fair to say that at some point in our lives we, or someone we've known, have probably had the experience of feeling like an unwelcome interruption when we needed compassion and concern. Be aware that patients, visitors, and other health-care workers are watching and listening. Be cognizant of the image you present. Never act as if drawing blood for a common study is unimportant. To those on the other end of the needle, it is very important, and how you behave will affect how they feel about the experience. Health care is a customer satisfaction industry blended with personal lives. It is important for each of us to respect that expectation of caring. Empower your coworkers, across all departments, to embrace a culture of caring by your informed example.

BIBLIOGRAPHY

Blood and Hemapoiesis. (n.d.). Retrieved from www.cmu.edu.cn/curriculum/upload/cell/e05.ppt

Blood basics. (2010). Retrieved from www.hematology.org/patients/blood-basics/5222.aspx

Blood volume. (n.d.). Retrieved from www.medical-dictionary.thefreedictionary.com/Blood+volume+determination

Bone marrow. (n.d.). Retrieved from www.sciencedaily.com/articles/b/bone_marrow.htm

Cavanaugh, B. (2003). Nurse's manual of laboratory and diagnostic tests (4th ed.). Philadelphia, PA: F.A. Davis.

Darrow, D., Soule, H., & Buckman, T. (1927). Blood volume in normal infants and children. Retrieved from www.ncbi.nlm.nih.gov/pmc/articles/PMC434708/pdf/jcinvest00515-0081.pdf

Drees, M., Kanapathippillai, N., & Zubrow, M. (2012, August 28). Bandemia with normal white blood cell counts associated with infection. Retrieved from www.ncbi.nlm.nih.gov/pubmed/22939096

Ernst, D. (2005). Applied phlebotomy. Philadelphia, PA: Lippincott Williams & Wilkins.

Jacobs, D., DeMott, W., & Oxley, D. (2001). Laboratory test handbook (5th ed.). Cleveland, OH: Lexi-Comp Inc.

Knowles, L. (n.d.). What are stem cells and where do they come from? Retrieved from www.stemcellschool.org/pdf/What-are-Stem-Cells-and-Where-do-They-Come-from.pdf

Krauss, J. (n.d.). The laboratory diagnosis of paroxysmal nocturnal hemoglobinuria (PNH). Retrieved from www.pnhdisease.org/modules.php?name=Downloads&d_op=viewdownload&cid=3&min=20&orderby=titleA&show=10

Lutz, C., & Przytulski, K. (2011). Nutrition and diet therapy (5th ed.). Philadelphia, PA: F.A. Davis.

Panchbhavi, V. (2011, July 5). Bone marrow anatomy. Retrieved from www.emedicine.medscape.com/article/1968326-overview#aw2aab6b5)

Ray, G. (Nov. 16, 2011). Plasma dilution. Retrieved from http://ahca.myflorida.com/MCHQ/Health_Facility_Regulation/Laboratory_Licensure/docs/organ_tissue/Advisory_Board/06082012_Meeting_Info/060812_AATB_Plasma_Dilution_2011.pdf

Thompson, G. (2013). Understanding anatomy and physiology. Philadelphia, PA: F.A. Davis.

Timby, B. (2009). Workbook to accompany introductory medical surgical nursing (10th ed.). Philadelphia, PA: Lippincott, Williams & Wilkins.

Van Leeuwen, A., and Bladh, M. (2015). Davis's comprehensive handbook of laboratory and diagnostic tests with nursing implications (6th ed.). Philadelphia, PA: F.A. Davis.

Yu, G. (2010, April 22). Retrieved from www.learnpediatrics.com/body-systems/hematology-oncology/pediatric-neutropenia/

Go to Section II of this book and http://www.davisplus.com for the Clinical Reasoning Tool and its case studies to provide you with a safe place to explore patient care situations. There are a total of 26 different case studies; 2 cases are presented for each of 13 body systems: One set of 13 cases are found in the Section II chapters, and a second set of 13 cases are available online at http://www.davisplus.com. Each case is designed with the specific goal of helping you to connect the dots of clinical reasoning. Cases are designed to reflect possible clinical scenarios; the outcomes may or may not be positive—you decide.

CHAPTER

3

Blood Studies: Hemostasis (Coagulation)

OVERVIEW

Hemostasis involves three components: blood vessel walls, platelets, and plasma coagulation proteins. Primary hemostasis has three major stages involving platelet adhesion, platelet activation, and platelet aggregation. Platelet adhesion is initiated by exposure of the endothelium as a result of damage to blood vessels (see Fig. 3.1). Exposed tissue factor–bearing cells trigger the simultaneous binding of von Willebrand factor to exposed collagen and circulating platelets. Activated platelets release a number of procoagulant factors from storage granules, including thromboxane, a very potent platelet activator. These factors enter the circulation and activate other platelets, and the cycle continues. The activated platelets aggregate at the site of vessel injury, and at this stage of hemostasis, the glycoprotein IIb/IIIa receptors on the activated platelets bind fibrinogen, causing the platelets to stick together and form a plug (see Fig. 3.2). There is a balance in health between the prothrombotic or clot formation process and the antithrombotic or clot disintegration process (see Figs. 3.3 and 3.4). Simultaneously, the coagulation process or secondary hemostasis occurs. In secondary hemostasis, the coagulation proteins respond to blood vessel injury in an overlapping chain of events. The contact activation (formerly known as the intrinsic pathway) and tissue factor (formerly known as the extrinsic pathway) pathways of secondary hemostasis are a series of reactions that involve the substrate protein fibrinogen, the coagulation factors (also known as *enzyme precursors* or *zymogens*), nonenzymatic cofactors (Ca^{2+}), and phospholipids. The factors were assigned Roman numerals in the order of their discovery, not their place in the coagulation sequence. Factor VI was originally thought to be a separate clotting factor. It was subsequently proven to be the same as a modified form of factor Va, and therefore the number is no longer used.

For many years it was believed that the intrinsic and extrinsic pathways operated equally, in parallel. A more modern concept of the coagulation process has replaced the traditional model (formerly called the coagulation cascade). The cellular-based model (see Fig. 3.5) includes four overlapping phases in the formation of thrombin: initiation, amplification, propagation, and termination. It is now known that the tissue factor pathway is the primary pathway for the initiation of blood coagulation. Tissue factor (TF) bearing cells (e.g., endothelial cells, smooth muscle cells, monocytes) can be induced to express TF and are the primary initiators of the coagulation cascade either by contact activation or trauma. The contact activation pathway is more related to inflammation, and although it plays an important role in the body's reaction to damaged endothelial surfaces, a deficiency in factor XII does not result in the development of a bleeding disorder, which demonstrates the minor role of the intrinsic pathway in the process of blood coagulation. Substances such as endotoxins, tumor necrosis factor alpha, and lipoproteins can also stimulate the expression of TF. TF, in combination with factor VII and calcium, forms a complex that then activates factors IX and X in the initiation phase. Activated factor X in the presence of factor II (prothrombin) leads to the formation of thrombin. TFPI quickly inactivates this stage of the pathway so that limited or trace amounts of thrombin are produced, and this results in the activation of factors VIII and V. Activated factor IX, assisted by activated factors V and VIII, initiate amplification and propagation of thrombin in the cascade. Thrombin activates factor XIII and begins converting fibrinogen into fibrin monomers, which spontaneously polymerize and then become cross-linked into a stable clot by activated factor XIII.

Qualitative and quantitative factor deficiencies can affect the function of the coagulation pathways. Factor V and factor II (prothrombin) mutations are examples

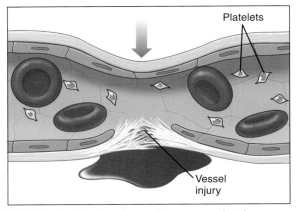

FIGURE 3.1 Blood vessel injury. *Used with permission, from Thompson, G. (2013). Understanding anatomy & physiology. FA Davis Company.*

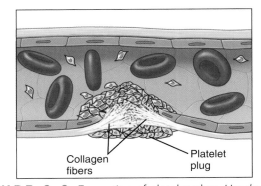

FIGURE 3.2 Formation of platelet plug. *Used with permission, from Thompson, G. (2013). Understanding anatomy & physiology. FA Davis Company.*

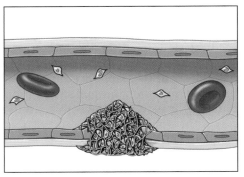

FIGURE 3.3 Blood clot formation and vessel repair. *Used with permission, from Thompson, G. (2013). Understanding anatomy & physiology. FA Davis Company.*

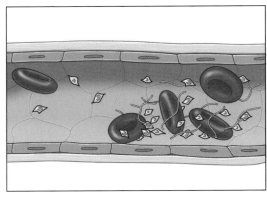

FIGURE 3.4 Dissolution of blood clot by fibrinolysis. *Used with permission, from Thompson, G. (2013). Understanding anatomy & physiology. FA Davis Company.*

Important Coagulation Factors

	Preferred Name	Synonym	Role in Modern Coagulation Cascade Model	Coagulation Test Responses in the Presence of Factor Deficiency
Factor I	Fibrinogen	N/A	Assists in the formation of the fibrin clot	PT prolonged, aPTT prolonged
Factor II	Prothrombin	Prethrombin	Assists factor Xa in formation of trace thrombin in the initiation phase and assists factors VIIIa, IXa, Xa, and Va to form thrombin in the propagation phase of hemostasis	PT prolonged, aPTT prolonged
Tissue factor (formerly known as factor III)	Tissue factor	Tissue thromboplastin	Assists factor VII and Ca^{2+} in the activation of factors IX and X during the initiation phase of hemostasis	PT prolonged, aPTT prolonged
Calcium (formerly known as factor IV)	Calcium	Ca^{2+}	Essential to the activation of multiple clotting factors	N/A

Important Coagulation Factors

	Preferred Name	Synonym	Role in Modern Coagulation Cascade Model	Coagulation Test Responses in the Presence of Factor Deficiency
Factor V	Proaccelerin	Labile factor, accelerator globulin (AcG)	Assists factors VIIIa, IXa, Xa, and II in the formation of thrombin during the amplification and propagation phases of hemostasis	PT prolonged, aPTT prolonged
Factor VII	Proconvertin	Stabile factor, serum prothrombin conversion accelerator, autoprothrombin I	Assists tissue factor and Ca^{2+} in the activation of factors IX and X	PT prolonged, aPTT normal
Factor VIII	Antihemophilic factor (AHF)	Antihemophilic globulin (AHG), antihemophilic factor A, platelet cofactor 1	Activated by trace thrombin during the initiation phase of hemostasis to amplify formation of additional thrombin	PT normal, aPTT prolonged
Factor IX	Plasma thromboplastin component (PTC)	Christmas factor, antihemophilic factor B, platelet cofactor 2	Assists factors Va and VIIIa in the amplification phase and factors VIIIa, Xa, Va, and II to form thrombin in the propagation phase	PT normal, aPTT prolonged
Factor X	Stuart-Prower factor	Autoprothrombin III, thrombokinase	Assists with formation of trace thrombin in the initiation phase and acts with factors VIIIa, IXa, Va, and II to form thrombin in the propagation phase	PT prolonged, aPTT prolonged
Factor XI	Plasma thromboplastin antecedent (PTA)	Antihemophilic factor C	Activated by thrombin produced in the extrinsic pathway to enhance production of additional thrombin inside the fibrin clot via the intrinsic pathway; this factor also participates in slowing the process of fibrinolysis	PT normal, aPTT prolonged
Factor XII	Hageman factor	Glass factor, contact factor	Contact activator of the kinin system (e.g., prekallikrein, and high molecular weight kininogen)	PT normal, aPTT prolonged
Factor XIII	Fibrin-stabilizing factor (FSF)	Laki-Lorand factor (LLF), fibrinase, plasma transglutaminase	Activated by thrombin and assists in formation of bonds between fibrin strands to complete secondary hemostasis	PT normal, aPTT normal
von Willebrand factor	von Willebrand factor	vWF	Assists in platelet adhesion and thrombus formation	Ristocetin cofactor decreased

of qualitative deficiencies and are the most common inherited predisposing factors for blood clots. Approximately 5% to 7% of Caucasians, 2% of Hispanics, 1% of African Americans and Native Americans, and 0.5% of Asians have the factor V Leiden mutation, and 2% to 3% of Caucasians and 0.3% of African Americans have a prothrombin mutation (see Figs. 3.6 and 3.7). Hemophilia A is an inherited deficiency of factor VIII and occurs at a prevalence of about 1 in 5,000 to 10,000 male births. Hemophilia B is an inherited deficiency of factor IX and occurs at a prevalence of about 1 in about 20,000 to 34,000 male births. Genetic testing is available for inherited mutations associated with inherited coagulopathies. The tests are performed on samples of whole blood. Counseling and informed written consent are generally required for genetic testing.

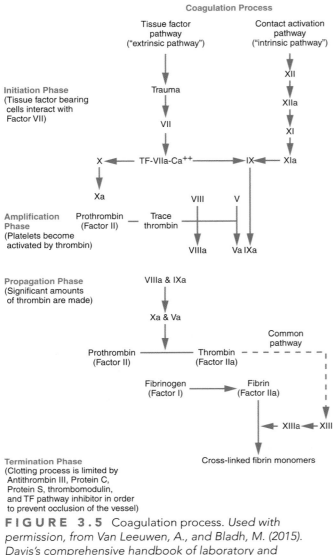

Coagulation Process

FIGURE 3.5 Coagulation process. *Used with permission, from Van Leeuwen, A., and Bladh, M. (2015). Davis's comprehensive handbook of laboratory and diagnostic tests with nursing implications (6th Ed.). FA Davis Company.*

Primary and secondary hemostasis must be kept in balance to prevent an injured vessel from becoming completely occluded. The antithrombotic process or termination phase of secondary hemostasis accomplishes this through the antithrombin and fibrinolytic systems. The antithrombin system involves neutralization of coagulation factors and of thrombin itself in several different ways. Antithrombin, also referred to as antithrombin III, is a potent anticoagulant. It inhibits a number of the coagulation factors such as IX, X, XI, XII, and II (thrombin). It is also known as heparin cofactor because the combined effect of heparin with antithrombin can increase the rate of factor inhibition by up to a thousand times. Further, the binding of thrombin to thrombomodulin receptors on damaged endothelial cells results in activation of Protein C and initiation of the activated Protein C anticoagulant

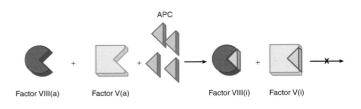

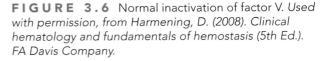

FIGURE 3.6 Normal inactivation of factor V. *Used with permission, from Harmening, D. (2008). Clinical hematology and fundamentals of hemostasis (5th Ed.). FA Davis Company.*

pathway. Protein C and its cofactor, Protein S, work together to inactivate factors V and VIII, which are critical factors in the formation of prothrombin. The fibrinolytic system involves the activation of plasminogen to plasmin. This conversion occurs mainly by the action of tissue plasminogen activator (tPA) and urokinase, which are believed to be released when the body recognizes that vessel damage has occurred and the modulation of hemostasis is required. Plasmin or fibrinolysin digests fibrinogen (fibrin's precursor) and fibrin (the blood clot's mesh-like network). It is also believed to inactivate factors V and VIII. Urokinase and recombinant tPA have both been used therapeutically for many years as thrombolytic agents in the treatment of MI and CVA; they are capable of destroying thrombi that have already formed. Urokinase has been used to treat DVT and PE. Heparin and warfarin (Coumadin) are two commonly used anticoagulant agents that act by interfering with the formation of clots. Heparin is the medication of choice for women who require anticoagulant therapy during pregnancy, because, unlike warfarin, heparin does not cross the placental barrier. Warfarin is known to be harmful to the fetus when it crosses the placenta because it may cause a fatal hemorrhage or cause congenital abnormalities in the developing fetus. Warfarin is not passed in breast milk and is safe for use in lactating females. A third group of anticoagulants are used therapeutically to protect the

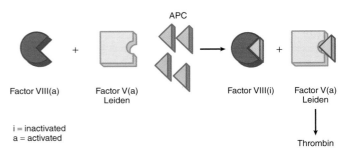

FIGURE 3.7 Factor V Leiden mutation alters binding site affecting coagulation pathway by preventing inactivation of factor V. *Used with permission, from Harmening, D. (2008). Clinical hematology and fundamentals of hemostasis (5th Ed.). FA Davis Company.*

cerebrovascular system of patients at risk of developing blood clots. They act against platelets to prevent aggregation or clumping, an important initial step in the formation of thrombi.

DISCUSSION POINT

Coagulation tests have some common factors that may impair the procedure or cause abnormal results:

- Review the results from other studies to help identify potentially confounding information. For example, a hematocrit level greater than 55% may affect results because of anticoagulant excess relative to plasma volume. Having this information in advance provides the opportunity, using established guidelines, to adjust the volume of anticoagulant in the tube prior to specimen collection, thus avoiding a potentially erroneous finding.
- Note that specimen collection technique has a significant impact on the validity of test results. Placement of the tourniquet for longer than 1 minute can result in venous stasis and changes in the concentration of the plasma proteins or platelets to be measured. Platelet activation may also occur under these conditions, resulting in erroneous measurements. Vascular injury caused during the venipuncture procedure can activate platelets and coagulation factors, causing erroneous, falsely decreased results. Evidence of this type of interference is evident in hemolyzed specimens, which must be rejected for analysis.
- When multiple specimens are drawn, collect the blue-top tube after the sterile (i.e., blood culture) tubes. Otherwise, when using a standard vacutainer system, the blue top is the first tube collected. When a butterfly is used and due to the added tubing, an extra red-top tube should be collected before the blue-top tube to ensure complete filling of the blue-top tube. Once the proper order of draw has been established, the venipuncture can be performed. The Clinical and Laboratory Standards Institute's recommendation for processed and unprocessed samples stored in unopened tubes is that testing should be completed within 1 to 4 hours of collection.
- Note that icteric or lipemic specimens interfere with optical testing methods, producing erroneous results.
- Be aware that certain specimens should be rejected for analysis, such as specimens with incompletely filled collection tubes, inadequately mixed specimens, specimens contaminated with heparin, clotted specimens, or unprocessed specimens not delivered to the laboratory within 1 to 2 hours of collection.

The aPTT measures the function of the contact activation pathway of coagulation and is used to monitor patients receiving heparin anticoagulant therapy. The PT/INR measures the function of the tissue factor pathway of coagulation and is used to monitor patients receiving warfarin or coumarin-derivative anticoagulant therapy. INR home testing is an available option as ordered by a health-care provider (HCP). Enrollment in the home testing program includes face-to-face training of patients by representatives for the instrument's manufacturer. The patient reports their INR results by telephone to the manufacturer. The manufacturer promptly communicates the results to the requesting HCP, who can then contact the patient directly to modify medication doses or implement other management strategies in a timely manner, between scheduled visits with the patient.

The major difficulties associated with the use of anticoagulants are hemorrhage and drug interaction. Observation of the patient for signs of internal and external spontaneous bleeding is also essential. Walking, leg exercises, elevation of the feet and legs, and the use of compression stockings are some effective interventions to avoid the development of blood clots. There is a wealth of information available to help educate patients receiving anticoagulant medications about dietary considerations or restrictions. Some foods are natural blood thinners because they are rich in salicylates, vitamin E, vitamin K, or act as blood thinners on their own. A few examples include blueberries (bilberry), cayenne pepper, cherries, cinnamon, clover (red and sweet), cranberries, curry powder, dill, fish oils, garlic, ginseng, grapes, grapefruit seed extract, kale, oregano, paprika, peppermint, raisins, senna, spinach, St. John's wort, strawberries, tangerines, thyme, and tumeric. These foods, when consumed regularly, may have a significant potentiating or inhibitory effect when combined with a regimen of anticoagulant medication. This could in turn put the patient at risk for thrombosis or bleeding. Patients must also be cautioned to consult with their HCP or pharmacist before taking any medications or over-the-counter herbal products in combination with an anticoagulant agent. Patients should be instructed in the prevention of accidental injury, basic first aid measures to control bleeding in the event of an accident, signs that warrant immediate medical attention, and finally assurance that bleeding can be controlled with the proper interventions. Women of childbearing age should receive counseling regarding the known effects of various contraception methods and risks for complications related to the coagulation system; the risk for potentially significant complications increases for women who have a medical condition requiring treatment with anticoagulants. Intrauterine devices can cause excessive endometrial bleeding, and estrogen-containing oral contraceptives have been associated with an increased risk for venous thromboembolism.

The information in the Part I studies is organized in a manner to help the student see how the five basic components of the nursing process (assessment, diagnosis, planning, implementation, and evaluation) can be applied to each phase of laboratory and diagnostic testing. The goal is to use nursing process to understand the integration of care (laboratory, diagnostic, nursing care) toward achieving a positive expected outcome.

- **Assessment** is the collection of information for the purpose of answering the question, "is there a problem?" Knowledge of the patient's health history, medications, complaints, and allergies as well as synonyms or alternate test names, common use for the procedure, specimen requirements, and normal ranges or interpretive comments provide the foundation for diagnosis.
- **Diagnosis** is the process of looking at the information gathered during assessment and answering the questions, "what is the problem?" and "what do I need to do about it?" Test indications tell us why the study has been requested, and potential diagnoses tell us the value or importance of the study relative to its clinical utility.
- **Planning** is a blueprint of the nursing care before the procedure. It is the process of determining how the nurse is going to partner with the patient to fix the problem (e.g., "the patient has a study ordered and this is what I should know before I successfully carry out the plan to have the study completed"). Knowledge of interfering factors, social and cultural issues, preprocedural restrictions, the need for written and informed consent, anxiety about the procedure, and concerns regarding pain are some considerations for planning a successful partnership.
- **Implementation** is putting the plan into action with an idea of what the expected outcome should be. Collaboration with the departments where the laboratory test or diagnostic study is to be performed is essential to the success of the plan. Implementation is where the work is done within each healthcare team member's scope of practice.
- **Evaluation** answers the question, "did the plan work or not?" Was the plan completely successful, partially successful, or not successful? If the plan did not work, evaluation is the process where you determine what needs to be changed to make the plan work better. This includes a review of all expected outcomes. Nursing care after the procedure is where information is gathered to evaluate the plan. Review of results, including critical findings, in relation to patient symptoms and other tests performed provides data that form a more complete picture of health or illness.
- **Expected Outcomes** are positive outcomes related to the test. They are the outcomes the nurse should expect if all goes well.

A number of pretest, intratest, and post-test universal points are presented in this overview section because the information applies to coagulation studies in general.

Universal Pretest Pearls (Planning)

- Obtain a history of the patient's complaints, including a list of known allergens, especially allergies or sensitivities to medications or latex so their use can be avoided or their effects mitigated if an allergy is present. Carefully evaluate all medications currently being taken by the patient. A list of the patient's current medications, prescribed and over the counter (including anticoagulants, aspirin and other salicylates, and dietary supplements), should also be obtained. Such products may be discontinued by medical direction for the appropriate number of days prior to the procedure. Ensure that all allergies are clearly noted in the medical record, and ensure that the patient is wearing an allergy and medical record armband. Report information that could interfere with, or delay proceeding with, getting the study to the HCP and laboratory.
- Obtain a history of the patient's affected body system, symptoms, and results of previously performed laboratory tests and diagnostic and surgical procedures. Previous test results will provide a basis of comparison between old and new data.
- An important aspect of planning is understanding the factors that may alter study findings or cause abnormal results. Interdepartmental communication is a key factor in the planning process. The inability of a patient to cooperate or remain still during the procedure because of age, significant pain, or mental status should be among the anticipated factors. Recent or past procedures, medications, or existing medical conditions that could complicate or interfere with test results should be noted.
- Review the steps of the study with the patient or caregiver. Expect patients to be nervous about the procedure itself and the pending results. Educating the patient on his or her role during the procedure and what to expect can facilitate this. The patient's role during the procedure is to remain still. The actual time required to complete each study will depend on a number of conditions, including the type of equipment being used and how well a patient will cooperate.
- Explain that specimen collection by venipuncture takes approximately 5 to 10 minutes. Bleeding or bruising can be prevented, once the needle has been removed, by applying direct pressure to the venipuncture site with dry gauze for a minute or two. The site should be observed/assessed for bleeding or hematoma formation, and then covered with a gauze and adhesive bandage.
- Address any concerns about pain, and explain or describe, as appropriate, the level and type of discomfort that may be expected. Advise the patient that some discomfort may be experienced during the venipuncture.

- Provide additional instructions and patient preparation regarding medication, diet, fluid intake, or activity, if appropriate. Unless specified in the individual study, there are no special instructions or restrictions.
- Always be sensitive to any cultural or psychosocial issues, including a concern for modesty before, during, and after the procedure.

Reminder

Ensure that a written and informed consent has been documented in the medical record prior to the study, if required. The consent must be obtained before medication is administered.

Universal Intratest Pearls (Implementation)

- Correct patient identification is crucial prior to any procedure. Positively identify the patient using two unique identifiers such as patient name, date of birth, Social Security number, or medical record number.
- Standard Precautions must be followed.
- Children and infants may be accompanied by a parent to calm them. Keep neonates and infants covered and in a warm room and provide a pacifier or gentle touch. The testing environment should be quiet, and the patient should be instructed, as appropriate, to remain still during the test as extraneous movements can affect results.
- Ensure that the patient has complied with pretesting instructions, including dietary, fluid, medication, and activity restrictions as given for the procedure.
- Before leaving the patient's side, appropriate specimen containers should always be labeled, with the corresponding patient demographics, initials of the person collecting the sample, collection date, time of collection, and applicable special notes, especially site location and laterality if appropriate, and then they should be promptly transported to the laboratory for processing and analysis.

Universal Post Test Pearls (Evaluation)

- Note that completed test results are made available to the requesting HCP, who will discuss them with the patient.
- Answer questions and address concerns voiced by the patient or family, and reinforce information given by the patient's HCP regarding further testing, treatment, or referral to another HCP. Recognize that patients will have anxiety related to test results. Provide teaching and information regarding the clinical implications of the test results on the patient's lifestyle as appropriate.

- Note that test results should be evaluated in context with the patient's signs, symptoms, and diagnosis. Depending on the results of the procedure, additional testing may be performed to evaluate or monitor progression of the disease process and determine the need for a change in therapy.
- Be aware that when a person goes through a traumatic event such as an illness or being given information that will impact his or her lifestyle, there are universal human reactions that occur. These include knowledge deficit, fear, anxiety, and coping; in some situations, grieving may occur. HCPs should always be aware of the human response and how it may affect the plan of care and expected outcomes.

DISCUSSION POINT

Regarding Post-Test Critical Findings: Timely notification of a critical finding for lab or diagnostic studies is a role expectation of the professional nurse. Notification processes will vary among facilities. Upon receipt of the critical finding, the information should be read back to the caller to verify accuracy. Most policies require immediate notification of the primary HCP, hospitalist, or on-call HCP. Reported information includes the patient's name, unique identifiers, critical finding, name of the person giving the report, and name of the person receiving the report. Documentation of notification should be made in the medical record with the name of the HCP notified, time and date of notification, and any orders received. Any delay in a timely report of a critical finding may require completion of a notification form with review by Risk Management.

STUDIES

- Complete Blood Count, Platelet Count
- Partial Thromboplastin Time, Activated
- Prothrombin Time and International Normalized Ratio

LEARNING OUTCOMES

Providing safe, effective nursing care (SENC) includes mastery of core competencies and standards of care. SENC is based on a judicious application of nursing knowledge in combination with scientific principles. The Art of Nursing lies in blending what you know with the ability to effectively apply your knowledge in a compassionate manner.

After reading/studying this chapter you will be able to:

Thinking

1. Name the three components of hemostasis.
2. State the primary purposes of anticoagulant therapy and identify its effects both on existing blood clots and in the prevention of blood clot development.

3. Identify which study is commonly used to monitor patients on heparin therapy and which study is used to monitor patients receiving warfarin or coumadin therapy.

Doing

1. Discuss the two types of hemostasis, primary and secondary hemostasis.
2. Discuss how a balance between repair of an injured vessel and complete vessel occlusion is accomplished.
3. Identify the major complications of anticoagulant therapy and some specific nursing interventions that can help prevent clot formation.

Caring

1. Recognize that perceiving how care is delivered though the patient's point of view is of value.

Complete Blood Count, Platelet Count

Quick Summary

SYNONYM ACRONYM: Thrombocytes.

COMMON USE: To assist in diagnosing and evaluating treatment for blood disorders such as thrombocytosis and thrombocytopenia and to evaluate preprocedure or preoperative coagulation status.

SPECIMEN: Whole blood from one full lavender-top (EDTA) tube.

NORMAL FINDINGS: (Method: Automated, computerized, multichannel analyzers)

Test Explanation

Platelets are nonnucleated, cytoplasmic, round or oval disks formed by budding off of large, multinucleated cells (megakaryocytes) (see Fig. 3.8). Platelets have an essential function in coagulation, hemostasis, and blood thrombus formation. Activated platelets release a number of procoagulant factors, including thromboxane, a very potent platelet activator, from storage granules. These factors enter the circulation and activate other platelets and the cycle continues. The activated platelets aggregate at the site of vessel injury, and at this stage of hemostasis the glycoprotein IIb/IIIa receptors on the activated platelets bind fibrinogen, causing the platelets to stick together and form a plug. Coagulation

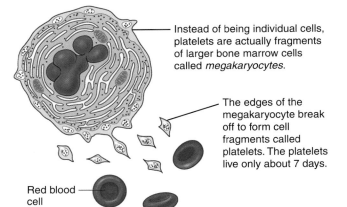

Instead of being individual cells, platelets are actually fragments of larger bone marrow cells called *megakaryocytes*.

The edges of the megakaryocyte break off to form cell fragments called platelets. The platelets live only about 7 days.

Red blood cell

FIGURE 3.8 Platelet formation. *Used with permission, from Thompson, G. (2013). Understanding anatomy & physiology. FA Davis Company.*

must be localized to the site of vessel wall injury, or the growing platelet plug would eventually occlude the affected vessel. The fibrinolytic system, under normal circumstances, begins to work, once fibrin begins to form, to ensure coagulation is limited to the appropriate site. *Thrombocytosis* is an increase in platelet count. In reactive thrombocytosis, the increase is transient and short lived, and it usually does not pose a health risk. One exception may be reactive thrombocytosis occurring after coronary bypass surgery. This circumstance has been identified as an important risk factor for postoperative infarction and thrombosis. The term *thrombocythemia* describes platelet increases associated with chronic myeloproliferative disorders; *thrombocytopenia* describes platelet counts of less than $140 \times 10^3/$microL. Decreased platelet counts occur whenever the body's need for platelets exceeds the rate of platelet production; this circumstance will arise if production rate decreases or platelet loss increases. The severity of bleeding is related to platelet count as well as platelet function. Platelet counts can be within normal limits, but the patient may exhibit signs of internal bleeding; this circumstance usually indicates an anomaly in platelet function. Abnormal findings by automated cell counters may indicate the need to review a smear of peripheral blood for platelet estimate. Abnormally large or giant platelets may result in underestimation of automated counts by 30% to 50%. A large discrepancy between the automated count and the estimate requires that a manual count be performed. Platelet clumping

Age	Platelet Count*	SI Units (Conventional Units × 1)	MPV (fL)	IPF (%)
Birth	150–450 × 10³/microL	150–450 × 10⁹/L	7.1–10.2	1.1–7.1
Child/Adult/Older adult	150–400 × 10³/microL	150–400 × 10⁹/L	7.1–10.2	1.1–7.1

Note: Platelet counts may decrease slightly with age. *Conventional units. MPV = mean platelet volume.

may result in the underestimation of the platelet count. Clumping may be detected by the automated cell counter or upon microscopic review of a blood smear. Perform a citrated platelet count, on a specimen collected in a blue-top tube, to obtain an accurate platelet count from patients who demonstrate platelet clumping in EDTA-preserved samples.

Thrombopoiesis or platelet production is reflected by the measurement of the immature platelet fraction (IPF). This parameter can be correlated to the total platelet count in the investigation of platelet disorders. A low platelet count with a low IPF can indicate a disorder of platelet production (e.g., drug toxicity, aplastic anemia, or bone marrow failure of another cause), whereas a low platelet count with an increased IPF might indicate platelet destruction or abnormally high platelet consumption (e.g., mechanical destruction, disseminated intravascular coagulation [DIC], idiopathic thrombocytopenic purpura [ITP], thrombotic thrombocytopenic purpura [TTP]).

Platelet size, reflected by mean platelet volume (MPV), and cellular age are inversely related; that is, younger platelets tend to be larger. An increase in MPV indicates an increase in platelet turnover. Therefore, in a healthy patient, the platelet count and MPV have an inverse relationship. Abnormal platelet size may also indicate the presence of a disorder. MPV and platelet distribution width (PDW) are both increased in ITP. MPV is also increased in May-Hegglin anomaly, Bernard-Soulier syndrome, myeloproliferative disorders, hyperthyroidism, and pre-eclampsia. MPV is decreased in Wiskott-Aldrich syndrome, septic thrombocytopenia, and hypersplenism.

Platelets have receptor sites that are essential for normal platelet function and activation. Drugs such as clopidogrel, abciximab (Reopro), eptifibatide (Integrilin), and tirofiban block these receptor sites and inhibit platelet function. Aspirin also can affect platelet function by the irreversible inactivation of a crucial cyclooxygenase (COX) enzyme. Medications like clopidogrel (Plavix) and aspirin are prescribed to prevent heart attack, stroke, and blockage of coronary stents. Studies have confirmed that up to 30% of patients receiving these medications may be nonresponsive. There are several commercial test systems that can assess platelet function and provide information that confirms platelet response. Platelet response testing helps ensure alternative or additional platelet therapy is instituted, if necessary. The test results can also be used preoperatively to determine whether antiplatelet medications have been sufficiently cleared from the patient's circulation such that surgery can safely be performed without risk of excessive bleeding. Thromboxane A2 is a potent stimulator of platelet activation. 11-Dehydrothromboxane B2 is the stable, inactive product of thromboxane A2 metabolism, released by activated platelets. Urine levels of 11-dehydrothromboxane B2 can be used to monitor response to aspirin therapy.

The metabolism of many commonly prescribed medications is driven by the cytochrome P450 (CYP450) family of enzymes. Genetic variants can alter enzymatic activity that results in a spectrum of effects ranging from the total absence of drug metabolism to ultrafast metabolism. Impaired drug metabolism can prevent the intended therapeutic effect or even lead to serious adverse drug reactions. Poor metabolizers (PMs) are at increased risk for drug-induced side effects due to accumulation of drug in the blood, while ultra-rapid metabolizers (UMs) require a higher than normal dosage because the drug is metabolized over a shorter duration than intended. Other genetic phenotypes used to report CYP450 results are intermediate metabolizer (IM) and extensive metabolizer (EM). CYP2C19 is a gene in the CYP450 family that metabolizes drugs such as clopidogrel (Plavix). Genetic testing can be performed on blood samples submitted to a laboratory. Testing for the most common genetic variants of CYP2C19 is used to predict altered enzyme activity and anticipate the most effective therapeutic plan. The test method commonly used is polymerase chain reaction. Counseling and informed written consent are generally required for genetic testing.

Nursing Implications

Assessment

Indications	Potential Nursing Problems
Confirm an elevated platelet count (thrombocytosis), which can cause increased clotting Confirm a low platelet count (thrombocytopenia), which can be associated with bleeding Identify the possible cause of abnormal bleeding, such as epistaxis, hematoma, gingival bleeding, hematuria, and menorrhagia Provide screening as part of a complete blood count (CBC) in a general physical examination, especially upon admission to a health-care facility or before surgery	• Bleeding • Cardiac Output • Confusion • Fatigue • Fear • Gas Exchange • Human Response • Injury Risk • Pain • Tissue Perfusion

Diagnosis: Clinical Significance of Test Results
INCREASED IN
Conditions that involve inflammation activate and increase the number of circulating platelets:

• Acute infections
• After exercise (transient)
• Anemias (posthemorrhagic, hemolytic, iron deficiency) *(bone marrow response to anemia; platelet formation is unaffected by iron deficiency)*

- Chronic heart disease
- Cirrhosis
- Essential thrombocythemia
- Leukemias (chronic)
- Malignancies (carcinoma, Hodgkin disease, lymphomas)
- Pancreatitis (chronic)
- Polycythemia vera *(hyperplastic bone marrow response in all cell lines)*
- Rebound recovery from thrombocytopenia *(initial response)*
- Rheumatic fever (acute)
- Rheumatoid arthritis
- Splenectomy (2 mo postprocedure) *(normal function of the spleen is to cull aging cells from the blood; without the spleen, the count increases)*
- Surgery (2 wk postprocedure)
- Trauma
- Tuberculosis
- Ulcerative colitis

DECREASED IN
DECREASED IN (AS A RESULT OF MEGAKARYOCYTIC HYPOPROLIFERATION)

- Alcohol toxicity
- Aplastic anemia
- Congenital states (Fanconi syndrome, May-Hegglin anomaly, Bernard-Soulier syndrome, Wiskott-Aldrich syndrome, Gaucher disease, Chédiak-Higashi syndrome)
- Drug toxicity
- Prolonged hypoxia

DECREASED IN (AS A RESULT OF INEFFECTIVE THROMBOPOIESIS)

- Ethanol misuse without malnutrition
- Iron-deficiency anemia
- Megaloblastic anemia (B_{12}/folate deficiency)
- Paroxysmal nocturnal hemoglobinuria
- Thrombopoietin deficiency
- Viral infection

DECREASED IN (AS A RESULT OF BONE MARROW REPLACEMENT)

- Lymphoma
- Granulomatous infections
- Metastatic carcinoma
- Myelofibrosis

INCREASED IN
INCREASED DESTRUCTION IN (AS A RESULT OF INCREASED LOSS/CONSUMPTION)

- Contact with foreign surfaces (dialysis membranes, artificial organs, grafts, prosthetic devices)
- Disseminated intravascular coagulation
- Extensive transfusion
- HELLP syndrome
- Severe hemorrhage
- Thrombotic thrombocytopenic purpura
- Uremia

INCREASED DESTRUCTION IN (AS A RESULT OF IMMUNE REACTION)

- Antibody/human leukocyte antigen reactions
- Hemolytic disease of the newborn *(target is platelets instead of RBCs)*
- Idiopathic thrombocytopenic purpura
- Refractory reaction to platelet transfusion

INCREASED DESTRUCTION IN (AS A RESULT OF IMMUNE REACTION SECONDARY TO INFECTION)

- Bacterial infections
- Burns
- Congenital infections (cytomegalovirus, herpes, syphilis, toxoplasmosis)
- Histoplasmosis
- Malaria
- Rocky Mountain spotted fever

INCREASED DESTRUCTION IN (AS A RESULT OF OTHER CAUSES)

- Radiation
- Splenomegaly caused by liver disease

Planning

Considerations for planning a successful partnership should include clear communication of what to expect during the test to decrease anxiety and improve cooperation. Before the procedure is performed, plan to review the steps with the patient. Address concerns about pain, and explain that there may be some discomfort during the venipuncture.

SPECIAL CONSIDERATIONS

An important aspect of planning is understanding the factors that may alter study findings or cause abnormal results. Interdepartmental communication is a key factor in the planning process. It should be noted when planning for this study that whenever possible, during the planning process, the appropriate timing for scheduling multiple studies should be taken into consideration. A baseline count should be obtained prior to x-ray studies as exposure to x-rays can decrease platelet counts.

It is also important to understand which medications or substances the patient may be exposed to in the health-care setting that can interfere with accurate testing:

- Drugs that may increase platelet counts include glucocorticoids.
- Drugs that may decrease platelet counts include acetohexamide, acetophenazine, amphotericin B, antazoline, anticonvulsants, antimony compounds,

apronalide, arsenicals, azathioprine, barbiturates, benzene, busulfan, butaperazine, chlordane, chlorophenothane, chlortetracycline, dactinomycin, dextromethorphan, diethylstilbestrol, ethinamate, ethoxzolamide, floxuridine, hexachlorobenzene, hydantoin derivatives, hydroflumethiazide, hydroxychloroquine, iproniazid, mechlorethamine, mefenamic acid, mepazine, miconazole, mitomycin, nitrofurantoin, novobiocin, nystatin, phenolphthalein, phenothiazine, pipamazine, plicamycin, procarbazine, pyrazolones, streptomycin, sulfonamides, tetracycline, thiabendazole, thiouracil, tolazamide, tolazoline, tolbutamide, trifluoperazine, and urethane.

DISCUSSION POINT

There are some circumstances in which platelet counts outside the normal range are expected. Platelet counts are normally decreased before menstruation and during pregnancy. Platelet counts normally increase under a variety of stressors, such as high altitudes or strenuous exercise. Counts may also be influenced by the patient's position, becoming decreased as a result of hemodilution when the patient is recumbent, and increased upon rising as a result of hemoconcentration.

● **Safety Tip**

The results of a CBC should be carefully evaluated during transfusion or acute blood loss because the body is not in a state of homeostasis and values may be misleading. Considerations for draw times after transfusion include the type of product, the amount of product transfused, and the patient's clinical situation. Generally, specimens collected an hour after transfusion will provide an acceptable reflection of the effects of the transfused product. Measurements taken during a massive transfusion are an exception, providing essential guidance for therapeutic decisions during critical care.

Implementation

Patient education is key to obtaining the patient's cooperation in following directions, and providing an explanation for the purpose of the procedure is an important part of this process. Inform the patient that this study can assist in diagnosing, evaluating, and monitoring bleeding disorders. Perform the venipuncture.

The specimen should be analyzed within 24 hours when stored at room temperature or within 48 hours if stored at a refrigerated temperature. If it is anticipated that the specimen will not be analyzed within 24 hours, two blood smears should be made immediately after the venipuncture and should be submitted with the blood sample. The smears can be used to make a platelet estimate.

Evaluation

Recognize anxiety related to test results, and discuss the implications of abnormal test results on the patient's lifestyle. Help patients who have a bleeding disorder understand the importance of taking precautions against bruising and bleeding. Provide education for

precautions to include the use of a soft-bristle toothbrush, the use of an electric razor, and avoiding constipation, salicylates (aspirin) and similar products, and intramuscular injections.

Inform the patient about the importance of periodic monitoring by means of laboratory testing if he or she is taking an anticoagulant. Patients should be encouraged to consume a variety of foods within the basic food groups, maintain a healthy weight, be physically active, limit salt intake, limit alcohol intake, and avoid the use of tobacco.

✅ *Critical Findings*

- Less than 30×10^3/microL (SI: Less than 30×10^9/L)
- Greater than $1,000 \times 10^3$/microL (SI: Greater than $1,000 \times 10^9$/L)

Consideration may be given to verifying the critical findings before action is taken. Policies vary among facilities and may include requesting immediate recollection and retesting by the laboratory.

Note and immediately report to the requesting health-care provider (HCP) any critical findings and related symptoms. A listing of these findings varies among facilities.

Critically low platelet counts can lead to brain bleeds or GI hemorrhage, which can be fatal. Some signs and symptoms of decreased platelet count include spontaneous nose bleeds or bleeding from the gums, bruising easily, prolonged bleeding from minor cuts and scrapes, or bloody stool. Possible interventions for decreased platelet count may include transfusion of platelets or changes in anticoagulant therapy.

✅ *Specific Complications*

There are a number of complications associated with performing a venipuncture. **Pain** is commonly associated with needles, and although the pain experienced during venipuncture is usually mild, on a rare occasion the needle may strike a nerve, causing permanent pain. Some patients experience a **vasovagal reaction** during the venipuncture procedure, evidenced by sweating, low blood pressure, fainting, or near fainting. The potential for a **fall injury** is a significant concern related to vasovagal reactions. Prolonged **bleeding** is a complication that occurs with patients who are taking blood thinners or who have coagulopathies such as hemophilia. A **hematoma** results when blood leaks into the tissue during or after a venipuncture, as evidenced by pain, bruising, and/or swelling at the venipuncture site. The swelling can cause injury by compression to surrounding nerves, which can be temporary or permanent. HCPs should watch for minor complications such as bruising and hematoma at the venipuncture site, which are fairly common. Hematomas occur more often in older adults or frail patients, or those with veins that are difficult to access. Bleeding or bruising can be prevented once the needle has been removed by applying direct pressure to the site with dry gauze for a minute or two. Some other more unusual complications of venipuncture include **cellulitis, phlebitis, inadvertent arterial puncture,** and **sepsis.** Sepsis can be caused by introduction of bacteria from the surface of the skin into the blood as the result of improper cleansing of the venipuncture site. Immunocompromised patients are at higher risk for developing this complication.

⊙ Related Tests

- Related tests include antidysrhythmic drugs (quinidine), biopsy bone marrow, bleeding time, blood groups and antibodies, clot retraction, coagulation factors, CBC, CBC RBC morphology and inclusions, CBC WBC count and differential, CT angiography, CT brain, FDP, fibrinogen, PTT, platelet antibodies, procalcitonin, PT/INR, and US pelvis.
- Refer to the Hematopoietic and Immune systems tables at the end of the book for related tests by body system.

Expected Outcomes

Expected outcomes associated with Complete Blood Count, Platelet Count, are:

- Understanding the importance of reporting any bleeding to HCP
- Absence of a transfusion reaction if a transfusion is required as a medical management modality

Partial Thromboplastin Time, Activated

Quick Summary

SYNONYM ACRONYM: aPTT, APTT.

COMMON USE: To assist in assessing coagulation disorders and monitor the effectiveness of therapeutic interventions.

SPECIMEN: Plasma collected in a completely filled blue-top (3.2% sodium citrate) tube. If the patient's hematocrit exceeds 55%, the volume of citrate in the collection tube must be adjusted.

NORMAL FINDINGS: (Method: Clot detection) 25 to 35 sec. The aPTT is slightly prolonged in infants and children and is slightly shortened in older adults. Reference ranges vary with respect to the equipment and reagents used to perform the assay. For the anticoagulated patient, therapeutic levels of heparin are achieved by adjusting the dosage so the aPTT value is 1.5 to 2.5 times the normal.

Test Explanation

The activated partial thromboplastin time (aPTT) test evaluates the function of the contact activation pathway, formerly known as intrinsic pathway (factors XII,

XI, IX, VIII, prekallikrein, and high molecular weight kininogen) and the common pathway (factors V, X, II, and I) of the coagulation sequence. The aPTT time represents the time required for formation of a firm fibrin clot after tissue thromboplastin reagents and calcium are added to a plasma specimen. The aPTT is abnormal in 90% of patients with coagulation disorders and is useful in monitoring effective inactivation of factor II (thrombin) by heparin therapy. The test is prolonged when there is a 30% to 40% deficiency in one of the factors required or when factor inhibitors (e.g., antithrombin III, protein C, or protein S) are present. The aPTT and prothrombin time (PT) tests assist in identifying the cause of or tendency for bleeding as related to coagulation defects. A comparison between the results of aPTT and PT tests can allow some inferences to be made that a factor deficiency exists. A normal aPTT with a prolonged PT can occur only with factor VII deficiency. A prolonged aPTT with a normal PT could indicate a deficiency in factors XII, XI, IX, VIII, and VIII:C (von Willebrand factor). Factor deficiencies can also be identified by correction or substitution studies using normal serum. These studies are easy to perform and are accomplished by adding plasma from a healthy patient to a sample from a patient suspected to be factor deficient. When the aPTT is repeated and is corrected, or is within the reference range, it can be assumed that the prolonged aPTT is caused by a factor deficiency. If the result remains uncorrected, the prolonged aPTT is most likely due to a circulating anticoagulant. (For more information on factor deficiencies, see the "Coagulation Factors" study.)

Nursing Implications

Assessment

Indications	Potential Nursing Problems
Detect congenital deficiencies in clotting factors, as seen in diseases such as hemophilia A (factor VIII) and hemophilia B (factor IX)	• Bleeding • Gas Exchange • Health Management • Human Response • Injury Risk • Liver • Nutrition • Tissue Perfusion
Evaluate response to anticoagulant therapy with heparin or coumarin derivatives	
Identify individuals who may be prone to bleeding during surgical, obstetric, dental, or invasive diagnostic procedures	
Identify the possible cause of abnormal bleeding, such as epistaxis, hematoma, gingival bleeding, hematuria, and menorrhagia	
Monitor the hemostatic effects of conditions such as liver disease, protein deficiency, and fat malabsorption	

Diagnosis: Clinical Significance of Test Results
PROLONGED IN

- Afibrinogenemia, dysfibrinoginemia, or hypofibrinogenemia *(related to insufficient levels of fibrinogen, which is required for clotting)*
- Circulating anticoagulants *(related to the presence of coagulation factor inhibitors, e.g., developed from long-term factor VIII therapy, or circulating anticoagulants associated with conditions like tuberculosis, systemic lupus erythematosus, rheumatoid arthritis, and chronic glomerulonephritis)*
- Circulating products of fibrin and fibrinogen degradation *(related to the presence of circulating breakdown products of fibrin)*
- Disseminated intravascular coagulation *(related to increased consumption of clotting factors)*
- Factor deficiencies *(related to insufficient levels of coagulation factors)*
- Hemodialysis patients *(related to the anticoagulant effect of heparin)*
- Severe liver disease *(insufficient production of clotting factors related to liver damage)*
- Vitamin K deficiency *(related to insufficient vitamin K levels required for clotting)*
- Von Willebrand disease *(related to a congenital deficiency of clotting factors)*

Planning

Considerations for planning a successful partnership should include clear communication of what to expect during the test to decrease anxiety and improve cooperation. Before the procedure is performed, plan to review the steps with the patient. Address concerns about pain, and explain that there may be some discomfort during the venipuncture.

SPECIAL CONSIDERATIONS

An important aspect of planning is understanding the factors that may alter study findings or cause abnormal results. Interdepartmental communication is a key factor in the planning process. The following should be noted when planning for this study:

- An elevated platelet count or inadequate centrifugation of the specimen prior to analysis will also result in decreased values.

It is also important to understand which medications or substances the patient may be exposed to in the healthcare setting that can interfere with accurate testing:

- Drugs and vitamins such as anistreplase, antihistamines, chlorpromazine, salicylates, and ascorbic acid may cause prolonged aPTT, as will anticoagulant therapy with heparin.
- Copper is a component of factor V, and severe copper deficiencies may affect the normal function of factor V, resulting in prolonged aPTT values.

Implementation

Patient education is key to obtaining the patient's cooperation in following directions, and providing an explanation for the purpose of the procedure is an important part of this process. Inform the patient that this study can assist in evaluating the effectiveness of blood clotting. Perform the venipuncture.

If delays in specimen transport and processing occur, it is important to consult with the testing laboratory. Whole blood specimens are stable at room temperature for up to 24 hours. Specimen stability requirements may also vary if the patient is receiving heparin therapy. Some laboratories require frozen plasma if testing will not be performed within 1 hour of collection.

Evaluation

Recognize anxiety related to test results, and discuss the implications of abnormal test results on the patient's lifestyle. Help patients who have a bleeding disorder understand the importance of taking precautions against bruising and bleeding. Instruct the patient to report severe bruising or bleeding from any areas of the skin or mucous membranes. Provide education for precautions to include the use of a soft-bristle toothbrush, the use of an electric razor, and avoiding constipation, salicylates and similar products, and intramuscular injections. Inform the patient about the importance of periodic laboratory testing to monitor aPTT levels while taking an anticoagulant.

Critical Findings

Adults & Children
Greater than 70 sec

Consideration may be given to verification of critical findings before action is taken. Policies vary among facilities and may include requesting immediate recollection and retesting by the laboratory or retesting using a rapid Point of Care testing instrument at the bedside, if available.

Note and immediately report to the requesting health-care provider (HCP) any critical findings and related symptoms. A listing of these findings varies among facilities.

Timely notification of critical findings for lab or diagnostic studies is a role expectation of the professional nurse. Notification processes will vary among facilities. Upon receipt of the critical finding the information should be read back to the caller to verify accuracy. Most policies require immediate notification of the primary HCP, Hospitalist, or on-call HCP. Reported information includes the patient's name, unique identifiers, critical finding, name of the person giving the report, and name of the person receiving the report. Documentation of notification should be made in the medical record with the name of the HCP notified, time and date of notification, and any orders received. Any delay in a timely report of a critical finding may require completion of a notification form with review by Risk Management.

Important signs to note are prolonged bleeding from cuts or gums, hematoma at a puncture site, bruising easily, blood in the stool, persistent epistaxis, heavy or prolonged menstrual flow, and shock. Monitor vital signs, PTT levels, unusual ecchymosis, occult blood, severe headache, unusual dizziness, and neurological changes until aPTT is within normal range.

✔ Specific Complications

There are a number of complications associated with performing a venipuncture. **Pain** is commonly associated with needles, and although the pain experienced during venipuncture is usually mild, on a rare occasion the needle may strike a nerve, causing permanent pain. Some patients experience a **vasovagal reaction** during the venipuncture procedure, evidenced by sweating, low blood pressure, fainting, or near fainting. The potential for a **fall injury** is a significant concern related to vasovagal reactions. Prolonged **bleeding** is a complication that occurs with patients who are taking blood thinners or who have coagulopathies such as hemophilia. A **hematoma** results when blood leaks into the tissue during or after a venipuncture, as evidenced by pain, bruising, and/or swelling at the venipuncture site. The swelling can cause injury by compression to surrounding nerves, which can be temporary or permanent. Health-care providers should watch for minor complications such as bruising and hematoma at the venipuncture site, which are fairly common. Hematomas occur more often in older adult or frail patients, or those with veins that are difficult to access. Bleeding or bruising can be prevented once the needle has been removed by applying direct pressure to the site with dry gauze for a minute or two. Some other more unusual complications of venipuncture include **cellulitis, phlebitis, inadvertent arterial puncture,** and **sepsis.** Sepsis can be caused by introduction of bacteria from the surface of the skin into the blood as the result of improper cleansing of the venipuncture site. Immunocompromised patients are at higher risk for developing this complication.

✔ Related Tests

Related tests include antithrombin III, bleeding time, coagulation factors, CBC, CBC platelet count, copper, D-dimer, FDP, plasminogen, protein C, protein S, PT/INR, and vitamin K.

Refer to the Hematopoietic and Hepatobiliary systems tables at the end of the book for related tests by body system.

Expected Outcomes

Expected outcomes associated with Partial Thromboplastin Time, Activated (aPTT), are:

- Establishing a compliant and successful therapeutic and monitoring regimen
- Cooperating with therapy to manage bleeding risk and adhering to recommendations to prevent injury

- Having a family that is supportive in creating a home environment that decreases injury risk
- Demonstrating positive coping skills in relation to underlying disease diagnosis

Prothrombin Time and International Normalized Ratio

Quick Summary

SYNONYM ACRONYM: Protime, PT.

COMMON USE: To assess and monitor coagulation status related to therapeutic interventions and disorders such as vitamin K deficiency.

SPECIMEN: Plasma collected in a completely filled blue-top (sodium citrate) tube. If the patient's hematocrit exceeds 55%, the volume of citrate in the collection tube must be adjusted.

NORMAL FINDINGS: (Method: Clot detection) 10 to 13 sec.

- International normalized ratio (INR) = 0.9–1.1 for patients not receiving anticoagulation therapy, 2 to 3 for patients receiving treatment for venous thrombosis, pulmonary embolism, and valvular heart disease.
- INR = 2.5 to 3.5 for patients with mechanical heart valves and/or receiving treatment for recurrent systemic embolism.
- For the anticoagulated patient, therapeutic levels of warfarin are achieved by adjusting the dosage so the PT value is 1.5 to 2.5 times longer than normal or so the INR is between 2 and 3.

Test Explanation

Prothrombin time (PT) is a coagulation test performed to measure the time it takes for a firm fibrin clot to form after tissue thromboplastin (factor III) and calcium are added to a sample of plasma. Coagulation factors in the patient's sample, including prothrombin (factor II) react with the reagents and complete the process of coagulation in proportion to the amount of available coagulation factors. The PT is used to evaluate the tissue factor pathway, formerly called the extrinsic pathway of the coagulation sequence in patients receiving oral warfarin (Coumadin) anticoagulants. Prothrombin is a vitamin K–dependent protein produced by the liver; measurement is reported as time in seconds or percentage of normal activity.

The goal of long-term anticoagulation therapy is to achieve a balance between in vivo thrombus formation and hemorrhage. It is a delicate clinical balance, and because of differences in instruments and reagents, there is a wide variation in PT results among laboratories. Worldwide concern for the need to provide more consistency in monitoring patients receiving anticoagulant therapy led to the development of an international committee. In the early 1980s, manufacturers of instruments and reagents began comparing their measurement systems with a single reference material provided by the World Health Organization (WHO). The international effort successfully developed an algorithm to provide comparable PT values regardless of differences in laboratory methodology. Reagent and instrument manufacturers compare their results to the WHO reference and derive a factor called an international sensitivity index (ISI) that is applied to a mathematical formula to standardize the results. Laboratories convert their PT values into an international normalized ratio (INR) by using the following formula:

$$INR = (patient\ PT\ result/normal\ patient\ average)^{(ISI)}$$

PT evaluation can now be based on an INR using a standardized thromboplastin reagent to assist in making decisions regarding oral anticoagulation therapy.

The metabolism of many commonly prescribed medications is driven by the cytochrome P450 (CYP450) family of enzymes. Genetic variants can alter enzymatic activity that results in a spectrum of effects ranging from the total absence of drug metabolism to ultrafast metabolism. Impaired drug metabolism can prevent the intended therapeutic effect or even lead to serious adverse drug reactions. Poor metabolizers (PMs) are at increased risk for drug-induced side effects due to accumulation of drug in the blood, whereas ultra-rapid metabolizers (UMs) require a higher-than-normal dosage because the drug is metabolized over a shorter duration than intended. In the case of prodrugs that require activation before metabolism, the opposite occurs: PMs may require a higher dose because the activated drug is becoming available more slowly than intended, and UMs may require less because the activated drug is becoming available sooner than intended. Other genetic phenotypes used to report CYP450 results are intermediate metabolizer (IM) and extensive metabolizer (EM). Genetic testing can be performed on blood samples submitted to a laboratory. The test method commonly used is polymerase chain reaction. Counseling and informed written consent are generally required for genetic testing. CYP2C9 is a gene in the CYP450 family that metabolizes prodrugs like the anticoagulant warfarin. Three major gene mutations, CYP2CP*2, CYP2C9*3, and VKORC1, are associated with warfarin response and are estimated to account for up to 45% of variations in warfarin dose response. CYP450 testing is available and should be used in conjunction with other factors, including all prescription and over-the-counter medications being used; mode of drug administration; use of tobacco products, foods, and supplements; age, weight, environment, activity level, and diseases with which the patient may be dealing.

Some inferences of factor deficiency can be made by comparison of results obtained from the activated partial thromboplastin time (aPTT) and PT tests. A normal aPTT with a prolonged PT can occur only with factor VII deficiency. A prolonged aPTT with a normal PT could indicate a deficiency in factors XII, XI, IX, and VIII as well as VIII:C (von Willebrand factor). Factor deficiencies can also be identified by correction or substitution studies using normal serum. These studies are easy to perform and are accomplished by adding plasma from a healthy patient to a sample from a suspected factor-deficient patient. When the PT is repeated and corrected, or within the reference range, it can be assumed that the prolonged PT is due to a factor deficiency (see study titled "Coagulation Factors"). If the result remains uncorrected, the prolonged PT is most likely due to a circulating anticoagulant.

Nursing Implications
Assessment

Indications	Potential Nursing Problems
Differentiate between deficiencies of clotting factors II, V, VII, and X, which prolong the PT, and congenital coagulation disorders such as hemophilia A (factor VIII) and hemophilia B (factor IX), which do not alter the PT Evaluate the response to anticoagulant therapy with coumadin derivatives and determine dosage required to achieve therapeutic results Identify individuals who may be prone to bleeding during surgical, obstetric, dental, or invasive diagnostic procedures Identify the possible cause of abnormal bleeding, such as epistaxis, hematoma, gingival bleeding, hematuria, and menorrhagia Monitor the effects of conditions such as liver disease, protein deficiency, and fat malabsorption on hemostasis Screen for prothrombin deficiency Screen for vitamin K deficiency	• Bleeding • Gas Exchange • Health Management • Human Response • Injury Risk • Nutrition • Tissue Perfusion

Diagnosis: Clinical Significance of Test Results
INCREASED IN
- Afibrinogenemia, dysfibrinogenemia, or hypofibrinogenemia *(related to insufficient levels of fibrinogen, which is required for clotting; its absence prolongs PT)*
- Alcohol use *(related to decreased liver function, which results in decreased production of clotting factors and prolonged PT)*

- Biliary obstruction *(related to poor absorption of fat-soluble vitamin K; vitamin K is required for clotting and its absence prolongs PT)*
- Disseminated intravascular coagulation *(related to increased consumption of clotting factors; PT is increased)*
- Hereditary deficiencies of factors II, V, VII, and X *(related to deficiency of factors required for clotting; their absence prolongs PT)*
- Liver disease (cirrhosis) *(related to decreased liver function, which results in decreased production of clotting factors and prolonged PT)*
- Massive transfusion of packed red blood cells (RBCs) *(related to dilutional effect of replacing a significant fraction of the total blood volume; there are insufficient clotting factors in plasma-poor, packed RBC products. Blood products contain anticoagulants, which compound the lack of adequate clotting factors in the case of massive transfusion)*
- Poor fat absorption *(tropical sprue, celiac disease, and chronic diarrhea are conditions that prevent absorption of fat-soluble vitamins, including vitamin K, which is required for clotting; its absence prolongs PT)*
- Presence of circulating anticoagulant *(related to the production of inhibitors of specific factors, e.g., developed from long-term factor VIII therapy or circulating anticoagulants associated with conditions like tuberculosis, systemic lupus erythematosus, rheumatoid arthritis, and chronic glomerulonephritis)*
- Salicylate intoxication *(related to decreased liver function)*
- Vitamin K deficiency *(related to dietary deficiency or disorders of malabsorption; vitamin K is required for clotting; its absence prolongs PT)*

DECREASED IN
- Increased absorption of Vitamin K *(related to dietary increases in fat, which enhances absorption of Vitamin K, or increases of green leafy vegetables that contain large amounts of Vitamin K)*
- Ovarian hyperfunction
- Regional enteritis or ileitis

Planning
Considerations for planning a successful partnership should include clear communication of what to expect during the test to decrease anxiety and improve cooperation. Before the procedure is performed, plan to review the steps with the patient. Address concerns about pain and explain that there may be some discomfort during the venipuncture.

SPECIAL CONSIDERATIONS
An important aspect of planning is understanding the factors that may alter study findings or cause abnormal results. Interdepartmental communication is a key factor in the planning process.

It is also important to understand which medications or substances the patient may be exposed to in the health-care setting that can interfere with accurate testing:

- Drugs that may increase the PT in patients receiving anticoagulation therapy include acetaminophen, acetylsalicylic acid, amiodarone, anabolic steroids, anisindione, anistreplase, antibiotics, antipyrine, carbenicillin, cathartics, chloral hydrate, chlorthalidone, cholestyramine, clofibrate, corticotropin, demeclocycline, dextrothyroxine, diazoxide, diflunisal, disulfiram, diuretics, doxycycline, erythromycin, ethyl alcohol, hydroxyzine, laxatives, mercaptopurine, miconazole, nalidixic acid, neomycin, niacin, oxyphenbutazone, phenytoin, quinidine, quinine, sulfachlorpyridazine, thyroxine, and tosylate bretylium.
- Drugs that may decrease the PT in patients receiving anticoagulation therapy include aminoglutethimide, amobarbital, anabolic steroids, antacids, antihistamines, barbiturates, carbamazepine, chloral hydrate, chlordane, chlordiazepoxide, cholestyramine, clofibrate, colchicine, corticosteroids, dichloralphenazone, diuretics, oral contraceptives, penicillin, primidone, raloxifene, rifabutin, rifampin, simethicone, spironolactone, tacrolimus, tolbutamide, and vitamin K.

● Safety Tip
Assessment for potential drug interactions is an important part of the planning process. One of the most significant negative patient outcomes for patients receiving anticoagulant therapy is related to adverse drug reactions. Patients are often unaware of the potentiating effects that occur between their anticoagulant and many common foods, medications, and over-the-counter products. Patients should be encouraged to speak with their HCP or pharmacist before taking additional medications.

Implementation
Patient education is key to obtaining the patient's cooperation in following directions, and providing an explanation for the purpose of the procedure is an important part of this process. Inform the patient that this study can assist in evaluating coagulation and in monitoring therapy. Perform the venipuncture.

Evaluation
DISCUSSION POINT
It should be noted that frequent monitoring of the PT/INR is very important. Concern with monitoring is mostly involved with elevated values. However, decreased PT results can indicate a risk for thrombosis. There are three factors, known as Virchow Triad, that increase the risk of developing a venous thrombus:

- Hypercoagulability, or a tendency for blood to coagulate at an abnormally rapid rate
- Venous stasis, or an impaired rate of blood flow through a vessel
- Vessel wall trauma or injury

Possible nursing interventions to decrease risk of thrombus include educating the patient regarding leg exercises, avoiding constrictive clothing (e.g., stockings or tight socks), or avoiding behaviors that might constrict blood flow, such as crossing the legs or maintaining a dependent position for long periods of time.

Recognize anxiety related to test results, and discuss the implications of abnormal test results on the patient's lifestyle. Help patients who have a bleeding disorder understand the importance of taking precautions against bruising and bleeding. Provide education for precautions to include the use of a soft-bristle toothbrush, the use of an electric razor, and avoiding constipation, salicylates (aspirin) and similar products, and intramuscular injections. Instruct the patient, as appropriate, in the use of home test kits for PT/INR approved by the U.S. Food and Drug Administration.

Nutritional Considerations: Foods high in vitamin K should be avoided by the patient on anticoagulant therapy. Foods that contain vitamin K include asparagus, beans, cabbage, cauliflower, chickpeas, egg yolks, green tea, pork, liver, milk, soybean products, tomatoes, mayonnaise, vegetable oils, and green leafy vegetables such as leaf lettuce, watercress, parsley, broccoli, brussels sprouts, kale, spinach, swiss chard, and collard, mustard, and turnip greens. Alcohol and alcohol products should be avoided while taking warfarin because the combination of the two increases the risk of gastrointestinal bleeding.

Critical Findings

INR
Greater than 5

Prothrombin Time
Greater than 27 sec

Consideration may be given to verification of critical findings before action is taken. Policies vary among facilities and may include requesting immediate recollection and retesting by the laboratory or retesting using a rapid Point of Care testing instrument at the bedside, if available.

Note and immediately report to the requesting health-care provider (HCP) any critical findings and related symptoms. A listing of these findings varies among facilities.

Important signs to note relate to bleeding in specific areas of the body and include prolonged bleeding from cuts or gums, hematoma at a puncture site, hemorrhage, blood in the stool, backache or flank pain, dark colored urine, joint pain, persistent epistaxis, heavy or prolonged menstrual flow, and shock. Monitor vital signs, unusual ecchymosis, occult blood, severe headache, unusual dizziness, and neurological changes until PT is within normal range. Intramuscular (IM) administration of vitamin K, an anticoagulant reversal agent, may be requested by the HCP.

Specific Complications

There are a number of complications associated with performing a venipuncture. **Pain** is commonly associated with needles, and although the pain experienced during venipuncture is usually mild, on a rare occasion the needle may strike a nerve causing permanent pain. Some patients experience a **vasovagal reaction** during the venipuncture procedure, evidenced by sweating, low blood pressure, fainting, or near fainting. The potential for a **fall injury** is a significant concern related to vasovagal reactions. Prolonged **bleeding** is a complication that occurs with patients who are taking blood thinners or who have coagulopathies such as hemophilia. A **hematoma** results when blood leaks into the tissue during or after a venipuncture, as evidenced by pain, bruising, and/or swelling at the venipuncture site. The swelling can cause injury by compression to surrounding nerves, which can be temporary or permanent. HCPs should watch for minor complications such as bruising and hematoma at the venipuncture site, which are fairly common. Hematomas occur more often in older adult or frail patients, or those with veins that are difficult to access. Bleeding or bruising can be prevented once the needle has been removed by applying direct pressure to the site with dry gauze for a minute or two. Some other more unusual complications of venipuncture include **cellulitis, phlebitis, inadvertent arterial puncture**, and **sepsis**. Sepsis can be caused by introduction of bacteria from the surface of the skin into the blood as the result of improper cleansing of the venipuncture site. Immunocompromised patients are at higher risk for developing this complication.

Related Tests

- Related tests include ALP, ALT, ANA, AT-III, AST, bilirubin, biopsy liver, bleeding time, calcium, coagulation factors, CBC, CBC platelet count, CT liver and biliary tract, cryoglobulin, D-dimer, fecal analysis, fecal fat, FDP, fibrinogen, GGT, gastric acid emptying scan, hepatitis antibodies (A, B, C, D), liver and spleen scan, lupus anticoagulant, aPTT, plasminogen, protein C, protein S, US abdomen, US liver, and vitamin K.
- Refer to the Cardiovascular, Hematopoietic, and Hepatobiliary systems tables at the end of the book for related tests by body system.

Expected Outcomes

Expected outcomes associated with Prothrombin Time and International Normalized Ratio (PT/INR) are:

- Recognizing the health risk of being deficient in vitamin K related to possible bleeding and injury
- Identifying foods that are high in vitamin K and making a list of them to incorporate into dietary choices
- Adhering to an HCP-recommended schedule to recheck the coagulation status to adjust anticoagulant therapy

REVIEW OF LEARNING OUTCOMES

Thinking

1. Name the three components of hemostasis. Answer: Hemostasis involves three components: blood vessel walls, platelets, and plasma coagulation proteins.

2. State the primary purposes of anticoagulant therapy and identify its effects both on existing blood clots and in the prevention of blood clot development. Answer: Anticoagulant therapy is used to prevent the formation of blood clots or thrombi in patients with conditions such as occlusive vascular disease or for patients who are immobilized or otherwise bedridden for a extended periods of time. Anticoagulant therapy is also used to dissolve thrombi that have already formed in patients with conditions such as pulmonary embolism (PE), myocardial infarction (MI), and cerebrovascular thrombosis. Urokinase and recombinant tPA have both been used therapeutically for many years as thrombolytic agents in the treatment of MI and cerebrovascular accident (CVA) as they are capable of destroying thrombi that have already formed. Urokinase has been used to treat deep vein thrombosis (DVT) and PE. Heparin and the coumarin compounds are anticoagulant agents that act by interfering with the formation of clots. A third group of anticoagulants, the antiplatelet drugs, is used therapeutically to protect the cerebrovascular system of patients at risk for developing blood clots like clopidogrel (Plavix) and salicylate (aspirin). They act against platelets to prevent aggregation or clumping, an important initial step in the formation of thrombi. The main therapeutic goal is to administer the lowest possible dose of anticoagulant needed to prevent clot formation while minimizing the risk of bleeding.

3. Identify which study is commonly used to monitor patients on heparin therapy and which study is used to monitor patients receiving warfarin or coumarin therapy. Answer: The aPTT is used to monitor patients on heparin therapy. The PT/INR is used to monitor patients receiving warfarin or coumarin therapy.

Doing

1. Discuss the two types of hemostasis, primary and secondary hemostasis. Answer: Primary hemostasis involves platelet activity in adhesion, activation, and aggregation to form a plug. Secondary hemostasis involves the action of the coagulation factors to form a stable fibrin clot that prevents bleeding.

2. Discuss how a balance between repair of an injured vessel and complete vessel occlusion is accomplished. Answer: Primary and secondary hemostasis must be kept in balance to prevent an injured vessel from becoming completely occluded. The antithrombotic process or termination phase of secondary hemostasis accomplishes this through the antithrombin and fibrinolytic systems. The antithrombin system involves neutralization of coagulation factors and of thrombin itself in several different ways. The fibrinolytic system involves the activation of plasminogen to plasmin.

3. Identify the major complications of anticoagulant therapy and some specific nursing interventions that can help prevent clot formation. Answer: The major difficulties associated with the use of anticoagulants are hemorrhage and drug interaction. Observation of the patient for signs of internal and external spontaneous bleeding is essential. Walking, leg exercises, elevation of the feet and legs, and the use of compression stockings are some effective interventions to avoid developing blood clots. There is a wealth of information available to help educate patients receiving anticoagulant medications regarding dietary considerations or restrictions. Some foods are natural blood thinners because they are rich in salicylates, vitamin E, vitamin K, or act as blood thinners on their own. A few examples include blueberries (bilberry), cayenne pepper, cherries, cinnamon, clover (red and sweet), cranberries, curry powder, dill, fish oils, garlic, ginseng, grapes, grapefruit seed extract, kale, oregano, paprika, peppermint, raisins, senna, spinach, St. John's wort, strawberries, tangerines, thyme, and tumeric. These foods, when consumed regularly, may have a significant potentiating or inhibitory effect when combined with a regimen of anticoagulant medication. This could in turn put the patient at risk for thrombosis or bleeding. Patients must also be cautioned to consult with their HCP or pharmacist before taking any medications or over-the-counter herbal products in combination with an anticoagulant agent. Patients should be instructed in the prevention of accidental injury, basic first aid measures to control bleeding in the event of an accident, signs that warrant immediate medical attention, and finally assurance that bleeding can be controlled with the proper interventions. Women of childbearing age should receive counseling regarding the known effects of various contraception methods and risks for complications related to the coagulation system; the risk for potentially significant complications increases for women who have a medical condition requiring treatment with anticoagulants. Intrauterine devices can cause excessive endometrial bleeding and estrogen containing oral

contraceptives have been associated with increased risk for venous thromboembolism. Heparin is the medication of choice for women who require anticoagulant therapy during pregnancy because, unlike warfarin, heparin does not cross the placental barrier. Warfarin is known to be harmful to the fetus when it crosses the placenta because it may cause a fatal hemorrhage or cause congenital abnormalities in the developing fetus. Warfarin is not passed in breast milk and is safe for use in lactating females.

Caring

1. Recognize that perceiving how care is delivered though the patient's point of view is of value. Answer: Fear is a universal reaction to being told that you have a medical problem. What seems simple to us, such as administering anticoagulants for a DVT, is devastating for others. Understanding your patients' point of view will help you provide direction about how to best meet their individual needs. Caring about what they feel and think is the only way to do that.

◖◗ Words OF Wisdom: There is an old nursery rhyme where a little girl sat down to three bowls of porridge. One bowl of porridge was too hot, one too cold, and one just right. Coagulation studies are like that. If our blood is too thin from altered clotting factors we can end up with internal bleeding, life-threatening syndromes, and multiorgan failure. If our altered clotting factors cause our blood to be too thick, we can end up with clots in the brain, heart, and lungs. These are also life-threatening events. It is the job of the nurse, physician, and pharmacist to partner together to ensure that the clotting factors of the patients blood are "just right." Do not make the mistake of taking this responsibility lightly. I know of a patient whose nurse did not and she ended up with a debilitating stoke. Be vigilant in monitoring all coagulation studies, trending them with prior results, and combining that information with patient assessment. Be active partners with the physician and pharmacist in coagulation management.

BIBLIOGRAPHY

Advance for medical laboratory professionals. (1999, January 25). Venipuncture after transfusion. Retrieved from www.laboratorian.advanceweb.com/Article/Venipuncture-After-Transfusion.aspx

Cavanaugh, B. (2003). Nurse's manual of laboratory and diagnostic tests. (4th ed.). Philadelphia, PA: F.A. Davis Company.

Lippi, G., Salvagno, G., Montagnana, M., & Guidi, G. (2005). Short term venous stasis influences routine coagulation testing. Blood Coagulation and Fibrinolysis, 16(6), 453-458. Retrieved from www.ncbi.nlm.nih.gov/pubmed/16093738

Moll, S. (2009). Antithrombin III deficiency. Retrieved from www.stoptheclot.org/News/article138.htm

Nogami, K., Shima. M., Matsumoto, T., Nishiya, K., Tanaka, I., & Yoshioka, A. (2006, December 21). Mechanisms of plasmin-catalyzed inactivation of Factor VIII. Journal of Biological Chemistry. doi 10.1074/jbc.M607816200

Nursing diagnoses for patients with coagulation abnormalities (n.d.). Retrieved from www.rnceus.com/coag/coagnd.html

PTT, aPTT, Partial thromboplastin time. (2013, March 3). Retrieved from www.clinlabnavigator.com/ptt-or-plasma thromboplastin time.html

Reik, R. (2008, August). How long should you wait after a unit of blood has been transfused before drawing a complete blood count, or doing other lab work, to ensure accurate test results? Retrieved from www.cap.org/apps/cap.portal?_nfpb=true&cntvwrPtlt_actionOverride=%2Fportlets%2FcontentViewer%2Fshow&cntvwrPtlt%7BactionForm.contentReference%7D=cap_today%2F0808%2F0808_qa.html&=cntvwr

Saiemaldahr, M. (n.d.). Fibrinolysis system. Retrieved from www.slideserve.com/matana/fibrinolsis-system

University of Illinois–Urbana/Champaign Carle Cancer Center Hematology Resource Page. (n.d.). Antithrombin III deficiency. Retrieved from www.med.illinois.edu/hematology/PtAntithrombin.htm

Van Leeuwen, A., and Bladh, M. (2015). Davis's comprehensive handbook of laboratory and diagnostic tests with nursing implications (6th ed.). Philadelphia, PA: F.A. Davis Company.

Wood-Moen, R. (2011). Herbal supplements contraindicated with blood thinners. Retrieved from www.livestrong.com/article/527837-herbal-supplements-contraindicated-with-blood-thinners/#ixzz2P8oLFgRh

Go to Section II of this book and http://www.davisplus.com for the Clinical Reasoning Tool and its case studies to provide you with a safe place to explore patient care situations. There are a total of 26 different case studies; 2 cases are presented for each of 13 body systems. One set of 13 cases are found in the Section II chapters, and a second set of 13 cases are available online at http://www.davisplus.com. Each case is designed with the specific goal of helping you to connect the dots of clinical reasoning. Cases are designed to reflect possible clinical scenarios; the outcomes may or may not be positive—you decide.

Blood Studies: Immunohematology (Blood Banking)

OVERVIEW

Immunohematology, also known as blood banking and transfusion medicine, is a special branch of immunology that studies antigens present on blood cell membranes and the corresponding development of circulating antibodies stimulated by the presence of red cell antigens during blood product transfusion or pregnancy. Immunohematologists prepare and select safe blood and plasma products for transfusion, such as leuko-reduced packed red blood cells, packed red blood cells, whole blood, platelets, cryoprecipitate, and fresh frozen plasma (see Figs. 4.1 and 4.2).

There are two terms commonly used to describe donated blood units: allogeneic (also known as homologous) and autologous. Allogeneic is the most common type of donated blood and is given by the donor to an unknown recipient. Autologous donations are made by a donor for their own use at a later date. Whole blood and blood products collected by apheresis for either type of donation are collected at a donation center. Allogeneic donations are usually made on a voluntary (unpaid) basis. The donor must sign an informed consent, complete a screening questionnaire, and undergo some general health tests such as blood pressure, pulse, body temperature, and hemoglobin level. These initial tests are crucial

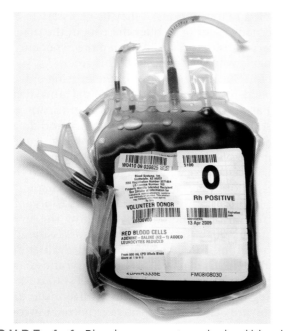

FIGURE 4.1 Blood component, packed red blood cells, for transfusion. *Copyright, Blood Systems. Used with permission.*

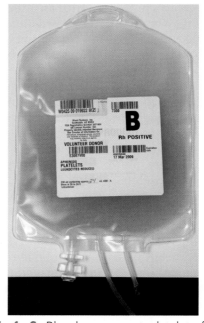

FIGURE 4.2 Blood component, platelets, for transfusion. *Copyright, Blood Systems. Used with permission.*

to selection of healthy blood donors. Donated blood products are tested for ABO group, Rh type, unexpected RBC antibodies, and transmissible infectious diseases that test for the presence of hepatitis B core antibody (antibodies directed against the hepatitis B core antigen), hepatitis B surface antigen, hepatitis B virus (viral DNA by nucleic acid testing [NAT]), hepatitis C antibody (viral RNA by NAT), HTLV I and II antibody, HIV 1 (viral RNA by NAT) and 2 antibody, and syphilis. Additional testing may be performed in cases of specific need to include cytomegalovirus antibody and IgA deficiency. Additional testing may also be performed for the presence of West Nile virus (viral RNA by NAT) or antibodies to *Trypanosoma cruzi* or Chagas disease when increased risk for transmission from a particular donor is suspected. All donated units receiving additional testing will be labelled with the results (positive or negative).

Another strategy for blood management is to reduce or eliminate the need for allogeneic blood transfusion through the use of perioperative blood recovery, a process by which blood is collected and mixed with an anticoagulant during or after a surgical procedure by specialized equipment such as a Cell Saver®. The equipment utilizes bar code technology that enables the user to collect and store information such as patient ID, user ID, and lot numbers for supplies. The blood is centrifuged, washed, and pumped into a transfer bag, where it can either be reinfused or stored for the patient's use at a later time. The specific time period that salvaged blood is usable is determined by the facility that provides transfusion services, and regulatory agencies such as the U.S. Food and Drug Administration (FDA) and AABB. Blood salvage is an option for patients undergoing a procedure with an anticipated need for two or more units of blood. Patients undergoing cardiac, gynecological, organ transplant, orthopedic, urologic, and vascular procedures might benefit from perioperative blood salvage.

An area of developing interest is hematopoietic therapy via stem cell transfusion. Bone marrow and umbilical cord blood contain hematopoietic stem cells that differentiate into the mature formed elements of blood: red blood cells, white blood cells, and platelets. Stem cells are pluripotent, meaning they have the capacity to develop into any cell type, even non-hematopoietic cell types. Stem cells also possess an unlimited capacity for self-renewal. Stem cells can be used to treat hematopoietic and immune system blood disorders, malignancies, and immunodeficiencies. Stem cell transplants can also be used therapeutically to restore bone marrow damaged by radiation or chemotherapy, as a mechanism to accomplish gene therapy for inherited disorders, and potentially to generate other types of tissue (e.g., heart, lung, liver, etc.) for organ repair.

SPECIAL CONSIDERATIONS

If blood units that match the patient's group and type are not available, a switch in ABO blood group is preferable to a change in Rh type. However, in extreme circumstances, Rh-positive blood can be issued to an Rh-negative recipient. It is very likely that the recipient will develop antibodies as the result of receiving Rh-positive red blood cells. Rh antibodies are highly immunogenic, and, once the antibodies are developed, the recipient can only receive Rh-negative blood for subsequent red blood cell transfusion.

Considerations may need to be given to patients who have religious or other objections to the transfusion of blood products. Jehovah's Witnesses are among those who may refuse based upon religious beliefs. The decision may vary by procedure and specific blood product. Even though autologous and homologous units of blood are generally considered unacceptable, perioperative blood recovery and the transfusion of plasma derivatives or components prepared from plasma, such as cryoprecipitate, may be acceptable. Most facilities have written guidelines for health-care providers (HCPs) about options for blood conservation as well as written policies for staff and patients regarding transfusions. Timely and good communication is key in order to avoid the refusal of transfusion at the time of an urgent need for blood or blood products. Some important documents to review at the time of admission to a facility include written Advance Directives, an executed health-care proxy, and institutional policies directing HCPs to ascertain in writing each patient's wishes regarding transfusion. Policies regarding a refusal of lifesaving blood transfusions also need to consider the needs of the HCPs who may object to caring for patients who object to transfusions. It may be necessary to arrange for alternative staff or to offer the patient the option of a voluntary transfer to a facility with more experience treating patients with special needs in this area.

The four basic components of the nursing process can be applied to each phase of laboratory and diagnostic testing as described in the Preface. The nursing process can also be incorporated into laboratory and diagnostic testing in a more general way by applying elements of assessment, diagnosis, planning, implementation, evaluation, and summary of expected outcomes to the specific test information as presented in this chapter.

The information in the Part I studies is organized in a manner to help the student see how the five basic components of the nursing process (assessment, diagnosis, planning, implementation, and evaluation) can be applied to each phase of laboratory and diagnostic testing. The goal is to use nursing process to understand the integration of care (laboratory, diagnostic, nursing care) toward achieving a positive expected outcome.

- **Assessment** is the collection of information for the purpose of answering the question, "is there a

● *Safety Tips*

Always follow the facility's transfusion policy and procedure; verify the transfusion order; conduct a physical assessment of the patient prior to transfusion for future comparison if changes occur; ensure the infusion rate is appropriate for the patient's age and treatment; positively identify the patient and the product to be transfused prior to administration; ensure the appropriate equipment is on hand to begin the infusion and to manage complications if they occur; if a pump is used, ensure the preventive maintenance sticker has not expired, indicating that the equipment should be taken out of use until its function checks have been certified (see Fig. 4.3). Most facilities require a special blood bank band to be placed on the recipient. The blood band is a safety feature that contains unique identifiers also used on the label of the recipient's blood product to ensure that the correct product is given to the intended recipient. Technology is available to utilize bar-coded bands and labels that can be scanned throughout the entire production cycle of the product up to administration at the bedside, providing a time stamp and tracking of products. Generally, two licensed nurses, one of whom is an RN, verify the order against the product and positively identify the patient prior to the administration of the product. The verification process is conducted in a similar manner to the read-back for critical findings in that it is interactive reading and verification by read-back of the information between the two nurses (see Fig. 4.4).

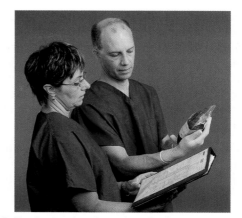

FIGURE 4.4 Blood product verification. *Used with permission, from Wilkinson, J., & Treas, L. (2010). Fundamentals of nursing (2nd Ed.). FA Davis Company.*

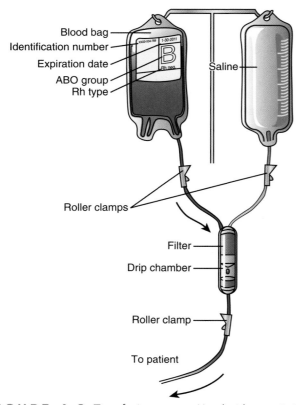

Blood bag
Identification number
Expiration date
ABO group
Rh type
Saline
Roller clamps
Filter
Drip chamber
Roller clamp
To patient

FIGURE 4.3 Transfusion set up. *Used with permission, from Burton, M. (2011). Fundamentals of nursing care: Concepts, connections, & skills. FA Davis Company.*

problem?" Knowledge of the patient's health history, medications, complaints, and allergies as well as synonyms or alternate test names, common use for the procedure, specimen requirements, and normal ranges or interpretive comments provide the foundation for diagnosis.

● **Diagnosis** is the process of looking at the information gathered during assessment and answering the questions, "what is the problem?" and "what do I need to do about it?" Test indications tell us why the study has been requested, and potential diagnoses tell us the value or importance of the study relative to its clinical utility.

● **Planning** is a blueprint of the nursing care before the procedure. It is the process of determining how the nurse is going to partner with the patient to fix the problem (e.g., "The patient has a study ordered and this is what I should know before I successfully carry out the plan to have the study completed"). Knowledge of interfering factors, social and cultural issues, preprocedural restrictions, the need for written and informed consent, anxiety about the procedure, and concerns regarding pain are some considerations for planning a successful partnership.

● **Implementation** is putting the plan into action with an idea of what the expected outcome should be. Collaboration with the departments where the laboratory test or diagnostic study is to be performed is essential to the success of the plan. Implementation is where the work is done within each healthcare team member's scope of practice.

● **Evaluation** answers the question, "did the plan work or not?" Was the plan completely successful, partially successful, or not successful? If the plan did not work, evaluation is the process used to determine what needs to be changed to make the plan work better. This includes a review of all expected outcomes. Nursing care after the procedure is where information is gathered to evaluate the plan. Review of results, including critical findings, in relation to patient symptoms and other tests performed, provides data that form a more complete picture of health or illness.

- **Expected Outcomes** are positive outcomes related to the test. They are the outcomes the nurse should expect if all goes well.

A number of pretest, intratest, and post-test universal points are presented in this overview section because the information applies to blood banking studies in general.

Universal Pretest Pearls (Planning)

- Obtain a history of the patient's complaints, including a list of known allergens, especially allergies or sensitivities to medications or latex so their use can be avoided or their effects mitigated if an allergy is present. Carefully evaluate all medications currently being taken by the patient. A list of the patient's current medications, prescribed and over the counter (including anticoagulants, aspirin and other salicylates, and dietary supplement), should also be obtained. Such products may be discontinued by medical direction for the appropriate number of days prior to the procedure. Ensure that all allergies are clearly noted in the medical record, and ensure that the patient is wearing an allergy and medical record armband. Report information that could interfere with, or delay proceeding with, the study to the HCP and laboratory.
- Obtain a history of the patient's affected body system, symptoms, and results of previously performed laboratory tests and diagnostic and surgical procedures. Previous test results will provide a basis of comparison between old and new data.
- An important aspect of planning is understanding the factors that may alter study findings or cause abnormal results. Interdepartmental communication is a key factor in the planning process. The inability of a patient to cooperate or remain still during the procedure because of age, significant pain, or mental status should be among the anticipated factors. Recent or past procedures, medications, or existing medical conditions that could complicate or interfere with test results should be noted.
- Review the steps of the study with the patient or caregiver. Expect patients to be nervous about the procedure and the pending results. Educating the patient on his or her role during the procedure and what to expect can help facilitate this. The patient's role during the procedure is to remain still. The actual time required to complete each study will depend on a number of conditions, including the type of equipment being used and how well a patient will cooperate.

- Explain that specimen collection by venipuncture takes approximately 5 to 10 minutes. Bleeding or bruising can be prevented, once the needle has been removed, by applying direct pressure to the venipuncture site with dry gauze for a minute or two. The site should be observed/assessed for bleeding or hematoma formation and then covered with a gauze and adhesive bandage.
- Address any concerns about pain and explain or describe, as appropriate, the level and type of discomfort that may be expected. Advise the patient that some discomfort may be experienced during the venipuncture.
- Address any concerns about pain during the transfusion and explain or describe, as appropriate, the level and type of discomfort that may be expected during the procedure. Explain that an IV line will be inserted prior to a blood product transfusion to allow the infusion of IV fluids such as blood products, normal saline, anesthetics, sedatives, or emergency medications. Advise the patient that some discomfort may be experienced during the insertion of the IV. Assure the patient that there should be no discomfort during the transfusion and instruct them to report any unusual symptoms during the transfusion, as described in the Blood Groups and Antibodies study in this chapter.
- Provide additional instructions and patient preparation regarding medication, diet, fluid intake, or activity if appropriate. Unless specified in the individual study, there are no special instructions or restrictions.
- Always be sensitive to any cultural or psychosocial issues, including a concern for modesty before, during, and after the procedure. Be prepared to address the patient's fears and concerns related to blood product transfusion. The patient's perceptions are often based upon information they have absorbed from various sources (e.g., media, Internet, word-of-mouth from friends or relatives) and most commonly involve topics that include the likelihood of disease transmission from the donated blood product, the chance of experiencing a transfusion reaction from getting the wrong blood, and having the ability to assert a religious right of refusal for transfusion.

Reminder

Ensure that a written and informed consent has been documented in the medical record prior to the study, if required. The consent must be obtained before medication or blood products are administered.

Universal Intratest Pearls (Implementation)

- Correct patient identification is crucial prior to any procedure. Positively identify the patient using two unique identifiers such as patient name, date of birth, Social Security number, or medical record number. Additional identification procedures for the administration of blood products are required. Protocols may vary by institution.
- Standard Precautions must be followed.
- Children and infants may be accompanied by a parent to calm them. Keep neonates and infants covered and in a warm room and provide a pacifier or gentle touch. The testing environment should be quiet, and the patient should be instructed, as appropriate, to remain still during the test as extraneous movements can affect results.
- Ensure that the patient has complied with pretesting instructions, including dietary, fluid, medication, and activity restrictions as given for the procedure.
- As appropriate, preparations for insertion of an IV line for infusion of fluids, blood products, antibiotics, anesthetics, or analgesics must be made. Inform the patient when prophylactic antibiotics will be administered before the procedure and assess for antibiotic allergy. Prior to the administration of any fluids or medications, verify that they are accurate for the study. Bleeding or bruising can be prevented, once the needle has been removed, by applying direct pressure to the injection site with dry gauze for a minute or two. The site should be observed/assessed for bleeding or hematoma formation, and then covered with a gauze and an adhesive bandage.
- Emergency equipment must be readily available.
- Baseline vital signs must be recorded, and monitoring continues throughout and after the procedure, according to organizational policy. A comparison should be made between the baseline and post-procedure vital signs and focused assessments. Protocols may vary among facilities.
- Before leaving the patient's side, appropriate specimen containers should always be labelled with the corresponding patient demographics, initials of the person collecting the sample, collection date, time of collection, and applicable special notes, especially site location and laterality if appropriate, and then promptly transported to the laboratory for processing and analysis.

Universal Post Test Pearls (Evaluation)

- Completed test results are made available to the requesting HCP, who will discuss them with the patient.

- Answer questions and address concerns voiced by the patient or family and reinforce information given by the patient's HCP regarding further testing, treatment, or referral to another HCP. Recognize that patients will have anxiety related to test results. Provide teaching and information regarding the clinical implications of the test results on the patient's lifestyle as appropriate.
- Note that test results should be evaluated in context with the patient's signs, symptoms, and diagnosis. Depending on the results of the procedure, additional testing may be performed to evaluate or monitor progression of the disease process and determine the need for a change in therapy.
- Be aware that when a person goes through a traumatic event such as an illness or being given information that will impact his or her lifestyle, there are universal human reactions that occur. These include knowledge deficit, fear, anxiety, and coping; in some situations, grieving may occur. HCPs should always be aware of the human response and how it may affect the plan of care and expected outcomes.

DISCUSSION POINT

Regarding Post-Test Critical Findings: Timely notification of a critical finding for lab or diagnostic studies is a role expectation of the professional nurse. Notification processes will vary among facilities. Upon receipt of the critical finding, the information should be read back to the caller to verify accuracy. Most policies require immediate notification of the primary HCP, hospitalist, or on-call HCP. Reported information includes the patient's name, unique identifiers, critical finding, name of the person giving the report, and name of the person receiving the report. Documentation of notification should be made in the medical record with the name of the HCP notified, time and date of notification, and any orders received. Any delay in a timely report of a critical finding may require completion of a notification form with review by Risk Management.

STUDIES

- Blood Groups and Antibodies (ABO, Rh & Antibody Screen)

LEARNING OUTCOMES

Providing safe, effective nursing care (SENC) includes mastery of core competencies and standards of care. SENC is based on a judicious application of nursing knowledge in combination with scientific principles. The Art of Nursing lies in blending what you know with the ability to effectively apply your knowledge in a compassionate manner.

After reading/studying this chapter you will be able to:

Thinking

1. Recognize the relationship between blood cell antigens in the ABO system to assignment of blood groups and presence or absence of Rh antigens to positive or negative blood type.
2. List the blood banking studies associated with compatibility testing and investigation of transfusion reactions.
3. List the blood banking studies associated with investigation of fetal maternal hemorrhage.

Doing

1. Engage every patient with equal respect and uniformity regardless of personal views.
2. Identify the most frequent cause of life-threatening ABO incompatibility and explain the importance of unique identifiers in providing safe patient care.
3. Describe signs and symptoms associated with a blood product transfusion reaction.
4. Discuss possible nursing interventions for transfusion reactions.

Caring

1. Value the ability of the individual in the prevention of errors.

Blood Groups and Antibodies

Quick Summary

SYNONYM ACRONYM: ABO group and Rh typing, blood group antibodies, type and screen, type and crossmatch.

COMMON USE: To identify ABO blood group and Rh type, typically for prenatal testing and transfusion purposes.

SPECIMEN: Serum collected in a red-top tube or whole blood collected in a lavender-top (EDTA) tube.

NORMAL FINDINGS: (Method: FDA-approved reagents with glass slides, glass tubes, gel, or automated systems) Compatibility (no clumping or hemolysis).

Test Explanation

Blood typing is a series of tests that include the ABO and Rh blood-group system performed to detect surface antigens on red blood cells (RBCs) by an agglutination test and compatibility tests to determine antibodies against these antigens. The major antigens in the ABO system are A and B, although AB and O are also common phenotypes. The patient with A antigens has group A blood; the patient with B antigens has group B blood. The patient with both A and B antigens has group AB

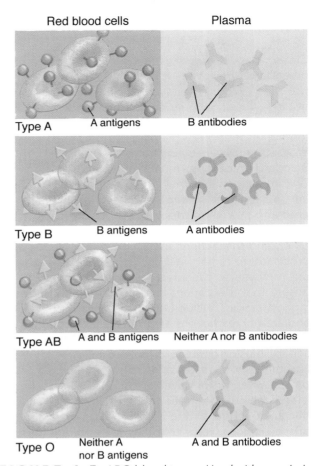

FIGURE 4.5 ABO blood types. *Used with permission, from Williams, L., & Hopper, P. (2010). Understanding medical surgical nursing (4th Ed.). FA Davis Company.*

blood (universal recipient); the patient with neither A nor B antigens has group O blood (universal donor) (see Fig. 4.5). Blood group and type are genetically determined. After 6 months of age, individuals develop serum antibodies that react with A or B antigen absent from their own RBCs. These are called *anti-A* and *anti-B* antibodies.

In ABO blood typing, the patient's RBCs mix with anti-A and anti-B sera, a process known as *forward grouping*. The process then reverses, and the patient's serum mixes with type A and B cells in *reverse grouping*.

Generally, only blood with the same ABO group and Rh type as the recipient is transfused because the anti-A and anti-B antibodies are strong agglutinins that cause a rapid, complement-mediated destruction of incompatible cells. However, blood donations have decreased nationwide, creating shortages in the available supply. Safe substitutions with blood of a different group and/or Rh type may occur depending on the inventory of available units. Many laboratories require consultation with the requesting HCP prior to issuing Rh-positive units to an Rh-negative individual.

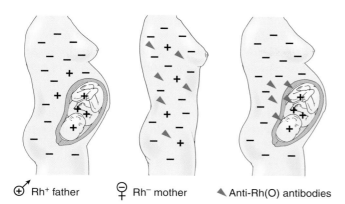

⊕ Rh⁺ father   ♀ Rh⁻ mother   ▲ Anti-Rh(O) antibodies

FIGURE 4.6 Rh isoimmunization process. *Used with permission, from Ward, S. (2009). Maternal-child nursing care: Optimizing outcomes for mothers, children, and families. FA Davis Company.*

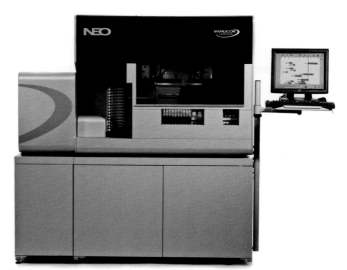

FIGURE 4.8 Automated blood type and screen equipment: Immucor Neo. *© 2011 Immucor, Inc. All rights reserved.*

ABO and Rh testing is also performed as a prenatal screen in pregnant women to identify the risk of hemolytic disease of the newborn. Although most of the anti-A and anti-B activity resides in the immunoglobulin M (IgM) class of immunoglobulins, some activity rests with immunoglobulin G (IgG). Anti-A and anti-B antibodies of the IgG class coat the RBCs without immediately affecting their viability and can readily cross the placenta, resulting in hemolytic disease of the newborn. Individuals with type O blood frequently have more IgG anti-A and anti-B than other people; thus, ABO hemolytic disease of the newborn will affect infants of type O mothers almost exclusively (unless the newborn is also type O).

Major antigens of the Rh system are D (or Rh$_O$), C, E, c, and e. Individuals whose RBCs possess D antigen are called Rh-positive; those who lack D antigen are called Rh-negative, no matter what other Rh antigens are present. Individuals who are Rh-negative produce anti-D antibodies when exposed to Rh-positive cells by

either transfusions or pregnancy. These anti-D antibodies cross the placenta to the fetus and can cause hemolytic disease of the newborn or transfusion reactions if Rh-positive blood is administered (see Fig. 4.6).

The type and screen (T&S) procedure is performed to determine the ABO/Rh and identify any antibodies that may react with transfused blood products (see Figs. 4.7 and 4.8). The T&S may take from 30 to 45 minutes or longer to complete depending on whether unexpected or unusual antibodies are detected. Every unit of product must be crossmatched against the intended recipient's serum and red blood cells for compatibility before transfusion. Knowing the ABO/Rh and antibody status saves time when the patient's sample is crossmatched against units of donated blood products. There are three crossmatch procedures. If no antibodies are identified in the T&S, it is permissible to use either an immediate spin crossmatch or an electronic crossmatch, either of which may take 5 to 10 minutes to complete. If antibodies are detected, the antiglobulin crossmatch procedure is performed, along with antibody identification testing, or the process is repeated, beginning with the selection of other units for compatibility testing. Typically, specimens for T&S can be held for 72 hours from the time of collection for use in future crossmatch procedures. This time frame may be extended for up to 14 days for patients with a reliably known history of no prior transfusions or pregnancy within the previous 3 months.

Febrile nonhemolytic reaction and urticarial/allergic reaction are the two most common types of reactions that occur in blood product transfusions. Many institutions have a policy that provides for premedication with acetaminophen and diphenhydramine to avoid initiation of mild transfusion reactions, where appropriate.

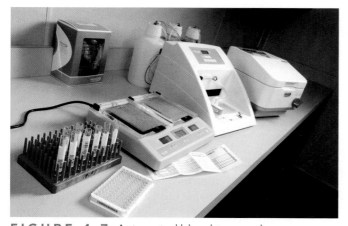

FIGURE 4.7 Automated blood type and screen equipment: Immucor Neo workstation. *© 2011 Immucor, Inc. All rights reserved.*

Nursing Implications

Assessment

Indications	Potential Nursing Problems
Determine ABO and Rh compatibility of donor and recipient before transfusion (type and screen or crossmatch). Determine anti-D antibody titer of Rh-negative mothers after sensitization by pregnancy with an Rh-positive fetus. Determine the need for a microdose of immunosuppressive therapy (e.g., with RhoGAM) during the first 12 wk of gestation or a standard dose after 12 wk of gestation for complications such as abortion, miscarriage, vaginal hemorrhage, ectopic pregnancy, or abdominal trauma. Determine Rh blood type and perform antibody screen of prenatal patients on initial visit to determine maternal Rh type and to indicate whether maternal RBCs have been sensitized by any antibodies known to cause hemolytic disease of the newborn, especially anti-D antibody. Rh blood type, antibody screen, and antibody titration (if an antibody has been identified) will be rechecked at 28 wk of gestation and prior to injection of prophylactic standard dose of Rh$_O$(D) immune globulin RhoGAM IM or Rhophylac IM or IV for Rh-negative mothers. These tests will also be repeated after delivery of an Rh-positive fetus to an Rh-negative mother and prior to injection of prophylactic standard dose of Rh$_O$(D) immune globulin (if maternal Rh-negative blood has not been previously sensitized with Rh-positive cells resulting in a positive anti-D antibody titer). A postpartum blood sample must be evaluated for fetal-maternal bleed on all Rh-negative mothers to determine the need for additional doses of Rh immune globulin. One in 300 cases will demonstrate hemorrhage greater than 15 mL of blood and require additional Rh$_O$(D) immune globulin. Identify donor ABO and Rh blood type for stored blood. Identify maternal and infant ABO and Rh blood types to predict risk of hemolytic disease of the newborn. Identify the patient's ABO and Rh blood type, especially before a procedure in which blood loss is a threat or blood replacement may be needed. Identify any unusual transfusion related antibodies in the patient's blood, especially before a procedure in which blood replacement may be needed.	• Activity • Airway • Breathing • Cardiac Output • Confusion • Fear • Fever • Fluid Volume • Gas Exchange • Human Response • Infection • Injury Risk **(related to transfusion reaction)** • Skin Integrity • Tissue Perfusion Breathing

Diagnosis: Clinical Significance of Test Results

- *Agglutination is graded from 1+ to 4+ in manual testing systems; with 4+ being the strongest degree of agglutination. Automated testing systems are capable of reporting 1+ to 4+ graded results, or providing images of the tested material so laboratory professionals can interpret the results, or providing computer assisted interpretation of the test results as positive or negative findings.*
- ABO system: A, B, AB, or O specific to person
- Rh system: positive or negative specific to person
- Crossmatching: compatibility between donor and recipient
- Incompatibility indicated by clumping (agglutination) of red blood cells

Group and Type	Incidence (%)	Alternative Transfusion Group and Type of Packed Cell Units in Order of Preference if Patient's Own Group and Type Not Available
O positive	37.4	O negative
O negative	6.6	O positive*
A positive	35.7	A negative, O positive, O negative
A negative	6.3	O negative, A positive,* O positive*
B positive	8.5	B negative, O positive, O negative
B negative	1.5	O negative, B positive,* O positive*
AB positive	3.4	AB negative, A positive, B positive, A negative, B negative, O positive, O negative
AB negative	0.6	A negative, B negative, O negative, AB positive,* A positive,* B positive,* O positive*
Rh Type		
Rh positive	85–90	
Rh negative	10–15	

*If blood units of exact match to the patient's group and type are not available, a switch in ABO blood group is preferable to a change in Rh type. However, in extreme circumstances, Rh-positive blood can be issued to an Rh-negative recipient. It is very likely that the recipient will develop antibodies as the result of receiving Rh-positive red blood cells. Rh antibodies are highly immunogenic, and, once the antibodies are developed, the recipient can only receive Rh-negative blood for subsequent red blood cell transfusion.

Planning

Considerations for planning a successful partnership should include clear communication of what to expect during the test to decrease anxiety and improve cooperation. Before the procedure is performed, plan to review the steps with the patient. Address any concerns about pain and explain that there may be some discomfort during the venipuncture.

Identification of ABO group and Rh blood type is an integral part of preparing donated blood units for storage and use in future transfusion. Determining ABO and Rh compatibility of donor and recipient before transfusion (type and screen or crossmatch) and identifying any unusual transfusion-related antibodies in the patient's blood (indirect Coombs antiglobulin test), especially before a procedure in which blood loss is a threat or blood replacement may be needed, is the first step in the immunohematology and blood banking process. Two questions need to be answered: (1) is the blood group compatible? and (2) is the Rh type compatible? For most adults, an ABO and Rh compatibility of the donor and recipient is identified before transfusion using a type and screen or crossmatch.

Any recent or past blood product transfusions should be noted as they could complicate or interfere with test results. A list of the patient's current medications (including dietary supplements) should also be obtained. This is an important step in the identification of any factors that may interfere with blood typing. A history of bone marrow transplant, cancer, or leukemia may cause discrepancy in ABO typing. Health-care providers (HCPs) should plan a careful review of the patient's medical record to evaluate for any of these interfering factors prior to obtaining a blood specimen.

● *Safety Tip*

Maternal and infant ABO and Rh blood types should be identified in the prenatal screen to predict risk of hemolytic disease of the newborn. HCPs should request a blood type and antibody screen prior to scheduling a procedure in which blood replacement may be needed because discovery of unusual antibodies in the patient's blood may significantly extend the amount of time required to identify compatible donated units.

Prenatal mothers may be concerned about blood collection from their newborn. Explain that a cord sample of blood taken from the infant at the time of delivery does not result in infant blood loss. Several phases of testing may be necessary for the prenatal patient. Prenatal patients may require Rh blood typing and an antibody screen during their initial visit to determine the maternal Rh type and to indicate whether maternal red blood cells have been sensitized by any antibodies known to cause hemolytic disease of the newborn, especially anti-D antibody. It may also be necessary to provide a microdose of immunosuppressive therapy (RhoGAM) during the first 12 weeks of gestation, or a standard dose after 12 weeks of gestation for complications such as abortion, miscarriage, vaginal hemorrhage, ectopic pregnancy, or abdominal trauma. If an antibody has been identified, a recheck consisting of an Rh blood typing, antibody screen, and antibody titration will be completed at 28 weeks of gestation. This evaluation should be completed prior to injection of a prophylactic standard dose of Rho(D), immune globulin RhoGAM intramuscular (IM), or Rhophylac IM or IV for Rh-negative mothers.

These tests will also be repeated after delivery of an Rh-positive fetus to an Rh-negative mother and prior to injection of prophylactic standard dose of $Rh_O(D)$ immune globulin (if maternal Rh-negative blood has not been previously sensitized with Rh-positive cells resulting in a positive anti-D antibody titer). A postpartum blood sample must be evaluated for fetal-maternal bleed on all Rh-negative mothers to determine the need for additional doses of Rh immune globulin. The Kleihauer-Betke test is used to determine the degree of fetal-maternal hemorrhage (FMH). One in 300 cases will demonstrate hemorrhage greater than 15 mL of blood and require additional $Rh_O(D)$ immune globulin.

DISCUSSION POINT

Most facilities require providing patients with education regarding blood transfusion choices before a transfusion is given. This education is not a replacement for informed consent but is given in addition to informed consent. Educational content generally focuses on the purpose of transfusions, transfusion choices, and transfusion risks. The Patient Education for Blood Transfusion Choices table is a sample of the type of information that may be provided in a pamphlet or other form by your facility.

Patient Education for Blood Transfusion Choices

Transfusion purpose	• To replace blood stores lost from trauma, surgery, or illness that causes acute or chronic blood loss • To prepare for anticipatory blood loss due to surgery
Transfusion choices	• Autologous blood—donating your own blood for future use such as for during surgery • Designated or directed donor—choosing relatives or friends with a compatible blood type to donate blood for your use • Volunteer donor—using blood that has been donated through the Red Cross or other agency for the use of any individual in need of a transfusion
Transfusion risks	• Donated blood is tested for the presence of transmissible disease prior to being made available for transfusion. However, there is always a risk that disease transmission can occur. Donated units are tested for HIV 1 and 2, hepatitis B, hepatitis C, syphilis, and human T-cell lymphotropic virus I and II. Additional testing may be performed in specific cases to include cytomegalovirus, West Nile virus, and *Trypanosoma cruzi* (Chagas disease). Transfusion reaction is another risk, resulting in fever, chills, headache, hives, itching, shortness of breath, anxiety, tachycardia, hypotension, or nausea and vomiting. Reactions are rare but they do occur.

See Appendix D online at Davis*Plus* for a more detailed description of transfusion reactions and potential nursing interventions and for further information regarding findings and potential nursing interventions associated with types of transfusion reactions.

SPECIAL CONSIDERATIONS

An important aspect of planning is understanding the factors that may alter the study or cause abnormal results. Interdepartmental communication is a key factor in the planning process. It should be noted when planning for this study that there is the possibility of false-negative findings in the presence of a weak antibody that is undetected during analysis.

It is also important to understand which medications or substances the patient may be exposed to in the healthcare setting that can interfere with accurate testing:

- A false-positive result in Rh typing and antibody screens may be caused by such drugs as levodopa, methyldopa, methyldopate hydrochloride, and cephalexin.
- The recent administration of blood, blood products, dextran, or an IV contrast medium may cause cellular aggregation that might falsely appear as agglutination in ABO typing.
- Procedural contrast material such as iodine, barium, gadolinium, or abnormal proteins, cold agglutinins, and bacteremia may also interfere with testing.

Make sure a written and informed consent has been signed prior to any transfusion of ABO- and Rh-compatible blood products.

Implementation

Correct patient identification is crucial when blood is collected for type and screen or type and crossmatch because clerical error is the most common cause of life-threatening ABO incompatibility. Patient safety requires that additional verification requirements are necessary, including two unique identifiers such as patient name, date of birth, Social Security number, medical record number, blood bank number on the wristband, and labels. Part of the verification process may include comparing wristband information with labels to match information and placing labels with the same information and blood bank number on blood sample tubes. To prevent errors, the HCP should strictly follow organizational guidelines in patient identification and transfusion verification.

Patient education is key to obtaining the patient's cooperation in following directions, and providing an explanation for the purpose of the procedure is an important part of this process. Inform the patient this study can assist in identification of blood group and type for prenatal screening and transfusion of blood products. Perform the venipuncture.

Evaluation

Recognize anxiety related to test results. When appropriate, inform the patient of his or her ABO blood and Rh type and advise storing the information on a card or other document routinely carried. Remind women who are designated as Rh-negative to inform the HCP of their Rh-negative status if they become pregnant or receive a blood or blood product transfusion.

◉ *Critical Findings*

Note and immediately report to the requesting HCP any signs and symptoms associated with a transfusion reaction. A listing of these findings varies among facilities.

Signs and symptoms of blood transfusion reaction range from mildly febrile to anaphylactic and may include chills, dyspnea, fever, headache, nausea, vomiting, palpitations and tachycardia, chest or back pain, apprehension, flushing, hives, angioedema, diarrhea, hypotension, oliguria, hemoglobinuria, acute kidney injury or chronic kidney disease, sepsis, shock, and jaundice. Complications from disseminated intravascular coagulation (DIC) may also occur.

Possible interventions in mildly febrile reactions include slowing the rate of infusion, then verifying and comparing patient identification, transfusion requisition, and blood bag label. The patient should be monitored closely for further development of signs and symptoms. Administration of epinephrine may be ordered.

Possible interventions in a more severe transfusion reaction may include immediately stopping the infusion, notifying the HCP, keeping the IV line open with saline or lactated Ringer solution, collecting red- and lavender-top tubes for post-transfusion work-up, collecting urine, monitoring vital signs every 5 minutes, ordering additional testing if DIC is suspected, maintaining patent airway and blood pressure, and administering mannitol. See Appendix D online at DavisPlus for a more detailed description of transfusion reactions and potential nursing interventions.

◉ *Study Specific Complications*

A transfusion reaction may occur in some patients. A transfusion reaction is also a critical finding. Signs, symptoms, and possible interventions are described in the Critical Findings section.

There are a number of complications associated with performing a venipuncture. **Pain** is commonly associated with needles and, although the pain experienced during venipuncture is usually mild, on a rare occasion the needle may strike a nerve, causing permanent pain. Some patients experience a **vasovagal reaction** during the venipuncture procedure, evidenced by sweating, low blood pressure, fainting, or near fainting. The potential for a **fall injury** is a significant concern related to vasovagal reactions. Prolonged **bleeding** is a complication that occurs with patients who are taking blood thinners or who have coagulopathies such as hemophilia. A **hematoma** results when blood leaks into the tissue during or after a venipuncture, as evidenced by pain, bruising, and/or swelling at the venipuncture site. The swelling can cause injury by compression to surrounding nerves, which can be temporary or permanent. HCPs should watch for minor complications such as bruising and hematoma at the venipuncture site, which are fairly common. Hematomas occur more often in older adult or frail patients, or those with veins that are difficult to access. Bleeding or bruising can be prevented once the needle has been removed by applying direct pressure to the site with dry gauze for a minute or two. Some other more unusual complications of venipuncture include **cellulitis, phlebitis, inadvertent arterial puncture, and sepsis.** Sepsis can be caused by introduction of bacteria from the surface of the skin into the blood as the result of improper cleansing of the venipuncture site. Immunocompromised patients are at higher risk for developing this complication.

Related Tests

- Related tests include Coomb antiglobulin, bilirubin, CBC, CBC hematocrit, CBC hemoglobin, CBC platelet count, CBC RBC count, cold agglutinin, FDP, fecal analysis, GI blood loss scan, haptoglobin, IgA, iron, Kleihauer-Betke, laparoscopy abdominal, Meckel diverticulum scan, and UA.
- Refer to Appendix E online at Davis*Plus* for further information regarding laboratory studies used in the investigation of transfusion reactions, findings, and potential nursing interventions associated with types of transfusion reactions.
- Refer to the Immune and Hematopoietic systems tables at the end of the book for related tests by body system.

Expected Outcomes

Expected outcomes associated with Blood Groups and Antibodies (ABO, Rh & Antibody Screen) are:

- Correctly labeling and transporting the sample for laboratory study
- Confirming informed consent prior to transfusion, with an acknowledgment of the risks and benefits of blood transfusion
- Correctly identifying the patient for transfusion
- Understanding the need to report itching, fever, or shortness of breath during or post-transfusion as this may indicate an allergic reaction
- Administering blood products without reaction followed by an improvement in patient status

REVIEW OF LEARNING OUTCOMES

Thinking

1. Recognize the relationship between blood cell antigens in the ABO system to assignment of blood groups and presence or absence of Rh antigens to positive or negative blood type. Answer: The major antigens in the ABO system are A and B, although AB and O are also common phenotypes. The presence or absence of antigens on the RBC determines the patient's blood group. Major antigens of the Rh system are D (or Rh$_O$), C, E, c, and e. Individuals whose red blood cells possess D antigen are called Rh-positive; those who lack D antigen are called Rh-negative, no matter what other Rh antigens are present. The patient with A antigens has group A blood. The patient with B antigens has group B blood. The patient with both A and B antigens has group AB blood (universal recipient). The patient with neither A nor B antigens has group O blood (universal donor).
2. List the blood banking studies associated with compatibility testing and investigation of transfusion reactions. Answer: ABO Blood Typing is also referred to as ABO group and Rh typing, blood group antibodies, type and screen, or type and crossmatch. This laboratory test is commonly used to identify ABO blood group and Rh type, typically for transfusion purposes. Coombs antiglobulin, indirect is also referred to as antibody screen, indirect antiglobulin testing, or IAT. This laboratory test is commonly used to check donor and recipient blood cells for antibodies prior to blood transfusion. Coombs anti-globulin, direct, is also referred to as direct antiglobulin testing or DAT. This laboratory test, along with repeat ABO group, Rh typing, and IAT, is commonly used to investigate transfusion reactions. See Appendix D for a more detailed description of tests used to investigate transfusion reactions.
3. List the blood banking studies associated with investigation of fetal maternal hemorrhage. Answer: The Kleihauer-Betke test is used to determine the degree of fetal-maternal hemorrhage (FMH).

Doing

1. Engage every patient with equal respect and uniformity regardless of personal views. Answer: The option to receive blood or blood products can be a very emotional issue for the patient, which engenders a lot of decisional conflict. Barriers to making a decision may be religious, cultural, or fear of harm. It is the nurse's role to provide accurate information in conjunction with the HCP's discussion of risks and benefits to assist in eliminating barriers to treatment. However, in the end, it is the patient's decision, not ours.
2. Identify the most frequent cause of life-threatening ABO incompatibility and explain the importance of unique identifiers in providing safe patient care. Answer: Correct patient

identification is crucial when blood is collected for type and screen or type and crossmatch because clerical error is the most common cause of life-threatening ABO incompatibility.

3. Describe signs and symptoms associated with a blood product transfusion reaction. Answer: A transfusion reaction may occur in some patients and should be immediately reported to the HCP. Signs and symptoms of blood transfusion reaction include fever, chills, dyspnea, headache, nausea, vomiting, palpitations, tachycardia, chest or back pain, apprehension, flushing, hives, angioedema, diarrhea, hypotension, oliguria, hemoglobinuria, acute kidney injury or chronic kidney disease, sepsis, shock, and jaundice. Complications from disseminated intravascular coagulation (DIC) may also occur.

4. Discuss possible nursing interventions for transfusion reactions. Answer: Possible interventions in mildly febrile reactions include slowing the rate of infusion, then verifying and comparing patient identification, transfusion requisition, and blood bag labeling. Blood transfusions should be stopped as appropriate. If this should occur, the patient should be monitored closely for further development of signs and symptoms. Administration of epinephrine may be ordered. Possible interventions in a more severe transfusion reaction may include the immediate cessation of infusion, notification of the HCP, keeping the IV line open with saline or lactated Ringer solution, the collection of red- and lavender-top tubes for post-transfusion work-up, the collection of urine, monitoring vital signs every 5 minutes, ordering additional testing if DIC is suspected, maintaining a patent airway and blood pressure, and administering mannitol.

Caring

1. Value the ability of the individual in the prevention of errors. Answer: Nurses are involved in all aspects of care. One very important aspect of care is to act as a protector against error. This action requires the nurse to be vigilant in validating that each laboratory study completed is correct for that specific patient. Imagine if your patient was to receive a blood transfusion but the type and crossmatch was drawn on someone else. The result could be a transfusion reaction that ends with the patient's death.

◖ *Words* OF *Wisdom:* Blood transfusion is a very emotional and personal experience for patients. For some, it is also a religious one. Think about it. You are asking them to put body fluids from a person they do not know into their own body. You are asking them to do this with the hope that there have been no errors that will result in transfusion reactions or disease transmission. Health care is run by human beings and even after all we have done to make transfusion safe, we cannot provide 100% assurance of that. What we can do to keep our patients safe is to strictly follow policy and protocol. Let our patients know of their alternatives to transfusion, and answer all questions honestly and openly. Once the transfusion has started, stay for a few minutes as the blood begins to go in to make sure all is well. That moment when they see the blood enter their body is the scariest part for them. Once they see that it will be all right, their stress level will decrease, and they will be very grateful to you for those minutes when you showed you cared. Your face is a memory they will carry in their hearts forever.

BIBLIOGRAPHY

AABB. (n.d.). Blood donation FAQs. Retrieved from www.aabb .org/tm/donation/Pages/donatefaqs.aspx)

AABB Primer of blood administration. (2010, September). Retrieved from www.bloodcenter.org/webres/File/Hospital% 20.pdf%20forms/AABB%20Primer%20of%20Blood%20 Administration.pdf

ABO blood group system. (2011, June 19). Retrieved from www .en.wikipedia.org/wiki/ABO_blood_group_system

California Department of Health Services. (2006). A patients guide to blood transfusion. Retrieved from www.cbbsweb.org/links/ cadhs_txguide_rev606.pdf

Canadian Blood Services Online Edition. (2011, February). Donor selection, transmissible disease testing, and pathogen reduction. Retrieved from www.transfusionmedicine.ca/resources/ clinical-guide-transfusion

Cavanaugh, B. (2003). Nurse's manual of laboratory and diagnostic tests (4th ed.). Philadelphia, PA: F.A. Davis Company.

Hemoglobinopathies. (n.d.). Retrieved from www.hawaii.edu (search on hemoglobinopathies)

Hemolytic disease of the fetus and newborn. (n.d.). Retrieved from www.ncabb.org/docs/ncabb-julie-jackson-20080423.pdf

Hillyer, C., Strauss, R., & Lubin, N. (Eds.). (2004). Neonatal testing. In Handbook of pediatric transfusion medicine (p. 198). Retrieved from www.books.google.com/books?id=MiuCNzmT AkEC&pg=PA198&dq=the+cord+blood+dat+may+be+only+w eakly+positive&hl=en&ei=M9lrTpmzN-7MsQKvzYnVBA&sa= X&oi=book_result&ct=result&resnum=1&ved=0CDkQ6AEwA A#v=onepage&q=the%20cord%20blood%20dat%20may%20 be%20only%20weakly%20positive&f=false

Kleihauer-Betke test. (2011, May 25). Retrieved from www .en.wikipedia.org/w/index.php?title=Kleihauer-Betke_test& action=history

LaCount, R. (n.d.). Lab investigations of transfusion reactions. Retrieved from www.scribd.com/doc/56819974/Transfusion-Reaction-Rachel-La-Count

Maryland Public Health Laboratory. (2015). Newborn screening provider page. Retrieved from http://dhmh.maryland.gov/ laboratories/SitePages/nbs_provider.aspx

Matrix gel system neonate group card. (n.d.). Retrieved from www .tulipgroup.com/Tulip_New/html/pack_inserts/Matrix%20 ABO-RhoD-AHG%20Neonate%20Group%20Card.pdf

Nova Scotia Provincial Blood Coordinating Program. (2010). Blood and blood product transfusion. Retrieved from www.gov.ns.ca/health/nspbcp/professionals.asp

Prenatal immunohematologic testing. (n.d.). Retrieved from www.clinlabnavigator.com/Transfusion/prenatal-immunohemato-logic-testing.html?letter=P

Prenatal hemorrhage. (n.d.). Retrieved from www.scribd.com/doc/2761938/NurseReviewOrg-Prenatal-hemorrhage

Silver, R., Varner, M., Reddy, U., Goldenberg, R., Robert M., Pinar, H., Conway, D., & Stoll, B. (2007, May). Work-up of stillbirth: A review of the evidence. American Journal of Obstetrics & Gynecology, 196(5), 433–444. doi 10.1016/j.ajog.2006.11.041

Van Leeuwen, A., and Bladh, M. (2015). Davis's comprehensive handbook of laboratory and diagnostic testing with nursing implications (6th ed.). Philadelphia, PA: F.A. Davis Company.

Go to Section II of this book and http://www.davisplus.com for the Clinical Reasoning Tool and its case studies to provide you with a safe place to explore patient care situations. There are a total of 26 different case studies; 2 cases are presented for each of 13 body systems. One set of 13 cases are found in the Section II chapters, and a second set of 13 cases are available online at http://www.davisplus.com. Each case is designed with the specific goal of helping you to connect the dots of clinical reasoning. Cases are designed to reflect possible clinical scenarios; the outcomes may or may not be positive—you decide.

Blood Studies: Immunology

OVERVIEW

Immunology is the laboratory subspecialty that deals with the immune system functions that protect the body from invasion by foreign elements. These elements range from microorganisms and allergens to chemical toxins, modified proteins, transfusion reactions, and transplanted organs. Laboratory tests can demonstrate many of the body's immune activities with remarkable sensitivity. Specific antibodies can be identified and quantitated from blood samples in the Serology laboratory using techniques such as immunoprecipitation, complement fixation, neutralization, particle agglutination/agglutination inhibition, immunofluorescence assay, enzyme immunoassay, and radioimmunoassay. Antibody identification and quantification in concentrations and titers are useful in diagnosing infectious diseases and in monitoring their progress once therapeutic measures have been implemented. Other specialty laboratories that study infectious agents for identification and treatment options include Virology, Microbiology, and Molecular Diagnostics laboratories.

Another area of active immunological research involves the development of tumor markers, which are defined as substances, usually proteins, produced in abnormal levels by either malignant (abnormal) or benign (normal) cells. They are detected by the examination of blood, body fluids, and tissue specimens. Tumor markers are used in the detection and identification of various types of cancer as well as in the monitoring and evaluation of therapeutic interventions. The main premise behind studies of immunological process is the concept of the body's ability to recognize "self" and distinguish it from harmful "foreign" elements. An antigen is any foreign substance that elicits an immune response. An antibody is a special protein called an *immunoglobulin* that is manufactured by cells of the immune system against specific antigens. There are two main categories of immune response: (1) the cell-mediated response (see Fig. 5.1) and (2) the humoral response (see Fig. 5.2). The hematology chapter discussed the five types of white blood cells (WBCs) and their various roles in providing a defensive system.

The cells responsible for immune reactivity are lymphocytes and macrophages. Lymphocytes can live weeks, months, or even many years given their role in immune response over an individual's lifetime of exposure to potentially harmful invaders (see Fig. 5.3). Lymphocytes can freely enter and leave the peripheral blood. Therefore, the normal number in circulation represents only a small fraction of the total number of available cells, with the majority being located in the spleen, lymph nodes, and other lymphatic tissues. Lymphocytes are divided into two major categories based on their immunologic activity: T lymphocytes and B lymphocytes. There also is a third and less prolific group of lymphocytes named null cells, so called because unlike the T and B cells, they lack any surface markers or membrane bound immunoglobulins. There are two types of null cells: killer cells and natural killer cells. Stimulated by the presence of antibodies, killer cells can directly attack certain cellular targets like bacteria, fungi, and parasites. Natural killer cells do not require the presence of antibodies to perform their function. Both cell types kill tumor or viral-infected cells, although not with the specificity of cytotoxic T cells.

The T lymphocytes are formed in the thymus during fetal development and are primarily responsible for cell-mediated immunity. The peripheral T lymphoid system is fully developed and functional at birth so that it is possible to remove the thymus after birth without impairment of the cell-mediated portion of the immune system. Two subsets of cytotoxic T lymphocytes, helper T cells and suppressor T cells, have been identified that balance cell-mediated activities

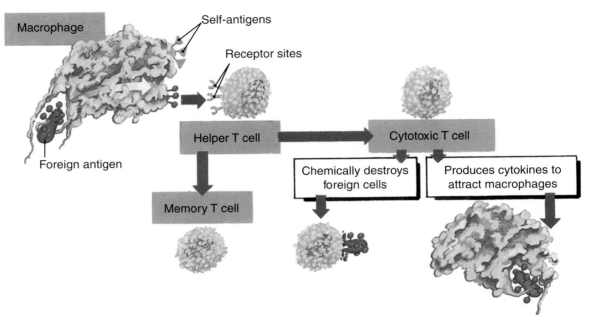

FIGURE 5.1 Cell mediated immunity. *Used with permission, from Scanlon, V., & Sanders, T. (2010). Essentials of anatomy and physiology (6th Ed.). FA Davis Company.*

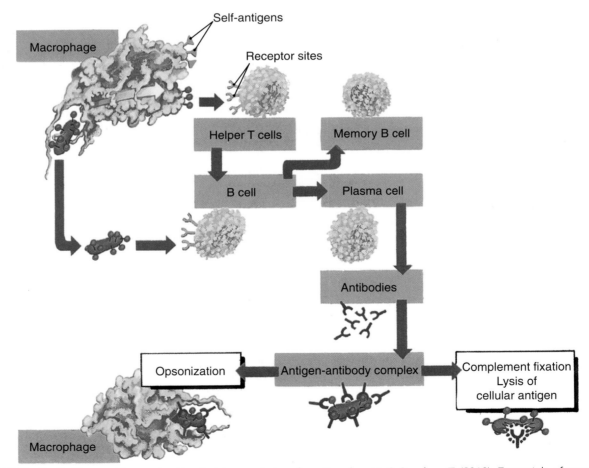

FIGURE 5.2 Humoral immunity. *Used with permission, from Scanlon, V., & Sanders, T. (2010). Essentials of anatomy and physiology (6th Ed.). FA Davis Company.*

under normal conditions. Helper T cells promote the proliferation of T lymphocytes, stimulate B lymphocyte activity, and activate macrophages. Suppressor T cells limit the magnitude of the immune response. The T lymphocyte memory cells have also been identified. These are cells that retain the ability to recognize antigens for rapid secondary immune response if ever

again challenged after the initial exposure (see Fig. 5.4). Examples of cell-mediated immune responses that require direct cell contact between the antigen and the lymphocyte include reactions against cells infected by pathogens such as bacteria, viruses, fungi, and protozoa. They also include reactions against positive skin tests (e.g., TB), contact dermatitis, solid organ transplant rejection, and the spontaneous destruction of malignant cells.

The B lymphocytes are responsible for humoral immunity through the production of antibodies. The actual production of antibodies (immunoglobulins) occurs in a differentiated form of B lymphocyte called the *plasma cell*. Five classes of immunoglobulins are currently identified: IgG, IgM, IgE, IgA, and IgD (see Fig. 5.5). Seventy-five percent of serum immunoglobulin is IgG, and it is the only immunoglobulin capable of crossing the placenta. IgG is also the most versatile of the immunoglobulins as it can fulfill the role of any of the immunoglobulins from acting as an opsonin by binding to cell membranes in the initiation of phagocytosis to activation of the complement cascade.

There are four subclasses of IgG. IgM is the largest immunoglobulin and the third most common serum antibody. The large size of the IgM molecule makes it good for impeding movement of foreign elements by agglutination. It is also very efficient in fixing complement and therefore very efficient in lysing foreign elements. IgE antibodies are responsible for hypersensitivity reactions described as atopic (allergic) or systemic

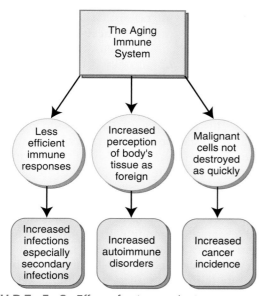

FIGURE 5.3 Effect of aging on the immune system. *Used with permission, from Williams, L., & Hopper, P. (2010). Understanding medical surgical nursing (4th Ed.). FA Davis Company.*

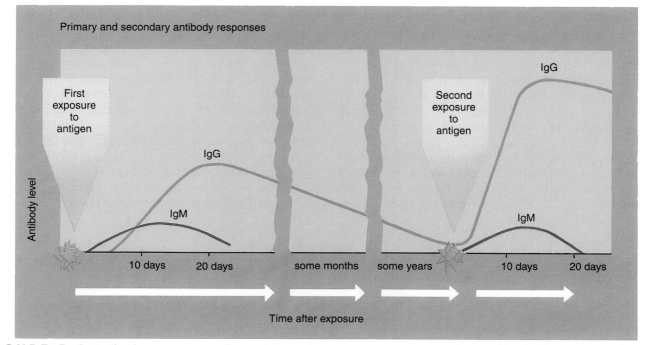

FIGURE 5.4 Antibody responses to a first and then subsequent exposure to a pathogen. *Used with permission, from Williams, L., & Hopper, P. (2010). Understanding medical surgical nursing (4th Ed.). FA Davis Company.*

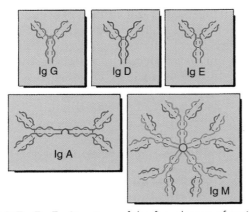

FIGURE 5.5 Structure of the five classes of antibodies

(anaphylactic). Examples of IgE-mediated allergic diseases include hay fever, asthma, and certain types of eczema. IgE-mediated anaphylactic responses are potentially fatal reactions to insect venoms and other drugs or chemicals. Almost all of the body's active IgE is bound to mast cells in the tissues with only small amounts in the circulating blood. When antigens come into contact with the tissue and bind to IgE, the interaction causes the mast cells to release histamine and other substances that promote vascular permeability.

IgA is the second most common immunoglobulin. It is found in secretions that lubricate mucosal tissue lining of the respiratory, gastrointestinal, and genitourinary systems, and is found in great quantities because of the very large amount of surface area covered by these tissue linings. It is believed to act by preventing invading organisms such as viruses from penetrating epithelial cell walls, accomplishing intracellular neutralization of viruses that do enter cells, and excreting deactivated virus particles from epithelial cells. There are two subclasses of IgA. The function of IgD is not completely understood. It is believed that IgD plays a role in the signalling of basophils, mast cells, and B lymphocytes to become activated for participation in defense.

Immune system activation is very complicated and interactive, requiring direct contact between antigen and immunoglobulin or specific lymphocyte surface immunoglobulins, as well as between B lymphocytes and helper T lymphocytes. The effects of humoral immunity provide many of the same results accomplished by cell-mediated immune functions and include the elimination of encapsulated bacteria, the neutralization of soluble toxins, and protection from various allergens, viruses, and parasites (see Fig. 5.6).

A final piece of the immune humoral response process is represented by complement. The "classical" complement pathway is a cascading system of individually inactive protein molecules: C1q, C1r, C1s, C4, C2, C3, C5, C6, C7, C8, and C9. These molecules become activated by IgG or IgM antigen-antibody complexes, aggregated IgA, certain naturally occurring polysaccharides and lipopolysaccharides, factors and products of the coagulation system, and bacterial endotoxins. The "alternate pathway" bypasses C1, C4, and C2 activation and begins directly with C3. The end result is an inflammatory response that destroys or damages cells. Activated B lymphocytes can also be transformed into memory cells similar to T lymphocyte memory cells, which retain the ability to recognize an antigen.

In both cellular and humoral immune responses, the initial exposure to specific antigens initiates the primary immune response. Depending on the quantity and type of antigen, it may take days, weeks, or months for the lymphocytes of either the cell-mediated or humoral system to mobilize, neutralize, and eliminate the antigen. Subsequent exposure to the same antigen, however, elicits the secondary (anamnestic) response much more rapidly than the primary response. In addition to proving protection, the immune system also helps remove damaged, abnormal, or old cells. Macrophages are responsible for performing this important maintenance function by engulfing particulate debris (phagocytosis). Macrophages also participate in mediation of the immune response by secreting enzymes, enzyme inhibitors, oxidizing agents, chemotactic agents, bioactive lipids (prostaglandins and related substances), complement components, and products that stimulate or inhibit multiplication of other cells. A third and critical function of macrophages is in the induction of the immune response. After phagocytosis and the processing of foreign elements, macrophages present processed antigen to lymphocytes for "memory and recognition" so that if the same antigen presents in the future, a more rapid immunologic reaction will occur.

FIGURE 5.6 Antibody reactivity against bacteria, viruses, and toxins. *Used with permission, from Williams, L., & Hopper, P. (2010). Understanding medical surgical nursing (4th Ed.). FA Davis Company.*

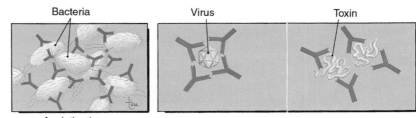

The information in the Part I studies is organized in a manner to help the student see how the five basic components of the nursing process (assessment, diagnosis, planning, implementation, and evaluation) can be applied to each phase of laboratory and diagnostic testing. The goal is to use nursing process to understand the integration of care (laboratory, diagnostic, nursing care) toward achieving a positive expected outcome.

- **Assessment** is the collection of information for the purpose of answering the question, "is there a problem?" Knowledge of the patient's health history, medications, complaints, and allergies as well as synonyms or alternate test names, common use for the procedure, specimen requirements, and normal ranges or interpretive comments provide the foundation for diagnosis.
- **Diagnosis** is the process of looking at the information gathered during assessment and answering the questions, "what is the problem?" and "what do I need to do about it?" Test indications tell us why the study has been requested, and potential diagnoses tell us the value or importance of the study relative to its clinical utility.
- **Planning** is a blueprint of the nursing care before the procedure. It is the process of determining how the nurse is going to partner with the patient to fix the problem (e.g., "The patient has a study ordered and this is what I should know before I successfully carry out the plan to have the study completed"). Knowledge of interfering factors, social and cultural issues, preprocedural restrictions, the need for written and informed consent, anxiety about the procedure, and concerns regarding pain are some considerations for planning a successful partnership.
- **Implementation** is putting the plan into action with an idea of what the expected outcome should be. Collaboration with the departments where the laboratory test or diagnostic study is to be performed is essential to the success of the plan. Implementation is where the work is done within each health-care team member's scope of practice.
- **Evaluation** answers the question, "did the plan work or not?" Was the plan completely successful, partially successful, or not successful? If the plan did not work, evaluation is the process where you determine what needs to be changed to make the plan work better. This includes a review of all expected outcomes. Nursing care after the procedure is where information is gathered to evaluate the plan. Review of results, including critical findings, in relation to patient symptoms and other tests performed provide data that form a more complete picture of health or illness.
- **Expected Outcomes** are positive outcomes related to the test. They are the outcomes the nurse should expect if all goes well.

A number of pretest, intratest, and post-test universal points are presented in this overview section because the information applies to immunology studies in general.

Universal Pretest Pearls (Planning)

- Obtain a history of the patient's complaints, including a list of known allergens, especially allergies or sensitivities to medications or latex so their use can be avoided or their effects mitigated if an allergy is present. Carefully evaluate all medications currently being taken by the patient. A list of the patient's current medications, prescribed and over the counter (including anticoagulants, aspirin and other salicylates, and dietary supplements), should also be obtained. Such products may be discontinued by medical direction for the appropriate number of days prior to the procedure. Ensure that all allergies are clearly noted in the medical record, and ensure that the patient is wearing an allergy and medical record armband. Report information that could interfere with, or delay proceeding with, the study to the health-care provider (HCP) and laboratory.
- Obtain a history of the patient's affected body system, symptoms, and results of previously performed laboratory tests and diagnostic and surgical procedures. Previous test results will provide a basis of comparison between old and new data.
- An important aspect of planning is understanding the factors that may alter study findings or cause abnormal results. Interdepartmental communication is a key factor in the planning process. The inability of a patient to cooperate or remain still during the procedure because of age, significant pain, or mental status should be among the anticipated factors. Recent or past procedures, medications, or existing medical conditions that could complicate or interfere with test results should be noted.
- Review the steps of the study with the patient or caregiver. Expect patients to be nervous about the procedure and the pending results. Educating the patient on his or her role during the procedure and what to expect can facilitate this. The patient's role during the procedure itself is to remain still. The actual time required to complete each study will depend on a number of conditions, including the type of equipment being used and how well a patient will cooperate.
- Explain that specimen collection by venipuncture takes approximately 5 to 10 minutes. Bleeding or bruising can be prevented, once the needle has been removed, by applying direct pressure to the venipuncture site with dry gauze for a minute or two. The site should be observed/assessed for

bleeding or hematoma formation, and then covered with a gauze and adhesive bandage.

- Address any concerns about pain and explain or describe, as appropriate, the level and type of discomfort that may be expected. Advise the patient that some discomfort may be experienced during the venipuncture.
- Provide additional instructions and patient preparation regarding medication, diet, fluid intake, or activity, if appropriate. Unless specified in the individual study, there are no special instructions or restrictions.
- Always be sensitive to any cultural or psychosocial issues, including a concern for modesty before, during, and after the procedure.

Reminder

Ensure that a written and informed consent has been documented in the medical record prior to the study, if required. The consent must be obtained before medication is administered.

Universal Intratest Pearls (Implementation)

- Correct patient identification is crucial prior to any procedure. Positively identify the patient using two unique identifiers such as patient name, date of birth, Social Security number, or medical record number.
- Standard Precautions must be followed.
- Children and infants may be accompanied by a parent to calm them. Keep neonates and infants covered and in a warm room and provide a pacifier or gentle touch. The testing environment should be quiet and the patient should be instructed, as appropriate, to remain still during the test as extraneous movements can affect results.
- Ensure that the patient has complied with pretesting instructions, including dietary, fluid, medication, and activity restrictions as given for the procedure.
- Before leaving the patient's side, appropriate specimen containers should always be labeled with the corresponding patient demographics, initials of the person collecting the sample, collection date, time of collection, and applicable special notes, especially site and laterality if appropriate, and then promptly transported to the laboratory for processing and analysis.

Universal Post Test Pearls (Evaluation)

- Note that completed test results are made available to the requesting HCP, who will discuss them with the patient.

- Answer questions and address concerns voiced by the patient or family and reinforce information given by the patient's HCP regarding further testing, treatment, or referral to another HCP. Recognize that patients will have anxiety related to test results. Provide teaching and information regarding the clinical implications of the test results on the patients lifestyle as appropriate.
- Note that test results should be evaluated in context with the patient's signs, symptoms, and diagnosis. Depending on the results of the procedure, additional testing may be performed to evaluate or monitor progression of the disease process and determine the need for a change in therapy.
- Be aware that when a person goes through a traumatic event such as an illness or being given information that will impact his or her lifestyle, there are universal human reactions that occur. These include knowledge deficit, fear, anxiety, and coping; in some situations, grieving may occur. HCPs should always be aware of the human response and how it may affect the plan of care and expected outcomes.

DISCUSSION POINT

Regarding Post-Test Critical Findings: Timely notification of a critical finding for lab or diagnostic studies is a role expectation of the professional nurse. Notification processes will vary among facilities. Upon receipt of the critical finding, the information should be read back to the caller to verify accuracy. Most policies require immediate notification of the primary HCP, hospitalist, or on-call HCP. Reported information includes the patient's name, unique identifiers, critical finding, name of the person giving the report, and name of the person receiving the report. Documentation of notification should be made in the medical record with the name of the HCP notified, time and date of notification, and any orders received. Any delay in a timely report of a critical finding may require completion of a notification form with review by Risk Management.

STUDIES

- Allergen-Specific Immunoglobulin E
- Antibodies, Antinuclear, Anti-DNA, Anticentromere, Antiextractable Nuclear Antigen, Anti-Jo, and Antiscleroderma
- Antibodies, Cardiolipin, Immunoglobulin A, Immunoglobulin G, and Immunoglobulin M
- Cancer Antigens: CA 15-3, CA 19-9, CA 125, and Carcinoembryonic
- Chlamydia Group Antibody, IgG and IgM

- Complement C3 and Complement C4
- Culture, Bacterial, Blood
- Immunoglobulin E
- Lupus Anticoagulant Antibodies
- Prostate-Specific Antigen
- Syphilis Serology

LEARNING OUTCOMES

Providing safe, effective nursing care (SENC) includes mastery of core competencies and standards of care. SENC is based on a judicious application of nursing knowledge in combination with scientific principles. The Art of Nursing is in blending what you know with the ability to effectively apply your knowledge in a compassionate manner.

After reading/studying this chapter you will be able to:

Thinking

1. Name the two types of immune response.
2. Name the white blood cell (WBC) type whose primary function is involved in the immune response.
3. Describe some examples of how the immune system functions to protect the body from invasion by foreign elements that range from microorganisms and allergens to chemical toxins, modified proteins, transfusion reactions, and transplanted organs.

Doing

1. Discuss the difference between the primary immune response and the secondary immune response.
2. Describe the appropriate assessment of patients with immune system disorders.
3. Describe some nursing interventions to care for patients with immune system disorders.

Caring

1. Recognize the value of nursing wisdom in relieving physical pain and emotional distress.

Allergen-Specific Immunoglobulin E

Quick Summary

SYNONYM ACRONYM: Allergen profile, radioallergosorbent test (RAST), ImmunoCAP® Specific IgE.

COMMON USE: To assist in identifying environmental allergens responsible for causing allergic reactions.

SPECIMEN: Serum collected in a gold-, red-, or red/gray-top tube.

NORMAL FINDINGS: (Method: Radioimmunoassay or fluorescence enzyme immunoassay)

RAST Scoring Method (Radioimmunoassay) and ImmunoCAP® Scoring Guide (Fluorescence Enzyme Immunoassay)	Conventional and SI Units Allergen-Specific IgE
Specific IgE Allergen Antibody Level	kU/L
Absent or undetectable allergy	Less than 0.35
Low allergy	0.35–0.7
Moderate allergy	0.71–3.5
High allergy	3.51–17.5
Very high allergy	17.6–50
Very high allergy	51–100
Very high allergy	Greater than 100

Test Explanation

Allergen-specific immunoglobulin E (IgE) is generally requested for groups of allergens commonly known to incite an allergic response in the affected individual. The test is based on the use of a radiolabeled or non-radiolabeled anti-IgE reagent to detect IgE in the patient's serum, produced in response to specific allergens. The panels include allergens such as animal dander, antibiotics, dust, foods, grasses, insects, trees, mites, molds, venom, and weeds. Allergen testing is useful for evaluating the cause of hay fever, extrinsic asthma, atopic eczema, respiratory allergies, and potentially fatal reactions to insect venom, penicillin, and other drugs or chemicals. RAST and non-radiolabeled methods are alternatives to skin test anergy and provocation procedures, which can be inconvenient, painful, and potentially hazardous to patients. ImmunoCAP® FEIA is a newer, nonradioactive technology with minimal interference from nonspecific binding to total IgE versus allergen-specific IgE.

A nasal smear can be examined for the presence of eosinophils to screen for allergic conditions. Either a single smear or smears of nasal secretions from each side of the nose should be submitted, at room temperature, for Hansel staining and evaluation. Normal findings vary by laboratory but generally, greater than 10% to 15% is considered eosinophilia or increased presence of eosonophils. Results may be invalid for patients already taking local or systemic corticosteroids.

Nursing Implications

Assessment

Indications	Potential Nursing Problems
Evaluate patients who refuse to submit to skin testing or who have generalized dermatitis or other dermatopathic conditions	• Airway (*related to allergen triggering bronchial edema and constriction*) • Breathing (*related to possible respiratory distress or failure*)

Continued

Table Continued

Indications	Potential Nursing Problems
Monitor response to desensitization procedures Test for allergens when skin testing is inappropriate, such as in infants Test for allergens when there is a known history of allergic reaction to skin testing Test for specific allergic sensitivity before initiating immunotherapy or desensitization shots Test for specific allergic sensitivity when skin testing is unreliable (patients taking long-acting antihistamines may have false-negative skin test)	• Health Management *(related to failure to comply with therapeutic regime)* • Human Response • Role Performance • Sleep • Skin *(related to rash)* • Socialization • Tissue Perfusion

Diagnosis: Clinical Significance of Test Results

Different scoring systems are used in the interpretation of RAST results.

INCREASED IN

Related to production of IgE, the antibody that primarily responds to conditions that stimulate an allergic response

- Allergic rhinitis
- Anaphylaxis
- Asthma (exogenous)
- Atopic dermatitis
- Echinococcus infection
- Eczema
- Hay fever
- Hookworm infection
- Latex allergy
- Schistosomiasis
- Visceral larva migrans

DECREASED IN
- Asthma (endogenous)
- Pregnancy
- Radiation therapy

Planning

Considerations for planning a successful partnership should include clear communication of what to expect during the test to decrease anxiety and improve cooperation. Before the procedure is performed, plan to review the steps with the patient. Explain that specimen collection takes approximately 5 to 10 minutes. Address concerns about pain and explain that there may be some discomfort during the venipuncture.

SPECIAL CONSIDERATIONS

An important aspect of planning is understanding the factors that may alter study findings or cause abnormal results. Interdepartmental communication is a key factor in the planning process. It should be noted when planning for this study that appropriate timing when scheduling multiple studies should be taken into consideration during the planning process as recent radioactive scans or radiation within 1 week of the test can invalidate test results when radioimmunoassay is the test method.

Implementation

Patient education is key to obtaining the patient's cooperation in following directions, and providing an explanation for the purpose of the procedure is an important part of this process. Inform the patient that this study can assist in identifying causal factors related to allergic reaction. Perform the venipuncture.

Evaluation

Recognize anxiety related to test results. Explain that lifestyle adjustments may be necessary, depending on the types of allergens found, and specific nutritional considerations may be recommended if food allergies are identified. Administer an allergy treatment if ordered. As appropriate, educate the patient in the proper technique for administering his or her own treatments as well as the safe handling and maintenance of treatment materials. Treatments may include eye drops, inhalers, nasal sprays, oral medications, or shots. Remind the patient about the importance of avoiding triggers and being in compliance with the recommended therapy, even if signs and symptoms disappear.

✓ Critical Findings

N/A

✓ Specific Complications

There are a number of complications associated with performing a venipuncture. **Pain** is commonly associated with needles, and although the pain experienced during venipuncture is usually mild, on a rare occasion the needle may strike a nerve causing permanent pain. Some patients experience a **vasovagal reaction** during the venipuncture procedure, evidenced by sweating, low blood pressure, fainting, or near fainting. The potential for a **fall injury** is a significant concern related to vasovagal reactions. Prolonged **bleeding** is a complication that occurs with patients who are taking blood thinners or who have coagulopathies such as hemophilia. A **hematoma** results when blood leaks into the tissue during or after a venipuncture, as evidenced by pain, bruising, and/or swelling at the venipuncture site. The swelling can cause injury by compression to surrounding nerves, which can be temporary or permanent. Health-care providers should watch for minor complications such as bruising and hematoma at the venipuncture site, which are fairly common. Hematomas occur more often in older adult or frail patients, or those with veins that are difficult to access. Bleeding or bruising can be prevented once the needle has been removed by applying direct pressure to the site with dry gauze for a minute or two. Some other more unusual complications of venipuncture include **cellulitis, phlebitis, inadvertent arterial puncture,** and **sepsis.** Sepsis can be caused by introduction of bacteria from the surface of the skin into the blood as the result of improper cleansing of the venipuncture site. Immunocompromised patients are at higher risk for developing this complication.

Related Tests

Related tests include arterial/alveolar oxygen ratio, blood gases, CBC, eosinophil count, fecal analysis, hypersensitivity pneumonitis, IgE, and PFT.

See the Immune and Respiratory systems tables at the end of the book for related tests by body system.

Expected Outcomes

Expected outcomes associated with Allergen-Specific IgE are:

- Successfully identifying allergens
- Administering appropriate therapy with a corresponding improvement in the patient's health and quality of life
- Maintaining a nonconstricted airway, which allows for ease of breathing
- Assisting in identifying allergens to prevent triggering other respiratory emergencies
- Managing anxiety to decrease the risk of triggering or worsening airway and breathing difficulties

Antibodies, Antinuclear, Anti-DNA, Anticentromere, Antiextractable Nuclear Antigen, Anti-Jo, and Antiscleroderma

Quick Summary

SYNONYM ACRONYM: Antinuclear antibodies (ANA), anti-DNA (anti-ds DNA), antiextractable nuclear antigens (anti-ENA, ribonucleoprotein [RNP], Smith [Sm], SS-A/Ro, SS-B/La), anti-Jo (antihistidyl transfer RNA [tRNA] synthase), and antiscleroderma (progressive systemic sclerosis [PSS] antibody, Scl-70 antibody, topoisomerase I antibody).

COMMON USE: To diagnose multiple systemic autoimmune disorders; primarily used for diagnosing systemic lupus erythematosus (SLE).

SPECIMEN: Serum collected in a red-top tube.

NORMAL FINDINGS: (Method: Indirect fluorescent antibody for ANA and anticentromere; Immunoassay multiplex flow for anti-DNA, ENA, Scl-70, and Jo-1)

ANA and anticentromere: Titer of 1:40 or less. Anti-ENA, Jo-1, and anti-Scl-70: Negative. Reference ranges for anti-DNA, anti-ENA, anti-Scl-70, and anti-Jo-1 vary widely due to differences in methods and the testing laboratory should be consulted directly.

Anti-DNA	
Negative	Less than 5 international units
Indeterminate	5–9 international units
Positive	Greater than 9 international units

Test Explanation

Antinuclear antibodies (ANA) are autoantibodies mainly located in the nucleus of affected cells. The presence of ANA indicates SLE, related collagen vascular diseases, and immune complex diseases. Antibodies against cellular DNA are strongly associated with SLE. Anticentromere antibodies are a subset of ANA. Their presence is strongly associated with CREST syndrome (*c*alcinosis, *R*aynaud phenomenon, *e*sophageal dysfunction, *s*clerodactyly, and *t*elangiectasia). Women are much more likely than men to be diagnosed with SLE. Jo-1 is an autoantibody found in the sera of some ANA-positive patients. Compared to the presence of other autoantibodies, the presence of Jo-1 suggests a more aggressive course and a higher risk of mortality. The clinical effects of this autoantibody include acute onset fever, dry and crackled skin on the hands, Raynaud phenomenon, and arthritis. The extractable nuclear antigens (ENAs) include ribonucleoprotein (RNP), Smith (Sm), SS-A/Ro, and SS-B/La antigens. ENAs and antibodies to them are found in various combinations in individuals with combinations of overlapping rheumatologic symptoms. The American College of Rheumatology's current criteria include a list of 11 signs and/or symptoms to assist in differentiating lupus from similar diseases. The patient should have four or more of these to establish suspicion of lupus; the symptoms do not have to manifest at the same time: malar rash (rash over the cheeks, sometimes described as a butterfly rash), discoid rash (red raised patches), photosensitivity (exposure resulting in development of or increase in skin rash), oral ulcers, nonerosive arthritis involving two or more peripheral joints, pleuritis or pericarditis, renal disorder (as evidenced by excessive protein in urine or the presence of casts in the urine), neurological disorder (seizures or psychosis in the absence of drugs known to cause these effects), hematological disorder (hemolytic anemia, leukopenia, lymphopenia, thrombocytopenia where the leukopenia or lymphopenia occurs on more than two occasions and the thrombocytopenia occurs in the absence of drugs known to cause it), positive ANA in the absence of a drug known to induce lupus, or immunological disorder (evidenced by positive anti-ds DNA, positive anti-Sm, positive antiphospholipid such as anticardiolipin antibody, positive lupus anticoagulant test, or a false-positive serological syphilis test, known to be positive for at least 6 months and confirmed to be falsely positive by a negative *Treponema pallidum* immobilization or FTA-ABS).

Nursing Implications

Assessment

Indications	Potential Nursing Problems
Assist in the diagnosis and evaluation of SLE Assist in the diagnosis and evaluation of suspected immune disorders, such as rheumatoid arthritis, systemic sclerosis, polymyositis, Raynaud syndrome, scleroderma, Sjögren syndrome, and mixed connective tissue disease Assist in the diagnosis and evaluation of idiopathic inflammatory myopathies	• Body Image • Fall • Grief (related to shortened life expectancy associated with the diagnosis) • Health Management • Human Response • Mobility • Noncompliance • Pain • Protection (related to alterations in autoimmune response) • Self-care (related to an actual or a perceived loss of independence associated with a decreasing ability to perform the activities of daily living) • Skin • Tissue Perfusion

Diagnosis: Clinical Significance of Test Results

ANA Pattern*	Associated Antibody	Associated Condition
Rim and/or homogeneous	Double-stranded DNA Single- or double-stranded DNA	SLE
Homogeneous	Histones	SLE
Speckled	Sm (Smith) antibody	SLE, mixed connective tissue disease, Raynaud scleroderma, Sjögren syndrome
	RNP*	Mixed connective tissue disease, various rheumatoid conditions
	SS-B/La, SS-A/Ro	Various rheumatoid conditions
Diffuse speckled with positive mitotic figures	Centromere	PSS with CREST, Raynaud syndrome
Nucleolar	Nucleolar, RNP	Scleroderma, CREST

*ANA patterns are helpful in that certain conditions are frequently associated with specific patterns. RNP = ribonucleoprotein.

INCREASED IN

- *Anti-Jo-1 is associated with dermatomyositis, idiopathic inflammatory myopathies, and polymyositis*
- *ANA is associated with drug-induced lupus erythematosus*
- *ANA is associated with lupoid hepatitis*
- *ANA is associated with mixed connective tissue disease*
- *ANA is associated with polymyositis*
- *ANA is associated with progressive systemic sclerosis*
- *ANA is associated with Raynaud syndrome*
- *ANA is associated with rheumatoid arthritis*
- *ANA is associated with Sjögren syndrome*
- *ANA and anti-DNA are associated with SLE*
- *Anti-RNP is associated with mixed connective tissue disease*
- *Anti-Scl 70 is associated with progressive systemic sclerosis and scleroderma*
- *Anti-SS-A and anti-SS-B are helpful in antinuclear antibody (ANA)–negative cases of SLE*
- *Anti-SS-A/ANA–positive, anti-SS-B–negative patients are likely to have nephritis*
- *Anti-SS-A/anti-SS-B–positive sera are found in patients with neonatal lupus*
- *Anti-SS-A–positive patients may also have antibodies associated with antiphospholipid syndrome*
- *Anti-SS-A/La is associated with primary Sjögren syndrome*
- *Anti-SS-A/Ro is a predictor of congenital heart block in neonates born to mothers with SLE*
- *Anti-SS-A/Ro–positive patients have photosensitivity*

DECREASED IN

N/A

Planning

Considerations for planning a successful partnership should include clear communication of what to expect during the test to decrease anxiety and improve cooperation. Before the procedure is performed, plan to review the steps with the patient. Address concerns about pain, and explain that there may be some discomfort during the venipuncture.

SPECIAL CONSIDERATIONS

An important aspect of planning is understanding the factors that may alter study findings or cause abnormal results. Interdepartmental communication is a key factor in the planning process. It should be noted when planning for this study that a patient can have lupus and test ANA-negative.

It is also important to understand which medications or substances the patient may be exposed to in the healthcare setting that can interfere with accurate testing:

- Drugs that may cause positive ANA results include acebutolol (diabetics), acetazolamide, anticonvulsants (increases with concomitant administration of multiple antiepileptic drugs), carbamazepine, chlorpromazine, ethosuximide, gemfibrozil, hydralazine, isoniazid, methyldopa, nitrofurantoin, oxyphenisatin, penicillins, phenytoin, primidone, procainamide, quinidine, and trimethadione.

Implementation

Patient education is key to obtaining the patient's cooperation in following directions, and providing an explanation for the purpose of the procedure is an important part of this process. Inform the patient that this study can assist in evaluating immune system function. Perform the venipuncture.

Evaluation

Recognize anxiety related to test results and stress the importance of compliance to the treatment regimen. Instruct the patient with SLE to contact the HCP immediately if new symptoms present, including vague or common symptoms such as fever. Educate the patient regarding lifestyle changes that must be implemented to protect him or her from an increased risk of infection and the development of cardiovascular disease. Patients with lupus should be advised to avoid direct exposure to sunlight or other sources of UV light, such as tanning beds *(related to the hypersensitivity of skin cells to UV light in people with lupus. The exact mechanism for this is not clearly understood, but it is believed that, in people with lupus, damaged or dead skin cells are not sloughed as efficiently as occurs in normal individuals. It is also believed that cell contents released from damaged or dead skin cells may instigate an immune response that leads to the development of a skin rash. Sun exposure is known to damage skin; therefore, avoiding direct exposure reduces the amount of damage incurred.).* Educate the patient regarding access to counseling services and provide contact information, if desired, for the American College of Rheumatology (www.rheumatology.org), the Lupus Foundation of America (www.lupus.org), or the Arthritis Foundation (www.arthritis.org).

DISCUSSION POINT

Patients wishing to become pregnant should discuss the possibility with their health-care provider (HCP). The stress of pregnancy and medication regimen may present significant risks to both mother and child; pregnancies should be carefully planned.

SPECIAL CONSIDERATIONS

Patients with lupus are at increased risk for infection and should discuss the need for vaccinations with their HCP. Recommendations may include receiving vaccines during periods of remission.

✓ Critical Findings

N/A

✓ Study Specific Complications

There are a number of complications associated with performing a venipuncture. **Pain** is commonly associated with needles, and although the pain experienced during venipuncture is usually mild, on a rare occasion the needle may strike a nerve causing permanent pain. Some patients experience a **vasovagal reaction** during the venipuncture procedure, evidenced by sweating, low blood pressure, fainting, or near fainting. The potential for a **fall injury** is a significant concern related to vasovagal reactions. Prolonged **bleeding** is a complication that occurs with patients who are taking blood thinners or who have coagulopathies such as hemophilia. A **hematoma** results when blood leaks into the tissue during or after a venipuncture, as evidenced by pain, bruising, and/or swelling at the venipuncture site. The swelling can cause injury by compression to surrounding nerves, which can be temporary or permanent. HCPs should watch for minor complications such as bruising and hematoma at the venipuncture site, which are fairly common. Hematomas occur more often in older adult or frail patients, or those with veins that are difficult to access. Bleeding or bruising can be prevented once the needle has been removed by applying direct pressure to the site with dry gauze for a minute or two. Some other more unusual complications of venipuncture include **cellulitis, phlebitis, inadvertent arterial puncture,** and **sepsis.** Sepsis can be caused by introduction of bacteria from the surface of the skin into the blood as the result of improper cleansing of the venipuncture site. Immunocompromised patients are at higher risk for developing this complication.

✓ Related Tests

Related tests include antibodies anticyclic citrullinated peptide, arthroscopy, biopsy kidney, biopsy skin, BMD, bone scan, chest x-ray, complement C3 and C4, complement total, CRP, creatinine, ESR, EMG, MRI musculoskeletal, procainamide, radiography bone, RF, synovial fluid analysis, and UA.

See the Immune and Musculoskeletal systems tables at the end of the book for related tests by body system.

Expected Outcomes

Expected outcomes associated with Antibodies, Antinuclear, Anti-DNA, Anticentromere, Antiextractable Nuclear Antigen, Anti-Jo, and Antiscleroderma are:

- Managing joint stiffness to enhance mobility and allow for participation in self-care activities
- Maintaining optimal tissue perfusion for clinical status
- Ensuring patient compliance with medication regimen and follow-up visits as ordered
- Observing patient demonstration of an understanding of and compliance with required lifestyle changes

Antibodies, Cardiolipin, Immunoglobulin A, Immunoglobulin G, and Immunoglobulin M

Quick Summary

SYNONYM ACRONYM: Antiphospholipid antibody, lupus anticoagulant, LA, ACA.

COMMON USE: To detect the presence of antiphospholipid antibodies, which can lead to the development of blood vessel problems and complications including stroke, heart attack, and miscarriage.

SPECIMEN: Serum collected in a red-top tube.

NORMAL FINDINGS: (Method: Immunoassay, enzyme-linked immunosorbent assay [ELIS])

IgA (APL = 1 unit IgA phospholipid)	IgG (GPL = 1 unit IgG phospholipid)	IgM (MPL = 1 unit IgM phospholipid)
Negative: 0–11 APL	Negative: 0–14 GPL	Negative: 0–12 MPL
Indeterminate: 12–19 APL	Indeterminate: 15–19 GPL	Indeterminate: 13–19 MPL
Positive: Greater than 80 APL	Positive: Greater than 80 GPL	Greater than 80 MPL

Test Explanation

Anticardiolipin (ACA) is one of several identified antiphospholipid antibodies. ACAs are of IgG, IgM, and IgA subtypes, which react with proteins in the blood that are bound to phospholipid and interfere with normal blood vessel function. The two primary types of problems they cause are narrowing and irregularity of the blood vessels and blood clots in the blood vessels. ACAs are found in individuals with lupus erythematosus, lupus-related conditions, infectious diseases, drug reactions, and sometimes fetal loss. ACAs are often found in association with lupus anticoagulant. Increased antiphospholipid antibody levels have been found in pregnant women with lupus who have had miscarriages. β_2 Glycoprotein 1, or apolipoprotein H, is an important facilitator in the binding of antiphospholipid antibodies like ACA. A normal level of β_2 glycoprotein 1 is 19 units or less when measured by ELISA assays. β_2 Glycoprotein 1 measurements are considered to be more specific than ACA because they do not demonstrate nonspecific reactivity as do ACA in sera of patients with syphilis or other infectious diseases. The combination of noninflammatory thrombosis of blood vessels, low platelet count, and history of miscarriage is termed *antiphospholipid antibody syndrome* and is documented as present if at least one of the clinical and one of the laboratory criteria are met.

Clinical Criteria

- Vascular thrombosis confirmed by histopathology or imaging studies

- Pregnancy morbidity defined as either one or more unexplained deaths of a morphologically normal fetus at or beyond the 10th week of gestation
- One or more premature births of a morphologically normal neonate before the 34th week of gestation due to eclampsia or severe pre-eclampsia
- Three or more unexplained consecutive spontaneous abortions before the 10th week of gestation

Laboratory Criteria (all measured by a standardized ELISA, according to recommended procedures)

- ACA IgG, or IgM, detectable at greater than 40 units on two or more occasions at least 12 weeks apart
- Lupus anticoagulant (LA) detectable on two or more occasions at least 12 weeks apart
- Anti-β_2 glycoprotein 1 antibody, IgG, or IgM detectable on two or more occasions at least 12 weeks apart

Nursing Implications

Assessment

Indications	Potential Nursing Problems
Assist in the diagnosis of antiphospholipid antibody syndrome	• Activity • Body Image • Confusion • Family • Fatigue • Fear • Grief • Health Maintenance • Human Response • Mobility • Noncompliance • Pain • Protection • Role Performance • Self-care • Self-esteem • Tissue Perfusion

Diagnosis: Clinical Significance of Test Results
INCREASED IN

While ACAs are observed in specific diseases, the exact mechanism of these antibodies in disease is unclear. In fact, the production of ACA can be induced by bacterial, treponemal, and viral infections. Development of ACA under this circumstance is transient and not associated with an increased risk of antiphospholipid antibody syndrome. Patients who initially demonstrate positive ACA levels should be retested after 6 to 8 weeks to rule out transient antibodies that are usually of no clinical significance.

- Antiphospholipid antibody syndrome
- Chorea
- Drug reactions

- Epilepsy
- Infectious diseases
- Mitral valve endocarditis
- Patients with lupus-like symptoms (often antinuclear antibody-negative)
- Placental infarction
- Recurrent fetal loss (strong association with two or more occurrences)
- Recurrent venous and arterial thromboses
- SLE

DECREASED IN

N/A

Planning

Considerations for planning a successful partnership should include clear communication of what to expect during the test to decrease anxiety and improve cooperation. Before the procedure is performed, plan to review the steps with the patient. Address concerns about pain, and explain that there may be some discomfort during the venipuncture.

SPECIAL CONSIDERATIONS

An important aspect of planning is understanding the factors that may alter study findings or cause abnormal results. Interdepartmental communication is a key factor in the planning process. The following should be noted when planning for this study:

- The presence of cardiolipin antibody can affect other tests by cross-reacting with those assays that use phospholipid reagents such as syphilis reagin antibody, lupus anticoagulant, and aPTT.
- False-positive syphilis results for the rapid plasma reagin method may occur in the presence of these antibodies.

It is also important to understand which medications or substances the patient may be exposed to in the healthcare setting that can interfere with accurate testing:

- Drugs that may increase anticardiolipin antibody levels include chlorpromazine, hydralazine, penicillin, procainamide, phenytoin, and quinidine.

Implementation

Patient education is key to obtaining the patient's cooperation in following directions, and providing an explanation for the purpose of the procedure is an important part of this process. Inform the patient that this study can assist in evaluating the amount of potentially harmful circulating antibodies associated with lupus and antiphospholipid antibody syndrome. Perform the venipuncture.

Evaluation

Recognize anxiety related to test results, and discuss the implications of abnormal test results on the patient's lifestyle. Provide teaching and information regarding the clinical implications of the test results as appropriate.

Educate the patient regarding access to counseling services. Provide contact information, if desired, for the Lupus Foundation of America (www.lupus.org).

✅ *Critical Findings*

N/A

✅ *Study Specific Complications*

There are a number of complications associated with performing a venipuncture. **Pain** is commonly associated with needles and, although the pain experienced during venipuncture is usually mild, on a rare occasion the needle may strike a nerve, causing permanent pain. Some patients experience a **vasovagal reaction** during the venipuncture procedure, evidenced by sweating, low blood pressure, fainting, or near fainting. The potential for a **fall injury** is a significant concern related to vasovagal reactions. Prolonged **bleeding** is a complication that occurs with patients who are taking blood thinners or who have coagulopathies such as hemophilia. A **hematoma** results when blood leaks into the tissue during or after a venipuncture, as evidenced by pain, bruising, and/or swelling at the venipuncture site. The swelling can cause injury by compression to surrounding nerves, which can be temporary or permanent. Healthcare providers should watch for minor complications such as bruising and hematoma at the venipuncture site, which are fairly common. Hematomas occur more often in older adult or frail patients, or those with veins that are difficult to access. Bleeding or bruising can be prevented once the needle has been removed by applying direct pressure to the site with dry gauze for a minute or two. Some other more unusual complications of venipuncture include **cellulitis, phlebitis, inadvertent arterial puncture,** and **sepsis.** Sepsis can be caused by introduction of bacteria from the surface of the skin into the blood as the result of improper cleansing of the venipuncture site. Immunocompromised patients are at higher risk for developing this complication.

✅ *Related Tests*

- Related tests include ANA, CBC, CBC platelet count, fibrinogen, lupus anticoagulant antibodies, protein C, protein S, and syphilis serology.
- See the Hematopoietic, Immune, and Reproductive systems tables at the end of the book for related tests by body system.

Expected Outcomes

Expected outcomes associated with Cardiolipin Antibodies are:

- Acknowledging the relationship between fatigue and the disease process
- Acknowledging the importance of achieving and maintaining disease remission
- Understanding that laboratory results can indicate a miscarriage risk related to the disease process

Cancer Antigens: CA 15-3, CA 19-9, CA 125, and Carcinoembryonic

Quick Summary

SYNONYM ACRONYM: Carcinoembryonic antigen (CEA), cancer antigen 125 (CA 125), cancer antigen 15-3 (CA 15-3), cancer antigen 19-9 (CA 19-9), cancer antigen 27.29 (CA 27.29).

COMMON USE: To identify the presence of various cancers, such as breast and ovarian, as well as to evaluate the effectiveness of cancer treatment.

SPECIMEN: Serum collected in a red-top tube. Care must be taken to use the same assay method if serial measurements are to be taken.

NORMAL FINDINGS: (Method: Electrochemiluminometric immunoassay)

Smoking Status	Conventional Units	SI Units (Conventional Units × 1)
CEA		
Smoker	Less than 5 ng/mL	Less than 5 mcg/L
Nonsmoker	Less than 2.5 ng/mL	Less than 2.5 mcg/L

Conventional Units	SI Units (Conventional Units × 1)
CA 125	
Less than 35 units/mL	Less than 35 kU/L
CA 15-3	
Less than 25 units/mL	Less than 25 kU/L
CA 19-9	
Less than 35 units/mL	Less than 35 kU/L
CA 27.29	
Less than 38.6 units/mL	Less than 38.6 kU/L

Test Explanation

Carcinoembryonic antigen (CEA) is a family of 36 different glycoproteins whose function is believed to be involved in cell adhesion. These structurally related proteins are part of the immunoglobulin superfamily. CEA is normally produced during fetal development and rapid multiplication of epithelial cells, especially those of the digestive system. A small amount of circulating CEA is detectable in the blood of normal adults; normal half-life is 7 days. The liver is the main site for metabolism of CEA. Because of the variability in CEA molecules, the test is not diagnostic for any specific disease and is not useful as a screening test for cancer. However, it is very useful for monitoring response to therapy in breast, liver, colon, and gastrointestinal cancer. Serial monitoring is also a useful indicator of recurrence or metastasis in colon or liver carcinoma. CEA levels are higher in the blood of smokers than in nonsmokers so most laboratories will have a normal range for each group.

CA 125 or Muc16 is a glycoprotein member of the mucin family and is present in normal endometrial tissue. It appears in the blood when natural endometrial protective barriers are destroyed, as occurs in cancer or endometriosis. CA 125 is most useful in monitoring the progression or recurrence of known ovarian cancer. It is not useful as a screening test because elevations can occur with numerous other conditions such as endometriosis, other diseases of the ovary, menstruation, pregnancy, and uterine fibroids. Persistently rising levels indicate a poor prognosis. Levels may also rise in pancreatic, liver, colon, breast, and lung cancers. Absence of detectable levels of CA 125 does not rule out the presence of tumor. Human epididymis protein 4 (HE4) is a newer protein marker associated with various types of cancer including ovarian cancer (OC). Significant or persistent elevations of HE4 may indicate the appearance, recurrence, or progression of epithelial OC. A significant elevation would be an increase of greater than 25% over normal findings. Normal findings for HE4 in premenopausal females is less than 70 pmol/L and less than 140 pmol/L in postmenopausal females.

CA 15-3 monitors patients for recurrence or metastasis of breast carcinoma.

CA 19-9 is a carbohydrate antigen used for posttherapeutic monitoring of patients with gastrointestinal, pancreatic, liver, and colorectal cancer.

CA 27.29 is a glycoprotein product of the muc-1 gene. It is most useful as a serial monitor for response to therapy or recurrence of breast carcinoma.

Nursing Implications

Assessment

Indications	Potential Nursing Problems
CEA	• Body Image
Determine stage of colorectal cancer and test for recurrence or metastasis	• Disturbed Sleep
Monitor response to treatment of breast and gastrointestinal cancers	• Family
CA 125	• Fatigue
Assist in the diagnosis of carcinoma of the cervix and endometrium	• Fear
Assist in the diagnosis of ovarian cancer	• Human Response
Monitor response to treatment of ovarian cancer	• Infection Risk
CA 15-3 and CA 27.29	• Pain
Monitor recurrent carcinoma of the breast	• Role Performance
CA 19-9	• Self-esteem
Monitor effectiveness of therapy	• Sexuality
Monitor gastrointestinal, head and neck, and gynecological carcinomas	• Skin
Predict recurrence of cholangiocarcinoma	
Predict recurrence of stomach, pancreatic, colorectal, gallbladder, liver, and urothelial carcinomas	

Diagnosis: Clinical Significance of Test Results
INCREASED IN
CEA

- Benign tumors, including benign breast disease
- Chronic tobacco smoking
- Cirrhosis
- Colorectal, pulmonary, gastric, pancreatic, breast, head and neck, esophageal, ovarian, and prostate cancer
- Inflammatory bowel disease
- Pancreatitis
- Radiation therapy (transient)

CA 125

- Breast, colon, endometrial, liver, lung, ovarian, and pancreatic cancer
- Endometriosis
- First-trimester pregnancy
- Menses
- Ovarian abscess
- Pelvic inflammatory disease
- Peritonitis

CA 15-3 AND CA 27.29

- Recurrence of breast carcinoma

CA 19-9

- Gastrointestinal, head and neck, and gynecologic carcinomas
- Recurrence of stomach, pancreatic, colorectal, gallbladder, liver, and urothelial carcinomas
- Recurrence of cholangiocarcinoma

DECREASED IN
- Effective therapy or removal of the tumor

Planning
Considerations for planning a successful partnership should include clear communication of what to expect during the test to decrease anxiety and improve cooperation. Before the procedure is performed, plan to review the steps with the patient. Address concerns about pain, and explain that there may be some discomfort during the venipuncture.

SPECIAL CONSIDERATIONS
An important aspect of planning is understanding the factors that may alter study findings or cause abnormal results. Interdepartmental communication is a key factor in the planning process. The following should be noted when planning for this study:

- Determine if the patient smokes because smokers may have elevations of CEA that are unrelated to the presence of cancer.

Implementation
Patient education is key to obtaining the patient's cooperation in following directions, and providing an explanation for the purpose of the procedure is an important part of this process. Inform the patient that this study can assist in monitoring the progress of various types of disease and can evaluate the response to therapy. Perform the venipuncture.

Evaluation
Recognize anxiety related to test results, and be supportive of a perceived loss of independence and fear of a shortened life expectancy. Discuss the implications of abnormal test results on the patients lifestyle. Provide teaching and information regarding the clinical implications of the test results as appropriate. Educate the patient regarding access to counseling services. Provide contact information, if desired, for the American Cancer Association (www.cancer.org).

Reinforce information given by the patient's healthcare provider (HCP) regarding further testing, treatment, or referral to another HCP. Answer any questions or address any concerns voiced by the patient or family.

DISCUSSION POINT
Decisions regarding the need for and frequency of breast self-examination, mammography, magnetic resonance imaging (MRI) of the breast, or other cancer screening procedures should be made after consultation between the patient and HCP. The American Cancer Society (ACS) recommends breast examinations be performed every 3 years for women between the ages of 20 and 39 years and annually for women over 40 years of age; annual mammograms should be performed on women 40 years and older as long as they are in good health. The ACS also recommends annual MRI testing for women at high risk of developing breast cancer. Genetic testing for inherited mutations (BRCA1 and BRCA2) associated with increased risk of developing breast cancer may be ordered for women at risk. The test is performed on a blood specimen. The most current guidelines for breast cancer screening of the general population as well as of individuals with increased risk are available from the American Cancer Society (www.cancer.org), the American College of Obstetricians and Gynecologists (ACOG) (www.acog.org), and the American College of Radiology (www.acr.org).

DISCUSSION POINT
Decisions regarding the need for and frequency of occult blood testing, colonoscopy, or other cancer screening procedures should be made after consultation between the patient and HCP. The ACS recommends regular screening for colon cancer, beginning at age 50 years for individuals without identified risk factors. Their recommendations for frequency of screening: annual for occult blood testing (fecal occult blood testing/FOBT and fecal immunochemical testing/FIT); every 5 years for flexible sigmoidoscopy, double contrast barium enema, and computed tomography (CT) colonography; and every 10 years for colonoscopy. There are both advantages and disadvantages

to the screening tests that are available today. Methods to use DNA testing of stool are being investigated and are awaiting FDA approval. The DNA test is designed to identify abnormal changes in DNA from the cells in the lining of the colon that are normally shed and excreted in stool. The DNA tests under development would use multiple markers to identify colon cancers with various, abnormal DNA changes and would be able to detect precancerous polyps. The most current guidelines for colon cancer screening of the general population as well as of individuals with increased risk are available from the American Cancer Society (www.cancer.org), U.S. Preventive Services Task Force (www.uspreventiveservicestaskforce.org), and the American College of Gastroenterology (www.gi.org).

✅ Critical Findings

N/A

✅ Study Specific Complications

There are a number of complications associated with performing a venipuncture. **Pain** is commonly associated with needles, and although the pain experienced during venipuncture is usually mild, on a rare occasion the needle may strike a nerve, causing permanent pain. Some patients experience a **vasovagal reaction** during the venipuncture procedure, evidenced by sweating, low blood pressure, fainting, or near fainting. The potential for a **fall injury** is a significant concern related to vasovagal reactions. Prolonged **bleeding** is a complication that occurs with patients who are taking blood thinners or who have coagulopathies such as hemophilia. A **hematoma** results when blood leaks into the tissue during or after a venipuncture, as evidenced by pain, bruising, and/or swelling at the venipuncture site. The swelling can cause injury by compression to surrounding nerves, which can be temporary or permanent. HCPs should watch for minor complications such as bruising and hematoma at the venipuncture site, which are fairly common. Hematomas occur more often in older adult or frail patients, or those with veins that are difficult to access. Bleeding or bruising can be prevented once the needle has been removed by applying direct pressure to the site with dry gauze for a minute or two. Some other more unusual complications of venipuncture include **cellulitis, phlebitis, inadvertent arterial puncture,** and **sepsis.** Sepsis can be caused by introduction of bacteria from the surface of the skin into the blood as the result of improper cleansing of the venipuncture site. Immunocompromised patients are at higher risk for developing this complication.

✅ Related Tests

Related tests include barium enema, biopsy breast, biopsy cervical, biopsy intestinal, biopsy liver, capsule endoscopy, colonoscopy, colposcopy, fecal analysis, HCG, liver and spleen scan, MRI breast, MRI liver, mammogram, stereotactic breast biopsy, proctosigmoidoscopy, radiofrequency ablation liver, US abdomen, US breast, and US liver.

Refer to the Gastrointestinal, Immune, and Reproductive systems tables at the end of the book for related tests by body system.

Expected Outcomes

Expected outcomes associated with Cancer Antigens are:

- Realistic expectations of the therapeutic interventions and longevity in relation to the stage of cancer diagnosed
- Ability to verbalize concerns regarding having children in the future based on the HCP prognosis
- Emotional and educational support are provided to the patient and family to assist in coping with the progression of the disease and treatment options
- Patient understanding and compliance with requests for follow-up testing and visits with the HCP

Chlamydia Group Antibody, IgG and IgM

Quick Summary

COMMON USE: To diagnose some of the more common chlamydia infections such as community-acquired pneumonia transmitted by *Chlamydophila pneumoniae* (formerly Chlamydia pneumoniae) and chlamydia disease that is sexually transmitted by *Chlamydia trachomatis.*

SPECIMEN: Serum collected in a red-top tube. Place separated serum into a standard transport tube within 2 hours of collection.

NORMAL FINDINGS: (Method: Enzyme immunofluorescent assay)

IgG	IgM
Less than 1:64	Less than 1:20

Test Explanation

Chlamydia, one of the most common sexually transmitted infections, is caused by *Chlamydia trachomatis.* These gram-negative bacteria are called *obligate cell parasites* because they require living cells for growth. There are three serotypes of *C. trachomatis.* One group causes lymphogranuloma venereum, with symptoms of the first phase of the disease appearing 2 to 6 weeks after infection; another causes a genital tract infection different from lymphogranuloma venereum, in which symptoms in men appear 7 to 28 days after intercourse (women are generally asymptomatic); and the third causes the ocular disease trachoma (incubation period, 7 to 10 days). *C. psittaci* is the cause of psittacosis in birds and humans. It is increasing in prevalence as a pathogen responsible for other significant diseases of the respiratory system. The incubation period for *C. psittaci* infections in humans is 7 to 15 days and is followed by chills, fever, and a persistent nonproductive cough. Another chlamydia, *C. pneumoniae* is a common cause of community-acquired pneumonia.

Chlamydia is difficult to culture and grow, so antibody testing has become the technology of choice. A limitation of antibody screening is that positive results may not distinguish past from current infection. The antigen used in many screening kits is not species specific and can confirm only the presence of *Chlamydia* species. Newer technology using nucleic acid amplification and DNA probes can identify the species. Assays that can specifically identify *C. trachomatis* require special collection and transport kits. They also have specific collection instructions, and the specimens are collected on swabs. The laboratory performing this testing should be consulted before specimen collection. Culture or liquid-based PAP test may also be requested for identification of chlamydia.

Nursing Implications
Assessment

Indications	Potential Nursing Problems
Establish Chlamydia as the cause of atypical pneumonia Establish the presence of chlamydial infection	• Activity • Airway • Fatigue • Gas Exchange • Health Maintenance • Human Response • Pain • Role Performance • Sexuality

Diagnosis: Clinical Significance of Test Results
POSITIVE FINDING IN
- Chlamydial infection
- Community-acquired pneumonia
- Infantile pneumonia *(related to transmission at birth from an infected mother)*
- Infertility *(related to scarring of ovaries or fallopian tubes from untreated chlamydial infection)*
- Lymphogranuloma venereum
- Ophthalmia neonatorum *(related to transmission at birth from an infected mother)*
- Pelvic inflammatory disease
- Urethritis

Planning
Considerations for planning a successful partnership should include clear communication of what to expect during the test to decrease anxiety and improve cooperation. Before the procedure is performed, plan to review the steps with the patient. Address concerns about pain, and explain that there may be some discomfort during the venipuncture.

SPECIAL CONSIDERATIONS
An important aspect of planning is understanding the factors that may alter study findings or cause abnormal results. Interdepartmental communication is a key factor in the planning process. The following should be noted when planning for this study:

- Positive results may demonstrate evidence of past infection and may not necessarily indicate current infection.
- Antibody testing methods may be affected by hemolysis or lipemia.

Implementation
Patient education is key to obtaining the patient's cooperation in following directions, and providing an explanation for the purpose of the procedure is an important part of this process. Inform the patient that this study can assist in diagnosing chlamydial infection and that several tests may be necessary to confirm diagnosis. Perform the venipuncture.

There are a number of other commonly used ways to diagnose chlamydial infection (see Ch. 19, the Skin Culture study) from samples containing a sufficient number of infected epithelial cells to include:

- Specimens collected in liquid-based PAP test kits, which can be "split" specifically for detection of Chlamydia trachomatis
- Specimens collected by cervical culture for females and urethral culture for males, which are followed by direct immunofluorescence, nucleic acid amplification, or DNA probe assays [e.g., Gen-Probe APTIMA]
- First-void urine specimens, which are followed by nucleic acid amplification or DNA probe assays [e.g., Gen-Probe APTIMA]
- Specimens collected by swab from other sites, such as the conjunctiva, posterior nasopharynx, throat, or rectum

DISCUSSION POINT
Chlamydia is an intracellular obligate pathogen. Culture of infected epithelial cells is considered the gold standard for the identification of chlamydia because of the higher sensitivity of nucleic acid amplification or DNA probe assays relative to antibody assays. Therefore, culture should always be the test of choice in cases of suspected or known child abuse.

Evaluation
Recognize anxiety related to test results and provide teaching and information regarding the clinical implications of the test results as appropriate. Any individual positive result should be repeated in 7 to 10 days to monitor a change in titer. Counsel the patient, as

appropriate, about the risk of sexual transmission, and educate the patient about proper prophylaxis. Discuss the implications of abnormal test results on the patient's lifestyle, and encourage the patient to persuade his or her sexual partner(s) to also receive testing as infection is frequently present without demonstrable signs or symptoms. Advise the patient to refrain from sexual activity until the results of the test have been discussed with the health-care provider (HCP). Inform the patient with positive *C. trachomatis* that findings must be reported to a local health department official who will question the patient regarding his or her sexual partners. Educate the patient regarding access to counseling services. Reinforce the importance of strict adherence to the treatment regimen.

SPECIAL CONSIDERATIONS

Social and Cultural Considerations: Offer support, as appropriate, to patients who may be the victim of rape or sexual assault. Educate the patient regarding access to counseling services. Provide a nonjudgmental, nonthreatening atmosphere for a discussion during which you explain the risks of sexually transmitted infections. It is also important to discuss emotions the patient may experience (guilt, depression, anger) as a victim of rape or sexual assault.

DISCUSSION POINT

Provide emotional support if the patient is pregnant and if results are positive. Inform the patient that chlamydial infection during pregnancy places the newborn at risk for pneumonia and conjunctivitis.

⚫ *Critical Findings*

N/A

⚫ *Study Specific Complications*

There are a number of complications associated with performing a venipuncture. **Pain** is commonly associated with needles and, although the pain experienced during venipuncture is usually mild, on a rare occasion the needle may strike a nerve, causing permanent pain. Some patients experience a **vasovagal reaction** during the venipuncture procedure, evidenced by sweating, low blood pressure, fainting, or near fainting. The potential for a **fall injury** is a significant concern related to vasovagal reactions. Prolonged **bleeding** is a complication that occurs with patients who are taking blood thinners or who have coagulopathies such as hemophilia. A **hematoma** results when blood leaks into the tissue during or after a venipuncture, as evidenced by pain, bruising, and/or swelling at the venipuncture site. The swelling can cause injury by compression to surrounding nerves, which can be temporary or permanent. HCPs should watch for minor complications such as bruising and hematoma at the venipuncture site, which are fairly common.

Hematomas occur more often in older adult or frail patients, or those with veins that are difficult to access. Bleeding or bruising can be prevented once the needle has been removed by applying direct pressure to the site with dry gauze for a minute or two. Some other more unusual complications of venipuncture include **cellulitis, phlebitis, inadvertent arterial puncture,** and **sepsis.** Sepsis can be caused by introduction of bacteria from the surface of the skin into the blood as the result of improper cleansing of the venipuncture site. Immunocompromised patients are at higher risk for developing this complication.

⚫ *Related Tests*

- Related tests include culture bacterial (anal, genital), culture viral, Gram stain, Pap smear, and syphilis serology.
- Refer to the Immune and Reproductive systems tables at the end of the book for related tests by body system.

Expected Outcomes

Expected outcomes associated with Chlamydia Group Antibody, IgG and IgM, are:

- Reporting feeling comfortable with the level of activity tolerance
- Reporting an absence of dyspnea at rest or with activity
- Understanding of and being compliant with lifestyle changes and the therapeutic regimen required to eliminate the infection
- Being compliant with prescribed medications, follow-up testing, and office visits as ordered

Complement C3 and Complement C4

Quick Summary

SYNONYM ACRONYM: C3 and C4.

COMMON USE: To assist in the diagnosis of immunological diseases, such as rheumatoid arthritis, and systemic lupus erythematosus (SLE), in which complement is consumed at an increased rate, or to detect inborn deficiency.

SPECIMEN: Serum collected in a red- or red/gray-top tube. Place separated serum into a standard transport tube within 2 hours of collection.

NORMAL FINDINGS: (Method: Immunoturbidimetric)

C3

Age	Conventional Units	SI Units (Conventional Units × 0.01)
Newborn	57–116 mg/dL	0.57–1.16 g/L
6 mo–adult	74–166 mg/dL	0.74–0.17 g/L
Adult	83–177 mg/dL	0.83–1.77 g/L

C4

Age	Conventional Units	SI Units (Conventional Units × 10)
Newborn	10–31 mg/dL	0.1–0.31 g/L
6 mo–6 yr	15–52 mg/dL	0.15–0.52 g/L
7–12 yr	19–40 mg/dL	0.19–0.4 g/L
13–15 yr	19–57 mg/dL	0.19–0.57 g/L
16–18 yr	19–42 mg/dL	0.19–0.42 g/L
Adult	12–36 mg/dL	0.12–0.36 g/L

Test Explanation

Complement is a system of 25 to 30 distinct cell membrane and plasma proteins, numbered C1 through C9. Once activated, the proteins interact with each other in a specific sequence called the *complement cascade*. The classical pathway is triggered by antigen-antibody complexes and includes participation of all complement proteins C1 through C9. The alternate pathway occurs when C3, C5, and C9 are activated without participation of C1, C2, and C4 or the presence of antigen-antibody complexes. Complement proteins act as enzymes that aid in the immunological and inflammatory response. The complement system is an important mechanism for the destruction and removal of foreign materials. Serum complement levels are used to detect autoimmune diseases. C3 and C4 are the most frequently assayed complement proteins, along with total complement.

Circulating C3 is synthesized in the liver and composes 70% of the complement system, but cells in other tissues can also produce C3. C3 is an essential activating protein in the classic and alternate complement cascades. It is decreased in patients with immunological diseases, in whom it is consumed at an increased rate. C4 is produced primarily in the liver but can also be produced by monocytes, fibroblasts, and macrophages. C4 participates in the classic complement pathway.

Nursing Implications
Assessment

Indications	Potential Nursing Problems
Detect genetic deficiencies Evaluate immunological diseases	• Body Image • Fatigue • Human Response • Mobility • Pain • Role Performance • Self-care • Skin

Diagnosis: Clinical Significance of Test Results

Normal C4 and decreased C3	Acute glomerulonephritis, membranous glomerulonephritis, immune complex diseases, SLE, C3 deficiency
Decreased C4 and normal C3	Immune complex diseases, cryoglobulinemia, C4 deficiency, hereditary angioedema
Decreased C4 and decreased C3	Immune complex diseases

INCREASED IN
Response to sudden increased demand

C3 AND C4

- Acute-phase reactions

C3

- Amyloidosis
- Cancer
- Diabetes
- Myocardial infarction
- Pneumococcal pneumonia
- Pregnancy
- Rheumatic disease
- Thyroiditis
- Viral hepatitis

C4

- Certain malignancies

DECREASED IN
Related to overconsumption during immune response

C3 AND C4

- Hereditary deficiency *(insufficient production)*
- Liver disease *(insufficient production related to damaged liver cells)*
- SLE

C3

- Chronic infection (bacterial, parasitic, viral)
- Post-membranoproliferative glomerulonephritis
- Post-streptococcal infection
- Rheumatic arthritis

C4

- Angioedema *(hereditary and acquired)*
- Autoimmune hemolytic anemia
- Autoimmune thyroiditis
- Cryoglobulinemia
- Glomerulonephritis
- Juvenile dermatomyositis
- Meningitis (bacterial, viral)

- Pneumonia
- Streptococcal or staphylococcal sepsis

Planning

Considerations for planning a successful partnership should include clear communication of what to expect during the test to decrease anxiety and improve cooperation. Before the procedure is performed, plan to review the steps with the patient. Address concerns about pain, and explain that there may be some discomfort during the venipuncture.

SPECIAL CONSIDERATIONS

An important aspect of planning is understanding the factors that may alter study findings or cause abnormal results. Interdepartmental communication is a key factor in the planning process.

It is also important to understand which medications or substances the patient may be exposed to in the healthcare setting that can interfere with accurate testing:

- Drugs that may increase C3 levels include cimetidine and cyclophosphamide. Drugs that may decrease C3 levels include danazol, methyldopa, and phenytoin.
- Drugs that may increase C4 levels include cimetidine, cyclophosphamide, and danazol. Drugs that may decrease C4 levels include dextran, methyldopa, and penicillamine.

Implementation

Patient education is key to obtaining the patient's cooperation in following directions, and providing an explanation for the purpose of the procedure is an important part of this process. Inform the patient that this study can assist in diagnosing diseases of the immune system. Perform the venipuncture.

Evaluation

Recognize anxiety related to test results and answer any questions or address any concerns voiced by the patient or family.

✔ Critical Findings

N/A

✔ Study Specific Complications

There are a number of complications associated with performing a venipuncture. **Pain** is commonly associated with needles, and although the pain experienced during venipuncture is usually mild, on a rare occasion the needle may strike a nerve, causing permanent pain. Some patients experience a **vasovagal reaction** during the venipuncture procedure, evidenced by sweating, low blood pressure, fainting, or near fainting. The potential for a **fall injury** is a significant concern related to vasovagal reactions. Prolonged **bleeding** is a complication that occurs with patients who are taking blood thinners or who have coagulopathies such as hemophilia. A **hematoma** results when blood leaks into the tissue during or after a venipuncture, as evidenced by pain, bruising, and/or swelling at the venipuncture site. The swelling can cause injury by compression to surrounding nerves, which can be temporary or permanent. Healthcare providers should watch for minor complications such as bruising and hematoma at the venipuncture site, which are fairly common. Hematomas occur more often in older adult or frail patients, or those with veins that are difficult to access. Bleeding or bruising can be prevented once the needle has been removed by applying direct pressure to the site with dry gauze for a minute or two. Some other more unusual complications of venipuncture include **cellulitis, phlebitis, inadvertent arterial puncture,** and **sepsis.** Sepsis can be caused by introduction of bacteria from the surface of the skin into the blood as the result of improper cleansing of the venipuncture site. Immunocompromised patients are at higher risk for developing this complication.

✔ Related Tests

Related tests include anticardiolipin antibody, ANA, complement total, cryoglobulin, and ESR.

Refer to the Immune System table at the end of the book for related tests by body system.

Expected Outcomes

Expected outcomes associated with Complement C3 and Complement C4 are:

- Ability to ambulate without joint pain
- Improved or eliminated fatigue

Culture, Bacterial, Blood

Quick Summary

COMMON USE: To identify pathogenic bacterial organisms in the blood as an indicator for appropriate therapeutic interventions for sepsis.

SPECIMEN: Whole blood collected in bottles containing standard aerobic and anaerobic culture media.

NORMAL FINDINGS: (Method: Growth of organisms in standard culture media identified by radiometric or infrared automation, by manual reading of subculture, or polymerase chain reaction [PCR].) Negative: no growth of pathogens.

Test Explanation

Pathogens can enter the bloodstream from soft-tissue infection sites, contaminated IV lines, or invasive procedures (e.g., surgery, tooth extraction, cystoscopy). Blood cultures are collected whenever bacteremia (bacterial infection of the blood) or septicemia (a condition of systemic infection caused by pathogenic organisms or their toxins) is suspected. Although mild bacteremia is found in many infectious diseases, a persistent, continuous, or recurrent bacteremia indicates a more serious condition that may require immediate treatment. Early detection of pathogens in the blood may aid in making clinical and etiological diagnoses.

Blood cultures can detect the presence of bacteria and fungi. Organisms can be classified in a number of ways; blood culture findings use oxygen requirements to categorize findings into one of two groups. Blood culture begins with the introduction of a blood specimen into two types of culture medium. The medium is designed to promote the growth of organisms; one group of organisms require oxygen (aerobic) and the other either requires sparing amounts to no oxygen at all (anaerobic). A blood culture may also be done with an antimicrobial removal device (ARD) if antibiotic therapy is initiated prior to specimen collection. This involves transferring some of the blood sample into a special vial containing absorbent resins that remove antibiotics from the sample before the culture is performed.

Traditional automated culture methods entail incubation of innoculated culture containers for a specific length of time, at a specific temperature, and under other conditions suitable for growth. If organisms are present, they will produce carbon dioxide as they metabolize the nutrients in the culture media. The presence of carbon dioxide in the culture is detected when the culture bottles are "read" by an instrument at specified intervals over a period of time. There are a number of automated blood culture systems with sophisticated computerized algorithms. The complex software allows for frequent monitoring of growth throughout the day and rapid interpretation of culture findings. With these systems as soon as a positive culture is detected, usually within 24–72 hours, the bottle can be removed from the system and a Gram stain performed to provide a preliminary identification of the bacteria present. This preliminary report provides an opportunity for the health-care provider (HCP) to initiate therapy. A sample from the positive blood culture bottle is then subcultured on the appropriate plated media for growth, isolation, and positive identification of the organism. The plated organisms are also used for sensitivity testing, if indicated. Sensitivity testing identifies the antibiotics to which the organisms are susceptible to ensure an effective treatment plan and can take several days. Negative cultures are generally removed from the automated culture system after 5 days and finalized as having "No Growth." The subspecialty of microbiology has been revolutionized by molecular diagnostics. Molecular diagnostics involves the identification of specific sequences of DNA. The application of molecular diagnostics techniques, such as PCR, has led to the development of automated instruments that can identify a single infectious agent or multiple pathogens from a small amount of blood in less than 2 hours. The instruments can detect the presence of gram-negative bacteria, gram-positive bacteria, and yeast commonly associated with bloodstream infections. The instruments can also detect mutations in the genetic material of specific pathogens that code for antibiotic resistance.

Nursing Implications
Assessment

Indications	Potential Nursing Problems
Determine sepsis in the newborn as a result of prolonged labor, early rupture of membranes, maternal infection, or neonatal aspiration	• Activity
	• Cardiac Output *(related to episodes of tachycardia)*
	• Confusion
	• Fatigue
Evaluate chills and fever in patients with infected burns, urinary tract infections, rapidly progressing tissue infection, postoperative wound sepsis, and indwelling venous or arterial catheter	• Fear
	• Fever
	• Fluid Volume
	• Gas Exchange *(related to episodes of tachypnea)*
	• Gastrointestinal *(altered perfusion)*
Evaluate intermittent or continuous temperature elevation of unknown origin	• Human Response
Evaluate persistent, intermittent fever associated with a heart murmur	• Infection *(related to an increase in the WBC count above previous levels and/ or a significant change in the differential; positive blood cultures; also, an increase in temperature, chills, and diaphoresis)*
Evaluate a sudden change in pulse and temperature with or without chills and diaphoresis	• Self-care
Evaluate suspected bacteremia after invasive procedures	• Tissue Perfusion
Identify the cause of shock in the postoperative period	• Urination *(altered related to renal damage associated with insufficient perfusion)*

Diagnosis: Clinical Significance of Test Results
POSITIVE FINDING IN

- Bacteremia or septicemia: Gram-negative organisms such as *Aerobacter, Bacteroides, Brucella, Escherichia coli* and other coliform bacilli, *Haemophilus influenzae, Klebsiella, Pseudomonas aeruginosa,* and *Salmonella.*
- Bacteremia or septicemia: Gram-positive organisms such as *Clostridium perfringens, Enterococci, Listeria monocytogenes, Staphylococcus aureus, S. epidermidis,* and β-hemolytic streptococci.
- Plague
- Malaria (by special request, a stained capillary smear would be examined)
- Typhoid fever

Note: Candida albicans is a yeast that can cause disease and can be isolated by blood culture.

Planning
Considerations for planning a successful partnership should include clear communication of what to expect during the test to decrease anxiety and improve cooperation. Before the procedure is performed, plan to review the steps with the patient. Address concerns about

pain, and explain that there may be some discomfort during the venipuncture. Explain that it may be necessary to collect a series of specimens. Assess whether the patient is taking any medications that will interfere with test results. The laboratory may be able to use an ARD to prevent interferences if there is notification of the need to take this step.

SPECIAL CONSIDERATIONS

An important aspect of planning is understanding the factors that may alter study findings or cause abnormal results. Interdepartmental communication is a key factor in the planning process. It should be noted when planning for this study that pretest factors can affect test results, including:

- Antimicrobial therapy begun prior to specimen collection, *related to delay or inhibition of growth*
- Contamination of the specimen by the skin's resident flora, *related to inability to differentiate skin surface flora from organisms circulating in the blood*
- An inadequate amount of blood or number of blood specimens drawn for examination, *related to undetectable levels of growth*
- Delay in transport of the specimen to the laboratory for more than 1 hour after collection, which may result in decreased growth or no growth of organisms, *related to delay in incubation at optimal temperature and other environmental elements required for growth*
- Collection of the specimen in an expired media tube, which will result in specimen rejection

Negative findings do not ensure the absence of infection.

● Safety Tips

If the patient has a history of severe allergic reaction to any of the materials in the iodine disinfectant solution, care should be taken to avoid the use of iodine disinfectant solutions. If the patient is sensitive to the iodine solution, a double alcohol scrub or green soap may be substituted.

Implementation

Patient education is key to obtaining the patient's cooperation in following directions, and providing an explanation for the purpose of the procedure is an important part of this process. Inform the patient that this study can assist in identifying the organism-causing infection. Perform the venipuncture.

The contamination of blood cultures by skin and other flora can also be dramatically reduced by careful preparation of the collection containers before specimen collection. Each container must be inspected prior to use. Containers with cracks, cloudiness of the medium, damaged (bulging or inverted) rubber stoppers,

or past expiration dates must be discarded. Remove the protective cover and cleanse the rubber stoppers of the collection containers with the appropriate disinfectant as recommended by the laboratory, allow to air-dry, and cleanse with 70% alcohol.

The collection site must also be carefully prepped in order to avoid contamination of the culture specimen with skin flora. Once the vein has been located by palpation, cleanse the site with 70% alcohol followed by swabbing with an iodine solution (or approved substitute). The iodine should be swabbed in a circular, concentric motion, moving outward or away from the puncture site. The iodine should be allowed to completely dry before the sample is collected. Avoid collecting the specimen from or above an existing IV site. Instead use the opposite arm or draw below the IV site. If collection is performed by directly drawing the sample into a culture tube, fill the aerobic culture tube first. If collection is performed using a syringe, transfer the blood sample directly into each culture bottle. Promptly transport the specimen to the laboratory for processing and analysis. More than three sets of cultures per day do not significantly add to the likelihood of pathogen capture. Capture rates are more likely affected by obtaining a sufficient volume of blood per culture. The use of ARDs or resin bottles is costly and controversial with respect to their effectiveness versus standard culture techniques. They may be useful in selected cases, such as when septicemia or bacteremia is suspected after antimicrobial therapy has been initiated. Cleanse the residual iodine from the collection site.

Disease Suspected	Recommended Collection
Bacterial pneumonia, fever of unknown origin, meningitis, osteomyelitis, sepsis	Two sets of cultures, each collected from a separate site, 30 minutes apart
Acute or subacute endocarditis	Three sets of cultures, each collected from a separate site, 30–40 minutes apart; if cultures are negative after 24–48 hours, repeat collections
Septicemia, fungal, or mycobacterial infection in immunocompromised patient	Two sets of cultures, each collected from a separate site, 30–60 minutes apart (the laboratory may use a lysis concentration technique to enhance recovery)
Septicemia, bacteremia after therapy has been initiated, or a request to monitor the effectiveness of antimicrobial therapy	Two sets of cultures, each collected from a separate site, 30–60 minutes apart (consider the use of ARD to enhance recovery)

Evaluation

Recognize anxiety related to test results, and inform the patient that preliminary results should be available in 24 to 72 hours, but that final results are not available for 5 to 7 days. Instruct the patient to report signs and symptoms of acute infection such as pain *related to tissue inflammation or irritation*, fever, and chills to the HCP. Instruct the patient to begin antibiotic therapy as prescribed and stress the importance of completing the entire course of antibiotic therapy even if no symptoms are present.

Emphasize the importance of reporting continued signs and symptoms of the infection. Provide information regarding vaccine-preventable diseases as indicated (e.g., *Haemophilus influenza* and meningococcal disease). Provide contact information, if desired, for the Centers for Disease Control and Prevention (www.cdc.gov/vaccines/vpd-vac).

Critical Findings

- Positive findings in any sterile body fluid such as blood

Note and immediately report to the HCP positive results and related symptoms.

It is essential that a critical finding be communicated immediately to the requesting HCP. A listing of these findings varies among facilities.

Assess for signs and symptoms of sepsis or development of septic shock to include change in body temperature (greater than 101.3°F/38.5°C or less than 95°F/35°C); decreased systolic blood pressure (less than 90 mm Hg); increased heart rate (greater than 90 beats per minute); sudden change in mental status (restlessness, agitation or confusion); significantly decreased urine output (less than 30 mL/hour); increased respirations (greater than 20 breaths per minute); change in extremities (pale, mottled, and/or cyanotic in appearance); and decreased or absent peripheral pulses. Note and immediately report to the health-care provider (HCP) positive results and related symptoms. Lists of specific organisms may vary among facilities; specific organisms are required to be reported to local, state, and national departments of health.

Study Specific Complications

There are a number of complications associated with performing a venipuncture. **Pain** is commonly associated with needles, and although the pain experienced during venipuncture is usually mild, on a rare occasion the needle may strike a nerve, causing permanent pain. Some patients experience a **vasovagal reaction** during the venipuncture procedure, evidenced by sweating, low blood pressure, fainting, or near fainting. The potential for a **fall injury** is a significant concern related to vasovagal reactions. Prolonged **bleeding** is a complication that occurs with patients who are taking blood thinners or who have coagulopathies such as hemophilia. A **hematoma** results when blood leaks into the tissue during or after a venipuncture, as evidenced by pain, bruising, and/or swelling at the venipuncture site. The swelling can cause injury by compression to surrounding nerves, which can be temporary or permanent. HCPs should watch for minor complications such as bruising and hematoma at the venipuncture site, which are fairly common. Hematomas occur more often in older adult or frail patients, or those with veins that are difficult to access. Bleeding or bruising can be prevented once the needle has been removed by applying direct pressure to the site with dry gauze for a minute or two. Some other more unusual complications of venipuncture include **cellulitis, phlebitis, inadvertent arterial puncture,** and **sepsis.** Sepsis can be caused by introduction of bacteria from the surface of the skin into the blood as the result of improper cleansing of the venipuncture site. Immunocompromised patients are at higher risk for developing this complication.

Related Tests

Related tests include bone scan, bronchoscopy, CBC, cultures (fungal, mycobacteria, throat, sputum, viral), CSF analysis, ESR, gallium scan, Gram stain, HIV-1/2 antibodies, MRI musculoskeletal, procalcitonin, PFT, radiography bone, and TB tests.

Refer to the Immune System table at the end of the book for related tests by body system.

Expected Outcomes

Expected outcomes associated with Culture, Bacterial, Blood, Culture are:

- Understanding to report changes that may indicate infection, such as fever, dizziness, and tachycardia
- Having urinary output that remains baseline normal
- Being compliant with the administration of appropriate medication to eliminate the infection, with a subsequent improvement in the patient's health status
- Verbalizing an understanding of the signs and symptoms of infection that are important to immediately report to the HCP
- Verbalizing an understanding of the risks and benefits of available immunizations

Immunoglobulin E

Quick Summary

SYNONYM ACRONYM: IgE.

COMMON USE: To assess immunoglobulin E (IgE) levels in order to identify the presence of an allergic or inflammatory immune response.

SPECIMEN: Serum collected in a gold-, red-, or red/gray-top tube. Place separated serum into a standard transport tube within 2 hours of collection.

NORMAL FINDINGS: (Method: Immunoassay)

Age	Conventional & SI Units
Newborn	Less than 12 International Units/L
Less than 1 yr	Less than 50 International Units/L
2–4 yr	Less than 200 International Units/L
5–9 yr	Less than 300 International Units/L
10 yr and older	Less than 100 International Units/L

Test Explanation

Immunoglobulin E (IgE) is an antibody whose primary response is to allergic reactions and parasitic infections. Most of the body's IgE is bound to specialized tissue cells; little is available in the circulating blood. IgE binds to the membrane of special granulocytes called *basophils* in the circulating blood and *mast cells* in the tissues. Basophil and mast cell membranes have receptors for IgE. Mast cells are abundant in the skin and the tissues lining the respiratory and alimentary tracts. When IgE antibody becomes cross-linked with antigen/allergen, the release of histamine, heparin, and other chemicals from the granules in the cells is triggered. A sequence of events follows activation of IgE that affects smooth muscle contraction, vascular permeability, and inflammatory reactions. The inflammatory response allows proteins from the bloodstream to enter the tissues. Helminths (worm parasites) are especially susceptible to immunoglobulin-mediated cytotoxic chemicals. The inflammatory reaction proteins attract macrophages from the circulatory system and granulocytes, such as eosinophils, from circulation and bone marrow. Eosinophils also contain enzymes effective against the parasitic invaders.

A nasal smear can be examined for the presence of eosinophils to screen for allergic conditions. Either a single smear or smears of nasal secretions from each side of the nose should be submitted, at room temperature, for Hansel staining and evaluation. Normal findings vary by laboratory but generally, greater than 10% to 15% is considered eosinophilia or increased presence of eosonophils. Results may be invalid for patients already taking local or systemic corticosteroids.

Nursing Implications

Assessment

Indications	Potential Nursing Problems
Assist in the evaluation of allergy and parasitic infection	• Airway • Anxiety • Breathing • Fear • Gastrointestinal • Human Response • Role Performance • Skin (*associated with itching, rash, and hives*) • Socialization

Diagnosis: Clinical Significance of Test Results

INCREASED IN

Conditions involving allergic reactions or infections that stimulate production of IgE.

- Alcoholism (*alcohol may play a role in the development of environmentally instigated IgE-mediated hypersensitivity*)
- Allergy
- Asthma
- Bronchopulmonary aspergillosis
- Dermatitis
- Eczema
- Hay fever
- IgE myeloma
- Parasitic infestation
- Rhinitis
- Sinusitis
- Wiskott-Aldrich syndrome

DECREASED IN

- Advanced carcinoma (*related to generalized decrease in immune system response*)
- Agammaglobulinemia (*related to decreased production*)
- Ataxia-telangiectasia (*evidenced by familial immunodeficiency disorder*)
- IgE deficiency

Planning

Considerations for planning a successful partnership should include clear communication of what to expect during the test to decrease anxiety and improve cooperation. Before the procedure is performed, plan to review the steps with the patient. Address concerns about pain, and explain that there may be some discomfort during the venipuncture.

SPECIAL CONSIDERATIONS

An important aspect of planning is understanding the factors that may alter study findings or cause abnormal results. Interdepartmental communication is a key factor in the planning process. It should be noted when planning for this study that normal IgE levels do not eliminate allergic disorders as a possible diagnosis.

It is also important to understand which medications or substances the patient may be exposed to in the health-care setting that can interfere with accurate testing:

- Drugs that may cause a decrease in IgE levels include phenytoin and tryptophan.

Implementation

Patient education is key to obtaining the patient's cooperation in following directions, and providing an explanation for the purpose of the procedure is an important part of this process. Inform the patient that this study can assist in identification of an allergic or inflammatory response. Perform the venipuncture.

Evaluation

Recognize anxiety related to test results. Acute hypersensitivity reactions are very frightening. Educate the patient with allergies to recognize signs of anaphylaxis. The patient should be encouraged to discuss interventions appropriate for her or his specific allergy with the health-care provider (HCP). Instruct the patient in the use of an Epipen, if appropriate.

NUTRITIONAL CONSIDERATIONS

Consideration should be given to diet if the patient has food allergies.

Discuss the use of a medical ID allergy alert band if appropriate. Teach the patient ways to recognize risk factors. For example, advise a patient with a food allergy to ask about the preparation of menu items as some foods may be prepared with oils containing the allergen and to pay close attention to food labels; advise the patient with an allergy to bee venom to avoid wearing perfumes when outside as they may attract insects.

Critical Findings

N/A

Study Specific Complications

There are a number of complications associated with performing a venipuncture. **Pain** is commonly associated with needles, and although the pain experienced during venipuncture is usually mild, on a rare occasion the needle may strike a nerve, causing permanent pain. Some patients experience a **vasovagal reaction** during the venipuncture procedure, evidenced by sweating, low blood pressure, fainting, or near fainting. The potential for a **fall injury** is a significant concern related to vasovagal reactions. Prolonged **bleeding** is a complication that occurs with patients who are taking blood thinners or who have coagulopathies such as hemophilia. A **hematoma** results when blood leaks into the tissue during or after a venipuncture, as evidenced by pain, bruising, and/or swelling at the venipuncture site. The swelling can cause injury by compression to surrounding nerves, which can be temporary or permanent. HCPs should watch for minor complications such as bruising and hematoma at the venipuncture site, which are fairly common. Hematomas occur more often in older adult or frail patients, or those with veins that are difficult to access. Bleeding or bruising can be prevented once the needle has been removed by applying direct pressure to the site with dry gauze for a minute or two. Some other more unusual complications of venipuncture include **cellulitis, phlebitis, inadvertent arterial puncture,** and **sepsis.** Sepsis can be caused by introduction of bacteria from the surface of the skin into the blood as the result of improper cleansing of the venipuncture site. Immunocompromised patients are at higher risk for developing this complication.

Related Tests

Related tests include allergen-specific IgE, alveolar/arterial gradient, biopsy intestine, biopsy liver, biopsy muscle, blood gases, carbon dioxide, CBC, CBC platelet count, CBC WBC count and differential, eosinophil count, fecal analysis, hypersensitivity pneumonitis, lung perfusion scan, and PFT.

Refer to the Immune and Respiratory systems tables at the end of the book for related tests by body system.

Expected Outcomes

Expected outcomes associated with Immunoglobulin E are:

- No evidence of air hunger with respiratory effort
- Respiratory rate that remains within normal limits, with no nasal flare or the use of accessory muscles
- Verbalization of an understanding of his or her allergy, allergy triggers, and the lifestyle changes required to successfully live with the condition

Lupus Anticoagulant Antibodies

Quick Summary

SYNONYM ACRONYM: Lupus inhibitor phospholipid type, lupus antiphospholipid antibodies, LA.

COMMON USE: To assess for systemic dysfunction related to anticoagulation and assist in diagnosing conditions such as lupus erythematosus and fetal loss.

SPECIMEN: Plasma collected in a completely filled blue-top (3.2% sodium citrate) tube. If the patient's hematocrit exceeds 55%, the volume of citrate in the collection tube must be adjusted.

NORMAL FINDINGS: (Method: Dilute Russell viper venom test time) Negative.

Test Explanation

Lupus anticoagulant (LA) antibodies are immunoglobulins, usually of the immunoglobulin G class. They are also called lupus antiphospholipid antibodies because they interfere with phospholipid-dependent coagulation tests such as activated partial thromboplastin time (aPTT) by reacting with the phospholipids in the test system. They are not associated with a bleeding disorder unless thrombocytopenia or antiprothrombin antibodies are already present. They are associated with an increased risk of thrombosis. The combination of noninflammatory thrombosis of blood vessels, low platelet count, and history of miscarriage is termed *antiphospholipid antibody syndrome* and is confirmed by the presence of at least one of the clinical criteria (vascular thrombosis confirmed by histopathology or imaging studies; pregnancy morbidity defined as either one or more unexplained deaths of a morphologically normal fetus at or beyond the 10th week of gestation, one or more premature births of a morphologically normal neonate before the 34th week of gestation due to eclampsia or severe pre-eclampsia, or three or more unexplained consecutive spontaneous abortions before the 10th week of gestation) and one of the laboratory criteria (ACA, IgG, or IgM, detectable at greater than 40 units on two or more occasions at least 12 weeks apart; or LA detectable on two or more occasions at least 12 weeks apart; or anti-β_2 glycoprotein 1 antibody, IgG, or IgM, detectable on two or more occasions at least 12 weeks apart, all measured by a standardized ELISA, according to recommended procedures).

Nursing Implications
Assessment

Indications	Potential Nursing Problems
Evaluate prolonged aPTT Investigate reasons for fetal death	• Activity • Body Image • Bleeding Risk *(related to thrombocytopenia)* • Fatigue • Fear *(related to miscarriage risk or premature birth)* • Health Management • Human Responses • Pain *(related to oxygen deficit in the occluded organ or blood vessel)* • Protection • Risk for Thrombosis • Socialization • Tissue Perfusion *(related to thrombus risk)*

Diagnosis: Clinical Significance of Test Results
POSITIVE FINDINGS IN
- Antiphospholipid antibody syndrome *(LA are nonspecific antibodies associated with this syndrome)*
- Fetal loss *(thrombosis associated with LA can form clots that lodge in the placenta and disrupt nutrition to the fetus)*
- Raynaud disease *(LA can be detected with this condition and can cause vascular inflammation)*
- Rheumatoid arthritis *(LA can be detected with this condition and can cause vascular inflammation)*
- Systemic lupus erythematosus *(related to formation of thrombi as a result of LA binding to phospholipids on cell walls)*
- Thromboembolism *(related to formation of thrombi as a result of LA binding to phospholipids on cell walls)*

NEGATIVE FINDINGS IN
N/A

Planning
Considerations for planning a successful partnership should include clear communication of what to expect during the test to decrease anxiety and improve cooperation. Before the procedure is performed, plan to review the steps with the patient. Address concerns about pain, and explain that there may be some discomfort during the venipuncture. Heparin therapy should be discontinued 2 days before specimen collection and Coumarin therapy should be discontinued 2 weeks before specimen collection, with medical direction.

SPECIAL CONSIDERATIONS
An important aspect of planning is understanding the factors that may alter study findings or cause abnormal results. Interdepartmental communication is a key factor in the planning process.

It is also important to understand which medications or substances the patient may be exposed to in the healthcare setting that can interfere with accurate testing:

- Drugs that may cause a positive LA test result include calcium channel blockers, chlorpromazine, heparin, hydralazine, hydantoin, isoniazid, methyldopa, phenytoin, phenothiazine, procainamide, quinine, quinidine, and Thorazine.

Implementation
Patient education is key to obtaining the patient's cooperation in following directions, and providing an explanation for the purpose of the procedure is an important part of this process. Inform the patient that this study can assist in the evaluation of antiphospholipid syndrome and thrombosis (the formation of blood clots). Perform the venipuncture.

When multiple specimens are drawn, the blue-top tube should be collected after sterile (i.e., blood culture) tubes. Otherwise, when using a standard vacutainer system, the blue-top tube is the first tube collected. When a butterfly is used, due to the added tubing, an extra red-top tube should be collected before the blue-top tube to ensure complete filling of the blue-top tube. The Clinical and Laboratory Standards Institute (CLSI) recommendation for processed and unprocessed samples stored in unopened tubes is that testing should be completed within 1 to 4 hours of collection.

Evaluation
Recognize anxiety related to test results and offer support. Provide teaching and information regarding the clinical implications of the test results as appropriate. It is also important to discuss feelings the mother and father may experience (e.g., guilt, depression, anger) if test results are abnormal. Educate the patient regarding access to counseling services. Provide contact information, if desired, for the Lupus Foundation of America (www.lupus.org). Explain that follow-up testing may

be required if anticoagulant therapy (aspirin, heparin, or warfarin) is ordered.

✓ Critical Findings

N/A

✓ Study Specific Complications

There are a number of complications associated with performing a venipuncture. **Pain** is commonly associated with needles and, although the pain experienced during venipuncture is usually mild, on a rare occasion the needle may strike a nerve, causing permanent pain. Some patients experience a **vasovagal reaction** during the venipuncture procedure, evidenced by sweating, low blood pressure, fainting, or near fainting. The potential for a **fall injury** is a significant concern related to vasovagal reactions. Prolonged **bleeding** is a complication that occurs with patients who are taking blood thinners or who have coagulopathies such as hemophilia. A **hematoma** results when blood leaks into the tissue during or after a venipuncture, as evidenced by pain, bruising, and/or swelling at the venipuncture site. The swelling can cause injury by compression to surrounding nerves, which can be temporary or permanent. Health-care providers should watch for minor complications such as bruising and hematoma at the venipuncture site, which are fairly common. Hematomas occur more often in older adult or frail patients, or those with veins that are difficult to access. Bleeding or bruising can be prevented once the needle has been removed by applying direct pressure to the site with dry gauze for a minute or two. Some other more unusual complications of venipuncture include **cellulitis, phlebitis, inadvertent arterial puncture,** and **sepsis.** Sepsis can be caused by introduction of bacteria from the surface of the skin into the blood as the result of improper cleansing of the venipuncture site. Immunocompromised patients are at higher risk for developing this complication.

✓ Related Tests

Related tests include antibody, anticardioligpin antibodies, anticyclic citrullinated peptide, ANA, arthroscopy, BMD, bone scan, CRP, ESR, FDP, MRI musculoskeletal, aPTT, protein S, PT/INR and mixing studies, radiography bone, RF, synovial fluid analysis, and US obstetric.

Refer to the Hematopoietic, Immune, Musculoskeletal, and Reproductive systems tables at the end of the book for related tests by body system.

Expected Outcomes

Expected outcomes associated with Lupus Anticoagulant Antibodies are:

- Acknowledging the relationship between fatigue and disease pathophysiology
- Identifying ways to reduce fatigue

- Being compliant with anticoagulant therapy and monitoring in order to prevent thrombosis
- Noting that the pregnant patient is provided with early identification and treatment for improved maternal and fetal/neonatal outcome by preventing fetal loss, pre-eclampsia, placental insufficiency, or premature birth

Prostate-Specific Antigen

Quick Summary

SYNONYM ACRONYM: PSA.

COMMON USE: To assess prostate health and assist in diagnosis of disorders such as prostate cancer, inflammation, and benign tumor and to evaluate effectiveness of medical and surgical therapeutic interventions.

SPECIMEN: Serum collected in a gold-, red-, or red/gray-top tube.

NORMAL FINDINGS: (Method: Immunoassay)

Gender	Free PSA ng/mL	Total PSA Conventional Units ng/mL [SI Units mcg/L (Conventional Units x 1)]		
Male (Ages)		Caucasians	African Americans	Asians
40–49 years	0–0.5	0–2.5	0–2	0–2
50–59 years	0–0.7	0–3.5	0–4	0–3
60–69 years	0–1	0–4.5	0–4.5	0–4
70 years and older	0–1.2	0–6.5	0–5.5	0–5
Post-radical prostatectomy (30–60 days)	Less than 0.1			
Female	Less than 0.5			

Test Explanation

Prostate-specific antigen (PSA) is produced exclusively by the epithelial cells of the prostate, periurethral, and perirectal glands. Used in conjunction with the digital rectal examination (DRE), PSA is a useful test for identifying and monitoring cancer of the prostate. Risk of diagnosis is higher in African American men, who are 61% more likely than Caucasian men to develop prostate cancer. Family history and age at diagnosis are other strong correlating factors. PSA circulates in both free and bound (complexed) forms. A low ratio of free to total PSA (i.e., less than 10%) is suggestive of prostate cancer; a ratio of greater than 30% is rarely associated with prostate cancer. PSA velocity, the rate of PSA increase over time, is being used to identify the potential aggressiveness of the cancer.

Estimated Risk for developing prostate cancer in men with a slightly elevated total PSA (between 4 and 10 ng/mL mcg/L).

Free PSA (%)	Probability of developing prostate cancer
Greater than 30%	8–20%
21–30%	16–19%
11–20%	20–25%
1–10%	40–50%
PSA velocity ng/mL	
Change of less than 0.75 per year	Low
Change of greater than 0.75 per year	Suspicious

Approximately 15% to 40% of patients who have had their prostate removed will encounter an increase in PSA. Patients treated for prostate cancer and who have had a PSA recurrence can still develop a metastasis for as long as 8 years after the postsurgical PSA level increased. The majority of prostate tumors develop slowly and require minimal intervention, but patients with an increase in PSA greater than 2 ng/mL in a year are more likely to have an aggressive form of prostate cancer with a greater risk of death.

The Prostate Health Index (PHI) is another multimarker strategy being used to improve the positive prediction rate of prostate cancer, especially when PSA levels are considered to be moderately increased (between 4 and 10 ng/mL). The PHI applies information provided by the results of prostate marker blood tests to a mathematical formula and offers additional information for clinical decision making. The three tests used in the formula are the total PSA, free PSA, and p2PSA (an isoform of PSA) where: PHI = p2PSA/(free PSA × total PSA). PHI less than 27% has a relatively low probability for prostate cancer, PHI between 27% and 55% predict a moderate probability for prostate cancer, and PHI greater than 55% has an increased risk for prostate cancer.

Personalized medicine provides a technology to predict the progression of prostate cancer, likelihood of recurrence, or development of related metastatic disease. New technology makes it possible to combine data such as analysis of molecular biomarkers and cellular structure specific to the individual's biopsy tissue, standard tissue biopsy results, Gleason score, number of positive tumor cores, tumor stage, presurgical and postsurgical PSA levels, and postsurgical margin status with computerized mathematical programs to create a personalized report that predicts the likelihood of post-prostatectomy disease progression. Serial measurements of PSA in the blood are often performed before and after surgery.

PSA is also produced in females, most notably in breast tissue. There is some evidence that elevated PSA levels in breast cancer patients are associated with positive estrogen and progesterone status.

Important note: When following patients using serial testing, the same method of measurement should be consistently used.

Nursing Implications
Assessment

Indications	Potential Nursing Problems
Evaluate the effectiveness of treatment for prostate cancer (prostatectomy): Levels decrease if treatment is effective; rising levels are associated with recurrence and a poor prognosis Investigate or evaluate an enlarged prostate gland, especially if prostate cancer is suspected Stage prostate cancer	• Fatigue *(related to exhaustion from treatment or the disease progression)* • Fear *(related to a potential diagnosis of cancer)* • Health Management • Human Response • Pain *(related to treatment or the disease progression)* • Role Performance • Sexuality *(Sexual dysfunction related to surgery, chemotherapy, or radiation therapy)* • Urination *(dysfunction related to obstruction due to prostate enlargement or tumor)*

Diagnosis: Clinical Significance of Test Results
INCREASED IN
A breach in the protective barrier between the prostatic lumen and the bloodstream due to significant disease will allow measurable levels of circulating PSA.

• Benign prostatic hypertrophy
• Prostate cancer
• Prostatic infarct
• Prostatitis
• Urinary retention

DECREASED IN
N/A

Planning
Considerations for planning a successful partnership should include clear communication of what to expect during the test to decrease anxiety and improve cooperation. Before the procedure is performed, plan to review the steps with the patient. Address concerns about pain and explain that there may be some discomfort during the venipuncture.

SPECIAL CONSIDERATIONS
An important aspect of planning is understanding the factors that may alter study findings or cause abnormal results. Interdepartmental communication is a key

factor in the planning process. The following should be noted when planning for this study:

- Increases may occur if ejaculation occurs within 24 hours prior to specimen collection.
- Increases can occur due to prostatic needle biopsy, cystoscopy, or prostatic infarction either by undergoing catheterization or the presence of an indwelling catheter; therefore, specimens should be collected prior to or 6 weeks after the procedure.
- There is conflicting information regarding the effect of DRE on PSA values, and some health-care providers (HCPs) may specifically request specimen collection prior to DRE.

It is also important to understand which medications or substances the patient may be exposed to in the health-care setting that can interfere with accurate testing:

- Drugs that decrease PSA levels include buserelin, dutasteride, finasteride, and flutamide.

Implementation

Patient education is key to obtaining the patient's cooperation in following directions, and providing an explanation for the purpose of the procedure is an important part of this process. Inform the patient that this study can assist in assessing prostate health. Perform the venipuncture.

Evaluation

Recognize anxiety related to test results and offer support. Counsel the patient, as appropriate, that sexual dysfunction related to altered body function, drugs, or radiation may occur. Discuss the implications of abnormal test results on the patient's lifestyle. Provide teaching and information regarding the clinical implications of the test results as appropriate. Educate the patient regarding access to counseling services. Decisions regarding the need for and frequency of routine PSA testing or other cancer screening procedures should be made after consultation between the patient and the HCP. Recommendations made by various medical associations and national health organizations regarding prostate cancer screening are moving away from routine PSA screening and toward informed decision making. The American Cancer Society's guidelines recommend that discussions about screening should begin at age 50 years for men at average risk, 45 years for men at high risk, and 40 years for men at the highest risk of developing prostate cancer. The most current guidelines for prostate cancer screening of the general population as well as of individuals with increased risk are available from the American Cancer Society (www.cancer.org) and the American Urological Association (www.aua.org).

SPECIAL CONSIDERATIONS
NUTRITIONAL CONSIDERATIONS

Assess nutritional status. There is growing evidence that inflammation and oxidation play key roles in the development of numerous diseases, including prostate cancer. Research also indicates that diets containing dried beans, fresh fruits and vegetables, nuts, spices, whole grains, and smaller amounts of red meats can increase the amount of protective antioxidants.

Assess for factors that cause limited mobility (e.g., pain, fatigue, nutritional deficit). Regular exercise, especially in combination with a healthy diet, can bring about changes in the body's metabolism that decrease inflammation and oxidation. Involve family in helping the patient with range-of-motion exercises, positioning, and walking. Encourage the use of assistive devices such as canes and walkers for patients with limited mobility. Describe ways the patient can regain good bladder control, including urinating at frequent intervals (every 2 to 3 hours), voiding in an upright position, stopping the intake of fluids at a certain point in the evening to avoid frequent voiding at night, and avoiding the consumption of caffeinated beverages. Instruct the patient regarding catheter care, if applicable. Patients receiving opioid medications for pain should receive instructions about strategies to prevent constipation. Encourage the patient to discuss alternative approaches and methods of sexual expression with the appropriate HCP. Educate the post-prostatectomy patient about ways to reduce pressure on the operative area, including avoiding prolonged sitting, standing, walking, or straining.

✓ Critical Findings

N/A

✓ Study Specific Complications

There are a number of complications associated with performing a venipuncture. **Pain** is commonly associated with needles, and although the pain experienced during venipuncture is usually mild, on a rare occasion the needle may strike a nerve, causing permanent pain. Some patients experience a **vasovagal reaction** during the venipuncture procedure, evidenced by sweating, low blood pressure, fainting, or near fainting. The potential for a **fall injury** is a significant concern related to vasovagal reactions. Prolonged **bleeding** is a complication that occurs with patients who are taking blood thinners or who have coagulopathies such as hemophilia. A **hematoma** results when blood leaks into the tissue during or after a venipuncture, as evidenced by pain, bruising, and/or swelling at the venipuncture site. The swelling can cause injury by compression to surrounding nerves, which can be temporary or permanent. HCPs should watch for minor complications such as bruising and hematoma at the venipuncture site, which are fairly common. Hematomas occur more often in older adult or frail patients, or those with veins that are difficult to access. Bleeding or bruising can be prevented once the needle has been removed by applying direct pressure to the site with dry gauze for a minute or two. Some other more unusual complications of venipuncture include **cellulitis, phlebitis, inadvertent arterial puncture,** and **sepsis.** Sepsis can be caused by introduction of bacteria from the surface of the skin into the blood as the result of improper cleansing of the venipuncture site. Immunocompromised patients are at higher risk for developing this complication.

✓ *Related Tests*

Related tests include biopsy prostate (with Gleason score), cystoscopy, cystourethrography voiding, PAP, retrograde ureteropyelography, semen analysis, and US prostate.

Refer to the Genitourinary System table at the end of the book for related tests by body system.

Expected Outcomes

Expected outcomes associated with PSA are:

- Expressing fear in realistic terms regarding a diagnosis of cancer
- Verbalizing an understanding of the illness, treatment options, and lifestyle changes required to cope with the condition
- Not having complications such as hemorrhage, infection, or obstruction of the bladder neck, and being able to name the signs or symptoms that must be reported to the HCP, such as bloody urine, passing blood clots, pain or burning near the catheter, urinary frequency, decreased urinary output, or an increased loss of bladder control
- Successfully regaining bladder control and noting the absence of urinary frequency, urgency, or bladder fullness
- Where applicable, demonstrating a satisfactory technique and understanding of catheter care; the patient does not develop an infection or report pain around the catheter
- Being compliant with the medication regimen, avoiding activities that aggravate or increase pain, and achieving good pain control
- Reporting improved physical and sexual activity

Syphilis Serology

Quick Summary

SYNONYM ACRONYM: Automated reagin testing (ART), fluorescent treponemal antibody testing (FTA-ABS), microhemagglutination–*Treponema pallidum* (MHA-TP), rapid plasma reagin (RPR), treponemal studies, Venereal Disease Research Laboratory (VDRL) testing.

COMMON USE: To indicate past or present syphilis infection.

SPECIMEN: Serum collected in a gold-, red-, or red/gray-top tube. Place separated serum into a standard transport tube within 2 hours of collection.

NORMAL FINDINGS: (Method: Dark-field microscopy, rapid plasma reagin, enzyme-linked immunosorbent assay [ELISA], microhemagglutination, fluorescence) Nonreactive or absence of treponemal organisms.

Test Explanation

Syphilis is a sexually transmitted infection (STI) with three stages. On average, symptoms start within 3 weeks of infection but can appear as soon as 10 days or as late as 90 days after infection. The primary stage of syphilis is usually marked by the appearance of a single sore, called a chancre, at the site where the organism entered the body. The chancre is small and round in appearance, is firm, and is usually painless. The chancre lasts 3 to 6 weeks and heals with or without treatment. If untreated, the infection progresses to the secondary stage as the chancre is healing or several weeks after the chancre has healed. The secondary stage is characterized by a skin rash and lesions of the mucous membranes. Other symptoms may include fever, swollen lymph glands, sore throat, patchy hair loss, headaches, weight loss, muscle aches, and fatigue. As with the primary stage, the signs and symptoms of secondary syphilis will resolve either with or without treatment. If untreated, the infection will progress to the latent or hidden stage in which the infection and ability to transmit infection is present even though the infected person is asymptomatic. The latent stage begins when the primary and secondary symptoms disappear, and it can last for years. About 15% of people in the latent stage, who have not been treated, will develop late-stage syphilis, which can appear 10 to 20 years after infection. Untreated disease at this stage can result in significant damage to the brain, nerves, eyes, heart, blood vessels, liver, bones, and joints—damage serious enough to cause death. Signs and symptoms of the late stage of syphilis include difficulty coordinating muscle movements, numbness, paralysis, blindness, and dementia.

There are numerous methods for detecting *Treponema pallidum*, the gram-negative spirochete bacterium known to cause syphilis. Syphilis serology is routinely ordered as part of a prenatal work-up and is required for evaluating donated blood units before release for transfusion. Selection of the proper testing method is important. Automated reagin testing (ART), rapid plasma reagin (RPR), and Venereal Disease Research Laboratory (VDRL) testing have traditionally been used for screening purposes. These nontreponemal assays detect antibodies directed against lipoidal antigens from damaged host cells. Nontreponemal assays can produce false-positive results, which are associated with older age or conditions unrelated to syphilis, such as autoimmune disorders or injection drug use, and require confirmation by a treponemal test method. Fluorescent treponemal antibody testing (FTA-ABS), microhemagglutination–*T. pallidum* (MHA-TP), and *T. pallidum* by particle agglutination (TP-PA) are confirmatory methods for samples that screen positive or reactive. Some laboratories have begun using a reverse-screening approach. Highly automated, rapid-testing treponemal enzyme immunoassays (EIA) and chemiluminescent assays (CIA) detect antibodies directed against *T. pallidum* proteins. These assays detect early primary infections as well as past treated infections. The problem with the EIAs and CIAs is that they are very sensitive but less specific; therefore, positive test results should be confirmed using a nontreponemal assay. If reverse screening is used, the Centers for Disease Control and Prevention recommends (1) positive EIA/CIA be confirmed using the RPR, and reactive RPR test results should be reported as the endpoint titer of reactivity; (2) a positive EIA/CIA followed by a nonreactive RPR should be tested by a direct treponemal assay such as the TP-PA or FTA-ABS to ensure a false-positive result is not reported and acted upon. Cerebrospinal fluid should be tested only by the FTA-ABS method. Cord blood should not be submitted for testing by any of the aforementioned methods; instead, the mother's serum should be tested to establish whether the infant should be treated.

Nursing Implications
Assessment

Indications	Potential Nursing Problems
Monitor effectiveness of treatment for syphilis Screen for and confirm the presence of syphilis	• Confusion **(related to brain damage in the latent period of the disease)** • Fear **(related to fetal infection in birth with associated deafness and deformities)** • Health Management • Human Response • Sensory Perception **(related to nerve damage in the latent period of the disease)** • Sexuality • Skin **(related to chancre sores and rash)**

Diagnosis: Clinical Significance of Test Results
POSITIVE FINDING IN
SYPHILIS

False-positive or false-reactive findings in screening (RPR, VDRL) tests

INFECTIOUS

- Bacterial endocarditis
- Chancroid
- Chickenpox
- HIV
- Infectious mononucleosis
- Leprosy

- Leptospirosis
- Lymphogranuloma venereum
- Malaria
- Measles
- Mumps
- Mycoplasma pneumonia
- Pneumococcal pneumonia
- Psittacosis
- Relapsing fever
- Rickettsial disease
- Scarlet fever
- Trypanosomiasis
- Tuberculosis
- Vaccinia (live or attenuated)
- Viral hepatitis

NONINFECTIOUS

- Advanced cancer
- Advancing age
- Chronic liver disease
- Connective tissue diseases
- IV drug use
- Multiple blood transfusions
- Multiple myeloma and other immunological disorders
- Narcotic addiction

PREGNANCY

False-positive or false-reactive findings in confirmatory (FTA-ABS, MHA-TP) tests

INFECTIOUS

- Infectious mononucleosis
- Leprosy
- Leptospirosis
- Lyme disease
- Malaria
- Relapsing fever

NONINFECTIOUS

- Systemic lupus erythematosus

False-positive findings in confirmatory (TP-PA) tests

INFECTIOUS

- Pinta
- Yaws

NEGATIVE FINDINGS IN
N/A

Planning
Considerations for planning a successful partnership should include clear communication of what to expect during the test to decrease anxiety and improve cooperation. Before the procedure is performed, plan to review the steps with the patient. Address concerns

about pain, and explain that there may be some discomfort during the venipuncture. Obtain a history of exposure.

SPECIAL CONSIDERATIONS

An important aspect of planning is understanding the factors that may alter study findings or cause abnormal results. Interdepartmental communication is a key factor in the planning process.

Implementation

Patient education is key to obtaining the patient's cooperation in following directions, and providing an explanation for the purpose of the procedure is an important part of this process. Inform the patient this study can assist in diagnosing syphilis. Perform the venipuncture.

Evaluation

Recognize anxiety related to test results and offer support. Counsel the patient, as appropriate, regarding the risk of transmission and proper prophylaxis, and reinforce the importance of strict adherence to the treatment regimen. Inform the patient that positive findings must be reported to local health department officials, who will question him or her regarding sexual partners. Provide teaching and information regarding the clinical implications of the test results as appropriate. Inform the patient that repeat testing may be needed at 3-month intervals for 1 year to monitor the effectiveness of treatment. Provide information regarding vaccine-preventable diseases where indicated (e.g., hepatitis A and B, HPV). Provide contact information, if desired, for the CDC (www.cdc.gov/vaccines/vpd-vac).

Offer support, as appropriate, to patients who may be the victim of rape or sexual assault. Educate the patient regarding access to counseling services. Provide a nonjudgmental, nonthreatening atmosphere for a discussion during which risks of sexually transmitted infections are explained. It is also important to discuss problems the patient may experience (e.g., guilt, depression, anger).

✔ Critical Findings

N/A

✔ Study Specific Complications

There are a number of complications associated with performing a venipuncture. **Pain** is commonly associated with needles and although the pain experienced during venipuncture is usually mild, on a rare occasion the needle may strike a nerve, causing permanent pain. Some patients experience a **vasovagal reaction** during the venipuncture procedure, evidenced by sweating, low blood pressure, fainting, or near fainting. The potential for a **fall injury** is a significant concern related to vasovagal reactions. Prolonged **bleeding** is a complication that occurs with patients who are taking blood thinners or who have coagulopathies such as hemophilia. A **hematoma** results when blood leaks into

the tissue during or after a venipuncture, as evidenced by pain, bruising, and/or swelling at the venipuncture site. The swelling can cause injury by compression to surrounding nerves, which can be temporary or permanent. Health-care providers should watch for minor complications such as bruising and hematoma at the venipuncture site, which are fairly common. Hematomas occur more often in older adult or frail patients, or those with veins that are difficult to access. Bleeding or bruising can be prevented once the needle has been removed by applying direct pressure to the site with dry gauze for a minute or two. Some other more unusual complications of venipuncture include **cellulitis, phlebitis, inadvertent arterial puncture,** and **sepsis.** Sepsis can be caused by introduction of bacteria from the surface of the skin into the blood as the result of improper cleansing of the venipuncture site. Immunocompromised patients are at higher risk for developing this complication.

✔ Related Tests

- Related tests include acid phosphatase, cerebrospinal fluid analysis, *Chlamydia* group antibody, culture bacterial anal, Gram stain, hepatitis B, hepatitis C, HIV, and β_2-microglobulin.
- Refer to the Immune and Reproductive systems tables at the end of the book for related tests by body system.

Expected Outcomes

Expected outcomes associated with Syphilis Serology are:

- Describing how to self-check for chancre sores associated with the disease
- Agreeing to adapt sexual encounters to prevent infecting others
- Being compliant with the treatment regimen and reporting resolution of the associated signs and symptoms

REVIEW OF LEARNING OUTCOMES

Thinking

1. Name the two types of immune response. Answer: There are two main categories of immune response: (1) cell-mediated response and (2) humoral response.
2. Name the white blood cell (WBC) type whose primary function is involved in the immune response. Answer: Lymphocytes are the primary WBC involved in the immune response. Lymphocytes are divided into two major categories based on their immunologic activity: T lymphocytes are responsible for cell-mediated immune response, and B lymphocytes are responsible for the humoral immune response by way of antibody production.

3. Describe some examples of how the immune system functions to protect the body from invasion by foreign elements that range from microorganisms and allergens to chemical toxins, modified proteins, transfusion reactions, and transplanted organs. Answer: Regarding cell-mediated responses, two subsets of cytotoxic T lymphocytes, helper T cells and suppressor T cells, have been identified that balance cell-mediated activities under normal conditions. Helper T cells promote the proliferation of T lymphocytes, stimulate B lymphocyte activity, and activate macrophages. Suppressor T cells limit the magnitude of the immune response. Examples of cell-mediated immune responses that require direct cell contact between the antigen and the lymphocyte include reactions against cells infected by pathogens such as bacteria, viruses, fungi, and protozoa; positive skin tests (e.g., TB); contact dermatitis; solid organ transplant rejection; and the spontaneous destruction of malignant cells. The effects of humoral immunity provide many of the same results accomplished by cell-mediated immune functions and include the elimination of encapsulated bacteria, the neutralization of soluble toxins, and protection from various allergens, viruses, and parasites. IgG is also the most versatile of the immunoglobulins as it can fulfill the role of any of the immunoglobulins from acting as an opsonin by binding to cell membranes in the initiation of phagocytosis to activation of the complement cascade. The large size of the IgM molecule makes it good for impeding movement of foreign elements by agglutination. It is also very efficient in fixing the complement and therefore is very efficient in lysing foreign elements. IgE antibodies are responsible for hypersensitivity reactions described as atopic (allergic) or systemic (anaphylactic). Examples of IgE-mediated allergic diseases include hay fever, asthma, and certain types of eczema.

Doing

1. Discuss the difference between the primary immune response and the secondary immune response. Answer: In both cellular and humoral immune responses, initial exposure to the specific antigens initiates the primary immune response. Depending on the quantity and type of the antigen, it may take days, weeks, or months for the lymphocytes of either the cell-mediated or humoral system to mobilize, neutralize, and eliminate the antigen. The T and B lymphocyte memory cells have been identified. These are cells that retain the ability to recognize antigens for rapid secondary immune response if challenged again after the initial exposure. Subsequent exposure to the same antigen, however, elicits the secondary (anamnestic) response much more rapidly than the primary response.

2. Describe the appropriate assessment of patients with immune system disorders. Answer: The most common types of immune system disorders fall into the categories of infection, allergy, host versus graft, autoimmune, or cancer. Objective assessment includes observation and examination of the patient for swollen or tender lymph nodes, fever, watery eyes, nasal stuffiness, or rash. Questions that might be asked of the patient include:

- Do you have a history of infections or incomplete or poor recovery from infection?
- How would you describe the level of stress in your daily life?
- Are you often fatigued?
- Have you suffered a loss of appetite?
- Would you describe your daily diet?
- Do you have any environmental allergies? Do you have any allergies to foods or medications? If so would you describe any allergic reactions you might have had?
- Are you taking immunosuppressant medications (e.g., drugs used for solid organ transplants, glucocorticoids used for the treatment of autoimmune diseases, and other drugs such as antibodies, interferons, and opioids)?

3. Describe some nursing interventions to care for patients with immune system disorders. Answer: It is important to take steps to reduce exposure to infection. Some suggestions of effective ways to reduce exposure to infection include frequent hand washing, the use of masks, and limiting direct contact with people who are ill. Monitor the patient's temperature and weight, and advise the patient to get adequate rest and to follow instructions for maintaining a healthy diet. Provide education regarding ways to avoid injuries that might provide a portal for infection (e.g., the use of electric razors, awareness of one's surroundings to avoid bumps and scrapes, and proper care of venipuncture sites after blood work is obtained).

Caring

1. Recognize the value of nursing wisdom in relieving physical pain and emotional distress. Answer: Physical pain is not the only way a patient can suffer. The long-range effects of a diagnosis can change a patient's life at every level. Always strive to be in tune with not just the physical pain but the emotional and spiritual pain your patient may be experiencing.

⟨ *Words* OF *Wisdom:* Nursing is a complex profession. We all strive to control our work environment. However, when that environment is centered around a living, breathing human being, control can be an illusion. In the end, the most we can do is to provide information, emotional and spiritual support, and clinical expertise in assisting the patient to meet his or her medical challenges. Collaboration with others, including the family and patient him- or herself is the only path to success. Center your care around your patient's wants and needs with consideration of the patient's individual circumstances. This may be your best approach to meet your goals.

BIBLIOGRAPHY

Cavanaugh, B. (2003). Nurse's manual of laboratory and diagnostic tests. (4th ed.). Philadelphia, PA: F.A. Davis Company.

Mayer, G. (2015). Immunoglobulins—Structure and function. Retrieved from http://www.microbiologybook.org/mayer/IgStruct2000.html

Null cell. (n.d.). Retrieved from www.medical-dictionary.thefreedictionary.com/null+cell

Null cells. (n.d.). Retrieved from www.immunologyden.blogspot.com/2012/11/null-cells.html

Van Leeuwen, A., & Bladh, M. (2015). Davis's comprehensive handbook of laboratory and diagnostic tests with nursing implications. (6th ed.). Philadelphia, PA: F.A. Davis Company.

Woof, J., & Kerr, M. (2006). The function of immunoglobulin A in immunity. Retrieved from www.ncbi.nlm.nih.gov/pubmed/16362985

Yan, H., Lamm, M., Björling, E, & Huang, Y. (2002, November). Multiple functions of immunoglobulin A in mucosal defense against viruses: an in vitro measles virus model. Journal of Virology, 76(21). doi 10.1128/JVI.76.21.10972-10979.2002

Go to Section II of this book and http://www.davisplus.com for the Clinical Reasoning Tool and its case studies to provide you with a safe place to explore patient care situations. There are a total of 26 different case studies; 2 cases are presented for each of 13 body systems. One set of 13 cases are found in the Section II chapters, and a second set of 13 cases are available online at http://www.davisplus.com. Each case is designed with the specific goal of helping you to connect the dots of clinical reasoning. Cases are designed to reflect possible clinical scenarios; the outcomes may or may not be positive—you decide.

Body Fluid Analysis Studies

OVERVIEW

The evaluation of blood, urine, and body fluids provides significant information regarding health and disease status. Body fluid studies are classified as the analysis of any fluid other than blood or urine. This chapter covers cerebrospinal fluid (CSF) analysis collected by lumbar puncture, amniotic fluid analysis collected by amniocentesis, and sputum culture collected by expectoration, tracheal suction, and bronchoscopy.

The collection of body fluids involves needle aspiration from a sterile body space under strict sterile conditions. The amount of fluid obtained depends on factors related to the purpose of the study as well as the minimum volume required for the laboratory to perform the requested studies. Testing should always be performed immediately after collection. This is to ensure that test results are obtained before rapid cellular degradation adversely affects clinical chemistry, hematology, microbiology, serology, or cytology findings. For this reason, body fluid studies are requested as the highest priority or STAT testing. If there is an anticipated delay, review the policy and ensure that preservation guidelines are followed.

The information in the Part I studies is organized in a manner to help the student see how the five basic components of the nursing process (assessment, diagnosis, planning, implementation, and evaluation) can be applied to each phase of laboratory and diagnostic testing. The goal is to use nursing process to understand the integration of care (laboratory, diagnostic, nursing care) toward achieving a positive expected outcome.

- **Assessment** is the collection of information for the purpose of answering the question, "is there a problem?" Knowledge of the patient's health history, medications, complaints, and allergies as well as synonyms or alternate test names, common use for

the procedure, specimen requirements, and normal ranges or interpretive comments provide the foundation for diagnosis.

- **Diagnosis** is the process of looking at the information gathered during assessment and answering the questions, "what is the problem?" and "what do I need to do about it?" Test indications tell us why the study has been requested, and potential diagnoses tell us the value or importance of the study relative to its clinical utility.
- **Planning** is a blueprint of the nursing care before the procedure. It is the process of determining how the nurse is going to partner with the patient to fix the problem (e.g., "The patient has a study ordered and this is what I should know before I successfully carry out the plan to have the study completed"). Knowledge of interfering factors, social and cultural issues, preprocedural restrictions, the need for written and informed consent, anxiety about the procedure, and concerns regarding pain are some considerations for planning a successful partnership.
- **Implementation** is putting the plan into action with an idea of what the expected outcome should be. Collaboration with the departments where the laboratory test or diagnostic study is to be performed is essential to the success of the plan. Implementation is where the work is done within each healthcare team member's scope of practice.
- **Evaluation** answers the question, "did the plan work or not?" Was the plan completely successful, partially successful, or not successful? If the plan did not work, evaluation is the process where you determine what needs to be changed to make the plan work better. This includes a review of all expected outcomes. Nursing care after the procedure is where information is gathered to evaluate the plan. Review of results, including critical findings, in relation to patient symptoms and other tests performed,

provides data that form a more complete picture of health or illness.

- **Expected Outcomes** are positive outcomes related to the test. They are the outcomes the nurse should expect if all goes well.

A number of pretest, intratest, and post-test universal points are presented in this overview section because the information applies to body fluid analysis studies in general.

Universal Pretest Pearls (Planning)

- Obtain a history of the patient's complaints, including a list of known allergens, especially allergies or sensitivities to medications or latex so that their use can be avoided or their effects mitigated if an allergy is present. Carefully evaluate all medications currently being taken by the patient. A list of the patient's current medications, prescribed and over the counter (including anticoagulants, aspirin and other salicylates, and dietary supplements), should also be obtained. Such products may be discontinued by medical direction for the appropriate number of days prior to the procedure. Ensure that all allergies are clearly noted in the medical record, and ensure that the patient is wearing an allergy and medical record armband. Report to the health-care provider (HCP) and laboratory any information that could interfere with or delay proceeding with the study.
- Obtain a history of the patient's affected body system, symptoms, and results of previously performed laboratory tests and diagnostic and surgical procedures. Previous test results will provide a basis of comparison between old and new data.
- An important aspect of planning is understanding the factors that may impair the procedure or cause abnormal results. Interdepartmental communication is a key factor in the planning process. The inability of a patient to cooperate or remain still during the procedure because of age, significant pain, or mental status should be among the anticipated factors. Recent or past procedures, medications, or existing medical conditions that could complicate or interfere with test results should be noted.
- Review the steps of the study with the patient or caregiver. Expect patients to be nervous about the procedure itself and the pending results. Educating the patient about his or her role during the procedure and what to expect can facilitate this. The patient's role during the procedure is to remain still. The actual time required to complete each study will depend on a number of conditions, including the type of equipment being used and how well a patient will cooperate.

- Address any concerns about pain, and explain or describe, as appropriate, the level and type of discomfort that may be expected during the procedure. Explain that an IV line may be inserted prior to some procedures to allow the infusion of fluids such as normal saline or medications. Advise the patient that some discomfort may be experienced during the insertion of the IV. Make the patient aware that there may be some mild discomfort during the procedure.
- Provide additional instructions and patient preparation regarding medication, diet, fluid intake, or activity if appropriate. Unless specified in the individual study, there are no special instructions or restrictions.
- Always be sensitive to any cultural or psychosocial issues, including a concern for modesty before, during, and after the procedure. For example, patients preparing for amniocentesis or lumbar puncture will be instructed to remove their clothes and wear the gown, robe, and slippers provided.

Reminder

Ensure that a written and informed consent has been documented in the medical record prior to the study, if required. The consent must be obtained before medication is administered.

Universal Intratest Pearls (Implementation)

- Correct patient identification is crucial prior to any procedure. Positively identify the patient using two unique identifiers, such as patient name, date of birth, Social Security number, or medical record number.
- Standard Precautions must be followed.
- Children and infants may be accompanied by a parent to calm them. Keep neonates and infants covered and in a warm room and provide a pacifier or gentle touch. The testing environment should be quiet, and the patient should be instructed, as appropriate, to remain still during the test as extraneous movements can affect results.
- Ensure that the patient has complied with pretesting instructions, including dietary, fluid, medication, and activity restrictions as given for the procedure. The number of days to withhold medication depends on the type of medication. Notify the HCP if pretesting instructions have not been followed (e.g., if patient anticoagulant therapy has not been withheld).
- The patient, as appropriate, should be prepared for insertion of an IV line for infusion of fluids, antibiotics, anesthetics, sedatives, analgesics, medications used in the procedure, or emergency medications. Prior to administration of any fluids

or medications, verify that they are accurate for the study. Bleeding or bruising can be prevented, once the needle has been removed, by applying direct pressure to the injection site with dry gauze for a minute or two. The site should be observed/assessed for bleeding or hematoma formation, and then covered with a gauze and adhesive bandage. Inform the patient when prophylactic antibiotics will be administered before the procedure and assess for antibiotic allergy.

- Emergency equipment must be readily available.
- Baseline vital signs must be recorded, and monitoring must continue throughout and after the procedure, according to organizational policy. A comparison should be made between the baseline and postprocedure vital signs and focused assessments. Protocols may vary among facilities.
- After the administration of general or local anesthesia, clippers are used to remove hair from the aspiration site if appropriate. The site is then cleansed with an antiseptic solution, and the area is draped with sterile towels.
- Before leaving the patient's side, appropriate specimen containers should always be labeled with the corresponding patient demographics, the initials of the person collecting the sample, collection date, time of collection, applicable special notes, especially site location and laterality, and then promptly transported to the laboratory for processing and analysis.

These include knowledge deficit, fear, anxiety, and coping; in some situations, grieving may occur. HCPs should always be aware of the human response and how it may affect the plan of care and expected outcomes.

DISCUSSION POINT

Regarding Post-Test Critical Findings: Timely notification of a critical finding for lab or diagnostic studies is a role expectation of the professional nurse. Notification processes will vary among facilities. Upon receipt of the critical finding, the information should be read back to the caller to verify accuracy. Most policies require immediate notification of the primary HCP, hospitalist, or on-call HCP. Reported information includes the patient's name, unique identifiers, critical finding, name of the person giving the report, and name of the person receiving the report. Documentation of notification should be made in the medical record with the name of the HCP notified, time and date of notification, and any orders received. Any delay in a timely report of a critical finding may require completion of a notification form with review by Risk Management.

STUDIES

- Amniotic Fluid Analysis and L/S Ratio
- Cerebrospinal Fluid Analysis
- Culture, Bacterial, Sputum

Universal Post Test Pearls (Evaluation)

- Note that completed test results are made available to the requesting HCP, who will discuss them with the patient.
- Answer questions and address concerns voiced by the patient or family and reinforce information given by the patient's HCP regarding further testing, treatment, or referral to another HCP. Recognize that patients will have anxiety related to test results. Provide teaching and information regarding the clinical implications of the test results on the patients lifestyle as appropriate.
- Note that test results should be evaluated in context with the patient's signs, symptoms, and diagnosis. Depending on the results of the procedure, additional testing may be performed to evaluate or monitor progression of the disease process and determine the need for a change in therapy.
- Be aware that when a person goes through a traumatic event such as an illness or being given information that will impact his or her lifestyle, there are universal human reactions that occur.

LEARNING OUTCOMES

Providing safe, effective nursing care (SENC) includes mastery of core competencies and standards of care. SENC is based on a judicious application of nursing knowledge in combination with scientific principles. The Art of Nursing is in blending what you know with the ability to effectively apply your knowledge in a compassionate manner.

After reading/studying this chapter you will be able to:

Thinking

1. Identify five tests commonly performed on amniotic fluid and their purpose.
2. Discuss differing alterations in CSF findings that might indicate bacterial versus viral meningitis.

Doing

1. Recognize that there can be instances where the patient's choices conflict with organizational policy and ethical standards of care.

Caring

1. Examine how the process of personal reflection on care practices can influence patient outcomes.

Amniotic Fluid Analysis and L/S Ratio

COMMON USE: To assist in identification of fetal gender, genetic disorders such as hemophilia and sickle cell anemia, chromosomal disorders such as Down syndrome, anatomical abnormalities such as spina bifida, and hereditary metabolic disorders such as cystic fibrosis. To assess for preterm infant fetal lung maturity to assist in evaluating for potential diagnosis of respiratory distress syndrome (RDS).

SPECIMEN: Amniotic fluid collected in a clean amber glass or plastic container.

NORMAL FINDINGS: (Method: Macroscopic observation of fluid for color and appearance, immunochemiluminometric assay [ICMA] for α_1-fetoprotein, electrophoresis for acetylcholinesterase, spectrophotometry for creatinine and bilirubin, chromatography for lecithin/sphingomyelin [L/S] ratio and phosphatidylglycerol, tissue culture for chromosome analysis, dipstick for leukocyte esterase, and automated cell counter for white blood cell count and lamellar bodies)

Test	Reference Value
Color	Colorless to pale yellow
Appearance	Clear
α_1-Fetoprotein	Less than 2 MoM*
Acetylcholinesterase	Absent
Creatinine	1.8–4 mg/dL (159.1–353.6 micromol/L)(SI Units = Conventional Units x 88.4) at term
Bilirubin	Less than 0.075 mg/dL (Less than 0.128 micromol/L)(SI Units = Conventional Units x 17.1) in early pregnancy
	Less than 0.025 mg/dL (Less than 0.428 micromol/L)(SI Units = Conventional Units x 17.1) at term
Bilirubin ΔA_{450}	Less than 0.048 ΔOD in early pregnancy
	Less than 0.02 ΔOD at term
L/S ratio	
Mature (nondiabetic)	Greater than 2:1 in the presence of phosphatidyl glycerol
Borderline	1.5 to 1.9:1
Immature	Less than 1.5:1
Phosphatidylglycerol	Present at term
Chromosome analysis	Normal karyotype
White blood cell count	None seen
Leukocyte esterase	Negative
Lamellar bodies	Findings and interpretive ranges vary depending on the type of instrument used

*MoM = Multiples of the median.

Test Explanation

Amniotic fluid is formed in the membranous sac that surrounds the fetus. The total volume of fluid at term is 500 to 2,500 mL. In amniocentesis, fluid is obtained by ultrasound-guided needle aspiration from the amniotic sac (see Fig. 6.1). This procedure is generally performed between 14 and 16 weeks' gestation for accurate interpretation of test results, but it also can be done between 26 and 35 weeks' gestation if fetal distress is suspected. Amniotic fluid is tested to identify genetic and neural tube defects, hemolytic diseases of the newborn, fetal infection, fetal renal malfunction, or maturity of the fetal lungs. Several rapid tests are also used to differentiate amniotic fluid from other body fluids in a vaginal specimen when premature rupture of membranes (PROM) is suspected. A vaginal swab obtained from the posterior vaginal pool can be used to perform a rapid, waived procedure to aid in the assessment of PROM. Nitrazine paper impregnated with an indicator dye will produce a color change indicative of vaginal pH. Normal vaginal pH is acidic (4.5 to 6), and the color of the paper will not change. Amniotic fluid has an alkaline pH (7.1 to 7.3), and the paper will turn a blue color. False-positive results occur in the presence of semen, blood, alkaline urine, vaginal infection, or if the patient is receiving antibiotics. The amniotic fluid crystallization or fern test is based on the observation of a fern pattern when amniotic fluid is placed on a glass slide and allowed to air dry. The fern pattern is due to the protein and sodium chloride content of the amniotic fluid. False-positive results occur in the presence of blood urine or cervical mucus. Both of these tests can produce false-negative results if only a small amount of fluid is leaked. The reliability of results

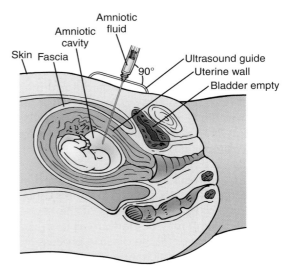

FIGURE 6.1 Amniocentesis. *Used with permission, from Ward, S. (2009). Maternal-child nursing care: Optimizing outcomes for mothers, children, and families. FA Davis Company.*

is also significantly diminished with the passage of time (greater than 24 hours). AmniSure is an immunoassay that can be performed on a vaginal swab sample. It is a rapid test that detects placental alpha microglobulin-1 protein (PAMG-1), which is found in high concentrations in amniotic fluid. AmniSure does not demonstrate the high frequency of false-positive and false-negative results inherent with the pH and fern tests.

Respiratory distress syndrome (RDS) is the most common problem encountered in the care of premature infants. RDS, also called hyaline membrane disease, results from a deficiency of phospholipid lung surfactants. The phospholipids in surfactant are produced by specialized alveolar cells and stored in granular lamellar bodies in the lung. In normally developed lungs, surfactant coats the surface of the alveoli. Surfactant reduces the surface tension of the alveolar wall during breathing. When there is an insufficient quantity of surfactant, the alveoli are unable to expand normally and gas exchange is inhibited. Amniocentesis, a procedure by which fluid is removed from the amniotic sac, is used to assess fetal lung maturity.

Lecithin is the primary surfactant phospholipid, and it is a stabilizing factor for the alveoli. It is produced at a low but constant rate until the 35th week of gestation, after which its production sharply increases. Sphingomyelin, another phospholipid component of surfactant, is also produced at a constant rate after the 26th week of gestation. Before the 35th week, the lecithin/sphingomyelin (L/S) ratio is usually less than 1.6:1. The ratio increases to 2 or greater when the rate of lecithin production increases after the 35th week of gestation. Other phospholipids, such as phosphatidyl glycerol (PG) and phosphatidyl inositol (PI), increase over time in amniotic fluid as well. The presence of PG indicates that the fetus is within 2 to 6 weeks of lung maturity (i.e., at full term). Simultaneous measurement of PG with the L/S ratio improves diagnostic accuracy. Production of phospholipid surfactant is delayed in diabetic mothers. Therefore, caution must be used when interpreting the results obtained from a diabetic patient, and a higher ratio is expected to predict maturity.

Nursing Implications

Assessment

Indications	Potential Nursing Problems
Assist in the diagnosis of (in utero) metabolic disorders, such as cystic fibrosis, or errors of lipid, carbohydrate, or amino acid metabolism Assist in the evaluation of fetal lung maturity when preterm delivery is being considered	• Airway (preterm newborn) • Breathing (preterm newborn)

Indications	Potential Nursing Problems
Detect infection secondary to ruptured membranes Detect fetal ventral wall defects Determine the optimal time for obstetric intervention in cases of threatened fetal survival caused by stresses related to maternal diabetes, toxemia, hemolytic diseases of the newborn, or postmaturity Determine fetal gender when the mother is a known carrier of a sex-linked abnormal gene that could be transmitted to male offspring, such as hemophilia or Duchenne muscular dystrophy Determine the presence of fetal distress in late-stage pregnancy Evaluate fetus in families with a history of genetic disorders, such as Down syndrome, Tay-Sachs disease, chromosome or enzyme anomalies, or inherited hemoglobinopathies Evaluate fetus in mothers of advanced maternal age (some of the aforementioned tests are routinely requested in mothers age 35 and older) Evaluate fetus in mothers with a history of miscarriage or stillbirth Evaluate known or suspected hemolytic disease involving the fetus in an Rh-sensitized pregnancy, indicated by rising bilirubin levels, especially after the 30th week of gestation Evaluate suspected neural tube defects, such as spina bifida or myelomeningocele, as indicated by elevated α_1-fetoprotein (see study titled "α_1-Fetoprotein" for information related to triple-marker testing) Identify fetuses at risk of developing RDS	• Caregiver • Conflicted Decision-making • Family • Fear • Gas Exchange (preterm newborn) • Human Response • Infection • Nutrition • Pain • Role Performance • Self-esteem • Spirituality

Diagnosis: Clinical Significance of Test Results

• Yellow, green, red, or brown fluid *indicates the presence of bilirubin, blood (fetal or maternal), or meconium, which indicate fetal distress or death, hemolytic disease, or growth retardation.*

• Elevated bilirubin levels *indicate fetal hemolytic disease or intestinal obstruction. Measurement of bilirubin is not usually performed before 20 to 24 weeks' gestation because no action can be taken before then. The severity of hemolytic disease is graded by optical density (OD) zones: A value of 0.28 to 0.46 OD at 28 to 31 weeks' gestation indicates mild hemolytic disease, which probably will not affect the fetus; 0.47 to 0.90 OD indicates a moderate effect on the fetus; and 0.91 to 1 OD indicates a significant effect on the fetus. A trend of increasing values with serial measurements may indicate the need for intrauterine transfusion or early delivery, depending on the fetal age. After 32 to 33 weeks' gestation, early delivery is preferred over intrauterine transfusion, because early delivery is more effective in providing the required care to the neonate.*

- Creatinine concentration greater than 2 mg/dL (greater than 176.8 micromol/L)(SI Units = Conventional Units × 88.4) *indicates fetal maturity (at 36 to 37 weeks) if maternal creatinine is also within the expected range. This value should be interpreted in conjunction with other parameters evaluated in amniotic fluid and especially with the L/S ratio, because normal lung development depends on normal kidney development.*

- An L/S ratio less than 2:1 and absence of phosphatidylglycerol at term *indicate fetal lung immaturity and possible respiratory distress syndrome. Other conditions that decrease production of surfactants include advanced maternal age, multiple gestation, and polyhydramnios. Conditions that may increase production of surfactant include hypertension, intrauterine growth retardation, malnutrition, maternal diabetes, placenta previa, placental infarction, and premature rupture of the membranes. The expected L/S ratio for the fetus of an insulin-dependent diabetic mother is higher (3.5:1).*

- *Lamellar bodies are specialized alveolar cells in which lung surfactant is stored.* They are approximately the size of platelets. Their presence in sufficient quantities is an indicator of fetal lung maturity.

- Elevated α_1-fetoprotein levels and presence of acetylcholinesterase *indicate a neural tube defect. Elevation of acetylcholinesterase is also indicative of ventral wall defects.*

- Abnormal karyotype *indicates genetic abnormality (e.g., Tay-Sachs disease, intellectual disability, chromosome or enzyme anomalies, and inherited hemoglobinopathies).*

- Elevated white blood cell count and positive leukocyte esterase *are indicators of infection.*

Planning

Considerations for planning a successful partnership should include clear communication of what to expect during the test to decrease anxiety and improve cooperation. Record the date of the last menstrual period and determine the pregnancy weeks' gestation and expected delivery date. Inquire about any family history of genetic disorders such as cystic fibrosis, Duchenne muscular dystrophy, hemophilia, sickle cell disease, Tay-Sachs disease, thalassemia, and trisomy 21. Before the procedure is performed, plan to review the steps with the patient. Maternal Rh type should be obtained and if Rh-negative, check for prior sensitization. Warn the patient that normal results do not guarantee a normal fetus. Assure the patient that precautions to avoid

injury to the fetus will be taken by localizing the fetus with ultrasound. If the patient is less than 20 weeks' gestation, instruct her to drink extra fluids 1 hour before the test and to refrain from urination. The full bladder assists in raising the uterus up and out of the way to provide better visualization during the ultrasound procedure. Patients who are at 20 weeks' gestation or beyond should void before the test because an empty bladder is less likely to be accidentally punctured during specimen collection. Inform the patient that specimen collection is performed by a health-care provider (HCP) specializing in this procedure and usually takes approximately 20 to 30 minutes to complete. Address concerns about pain, and explain that during the transabdominal procedure, any discomfort with a needle biopsy will be minimized with local anesthetics. Encourage relaxation and controlled breathing during the procedure to aid in reducing any mild discomfort. A standard dose of $Rh_o(D)$ immune globulin RhoGAM IM or Rhophylac IM or IV is indicated after amniocentesis; repeat doses should be considered if repeated amniocentesis is performed.

CONTRAINDICATIONS

Amniocentesis is contraindicated in women with a history of premature labor, incompetent cervix, or in the presence of placenta previa or abruptio placentae.

- There is some risk to having an amniocentesis performed, and this should be weighed against the need to obtain the desired diagnostic information. A small percentage (0.5%) of patients have experienced complications, including premature rupture of the membranes, premature labor, spontaneous abortion, and stillbirth.

SPECIAL CONSIDERATIONS

An important aspect of planning is understanding the factors that may impair the procedure or cause abnormal results. Interdepartmental communication is a key factor in the planning process. The following should be noted when planning for this study:

- L/S ratio, α_1-fetoprotein and acetylcholinesterase may be falsely elevated if the sample is contaminated with fetal blood.
- Exposure of the specimen to light may cause falsely decreased bilirubin or L/S values.
- Bilirubin may be falsely elevated if maternal hemoglobin or meconium is present in the sample; fetal acidosis may also lead to falsely elevated bilirubin levels.
- Contamination of the sample with blood or meconium or complications in pregnancy may yield inaccurate L/S ratios.
- Bilirubin may be falsely decreased if the sample is exposed to light or if amniotic fluid volume is excessive.
- Maternal serum creatinine should be measured simultaneously for comparison with amniotic fluid

creatinine for proper interpretation. Even in circumstances in which the maternal serum value is normal, the results of the amniotic fluid creatinine may be misleading. A high fluid creatinine value in the fetus of a diabetic mother may reflect the increased muscle mass of a larger fetus. If the fetus is big, the creatinine may be high, and the fetus may still have immature kidneys.

- Karyotyping cannot be performed under the following conditions: (1) failure to promptly deliver samples for chromosomal analysis to the laboratory performing the test, or (2) improper incubation of the sample, which causes cell death.

● Safety Tip

Make sure a written and informed consent has been signed prior to the procedure and before administering any medications.

Implementation

Patient education is key to obtaining the patient's cooperation in following directions, and providing an explanation for the purpose of the procedure is an important part of this process. Inform the patient that this study can assist in providing a sample of fluid that will allow for the evaluation of fetal well-being.

Ensure that the patient has a full bladder before the procedure if gestation is 20 weeks or fewer; have the patient void before the procedure if gestation is 21 weeks or more. Have emergency equipment readily available. Have the patient remove clothes below the waist. Assist the patient to a supine position on the examination table with abdomen exposed. Drape the patient's legs, leaving the abdomen exposed. Raise her head or legs slightly to promote comfort and to relax abdominal muscles. If the uterus is large, place a pillow or rolled blanket under the patient's right side to prevent hypertension caused by great-vessel compression. Direct the patient to breathe normally and to avoid unnecessary movement during the administration of the local anesthetic and the procedure. Record maternal and fetal baseline vital signs and continue to monitor throughout the procedure. Monitor for uterine contractions. Monitor fetal vital signs using ultrasound. Protocols may vary among facilities.

Assess the position of the amniotic fluid, fetus, and placenta using ultrasound. Assemble the necessary equipment, including an amniocentesis tray with solution for skin preparation, local anesthetic, 10- or 20-mL syringe, needles of various sizes (including a 22-gauge, 5-inch spinal needle), sterile drapes, sterile gloves, and foil-covered or amber-colored specimen collection containers. Cleanse the suprapubic area with an antiseptic solution and protect with sterile drapes. Explain that the administration of local anesthetic may cause a stinging sensation. Administer local anesthetic. A 22-gauge, 5-inch spinal needle is inserted through the abdominal and uterine walls. Explain that a sensation of pressure may be experienced when the needle is inserted. Explain to the patient how to use focused and controlled breathing for relaxation during the procedure. After the fluid is collected and the needle is withdrawn, apply slight pressure to the site. If there is no evidence of bleeding or other drainage, apply a sterile adhesive bandage to the site. Monitor the patient for complications related to the procedure (e.g., premature labor, allergic reaction, anaphylaxis).

Evaluation

Recognize anxiety related to test results and, after the procedure, fetal heart rate and maternal life signs (e.g., heart rate, blood pressure, pulse, and respiration) should be compared with baseline values and closely monitored every 15 minutes for 30 to 60 minutes after the amniocentesis procedure. Protocols may vary among facilities. Observe/assess for delayed allergic reactions, such as rash, urticaria, tachycardia, hyperpnea, hypertension, palpitations, nausea, or vomiting. Immediately report symptoms to the appropriate HCP. Observe/assess the amniocentesis site for bleeding, inflammation, or hematoma formation. Instruct the patient about the care and assessment of the amniocentesis site. Instruct the patient to report any redness, edema, bleeding, or pain at the amniocentesis site. Instruct the patient to expect mild cramping, leakage of small amounts of amniotic fluid, and vaginal spotting for up to 2 days following the procedure. Instruct the patient to report moderate-to-severe abdominal pain or cramps, a change in fetal activity, increased or prolonged leaking of amniotic fluid from abdominal needle site, vaginal bleeding that is heavier than spotting, and either chills or fever. Instruct the patient to rest until all symptoms have disappeared before resuming normal levels of activity. Administer standard RhoGAM dose, as ordered, to maternal Rh-negative patients to prevent maternal Rh sensitization should the fetus be Rh-positive.

Discuss the implications of abnormal test results on the patient's lifestyle. Provide teaching and information regarding the clinical implications of the test results as appropriate. Encourage the family to seek appropriate counseling if concerned with pregnancy termination and to seek genetic counseling if a chromosomal abnormality is determined. Decisions regarding elective abortion should take place in the presence of both parents. Provide a nonjudgmental, nonthreatening atmosphere for discussing the risks and difficulties of delivering and raising a developmentally challenged infant as well as for exploring other options (termination of pregnancy or adoption). It is also important to discuss problems the mother and father may experience (e.g., guilt, depression, anger) if fetal abnormalities are detected. Inform the patient that it may be 2 to 4 weeks before all results are available. Answer any questions or address any concerns voiced by the patient or family. Instruct the patient about the use of any ordered medications. Explain the importance of adhering to the therapy regimen. As appropriate, instruct the patient about significant side effects and systemic reactions associated with the prescribed medication. Encourage her to review corresponding literature provided by a pharmacist.

✓ Critical Findings

An L/S ratio less than 1.5:1 is predictive of RDS at the time of delivery.

Note and immediately report to the requesting HCP any critical findings and related symptoms. A listing of these findings varies among facilities.

Infants known to be at risk for RDS can be treated with surfactant by intratracheal administration at birth.

✓ Study Specific Complications

Hemorrhage from highly vascular tissue or infection may result following amniocentesis. Instruct the patient to look for excessive bleeding, redness of skin, fever or chills, and to notify her HCP if these symptoms occur. An additional risk with amniocentesis is maternal Rh sensitization by fetal RBCs in the case of an Rh-negative mother carrying an Rh-positive fetus. RhIG (Rh immune globulin) or RhoGam may be administered after amniocentesis to Rh-negative mothers to prevent the formation of Rh antibodies.

There are a number of complications associated with performing specimen collection by needle aspiration. Pain is commonly associated with needles, and although the pain experienced during venipuncture is usually mild, on a rare occasion the needle may strike a nerve, causing permanent pain. Prolonged bleeding is a complication that occurs with patients who are taking blood thinners or who have coagulopathies such as hemophilia. A hematoma results when blood leaks into the tissue during or after a skin puncture, as evidenced by pain, bruising, and/or swelling at the puncture site. The swelling can cause injury by compression to surrounding nerves, which can be temporary or permanent. HCPs should watch for minor complications such as bruising and hematoma at the puncture site, which are fairly common. Bleeding or bruising can be prevented once the needle has been removed by applying direct pressure to the site with dry gauze for a minute or two. Some other more unusual complications of skin puncture include cellulitis, phlebitis, inadvertent arterial puncture, and sepsis. Sepsis can be caused by the introduction of bacteria from the surface of the skin into the blood as the result of improper cleansing of the puncture site. Immunocompromised patients are at higher risk for developing this complication.

✓ Related Tests

- Related tests include α_1-fetoprotein, antibodies anticardiolipin, blood groups and antibodies, chromosome analysis, fetal fibronectin, glucose, ketones, Kleihauer-Betke test, lupus anticoagulant antibodies, newborn screening, potassium, US biophysical profile obstetric, and UA.
- Refer to the Reproductive System table at the end of the book for related tests by body system.

Expected Outcomes

Expected outcomes associated with Amniotic Fluid Analysis and L/S Ratio are:

- Understanding the risks and benefits of obtaining an amniotic fluid specimen
- Preparing emotionally for the results of the amniotic fluid analysis
- Accepting the gender of the fetus
- Agreeing to attend a support group for parents with a special needs child
- Discussing the options of pregnancy viability with HCP
- Not having retractions or nasal flare with respirations in the newborn
- Having newborn respirations that remain within normal limits
- Expressing fear in relation to diagnosis and observable symptoms
- Being compliant with the therapeutic regime recommended by the HCP

Cerebrospinal Fluid Analysis

Quick Summary

SYNONYM ACRONYM: CSF analysis.

COMMON USE: To assist in the differential diagnosis of infection or hemorrhage of the brain. Also used in the evaluation of other conditions with significant neuromuscular effects, such as multiple sclerosis.

SPECIMEN: CSF collected in three or four separate plastic conical tubes. Tube 1 is used for chemistry and serology testing, tube 2 is used for microbiology, tube 3 is used for cell count, and tube 4 is used for miscellaneous testing.

NORMAL FINDINGS: (Method: Macroscopic evaluation of appearance; spectrophotometry for glucose, lactic acid, and protein; immunoassay for myelin basic protein; nephelometry for immunoglobulin G [IgG]; electrophoresis for oligoclonal banding; Gram stain, India ink preparation, and culture or polymerase chain reaction (PCR) for microbiology; microscopic examination of fluid for cell count; flocculation for Venereal Disease Research Laboratory [VDRL])

Lumbar Puncture	Conventional Units	SI Units
Color and appearance	Crystal clear	
(Conventional Units × 10)		
Protein		
0–1 mo	Less than 150 mg/dL	Less than 1,500 mg/L
1–6 mo	30–100 mg/dL	300–1,000 mg/L
7 mo–adult	15–45 mg/dL	150–450 mg/L
Older adult	15–60 mg/dL	150–600 mg/L
(Conventional Units × 0.0555)		
Glucose		
Infant or child	60–80 mg/dL	3.3–4.4 mmol/L
Adult/older adult	40–70 mg/dL	2.2–3.9 mmol/L
(Conventional Units × 0.111)		
Lactic acid		
Neonate	10–60 mg/dL	1.1–6.7 mmol/L
3–10 days	10–40 mg/dL	1.1–4.4 mmol/L
Adult	Less than 25.2 mg/dL	Less than 2.8 mmol/L
(Conventional Units × 1)		
Myelin basic protein	Less than 4 ng/mL	Less than 4 mcg/L
Oligoclonal bands	Absent	
(Conventional Units × 10)		
IgG	Less than 3.4 mg/dL	Less than 34 mg/L
Gram stain	Negative	
India ink	Negative	
Culture	No growth	
RBC count	0	0
(Conventional Units × 1)		
WBC count		
Neonate–1 mo	0–30 /microL	0–30 × 10⁶/L
1 mo–1 yr	0–10 /microL	0–10 × 10⁶/L
1–5 yr	0–8 /microL	0–8 × 10⁶/L
5 yr–adult	0–5 /microL	0–5 × 10⁶/L
VDRL	Nonreactive	
Cytology	No abnormal cells seen	

CSF glucose should be 60% to 70% of plasma glucose level. RBC = red blood cell; VDRL = Venereal Disease Research Laboratory; WBC = white blood cell. Color should be assessed after sample is centrifuged.

WBC Differential	Adult	Children
Lymphocytes	40%–80%	5%–13%
Monocytes	15%–45%	50%–90%
Neutrophils	0%–6%	0%–8%

Test Explanation

Cerebrospinal fluid (CSF) circulates in the subarachnoid space and has a twofold function: to protect the brain and spinal cord from injury and to transport products of cellular metabolism and neurosecretion. The total volume of CSF is 90 to 150 mL in adults and 60 mL in infants. CSF analysis helps determine the presence and cause of bleeding and assists in diagnosing cancer, infections, and degenerative and autoimmune diseases of the brain and spinal cord. Specimens for analysis are most frequently obtained by lumbar puncture and sometimes by ventricular or cisternal puncture. Lumbar puncture can also have therapeutic uses, including injection of drugs and anesthesia (see Fig. 6.2). The subspeciality of microbiology has been revolutionized by molecular diagnostics. Molecular diagnostics involves the identification of specific sequences of DNA. The application of molecular diagnostics techniques, such as PCR, has led to the development of automated instruments that can identify a single infectious agent or multiple pathogens from a cerebrospinal fluid sample in less than 2 hours. The instruments can detect the presence of bacteria, viruses, and yeast commonly associated with meningitis and encephalitis.

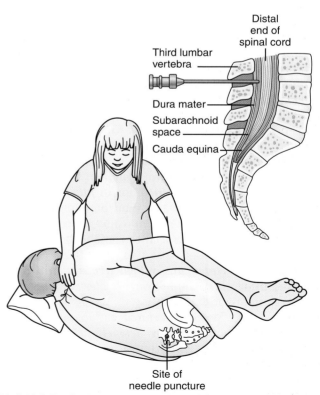

FIGURE 6.2 Lumbar puncture. *Used with permission, from Burton, M. (2011). Fundamentals of nursing care: Concepts, connections, & skills. FA Davis Company.*

Nursing Implications

Assessment

Indications	Potential Nursing Problems
Assist in the diagnosis and differentiation of subarachnoid or intracranial hemorrhage Assist in the diagnosis and differentiation of viral or bacterial meningitis or encephalitis Assist in the diagnosis of diseases such as multiple sclerosis, autoimmune disorders, or degenerative brain disease Assist in the diagnosis of neurosyphilis and chronic central nervous system (CNS) infections Detect obstruction of CSF circulation due to hemorrhage, tumor, or edema Establish the presence of any condition decreasing the flow of oxygen to the brain Monitor for metastases of cancer into the CNS Monitor severe brain injuries	• Activity • Airway • Body Image • Communication • Family • Fatigue • Human Response • Infection • Mobility • Nutrition • Role Performance • Self-care • Sexuality

Diagnosis: Clinical Significance of Test Results
INCREASED IN

- Color and appearance *(xanthochromia is any pink, yellow, or orange color; bloody—hemorrhage; xanthochromic—old hemorrhage, red blood cell [RBC] breakdown, methemoglobin, bilirubin [greater than 6 mg/dL (SI: 102.6 micromol/L)], increased protein [greater than 150 mg/dL (SI: 1,500 mg/L)], melanin [meningeal melanosarcoma], carotene [systemic carotenemia]; hazy—meningitis; pink to dark yellow—aspiration of epidural fat; turbid—cells, microorganisms, protein, fat, or contrast medium)*
- Protein *(related to alterations in blood-brain barrier that allow permeability to proteins)*: Type 2 diabetes *(related to relative increase in plasma glucose)*, encephalitis, Guillain-Barré syndrome (elevated protein with normal WBC count—also referred to as albuminocytological dissociation), meningitis, trauma, tumors
- Lactic acid *(related to cerebral hypoxia and correlating anaerobic metabolism)*: bacterial, tubercular, fungal meningitis
- Myelin basic protein *(related to accumulation as a result of nerve sheath demyelination)*: trauma, stroke, tumor, multiple sclerosis, subacute sclerosing panencephalitis
- IgG and oligoclonal banding *(related to autoimmune or inflammatory response)*: multiple sclerosis, CNS syphilis, and subacute sclerosing panencephalitis

- Gram stain: *Meningitis due to Escherichia coli, Streptococcus agalactiae, S. pneumoniae, Haemophilus influenzae, Mycobacterium avium-intracellulare, M. leprae, M. tuberculosis, Neisseria meningitidis, or Cryptococcus neoformans*
- India ink preparation: *Meningitis due to C. neoformans*
- Culture: *Encephalitis or meningitis due to herpes simplex virus, S. pneumoniae, H. influenzae, N. meningitidis, or C. neoformans*
- RBC count: *Hemorrhage*
- White blood cell (WBC) count:
  - *General increase—injection of contrast media or anticancer drugs in subarachnoid space; CSF infarct; metastatic tumor in contact with CSF; reaction to repeated lumbar puncture*
  - *Elevated WBC count with a predominance of neutrophils indicative of abscess, bacterial meningitis, tubercular meningitis*
  - *Elevated WBC count with a predominance of lymphocytes indicative of viral, tubercular, parasitic, or fungal meningitis; multiple sclerosis*
  - *Elevated WBC count with a predominance of monocytes indicative of chronic bacterial meningitis, amebic meningitis, multiple sclerosis, or toxoplasmosis*
  - *Increased plasma cells indicative of acute viral infections, demyelinating diseases, multiple sclerosis, neurosyphilis, sarcoidosis, syphilitic meningoencephalitis, subacute sclerosing panencephalitis, tubercular meningitis, parasitic infections, or Guillain-Barré syndrome*
  - *Presence of eosinophils indicative of parasitic and fungal infections, acute polyneuritis, idiopathic hypereosinophilic syndrome, reaction to drugs, or a shunt in CSF*
- VDRL: *Syphilis*

POSITIVE FINDING IN

- Cytology: *Malignant cells*

DECREASED IN
- Glucose: *Bacterial and tubercular meningitis*

Planning

Considerations for planning a successful partnership should include clear communication of what to expect during the test to decrease anxiety and improve cooperation. Before the procedure is performed, plan to review the steps with the patient. Perform a basic neurological examination; assess the patient's gait and leg muscle strength prior to the procedure. Explain that the procedure will be performed by a trained healthcare provider (HCP) and will take approximately 20 minutes. Discuss the discomfort that may be felt during the procedure. The HCP will inject a local anesthetic at the site causing a stinging sensation. Encourage the patient to report any pain or other sensations that may require repositioning of the spinal needle. Patients will be assisted to remain still and in the correct position because it is somewhat awkward. Reinforce with the patient that his or her role is to lie still and breath normally throughout the procedure.

CONTRAINDICATIONS

This procedure is contraindicated if infection is present at the needle insertion site.

- It may also be contraindicated in patients with degenerative joint disease or coagulation defects and in patients who are uncooperative during the procedure.
- Use with extreme caution in patients with increased intracranial pressure because overly rapid removal of CSF can result in herniation.

SPECIAL CONSIDERATIONS

An important aspect of planning is understanding the factors that may impair the procedure or cause abnormal results. Interdepartmental communication is a key factor in the planning process. The following should be noted when planning for this study:

- RBC count may be falsely elevated with a traumatic spinal tap.
- Delays in analysis may present a false-positive appearance of xanthochromia due to RBC lysis that begins within 4 hours of a bloody tap.

It is also important to understand which medications or substances the patient may be exposed to in the healthcare setting that can interfere with accurate testing:

- Drugs that may decrease CSF protein levels include cefotaxime and dexamethasone.
- Drugs that may increase CSF glucose levels include cefotaxime and dexamethasone. Interferon-β may increase myelin basic protein levels.

● *Safety Tip*

Make sure a written and informed consent has been signed prior to the procedure and before administering any medications.

Implementation

Patient education is key to obtaining the patient's cooperation in following directions, and providing an explanation for the purpose of the procedure is an important part of this process. Inform the patient that this study can assist in evaluating health by providing a sample of fluid from around the spinal cord to be tested for disease and infection. Ensure that anticoagulant therapy has been withheld for the appropriate number of days prior to the procedure; the number of days to withhold medication is dependent on the type of anticoagulant. Notify the HCP if patient anticoagulant therapy has

not been withheld. Have emergency equipment readily available.

Record baseline vital signs and assess neurological status. Protocols may vary among facilities. To perform a lumbar puncture, position the patient in the knee-chest position at the side of the bed, bending the neck and chest to the knees; an alternative is to place the patient in a sitting position. Provide pillows to support the spine or for the patient to grasp. Prepare the site (usually between L3 and L4 or L4 and L5) with povidone-iodine, drape the area, and administer a local anesthetic by injection. Using sterile technique, the HCP inserts the spinal needle through the spinous processes of the vertebrae and into the subarachnoid space (see Fig. 6.3). Larger-gauge spinal needles have been shown to play a significant role in the predictable incidence of postpuncture headache However, the smaller the bevel, the more time is required to collect a sufficient volume of fluid; usually a 22-gauge needle is used. The stylet is removed. CSF drips from the needle if it is properly placed. Attach the stopcock and manometer, and measure initial CSF pressure. Normal pressure for an adult in the lateral recumbent position is 60 to 200 mm H_2O, and 10 to 100 mm H_2O for children younger than 8 years. These values depend on the body position and are different in a horizontal or sitting position. CSF pressure may be elevated if the patient is anxious, holding his or her breath, tensing muscles, or if the patient's knees are flexed too firmly against the abdomen. CSF pressure may be significantly elevated in patients with intracranial tumors or space occupying pockets of infection as seen in meningitis. If the initial pressure is elevated, the HCP may perform Queckenstedt test. To perform this test, apply pressure to the jugular vein for about 10 sec. CSF pressure usually rises in response to the occlusion, then rapidly returns to normal within 10 sec after the

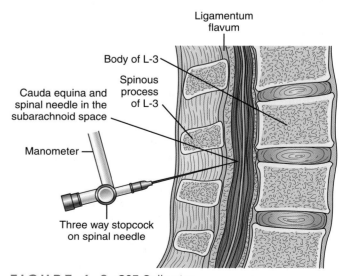

FIGURE 6.3 CSF Collection

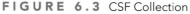

pressure is released. Sluggish response may indicate CSF obstruction. Obtain four (or five) vials of fluid, according to the HCP's request, in separate tubes (1 to 3 mL in each), and label them numerically (1 to 4 or 5) in the order they were filled. Take a final pressure reading, and remove the needle. Clean the puncture site with an antiseptic solution, and apply direct pressure with dry gauze to stop bleeding or CSF leakage. Observe/assess puncture site for bleeding, CSF leakage, or hematoma formation, and secure gauze with adhesive bandage.

Evaluation

Recognize anxiety related to test results, and monitor vital signs and neurological status and for headache every 15 minutes for 1 hour, then every 2 hours for 4 hours, and then as ordered by the HCP. Compare with baseline values. Notify the HCP if temperature is elevated. Protocols may vary among facilities.

Administer fluids if permitted, especially fluids containing caffeine, to replace lost CSF and to help prevent or relieve headache, which is a side effect of lumbar puncture. The use of a flexible straw facilitates intake of fluids while remaining flat. Advise the patient that headache may begin within a few hours up to 2 days after the procedure and may be associated with dizziness, nausea, and vomiting. The length of time for the headache to resolve varies considerably. Observe/assess the puncture site for leakage, and frequently monitor body signs, such as temperature and blood pressure. Position the patient flat, either on the back or abdomen following the HCP's instructions; some HCPs allow 30 degrees of elevation. Maintain this position for 8 hours. Changing position is acceptable as long as the body remains horizontal. Observe/assess the patient for neurological changes, such as an altered level of consciousness, a change in pupils, reports of tingling or numbness, and irritability.

Discuss the implications of abnormal test results on the patient's lifestyle. Provide teaching and information regarding the clinical implications of the test results as appropriate. Provide information regarding vaccine preventable diseases when indicated (encephalitis, influenza, meningococcal diseases). Provide contact information, if desired, for the Centers for Disease Control and Prevention (www.cdc.gov/vaccines/vpd-vac). Answer any questions or address any concerns voiced by the patient or family. Instruct the patient about the use of any ordered medications. Explain the importance of adhering to the therapy regimen. As appropriate, instruct the patient about significant side effects and systemic reactions associated with the prescribed medication. Encourage him or her to review corresponding literature provided by a pharmacist.

⊘ Critical Findings

- Positive Gram stain, India ink preparation, or culture
- Presence of malignant cells or blasts

- Elevated WBC count
- Adults: Glucose less than 37 mg/dL (SI: Less than 2.1 mmol/L); greater than 440 mg/dL (SI: Greater than 24.4 mmol/L)
- Children: Glucose less than 31 mg/dL (SI: Less than 1.7 mmol/L); greater than 440 mg/dL (SI: Greater than 24.4 mmol/L)

Note and immediately report to the requesting HCP any critical findings and related symptoms. A listing of these findings varies among facilities.

Important signs to note include allergic or other reaction to the anesthesia, bleeding or CSF drainage at the puncture sight, changes in level of consciousness, changes to or inequality of pupil size, or respiratory failure.

⊘ Study Specific Complications

Headache is a common minor complication experienced after lumbar puncture and is caused by leakage of the spinal fluid from around the puncture site. On a rare occasion, the headache may require treatment with an epidural blood patch in which an anesthesiologist or pain management specialist injects a small amount of the patient's blood in the epidural space of the puncture site. The blood patch forms a clot and seals the puncture site to prevent further leakage of CSF and provides relief within 30 minutes. Other complications include lower back pain after the procedure or brain stem herniation due to increased intracranial pressure.

There are a number of complications associated with performing a procedure involving specimen collection by needle aspiration. Pain is commonly associated with needles, and although the pain experienced during skin puncture is usually mild, on a rare occasion the needle may strike a nerve causing permanent pain. Prolonged bleeding is a complication that occurs with patients who are taking blood thinners or who have coagulopathies such as hemophilia. A hematoma results when blood leaks into the tissue during or after a skin puncture, as evidenced by pain, bruising, and/or swelling at the puncture site. The swelling can cause injury by compression to surrounding nerves, which can be temporary or permanent. HCPs should watch for minor complications such as bruising and hematoma at the puncture site, which are fairly common. Hematomas occur more often in older adult or frail patients, or those with veins that are difficult to access. Bleeding or bruising can be prevented once the needle has been removed by applying direct pressure to the site with dry gauze for a minute or two. Some other more unusual complications of skin puncture include cellulitis and sepsis. Sepsis can be caused by introduction of bacteria from the surface of the skin into the blood as the result of improper cleansing of the puncture site. Immunocompromised patients are at higher risk for developing this complication.

Related Tests

- Related tests include CBC, CT brain, culture for appropriate organisms (blood, fungal, mycobacteria, sputum, throat, viral, wound), EMG, evoked brain potentials, Gram stain, MRI brain, PET brain, and syphilis serology.
- Refer to the Immune and Musculoskeletal systems tables at the end of the book for related tests by body system.

Expected Outcomes

Expected outcomes associated with Cerebrospinal Fluid Analysis are:

- Agreeing to take precautions to prevent injury from altered mobility
- Adapting to the use of devices necessary to support adequate nutrition related to ongoing spasticity
- Receiving test results that are negative for infection
- Stating that headache has been relieved
- Verbalizing an understanding of the disease process
- Not having photophobia

Culture, Bacterial, Sputum

Quick Summary

SYNONYM ACRONYM: Routine culture of sputum.

COMMON USE: To identify pathogenic bacterial organisms in the sputum as an indicator for appropriate therapeutic interventions for respiratory infections.

SPECIMEN: Sputum.

NORMAL FINDINGS: (Method: Aerobic culture on selective and enriched media; microscopic examination of sputum by Gram stain.) The presence of normal upper respiratory tract flora should be expected. Tracheal aspirates and bronchoscopy samples can be contaminated with normal flora, but transtracheal aspiration specimens should show no growth. Normal respiratory flora include *Neisseria catarrhalis*, *Candida albicans*, diphtheroids, α-hemolytic streptococci, and some staphylococci. The presence of normal flora does not rule out infection. A normal Gram stain of sputum contains polymorphonuclear leukocytes, alveolar macrophages, and a few squamous epithelial cells.

Test Explanation

This test involves collecting a sputum specimen so the pathogen can be isolated and identified (see Figs. 6.4 and 6.5). The test results will reflect the type and number of organisms present in the specimen as well as the antibiotics to which the identified pathogenic organisms are susceptible. Sputum collected by expectoration or suctioning with catheters and by bronchoscopy cannot be cultured for anaerobic organisms; instead, transtracheal aspiration or lung biopsy must be used.

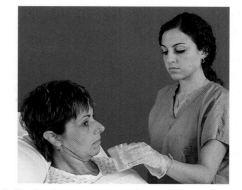

FIGURE 6.4 Expectorated sputum collection. *Used with permission, from Wilkinson, J., & Treas, L. (2010). Fundamentals of nursing (2nd Ed.). FA Davis Company.*

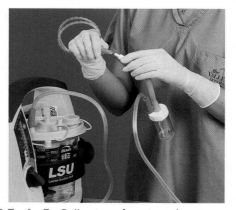

FIGURE 6.5 Collection of suctioned sputum specimens. *Used with permission, from Wilkinson, J., & Treas, L. (2010). Fundamentals of nursing (2nd Ed.). FA Davis Company.*

The laboratory will initiate antibiotic sensitivity testing if indicated by test results. Sensitivity testing identifies antibiotics to which the organisms are susceptible to ensure an effective treatment plan.

Nursing Implications

Assessment

Indications	Potential Nursing Problems
Culture • Assist in the diagnosis of respiratory infections, as indicated by the presence or absence of organisms in culture **Gram Stain** • Assist in the differentiation of gram-positive from gram-negative bacteria in respiratory infection • Assist in the differentiation of sputum from upper respiratory tract secretions, the latter being indicated by excessive squamous cells or absence of polymorphonuclear leukocytes	• Activity • Airway • Breathing • Gas Exchange • Human Response • Infection • Self-care

Diagnosis: Clinical Significance of Test Results

The major difficulty in evaluating results is in distinguishing organisms infecting the lower respiratory tract from organisms that have colonized but not infected the lower respiratory tract. Review of the Gram stain assists in this process. The presence of greater than 25 squamous epithelial cells per low-power field (lpf) indicates oral contamination, and the specimen should be rejected. The presence of many polymorphonuclear neutrophils and few squamous epithelial cells indicates that the specimen was collected from an area of infection and is satisfactory for further analysis.

Bacterial pneumonia can be caused by *Streptococcus pneumoniae*, *Haemophilus influenzae*, staphylococci, and some gram-negative bacteria. Other pathogens that can be identified by culture are *Corynebacterium diphtheriae*, *Klebsiella pneumoniae*, and *Pseudomonas aeruginosa*. Some infectious agents, such as *C. diphtheriae*, are more fastidious in their growth requirements and cannot be cultured and identified without special treatment. Suspicion of infection by less commonly identified and/or fastidious organisms must be communicated to the laboratory to ensure selection of the proper procedure required for identification.

Planning

Considerations for planning a successful partnership should include clear communication of what to expect during the test to decrease anxiety and improve cooperation. Before the procedure is performed, plan to review the steps with the patient. Reassure the patient that he or she will be able to breathe during the procedure if the sputum specimen is collected by tracheal suction method. There are no food or fluid restrictions for specimens to be collected by expectoration or tracheal suction, unless by medical direction. Ensure that oxygen has been administered 20 to 30 minutes before the procedure if the specimen is to be obtained by tracheal suction. Address concerns about pain related to the procedure. Atropine is usually given before bronchoscopy examinations to reduce bronchial secretions and prevent vagally induced bradycardia. Meperidine (Demerol) or morphine may be given as a sedative. Lidocaine is sprayed in the patient's throat to reduce discomfort caused by the presence of the tube. Explain to the patient that the time it takes to collect a proper specimen varies according to the level of cooperation of the patient and the specimen collection site. Emphasize that sputum and saliva are not the same. Inform the patient that multiple specimens may be required.

SPECIAL CONSIDERATIONS

An important aspect of planning is understanding the factors that may impair the procedure or cause abnormal results. Interdepartmental communication is a key factor in the planning process. It should be noted when planning for this study that contamination with oral flora may invalidate results.

It is also important to understand which medications or substances the patient may be exposed to in the health-care setting that can interfere with accurate testing. Specimen collection after antibiotic therapy has been initiated may result in an inhibited growth or no growth of organisms.

PROCEDURES REQUIRING ANESTHESIA

- Patients undergoing bronchoscopy should be informed of the risks associated with general anesthesia as part of the informed consent. These risks can include possible dental injuries from intubation as well as serious complications. Although these risks of serious complications are low, they can include heart attack, stroke, brain damage, and death. These risks depend in part on the patient's age, sex, weight, allergies, general health, and history of smoking, alcohol or drug use.
- Patients on beta blockers before the surgical procedure should be instructed to take their medication as ordered during the perioperative period. Protocols may vary among facilities.
- Inform the patient that it may be necessary to remove hair from the site before the procedure.
- Sedation and pain concerns often cause patients to exhibit anxiety. Patients may be given sedatives or analgesia for minimal to conscious sedation. Local anesthesia or general anesthesia for a drug-induced loss of consciousness is considered for some laboratory and diagnostic procedures. General anesthesia is intended to bring about five states during a surgical procedure:

1. Analgesia, or pain relief
2. Loss of consciousness
3. Weakening of the autonomic responses
4. Achievement of a motionless state
5. Amnesia, or loss of memory of the procedure

- Preoperative dietary restrictions are an important part of ensuring as safe a surgical experience as possible. They are intended to minimize the possibility of aspirating (inhaling) stomach contents into the lungs, a rare but potentially serious complication of anesthesia, and to reduce the likelihood of postoperative nausea. The American Society of Anesthesiologists has fasting guidelines for risk levels according to patient status. More information can be located at www.asahq.org. The preoperative fasting guidelines of the American Society of Anesthesiologists for scheduled surgery are as follows:
  - No solid food for 6 hours prior to an elective surgery
  - No milk or milk products for 8 hours prior to an elective surgery
  - No clear liquids for 2 hours before an elective surgery

The absence of a gag reflex and the inability to swallow easily are considered risks for aspiration. Following the use of anesthesia, ensure the patient is fully awake before swallowing clear liquids.

Implementation

Patient education is key to obtaining the patient's cooperation in following directions, and providing an explanation for the purpose of the procedure is an important part of this process. Inform the patient that this study can assist in identification of the organism-causing infection.

Observe standard precautions and positively identify the patient.

SPECIMEN COLLECTION BY EXPECTORATION

Inform the patient that additional liquids the night before may assist in liquefying secretions during expectoration the following morning. Assist the patient with oral cleaning before sample collection to reduce the amount of sample contamination by organisms that normally inhabit the mouth. Instruct the patient not to touch the edge or inside of the specimen container with the hands or mouth. Ask the patient to sit upright, with assistance and support (e.g., with an over-bed table) as needed. Ask the patient to take two or three deep breaths and cough deeply. Any sputum raised should be expectorated directly into a sterile sputum collection container. If the patient is unable to produce the desired amount of sputum, several strategies may be attempted. One approach is to have the patient drink two glasses of water, and then assume the position for postural drainage of the upper and middle lung segments. Effective coughing may be assisted by placing either the hands or a pillow over the diaphragmatic area and applying slight pressure. Another approach is to place a vaporizer or other humidifying device at the bedside. After sufficient exposure to adequate humidification, postural drainage of the upper and middle lung segments may be repeated before attempting to obtain the specimen. Other methods may include obtaining an order for an expectorant to be administered with additional water approximately 2 hours before attempting to obtain the specimen. Chest percussion and postural drainage of all lung segments may also be employed. If the patient is still unable to raise sputum, the use of an ultrasonic nebulizer ("induced sputum") may be necessary; this is usually done by a respiratory therapist. Generally, a series of three to five early morning sputum samples are collected in sterile containers.

SPECIMEN COLLECTION BY TRACHEAL SUCTION

Assist the patient by providing extra fluids, unless contraindicated, and proper humidification to decrease tenacious secretions. Inform the patient that increasing fluid intake before retiring on the night before the test aids in liquefying secretions and may make it easier to expectorate in the morning. Also explain that humidifying inspired air also helps liquefy secretions. Obtain the necessary equipment, including a suction device, suction kit, and Lukens tube or in-line trap. Position the patient with head elevated as high as tolerated. Put on sterile gloves. Maintain the dominant hand as sterile and the nondominant hand as clean. Using the sterile hand, attach the suction catheter to the rubber tubing of the Lukens tube or in-line trap. Then attach the suction tubing to the male adapter of the trap with the clean hand. Lubricate the suction catheter with sterile saline. Tell nonintubated patients to protrude the tongue and to take a deep breath as the suction catheter is passed through the nostril. When the catheter enters the trachea, a reflex cough is stimulated; immediately advance the catheter into the trachea and apply suction. Maintain suction for approximately 10 sec, but never longer than 15 sec. Withdraw the catheter without applying suction. Separate the suction catheter and suction tubing from the trap, and place the rubber tubing over the male adapter to seal the unit. For intubated patients or patients with a tracheostomy, the previous procedure is followed except that the suction catheter is passed through the existing endotracheal or tracheostomy tube rather than through the nostril. The patient should be hyperoxygenated before and after the procedure in accordance with standard protocols for suctioning these patients.

SPECIMEN COLLECTION BY BRONCHOSCOPY

Ensure that the patient undergoing bronchoscopy has complied with dietary and medication restrictions prior to the bronchoscopy procedure. Have the patient remove dentures, contact lenses, eyeglasses, and jewelry. Notify the health-care provider (HCP) if the patient has permanent crowns on teeth. Have the patient remove clothing and change into a gown for the procedure. Have emergency equipment readily available. Keep resuscitation equipment on hand in case of respiratory impairment or laryngospasm after the procedure. Avoid using morphine sulfate in patients with asthma or other pulmonary disease. This drug can further exacerbate bronchospasms and respiratory impairment. Record baseline vital signs. The patient is positioned in relation to the type of anesthesia being used. If local anesthesia is used, the patient is seated and the tongue and oropharynx are sprayed and swabbed with anesthetic before the bronchoscope is inserted. Assist the patient to a comfortable position, and direct the patient to breathe normally during the beginning of the local anesthesia and to avoid unnecessary movement during the local anesthetic and the procedure. Instruct the patient to cooperate fully and to follow directions. For general anesthesia, the patient is placed in a supine position with the neck hyperextended. After inspection, the samples are collected from suspicious sites by bronchial brush or biopsy forceps. After anesthesia, the patient is kept in supine or shifted to a side-lying position and the bronchoscope is inserted.

GENERAL INSTRUCTIONS

Label the appropriate collection container with the corresponding patient demographics, the date and time of collection, the method of specimen collection, applicable laterality, and any medication the patient is taking that may interfere with test results (e.g., antibiotics). If leprosy is suspected, obtain a smear from nasal scrapings or a biopsy specimen from lesions in a sterile container. Promptly transport the specimen to the laboratory for processing and analysis.

Evaluation

Recognize anxiety related to test results. Monitor the patient for complications related to the procedure (e.g., allergic reaction, anaphylaxis, bronchospasm). Inform the patient that he or she may experience some throat soreness and hoarseness. The absence of a gag reflex and the inability to swallow easily are considered risks for aspiration. Following the use of anesthesia, ensure the patient is fully awake before swallowing clear liquids. Instruct the patient to treat throat discomfort with lozenges and warm gargles when the gag reflex returns. Monitor vital signs and compare with baseline values every 15 minutes for 1 hour, then every 2 hours for 4 hours, and then as ordered by the HCP. Monitor the patient's temperature every 4 hours for 24 hours. Notify the HCP if temperature is elevated. Protocols may vary among facilities. Emergency resuscitation equipment should be readily available if the vocal cords become spastic after intubation. Observe for delayed allergic reactions, such as rash, urticaria, tachycardia, hyperpnea, hypertension, palpitations, nausea, or vomiting. Observe the patient for hemoptysis, difficulty breathing, cough, air hunger, excessive coughing, pain, or absent breathing sounds over the affected area. Report any symptoms to the HCP. Evaluate the patient for symptoms indicating the development of pneumothorax, such as dyspnea, tachypnea, anxiety, decreased breathing sounds, or restlessness. A chest x-ray may be ordered to check for the presence of this complication. Evaluate the patient for symptoms of empyema, such as fever, tachycardia, malaise, or an elevated white blood cell count. Administer antibiotic therapy if ordered. Remind the patient of the importance of completing the entire course of antibiotic therapy, even if signs and symptoms disappear before the completion of therapy.

Discuss the implications of abnormal test results on the patient's lifestyle. Provide teaching and information regarding the clinical implications of the test results, as appropriate. Educate the patient regarding access to counseling services as appropriate. Provide information regarding vaccine-preventable diseases where indicated (e.g., H1N1 flu, H*aemophilus influenzae*, seasonal influenza, pertussis, pneumococcal disease). Provide contact information, if desired, for the Centers for Disease Control and Prevention (www.cdc.gov/vaccines/vpd-vac). Reinforce information given by the patient's HCP regarding further testing, treatment, or referral to another HCP. Instruct the patient to use lozenges or gargle for throat discomfort. Inform the patient of smoking cessation programs as appropriate. The importance of following the prescribed diet should be stressed to the patient/caregiver. Educate the patient regarding access to counseling services, as appropriate. Answer any questions or address any concerns voiced by the patient or family. Instruct the patient in the use of any ordered medications. Explain the importance of adhering to the therapy regimen. As appropriate, instruct the patient about significant side effects and systemic reactions associated with the prescribed medication. Encourage him or her to review corresponding literature provided by a pharmacist.

NUTRITIONAL CONSIDERATIONS: Malnutrition is commonly seen in patients with severe respiratory disease for numerous reasons, including fatigue, lack of appetite, and gastrointestinal distress. Adequate intake of Vitamins A and C are also important to prevent pulmonary infection and to decrease the extent of lung tissue damage.

✅ *Critical Findings*

- *C. diphtheriae*
- *Legionella*

Note and immediately report to the requesting HCP any critical findings and related symptoms. Lists of specific organisms may vary among facilities; specific organisms are required to be reported to local, state, and national departments of health.

✅ *Study Specific Complications*

Complications associated with bronchoscopy are rare but may include bleeding, bronchial perforation, bronchospasm, infection, laryngospasm, and pneumothorax.

✅ *Related Tests*

- Related tests include antibodies, anti-glomerular basement membrane, arterial/alveolar oxygen ratio, biopsy lung, blood gases, bronchoscopy, chest x-ray, CBC, CT thoracic, culture (fungal, mycobacterium, throat, viral), cytology sputum, gallium scan, Gram stain/acid-fast stain, HIV-1/2 antibodies, lung perfusion scan, lung ventilation scan, MRI chest, mediastino-scopy, pleural fluid analysis, PFT, and TB tests.
- Refer to the Immune and Respiratory systems tables at the end of the book for related tests by body system.

Expected Outcomes

Expected outcomes associated with Culture, Bacterial, Sputum are:

- An understanding of the importance of providing a timely specimen to identify the infecting organism
- An absence of respiratory distress

- Attempts by the nurse to collect sputum specimen prior to beginning antibiotic therapy
- Sensitivity results that are reported to HCP in a timely manner, assuring that the correct antibiotic is being used to kill the identified organism

REVIEW OF LEARNING OUTCOMES

Thinking

1. Identify five tests commonly performed on amniotic fluid and their purpose. Answer: α_1-Fetoprotein (birth defect), L/S ratio (fetal lung maturity), chromosome analysis (genetic abnormality), WBC count (infection), bilirubin (hemolytic disease of the newborn).
2. Discuss differing alterations in CSF findings that might indicate bacterial versus viral meningitis. Answer: Bacterial meningitis is associated with an elevated WBC count with predominance of neutrophils, decreased glucose, and a positive Gram stain. Viral meningitis is associated with an elevated WBC count with a predominance of lymphocytes, normal glucose, and a negative Gram stain.

Doing

1. Recognize that there can be instances where the patient's choices conflict with organizational policy and ethical standards of care Answer: Health care is filled with emotional land mines. Choices made by a pregnant woman, a new parent, a couple seeking assistance to have children, and children of a person with Alzheimer disease may not be the choices you believe they should make morally or ethically, depending on your point of view. This can create tension with the nurse, other HCPs, and the organization as a whole. It is important to separate your personal beliefs from the care that you give. What seems normal and appropriate to you based on your point of view may not be acceptable to the patient through his or her point of view.

Caring

1. Examine how the process of personal reflection on care practices can influence patient outcomes. Answer: Becoming a nurse requires serious contemplation of how your day has gone. How effective have you been? Did you send the sputum specimen before you started the antibiotic? If not, why not? What could you have done to obtain that specimen, what were your alternatives, and who were your resources? Becoming a nurse is very much a "learn as you go" job that is built on scientific principles. Think about the choices you made today and consider what you could have done better. Doing this will allow you to make better choices in the future, leading to improved patient outcomes.

Words OF Wisdom: What do you say to a woman who has been trying to have a baby for the past 10 years and is now in premature labor and at risk of losing another child? What do you say to a parent whose child is critically ill with a respiratory disease, or a child of a beloved parent with Alzheimer disease? Part of your role of the nurse is to provide emotional support without becoming overcome with emotional distress. It is not easy, but it is what is required of us. Go back to the question of how to help your patient. You help your patient by providing her or him with all of the information she or he needs in order to have a clear understanding of what is going on. Sometimes all it requires is some clarification from you; sometimes you need to find an expert and have the expert help. Your job is to Figure out what is needed and make it happen. By the way, it is okay to cry; we are human after all. Just try not to do it in such a way that the family is taking care of you instead of you taking care of them.

BIBLIOGRAPHY

Ahmed, S., Jayawarna, C., & Jude, E. (2006). Post lumber puncture headache: diagnosis and management. Retrieved from www.ncbi.nlm.nih.gov/pmc/articles/PMC2660496/

Mayo Clinic Staff. (2012). Amniocentesis. Retrieved from www.mayoclinic.com/health/amniocentesis/MY00155/DSECTION=risks

Mundt, L., & Shanahan, K. (2010). Graff's textbook of urinalysis and body fluids (2nd ed.). Philadelphia, PA: Lippincott Williams & Wilkins.

Van Leeuwen, A., & Bladh, M. (2015). Davis's comprehensive handbook of laboratory and diagnostic tests with nursing implications (6th ed.). Philadelphia, PA: F.A. Davis Company.

Go to Section II of this book and http://www.davisplus.com for the Clinical Reasoning Tool and its case studies to provide you with a safe place to explore patient care situations. There are a total of 26 different case studies; 2 cases are presented for each of 13 body systems. One set of 13 cases are found in the Section II chapters, and a second set of 13 cases are available online at http://www.davisplus.com. Each case is designed with the specific goal of helping you to connect the dots of clinical reasoning. Cases are designed to reflect possible clinical scenarios; the outcomes may or may not be positive—you decide.

Computed Tomography Studies

OVERVIEW

Tomography is an imaging technique that produces cross-sectional views of an anatomical area of interest. Many applications of tomography have been developed for specific medical uses. Cross-sectional images can also be viewed in other modalities of diagnostic testing such as with nuclear medicine, magnetic resonance imaging (MRI), and ultrasound (US) techniques. Advances have been made in the development of different types of tomography methods, with and without radiographical exposure, including helical or spiral computed, optical coherence (OCT), positron emission (PET), single photon emission computed (SPECT), ultrafast computed, and xenon-enhanced computed.

Computed axial tomography, also known as the CAT scan, is a diagnostic imaging tool that came into use in the 1970s and 1980s. With the advent of sophisticated computer software, three-dimensional imaging, and the ability to scan in multiple planes of the body, such as the coronal, horizontal, or sagittal planes, the "axial" was dropped from the title, and this scanning process is now known as computed tomography or CT scanning. Newer scanners have been designed to collect multiple "slices," such that hundreds of slices can be collected in a matter of seconds. Scanners have also been developed to combine techniques so that CT and PET scans or MR and PET scans can be performed simultaneously. The images can be used diagnostically to create a surgical plan. They can also be used to perform alternative, nonsurgical procedures such as CT-guided tissue biopsy or CT-guided catheter insertion for arteriograms or the removal of fluids. CT is also used in radiation oncology to differentiate normal tissue from diseased tissue. Radiation therapy plans can be facilitated with CT images taken through the treatment fields while the patient is in the treatment position. The quality and accuracy of radiation therapy have been significantly improved with the integration of real-time CT imaging during treatments.

In standard radiographic CT, the objective of producing a clear image is accomplished by movement of the x-ray tube and detector in opposite directions. The orientation of the components in a CT unit has the effect of obscuring overlapping structures above and below the selected focal plane. Captured scanned images are sent to a computer that transcribes them into a digital form to be viewed and saved for future use. Visually, a CT image looks like a black-and-white photograph. The density of items in the photograph is seen as varying shades of black (air, no density) and white (solid density, like bone), to gray shades (tissue). Contrast media (iodine, barium) can be used to enhance visualization of organs or structures under clinical investigation, such as tumor identification. After comparison to a reference material, which is arbitrarily assigned a value of zero, the densities of various anatomical structures are assigned different CT numbers (also known as Hounsfield units, or HUs); tissues with less density than the reference material are given negative CT numbers, and tissues with more density are given positive CT numbers. Water is used as the reference material for CT studies due to its uniform density and abundance in the tissues and organs of the human body.

The goal of CT is to allow us to look inside the patient's body and come to a clinical decision about "what is going on." Areas of inquiry facilitated by CT scanning move from general examination to specifically targeted goals. Generally, a CT scan may be used as an investigative tool related to the extremities, neck, head, abdomen, spine, pelvis, and chest. CT scans can be used to assess body organs and cavities for areas of fluid, blood, or fat accumulation, and to identify mass and tumor. Specifically, CT scanning can be used to target an identified organ or area. Examples include using CT scans to assess skull fracture or bleeding after head trauma, disk herniation, or craniofacial and spinal fractures. CT scans can be used to identify and evaluate specific tumors, other cancers, and to differentiate between ischemic and hemorrhagic stroke. CT scans are an invaluable tool in staging tumors.

The most common requests for CT scanning are for the head, chest, and abdomen. Interventional radiologists will use CT scans to assist with abscess drainage, tissue biopsy, and cyst aspiration. In addition, CT scans are used during radiofrequency ablations and cryoablations of tumors. Serial CT scans can provide information about whether or not a chosen diagnostic treatment is working. An example is a cancer patient being treated with radiation and chemotherapy. If the tumor continues to grow, the chosen treatment may need to be changed.

Technology in CT scanning continues to develop and includes the following modalities:

DYNAMIC CT SCAN

- Takes rapid sequential pictures during dye injection to evaluate the blood flow and vascularity of a particular organ
- Assesses, for example, for an aortic aneurysm

HELICAL CT SCAN

- Takes faster and more accurate large data images over about 30 seconds
- Takes between 200 and 500 individual 1-mm to 5-mm very slim images that can be reconstructed into three dimensions
- Decreases the potential for misinterpretation from breathing or movement

HELICAL VIRTUAL ANGIOGRAPHY

- Creates images of the arteries of any chosen organ

VIRTUAL ANGIOGRAPHY

- Assists the clinician to identify areas of stenosis

THREE-DIMENSIONAL (3D) SCAN

- Allows for a virtual exploration of chosen areas as an option to a more invasive procedure
- Allows, for example, the clinician to look inside the colon using a virtual colonoscopy. The clinician can evaluate for disease before deciding if the more invasive colonoscopy is needed
- Offers a more comfortable and less stressful option for the patient

The value of CT scans is in the quality of the images that assist in early diagnosis and treatment of multiple medical problems. The ability to image anatomy has been the benefit of CT scans since their inception. Now, through the use of fusion imaging, CT/PET scans can also provide physiologic information. **Fusion CT** and **positron emission tomography (PET) scans**

- Can determine if an abnormality is malignant or benign
- Often saves the patient from an invasive biopsy

CT SYSTEM COMPONENTS: There are three major system components to a CT scanner:

- Computer, which provides the link between the CT technologist and the other components of the imaging system.
- Gantry, which is a circular device that houses the x-ray tube and detectors. The opening in the gantry is called the aperture and most are about 28 inches wide to accommodate a variety of patient sizes as the table advances through it.
- Table, which is an automated device linked to the gantry and computer. The table is an extremely important part of a CT scanner and can be programmed to move in and out of the gantry during the exam. Most CT tables have a weight limit from the manufacturer from 300 to 600 pounds (see Fig. 7.1).

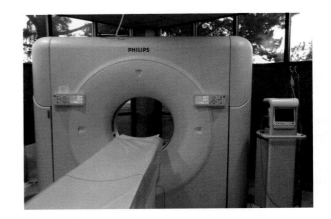

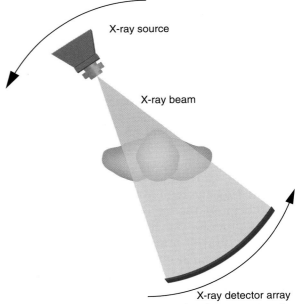

FIGURE 7.1 CT scanner. *Used with permission, from Weber, E., Vilensky, J., & Fog, A. (2013). Practical radiology: A system-based approach. FA Davis Company.*

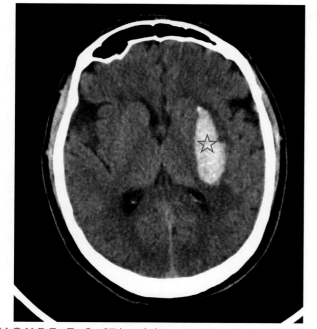

FIGURE 7.2 CT head demonstrating intracerebral hemorrhage. *Used with permission, from Weber, E., Vilensky, J., & Fog, A. (2013). Practical radiology: A system-based approach. FA Davis Company.*

DISCUSSION POINT

CONTRAST MEDIA: Contrast media can be used to assist in differentiating between normal anatomy and disease pathology. Contrast media can be given to the patient intravenously (IV), orally, or rectally. Nonionic contrast media is used by some facilities due to the deceased reaction risk. IV contrasts are useful for showing tumors that are very vascular in addition to visualizing other vascular structures in the body. Figure 7.2 shows an acute intracerebral hemorrhage that can result from nontraumatic causes, such as bleeding disorders (e.g., sickle cell anemia) (see Fig. 7.2). IV contrast should be used only with approval of the radiologist. Before the patient has a CT scan, the patient's medical and allergy history should be assessed. Renal function should be evaluated before iodinated contrast material is given. The serum creatinine level and glomerular filtration rate are a good way to assess renal function. Many CT examinations can be performed without IV contrast, if necessary; however, the amount of diagnostic information can be limited.

Oral contrast media must be given for imaging the abdomen and pelvis. When given orally, the contrast material in the gastrointestinal tract helps differentiate between loops of bowel and other structures within the abdomen. An oral contrast medium is generally a 2% barium mixture, which has a low concentration and prevents contrast artifacts while still allowing for good visualization of the stomach and intestinal tract. Rectal contrast media is often requested as part of an abdominal or pelvic protocol and is useful in showing the distal colon relative to the bladder and other structures of the pelvic cavity.

● *Safety Tip*

Radiation Safety Typically, radiation received during radiologic examinations comes from a fixed source with delivery in one or two places. These exposures produce a much higher skin entrance dose than the exit skin dose. In contrast, CT exposures come from an essentially continuous source that rotates 360° around the patient and results in a radially symmetric radiation dose within the patient. The patient dose must be a part of the permanent record for each examination in CT.

Pediatric CT Scans Millions of CT examinations are performed each year on children within the United States. Concerns regarding the use of CT scan in children fall into three areas; sensitivity, life expectancy, and the radiation dose. Children are more sensitive to radiation exposure than adults. Radiation risk is higher in young patients as they have more rapidly dividing cells than adults. The younger the patient, the more sensitive to radiation he or she is. As part of the normal aging process, children live longer than adults. Exposure to radiation at a younger age increases the likelihood to develop disease as a result of that exposure. Children's longevity increases the possibility of developing diseases such as brain tumor and leukemia due to cumulative CT radiation doses. This cumulative effect is dependent upon the age of the child, the number of scans, and the amount of radiation exposure and milligray absorption (unit of the absorbed dose). There are recommendations to decrease the risk to children with CT scans. First, clinicians should consider other diagnostic options before using CT scan. If CT scanning is necessary, radiologists are encouraged to use the lowest dose of radiation necessary for a successful scan. Thought should be given to adjusting the amount of radiation to the size and weight of the child. Scanning when performed on children should be limited to medically necessary areas. The creation of pediatric standardized scanning protocols with defined exposure settings can also be beneficial. The Image Gently Campaign was launched in 2008 to raise awareness of safety concerns related to radiation exposure from diagnostic procedures. It has grown into a national coalition of more than 40 organizations whose goal is to provide education to individuals and institutions, promoting awareness of safe pediatric imaging practices. Information for patients, parents, and health-care providers (HCPs), about the Image Gently Campaign, can be found at www.imagegently.org.

Encourage parents to ask questions and then point them to this page, http://www.pedrad.org/associations/5364/ig/?page=595 which contains two informational brochures–What Parents Should Know About CT Scans for Children and What Parents Should Know About Medical Radiation Safety–which discuss the issue in greater depth.

The information in the Part I studies is organized in a manner to help the student see how the five basic components of the nursing process (assessment, diagnosis, planning, implementation, and evaluation) can be applied to each phase of laboratory and diagnostic testing. The goal is to use nursing process to understand the integration of care (laboratory, diagnostic, nursing care) toward achieving a positive expected outcome.

- **Assessment** is the collection of information for the purpose of answering the question, "is there a problem?" Knowledge of the patient's health history, medications, complaints, and allergies as well as synonyms or alternate test names, common use for the procedure, specimen requirements, and normal ranges or interpretive comments provide the foundation for diagnosis.
- **Diagnosis** is the process of looking at the information gathered during assessment and answering the questions, "what is the problem?" and "what do I need to do about it?" Test indications tell us why the study has been requested, and potential diagnoses tell us the value or importance of the study relative to its clinical utility.
- **Planning** is a blueprint of the nursing care before the procedure. It is the process of determining how the nurse is going to partner with the patient to fix the problem (e.g., "The patient has a study ordered and this is what I should know before I successfully carry out the plan to have the study completed."). Knowledge of interfering factors, social and cultural issues, preprocedural restrictions, the need for written and informed consent, anxiety about the procedure, and concerns regarding pain are some considerations for planning a successful partnership.
- **Implementation** is putting the plan into action with an idea of what the expected outcome should be. Collaboration with the departments where the laboratory test or diagnostic study is to be performed is essential to the success of the plan. Implementation is where the work is done within each health-care team member's scope of practice.
- **Evaluation** answers the question, "did the plan work or not?" Was the plan completely successful, partially successful, or not successful? If the plan did not work, evaluation is the process where you determine what needs to be changed to make the plan work better. This includes a review of all expected outcomes. Nursing care after the procedure is where information is gathered to evaluate the plan. Review of results, including critical findings, in relation to patient symptoms and other tests performed, provides data that form a more complete picture of health or illness.
- **Expected Outcomes** are positive outcomes related to the test. They are the outcomes the nurse should expect if all goes well.

A number of pretest, intratest, and post-test universal points are presented in this overview section because the information applies to CT studies in general.

Universal Pretest Pearls (Planning)

- Obtain a history of the patient's complaints, including a list of known allergens, especially allergies or sensitivities to medications or latex so that their use can be avoided or their effects mitigated if an allergy is present. Carefully evaluate all medications currently being taken by the patient. A list of the patient's current medications, prescribed and over the counter (including anticoagulants, aspirin and other salicylates, herbs, nutritional supplements, and neutraceuticals), should also be obtained. Such products may be discontinued by medical direction for the appropriate number of days prior to the procedure. Ensure that all allergies are clearly noted in the medical record, and ensure that the patient is wearing an allergy and medical record armband. Report information that could interfere with, or delay proceeding with, the study to the health-care provider (HCP) and laboratory.
- Obtain a history of the patient's affected body system, symptoms, and results of previously performed laboratory tests and diagnostic and surgical procedures. Previous test results will provide a basis of comparison between old and new data.
- An important aspect of planning is understanding the factors that may alter study findings or cause abnormal results. Interdepartmental communication is a key factor in the planning process. The inability of a patient to cooperate or remain still during the procedure because of age, significant pain, or mental status should be among the anticipated factors. Recent or past procedures, medications, or existing medical conditions that could complicate or interfere with test results should be noted.
- Review the steps of the study with the patient or caregiver. Expect patients to be nervous about the procedure and the pending results. Educating the patient on his or her role during the procedure and what to expect can facilitate this. The patient's role during the procedure is to remain still. The actual time required to complete each study will depend on a number of conditions, including the type of equipment being used and how well a patient will cooperate.
- Address any concerns about pain, and explain or describe, as appropriate, the level and type of discomfort that may be expected. Explain that an IV line may be inserted prior to some procedures to allow the infusion of IV fluids such as normal saline, contrast medium, or medications. Advise the patient that some discomfort may be experienced during the insertion of the IV. Make the patient aware that there may be some mild discomfort during the procedure.

- Provide additional instructions and patient preparation regarding medication, diet, fluid intake, or activity, if appropriate. Unless specified in the individual study, there are no special instructions or restrictions.
- Always be sensitive to any cultural or psychosocial issues, including a concern for modesty before, during, and after the procedure.

Reminder

Ensure that a written and informed consent has been documented in the medical record prior to the study, if required. The consent must be obtained before medication is administered.

Universal Intratest Pearls (Implementation)

- Correct patient identification is crucial prior to any procedure: Positively identify the patient using two unique identifiers, such as patient name, date of birth, Social Security number, or medical record number.
- Standard Precautions must be followed.
- Children and infants may be accompanied by a parent to calm them. Keep neonates and infants covered and in a warm room and provide a pacifier or gentle touch. The testing environment should be quiet and the patient should be instructed, as appropriate, to remain still during the test as extraneous movements can affect results.
- Ensure that the patient has complied with pretesting instructions, including dietary, fluid, medication, and activity restrictions as given for the procedure is necessary. The number of days to withhold medication depends on the type of medication. Notify the HCP if pretesting instructions have not been followed (e.g., if patient anticoagulant therapy has not been withheld).
- The patient, as appropriate, should be prepared for insertion of an IV line for infusion of IV fluids, contrast medium, antibiotics, anesthetics, analgesics, medications used in the procedure, or emergency medications. Inform the patient when prophylactic antibiotics will be administered before the procedure, and assess for antibiotic allergy. Prior to administration of any fluids or medications, verify that they are accurate for the study. Bleeding or bruising can be prevented, once the needle has been removed, by applying direct pressure to the injection site with dry gauze for a minute or two. The site should be observed/assessed for bleeding or hematoma formation, and then covered with a gauze and adhesive bandage.
- Emergency equipment should be readily available.

- Baseline vital signs must be recorded and monitored throughout and after the procedure, according to organizational policy. A comparison should be made between the baseline and postprocedure vital signs and focused assessments. Protocols may vary among facilities.
- Before leaving the patient's side, appropriate specimen containers should always be labeled with the corresponding patient demographics, initials of the person collecting the sample, collection date, time of collection, applicable special notes, especially site location and laterality, and then promptly transported to the laboratory for processing and analysis. Place tissue samples for standard biopsy examination in properly labeled specimen containers containing formalin solution, place tissue samples for molecular diagnostic studies in properly labeled specimen containers, and promptly transport the specimen to the laboratory for processing and analysis.

Universal Post Test Pearls (Evaluation)

- Note that completed test results are made available to the requesting HCP, who will discuss them with the patient.
- Answer questions and address concerns voiced by the patient or family and reinforce information given by the patient's HCP regarding further testing, treatment, or referral to another HCP. Recognize that patients will have anxiety related to test results. Provide teaching and information regarding the clinical implications of the test results on the patient's lifestyle as appropriate.
- Note that test results should be evaluated in context with the patient's signs, symptoms, and diagnosis. Depending on the results of the procedure, additional testing may be performed to evaluate or monitor progression of the disease process and determine the need for a change in therapy.
- Be aware that when a person goes through a traumatic event such as an illness or is being given information that will impact his or her lifestyle, there are universal human reactions that occur. These include knowledge deficit, fear, anxiety, and coping; in some situations, grieving may occur. HCPs should always be aware of the human response and how it may affect the plan of care and expected outcomes.

DISCUSSION POINT

Regarding Post-Test Critical Findings: Timely notification of a critical finding for lab or diagnostic studies is a role expectation of the professional nurse. Notification

processes will vary among facilities. Upon receipt of the critical finding, the information should be read back to the caller to verify accuracy. Most policies require immediate notification of the primary HCP, hospitalist, or on-call HCP. Reported information includes the patient's name, unique identifiers, critical finding, name of the person giving the report, and name of the person receiving the report. Documentation of notification should be made in the medical record with the name of the HCP notified, time and date of notification, and any orders received. Any delay in a timely report of a critical finding may require completion of a notification form with review by Risk Management.

STUDIES

- Computed Tomography, Abdomen
- Computed Tomography, Biliary Tract and Liver
- Computed Tomography, Brain
- Computed Tomography, Pancreas

LEARNING OUTCOMES

Providing safe, effective nursing care (SENC) includes mastery of core competencies and standards of care. SENC is based on a judicious application of nursing knowledge in combination with scientific principles. The Art of Nursing lies in blending what you know with the ability to effectively apply your knowledge in a compassionate manner.

After reading/studying this chapter you will be able to:

Thinking

1. Recognize that human beings are imperfect, and failure to follow policy and standards of care, or participate in work-arounds can place a patient at risk.
2. Examine the scope of practice related to specific aspects of care such as information management; evidence-based education; and organizational, patient, family, and ancillary communication.

Doing

1. Recognize that memory can be imperfect, and the use of assistive resources (checklists, electronic tablets, etc.) can reduce care errors.
2. Identify barriers that prevent the patient from participating in health and wellness.

Caring

1. Value the ability of the individual in the prevention of errors.
2. Recognize that perceiving how care is delivered though the patient's point of view is of value.

Computed Tomography, Abdomen

Quick Summary

SYNONYM ACRONYM: Computed axial tomography (CAT), computed transaxial tomography (CTT), abdominal CT, helical/spiral CT.

COMMON USE: To visualize and assess abdominal structures and to assist in diagnosing tumors, bleeding, and abscess. Used as an evaluation tool for surgical, radiation, and medical therapeutic interventions.

AREA OF APPLICATION: Abdomen.

NORMAL FINDINGS: Normal size, position, and shape of abdominal organs and vascular system

Test Explanation

Abdominal computed tomography (CT) is a noninvasive procedure used to enhance certain anatomic views of the abdominal structures. It becomes invasive when contrast medium is used. During the procedure, the patient lies on a motorized table. The table is moved in and out of a circular opening in a doughnut-like device called a *gantry,* which houses the x-ray tube and associated electronics. A beam of x-rays irradiates the patient as the table moves in and out of the scanner in a series of phases. The x-rays penetrate liquids and solids of different densities by varying degrees. Multiple detectors rotate around the patient to collect numeric data associated with the density coefficients assigned to each degree of tissue density. The imaging system's computer converts the numeric data obtained from the scanner into digital images. Air appears black, bone appears white, and body fluids, fat, and soft tissue structures are represented in various shades between black and white. The cross-sectional views or slices of the liver, biliary tract, gallbladder, pancreas, kidneys, adrenal glands, spleen, intestines, and associated vascular system can be reviewed individually or as a three-dimensional image to allow differentiations of solid, cystic, inflammatory, or vascular lesions, as well as identification of suspected hematomas and aneurysms. The scan may be repeated after administration of contrast medium given orally, by IV, or rectally. Contrast is used to differentiate, enhance, or "light up" areas of interest depending on the type of study to be performed, type of contrast medium to be used, and method of administration. The medium works by creating a contrast between areas of interest based on density; penetration of the x-rays is weaker in areas where the contrast medium is detected by the scanner showing the blood vessels, organs, and tissue as whitish areas that either outline the area of interest or completely fill it. Oral ingestion of contrast medium can be used for opacification to distinguish the bowel, adjacent abdominal organs, other types of tissue, and blood vessels as the medium moves through the digestive tract.

Intravenous injection of contrast medium is used for evaluation of blood flow through vessels and greater enhancement of tissue density and organ visualization. In some cases scans may be repeated after multiple types of contrast are administered. Multislice or multi-detector CT (MDCT) scanners continuously collect images in a helical or spiral fashion instead of a series of individual images as with standard scanners. Helical CT is capable of collecting many images over a short period of time (seconds), is very sensitive in identifying small abnormalities, and produces high-quality images. Positron emission tomography (PET) and single photon emission tomography (SPECT) are types of nuclear medicine studies that offer insights into functionality such as movement of blood flow or uptake and distribution of metabolites into tumors. PET/CT and SPECT/CT are imaging applications that superimpose PET or SPECT and CT findings. The images are collected and produced by a single gantry system. The co-registered or image fusion of PET/CT or SPECT/CT findings are capable of providing a very detailed combination of anatomical and functional images. Images can be recorded on photographic or x-ray film, or stored in digital format as digitized computer data. The CT scan can be used to guide biopsy needles into areas of suspected tumors to obtain tissue for laboratory analysis and to guide placement of catheters for drainage of cysts or abscesses. Tumor staging and progression, before and after therapy, and effectiveness of medical interventions may be monitored by PET/CT or SPECT/CT scanning. The images can be reevaluated and manipulated for further, detailed examination without having to repeat the procedure (see Fig. 7.3).

Nursing Implications

Assessment

Indications	Potential Nursing Problems
Assist in differentiating between benign and malignant tumors	• Bleeding
Detect aortic aneurysms	• Breathing
Detect tumor extension of masses and metastasis into the abdominal area	• Cardiac Output
Differentiate aortic aneurysms from tumors near the aorta	• Fear
Differentiate between infectious and inflammatory processes	• Fever
Evaluate cysts, masses, abscesses, renal calculi, gastrointestinal (GI) bleeding and obstruction, and trauma	• Gas Exchange
Evaluate retroperitoneal lymph nodes	• Human Response
Monitor and evaluate the effectiveness of medical, radiation, or surgical therapies	• Injury Risk
	• Pain
	• Renal
	• Shock
	• Tissue Perfusion

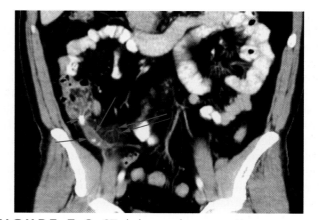

FIGURE 7.3 CT abdomen demonstrating acute appendicitis. *Used with permission, from Weber, E., Vilensky, J., & Fog, A. (2013). Practical radiology: A system-based approach. FA Davis Company.*

Diagnosis: Clinical Significance of Test Results
ABNORMAL FINDING

Identification of abnormal findings is assisted by comparison of parameters such as size, shape, symmetry, density, and location; for example, areas of altered density in either an expected or unexpected location may indicate enlargement of an organ or the presence of blood or other fluids, tumors, or cysts. Comparison by type of abnormal findings may also assist in evaluating areas of altered density; for example, well-defined round or oval areas, smaller in size and having lower density than a primary tumor, may indicate a cyst.

- Abdominal abscess
- Abdominal aortic aneurysm
- Abnormal accumulations of blood, fat, or body fluid
- Adrenal tumor or hyperplasia
- Appendicitis
- Bowel obstruction
- Bowel perforation
- Cirrhosis
- Dilation of the common hepatic duct, common bile duct, or gallbladder
- Diverticulitis or irritable bowel
- Gallstones
- GI bleeding
- Hematomas, diverticulitis, gallstones
- Hemoperitoneum
- Hepatic cysts or abscesses
- Infarction
- Infection
- Pancreatic pseudocyst
- Primary and metastatic neoplasms in bone, organs, glands, ducts, or ligaments
- Renal calculi
- Splenic laceration, tumor, infiltration, and trauma
- Trauma

Planning

Considerations for planning a successful partnership should include clear communication of what to expect during the test to decrease anxiety and improve cooperation. Before the procedure is performed, plan to review the steps with the patient. Ensure that the results of coagulation testing are obtained and recorded prior to the procedure; BUN and creatinine results are also needed if contrast medium is to be used. Note any recent procedures that can interfere with test results, including examinations using barium- or iodine-based contrast medium. Ensure that barium studies were performed more than 4 days before the CT scan. Record the date of the last menstrual period, and determine the possibility of pregnancy in perimenopausal women. Explain that minimal discomfort should be experienced during the exam, and inform the patient that the procedure is performed in a CT suite by a CT technologist and takes approximately 15–30 minutes. Remind the patient that she or he should remain still during the procedure, and instruct the patient to remove all metal in the area to be examined. Inform the patient as appropriate that CT studies performed without contrast usually do not require the patient to fast before the procedure. Instruct the patient, if required, to fast and restrict fluids for the specified time period, prior to the procedure; fasting is required for several hours prior to contrast enhanced studies as a precaution against pulmonary aspiration of stomach contents during the procedure. Instruct the patient to avoid taking anticoagulant medication or to reduce dosage as ordered prior to the procedure; due to increased risk of bleeding at the IV insertion site. Protocols may vary among facilities. Explain that she or he may be required to drink approximately 450 mL of a dilute barium solution (approximately 1% barium) or water-soluble contrast before the examination; the oral contrast is given at a specified time period, prior to the study. This is administered to distinguish GI organs from the other abdominal organs. Inquire about previous allergies and contrast reactions. If iodinated contrast medium is scheduled to be used in patients receiving metformin (Glucophage) for non-insulin-dependent (type 2) diabetes, the drug should be discontinued on the day of the test and continue to be withheld for 48 hours after the test. Iodinated contrast can temporarily impair kidney function, and failure to withhold metformin may indirectly result in drug-induced lactic acidosis, a dangerous and sometimes fatal adverse effect of metformin *related to renal impairment that does not support sufficient excretion of metformin.* Explain that an IV line may be inserted to allow the infusion of IV fluids (e.g., normal saline), anesthetics, contrast medium, or sedatives. Inform the patient that she or he may experience nausea, a feeling of warmth, a flushed sensation, a salty or metallic taste, or may notice a transient headache if IV contrast is used, and that these reactions are considered normal.

CONTRAINDICATIONS

- Patients who are pregnant or are suspected of being pregnant, unless the potential benefits of the procedure far outweigh the risk of radiation exposure to the fetus and mother
- Patients who are claustrophobic
- Conditions associated with adverse reactions to the contrast medium (e.g., asthma, food allergies, or allergy to the contrast medium). Although patients are still asked specifically if they have a known allergy to iodine or shellfish, it has been well established that the reaction is not to iodine; in fact, an actual iodine allergy would be very problematic because iodine is required for the production of thyroid hormones. In the case of shellfish, the reaction is to a muscle protein called *tropomyosin*; in the case of iodinated contrast medium, the reaction is to the noniodinated part of the contrast molecule. Patients with a known hypersensitivity to the medium may benefit from premedication with corticosteroids and diphenhydramine. The use of nonionic contrast or an alternative noncontrast imaging study, if available, may be considered for patients who have severe asthma or who have experienced moderate to severe reactions to ionic contrast medium.
- Conditions associated with preexisting renal insufficiency (e.g., chronic kidney disease, single kidney transplant, nephrectomy, diabetes, multiple myeloma, treatment with aminoglycosides and NSAIDs) *because iodinated contrast is nephrotoxic*
- Older adults and compromised patients who are chronically dehydrated before the test *because of their risk of contrast-induced acute kidney injury*
- Patients with pheochromocytoma, *because iodinated contrast may cause a hypertensive crisis*
- Patients with bleeding disorders receiving an arterial or venous puncture (angiography) *because the site may not stop bleeding*

SPECIAL CONSIDERATIONS

An important aspect of planning is understanding the factors that may alter study findings or cause abnormal results. Interdepartmental communication is a key factor in the planning process. The following should be noted when planning for this study:

- Gas or feces in the gastrointestinal (GI) tract resulting from inadequate cleansing or failure to restrict food intake before the study may result in unclear images.
- Retained barium from a previous radiological procedure may cause unclear images.
- Patients who are very obese may exceed the weight limit for the equipment.

- Metallic objects within the examination field (e.g., jewelry, body rings) may inhibit organ visualization and cause unclear images.
- Patients with extreme claustrophobia, unless sedation is given before the study, may be unable to cooperate or remain still during the procedure.
- Patients may be unable to cooperate or remain still during the procedure because of age, significant pain, or mental status, and this may cause unclear images.
- The occurrence of chest pain or severe cardiac dysrhythmias may require termination of the procedure.
- Failure to follow dietary restrictions and other pretesting preparations may lead to cancellation or rescheduling of the procedure

● Safety Tip

Consultation with a health-care provider (HCP) should occur before the procedure for radiation safety concerns regarding younger patients or patients who are lactating. **Pediatric Considerations** Information on the Image Gently Campaign can be found at the Alliance for Radiation Safety in Pediatric Imaging (www.pedrad.org/ associations/5364/ig/). Risks associated with radiation overexposure can result from frequent x-ray procedures. Personnel in the examination room with the patient should wear a protective lead apron, stand behind a shield, or leave the area while the examination is being done. Personnel working in the examination area should wear badges to record their level of radiation exposure.

● Safety Tip

Make sure a written and informed consent has been signed prior to the procedure if a biopsy is planned and before administering any medications.

Implementation

Patient education is key to obtaining the patient's cooperation in following directions, and providing an explanation for the purpose of the procedure is an important part of this process. Inform the patient that this study can assist in assessing for disorders of the abdomen, including organs and vessels. Ensure that the patient is in compliance with pretesting instructions. Record baseline vital signs, and continue to monitor throughout the procedure. Protocols may vary among facilities. Establish an IV fluid line for the injection of contrast, emergency drugs, and sedatives. Administer an antianxiety agent, as ordered, if the patient has claustrophobia. Administer a sedative to a child or to an uncooperative adult, as ordered.

Position the patient in a supine position on the CT table with the patient's arms above her or his head. The table is moved into the gantry and the area between the dome of the diaphragm, and the iliac crest is scanned with 0.5-mm transverse images. IV contrast is injected, if ordered, following completion of the first set of images, and the entire series is repeated. The images are reviewed by the technologist on a special viewing monitor in the scanning room and then recorded digitally for radiologist interpretation. Monitor the patient for complications related to the procedure (e.g., allergic reaction, anaphylaxis, bronchospasm) if contrast is used. Following completion of the scans, remove the IV needle and cover with a sterile dressing. Observe the patient for any signs of an allergic reaction to the contrast.

Evaluation

Recognize anxiety related to test results and be supportive of impaired activity related to a perceived loss of independence. Instruct the patient to resume his or her usual diet, fluids, medications, and activity as directed by the HCP. Renal function should be assessed before metformin is resumed, if contrast was used. Monitor vital signs and the neurological status every 15 minutes for 1 hour, then every 2 hours for 4 hours, and then as ordered by the HCP. Monitor patient temperature every 4 hours for 24 hours. Monitor intake and output at least every 8 hours. Compare all of these with baseline values. Notify the HCP if temperature is elevated. Protocols may vary from facility to facility. If contrast was used, observe for delayed allergic reactions, such as rash, urticaria, tachycardia, hyperpnea, hypertension, palpitations, nausea, or vomiting. Instruct the patient to immediately report symptoms such as a fast heart rate, difficulty breathing, skin rash, itching, chest pain, persistent right shoulder pain, or abdominal pain. Immediately report symptoms to the appropriate HCP. Antihistamines or steroids may be administered if needed. Observe/assess the needle insertion site for bleeding, inflammation, or hematoma formation. Discuss the implications of abnormal test results on the patient's lifestyle. Provide teaching and information regarding the clinical implications of the test results as appropriate. Answer any questions or address any concerns voiced by the patient or family. Educate the patient regarding access to counseling services.

Inform the patient that following the ingestion of an oral contrast, she or he may experience diarrhea, and encourage the patient to drink fluids to promote contrast excretion. Instruct the patient in the care and assessment of the site. Instruct the patient to apply cold compresses to the insertion site as needed to reduce discomfort or edema.

✓ Critical Findings

- Abscess
- Acute GI bleed
- Aortic aneurysm
- Appendicitis
- Aortic dissection
- Bowel perforation
- Bowel obstruction
- Mesenteric torsion
- Tumor with significant mass effect
- Visceral injury; significant solid organ laceration

Note and immediately report to the requesting health-care provider (HCP) any critical findings and related symptoms. A listing of these findings varies among facilities.

Study Specific Complications

Injection of the contrast through IV tubing into a blood vessel is an invasive procedure. Complications are rare but do include the risk of allergic reaction *related to contrast reaction*. It is important to have oxygen and endotracheal equipment in the vicinity for immediate use. In the event of an anaphylactic reaction, epinephrine, diphenhydramine and steroids are included with resuscitative efforts.

Contrast Reactions: Signs, Symptoms, and Treatment

	Minor	Intermediate	Life-Threatening
Signs, Symptoms	Nausea, vomiting, urticaria, sneezing	Bronchospasms; chills and fever; chest pain, laryngeal or tongue edema	Hypotension, cardiac dysrhythmias; seizures; loss of bowel/bladder control; laryngeal and pulmonary edema
Interventions	Antihistamines	Antihistamines, steroids, bronchodilators, IV fluids and observation	All intermediate interventions plus: intubation and ventilation, pressors and antiseizure medications

Other complications related to the procedure may include:

- Cardiac dysrhythmias may occur.
- Acute kidney injury may occur as a result of contrast infusion; hydration prior to the study can reduce the likelihood of this complication.
- Acidosis or hypoglycemia may occur in patients taking metformin when receiving iodinated contrast; metformin should be withheld for 48 hours prior to the study
- Bruising, hematoma *related to blood leakage into the tissue following insertion of the IV needle*, infection or sepsis *which might occur if bacteria from the skin surface is introduced at the IV needle insertion site*, pain, prolonged bleeding, swelling, and vasovagal reactions are associated with venipuncture. Infections can occur as a result of any invasive procedure. Antibiotic therapy should be ordered if this occurs. Elevated temperatures, abnormal-colored sputum, changes in breathing patterns, chills, and hypotension can all indicate infection or sepsis.
- Hemorrhage from highly vascular tissue or infection may also occur following a CT-guided biopsy. Instruct the patient to look for excessive bleeding, skin redness, and fever or chills, and to notify her or his HCP if these symptoms occur.

Related Tests

Related tests include ACTH and challenge tests, amylase, angiography abdomen, biopsy intestinal, BUN, calculus kidney stone panel, CBC, CBC hematocrit, CBC hemoglobin, cortisol and challenge tests, creatinine, cystoscopy, hepatobiliary scan, IVP, KUB studies, MRI abdomen, peritoneal fluid analysis, PT/INR, renogram, US abdomen, and US pelvis.

Refer to the Gastrointestinal and Hepatobiliary systems tables at the end of the book for related tests by body system.

Expected Outcomes

Expected outcomes associated with Computed Tomography, Abdomen, are

- Blood pressure that remains within normal limits
- Normal breathing pattern
- Verbalizing an understanding of activities that place them at risk for disease
- Collaborating with the HCP to devise an appropriate treatment plan

Computed Tomography, Biliary Tract and Liver

Quick Summary

SYNONYM ACRONYM: Computed axial tomography (CAT), computed transaxial tomography (CTT), abdominal CT, helical/spiral CT.

COMMON USE: To visualize and assess the structure of the liver and biliary tract toward the diagnosis of tumor, obstruction, bleeding, and infection. Used as an evaluation tool for surgical, radiation, and medical therapeutic interventions.

AREA OF APPLICATION: Liver, biliary tract, and adjacent structures.

NORMAL FINDINGS: Normal size, position, and contour of the liver and biliary ducts

Test Explanation

Computed tomography (CT) of the liver and biliary tract is a noninvasive procedure that enhances certain anatomic views of these structures. It becomes invasive with the use of contrast medium. During the procedure, the patient lies on a motorized table. The table is moved in and out of a circular opening in a doughnut-like device called a *gantry,* which houses the x-ray tube and associated electronics. A beam of x-rays irradiates the patient as the table moves in and out of the scanner in a series of phases. The x-rays penetrate liquids and solids of different densities by varying degrees. Multiple detectors rotate around the patient to collect numeric data associated with the density coefficients assigned to each degree of tissue density. The imaging system's computer converts the numeric data obtained from the scanner into digital images. Air appears black, bone appears white, and body fluids, fat, and soft tissue structures are represented in various shades between black and white. The cross-sectional views or slices of the liver, biliary tract, and associated vascular system can be reviewed individually or as a three-dimensional image to allow differentiations of solid, cystic, inflammatory, or vascular lesions, as well as identification of suspected hematomas. The scan may be repeated after administration of contrast medium given orally or by IV. Contrast is used to differentiate, enhance, or "light up" areas of interest depending on the type of study to be performed, type of contrast medium to be used, and method of administration. The medium works by creating a contrast between areas of interest based on density; penetration of the x-rays is weaker in areas where the contrast medium is detected by the scanner showing the blood vessels, organs, and tissue as whitish areas that either outline the area of interest or completely fill it. Oral ingestion of contrast medium can be used for opacification to distinguish the bowel, adjacent abdominal organs, other types of tissue, and blood vessels as the medium moves through the digestive tract. Intravenous injection of contrast medium is used for evaluation of blood flow through vessels and greater enhancement of tissue density and organ visualization. In some cases scans may be repeated after both types of contrast are administered. Multislice or multidetector CT (MDCT) scanners continuously collect images in a helical or spiral fashion instead of a series of individual images as with standard scanners. Helical CT is capable of collecting many images over a short period of time (seconds), is very sensitive in identifying small abnormalities, and produces high-quality images. Positron emission tomography (PET) and single photon emission tomography (SPECT) are types of nuclear medicine studies that offer insights into functionality such as movement of blood flow or uptake and distribution of metabolites into tumors. PET/CT and SPECT/CT are imaging applications that superimpose PET or SPECT and CT findings. The images are collected and produced by a single gantry system. The co-registered or image fusion of PET/CT or SPECT/CT findings are capable of providing a very detailed combination of anatomical and functional images. Images can be recorded on photographic or x-ray film or stored in digital format as digitized computer data. The CT scan can be used to guide biopsy needles into areas of suspected tumors to obtain tissue for laboratory analysis and to guide placement of catheters for drainage of cysts or abscesses. Tumor staging and progression, before and after therapy, and effectiveness of medical interventions may be monitored by PET/CT or SPECT/CT scanning. The images can be reevaluated and manipulated for further, detailed examination without having to repeat the procedure.

Nursing Implications
Assessment

Indications	Potential Nursing Problems
Assist in differentiating between benign and malignant tumors Detect dilation or obstruction of the biliary ducts with or without calcification or gallstone Detect liver abnormalities, such as cirrhosis with ascites and fatty liver Detect tumor extension of masses and metastasis into the hepatic area Differentiate aortic aneurysms from tumors near the aorta Differentiate between obstructive and nonobstructive jaundice Differentiate infectious from inflammatory processes Evaluate hepatic cysts, masses, abscesses, and hematomas, or hepatic trauma Monitor and evaluate effectiveness of medical, radiation, or surgical therapies	• Airway • Breathing • Confusion • Fluid Volume • Gastrointestinal • Human Response • Injury Risk • Nutrition • Pain • Powerlessness

Diagnosis: Clinical Significance of Test Results
ABNORMAL FINDING

Identification of abnormal findings is assisted by comparison of parameters such as size, shape, symmetry, density, and location, for example areas of altered density in either an expected or unexpected location may indicate enlargement of an organ or the presence of blood or other fluids, tumors, or cysts; a crescent shaped area of abnormal density that alters the proximity of the liver to the Glisson's capsule may indicate a hematoma; areas of less than normal density may indicate hepatic lesions; or dilation of the associated ducts may indicate an obstruction. Comparison by type of abnormal findings may also assist in evaluating areas of altered density, for example well defined round or oval areas, smaller in size and having lower density than a primary tumor may indicate a cyst.

- Dilation of the common hepatic duct, common bile duct, or gallbladder
- Gallstones
- Hematomas
- Hepatic cysts or abscesses
- Jaundice (obstructive or nonobstructive)
- Primary and metastatic neoplasms

Planning

Considerations for planning a successful partnership should include clear communication of what to expect during the test to decrease anxiety and improve cooperation. Before the procedure is performed, plan to review the steps with the patient. Ensure that the results of coagulation testing are obtained and recorded prior to the procedure; BUN and creatinine results are also needed if contrast medium is to be used. Note any recent procedures that can interfere with test results, including examinations using barium- or iodine-based contrast medium. Ensure that barium studies were performed more than 4 days before the CT scan. Record the date of the last menstrual period, and determine the possibility of pregnancy in perimenopausal women. Explain that minimal discomfort should be experienced during the exam, and inform the patient that the procedure is performed in a CT suite by a CT technologist and takes approximately 15–30 minutes depending on factors such as the type of study ordered, whether contrast will be used, and the type of contrast used. Remind the patient that she or he should remain still during the procedure, and instruct the patient to remove all metal in the area to be examined. Inform the patient as appropriate that CT studies performed without contrast usually do not require the patient to fast before the procedure. Instruct the patient, if required, to fast and restrict fluids for the specified time period, prior to the procedure; fasting is required for several hours prior to contrast enhanced studies as a precaution against pulmonary aspiration of stomach contents during the procedure. Instruct the patient to avoid taking anticoagulant medication or to reduce the dosage as ordered prior to the procedure due to increased risk of bleeding at the IV insertion site. Protocols may vary among facilities. Explain that she or he may be required to drink approximately 450 mL of a dilute barium solution (approximately 1% barium) or water-soluble contrast before the examination; the oral contrast is given at a specified time period, prior to the study. This is administered to distinguish GI organs from the other abdominal organs. Inquire about previous allergies and contrast reactions. If iodinated contrast medium is scheduled to be used in patients receiving metformin (Glucophage) for non-insulin-dependent (type 2) diabetes, the drug should be discontinued on the day of the test and continue to be withheld for 48 hours after the test. Iodinated contrast can temporarily impair kidney function, and failure to withhold metformin may indirectly result in drug-induced lactic acidosis, a dangerous and sometimes fatal adverse effect of metformin *related to renal impairment that does not support sufficient excretion of metformin.* Explain that an IV line may be inserted to allow the infusion of IV fluids (e.g., normal saline), anesthetics, contrast medium, or sedatives. Inform the patient that she or he may experience nausea, a feeling of warmth, a flushed sensation, a salty or metallic taste, or may notice a transient headache if IV contrast is used and that these reactions are considered normal.

CONTRAINDICATIONS

- Patients who are pregnant or suspected of being pregnant, unless the potential benefits of the procedure far outweigh the risk of radiation exposure to the fetus and mother
- Patients who are claustrophobic
- Conditions associated with adverse reactions to the contrast medium (e.g., asthma, food allergies, or allergy to the contrast medium) Although patients are still asked specifically if they have a known allergy to iodine or shellfish, it has been well established that the reaction is not to iodine; in fact, an actual iodine allergy would be very problematic because iodine is required for the production of thyroid hormones. In the case of shellfish, the reaction is to a muscle protein called *tropomyosin*; in the case of iodinated contrast medium, the reaction is to the noniodinated part of the contrast molecule. Patients with a known hypersensitivity to the medium may benefit from premedication with corticosteroids and diphenhydramine. The use of nonionic contrast or an alternative noncontrast imaging study, if available, may be considered for patients who have severe asthma or who have experienced moderate to severe reactions to ionic contrast medium.
- Conditions associated with preexisting renal insufficiency (e.g., chronic kidney disease, single kidney transplant, nephrectomy, diabetes, multiple myeloma, treatment with aminoglycosides and NSAIDs) *because iodinated contrast is nephrotoxic*
- Older adult and compromised patients who are chronically dehydrated before the test, *because of their risk of contrast-induced acute kidney injury*
- Patients with pheochromocytoma, *because iodinated contrast may cause a hypertensive crisis*
- Patients with bleeding disorders receiving an arterial or venous puncture (angiography), *because the site may not stop bleeding*

SPECIAL CONSIDERATIONS

An important aspect of planning is understanding the factors that may alter study findings or cause abnormal results. Interdepartmental communication is a key factor in the planning process. The following should be noted when planning for this study:

- Gas or feces in the gastrointestinal (GI) tract resulting from inadequate cleansing or failure to restrict food intake before the study may result in unclear images.
- Retained barium from a previous radiological procedure may cause unclear images.
- Weight limits for the equipment may be exceeded by patients who are very obese.
- Metallic objects within the examination field (e.g., jewelry, body rings) may inhibit organ visualization and cause unclear images.
- Extreme claustrophobia may cause a patient to be unable to cooperate or remain still during the procedure unless sedation is given before the study.
- Age, significant pain, or mental status may cause a patient to be unable to cooperate or remain still during the procedure, producing unclear images.
- The occurrence of chest pain or severe cardiac dysrhythmias may require termination of the procedure.
- Failure to follow dietary restrictions and other pretesting preparations may cause the procedure to be canceled or repeated.

● Safety Tip

Consultation with a health-care provider (HCP) should occur before the procedure for radiation safety concerns regarding younger patients or patients who are lactating. **Pediatric Considerations** Information on the Image Gently Campaign can be found at the Alliance for Radiation Safety in Pediatric Imaging (www.pedrad.org/associations/5364/ig/). Risks associated with radiation overexposure can result from frequent x-ray procedures. Personnel in the examination room with the patient should wear a protective lead apron, stand behind a shield, or leave the area while the examination is being done. Personnel working in the examination area should wear badges to record their level of radiation exposure.

● Safety Tip

Make sure a written and informed consent has been signed prior to the procedure if a biopsy is planned and before administering any medications.

Implementation

Patient education is key to obtaining the patient's cooperation in following directions, and providing an explanation for the purpose of the procedure is an important part of this process. Inform the patient that this study can assist in assessing for disorders of the liver and biliary tract. Ensure that the patient is in compliance with pretesting instructions. Record baseline vital signs,

and continue to monitor them throughout the procedure. Protocols may vary among facilities. Establish an IV fluid line for the injection of contrast, emergency drugs, and sedatives. Administer an antianxiety agent, as ordered, if the patient has claustrophobia. Administer a sedative to a child or to an uncooperative adult, as ordered. If protocol dictates, the patient may be asked to drink a glass of oral contrast prior to the start of the study to differentiate the gastrointestinal structures from abdominal organs.

Position the patient in a supine position on the CT table with the patient's arms above her or his head. The table is moved into the gantry, and the area between the dome of the diaphragm and the iliac crest is scanned with 0.5-mm transverse images. IV contrast is injected, if ordered, following completion of the first set of images, and the entire series is repeated. The images are reviewed by the technologist on a special viewing monitor in the scanning room and then recorded digitally for radiologist interpretation. Monitor the patient for complications related to the procedure (e.g., allergic reaction, anaphylaxis, bronchospasm) if contrast is used. Following completion of the scans, remove the IV needle and cover with a sterile dressing. Observe the patient for any signs of an allergic reaction to the contrast.

Evaluation

Recognize anxiety related to test results and be supportive of impaired activity related to abnormal liver function. Instruct the patient to resume his or her usual diet, fluids, medications, and activity as directed by the HCP. Renal function should be assessed before metformin is resumed, if contrast was used. Monitor vital signs and neurological status every 15 minutes for 1 hour, then every 2 hours for 4 hours, and then as ordered by the HCP. Monitor temperature every 4 hours for 24 hours. Monitor intake and output at least every 8 hours. Compare all of these with baseline values. Notify the HCP if temperature is elevated. Protocols may vary from facility to facility. If contrast was used, observe for delayed allergic reactions, such as rash, urticaria, tachycardia, hyperpnea, hypertension, palpitations, nausea, or vomiting. Instruct the patient to immediately report symptoms such as fast heart rate, difficulty breathing, skin rash, itching, chest pain, persistent right shoulder pain, or abdominal pain. Immediately report symptoms to the appropriate HCP. Antihistamines or steroids may be administered if needed. Observe/assess the needle insertion site for bleeding, inflammation, or hematoma formation. Discuss the implications of abnormal test results on the patient's lifestyle. Hepatitis C, fatty liver, and alcohol abuse are the most common causes of cirrhosis of the liver in the United States, but anything that damages the liver can cause cirrhosis, including fatty liver associated with obesity and diabetes, chronic viral infections of the liver (hepatitis types B,

C, and D), and blockage of the bile duct, which carries bile formed in the liver to the intestines. In babies, this can be caused by biliary atresia in which bile ducts are absent or damaged, causing bile to back up in the liver. Provide teaching and information regarding the clinical implications of the test results as appropriate. Answer any questions or address any concerns voiced by the patient or family. Educate the patient regarding access to counseling services. Provide contact information, if desired, for the National Digestive Diseases Information Clearinghouse (NDDIC) found at http://digestive .niddk.nih.gov/ddiseases/pubs/cirrhosis_ez/.

Inform the patient that following the ingestion of an oral contrast, she or he may experience diarrhea, and encourage the patient to drink fluids to promote contrast excretion. Instruct the patient in the care and assessment of the site. Instruct the patient to apply cold compresses to the insertion site as needed to reduce discomfort or edema.

✓ Critical Findings

N/A

✓ Study Specific Complications

Injection of the contrast through IV tubing into a blood vessel is an invasive procedure. Complications are rare but do include risk of allergic reaction **related to contrast reaction**. It is important to have oxygen and endotracheal equipment in the vicinity for immediate use. In the event of an anaphylactic reaction, epinephrine, diphenhydramine, and steroids are included with resuscitative efforts.

Contrast Reactions: Signs, Symptoms, and Treatment

	Minor	Intermediate	Life-Threatening
Signs, Symptoms	Nausea, vomiting, urticaria, sneezing	Bronchospasms; chills and fever; chest pain, laryngeal or tongue edema	Hypotension, cardiac dysrhythmias; seizures; loss of bowel/bladder control; laryngeal and pulmonary edema
Interventions	Antihistamines	Antihistamines, steroids, bronchodilators, IV fluids and observation	All intermediate interventions plus: intubation and ventilation, pressors and antiseizure medications

Other complications related to the procedure may include

- Cardiac dysrhythmias may occur.
- Acute kidney injury may occur as a result of contrast infusion; hydration prior to the study can reduce the likelihood of this complication.
- Acidosis or hypoglycemia may occur in patients taking metformin when receiving iodinated contrast; metformin should be withheld for 48 hours prior to the study.
- Bruising, hematoma **related to blood leakage into the tissue following insertion of the IV needle**, infection or sepsis **which might occur if bacteria from the skin surface is introduced at the IV needle insertion site**, pain, prolonged bleeding, swelling, and vasovagal reactions are associated with venipuncture. Infections can occur as a result of any invasive procedure. Antibiotic therapy should be ordered if this occurs. Elevated temperatures, abnormal-colored sputum, changes in breathing patterns, chills, and hypotension can all indicate infection or sepsis.
- Hemorrhage from highly vascular tissue or infection may also occur following a CT-guided biopsy. Instruct the patient to look for excessive bleeding, skin redness, fever, or chills, and to notify her or his HCP if these symptoms occur.

✓ Related Tests

Related tests include ALT, AST, bilirubin, biopsy liver, BUN, CBC, CBC hematocrit, CBC hemoglobin, creatinine, GGT, hepatobiliary scan, KUB, liver and spleen scan, MRI abdomen, PT/INR, and US liver.

Refer to the Hepatobiliary System table at the end of the book for related tests by body system.

Expected Outcomes

Expected outcomes associated with Computed Tomography, Biliary Tract and Liver, are

- Making his or her own choices for end-of-life care
- Freedom from discomfort and emotional distress while dying
- Taking an active interest in making end-of-life decisions

Computed Tomography, Brain and Head

Quick Summary

SYNONYM ACRONYM: Computed axial tomography (CAT) of the head, computed transaxial tomography (CTT) of the head, brain CT, helical/spiral CT.

COMMON USE: To visualize and assess the brain to assist in diagnosing tumor, bleeding, infarct, infection, structural changes, and edema. Also valuable in evaluation of medical, radiation, and surgical interventions.

AREA OF APPLICATION: Brain.

NORMAL FINDINGS: Normal size, position, and shape of intracranial, head, and neck structures and associated vascular system

Test Explanation

Computed tomography (CT) of the brain is a noninvasive procedure used to assist in diagnosing abnormalities of the head, brain tissue, cerebrospinal fluid, and blood circulation. It becomes invasive if contrast medium is used. During the procedure, the patient lies on a motorized table. The table is moved in and out of a circular opening in a doughnut-like device called a *gantry*, which houses the x-ray tube and associated electronics. A beam of x-rays irradiates the patient as the table moves in and out of the scanner in a series of phases. The x-rays penetrate liquids and solids of different densities by varying degrees. Multiple detectors rotate around the patient to collect numeric data associated with the density coefficients assigned to each degree of tissue density. The imaging system's computer converts the numeric data obtained from the scanner into digital images. Air appears black, bone appears white, and body fluids, fat, and soft tissue structures are represented in various shades between black and white. The cross-sectional views or slices of the head, brain, neck, thyroid gland, and associated vascular system can be reviewed individually or as a three-dimensional image to allow differentiations of solid, cystic, inflammatory, or vascular lesions, as well as identification of suspected aneurysms, intracranial bleeds, and subdural or epidural hematomas. The scan may be repeated after administration of contrast medium given by IV. Contrast is used to differentiate, enhance, or "light up" areas of interest depending on the type of study to be performed, type of contrast medium to be used, and method of administration. The medium works by creating a contrast between areas of interest based on density; penetration of the x-rays is weaker in areas where the contrast medium is detected by the scanner showing the blood vessels, organs, and tissue as whitish areas that either outline the area of interest or completely fill it. Intravenous injection of contrast medium is used for evaluation of blood flow through vessels and greater enhancement of tissue density and organ visualization. Multislice or multidetector CT (MDCT) scanners continuously collect images in a helical or spiral fashion instead of a series of individual images as with standard scanners. Helical CT is capable of collecting many images over a short period of time (seconds), is very sensitive in identifying small abnormalities, and produces high-quality images. Positron emission tomography (PET) and single photon emission tomography

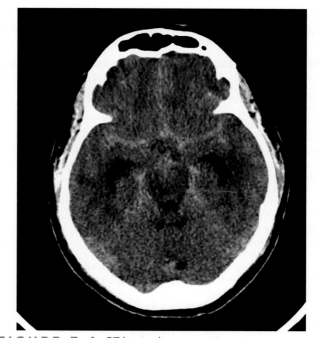

FIGURE 7.4 CT brain demonstrating acute subarachnoid hemorrhage (*e.g., stroke*). *Used with permission, from Weber, E., Vilensky, J., & Fog, A. (2013). Practical radiology: A system-based approach. FA Davis Company.*

(SPECT) are types of nuclear medicine studies that offer insights into functionality such as movement of blood flow or uptake and distribution of metabolites into tumors. PET/CT and SPECT/CT are imaging applications that superimpose PET or SPECT and CT findings. The images are collected and produced by a single gantry system. The co-registered or image fusion of PET/CT or SPECT/CT findings are capable of providing a very detailed combination of anatomical and functional images. Images can be recorded on photographic or x-ray film or stored in digital format as digitized computer data. The CT scan can be used to guide biopsy needles into areas of suspected tumors to obtain tissue for laboratory analysis and to guide placement of catheters for drainage of cysts or abscesses. Tumor staging and progression, before and after therapy, and effectiveness of medical interventions may be monitored by PET/CT, SPECT/CT, or FDG PET scanning. The images can be reevaluated and manipulated for further, detailed examination without having to repeat the procedure (see Fig. 7.4). Xenon-enhanced CT scanning is an imaging method used to assess cerebral blood flow. Xenon-133 is an odorless, colorless, radioactive gas that can either be inhaled or injected. The isotope moves rapidly through the blood into the brain. The diffused gas demonstrates how much blood goes to each area of the brain. Sensitivity of stroke detection in the acute phase is increased by using Xenon.

Nursing Implications

Assessment

Indications	Potential Nursing Problems
Detect brain infection, abscess, or necrosis, as evidenced by decreased density on the image	• Body Image
Detect ventricular enlargement or displacement by increased cerebrospinal fluid	• Communication • Confusion
Determine benign and cancerous tumors and cyst formation, as evidenced by changes in tissue densities	• Family • Human Response • Mobility
Determine cause of increased intracranial pressure	• Nutrition • Pain
Determine presence and type of hemorrhage in infants and children experiencing signs and symptoms of intracranial trauma or congenital conditions such as hydrocephalus and arteriovenous malformations (AVMs)	• Role Performance • Skin • Swallowing • Tissue Integrity
Determine presence of multiple sclerosis, as evidenced by sclerotic plaques	
Determine lesion size and location causing infarct or hemorrhage	
Differentiate hematoma location after trauma (e.g., subdural, epidural, cerebral) and determine extent of edema, as evidenced by higher blood densities	
Differentiate between cerebral infarction and hemorrhage	
Evaluate abnormalities of the middle ear ossicles, auditory nerve, and optic nerve	
Evaluate for thyroid cancer	
Monitor and evaluate the effectiveness of medical, radiation, or surgical therapies	

Diagnosis: Clinical Significance of Test Results

Identification of abnormal findings is assisted by comparison of parameters such as size, shape, symmetry, density, and location; for example, areas of altered density in either an expected or unexpected location may indicate abnormal anatomical enlargement or the presence of blood or other fluids, tumors, or cysts. Comparison by type of abnormal findings may also assist in evaluating areas of altered density; for example, well-defined round or oval areas, smaller in size and having lower density than a primary tumor, may indicate a cyst.

- Abscess
- Alzheimer disease
- Aneurysm

- AVMs
- Cerebral atrophy
- Cerebral edema
- Cerebral infarction
- Congenital abnormalities
- Craniopharyngioma
- Cysts
- Foreign body
- Hematomas (e.g., epidural, subdural, intracerebral)
- Hemorrhage
- Hydrocephaly
- Increased intracranial pressure or trauma
- Infarction
- Infection
- Pheochromocytoma
- Sclerotic plaques suggesting multiple sclerosis
- Sinusitis
- Trauma
- Tumor
- Ventricular or tissue displacement or enlargement

Planning

Considerations for planning a successful partnership should include clear communication of what to expect during the test to decrease anxiety and improve cooperation. Before the procedure is performed, plan to review the steps with the patient. Ensure that the results of coagulation testing are obtained and recorded prior to the procedure; BUN and creatinine results are also needed if contrast medium is to be used. Note any recent procedures that can interfere with test results, including examinations using barium- or iodine-based contrast medium. Ensure that barium studies were cord the date of the last menstrual period, and determine the possibility of pregnancy in perimenopausal women. Explain that minimal discomfort should be experienced during the exam, and inform the patient that the procedure is performed in a CT suite by a CT technologist and takes approximately 15–30 minutes depending on factors such as the type of study ordered, whether contrast will be used, and the type of contrast used. Remind the patient that she or he should remain still during the procedure, and instruct the patient to remove all metal in the area to be examined. Inform the patient as appropriate that CT studies performed without contrast usually do not require the patient to fast before the procedure. Instruct the patient, if required, to fast and restrict fluids for the specified time period, prior to the procedure; fasting is required for several hours prior to contrast enhanced studies as a precaution against pulmonary aspiration of stomach contents during the procedure. Instruct the patient to avoid taking anticoagulant medication or to reduce the dosage as ordered prior to the procedure due to increased risk of bleeding at the IV insertion site. Protocols may vary among facilities. Explain that she or he may be required to drink approximately 450 mL of a dilute barium solution (approximately 1% barium) or water-soluble contrast before the examination; the oral contrast is given at a specified time period, prior to the study. This is administered to distinguish GI organs from the other abdominal organs. Inquire about previous allergies and contrast reactions. If iodinated contrast medium is scheduled to be used in patients receiving metformin (Glucophage) for non-insulin-dependent (type 2) diabetes, the drug should be discontinued on the day of the test and continue to be withheld for 48 hours after the test. Iodinated contrast can temporarily impair kidney function, and failure to withhold metformin may indirectly result in drug-induced lactic acidosis, a dangerous and sometimes fatal adverse effect of metformin *related to renal impairment that does not support sufficient excretion of metformin.* Explain that an IV line may be inserted to allow the infusion of IV fluids (e.g., normal saline), anesthetics, contrast medium, or sedatives. Inform the patient that she or he may experience nausea, a feeling of warmth, a flushed sensation, a salty or metallic taste, or may notice a transient headache if IV contrast is used, and that these reactions are considered normal.

CONTRAINDICATIONS

- Patients who are pregnant or suspected of being pregnant, unless the potential benefits of the procedure far outweigh the risk of radiation exposure to the fetus and mother
- Patients who are claustrophobic
- Conditions associated with adverse reactions to contrast medium (e.g., asthma, food allergies, or allergy to contrast medium). Although patients are still asked specifically if they have a known allergy to iodine or shellfish, it has been well established that the reaction is not to iodine; in fact, an actual iodine allergy would be very problematic because iodine is required for the production of thyroid hormones. In the case of shellfish, the reaction is to a muscle protein called *tropomyosin*; in the case of iodinated contrast medium, the reaction is to the noniodinated part of the contrast molecule. Patients with a known hypersensitivity to the medium may benefit from premedication with corticosteroids and diphenhydramine; the use of nonionic contrast or an alternative noncontrast imaging study, if available, may be considered for patients who have severe asthma or who have experienced moderate to severe reactions to ionic contrast medium.
- Conditions associated with preexisting renal insufficiency (e.g., chronic kidney disease, single kidney transplant, nephrectomy, diabetes, multiple myeloma,

treatment with aminoglycosides and NSAIDs) *because iodinated contrast is nephrotoxic*
- Older adult and compromised patients who are chronically dehydrated before the test *because of their risk of contrast-induced acute kidney injury*
- Patients with pheochromocytoma *because iodinated contrast may cause a hypertensive crisis*
- Patients with bleeding disorders receiving an arterial or venous puncture (angiography) *because the site may not stop bleeding*

SPECIAL CONSIDERATIONS

An important aspect of planning is understanding the factors that may alter study findings or cause abnormal results. Interdepartmental communication is a key factor in the planning process. The following should be noted when planning for this study:

- Gas or feces in the gastrointestinal (GI) tract resulting from inadequate cleansing or failure to restrict food intake before the study may result in unclear images.
- Retained barium from a previous radiological procedure may cause unclear images.
- The weight limit for the equipment may be exceeded by patients who are very obese.
- Metallic objects within the examination field (e.g., jewelry, body rings) may inhibit organ visualization and cause unclear images.
- Extreme claustrophobia may cause the patient to be unable to cooperate or remain still during the procedure unless sedation is given before the study.
- Age, significant pain, or mental status may cause the patient to be unable to cooperate or remain still during the procedure, which may produce unclear images.
- The occurrence of chest pain or severe cardiac dysrhythmias may require termination of the procedure.
- Failure to follow dietary restrictions and other pretesting preparations may cause the procedure to be canceled or repeated.

● *Safety Tip*

Consultation with a health-care provider (HCP) should occur before the procedure for radiation safety concerns regarding younger patients or patients who are lactating. **Pediatric Considerations** Information on the Image Gently Campaign can be found at the Alliance for Radiation Safety in Pediatric Imaging (www.pedrad.org/associations/5364/ig/). Risks associated with radiation overexposure can result from frequent x-ray procedures. Personnel in the examination room with the patient should wear a protective lead apron, stand behind a shield, or leave the area while the examination is being done. Personnel working in the examination area should wear badges to record their level of radiation exposure.

● **Safety Tip**

Make sure a written and informed consent has been signed prior to the procedure and before administering any medications.

Implementation

Patient education is key to obtaining the patient's cooperation in following directions, and providing an explanation for the purpose of the procedure is an important part of this process. Inform the patient that this study can assist in assessing for disorders of the brain, head, and neck, including blood vessels. Ensure that the patient is in compliance with pretesting instructions. Record baseline vital signs and continue to monitor them throughout the procedure. Protocols may vary among facilities. Establish an IV fluid line for the injection of contrast, emergency drugs, and sedatives. Administer an antianxiety agent, as ordered, if the patient has claustrophobia. Administer a sedative to a child or to an uncooperative adult, as ordered. If protocol dictates, the patient may be asked to drink a glass of oral contrast prior to the start of the study to differentiate the gastrointestinal structures from abdominal organs.

Position the patient in a supine position on the CT table with the patient's arms above her or his head. The table is moved into the gantry and the area between the dome of the diaphragm, and the iliac crest is scanned with 0.5-mm transverse images. IV contrast is injected, if ordered, following completion of the first set of images, and the entire series is repeated. The images are reviewed by the technologist on a special viewing monitor in the scanning room and then recorded digitally for radiologist interpretation. Monitor the patient for complications related to the procedure (e.g., allergic reaction, anaphylaxis, bronchospasm) if contrast is used. Following completion of the scans, remove the IV needle and cover with a sterile dressing. Observe the patient for any signs of an allergic reaction to the contrast.

Evaluation

Recognize anxiety related to test results and be supportive of impaired activity related to a perceived loss of independence. Instruct the patient to resume his or her usual diet, fluids, medications, and activity, as directed by the HCP. Renal function should be assessed before metformin is resumed, if contrast was used. Monitor vital signs and the neurological status every 15 minutes for 1 hour, then every 2 hours for 4 hours, and then as ordered by the HCP. Monitor temperature every 4 hours for 24 hours. Monitor intake and output at least every 8 hours. Compare all of these with baseline values. Notify the HCP if temperature is elevated. Protocols may vary from facility to facility. If contrast was used, observe for delayed allergic reactions, such as rash, urticaria, tachycardia, hyperpnea, hypertension, palpitations, nausea, or vomiting. Instruct the patient to immediately report symptoms such as fast heart rate, difficulty breathing, skin rash, itching, chest pain, persistent right shoulder pain, or abdominal pain. Immediately report symptoms to the appropriate HCP. Antihistamines or steroids may be administered if needed. Observe/assess the needle insertion site for bleeding, inflammation, or hematoma formation. Discuss the implications of abnormal test results on the patient's lifestyle. Provide teaching and information regarding the clinical implications of the test results as appropriate. Answer any questions or address any concerns voiced by the patient or family. Patients experiencing a stroke or hemorrhage often exhibit severe anxiety and confusion. People who have had strokes may have more difficulty controlling their emotions, or they may develop depression. Educate the patient regarding access to counseling services. Provide patients with information, if desired, such as *Life After Stroke: Resources and Information* retrieved at http://www.stroke.org/site/PageServer?pagename=LAS. Educate the patient regarding access to counseling services.

Instruct the patient in the care and assessment of the site. Instruct the patient to apply cold compresses to the insertion site as needed, to reduce discomfort or edema.

✓ Critical Findings

- Abscess
- Acute hemorrhage
- Aneurysm
- Infarction
- Infection
- Tumor with significant mass effect

Note and immediately report to the requesting HCP any critical findings and related symptoms. A listing of these findings varies among facilities.

✓ Study Specific Complications

Injection of the contrast through IV tubing into a blood vessel is an invasive procedure. Complications are rare but do include risk of allergic reaction ***related to contrast reaction***. It is important to have oxygen and endotracheal equipment in the vicinity for immediate use. In the event of an anaphylactic reaction, epinephrine, diphenhydramine and steroids are included with resuscitative efforts.

Contrast Reactions: Signs, Symptoms, and Treatment

	Minor	Intermediate	Life-Threatening
Signs, Symptoms	Nausea, vomiting, urticaria, sneezing	Bronchospasms; chills and fever; chest pain, laryngeal or tongue edema	Hypotension, cardiac dysrhythmias; seizures; loss of bowel/bladder control; laryngeal and pulmonary edema
Interventions	Antihistamines	Antihistamines, steroids, bronchodilators, IV fluids and observation	All intermediate interventions plus: intubation and ventilation, pressors and antiseizure medications

Other complications related to the procedure may include

- Cardiac dysrhythmias may occur.
- Acute kidney injury may occur as a result of contrast infusion; hydration prior to the study can reduce the likelihood of this complication.
- Acidosis or hypoglycemia may occur in patients taking metformin when receiving iodinated contrast; metformin should be withheld for 48 hours prior to the study.
- Bruising, hematoma *related to blood leakage into the tissue following insertion of the IV needle*, infection or sepsis *which might occur if bacteria from the skin surface is introduced at the IV needle insertion site*, pain, prolonged bleeding, swelling, and vasovagal reactions are associated with venipuncture. Infections can occur as a result of any invasive procedure. Antibiotic therapy should be ordered if this occurs. Elevated temperatures, abnormal-colored sputum, changes in breathing patterns, chills, and hypotension can all indicate infection or sepsis.
- Hemorrhage from highly vascular tissue or infection may also occur following a CT-guided biopsy. Instruct the patient to look for excessive bleeding, skin redness, fever, or chills, and to notify her or his HCP if these symptoms occur.

✅ Related Tests

Related tests include angiography carotid, audiometry hearing loss, BUN, CSF analysis, CBC, CBC hematocrit, CBC hemoglobin, CT angiography, creatinine, EEG, EMG, evoked brain potentials, MR angiography, MRI brain, nerve fiber analysis, otoscopy, PET brain, PT/INR, spondee speech reception threshold, and tuning fork tests.

Refer to the Musculoskeletal System table at the end of the book for related tests by body system.

Expected Outcomes

Expected outcomes associated with Computed Tomography, Brain, are

- Interacting appropriately with the environment
- Being able to express one's self without frustration

- Adapting to cognitive deficits with the support of family or significant others
- Recognizing that role performance will need to be altered to meet the patient's new reality

Computed Tomography, Pancreas

Quick Summary

SYNONYM ACRONYM: Computed axial tomography (CAT), computed transaxial tomography (CTT), abdominal CT, helical/spiral CT.

COMMON USE: To visualize and assess the pancreas toward assisting in diagnosing tumors, masses, cancer, bleeding, infection, and abscess. Used as an evaluation tool for surgical, radiation, and medical therapeutic interventions.

AREA OF APPLICATION: Pancreas.

NORMAL FINDINGS: Normal size, position, and contour of the pancreas, which lies obliquely in the upper abdomen

Test Explanation

Computed tomography (CT) is a noninvasive procedure used to enhance certain anatomic views of the abdominal structures. It becomes an invasive procedure when contrast medium is used. CT of the pancreas aids in the diagnosis or evaluation of pancreatic cysts, pseudocysts, inflammation, tumors, masses, metastases, abscesses, and trauma. In all but the thinnest or most emaciated patients, the pancreas is surrounded by fat that clearly defines its margins. During the procedure, the patient lies on a motorized table. The table is moved in and out of a circular opening in a doughnut-like device called a *gantry.* The x-rays penetrate liquids and solids of different densities by varying degrees. Multiple detectors rotate around the patient to collect numeric data associated with the density coefficients assigned to each degree of tissue density. The imaging system's computer converts the numeric data obtained from the scanner into digital images. Air appears black, bone appears white, and body fluids, fat, and soft tissue structures are represented in various shades between black and white. The cross-sectional views or slices of the pancreas can be reviewed individually or as a three-dimensional image to allow differentiations of solid, cystic, inflammatory, or vascular lesions, as well as identification of suspected areas of enlargement, atrophy, or obstructed ducts. The scan may be repeated after administration of contrast medium given orally, by IV, or rectally. Contrast is used to differentiate, enhance, or "light up" areas of interest depending on the type of study to be performed, type of contrast medium to be used, and method of administration. The medium works by creating a contrast between areas of interest based on density; penetration of the x-rays is weaker in areas where the contrast medium is detected by the scanner showing the blood vessels, organs, and tissue as whitish areas that either outline the area of interest or completely fill it. Oral ingestion of contrast medium can be used for opacification to distinguish the bowel, adjacent abdominal organs, other types of tissue, and blood vessels as the medium moves through the digestive tract. Intravenous injection of contrast medium is used for evaluation of blood flow through vessels and greater enhancement of tissue density and organ visualization. In some cases scans may be repeated after multiple types of contrast are administered. Multislice or multidetector CT (MDCT) scanners continuously collect images in a helical or spiral fashion instead of a series of individual images as with standard scanners. Helical CT is capable of collecting many images over a short period of time (seconds), is very sensitive in identifying small abnormalities, and produces high-quality images. PET/CT is an imaging application that superimposes PET and CT findings. The images are collected and produced by a single gantry system. The co-registered or image fusion PET/CT findings are capable of providing a very detailed combination of anatomical and functional images. Images can be recorded on photographic or x-ray film or stored in digital format as digitized computer data. The CT scan can be used to guide biopsy needles into areas of suspected tumors to obtain tissue for laboratory analysis and to guide placement of catheters for drainage of abscesses. Tumor staging and progression, before and after therapy, and effectiveness of medical interventions may be monitored by CT scanning. The images can be reevaluated and manipulated for further, detailed examination without having to repeat the procedure (see Fig. 7.5).

Nursing Implications

Assessment

Indications	Potential Nursing Problems
Detect dilation or obstruction of the pancreatic ducts	• Breathing
Differentiate between pancreatic disorders and disorders of the retroperitoneum	• Fluid Volume
	• Gas Exchange
Evaluate benign or cancerous tumors or metastasis to the pancreas	• Human Response
	• Infection
Evaluate pancreatic abnormalities (e.g., bleeding, pancreatitis, pseudocyst, abscesses)	• Injury Risk
	• Nutrition
Evaluate unexplained weight loss, jaundice, and epigastric pain	• Pain
Monitor and evaluate effectiveness of medical or surgical therapies	

Diagnosis: Clinical Significance of Test Results
ABNORMAL FINDINGS

Identification of abnormal findings is assisted by comparison of parameters such as size, shape, symmetry, density, and location; for example, areas of altered density in either an expected or unexpected location may indicate enlargement of an organ or the presence of blood or other fluids, tumors, or cysts. Comparison by type of abnormal findings may also assist in evaluating areas of altered density; for example, well-defined round or oval areas, smaller in size and having lower density than a primary tumor, may indicate a cyst.

- Acute or chronic pancreatitis
- Obstruction of the pancreatic ducts
- Pancreatic abscesses
- Pancreatic carcinoma
- Pancreatic pseudocyst
- Pancreatic tumor

Planning

Considerations for planning a successful partnership should include clear communication of what to expect during the test to decrease anxiety and improve

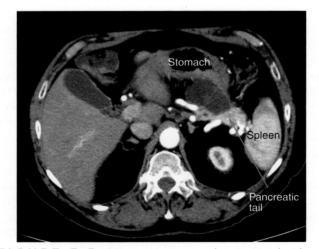

FIGURE 7.5 CT pancreatic pseudocyst. *Used with permission, from Weber, E., Vilensky, J., & Fog, A. (2013). Practical radiology: A system-based approach. FA Davis Company.*

cooperation. Before the procedure is performed, plan to review the steps with the patient. Ensure results of coagulation testing are obtained and recorded prior to the procedure; BUN and creatinine results are also needed if contrast medium is to be used. Note any recent procedures that can interfere with test results, including examinations using barium- or iodine-based contrast medium. Ensure that barium studies were performed more than 4 days before the CT scan. Record the date of the last menstrual period, and determine the possibility of pregnancy in perimenopausal women. Explain that minimal discomfort should be experienced during the exam, and inform the patient that the procedure is performed in a CT suite by a CT technologist and takes approximately 15–30 minutes depending on factors such as the type of study ordered, whether contrast will be used, and the type of contrast used. Remind the patient that she or he should remain still during the procedure, and instruct the patient to remove all metal in the area to be examined. Inform the patient as appropriate that CT studies performed without contrast usually do not require the patient to fast before the procedure. Instruct the patient, if required, to fast and restrict fluids for the specified time period, prior to the procedure; fasting is required for several hours prior to contrast enhanced studies as a precaution against pulmonary aspiration of stomach contents during the procedure. Instruct the patient to avoid taking anticoagulant medication or to reduce dosage as ordered prior to the procedure due to increased risk of bleeding at the IV insertion site. Protocols may vary among facilities. Explain that she or he may be required to drink approximately 450 mL of a dilute barium solution (approximately 1% barium) or water-soluble contrast before the examination; the oral contrast is given at a specified time period, prior to the study. This is administered to distinguish gastrointestinal (GI) organs from the other abdominal organs. Inquire about previous allergies and contrast reactions. If iodinated contrast medium is scheduled to be used in patients receiving metformin (Glucophage) for non-insulin-dependent (type 2) diabetes, the drug should be discontinued on the day of the test and continue to be withheld for 48 hours after the test. Iodinated contrast can temporarily impair kidney function, and failure to withhold metformin may indirectly result in drug-induced lactic acidosis, a dangerous and sometimes fatal adverse effect of metformin *related to renal impairment that does not support sufficient excretion of metformin.* Explain that an IV line may be inserted to allow infusion of IV fluids (e.g., normal saline), anesthetics, contrast medium, or sedatives. Inform the patient that she or he may experience nausea, a feeling of warmth, a flushed sensation, a salty or metallic taste, or may notice a transient headache if IV contrast is used and that these reactions are considered normal.

CONTRAINDICATIONS

- Patients who are pregnant or suspected of being pregnant, unless the potential benefits of the procedure far outweigh the risk of radiation exposure to the fetus and mother
- Patients who are claustrophobic
- Conditions associated with adverse reactions to contrast medium (e.g., asthma, food allergies, or allergy to contrast medium)Although patients are still asked specifically if they have a known allergy to iodine or shellfish, it has been well established that the reaction is not to iodine; in fact, an actual iodine allergy would be very problematic because iodine is required for the production of thyroid hormones. In the case of shellfish, the reaction is to a muscle protein called *tropomyosin*; in the case of iodinated contrast medium, the reaction is to the noniodinated part of the contrast molecule. Patients with a known hypersensitivity to the medium may benefit from premedication with corticosteroids and diphenhydramine; the use of nonionic contrast or an alternative noncontrast imaging study, if available, may be considered for patients who have severe asthma or who have experienced moderate to severe reactions to ionic contrast medium.
- Conditions associated with preexisting renal insufficiency (e.g., chronic kidney disease, single kidney transplant, nephrectomy, diabetes, multiple myeloma, treatment with aminoglycocides and NSAIDs) *because iodinated contrast is nephrotoxic*
- Older adult and compromised patients who are chronically dehydrated before the test *because of their risk of contrast-induced acute kidney injury*
- Patients with pheochromocytoma *because iodinated contrast may cause a hypertensive crisis*
- Patients with bleeding disorders receiving an arterial or venous puncture (angiography) *because the site may not stop bleeding*

SPECIAL CONSIDERATIONS

An important aspect of planning is understanding the factors that may alter study findings or cause abnormal results. Interdepartmental communication is a key factor in the planning process. The following should be noted when planning for this study:

- Gas or feces in the GI tract resulting from inadequate cleansing or failure to restrict food intake before the study may result in unclear images.
- Retained barium from a previous radiological procedure may cause unclear images.
- The weight limit for the equipment may be exceeded by patients who are very obese.
- Metallic objects within the examination field (e.g., jewelry, body rings) may inhibit organ visualization and cause unclear images.

- Extreme claustrophobia may cause patients to be unable to cooperate or remain still during the procedure unless sedation is given before the study.
- Age, significant pain, or mental status may cause the patient to be unable to cooperate or remain still during the procedure, which may produce unclear images.
- The occurrence of chest pain or severe cardiac dysrhythmias may require termination of the procedure.
- Failure to follow dietary restrictions and other pretesting preparations may cause the procedure to be canceled or repeated.

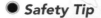

● Safety Tip

Consultation with a health-care provider (HCP) should occur before the procedure for radiation safety concerns regarding younger patients or patients who are lactating. **Pediatric Considerations** Information on the Image Gently Campaign can be found at the Alliance for Radiation Safety in Pediatric Imaging (www.pedrad.org/associations/5364/ig/). Risks associated with radiation overexposure can result from frequent x-ray procedures. Personnel in the examination room with the patient should wear a protective lead apron, stand behind a shield, or leave the area while the examination is being done. Personnel working in the examination area should wear badges to record their level of radiation exposure.

● Safety Tip

Make sure a written and informed consent has been signed prior to the procedure if a biopsy is planned and before administering any medications.

Implementation

Patient education is key to obtaining the patient's co-operation in following directions, and providing an explanation for the purpose of the procedure is an important part of this process. Inform the patient that this study can assist in assessing for disorders of the pancreas. Ensure that the patient is in compliance with pretesting instructions. Record baseline vital signs and continue to monitor throughout the procedure. Protocols may vary among facilities. Establish an IV fluid line for the injection of contrast, emergency drugs, and sedatives. Administer an antianxiety agent, as ordered, if the patient has claustrophobia. Administer a sedative to a child or to an uncooperative adult, as ordered. If protocol dictates, the patient may be asked to drink a glass of oral contrast prior to the start of the study to differentiate the GI structures from abdominal organs.

Position the patient in a supine position on the CT table with the patient's arms above her or his head. The table is moved into the gantry, and the area between the dome of the diaphragm and the iliac crest is scanned with 0.5-mm transverse images. IV contrast is injected, if ordered, following completion of the first set of images, and the entire series is repeated. The images are reviewed by the technologist on a special viewing monitor in the scanning room and then recorded digitally for radiologist interpretation. Monitor the patient for complications related to the procedure (e.g., allergic reaction, anaphylaxis, bronchospasm) if contrast is used. Following completion of the scans, remove the IV needle and cover with a sterile dressing. Observe the patient for any signs of an allergic reaction to the contrast.

Evaluation

Recognize anxiety related to test results and be supportive of impaired activity related to a perceived loss of independence. Instruct the patient to resume usual diet, fluids, medications, and activity, as directed by the HCP. Renal function should be assessed before metformin is resumed, if contrast was used. Monitor vital signs and neurological status every 15 minutes for 1 hour, then every 2 hours for 4 hours, and then as ordered by the HCP. Monitor temperature every 4 hours for 24 hours. Monitor intake and output at least every 8 hours. Compare with baseline values. Notify the HCP if temperature is elevated. Protocols may vary from facility to facility. If contrast was used, observe for delayed allergic reactions, such as rash, urticaria, tachycardia, hyperpnea, hypertension, palpitations, nausea, or vomiting. Instruct the patient to immediately report symptoms such as fast heart rate, difficulty breathing, skin rash, itching, chest pain, persistent right shoulder pain, or abdominal pain. Immediately report symptoms to the appropriate HCP. Antihistamines or steroids may be administered if needed. Observe/assess the needle insertion site for bleeding, inflammation, or hematoma formation. Discuss the implications of abnormal test results on the patient's lifestyle. Provide teaching and information regarding the clinical implications of the test results as appropriate. Answer any questions or address any concerns voiced by the patient or family. Educate the patient regarding access to counseling services.

Inform the patient that following the ingestion of an oral contrast, she or he may experience diarrhea, and encourage the patient to drink fluids to promote contrast excretion. Instruct the patient in the care and assessment of the site. Instruct the patient to apply cold compresses to the insertion site as needed, to reduce discomfort or edema.

Recognize anxiety related to test results, and be supportive of pancreas abnormalities and a perceived loss of independence. Discuss the implications of abnormal test results on the patient's lifestyle. Provide teaching and information regarding the clinical implications of the test results as appropriate. Answer any questions or address any concerns voiced by the patient or family.

Provide contact information, if desired, for the online booklet "What You Need To Know About Cancer of the Pancreas" found at http://www.cancer.gov/cancertopics/wyntk/pancreas to learn about pancreatic cancer symptoms, diagnosis, treatment, and questions to ask the HCP. Educate the patient regarding access to counseling services.

Critical Findings

N/A

Study Specific Complications

Injection of the contrast through IV tubing into a blood vessel is an invasive procedure. Complications are rare but do include risk of allergic reaction *related to contrast reaction*. It is important to have oxygen and endotracheal equipment in the vicinity for immediate use. In the event of an anaphylaxic reaction, epinephrine, diphenhydramine, and steroids are included with resuscitative efforts.

Contrast Reactions: Signs, Symptoms, and Treatment

	Minor	Intermediate	Life-Threatening
Signs, Symptoms	Nausea, vomiting, urticaria, sneezing	Bronchospasms; chills and fever; chest pain, laryngeal or tongue edema	Hypotension, cardiac dysrhythmias; seizures; loss of bowel/bladder control; laryngeal and pulmonary edema
Interventions	Antihistamines	Antihistamines, steroids, bronchodilators, IV fluids and observation	All intermediate interventions plus: intubation and ventilation, pressors and antiseizure medications

Other complications related to the procedure may include

- Cardiac dysrhythmias may occur.
- Acute kidney injury may occur as a result of contrast infusion; hydration prior to the study can reduce the likelihood of this complication.
- Acidosis or hypoglycemia may occur in patients taking metformin when receiving iodinated contrast; metformin should be withheld for 48 hours prior to the study.
- Bruising, hematoma *related to blood leakage into the tissue following insertion of the IV needle*, infection or sepsis *which might occur if bacteria from the skin surface is introduced at the IV needle insertion site*, pain, prolonged bleeding, swelling, and vasovagal reactions are associated with venipuncture. Infections can occur as a result of any invasive procedure. Antibiotic therapy should be ordered if this occurs. Elevated temperatures, abnormal-colored sputum, changes in breathing patterns, chills, and hypotension can all indicate infection or sepsis.
- Hemorrhage from highly vascular tissue or infection may also occur following a CT-guided biopsy. Instruct the patient to look for excessive bleeding, skin redness, fever, or chills, and to notify her or his HCP if these symptoms occur.

Related Tests

Related tests include amylase, angiography of the abdomen, biopsy intestinal, BUN, cancer antigens, CBC hemoglobin, creatinine, ERCP, lipase, MRI abdomen, PT/INR, and US pancreas.

Refer to the Gastrointestinal and Hepatobiliary systems tables at the end of the book for related tests by body system.

Expected Outcomes

Expected outcomes associated with Computed Tomography, Pancreas, are

- Maintaining normal fluid volume
- Clearing bilateral breath sounds
- Maintaining an adequate diet that supports baseline body functioning and a normal weight

REVIEW OF LEARNING OUTCOMES

Thinking

1. Recognize that human beings are imperfect, and failure to follow policy and standards of care, or participate in work-arounds can place a patient at risk. Answer: Keeping the patient safe in the health-care environment is a primary role of the nurse. Accurate screening of the patient for contraindications to CT scanning, such as renal insufficiency with CT contrast, iodine allergy, and extreme obesity, are concerns that should be reported before the patient is scanned. Insufficient hand-off communication and patient identification can occur with the most vigilant nurse. Unsafe practice occurs when the nurse fails to follow established protocols that have been put in place to enhance patient safety.

2. Examine the scope of practice related to specific aspects of care such as information management; evidence-based education; and organizational, patient, family, and ancillary communication. Answer: The nurse's role is to coordinate the care of the patient in relation to all other disciplines that are involved in care. What this means is that you need to make a decision about whether or not the study can go forward based on your assessment of the patient's condition and overall clinical appearance. If there is some impediment to completing the study, the HCP needs to be notified immediately.

Doing

1. Recognize that memory can be imperfect and the use of assistive resources (checklists, electronic tablets, etc.) can reduce care errors. Answer: The nurse's role is to prevent harm. Strategies to prevent harm include clear communication with the physician and CT department, and strict adherence to policy, procedure, and protocols that have been put in place to protect the patient and prevent harm. If you have a question, do not be afraid to ask: It is the unasked questions that often cause the most harm.

2. Identify barriers that prevent the patient from participating in health and wellness. Answer: If you ask a patient why he or she refuses the recommended diagnostic procedure, it is usually for a couple or reasons: The patient is afraid of pain or the patient is afraid of the results and what that will mean for the patient and the patient's family. As the nurse, you need to look at the situation from the patient's point of view and frame the conversation in a way that is meaningful and supportive of him or her. Once you have done all that you can to provide the patient with all the information to make an informed decision, you must respect that decision. Regardless of all else, the patient has the right to refuse.

Caring

1. Value the ability of the individual in the prevention of errors. Answer: A near miss is an error that almost happened. Your role in the provision of care is to protect the patient from both a near miss and an error. Either of these can cause harm. Errors occur when nurses believe they are too busy to follow the safety protocols based organizational policy, the standards of practice, and evidence-based care. Take time to make the right choices: It is much easier to make the right choice than to correct a mistake that both you and your patient will regret.

2. Recognize that perceiving how care is delivered though the patients point of view is of value.

Answer: There is a saying about needing to walk a day in the shoes of another to truly understand the situation from his or her perspective. Letting the patient make the decisions is difficult for some nurses. Ask yourself if you would like someone who has just barely met you to make your healthcare decisions. Of course not! Look at the situation through the patient's eyes, and empathize with how decisions made will effect his or her life. Once the patient sees that you care, that you get it, you have a better chance of being successful in your endeavors.

Words OF Wisdom: People equate these types of diagnostic studies with "bad news." Many have put off seeking medical intervention hoping that whatever symptoms they are experiencing will go away. Now that the time has come to face the reality of their situation, many are not emotionally prepared. Oftentimes it is the nurse who is left to help the patient really understand just what the physician has told him or her. Be conscious of the level of literacy of your patient and the patient's family culture. Make sure that explanations are not couched in even basic medical terminology; there is so much confusion that can occur through misunderstandings. Assistance can be given by simply asking them, "Tell me what you understood the doctor to say," followed by "What questions do you have about that?" Don't worry about not knowing the answer— you don't have to know everything. However, you do need to know how to find the answers necessary to put your patient at ease. Part of the professional nursing role is knowing your resources and how to use them on behalf of your patient.

BIBLIOGRAPHY

Agatston, A., Are you a cardiac time bomb? A simple heart scan can tell. (2013). Retrieved from www.huffingtonpost.com/arthur-agatston-md/heart-month_b_2598365.html

The American Association for the Surgery of Trauma. (2015). Splenic injury grading. Retrieved from http://www.aast.org/library/traumatools/injuryscoringscales.aspx#spleen

American College of Radiology (2014). About imaging agents or tracers. Retrieved from www.acrin.org/PATIENTS/ABOUTIMAGINGEXAMSANDAGENTS/ABOUTIMAGINGAGENTSORTRACERS.aspx

American College of Radiology (2013). ACR Manual on Contrast Media. Retrieved from http://www.acr.org/quality-safety/resources/~/media/37D84428BF1D4E1B9A3A2918DA9E27A3.pdf/

Barnhart, K. Ectopic pregnancy. (2009). New England Journal of Medicine, 361, 379–387.

Conditions which may contraindicate the use of IV iodinated contrast. (n.d.). Retrieved from http://www.fda.gov/MedicalDevices/ProductsandMedicalProcedures/InVitroDiagnostics/ucm301431.htm

CT Colonography. (2013). Retrieved from www.radiologyinfo.org/en/info.cfm?pg=ct_colo

Frank, E., Long, B., & Smith, B. (2012). Merrill's atlas of radiographic positioning and procedures. (12th Ed.). Mosby-Elsevier: St. Louis, MO.

Furukawa, A., Yamasaki, M., Furuichi, K., Yokoyama, K., Nagata, T., Takahashi, M., Murata, K., & Sakamoto, T. (2001). Helical CT in the diagnosis of small bowel obstruction. Retrieved from http://medical-imaging.utoronto.ca/Assets/Medical%2BImaging%2BDigital%2BAssets/resident/edu/jaffer/jaffer3.pdf

Goergen, S., Revell, A., & Walker, C. (2009). Iodine-containing contrast medium (ICCM). Retrieved from http://www.insideradiology.com.au/pages/view.php?T_id=21

Gonzalez, R. Stroke CT angiography (CTA). (2012). Retrieved from http://www.mc.vanderbilt.edu/documents/NeuroICU/files/Stroke%20CTA.pdf

Horton, K., & Fishman, E. (2010). CT angiography of the mesenteric circulation. Radiologic Clinics of North America, 48(2), 331–345.

Imaging pediatrics and small patients. (2008). Retrieved from www.gehealthcare.com/usen/ct/docs/pedschapterinOM.pdf

Khan, A. (2013). Chronic pancreatitis imaging. Retrieved from http://emedicine.medscape.com/article/371772-overview

Liu, P.S., & Platt, J.F. (2010). CT angiography of the renal circulation. Radiologic Clinics of North America, 48(2), 347–365.

Maddox, T. (2002). Adverse reactions to contrast material: Recognition, prevention, and treatment. Retrieved fromhttp://www.aafp.org/afp/2002/1001/p1229.html

Cavanaugh, B. (2003). Nurse's manual of laboratory and diagnostic tests (4th ed.). Philadelphia, PA: F.A. Davis Company.

Pearce, M., Salottim, J., Little, M., McHugh, K., Lee, C., Kim, K., Howe, N., Ronckers, C., Rajaraman, P., Craft, A., Parker, L., & Berrington de Gonzlez, A. (2012). Radiation exposure from CT scans in childhood and subsequent risk of leukaemia and brain tumors: A retrospective short study. Retrieved from www.ncbi.nlm.nih.gov/pmc/articles/PMC3418594/

Poulis, P., & Beaulieu, C. (2012). Current techniques in the performance, interpretation, and reporting of CT colonography. Gastrointestinal Endoscopy Clinics, 20(2), 169–192.

Radiation risks and pediatric computed tomography (CT): A guide for health care providers. (2012). Retrieved from www.cancer.gov/about-cancer/causes-prevention/risk/radiation/pediatric-ct-scans/

RadiologyInfo. (2014). Retrieved from www.radiologyinfo.org/

Rothrock, S. (2013). Myth of shellfish, iodine, and CT contrast allergy link debunked. Retrieved from www.compactmedicalguides.com/blog/post/myth-of-shellfish-iodine-and-ct-contrast-allergy-link-debunked

Rubin, G., Firlik, A., Levy E., Pindzola R., & Yonas, H. (1999). Xenon-enhanced computed tomography cerebral blood flow measurements in acute cerebral ischemia: Review of 56 cases. Retrieved from www.ncbi.nlm.nih.gov/pubmed/17895194

Seeran, E. (2009). Computed tomography, physical principles, clinical applications, and quality control. (3rd ed.). St. Louis, MO: Saunders-Elsevier.

Singh, J., Steward, M. Booth, T., Mukhtar, H., & Murray. D. (2010). Evolution of imaging for abdominal perforation. Retrieved from www.ncbi.nlm.nih.gov/pmc/articles/PMC3080072/

Van Leeuwen, A., and Bladh, M. (2015). Davis's comprehensive handbook of laboratory and diagnostic testing with nursing implications (6th ed.). Philadelphia, PA: F.A. Davis Company.

Venes, D. (Ed.). (2009). Taber's cyclopedic medical dictionary (21st ed.). Philadelphia, PA: F.A. Davis Company.

Vidalink. (2007). The IV Contrast/Iodine Allergy Myth. Retrieved from http://www.ct-scan-info.com/ctcontrast.html

What do studies tell us about small unruptured aneurysms bleeding. (n.d.). Retrieved from www.avmsurgeon.com/unrupturedaneurysms.html

Xenon enhanced CT. (2014). Retrieved from http://en.wikipedia.org/wiki/Xenon-enhanced_computed_tomography

Go to Section II of this book and www.davisplus.com for the Clinical Reasoning Tool and its case studies to provide you with a safe place to explore patient care situations. There are a total of 26 different case studies; 2 cases are presented for each of 13 body systems. One set of 13 cases are found in the Section II chapters, and a second set of 13 cases are available online at www.davisplus.com. Each case is designed with the specific goal of helping you to connect the dots of clinical reasoning. Cases are designed to reflect possible clinical scenarios; the outcomes may or may not be positive—you decide.

Electrophysiologic Studies

OVERVIEW

Electrophysiologic studies use both electric and electronic devices to assist in diagnosing tissue and organ pathology related to a disease process. The goal is to obtain an indirect measure of an organ's structure and function during an electric event. Electrophysiologic studies are used to assess the effects of electric stimulation on tissues and the production of electric currents by organs and tissues. Studies are performed by attaching electrodes to the body close to the organ or tissue being investigated. The electrodes measure the electrical current or activity of the chosen area of inquiry. Results of the study are seen visually as a graphic drawing called an *electrogram*. The electrogram is used by the health-care provider (HCP) as a diagnostic tool to identify a disease process. Current results are also used by the HCP to compare against earlier results to validate the success of the chosen treatment plan. Electrophysiologic studies are used most often to assess for disease of the heart, muscles, or nerves. Studies can be performed in both inpatient and outpatient locations. Physicians may perform some of these studies in their office, some can be performed in the patient's room, and others will need to be performed in a specialty lab. Depending on the invasiveness of the study, it may be performed by a trained technician, physician, or radiologist. A signed consent is not required for noninvasive electrophysiological studies. Patients who are having their heart evaluated will be asked to withhold taking antidysrhythmic medications for up to 24 hours before the study begins.

Electrical impulses run continuously through the cells, tissues, and organs involved in any type of metabolic process. A few examples include the musculoskeletal, cardiovascular, and nervous systems. The impulses are conducted and sustained through complex chain reactions involving electrolytes such as sodium, potassium, calcium, and magnesium. The ability of tissues to conduct or prevent the passage of electrical energy varies with changes in the concentration of electrolytes in intra- and extracellular fluids, changes in cell membrane permeability, cellular composition, and water content. When an electric current is passed through the body, it is conducted through the intra- and extracellular fluids containing water and electrolytes. Lean tissue contains more water than fatty tissue; therefore, the flow of current occurs easily through muscle but is impeded by fat, which is the basis for bioelectric impedance analysis. Bioelectric impedance measurements are a reflection of the structure, composition, and function of specific tissues.

Measurements of the electrical properties of normal tissue have been expanded to explore tissue profiles along a continuum of cellular change from damaged to expired. These advances may make it possible to diagnose diseases earlier, predict survival, and guide the progress of therapeutic interventions. The technology has appeal because it is simple, portable, noninvasive, relatively inexpensive, and has rapid turnaround to results. In practice, it is usually conducted by contact with electrodes at the site of interest such as the trunk, wrist to ankle, hand to hand, or other combinations of trunk and limbs. Estimates of body fat percentage are derived from the measurements set against formulas that consider a person's height, weight, and gender. The development of medical applications based on bioelectric impedance analysis (BIA) include impedance plethysmography; electroencephalography; hydration management for patients with hemodynamic disturbances; nutritional interventions for malnourished, critically ill patients; and assessment of body composition as a risk factor for developing diseases such as heart disease, diabetes, hypertension, and some types of cancer. Nutritionists, athletic club trainers, and members of sports organizations are using BIA to assess health and assist patients in successful weight management. Health assessment has become part of some employee wellness programs. Participation in health assessment is also tied to some employer-sponsored health insurance plans that offer discounts to employees who participate and penalties for those who do not participate. Drawbacks to some of the simpler equipment used to measure body composition in normal subjects are inconsistent readings due to variations in hydration level, skin temperature, and testing environment, as well as the skill level of the person administering the measurements.

The information in the Part I studies is organized in a manner to help the student see how the five basic components of the nursing process (assessment, diagnosis, planning, implementation, and evaluation) can be applied to each phase of laboratory and diagnostic testing. The goal is to use nursing process to understand the integration of care (laboratory, diagnostic, nursing care) toward achieving a positive expected outcome.

- **Assessment** is the collection of information for the purpose of answering the question, "is there a problem?" Knowledge of the patient's health history, medications, complaints, and allergies as well as synonyms or alternate test names, common use for the procedure, specimen requirements, and normal ranges or interpretive comments provide the foundation for diagnosis.
- **Diagnosis** is the process of looking at the information gathered during assessment and answering the questions, "what is the problem?" and "what do I need to do about it?" Test indications tell us why the study has been requested, and potential diagnoses tell us the value or importance of the study relative to its clinical utility.
- **Planning** is a blueprint of the nursing care before the procedure. It is the process of determining how the nurse is going to partner with the patient to fix the problem (e.g., "The patient has a study ordered and this is what I should know before I successfully carry out the plan to have the study completed."). Knowledge of interfering factors, social and cultural issues, preprocedural restrictions, the need for written and informed consent, anxiety about the procedure, and concerns regarding pain are some considerations for planning a successful partnership.
- **Implementation** is putting the plan into action with an idea of what the expected outcome should be. Collaboration with the departments where the laboratory test or diagnostic study is to be performed is essential to the success of the plan. Implementation is where the work is done within each healthcare team member's scope of practice.
- **Evaluation** answers the question, "did the plan work or not?" Was the plan completely successful, partially successful, or not successful? If the plan did not work,

evaluation is the process where you determine what needs to be changed to make the plan work better. This includes a review of all expected outcomes. Nursing care after the procedure is where information is gathered to evaluate the plan. Review of results, including critical findings, in relation to patient symptoms and other tests performed, provides data that form a more complete picture of health or illness.

- **Expected Outcomes** are positive outcomes related to the test. They are the outcomes the nurse should expect if all goes well.

A number of pretest, intratest, and post-test universal points are presented in this overview section because the information applies to electrophysiologic studies in general.

Universal Pretest Pearls (Planning)

- Obtain a history of the patient's complaints, including a list of known allergens, especially allergies or sensitivities to medications or latex so that their use can be avoided or their effects mitigated if an allergy is present. Carefully evaluate all medications currently being taken by the patient. A list of the patient's current medications, prescribed and over the counter (including anticoagulants, aspirin and other salicylates, and dietary supplements), should also be obtained. Such products may be discontinued by medical direction for the appropriate number of days prior to the procedure. Ensure that all allergies are clearly noted in the medical record, and ensure that the patient is wearing an allergy and medical record armband. Report information that could interfere with, or delay proceeding with, the study to the HCP and laboratory.
- Obtain a history of the patient's affected body system, symptoms, and results of previously performed laboratory tests and diagnostic and surgical procedures. Previous test results will provide a basis of comparison between old and new data.
- An important aspect of planning is understanding the factors that may alter study findings or cause abnormal results. Interdepartmental communication is a key factor in the planning process. The inability of a patient to cooperate or remain still during the procedure because of age, significant pain, or mental status should be among the anticipated factors. Recent or past procedures, medications, or existing medical conditions that could complicate or interfere with test results should be noted.
- Review the steps of the study with the patient or caregiver. Expect patients to be nervous about the procedure and the pending results. Educating the patient on his or her role during the procedure and

what to expect can facilitate this. The patient's role during the procedure itself is to remain still. The actual time required to complete each study will depend on a number of conditions, including the type of equipment being used and how well a patient will cooperate.

- Address any concerns about pain, and explain or describe, as appropriate, the level and type of discomfort that may be expected.
- Provide additional instructions and patient preparation regarding medication, diet, fluid intake, or activity, if appropriate. Unless specified in the individual study, there are no special instructions or restrictions.
- Always be sensitive to any cultural or psychosocial issues, including a concern for modesty before, during, and after the procedure.

Reminder

Ensure that a written and informed consent has been documented in the medical record prior to the study, if required. The consent must be obtained before medication is administered.

Universal Intratest Pearls (Implementation)

- Correct patient identification is crucial prior to any procedure: Positively identify the patient using two unique identifiers, such as patient name, date of birth, Social Security number, or medical record number.
- Standard Precautions must be followed.
- Children and infants may be accompanied by a parent to calm them. Keep neonates and infants covered and in a warm room and provide a pacifier or gentle touch. The testing environment should be quiet and the patient should be instructed, as appropriate, to remain still during the test as extraneous movements can affect results.
- Ensure that the patient has complied with pretesting instructions, including dietary, fluid, medication, and activity restrictions as given for the procedure. The number of days to withhold medication depends on the type of medication. Notify the HCP if pretesting instructions have not been followed (e.g., if applicable, if patient anticoagulant therapy has not been withheld).
- Baseline vital signs must be monitored and continue to be monitored throughout and after the procedure, according to organizational policy. A comparison should be made between the baseline and postprocedure vital signs and focused assessments. Protocols may vary among facilities.

Universal Post Test Pearls (Evaluation)

- Note that completed test results are made available to the requesting HCP, who will discuss them with the patient.
- Answer questions and address concerns voiced by the patient or family and reinforce information given by the patient's HCP regarding further testing, treatment, or referral to another HCP. Recognize that patients will have anxiety related to test results. Provide teaching and information regarding the clinical implications of the test results on the patient's lifestyle as appropriate.
- Note that test results should be evaluated in context with the patient's signs, symptoms, and diagnosis. Depending on the results of the procedure, additional testing may be performed to evaluate or monitor progression of the disease process and determine the need for a change in therapy.
- Be aware that when a person goes through a traumatic event such as an illness or is being given information that will impact his or her lifestyle, there are universal human reactions that occur. These include knowledge deficit, fear, anxiety, and coping; in some situations, grieving may occur. HCPs should always be aware of the human response and how it may affect the plan of care and expected outcomes.

DISCUSSION POINT

Regarding Post-Test Critical Findings: Timely notification of a critical finding for lab or diagnostic studies is a role expectation of the professional nurse. Notification processes will vary among facilities. Upon receipt of the critical finding, the information should be read back to the caller to verify accuracy. Most policies require immediate notification of the primary HCP, hospitalist, or on-call HCP. Reported information includes the patient's name, unique identifiers, critical finding, name of the person giving the report, and name of the person receiving the report. Documentation of notification should be made in the medical record with the name of the HCP notified, time and date of notification, and any orders received. Any delay in a timely report of a critical finding may require completion of a notification form with review by Risk Management.

STUDIES

- Electrocardiogram
- Electroencephalography
- Evoked Brain Potentials

LEARNING OUTCOMES

Providing safe, effective nursing care (SENC) includes mastery of core competencies and standards of care. SENC is based on a judicious application of nursing knowledge in combination with scientific principles. The Art of Nursing lies in blending what you know with the ability to effectively apply your knowledge in a compassionate manner.

After reading/studying this chapter you will be able to:

Thinking

1. Identify barriers that prevent the patient from participating in health and wellness.

Doing

1. Evaluate for the existence and severity of the patient's pain and distress.

Caring

1. Recognize the merit of collaborating with patient, family, and significant others to design, implement, and evaluate the plan of care.

Electrocardiogram

Quick Summary

SYNONYM ACRONYM: ECG, EKG.

COMMON USE: To evaluate the electrical impulses generated by the heart during the cardiac cycle to assist with diagnosis of cardiac dysrhythmias, blocks, damage, infection, or enlargement.

AREA OF APPLICATION: Heart.

Normal Resting Heart Rate by Age	
Age	Beats/Min
Newborns (0–1 mo)	70–180
Infants (2–11 mo)	80–160
1–2 yr	80–130
3–4 yr	75–140
5–7 yr	70–130
8–9 yr	70–120
10 years and older, adults, older adults	60–100

• Normal, regular rhythm and wave deflections with normal measurement of ranges of cycle components and height, depth, and duration of complexes as follows:
  • P wave: 0.12 seconds or three small blocks with amplitude of 2.5 mm
  • Q wave: less than 0.04 mm
  • R wave: 5 to 27 mm amplitude, depending on lead
  • T wave: 1 to 13 mm amplitude, depending on lead
  • QRS complex: 0.1 seconds or two and a half small blocks
  • ST segment: 1 mm

Test Explanation

The cardiac muscle consists of three layers of cells: the inner *endocardium*, the middle *myocardium*, and the outer *epicardium*. The systolic phase of the cardiac cycle reflects the contraction of the myocardium, whereas the diastolic phase takes place when the heart relaxes to allow blood to rush in. All muscle cells have a characteristic rate of contraction called *depolarization*. Therefore, the heart will maintain a predetermined heart rate unless other stimuli are received.

The monitoring of pulse and blood pressure evaluates only the mechanical activity of the heart. The electrocardiogram (ECG), a noninvasive study, measures the electrical currents or impulses that the heart generates during a cardiac cycle. Electrical impulses travel through a conduction system beginning with the sinoatrial (SA) node, moving to the atrioventricular (AV) node via internodal pathways. From the AV node, the impulses travel to the bundle of His and onward to the right and left bundle branches. These bundles are located within the right and left ventricles. The impulses continue to the cardiac muscle cells by terminal fibers called *Purkinje fibers*. The ECG is a graphic display of the electrical activity of the heart, which is analyzed by time intervals and segments. Continuous tracing of the cardiac cycle activity is captured as heart cells are electrically stimulated, causing depolarization and movement of the activity through the cells of the myocardium.

The ECG study is completed by using 12, 15, or 18 electrodes attached to the skin surface to obtain the total electrical activity of the heart. Each lead records the electrical potential between the limbs or between the heart and limbs. The ECG machine records and marks the 12 leads (most common system used) on the strip of paper in the machine in proper sequence, usually 6 inches of the strip for each lead. Leads I, II, and III, known as extremity leads in a 12-lead ECG, form a triangle known as Einthoven triangle when placed on the body (see Fig. 8.1). The ECG pattern, called a *heart rhythm*, is recorded by a machine as a series of waves, intervals, and segments, each of which pertains to a specific occurrence during the contraction of the heart. The ECG tracings are recorded on graph paper using vertical and horizontal lines for analysis and calculations of time, measured by the vertical lines (1 mm apart and 0.04 seconds per line), and of voltage, measured by the horizontal lines (1 mm apart and 0.5 mV per five squares) (see Fig. 8.2). A pulse rate can be calculated from the ECG strip to obtain the beats per minute. The P wave represents the depolarization

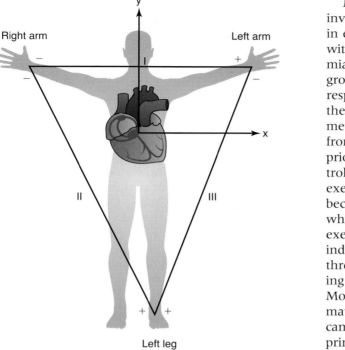

FIGURE 8.1 Einthoven triangle

of the atrial myocardium; the QRS complex represents the depolarization of the ventricular myocardium; the P-R interval represents the time from beginning of the excitation of the atrium to the beginning of the ventricular excitation; and the ST segment has no deflection from baseline, but in an abnormal state may be elevated or depressed. An abnormal rhythm is called an *dysrhythmia*.

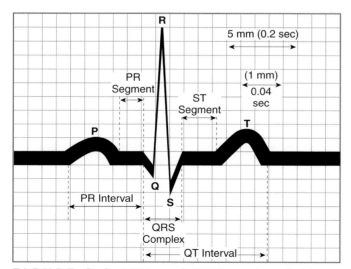

FIGURE 8.2 QRS interval. *QRS interval, used with permission, from Van Leeuwen, A., Bladh, M., & Poelhuis-Leth, D. (2013). Davis's comprehensive handbook of laboratory and diagnostic tests with nursing implications (5th ed.). FA Davis Company.*

Microvolt T wave alternans (MTWA) is a type of non-invasive testing that identifies variations or alterations in electrical activity of the T wave which are associated with sudden cardiac death from ventricular dysrhythmias. Specialized electrodes are used to reduce background noise from natural internal movement such as respirations or external movement such as caused by the friction of electrodes on skin. There are two main methods of interpreting the beat to beat data collected from electrodes placed on the patient's chest at rest prior to a period of activity: during an interval of controlled exercise, and during the recovery period after exercise. Research has shown that the extent of MTWA becomes more demonstrable as heart rate increases, which is why the test includes a period of controlled exercise. MTWA occurs at a rate that is specific to each individual and is reproducible at a rate above the initial threshold for an individual. The methods for interpreting the ECG T wave data are known as the Spectral and Modified Moving Average methods; both use sensitive mathematical algorithms. Either of the two methods can be combined with a computer program to produce printable reports from the study results which are interpreted by a cardiologist as positive, negative, or indeterminate. Spectral analysis is considered the preferred method for measurement and comparison of T wave activity based on the availability of documented studies using spectral analysis.

Another modification of the ECG, used to evaluate for ventricular dysrhythmias, is the signal-averaged ECG. Heart rhythms in patients who have CAD, are recovering from a MI, have nonischemic dilated cardiomyopathy, left ventricular aneurysm, ventricular tachycardia, or have healed ventricular incisions may demonstrate abnormally slow electrical conduction through the heart, called *late potentials*. The late potentials are believed to be the result of delayed conduction through areas of plaque, fibrous scarring, or inflammation and can reliably predict significant and sudden ventricular dysrhythmias. The abnormal changes in conduction are too small to be detected by standard ECG equipment and require specially designed computer software. The test takes 15–20 minutes and analyses hundreds of cardiac cycles to detect the presence of late potentials.

The ankle-brachial index (ABI) can also be assessed during this study. This noninvasive, simple comparison of blood pressure measurements in the arms and legs can be used to detect peripheral arterial disease (PAD). A Doppler stethoscope is used to obtain the systolic pressure in either the dorsalis pedis or the posterior tibial artery. This ankle pressure is then divided by the highest brachial systolic pressure acquired after taking the blood pressure in both arms of the patient. This index should be greater than 1. When the index falls below 0.5, blood flow impairment is considered significant. Patients should be scheduled for a vascular consult for an abnormal ABI. Patients with diabetes or kidney disease, as well as some older adult patients, may have a falsely elevated ABI due to calcifications of the vessels in the ankle causing an increased systolic pressure. The ABI test approaches 95% accuracy in detecting PAD. However, a normal ABI value does not absolutely rule out the possibility of PAD for some individuals, and additional tests should be done to evaluate symptoms.

Nursing Implications
Assessment

Indications	Potential Nursing Problems
Assess the extent of congenital heart disease	• Cardiac Output
Assess the extent of myocardial infarction (MI) or ischemia, as indicated by abnormal ST segment, interval times, and amplitudes	• Fear
	• Health Management
Assess the function of heart valves	• Human Response
Assess global cardiac function	• Pain
Detect dysrhythmias, as evidenced by abnormal wave deflections	• Role Performance
Detect peripheral arterial disease (PAD)	• Tissue Perfusion
Detect pericarditis, shown by ST segment changes or shortened P-R interval	• Self-Care
	• Self-Esteem
Determine electrolyte imbalances, as evidenced by short or prolonged Q-T interval	• Sexuality
Determine hypertrophy of the chamber of the heart or heart hypertrophy, as evidenced by P or R wave deflections	
Evaluate and monitor cardiac pacemaker function	
Evaluate and monitor the effect of drugs, such as digoxin, dysrhythmics, or vasodilating agents	
Monitor ECG changes during an exercise test	
Monitor rhythm changes during the recovery phase after an MI	

Diagnosis: Clinical Significance of Test Results
ABNORMAL FINDINGS
- Atrial or ventricular hypertrophy
- Bundle branch block
- Dysrhythmias
- Electrolyte imbalances
- Heart rate of 40 to 60 beats/min in adults
- Ischemia or MI
- PAD
- Pericarditis
- Pulmonary infarction

- P wave: An enlarged P wave deflection could indicate atrial enlargement; an absent or altered P wave could suggest that the electrical impulse did not come from the SA node.
- P-R interval: An increased interval could imply a conduction delay in the AV node.
- QRS complex: An enlarged Q wave may indicate an old infarction; an enlarged deflection could indicate ventricular hypertrophy; and increased time duration may indicate a bundle branch block.
- ST segment: A depressed ST segment indicates myocardial ischemia; an elevated ST segment may indicate an acute MI or pericarditis; and a prolonged ST segment (or prolonged QT) may indicate hypocalcemia. A shortened ST segment may indicate hypokalemia.
- Tachycardia greater than 120 beats/min
- T wave: A flat or inverted T wave may indicate myocardial ischemia, infarction, or hypokalemia; a tall, peaked T wave with a shortened QT interval may indicate hyperkalemia.

Planning
Considerations for planning a successful partnership should include clear communication of what to expect during the test to decrease anxiety and improve cooperation. Before the procedure is performed, plan to review the steps with the patient. Explain that no discomfort should be experienced during the exam, and inform the patient that the procedure is performed in a special room or bedside by a health-care provider (HCP), and takes approximately 15 minutes. Explain that electrocardiography does not use radiation and is considered safe.

SPECIAL CONSIDERATIONS
An important aspect of planning is understanding the factors that may alter study findings or cause abnormal results. Interdepartmental communication is a key factor in the planning process. The following should be noted when planning for this study:

- Anatomic variation of the heart (i.e., the heart may be rotated in both the horizontal and frontal planes)
- Distortion of cardiac cycles due to age, gender, weight, or a medical condition (e.g., infants, women [may exhibit slight ST segment depression], patients who are obese, patients who are pregnant, patients with ascites)
- ECG machine malfunction or interference from electromagnetic waves in the vicinity
- Increased patient anxiety, which causes hyperventilation or deep respirations
- Strenuous exercise before the procedure
- Inability of the patient to remain still during the procedure, because movement, muscle tremor, or twitching can affect accurate test recording

- Improper placement of electrodes or inadequate contact between skin and electrodes because of insufficient conductive gel or poor placement, which can cause ECG tracing problems
- High intake of carbohydrates or electrolyte imbalances of potassium or calcium

It is also important to understand which medications or substances the patient may be exposed to in the healthcare setting that can interfere with accurate testing:

- Barbiturates, digoxin, and quinidine may cause alterations in cardiac cycles which can affect test results

Implementation

Note that patient education is key to obtaining the patient's cooperation in following directions, and providing an explanation for the purpose of the procedure is an important part of this process. Inform the patient that this study can assist in assessing for disorders of the heart.

Position the patient in a supine position on the examination table and drape appropriately. Prepare the patient's skin using alcohol swabs to remove skin oil. Electrodes with electropaste are strapped to all four extremities with the color-coded wires inserted into the correct leads. Arm electrodes should be placed on the upper arm to minimize detection of muscle tremors. The placement of the electrocardiographic leads (ECG) on the chest depends on the type of ECG machine used and can be done one at a time, three at a time, or six at a time. If the patient has a large amount of hair on the chest, clip hair from the area of lead placements.

Position the leads as follows (see Fig. 8.3):

- V_1 in the fourth intercostal space (4ICS) at the right sternal border
- V_2 in the 4ICS at the left sternal border
- V_3 halfway between V_2 and V_4
- V_4 in the 5ISC at the midclavicular line
- V_5 at the left anterior axillary line at the level of V_4 horizontally

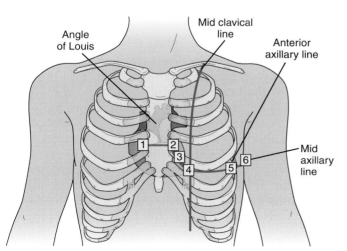

FIGURE 8.3 ECG lead placement

- V_6 at the left midaxillary line at the level of V_4 horizontally

Instruct the patient to tell you if he or she experiences any chest pain during the study, and mark the ECG paper at the time of pain. Following completion of the ECG recording, remove all leads and wipe the gel from the patient's chest and extremities.

Evaluation

Recognize anxiety related to test results, and be supportive of impaired activity related to cardiac dysrhythmia and a perceived loss of independence. Discuss the implications of abnormal test results on the patient's lifestyle. Provide teaching and information regarding the clinical implications of the test results as appropriate. Answer any questions or address any concerns voiced by the patient or family. Educate the patient regarding access to counseling services and provide contact information, if desired, for the American Heart Association (www.americanheart.org), the National Heart, Lung, and Blood Institute (NHLBI) (www.nhlbi.nih.gov), Institute of Medicine of the National Academies (www.iom.edu) or the USDA's resource for nutrition (http://www.choosemyplate.gov/), or the Legs for Life (www.legsforlife.org).

SPECIAL CONSIDERATIONS

Numerous studies point to the prevalence of excess body weight in American children and adolescents. Experts estimate that obesity is present in 25% of the population ages 6 to 11 years. The medical, social, and emotional consequences of excess body weight are significant. Special attention should be given to instructing the child and caregiver regarding health risks and weight-control education.

NUTRITIONAL CONSIDERATIONS FOR THE CARDIAC PATIENT: Abnormal findings may be associated with cardiovascular disease. Nutritional therapy is recommended for the patient identified to be at risk for developing CAD or for individuals who have specific risk factors and/or existing medical conditions (e.g., elevated LDL cholesterol levels, low HDL cholesterol levels, other lipid disorders, insulin-dependent diabetes, insulin resistance, or metabolic syndrome). Other changeable risk factors that warrant patient education include strategies to encourage patients, especially those who are overweight and with high blood pressure, to safely decrease sodium intake, achieve a normal weight, ensure regular participation of moderate aerobic physical activity three to four times per week, eliminate tobacco use, and adhere to a heart-healthy diet. If triglycerides also are elevated, the patient should be advised to eliminate or reduce alcohol. A variety of dietary patterns are beneficial for people with CAD and there are many meal-planning approaches with nutritional goals endorsed by the American Diabetes Association (ADA). The *Guideline on*

Lifestyle Management to Reduce Cardiovascular Risk, published by the American College of Cardiology (ACC) and the American Heart Association (AHA) in conjunction with the National Heart, Lung, and Blood Institute (NHLBI) recommends a "Mediterranean"-style diet rather than a low-fat diet. The guideline emphasizes inclusion of vegetables, whole grains, fruits, low-fat dairy, nuts, legumes, and nontropical vegetable oils (e.g., olive, canola, peanut, sunflower, flaxseed) along with fish and lean poultry. A similar dietary pattern known as the Dietary Approaches to Stop Hypertension (DASH) diet makes additional recommendations for the reduction of dietary sodium. Both dietary styles emphasize a reduction in consumption of red meats, which are high in saturated fats and cholesterol, and other foods containing sugar, saturated fats, trans fats, and sodium. The ADA also includes a vegetarian diet as well as other potential weight loss diets, such as Weight Watchers. The nutritional needs of each patient need to be determined individually (especially during pregnancy) with the appropriate HCPs, particularly professionals educated in nutrition.

✓ Critical Findings

ADULT

- Acute changes in ST elevation are usually associated with acute MI or pericarditis.
- Asystole
- Heart block, second and third degree with bradycardia less than 60 beats/min
- Pulseless electrical activity
- Pulseless ventricular tachycardia
- Premature ventricular contractions (PVCs) greater than three in a row, pauses greater than 3 seconds, or identified blocks
- Unstable tachycardia
- Ventricular fibrillation

PEDIATRIC

- Asystole
- Bradycardia less than 60 beats/min
- Pulseless electrical activity
- Pulseless ventricular tachycardia
- Supraventricular tachycardia
- Ventricular fibrillation

Note and immediately report to the requesting HCP any critical findings and related symptoms. A listing of these findings varies among facilities.

✓ Study Specific Complications

N/A

✓ Related Tests

- Related tests include antidysrhythmic drugs, apolipoprotein A and B, AST, atrial natriuretic peptide, BNP,

blood gases, blood pool imaging, calcium, chest x-ray, cholesterol (total, HDL, LDL), CT cardiac scoring, CT thorax, CRP, CK and isoenzymes, echocardiography, echocardiography transesophageal, exercise stress test, glucose, glycated hemoglobin, Holter monitor, homocysteine, ketones, LDH and isos, lipoprotein electrophoresis, lung perfusion scan, magnesium, MRI chest, MI infarct scan, myocardial perfusion heart scan, myoglobin, PET heart, potassium, pulse oximetry, sodium, triglycerides, and troponin.

- Refer to the Cardiovascular System table at the end of the book for related tests by body system.

Expected Outcomes

Expected outcomes associated with Electrocardiogram are

- Heart sounds that are normal
- Agreement to the therapeutic regime in order to control cardiac dysrhythmia
- Understanding of the importance of reporting chest pain in a timely manner
- Verbalization of fear associated with the diagnosis of serious cardiac disease

Electroencephalography

Quick Summary

SYNONYM ACRONYM: Electrical activity (for sleep disturbances), EEG.

COMMON USE: To assess the electrical activity in the brain toward assisting in diagnosis of brain death, injury, infection, and bleeding.

AREA OF APPLICATION: Brain.

- Normal occurrences of alpha, beta, theta, and delta waves (rhythms varying depending on the patient's age)
- Normal frequency, amplitude, and characteristics of brain waves

Test Explanation

Electroencephalography (EEG) is a noninvasive study that measures the brain's electrical activity and records that activity on graph paper. These electrical impulses arise from the brain cells of the cerebral cortex. Electrodes, placed on the patient's scalp according to the International 10/20 system, transmit the different frequencies and amplitudes of the brain's electrical activity to the EEG equipment, which records the results in graph form on a moving paper strip or a computerized system for retrieval, review, or comparison, at a later date. Guidelines for the performance and evaluation of an EEG are set by the American Clinical Neurophysiology Society. The EEG can evaluate responses to various stimuli, such as flickering light, hyperventilation, auditory signals, or somatosensory signals generated by skin electrodes. The procedure is usually performed in a room designed to eliminate electrical interference and minimize distractions. An EEG can be done at the bedside, and a health-care provider (HCP) analyzes the waveforms. The test is used to detect epilepsy, intracranial abscesses, or tumors; to evaluate cerebral involvement due to head injury or meningitis; and to monitor for cerebral tissue ischemia during surgery when cerebral vessels must be occluded (e.g., carotid endarterectomy). EEG is also used to confirm brain death, which can be defined as absence of electrical activity in the brain. To evaluate abnormal EEG waves further, the patient may be connected to an ambulatory EEG system similar to a Holter monitor for the heart.

Nursing Implications

Assessment

Indications	Potential Nursing Problems
Confirm brain death Confirm suspicion of increased intracranial pressure caused by trauma or disease Detect cerebral ischemia during endarterectomy Detect intracranial cerebrovascular lesions, such as hemorrhages and infarcts Detect seizure disorders and identify focus of seizure and seizure activity, as evidenced by abnormal spikes and waves recorded on the graph Determine the presence of tumors, abscesses, or infection Evaluate the effect of drug intoxication on the brain Evaluate sleeping disorders, such as sleep apnea and narcolepsy Identify area of abnormality in dementia (e.g. Alzheimer Disease)	• Bleeding • Communication • Conflicted Decision Making • Confusion • Fear • Family • Human Response • Memory • Mobility • Role Performance

Diagnosis: Clinical Significance of Test Results
ABNORMAL FINDINGS
- Abscess
- Alzheimer disease
- Brain death
- Cerebral infarct
- Encephalitis
- Glioblastoma and other brain tumors
- Head injury
- Hematoma
- Hypocalcemia or hypoglycemia
- Infarct
- Intracranial hemorrhage
- Meningitis
- Migraine headaches

- Narcolepsy
- Parkinson disease
- Seizure disorders (epilepsy, grand mal, focal, temporal lobe, myoclonic, petit mal)
- Sleep apnea

Planning
Considerations for planning a successful partnership should include clear communication of what to expect during the test to decrease anxiety and improve cooperation. Before the procedure is performed, plan to review the steps with the patient. Address concerns about pain related to the procedure, and assure the patient that there is no discomfort during the procedure, but if needle electrodes are used, a slight pinch may be felt. Explain that, during the procedure, electricity flows from the patient's body, not into the body, and that the procedure reveals brain activity only, not thoughts, feelings, or intelligence. Inform the patient that the procedure is performed in a quiet room or bedside by a HCP, and takes approximately 30–120 minutes, depending on the purpose of the study. Explain that electroencephalography does not use radiation and is considered safe. Inform the patient that he or she may be asked to do the following: alter his or her breathing pattern; follow simple commands such as opening or closing eyes, blinking, or swallowing; be stimulated with bright light; or be given a sedative to promote sleep at the beginning of the examination. Instruct the patient to avoid caffeine and alcohol for 8 hours, and to avoid stimulants, anticonvulsants, and sedative for 24–48 hours before the exam because they may alter electroencephalographic activity. If a sleep-deprived exam is performed, which can evaluate seizures or sleep disorders, instruct the patient not to sleep the night before the exam. The patient should also be instructed not to fast, as hypoglycemia may alter the study findings.

DISCUSSION POINT
When an EEG is performed on a child or an infant, the presence of the parent in the room may help to calm him or her. If the child has a favorite blanket or special stuffed animal, instruct the parent to bring it with him or her, but do not allow the parent to bring any toys or games that involve movement or interaction into the testing area. Children are studied for approximately 1 to 2 hours as outpatients and, occasionally, it may be necessary to sedate a child with a mild medication to obtain sleep. Patients older than 8 years should receive 4 hours of sleep only, between midnight and 4:00 a.m. Younger children should sleep one-half their normal sleep hours and be awakened at 4:00 a.m., and infants (younger than 1 year of age) do not need to be sleep deprived the night before unless the test is scheduled at 8:00 a.m. In this case, the child should be awakened early so that she or he will be tired by 9:00 a.m. Infants and children who take naps should be deprived of naps on the day of the test.

SPECIAL CONSIDERATIONS

An important aspect of planning is understanding the factors that alter study findings or cause abnormal results. Interdepartmental communication is a key factor in the planning process. The following should be noted when planning for this study:

- Dirty or oily hair; hair with hair spray or other products that can affect electrode placement and contact
- Hypoglycemia or hypothermia
- Inability of the patient to remain still during the study (muscle contractions or body movements)

It is also important to understand which medications or substances the patient may be exposed to in the healthcare setting that can interfere with accurate testing:

- Alcohol or medications such as sedatives, anticonvulsants, or antiaxolytics may alter the results of the study
- Beverages containing caffeine or other stimulants may alter the results of the study

● **Safety Tip**

Make sure a written and informed consent has been signed prior to the procedure or administering any medications.

Implementation

Patient education is key to obtaining the patient's cooperation in following directions, and providing an explanation for the purpose of the procedure is an important part of this process. Inform the patient that this study can assist in assessing for disorders of the brain. Verify that the patient has complied with medication and sleep restrictions.

● **Safety Tip**

Bedside rails must be put in the raised position for safety.

Position the patient in a reclining chair or in a supine position on the bed and provide warm blankets for comfort. The test should be conducted in a special room protected from any noise or electrical interferences that could affect the tracings. Apply the electrodes to the scalp in a set pattern, on the pre-frontal, frontal, temporal, parietal, and occipital areas of both sides of the head, with a conductive gel to improve reception of the brain waves (see Fig. 8.4). Connect the electrode wires to an amplifier and a recording device. Instruct the patient to remain still, and to not talk or move her head. Dim the lights and begin the recording, which may take up to 120 minutes. Procedures may be done to bring out abnormal electrical activity or other brain abnormalities, including stroboscopic light stimulation, hyperventilation to induce alkalosis, and sleep induction by administration of sedative to detect abnormalities that occur only during sleep. Observations for

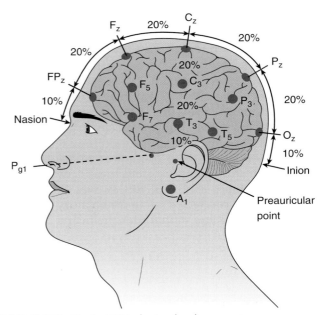

FIGURE 8.4 EEG electrode placement

seizure activity are carried out during the study, and a description and time of activity is noted by the HCP. If a sedative was given during the test, allow the patient to recover. Following completion of the EEG, remove the electrodes from the scalp and clean the hair and scalp using a cleanser, and instruct the patient to wash his or her hair at home to remove any residual paste.

Evaluation

Recognize anxiety related to test results, and be supportive of impaired activity related to abnormal brain activity and a perceived loss of independence. Discuss the implications of abnormal test results on the patient's lifestyle. Provide teaching and information regarding the clinical implications of the test results as appropriate. Answer any questions or address any concerns voiced by the patient or family. Educate the patient regarding access to counseling services and provide contact information, if desired, for additional information concerning the diagnosis. Refer the patient or family to websites to obtain additional information, such as the Epilepsy Foundation (www.epilepsyfoundation.org/), Alzheimer's Association of America (www.alzfdn.org), or the U.S. Government Information on Organ and Tissue Donation and Transplantation (http://www.organdonor.gov/index.html).

✓ **Critical Findings**

- Abscess
- Brain death
- Head injury
- Hemorrhage
- Intracranial hemorrhage

Note and immediately report to the requesting HCP any critical findings and related symptoms. A listing of these findings varies among facilities.

Study Specific Complications

N/A

Related Tests

- Related tests include CSF analysis, CT brain, evoked brain potentials (SER, VER), MRI brain, and PET brain.
- Refer to the Musculoskeletal System table at the end of the book for related tests by body system.

Expected Outcomes

Expected outcomes associated with electroencephalography are

- Recognition of a baseline memory that remains intact
- Adaptation to alterations in role performance
- Verbalization by the family or surrogate of an understanding of end-of-life information provided by HCP related to brain death
- Agreement by the family or surrogate to consider organ donation upon the confirmation of brain death

Evoked Brain Potentials

Quick Summary

SYNONYM ACRONYM: Brainstem auditory-evoked potentials (BAEPs), brainstem auditory-evoked responses (BAERs), EP studies.

COMMON USE: To assist in diagnosing sensory deficits related to nervous system lesions manifested by visual defects, hearing defects, neuropathies, and cognitive disorders.

AREA OF APPLICATION: Brain.

- ***VER and ABR:*** Normal latency in recorded cortical and brainstem waveforms depending on age, gender, and stature
- ***ERP:*** Normal recognition and attention span
- ***SER:*** No loss of consciousness or presence of weakness

Test Explanation

Evoked brain potentials, also known as evoked potential (EP) responses, are electrophysiological studies performed to measure the brain's electrical responses to various visual, auditory, and somatosensory stimuli. EP studies help diagnose lesions of the nervous system by evaluating the integrity of the visual, somatosensory, and auditory nerve pathways. Three response types are measured: visual-evoked response (VER), auditory brainstem response (ABR), and somatosensory-evoked response (SER). The stimuli activate the nerve tracts that connect the stimulated (receptor) area with the cortical (visual and somatosensory) or midbrain (auditory) sensory area. A number of stimuli are given, and then responses are electronically displayed in waveforms, recorded, and computer analyzed. Abnormalities are determined by a delay in time, measured in milliseconds, between the stimulus and the response. This

is known as ***increased latency.*** VER provides information about visual pathway function to identify lesions of the optic nerves, optic tracts, and demyelinating diseases such as multiple sclerosis. ABR provides information about auditory pathways to identify hearing loss and lesions of the brainstem. SER provides information about the somatosensory pathways to identify lesions at various levels of the central nervous system (spinal cord and brain) and peripheral nerve disease. EP studies are especially useful in patients with problems related to the nervous system and those unable to speak or respond to instructions during the test, because these studies do not require voluntary cooperation or participation in the activity. This allows collection of objective diagnostic information about visual or auditory disorders affecting infants and children and allows differentiation between organic brain and psychological disorders in adults. EP studies are also used to monitor the progression of or the effectiveness of treatment for deteriorating neurological diseases such as multiple sclerosis.

Nursing Implications

Assessment

Indications	Potential Nursing Problems
VER (potentials) Detect cryptic or past retrobulbar neuritis Detect lesions of the eye or optic nerves Detect neurological disorders such as multiple sclerosis, Parkinson disease, and Huntington chorea Evaluate binocularity in infants Evaluate optic pathway lesions and visual cortex defects	• Activity • Communication • Confusion • Fall Risk • Human Response • Mobility • Sensory Perception (auditory, visual) • Socialization • Swallowing
ABR (potentials) Detect abnormalities or lesions in the brainstem or auditory nerve areas Detect brainstem tumors and acoustic neuromas Screen or evaluate neonates, infants, children, and adults for auditory problems EP studies may be indicated when a child falls below growth chart norms Evaluate patients in comatose states	
SER (potentials) Detect multiple sclerosis and Guillain-Barré syndrome Detect sensorimotor neuropathies and cervical pathology Evaluate spinal cord and brain injury and function Monitor sensory potentials to determine spinal cord function during a surgical procedure or medical regimen	
ERP (potentials) Detect suspected psychosis or dementia Differentiate between organic brain disorder and cognitive function abnormality	

Diagnosis: Clinical Significance of Test Results

ABNORMAL FINDINGS

- VER (extended latencies):
  - Absence of binocular vision
  - Amblyopias
  - Blindness
  - Demyelinating diseases such as multiple sclerosis
  - Huntington chorea
  - Lesions or disease of the optic nerve and eye (e.g., anterior optic chiasm, neuritis)
  - Lesions or disease of the optic tract
  - Optic nerve neuritis
  - Parkinson disease
  - Visual field defects
- ABR (extended latencies):
  - Acoustic neuroma
  - Auditory nerve or brain stem damage or disease
  - Cerebrovascular accidents
  - Demyelinating diseases such as multiple sclerosis
- SER (extended latencies):
  - Abnormal upper limb latencies suggest cervical spondylosis or intracerebral lesions.
  - Abnormal lower limb latencies suggest peripheral nerve root disease such as Guillain-Barré syndrome, multiple sclerosis, transverse myelitis, or traumatic spinal cord injuries.

Planning

DISCUSSION POINT

Approximately 3 in 1,000 babies are born with permanent hearing loss, making hearing loss one of the most common birth defects in the United States. Left undetected, mild or unilateral hearing loss can result in delayed speech and language acquisition, social-emotional or behavioral problems, and lags in academic achievement. The purpose of auditory-evoked potentials testing in pediatric cases is to identify the lowest sound level that causes a reaction in the ear. Because auditory-evoked potentials testing is not a direct measure of the baby's ability to hear, follow-up evaluations are scheduled to confirm findings.

Considerations for planning a successful partnership should include clear communication of what to expect during the test to decrease anxiety and improve cooperation. Before the procedure is performed, plan to review the steps with the patient or parent and explain that the test measures the electrical activity of the brain. Explain that no discomfort should be experienced during the test, and inform the patient that the procedure is performed in a special room by a neurologist or specially trained technician, and takes approximately 20 to 30 minutes. Instruct the patient to wash his or her hair the night before the test, and to not use conditioner or apply any hair spray or other hair products because electrodes will be attached to the scalp. Remind the patient that all jewelry and other metal objects must be removed.

When this study is performed on a child or an infant, the presence of the parent in the room may help to calm the child. If the child has a favorite blanket or special stuffed animal, instruct the parent to bring it with him or her, but do not bring any toys or games that involve movement or interaction into the testing area.

SPECIAL CONSIDERATIONS

An important aspect of planning is understanding the factors that may alter study findings or cause abnormal results. Interdepartmental communication is a key factor in the planning process. The following should be noted when planning for this study:

- Severe nearsightedness
- Presence of earwax or inflammation of the middle ear
- Severe hearing impairment
- Muscle spasms in the head or neck
- Obesity or edema

● Safety Tip

Make sure a written and informed consent has been signed prior to the procedure if a biopsy is planned and before administering any medications.

Implementation

Patient education is key to obtaining the patient's cooperation in following directions, and providing an explanation for the purpose of the procedure is an important part of this process. Inform the patient that this study can assist in assessing for disorders of the brain and provide simple instructions to the patient to relax, breathe normally, and avoid unnecessary movement.

VISUAL-EVOKED POTENTIALS: Place the patient in a reclining chair or lying on a bed. If a visual-evoked potential is planned, attach electrodes to the patient's scalp at the occipital, parietal, and vertex sites. Placement of electrodes for VER generally follows the 10–20 International System. An additional electrode, a reference electrode, is placed on the ear or the midfrontal area of the head. Cover one eye and position the patient 3 ft from the pattern stimulator. Instruct the patient to focus his or her gaze on the dot in the center of the screen as the checkerboard pattern is reversed 100 times, once or twice per second. The brain's responses to each stimulus are amplified and averaged, and the results are plotted as a waveform. When one eye is completed, switch the eye patch and repeat on the second eye. Remove the electrodes when completed, and cleanse the areas to remove the paste.

SOMATOSENSORY-EVOKED POTENTIALS: When performing a somatosensory-evoked potential, electrodes are placed over sematosensory pathways such as the knee, ankle, and wrist. This allows for stimulation of the peripheral nerves. Place the recording electrodes over the sensory cortex on the scalp opposite the extremity to be examined. Additional recording electrodes may be placed on other areas of the body, such as the lower lumbar, the second cervical vertebra, or above the clavicle over the brachial plexus (Erb point). Rapid-rate electrical stimulus is delivered to the peripheral nerve through the electrode at an intensity that will produce a small muscle response, such as a thumb twitch. These electrical stimuli are then delivered for a minimum of 500 times at a rate of 5/sec. The time it takes for the electric current to reach the cortex is measured and averaged by the computer, and the results are recorded as waveforms measured in milliseconds (msec). When completed, the test is repeated to verify the results before placing the electrodes on the other side of the body. The entire procedure is then repeated. Remove the electrodes when completed, and cleanse the areas to remove the paste.

AUDITORY-EVOKED POTENTIALS: When performing an auditory-evoked potential, place the patient in a comfortable position and secure the electrodes on each earlobe and at the scalp on the vertex lobe. Provide the patient with earphones to place in the ears and begin with a clicking stimulus in one ear while a continuous tone is delivered to the other ear. The response to the stimuli is recorded as waveforms for analysis. Remove the electrodes when completed, and cleanse the areas to remove the paste.

Evaluation

Recognize anxiety related to test results and be supportive of impaired activity related to brain abnormalities and a perceived loss of independence. Discuss the implications of abnormal test results on the patient's lifestyle. Provide teaching and information regarding the clinical implications of the test results as appropriate. Answer any questions or address any concerns voiced by the patient or family. Educate the patient regarding access to counseling services, and provide contact information, if desired, for additional information concerning the diagnosis. Patients should be directed to websites such as the National Multiple Sclerosis Society at http://www.nationalmssociety.org/about-multiple-sclerosis/what-we-know-about-ms/what-is-ms/index.aspx or Facts about Pediatric Hearing Loss at http://www.asha.org/aud/Facts-about-Pediatric-Hearing-Loss/ for additional information depending on the test results.

⊘ Critical Findings

N/A

⊘ Study Specific Complications

N/A

⊘ Related Tests

- Related tests include acetylcholine receptor antibody, Alzheimer disease markers, biopsy muscle, CSF analysis, CT brain, CK, EEG, ENG, MRI brain, plethysmography, and PET brain.
- Refer to the Musculoskeletal System table at the end of the book for related tests by body system.

Expected Outcomes

Expected outcomes associated with evoked brain potentials are

- Demonstration of the desire to initiate movement
- Agreement to facial and tongue exercises to improve communication and prevent choking
- Demonstration of alternate communication techniques, ensuring that needs and wants are met
- Verbalization of an understanding of the fall risk associated with an alteration in senses

REVIEW OF LEARNING OUTCOMES

Thinking

1. Identify barriers that prevent the patient from participating in health and wellness. Answer: When a patient refuses to participate in improving his or her health, it is important to ask yourself why. It is easy to fall into the trap of viewing your patient as a diagnosis rather than as a person. Take into consideration the person in the bed and you will probably be able to discover why he or she is refusing. For example, consider Mari, who was recently diagnosed with neurologic disease that will require expensive medication and follow-up care. Mari refuses and you wonder why. Consider Mari from a different perspective. Mari has no insurance, is a single mother, and has a job that pays minimum wage. She is not thinking about her health, she is thinking about her family, and the debt she cannot afford. This is the difference between treating the disease and treating the person.

Doing

1. Evaluate for the existence and severity of the patients pain and distress. Answer: Pain management is the one of the aspects of care we are worst at. Why? Some nurses believe that unless you see writhing and crying, the pain the patient reports is imagined. Some believe that the patient is asking for medication just because they want it and not because they need it to manage their pain. Look beyond the obvious. Individuals from different cultures display pain in different ways. This must always be a part of your pain assessment.

Emotional suffering can be worse than physical pain. Those who receive devastating diagnoses will need your help personally, professionally, and as a way to access resources to help them cope.

Caring

1. Recognize the merit of collaborating with patient, family, and significant others to design, implement, and evaluate the plan of care. Answer: Active participation by the patient, family, or surrogate is the only way to achieve goals. There is an old saying that "You can lead a horse to water but you can't make them drink." You can't make patients do anything; you can only persuade them that the course of action you suggest will help them to achieve their goal. What is their goal? That is a discussion you need to have with the patient. The patient's goals may be completely different from yours.

( ) **Words OF Wisdom:** Health-care issues derived from these studies can be "game changers" for patients. That means that everything about how they had planned to live their lives may now have to be revised. Imagine a single mother who has two small children and no family support who is newly diagnosed with a disease that will result in progressive disability, or one that will require expensive treatment over a long period of time. Does she choose between her health and the welfare of her family? How will you, as the nurse, identify the issues surrounding these type of situations? It is the nursing role to manage all aspects of care. Getting assigned tasks completed is a part of that but so is accessing resources to assist the patient in meeting health-care goals.

BIBLIOGRAPHY

Auditory evoked potentials testing. (2014). Retrieved from www.memphis.edu/mshc/aeptesting.htm

Benbadis, S. (2013). Focal (nonepileptic) abnormalities on EEG. Retrieved from http://emedicine.medscape.com/article/1140635-overview

Comer, S. (2005). Critical care nursing care plans (2nd ed.). Clifton Park, NY: Thomson Delmar Learning.

Electroencephalogram–EEG–for migraine diagnosis. (2014). Retrieved from http://migraine.com/migraine-diagnosis/electroencephalogram/

Electroencephalogram (EEG) (Electroencephalography, brain wave test). (n.d.). Retrieved from www.hopkinsmedicine.org/healthlibrary/test_procedures/neurological/electroencephalogram_eeg_92,P07655/

Electroencephalograms. (2014). Retrieved from www.childrenshospital.org/health-topics/procedures/electroencephalograms

Ellison, D. (2009). Electrodiagnostic studies. Critical Care Nursing Clinics of North America, 22(1), 1–18.

Evans, A. Clinical utility of evoked potentials. (2014). Retrieved from http://emedicine.medscape.com/article/1137451-overview

Evoked potentials studies. (n.d.). Retrieved from www.hopkinsmedicine.org/healthlibrary/test_procedures/neurological/evoked_potentials_studies_92,P07658/

Fishbach, F., & Dunning, M. (2009). A manual of laboratory and diagnostic tests (8th ed.). Philadelphia, PA: Lippencott Williams & Wilkins.

Goldberg, A., & Litt, H. (2010). Evaluation of the patient with acute chest pain. Radiologic Clinics of North America, 48(4), 745–755.

Kee, J. (2009). Prentice Hall handbook of laboratory and diagnostic tests with nursing implications (6th ed.). Upper Saddle River, NJ: Pearson Prentice Hall.

Malarkey, L., & McMorrow, M. (2012). Saunders guide to laboratory and diagnostic tests (2nd ed). St. Louis, MO: Elsevier Saunders.

O'Connor, M., & McDaniel, N. (2008). The pediatric electrocardiogram: Age-related interpretation. Retrieved from www.ncbi.nlm.nih.gov/pubmed/18272106

Pagana, K., & Pagana, T. (2010). Mosby's manual of diagnostic and laboratory tests (4th ed.). St. Louis, MO: Mosby Elsevier.

Stachowiak, J. (2009). Evoked potentials for diagnosis of multiple sclerosis: What are these tests and why are they used? Retrieved from http://ms.about.com/od/multiplesclerosis101/a/evoked_pot_utd.htm.

Van Leeuwen, A., and Bladh, M. (2015). Davis's comprehensive handbook of laboratory and diagnostic testing with nursing implications (6th ed.). Philadelphia, PA: F.A. Davis Company.

Venes, D. (Ed.). (2009). Taber's cyclopedic medical dictionary (21st ed.). Philadelphia, PA: F.A. Davis Company.

Go to Section II of this book and www.davisplus.com for the Clinical Reasoning Tool and its case studies to provide you with a safe place to explore patient care situations. There are a total of 26 different case studies; 2 cases are presented for each of 13 body systems. One set of 13 cases are found in the Section II chapters, and a second set of 13 cases are available online at www.davisplus.com. Each case is designed with the specific goal of helping you to connect the dots of clinical reasoning. Cases are designed to reflect possible clinical scenarios; the outcomes may or may not be positive—you decide.

Endoscopic Studies

OVERVIEW

Endoscopy is the general term applied to the visual examination and inspection of body organs or cavities. Endoscopy may be performed for many different reasons, such as evaluating known or suspected esophageal or bowel symptoms, or assessing bleeding, pain, difficulty swallowing, or a change in bowel habits. Endoscopes can be rigid metal scopes or flexible fiberoptic scopes. Each uses a light source to assist in visual examination. Endoscopes can be inserted through a body orifice or an incision. The type of scope selected depends on the purpose of the exam and areas to be visualized. A rigid scope may be selected for body areas that need a larger scope. A flexible fiberoptic scope may be chosen because it is better at sending light around curves. This makes it easier to visualize areas that a rigid scope cannot reach. Flexible scopes are also more comfortable for patients. Endoscopes vary in size and length and are capable of accommodating special instruments that are designed to obtain specimens, remove objects, facilitate photos for examination, and cauterize bleeding. Endoscopes also allow for administration of medication and insertion of suctioning. The size, length, type of scope, and special features selected are dependent upon the goals of the endoscopy and size of the patient (see Figs. 9.1 and 9.2). Video documentation and endoscopic sonography can be used to assist in diagnosing cancer and staging cancer. Endoscopic procedures are invasive and require informed consent from the patient or the parent of a minor child. Sedation is used in the performance of these studies, which are typically performed in a special department. Some procedures can be completed in the patient's room if necessary and appropriate. Only health-care providers (HCPs) with special training can perform these procedures.

There are many types of endoscopes, each one named according to the organs or areas being examined. The following are examples of endoscopic types:

- Arthroscope: Used to visualize the joints
- Bronchoscope: Used to visualize the lungs
- Cystoscope: Used to visualize the inside of the urinary bladder
- Laparoscope: Used to visualize the ovaries, appendix, or other abdominal organs

The information in Part I studies is organized in a manner to help the student see how the five basic components of the nursing process (assessment, diagnosis, planning, implementation, and evaluation) can be applied to each phase of laboratory and diagnostic testing. The goal is to use the nursing process to understand the integration of care (laboratory,

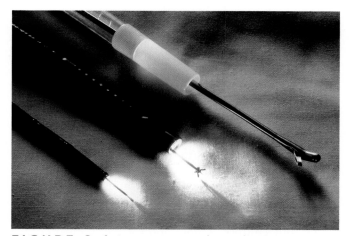

FIGURE 9.1 Instruments used in endoscopy. *Endoscopy, released into public domain by the National Cancer Institute. Photograph by Linda Bartlett. Accessed at http://commons.wikimedia.org/wiki/File:Endoscopy.jpg*

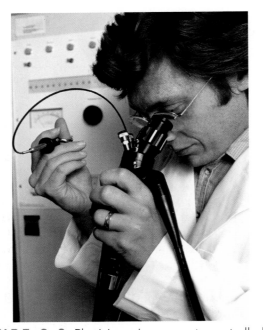

FIGURE 9.2 Physician using a remote-controlled endoscope. *Physician using a remote controlled endoscope, released into public domain by the National Cancer Institute. Photograph by Linda Bartlett. Accessed at http://commons .wikimedia.org/wiki/File:Endoscopy_nci-vol-1982-300.jpg*

diagnostic, nursing care) toward achieving a positive expected outcome.

- **Assessment** is the collection of information for the purpose of answering the question, "is there a problem?" Knowledge of the patient's health history, medications, complaints, and allergies as well as synonyms or alternate test names, common use for the procedure, specimen requirements, and normal ranges or interpretive comments provide the foundation for diagnosis.
- **Diagnosis** is the process of looking at the information gathered during assessment and answering the questions "what is the problem?" and "what do I need to do about it?" Test indications tell us why the study has been requested, and potential diagnoses tell us the value or importance of the study relative to its clinical utility.
- **Planning** is a blueprint of the nursing care before the procedure. It is the process of determining how the nurse is going to partner with the patient to fix the problem (e.g., "The patient has a study ordered and this is what I should know before I successfully carry out the plan to have the study completed."). Knowledge of interfering factors, social and cultural issues, preprocedural restrictions, the need for written and informed consent, anxiety about the procedure, and concerns regarding pain are some considerations for planning a successful partnership.

- **Implementation** is putting the plan into action with an idea of what the expected outcome should be. Collaboration with the departments where the laboratory test or diagnostic study is to be performed is essential to the success of the plan. Implementation is where the work is done within each health-care team member's scope of practice.
- **Evaluation** answers the question "did the plan work or not?" Was the plan completely successful, partially successful, or not successful? If the plan did not work, evaluation is the process where you determine what needs to be changed to make the plan work better. This includes a review of all expected outcomes. Nursing care after the procedure is where information is gathered to evaluate the plan. Review of results, including critical findings, in relation to patient symptoms and other tests performed, provide data that form a more complete picture of health or illness.
- **Expected Outcomes** are positive outcomes related to the test. They are the outcomes the nurse should expect if all goes well.

A number of pretest, intratest, and post-test universal points are presented in this overview section because the information applies to endoscopic studies in general.

Universal Pretest Pearls (Planning)

- Obtain a history of the patient's complaints, including a list of known allergens, especially allergies or sensitivities to medications or latex so their use can be avoided or their effects mitigated if an allergy is present. Carefully evaluate all medications currently being taken by the patient. A list of the patient's current medications, prescribed and over the counter (including anticoagulants, aspirin and other salicylates, and dietary supplements), should also be obtained. Such products may be discontinued by medical direction for the appropriate number of days prior to the procedure. Ensure that all allergies are clearly noted in the medical record, and ensure that the patient is wearing an allergy and medical record armband. Report information that could interfere with, or delay proceeding with, the study to the HCP and laboratory.
- Obtain a history of the patient's affected body system, symptoms, and results of previously performed laboratory tests and diagnostic and surgical procedures. Previous test results will provide a basis of comparison between old and new data.
- An important aspect of planning is understanding the factors that may alter study findings or cause abnormal results. Interdepartmental communication is

a key factor in the planning process. The inability of a patient to cooperate or remain still during the procedure because of age, significant pain, or mental status should be among the anticipated factors. Recent or past procedures, medications, or existing medical conditions that could complicate or interfere with test results should be noted.

- Review the steps of the study with the patient or caregiver. Expect patients to be nervous about the procedure and the pending results. Educating the patient on his or her role during the procedure and what to expect can facilitate this. The patient's role during the procedure is to remain still. The actual time required to complete each study will depend on a number of conditions, including the type of equipment being used and how well a patient will cooperate.
- Address any concerns about pain, and explain or describe, as appropriate, the level and type of discomfort that may be expected during the procedure. Explain that an IV line may be inserted prior to some procedures to allow infusion of IV fluids such as normal saline, anesthetics, sedatives, medications used in the procedure, or emergency medications. Advise the patient that some discomfort may be experienced during the insertion of the IV. Make the patient aware that there may be some mild discomfort during the procedure.
- Provide additional instructions and patient preparation regarding medication, diet, fluid intake, or activity, if appropriate. Unless specified in the individual study, there are no special instructions or restrictions.
- Always be sensitive to any cultural or psychosocial issues, including a concern for modesty before, during, and after the procedure.

Reminder

Ensure that a written and informed consent has been documented in the medical record prior to the study, if required. The consent must be obtained before medication is administered.

Universal Intratest Pearls (Implementation)

- Correct patient identification is crucial prior to any procedure. Positively identify the patient using two unique identifiers, such as patient name, date of birth, Social Security number, or medical record number.
- Standard Precautions must be followed.
- Children and infants may be accompanied by a parent to calm them. Keep neonates and infants covered and in a warm room and provide a pacifier or gentle touch. The testing environment should be quiet and the patient should be instructed, as

appropriate, to remain still during the test as extraneous movements can affect results.

- Ensure the patient has complied with pretesting instructions, including dietary, fluid, medication, and activity restrictions as given for the procedure. The number of days to withhold medication depends on the type of medication. Notify the HCP if pretesting instructions have not been followed (e.g., if patient anticoagulant therapy has not been withheld).
- The patient, as appropriate, should be prepared for insertion of an IV line for infusion of IV fluids, contrast medium, antibiotics, anesthetics, or analgesics must be made. Inform the patient when prophylactic antibiotics will be administered before the procedure and assess for antibiotic allergy. Prior to administration of any fluids or medications, verify that they are accurate for the study. Bleeding or bruising can be prevented, once the needle has been removed, by applying direct pressure to the injection site with dry gauze for a minute or two. The site should be observed/assessed for bleeding or hematoma formation, and then covered with a gauze and adhesive bandage.
- Emergency equipment must be readily available.
- Baseline vital signs must be recorded, and monitoring must continue throughout and after the procedure, according to organizational policy. A comparison should be made between the baseline and postprocedure vital signs and focused assessments. Protocols may vary among facilities.
- After the administration of general or local anesthesia, clippers should be used to remove hair from the surgical site if appropriate, the site must be cleaned with an antiseptic solution, and the area must be draped with sterile towels.
- Before leaving the patient's side, appropriate specimen containers should always be labeled with the corresponding patient demographics, initials of the person collecting the sample, collection date, time of collection, and applicable special notes, especially site location and laterality, if appropriate, and then promptly transported to the laboratory for processing and analysis. Place tissue samples for standard biopsy examination in properly labeled specimen containers containing formalin solution, place tissue samples for molecular diagnostic studies in properly labeled specimen containers, and promptly transport the specimen to the laboratory for processing and analysis.

Universal Post Test Pearls (Evaluation)

- Note that completed test results are made available to the requesting HCP, who will discuss them with the patient.

- Answer questions and address concerns voiced by the patient or family, and reinforce information given by the patient's HCP regarding further testing, treatment, or referral to another HCP. Recognize that patients will have anxiety related to test results. Provide teaching and information regarding the clinical implications of the test results on the patient's lifestyle as appropriate.

- Note that test results should be evaluated in context with the patient's signs, symptoms, and diagnosis. Depending on the results of the procedure, additional testing may be performed to evaluate or monitor progression of the disease process and determine the need for a change in therapy.

- Be aware that when a person goes through a traumatic event such as an illness or being given information that will impact his or her lifestyle, there are universal human reactions that occur. These include knowledge deficit, fear, anxiety, and coping; in some situations, grieving may occur. HCPs should always be aware of the human response and how it may affect the plan of care and expected outcomes.

DISCUSSION POINT

Regarding Post-Test Critical Findings: Timely notification of a critical finding for lab or diagnostic studies is a role expectation of the professional nurse. Notification processes will vary among facilities. Upon receipt of the critical finding, the information should be read back to the caller to verify accuracy. Most policies require immediate notification of the primary HCP, hospitalist, or on-call HCP. Reported information includes the patient's name, unique identifiers, critical finding, name of the person giving the report, and name of the person receiving the report. Documentation of notification should be made in the medical record with the name of the HCP notified, time and date of notification, and any orders received. Any delay in a timely report of a critical finding may require completion of a notification form with review by Risk Management.

SPECIAL CONSIDERATIONS
PROCEDURES REQUIRING ANESTHESIA

- As part of the informed consent, patients undergoing endoscopy procedures requiring anesthesia should be informed of the risks associated with general anesthesia. These risks can include possible dental injuries from intubation as well as serious complications. Although these risks of serious complications are low, they can include heart attack, stroke, brain damage, and death. These risks depend in part on the patient's age, sex, weight, allergies, general health, and history of smoking, alcohol, or drug use.

- Patients on beta blockers before the surgical procedure should be instructed to take their medication as ordered during the perioperative period. Protocols may vary among facilities.

- Patients should be informed that it may be necessary to remove hair from the site before the procedure.

- Patients may exhibit anxiety due to concerns about sedation and pain. Patients may be given sedatives or analgesia for minimal to conscious sedation. Local anesthesia or general anesthesia for drug-induced loss of consciousness is considered for some laboratory and diagnostic procedures. General anesthesia is intended to bring about five states during a surgical procedure:

1. Analgesia, or pain relief
2. Loss of consciousness
3. Weakening of the autonomic responses
4. Achievement of a motionless state
5. Amnesia, or loss of memory of the procedure

- Patients should be aware that preoperative dietary restrictions are an important part of ensuring as safe a surgical experience as possible. They are intended to minimize the possibility of aspirating (inhaling) stomach contents into the lungs, a rare but potentially serious complication of anesthesia, and to reduce the likelihood of postoperative nausea. The American Society of Anesthesiologists has fasting guidelines for risk levels according to patient status. More information can be located at www.asahq.org. The preoperative fasting guidelines of the American Society of Anesthesiologists for scheduled surgery are as follows:

  - No solid food for 6 hours prior to an elective surgery
  - No milk or milk products for 6 hours prior to an elective surgery
  - No clear liquids for 2 hours before an elective surgery

The absence of a gag reflex and the inability to swallow easily are considered risks for aspiration. Following the use of anesthesia, ensure the patient is fully awake before swallowing clear liquids.

SPECIAL CONSIDERATIONS

Malignant hyperthermia is a rare, life-threatening condition that occurs following the administration of general anesthesia in susceptible individuals. It is an inherited disorder involving rapid escalation of cellular activities and accumulation of calcium in the skeletal muscle to a hypermetabolic state that occurs upon exposure to certain anesthetic gases such as halothane, isoflurane, sevoflurane, desflurane, and enflurane, either alone or in conjunction with the muscle relaxant succinylcholine. Early manifestations of the syndrome usually occur in the operating room and include acidosis, hypercapnia, tachycardia, muscle rigidity, tachypnea, and hyperkalemia; as the process continues, the patient demonstrates an extreme increase in fever *(related to increased* metabolic state), myoglobinuria *(related to release of large amounts of myoglobin from damages skeletal muscle)*, and multiorgan failure that often results in death. There is also some evidence that excessive exercise and exposure to climates with high ambient temperatures may also trigger malignant hyperthermia. Fatalities can be avoided by rapid recognition of the syndrome and immediate administration of dantrolene, which will usually reverse the progression of excessive metabolic rate. A confounding factor in the identification of individuals at risk for developing malignant hyperthermia is that the triggers are inconsistent in initiating the condition; that is, a susceptible individual may undergo anesthesia that includes the suspected trigger medications on a single or even multiple occasions without reaction and on a subsequent exposure will experience a life-threatening reaction. The incidence of gene abnormalities that result in malignant hyperthermia is unknown because universal reporting is not required in the United States and also because many people have not yet been exposed to the triggering chemicals. Methods used to identify susceptible individuals include molecular genetic testing and the caffeine halothane contracture test performed on tissue obtained by muscle biopsy.

STUDIES

- Arthroscopy
- Cholangiopancreatography, Endoscopic Retrograde
- Cystoscopy
- Laparoscopy, Gynecologic

LEARNING OUTCOMES

Providing safe, effective nursing care (SENC) includes mastery of core competencies and standards of care. SENC is based on a judicious application of nursing knowledge in combination with scientific principles. The Art of Nursing lies in blending what you know with the ability to effectively apply your knowledge in a compassionate manner.

After reading/studying this chapter, you will be able to

Thinking

1. Describe safety risks associated with endoscopic procedures.
2. Select and discuss potential nursing diagnoses commonly encountered when interacting with older adult patients undergoing endoscopic studies that utilize contrast medium.

Doing

1. Incorporate elements of care using an integrated multidisciplinary approach.

2. Apply safe nursing practices in follow-up patient care.
3. Ensure clear communication of patient preferences to ancillaries who are providing care.
4. Develop and implement an individualized plan of care based on patient preferences and specific health-care needs.

Caring

1. Recognize the merit of collaborating with patient, family, and significant others to design, implement, and evaluate the plan of care.

Arthroscopy

Quick Summary

COMMON USE: To obtain direct visualization of a specific joint to assist in diagnosis of joint injury or disease, and assessment of response to treatment.

AREA OF APPLICATION: Joints.

- Normal muscle, ligament, cartilage, synovial, and tendon structures of the joint, which is lined with a smooth, finely vascularized synovial membrane. The normal appearance of the cable-like ligaments and tendons visible in joints is smooth and silvery; the cartilage appears smooth and white.

Test Explanation

Arthroscopy provides direct visualization of a joint, usually a major joint such as the ankle, knee, hip, or shoulder, through the use of a fiberoptic endoscope. The arthroscope has a light, fiberoptics, and lenses; it connects to a monitor, and the images are recorded for future study and comparison. This procedure is used for inspection of joint structures, performance of a biopsy, and surgical repairs to the joint. Meniscus removal, spur removal, and ligamentous repair are some of the surgical procedures that may be performed.

Nursing Implications

Assessment

Indications	Potential Nursing Problems
Detect torn ligament or tendon	• Activity
Evaluate joint pain and damaged cartilage	• Body Image
Evaluate meniscal, patellar, condylar, extrasynovial, and synovial injuries or diseases of the knee	• Human Reaction
	• Infection
	• Mobility
Evaluate the extent of arthritis	• Pain
Evaluate the presence of gout	• Safety (fall risk)
Monitor effectiveness of therapy	• Self-care
Remove loose objects	• Skin

Diagnosis: Clinical Significance of Test Results

ABNORMAL FINDINGS

- Arthritis
- Chondromalacia
- Cysts
- Degenerative joint changes
- Fractures
- Ganglion or Baker cyst
- Gout or pseudogout
- Hemarthrosis
- Infection
- Joint tumors
- Loose bodies
- Meniscal disease
- Osteoarthritis
- Osteochondritis
- Rheumatoid arthritis
- Subluxation, fracture, or dislocation
- Synovial rupture
- Synovitis
- Torn cartilage
- Torn ligament
- Torn rotator cuff
- Trapped synovium

Planning

Considerations for planning a successful partnership should include clear communication of what to expect during the test to decrease anxiety and improve cooperation. Before the procedure is performed, plan to review the steps with the patient. Explain that the procedure is usually performed in an operating room by a health-care professional (HCP), and takes approximately 60 to 120 minutes, depending on the joint studied. The risk of surgical site infection (SSI) is approximately 1% to 3% for elective clean surgery. Arthroscopies harbor the absolute lowest SSI rates, but apart from patient endogenous factors, the role of external risk factors in the pathogenesis of SSI is well recognized. However, among the many measures to prevent SSI, only some are based on strong evidence, for example, the adequate perioperative administration of prophylactic antibiotics given 30 minutes prior to the incision. The joint area and the areas 5 to 6 inches above and below the joint are clipped and prepared for the procedure. Complications from hair removal develop in 2% to 5% of patients operated on each year. The Surgical Care Improvement Project (SCIP), a national quality partnership of organizations focused on improving surgical care by reducing surgical complications, has developed recommendations for hair removal methods that can help reduce the occurrence of surgical site infections. Razors can rapidly remove hair from the surgical field, but this method may result in small cuts and abrasions to the patient's skin. An alternative to using razors is powered surgical clippers. Clippers mechanically trim the hair close to the skin, effectively removing it from the field, and avoid the skin trauma caused by the sharp blade of a razor.

Food, fluid, or medication should be withheld, as ordered after midnight the day of the test because general anesthesia may be required. Explain to patients receiving local anesthesia that some discomfort may be experienced from the injections, and a thumping sensation may occur when the arthroscope is inserted. Many people are fearful of pain when faced with an unknown situation, so it is important to clearly communicate any potential discomfort the patient may experience.

SPECIAL CONSIDERATIONS

An important aspect of planning is understanding the factors that may alter study findings or cause abnormal results. Interdepartmental communication is a key factor in the planning process. The following should be noted when planning for this study:

- Impaired maneuvering of the scope may be experienced when the procedure is performed on a joint with flexion of less than 50°, as may be experienced in patients with ankylosis.
- Difficulty may also be encountered when the study is attempted in patients who have had a recent arthrogram due to residual inflammation from the contrast.
- In some cases, the procedure may get cancelled due to a significant contraindication. An example is a known skin infection near the arthroscope insertion site, which can be introduced into the joint by the contaminated arthroscope.

● Safety Tip

Make sure a written and informed consent has been signed prior to the procedure and before administering any medications.

Implementation

Patient education is key to obtaining the patient's cooperation in following directions, and providing an explanation for the purpose of the procedure is an important part of this process. Inform the patient that this study can assist in assessing for disorders of the joints. Inquire at this time if the patient has complied with dietary restrictions and remind the patient that the procedure may be cancelled for safety reasons if he or she is not in compliance.

Prior to the procedure, the extremity is scrubbed, elevated, and wrapped with an elastic bandage from the distal portion of the extremity to the proximal portion to drain as much blood from the limb as possible. A pneumatic tourniquet placed around the proximal portion of the limb is inflated, and the elastic bandage is removed. As an alternative to a tourniquet, a mixture of lidocaine with epinephrine and sterile normal saline may be instilled into the joint to help reduce bleeding. The joint is placed in a 45° angle, and a local anesthetic is administered. During the arthroscopy, a small incision is made and fluid can be aspirated from the joint space at this time. The diameter of the scope used depends on the joint being examined and the purpose of the procedure. The arthroscope is inserted within the joint following the injection of saline to distend the joint, and the scope is maneuvered to visualize the joint structures. In some instances, additional punctures are necessary for better visualization or surgical maneuvers, and, if required, cultures, biopsy, surgical repair, and the removal of loose bodies can then be completed. The joint is irrigated prior to the removal of the scope, and steroids are injected to help decrease inflammation in some cases. The wounds are closed with a single suture or Steri-Strips® and a sterile dressing is applied and the joint immobilized.

Evaluation

Recognize anxiety related to test results, and be supportive of impaired activity related to a perceived loss of independence. Monitor the patient's circulation and sensations in the joint area. HCPs should look for signs of infection, hemarthrosis, hematoma, swelling, thrombophlebitis, and synovial rupture, which are the most common potential complications. Assess vital signs, and instruct the patient to elevate the knee to minimize swelling. Educate the patient about signs of bleeding into the joint. Instruct the patient to immediately report symptoms such as fever, excessive bleeding, difficulty breathing, incision site redness, coldness, numbness, tingling, swelling, change in skin color (blue or dusky), and tenderness. Ice bags may be used to reduce postprocedure swelling. Instruct the patient to elevate the joint when sitting and to avoid overbending of the joint to reduce swelling and formation of blood clots. Analgesics for pain, anticoagulants to prevent new clots, and antibiotics for infection may be necessary. Inform the patient to shower after 48 hours but to avoid a tub bath until after his or her appointment with the HCP.

SPECIAL CONSIDERATIONS

Discuss the implications of abnormal test results on the patient's lifestyle. Provide teaching and information regarding the clinical implications of the test results as appropriate. Provide contact information, if desired, for the American College of Rheumatology (www .rheumatology.org) or for the Arthritis Foundation (www.arthritis.org). Patients may need to be taught how to walk with crutches because of impaired mobility and should be instructed not to drive until approved by the HCP. Refer the patient for physical therapy if instructed by the HCP.

✅ Critical Findings

N/A

✅ Study Specific Complications

Venipuncture	Endoscopic Procedures	Tracheal Anesthesia
Bruising, hematomas, infection, pain, prolonged bleeding, sepsis, swelling, vasovagal reactions	Black tarry stools, hematemesis, hypotension, perforation, persistent bleeding, tachycardia	Abnormal gag reflex, aspiration

Infections can occur as a result of any invasive procedure. Antibiotic therapy should be ordered if this occurs. Elevated temperatures, abnormal-colored sputum, changes in breathing patterns, chills, and hypotension can all indicate infection or sepsis.

Phlebitis is a possible complication in patients immobilized by joint pain, and patients should be educated to observe for this. Swelling, fever, pain, and redness are all indications that this may be occurring. Inform the patient that ice should be applied to the joint to minimize normal swelling, and that elevating the affected leg can also assist in swelling reduction.

✅ Related Tests

- Related tests include anti-cyclic citrullinated peptide, ANA, arthrogram, BMD, bone scan, CBC, CRP, ESR, MRI musculoskeletal, radiography of the bone, RF, synovial fluid analysis, and uric acid.
- Refer to the Musculoskeletal System table at the end of the book for related tests by body system.

Expected Outcomes

Expected outcomes associated with Arthroscopy are

- Ability to be mobile within disease limitations
- Adaptation to mobility and activity limitations
- Performance of self-care as best able
- Acceptance of diagnostic results related to physical limitations
- Verbalization of the importance of results to lifestyle choices

Cholangiopancreatography, Endoscopic Retrograde

Quick Summary

SYNONYM ACRONYM: ERCP.

COMMON USE: To visualize and assess the pancreas and common bile ducts for occlusion or stricture.

AREA OF APPLICATION: Gallbladder, bile ducts, pancreatic ducts.

- Normal appearance of the duodenal papilla
- Patency of the pancreatic and common bile ducts

Test Explanation

Endoscopic retrograde cholangiopancreatography (ERCP) allows direct visualization of the pancreatic and biliary ducts with a flexible endoscope and, after injection of contrast material, with x-rays. It allows the health-care provider (HCP) performing the procedure to view the pancreatic, hepatic, and common bile ducts and the ampulla of Vater. ERCP and percutaneous transhepatic cholangiography (PTC) are the only procedures that allow direct visualization of the biliary and pancreatic ducts. ERCP is less invasive and has less morbidity than PTC. It is useful in the evaluation of patients with jaundice, because the ducts can be visualized even when the patient's bilirubin level is high. (In contrast, oral cholecystography and IV cholangiography cannot visualize the biliary system when the patient has high bilirubin levels.) With endoscopy, the distal end of the common bile duct can be widened, and gallstones can be removed and stents placed in narrowed bile ducts to allow bile to be drained in jaundiced patients. During the endoscopic procedure, specimens of suspicious tissue can be taken for pathological review, and manometry pressure readings can be obtained from the bile and pancreatic ducts. ERCP is used in the diagnosis and follow-up of pancreatic disease; it can also be used therapeutically to remove small lesions called choleliths, perform sphincterotomy (biliary or pancreatic repair for stenosis), perform stent placement, repair stenosis using dilation balloons, or accomplish the extraction of stones using dilation balloons.

Nursing Implications

Assessment

Indications	Potential Nursing Problems
Assess jaundice of unknown cause to differentiate biliary tract obstruction from liver disease	• Bleeding
Collect specimens for cytology	• Fluid Volume
Identify obstruction caused by calculi, cysts, ducts, strictures, stenosis, and anatomic abnormalities	• Grief • Health Management • Human Reaction
Retrieve calculi from the distal common bile duct and release strictures	• Infection • Nutrition
Perform therapeutic procedures, such as sphincterotomy and placement of biliary drains	• Pain • Self-Perception

Diagnosis: Clinical Significance of Test Results
ABNORMAL FINDINGS
- Anatomical deviations of biliary or pancreatic ducts
- Biliary cirrhosis
- Cancer of the bile ducts
- Duodenal papilla tumors
- Gallstones
- Pancreatic cancer
- Pancreatic cysts or pseudocysts
- Pancreatic fibrosis
- Pancreatitis
- Sclerosing cholangitis
- Stenosis of biliary or pancreatic ducts

Planning

Considerations for planning a successful partnership should include clear communication of what to expect during the test to decrease anxiety and improve cooperation. Before the procedure is performed, plan to review the steps with the patient. Explain to your patient that the procedure is usually performed in a specialized department by a HCP and takes approximately 30 to 60 minutes. The patient should fast and withhold fluids for 6 hours prior to the procedure, and should either avoid taking anticoagulant medication or reduce the dosage as ordered prior to the procedure. If iodinated contrast medium is scheduled to be used in patients receiving metformin (Glucophage) for non-insulin-dependent (type 2) diabetes, the drug should be discontinued on the day of the test and continue to be withheld for 48 hours after the test. Iodinated contrast can temporarily impair kidney function, and failure to withhold metformin may indirectly result in drug-induced lactic acidosis, a dangerous and sometimes fatal side effect of metformin *related to renal impairment that does not support sufficient excretion of metformin.*

CONTRAINDICATIONS
- Patients who are pregnant or suspected of being pregnant, unless the potential benefits of a procedure using radiation far outweigh the risk of radiation exposure to the fetus and mother
- Conditions associated with adverse reactions to contrast medium (e.g., asthma, food allergies, or allergy to contrast medium). Although patients are still asked specifically if they have a known allergy to iodine or shellfish, it has been well established that the reaction is not to iodine; in fact, an actual iodine allergy would be very problematic because iodine is required for the production of thyroid hormones. In the case of shellfish, the reaction is to a muscle protein called tropomyosin; in the case of iodinated contrast medium, the reaction is to the noniodinated part of the contrast molecule. Patients with a known hypersensitivity to the medium may benefit from premedication with corticosteroids and diphenhydramine; the use of nonionic contrast or an alternative noncontrast imaging study, if available, may be considered for patients who have severe asthma or who have experienced moderate to severe reactions to ionic contrast medium.
- Conditions associated with preexisting renal insufficiency (e.g., kidney injury, kidney disease, single kidney transplant, nephrectomy, diabetes, multiple

myeloma, treatment with aminoglycocides and NSAIDs) because iodinated contrast is nephrotoxic

- Older adult and compromised patients who are chronically dehydrated before the test, because of their risk of contrast-induced acute kidney injury
- Patients with bleeding disorders because the puncture site may not stop bleeding
- Patients with an acute infection of the biliary system, pharyngeal or esophageal obstruction (e.g., Zenker diverticulum), or possible pseudocyst of the pancreas

SPECIAL CONSIDERATIONS

An important aspect of planning is understanding the factors that may alter study findings or cause abnormal results. Interdepartmental communication is a key factor in the planning process. The following should be noted when planning for this study:

- Gas or feces in the gastrointestinal (GI) tract resulting from inadequate cleansing or failure to restrict food intake before the study
- Retained barium from a previous radiological procedure
- Previous surgery involving the stomach or duodenum, which can make locating the duodenal papilla difficult
- Incorrect positioning of the patient, which may produce poor visualization of the area to be examined
- Inability of the patient to cooperate or remain still during the procedure because of age, significant pain, or mental status
- Occurrence of chest pain or severe cardiac dysrhythmias, in which case the procedure may be terminated
- Unstable cardiopulmonary status, blood coagulation defects, or cholangitis (the test may have to be rescheduled unless the patient received antibiotic therapy before the test)
- Failure to follow dietary restrictions and other pretesting preparations, which may cause the procedure to be canceled or repeated
- Blood specimens for bilirubin, amylase, or lipase, if ordered, should be collected before the procedure; results will be elevated after the procedure.

● *Safety Tip*

Consultation with a HCP should occur before the procedure for radiation safety concerns regarding younger patients or patients who are lactating. **Pediatric Considerations** Information on the Image Gently Campaign can be found at the Alliance for Radiation Safety in Pediatric Imaging (www.pedrad.org/associations/5364/ig/). Risks associated with radiation overexposure can result from frequent x-ray procedures. Personnel in the examination room with the patient should wear a protective lead apron, stand behind a shield, or leave the area while the examination is being done. Personnel working in the examination area should wear badges to record their level of radiation exposure.

● *Safety Tip*

Make sure a written and informed consent has been signed prior to the procedure and before administering any medications.

Implementation

Patient education is key to obtaining the patient's cooperation in following directions, and providing an explanation for the purpose of the procedure is an important part of this process. Inform the patient that this study can assist in assessing for disorders of the biliary and pancreatic ducts. Explain that an IV line may be inserted to allow the infusion of contrast, medications, or IV fluids. Bleeding or bruising can be prevented, once the needle has been removed, by applying direct pressure to the injection site with dry gauze for a minute or two while observing/assessing for bleeding or hematoma formation. The injection site can then be covered with a gauze and adhesive bandage.

Administer ordered prophylactic steroids or antihistamines before the procedure. Ensure that the HCP performing the procedure is aware of the allergy concerns as it may be necessary to use a nonionic contrast medium for the procedure. Explain to the patient that he or she will receive ordered sedation and will have an x-ray of the abdomen taken to determine if any residual contrast medium is present from previous studies. Ensure the patient understands that once the procedure begins, the oropharynx (back of the throat) is sprayed or swabbed with a topical local anesthetic. The patient will then be placed on an examination table in the left lateral position with his or her left arm behind the back and his or her right hand at the side, slightly flexing the neck. Let the patient know that a protective guard will be placed into his or her mouth to cover the teeth. A bite block can also be placed in the mouth to maintain an adequate opening. Explain that the endoscope is first passed through the mouth with a dental suction device in place to drain secretions. Then a side-viewing flexible fiberoptic endoscope is passed into the duodenum, and a small cannula is inserted into the duodenal papilla (ampulla of Vater). Tell the patient that he or she will be rolled into a prone position and the duodenal papilla is visualized and cannulated with a catheter. Occasionally, the patient can be turned slightly to the right side to aid in visualization of the papilla. Atrophine sulfate and glucagon or anticholinergics can be administered to minimize duodenal spasm and to facilitate visualization of the ampulla of Vater. ERCP manometry can be done at this time to measure the pressure in the bile duct, the pancreatic duct, and the sphincter of Oddi at the papilla area via the catheter as it is placed in the area before the contrast medium is injected. Ensure the patient understands that contrast medium is injected through the catheter into the pancreatic and biliary ducts. Fluoroscopic images are taken and biopsy specimens for cytological analysis may be obtained and placed in appropriate containers, labeled properly, and promptly transported to the laboratory. Explain that once the examination is concluded, the dental suction device is removed and the endoscope is withdrawn (see Fig. 9.3).

Evaluation

Recognize anxiety related to test results. Discuss the implications of abnormal test results on the patient's lifestyle. Provide teaching and information regarding the clinical implications of the test results, as appropriate. Monitor the patient's vital signs and neurological status every 15 minutes for 1 hour, then every 2 hours for 4 hours, then every 4 hours for 24 hours, and monitor intake and output every 8 hours. Compare all results with the baseline values and document. Do not allow the patient to eat or drink until the gag reflex returns, after which the patient is permitted to eat lightly for 12 to 24 hours. Instruct the patient to resume his or her usual diet, fluids, medications, and activity after 24 hours, or as directed by the HCP. If contrast was used, renal function should be assessed before metformin is resumed, and the patient should be monitored for reactions, including rash, urticaria, tachycardia, hyperpnea, hypertension, palpitations, nausea, and vomiting.

Inform the patient to expect some throat soreness and possible hoarseness. Encourage him to use warm gargles, lozenges, ice packs to the neck, or cool fluids to alleviate throat discomfort. Explain that any belching, bloating, or flatulence is the result of air insufflation and is normal. Instruct the patient to immediately report symptoms to the appropriate HCP, such as a fast heart rate, difficulty breathing, skin rash, itching, chest pain, persistent right shoulder pain, or abdominal pain.

✔ Critical Findings

N/A

✔ Study Specific Complications

Venipuncture	Endoscopic Procedures	Tracheal Anesthesia
Bruising, hematomas, infection, pain, prolonged bleeding, sepsis, swelling, vasovagal reactions	Black tarry stools, hematemesis, hypotension, perforation, persistent bleeding, tachycardia	Abnormal gag reflex, aspiration

Infections can occur as a result of any invasive procedure. Antibiotic therapy should be ordered if this occurs. Elevated temperatures, abnormal colored sputum, changes in breathing patterns, chills, and hypotension can all indicate infection or sepsis.

Perforation of the pharynx or esophagus indicated by neck or chest pain, hemoptysis, or changes in vital signs for potential hypovolemia.

Pancreatitis and respiratory depression are other possible complications related to ERCP.

✔ Related Tests

- Related tests include amylase, CT abdomen, hepatobiliary scan, KUB studies, lipase, MRI abdomen, peritoneal fluid analysis, pleural fluid analysis, and US liver and biliary system.
- Refer to the Gastrointestinal and Hepatobiliary systems tables at the end of the book for related tests by body system.

Expected Outcomes

Expected outcomes associated with Cholangiopancreatography, Endoscopic Retrograde, (ERCP) are

- Skin that is intact with an absence of jaundice
- No risk of bleeding or infection related to an invasive procedure
- Remaining nonvolemic
- Participation in care decisions, which increases one's sense of control
- Open expression of feelings, which promotes an acceptance of the diagnosis
- Recognition of the importance of reporting any fever

Cystoscopy

Quick Summary

SYNONYM ACRONYM: Cystoureterography, prostatography.

COMMON USE: To assess the urinary tract for bleeding, cancer, tumor, and prostate health.

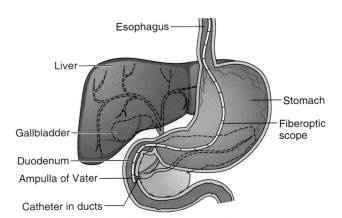

FIGURE 9.3 Endoscopic retrograde cholangiopancreatography (ERCP). *ERCP, used with permission, from Williams, L., & Hopper, P. (2010). Understanding medical surgical nursing (4th ed.). FA Davis Company.*

AREA OF APPLICATION: Bladder, urethra, ureteral orifices.
- Normal ureter, bladder, and urethral structure

Test Explanation

Cystoscopy provides direct visualization of the urethra, urinary bladder, and ureteral orifices—areas not usually visible with x-ray procedures. This procedure is also used to obtain specimens and treat pathology associated with the aforementioned structures. Cystoscopy is accomplished by transurethral insertion of a cystoscope into the bladder. Rigid cystoscopes contain an obturator and a telescope with a lens and light system; there are also flexible cystoscopes, which use fiberoptic technology. The procedure may be performed during or after ultrasonography or radiography, or during urethroscopy or retrograde pyelography.

Nursing Implications
Assessment

Indications	Potential Nursing Problems
Coagulate bleeding areas	• Conflicted Decision Making
Determine the possible source of persistent urinary tract infections	• Grieving
Determine the source of hematuria of unknown cause	• Human Reactions
Differentiate, through tissue biopsy, between benign and cancerous lesions involving the bladder	• Incontinence
Dilate the urethra and ureters	• Infection
Evacuate blood clots and perform fulguration of bleeding sites within the lower urinary tract	• Pain
Evaluate changes in urinary elimination patterns	• Self-Perception
Evaluate the extent of prostatic hyperplasia and degree of obstruction	• Sexuality
Evaluate the function of each kidney by obtaining urine samples via ureteral catheters	• Urgency
Evaluate urinary tract abnormalities such as dysuria, frequency, retention, inadequate stream, urgency, and incontinence	• Urination
Identify and remove polyps and small tumors (including by fulguration) from the bladder	
Identify and remove foreign body	
Identify congenital anomalies, such as duplicate ureters, ureteroceles, urethral or ureteral strictures, and areas of inflammation or ulceration	
Implant radioactive seeds	
Place ureteral catheters to drain urine from the renal pelvis or for retrograde pyelography	
Place ureteral stents and resect prostate gland tissue (transurethral resection of the prostate)	
Remove renal calculi from the bladder or ureters	
Resect small tumors	

Diagnosis: Clinical Significance of Test Results
ABNORMAL FINDINGS
- Bladder cancer
- Diverticulum of the bladder, fistula, stones, and strictures
- Foreign body
- Inflammation or infection
- Obstruction
- Polyps
- Prostatic hypertrophy or hyperplasia
- Prostatitis
- Tumors
- Ureteral calculi
- Ureteral reflux
- Ureteral or urethral stricture
- Ureterocele
- Urinary fistula
- Urinary tract malformation and congenital anomalies

Planning

Considerations for planning a successful partnership should include clear communication of what to expect during the test to decrease anxiety and improve cooperation. Before the procedure is performed, plan to review the steps with the patient. Explain that the procedure is usually performed in a special cystoscopy suite near or in the surgery unit by a health-care provider (HCP), and takes approximately 10 to 30 minutes. The procedure can also be performed on adults in a urologist's office; pediatric cystoscopy is performed in the surgery unit. Inform the patient that a cystoscope will be inserted through the urethra, and address concerns about pain. Restrict food and fluids for 6 hours if the patient is having general or spinal anesthesia, and allow only clear liquids 2 hours before the procedure for local anesthesia.

CONTRAINDICATIONS
- Patients who are pregnant or suspected of being pregnant, unless the potential benefits of a procedure using radiation far outweigh the risks to the fetus and mother
- Patients with bleeding disorders because instrumentation may lead to excessive bleeding from the lower urinary tract
- Patients with acute cystitis or urethritis because instrumentation could allow bacteria to enter the bloodstream, resulting in septicemia

● **Safety Tip**

Make sure a written and informed consent has been signed prior to the procedure and before administering any medications.

Implementation

Patient education is key to obtaining the patient's cooperation in following directions, and providing an explanation for the purpose of the procedure is an important

part of this process. Inform the patient that this study can assist in assessing for disorders of the urethra, bladder, ureters, and prostate gland. Ensure the patient has complied with pretesting instructions. Explain that required general or spinal anesthesia should be administered before the position is positioned on the procedure table. Once on the table, his or her legs will be placed in stirrups. Assure the patient that he or she will be draped, keeping in mind privacy concerns. Explain that as the procedure begins, the external genitalia will be cleansed with an antiseptic solution. If a local anesthetic is used, it is instilled into the urethra and retained for 5 to 10 minutes. A penile clamp may be used in male patients to aid in retention of the anesthetic. Explain that the HCP will then insert a cystoscope or a urethroscope to examine the urethra before performing the cystoscopy. The urethroscope has a sheath that may be left in place, and the cystoscope is inserted through it, avoiding multiple instrumentations.

After insertion of the cystoscope, a sample of residual urine may be obtained for culture or other analysis. The bladder is irrigated via an irrigation system attached to the scope because the irrigation fluid aids in bladder visualization. If a prostatic tumor is found, a biopsy specimen may be obtained by means of a cytology brush or biopsy forceps inserted through the scope. If the tumor is small and localized, it can be excised and fulgurated. This procedure is termed *transurethral resection of the bladder* (TURB) (see Fig. 9.4). Upon completion of the examination and related procedures, the cystoscope is withdrawn. Specimens obtained should be placed in proper containers, labeled properly, and immediately transported to the laboratory.

Evaluation

Recognize anxiety related to test results. Discuss the implications of abnormal test results on the patient's lifestyle. Provide teaching and information regarding the clinical implications of the test results, as appropriate. Monitor the patient's vital signs and neurological status every 15 minutes for 1 hour, then every 2 hours for 4 hours, and monitor intake and output at least every 8 hours. Compare all results with the baseline values and document. Observe the patient until the effects of the sedation, if ordered, have worn off. Assess for normal voiding patterns and the appearance of the urine. If the patient experiences bladder spasms, administer an anticholinergic.

If a biopsy was performed, inform the patient that a discharge may persist for a few days to a few weeks and to expect slight bleeding for 2 days after removal of biopsy specimens. Emphasize that persistent abdominal pain, persistent bloody urine, difficulty or change in the urinary pattern, or fever must be reported to the HCP immediately.

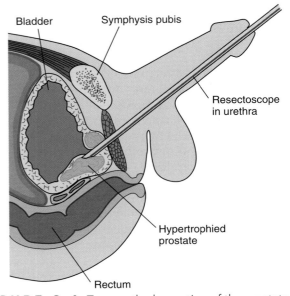

FIGURE 9.4 Transurethral resection of the prostate. *Used with permission, from Williams, L., & Hopper, P. (2010). Understanding medical surgical nursing (4th ed.). FA Davis Company.*

⊘ Critical Findings

N/A

⊘ Study Specific Complications

Venipuncture	Endoscopic Procedures	Tracheal Anesthesia
Bruising, hematomas, infection, pain, prolonged bleeding, sepsis, swelling, vasovagal reactions	Black tarry stools, hematemesis, hypotension, perforation, persistent bleeding, tachycardia	Abnormal gag reflex, aspiration

Infections can occur as a result of any invasive procedure. Antibiotic therapy should be ordered if this occurs. Elevated temperatures, abnormal-colored sputum, changes in breathing patterns, chills, and hypotension can all indicate infection or sepsis.

Other complications may include

- Urinary tract infection (UTI) as evidenced by burning on urination, voiding frequency, positive culture results, or chills and fever
- Bladder perforation noted by suprapubic pain or excessive hematuria
- Urinary retention which may require catheterization and increased fluid intake

- Hemorrhage indicated by excessive and persistent hematuria with changes in vital signs indicating hypovolemia if a biopsy was performed

Related Tests

- Related tests include biopsy kidney, biopsy prostate, calculus kidney stone panel, *Chlamydia* group antibody, CT pelvis, culture urine, cytology urine, IVP, MRI pelvis, PSA, US pelvis, and UA.
- Refer to the Genitourinary System table at the end of the book for related tests by body system.

Expected Outcomes

Expected outcomes associated with Cystoscopy are

- Absence of bleeding or infection related to an invasive procedure
- Absence of procedure-related complications
- Understanding of the altered pathophysiology related to urinary elimination difficulties
- Demonstration of unobstructed urinary flow
- Expression of concerns about potential sexual dysfunction

Laparoscopy, Gynecologic

Quick Summary

SYNONYM ACRONYM: Gynecologic pelviscopy, gynecologic laparoscopy, pelvic endoscopy, peritoneoscopy.

COMMON USE: To visualize and assess the ovaries, fallopian tubes, and uterus toward diagnosing inflammation, malformations, cysts, and fibroids and to evaluate causes of infertility.

AREA OF APPLICATION: Pelvis.

- Normal appearance of uterus, ovaries, fallopian tubes, and other pelvic contents

Test Explanation

Gynecologic laparoscopy provides direct visualization of the internal pelvic contents, including the ovaries, fallopian tubes, and uterus, after insufflation of carbon dioxide (CO_2). It is done to diagnose and treat pelvic organ disorders as well as to perform surgical procedures on the organs. In this procedure, a rigid laparoscope is introduced into the body cavity through a 1- to 2-cm periumbilical incision. The endoscope has a microscope to allow visualization of the organs, and it can be used to insert instruments for performing procedures such as biopsy (e.g., biopsy of suspected endometrial lesions) and tumor resection. Under general or local anesthesia, the peritoneal cavity is inflated with 2 to 3 L of CO_2. The gas distends the abdominal wall so that the instruments can be inserted safely. Advantages of this procedure compared to an open laparotomy include reduced pain, reduced length of stay at the hospital or surgical center, and reduced time off from work.

Nursing Implications
Assessment

Indications	Potential Nursing Problems
Detect ectopic pregnancy and determine the need for surgery	• Bleeding
Detect pelvic inflammatory disease or abscess	• Communication
Detect uterine fibroids, ovarian cysts, and uterine malformations (ovarian cysts may be aspirated during the procedure)	• Family • Grief • Human Reactions
Evaluate amenorrhea and infertility	• Infection
Evaluate fallopian tubes and anatomic defects to determine the cause of infertility	• Pain • Self-Esteem
Evaluate known or suspected endometriosis, salpingitis, and hydrosalpinx	• Self-Perception
Evaluate pelvic pain or masses of unknown cause	• Sexuality
Evaluate reproductive organs after therapy for infertility	• Tissue Integrity
Obtain biopsy specimens to confirm suspected pelvic malignancies or metastasis	
Perform tubal sterilization and ovarian biopsy	
Perform vaginal hysterectomy	
Remove adhesions or foreign bodies such as intrauterine devices	
Treat endometriosis through electrocautery or laser vaporization	

Diagnosis: Clinical Significance of Test Results
ABNORMAL FINDINGS

- Abscesses
- Adhesions or scar tissue
- Ascites
- Cancer staging
- Ectopic pregnancy
- Endometriosis
- Enlarged fallopian tubes
- Infection
- Ovarian cyst
- Ovarian tumor
- Pelvic adhesions
- Pelvic inflammatory disease
- Pelvic tumor
- Salpingitis
- Uterine fibroids

Planning

Considerations for planning a successful partnership should include clear communication of what to expect during the test to decrease anxiety and improve cooperation. Before the procedure is performed, plan to review the steps with the patient. Address concerns

about pain, and explain that no discomfort will be experienced during the test. Explain that the procedure is usually performed in a specialized department by a health-care provider (HCP), and it takes approximately 30 to 60 minutes. Inform the patient that a laxative and cleansing enema may be needed the day before the procedure, with cleansing enemas on the morning of the procedure, depending on the institution's policy, and instruct the patient to fast and restrict fluids for 6 hours prior to the procedure.

CONTRAINDICATIONS

- Are pregnant or suspected of being pregnant, unless the potential benefits of the procedure far outweigh the risk to the fetus and mother
- Have bleeding disorders, especially those associated with uremia and cytotoxic chemotherapy
- Have cardiac conditions dysrhythmias, advanced respiratory or cardiovascular disease
- Have intestinal obstruction, abdominal mass, abdominal hernia, or suspected intra-abdominal hemorrhage
- Have a history of peritonitis or multiple abdominal operations that cause dense adhesions

An important aspect of planning is understanding the factors that may alter study findings or cause abnormal results. Interdepartmental communication is a key factor in the planning process. The following should be noted when planning for this study:

- Gas or feces in the gastrointestinal (GI) tract resulting from inadequate cleansing or failure to restrict food intake before the study
- Retained barium from a previous radiological procedure
- Metallic objects (e.g., jewelry, body rings) within the examination field, which may inhibit organ visualization and cause unclear images
- Inability of the patient to cooperate or remain still during the procedure because of age, significant pain, or mental status
- Occurrence of chest pain or severe cardiac dysrhythmias, which will cause termination of the procedure
- A hypoxemic or hypercapnic state, which will require continuous oxygen administration to the patient
- Failure to follow dietary restrictions and other pretesting preparations, which may cause the procedure to be canceled or repeated

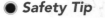

● *Safety Tip*

Make sure a written and informed consent has been signed prior to the procedure and before administering any medications.

Implementation

Patient education is key to obtaining the patient's cooperation in following directions, and providing an explanation for the purpose of the procedure is an important part of this process. Inform the patient that this study can assist in assessing for disorders of the ovaries, uterus, and fallopian tubes. Explain that an IV line may be inserted to allow infusion of contrast or IV fluids.

Ensure medications to reduce discomfort and to promote relaxation and sedation are administered, as ordered, and the patient is in compliance with pretesting instructions. Explain to the patient that she will be placed on the laparoscopy table and if general anesthesia is to be used, it is administered at this time. Tell the patient that after being placed in a modified lithotomy position with the head tilted downward, the abdomen will be cleansed with an antiseptic solution, and draped. A catheter may be placed if ordered. Explain that once the procedure is ready to begin the HCP will identify the site for the scope insertion and administer a local anesthesia, if that is to be used (see Fig. 9.5). After deeper layers are anesthetized, a pneumoperitoneum needle is placed between the visceral and parietal peritoneum. CO_2 is insufflated through the pneumoperitoneum needle to separate the abdominal wall from the viscera and to aid in visualization of the pelvic structures. The pneumoperitoneum needle is removed, and the trocar and laparoscope are inserted through the incision. Explain that the HCP inserts a uterine manipulator through the vagina and cervix and into the uterus so that the uterus, fallopian tubes, and ovaries can be moved to permit better visualization. After the examination, collection of tissue samples, and performance of therapeutic procedures (e.g., tubal ligation), the scope is withdrawn. All possible CO_2 is evacuated via the trocar, which is then removed. Tell the patient that the skin incision is closed with sutures, clips, or sterile strips, and a small dressing or adhesive strip is applied. After the perineum is cleansed, the uterine manipulator is removed and a sterile pad is applied.

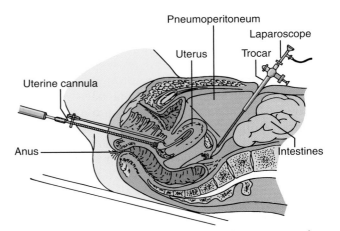

FIGURE 9.5 Laparoscopy. *Used with permission, from Williams, L., & Hopper, P. (2010). Understanding medical surgical nursing (4th ed.). FA Davis Company.*

Evaluation

Recognize anxiety related to test results, and discuss the implications of abnormal test results on the patient's lifestyle. Provide teaching and information regarding the clinical implications of the test results as appropriate. Monitor vital signs and neurological status every 15 minutes for 1 hour, then every 2 hours for 4 hours, and then every 4 hours for 24 hours. Monitor intake and output at least every 8 hours. Compare all results with baseline values. Notify the HCP if temperature is elevated, and instruct the patient to restrict activity for 2 to 7 days after the procedure. Instruct the patient in the care and assessment of the incision site and, if indicated, inform the patient of a follow-up appointment for the removal of sutures. Inform the patient that shoulder discomfort may be experienced for 1 or 2 days after the procedure as a result of abdominal distention caused by insufflation of CO_2 into the abdomen and that mild analgesics and cold compresses, as ordered, can be used to relieve the discomfort. Emphasize that any persistent shoulder pain, abdominal pain, vaginal bleeding, fever, redness, or swelling of the incisional area must be reported to the HCP immediately.

✓ *Critical Findings*

- Ectopic pregnancy
- Foreign body
- Tumor with significant mass effect

Note and immediately report to the requesting HCP any critical findings and related symptoms. A listing of these findings varies among facilities.

✓ *Study Specific Complications*

Venipuncture	Endoscopic Procedures	Tracheal Anesthesia
Bruising, hematomas, infection, pain, prolonged bleeding, sepsis, swelling, vasovagal reactions	Black tarry stools, hematemesis, hypotension, perforation, persistent bleeding, tachycardia	Abnormal gag reflex, aspiration

Patients with acute infection or advanced malignancy involving the abdominal wall are at increased risk for infection because organisms may be introduced into the normally sterile peritoneal cavity. Infections can occur as a result of any invasive procedure. Antibiotic therapy should be ordered if this occurs. Elevated temperatures, abnormal-colored sputum, changes in breathing patterns, chills, and hypotension can all indicate infection or sepsis.

Hemorrhage from the trocar site and umbilical hernia from an inadequate hole in the fascia are other complications that may occur with laparoscopy.

✓ *Related Tests*

- Related tests include cancer antigens, Chlamydia group antibody, CT abdomen, CT pelvis, HCG, MRI pelvis, Pap smear, progesterone, US pelvis, and uterine fibroid embolization.
- Refer to the Reproductive System table at the end of the book for related tests by body system.

Expected Outcomes

Expected outcomes associated with Laparoscopy, Gynecologic, are

- No complications associated with invasive procedure, infection, bleeding, and pain
- No hemorrhage from the trocar site, no perforation of the bowel, and no umbilical hernia from an inadequate hole in the fascia
- Improvement in the potential for carrying a viable fetus
- Acceptance of diagnosed infertility
- Verbalization of acceptance about the loss of potential future children
- Reporting of an ability to move and walk without pain
- Coping with anxiety in dealing with the unknown

REVIEW OF LEARNING OUTCOMES

Thinking

1. Describe safety risks associates with endoscopic procedures. Answer: Complications can occur when doing endoscopic procedures. Risks are most commonly those associated with venipuncture, the perforation of cavities, persistent bleeding, or infections.
2. Select and discuss potential nursing diagnoses commonly encountered when interacting with older adult patients undergoing endoscopic studies utilizing contrast medium. Answer: Injury risk (delayed allergic reactions), anxiety, skin (urticaria), fear, nausea, vomiting, and cardiac output (tachycardia).

Doing

1. Incorporate elements of care using an integrated multidisciplinary approach. Answer: Patients should be screened for the interference of medications or substances that alter exam results. Pregnancy should be determined along with prior diagnostic examinations that may contraindicate a study.
2. Apply safe nursing practices in follow-up patient care. Answer: Initiate education, emotional support, and counseling for positive results. Observe the patient for possible reactions and assure that patients understand the follow-up care needed.

3. Ensure clear communication of patient preferences to ancillaries who are providing care. Answer: Communication is the key to the coordination of care. It is the nurse's responsibility to make sure that everyone is on board with the plan of care to assure its success.

4. Develop and implement an individualized plan of care based on patient preferences and specific health-care needs. Answer: Everybody is different. Acknowledging and accepting your patients' culture and values is essential to understanding the frame of reference he or she uses to make health-care decisions. This will allow you to move forward as a team in the development of a usable plan of care, which will help to address the patient's problems in a way that is meaningful and will allow for clear communication of priorities and acceptable interventions.

Caring

1. Recognize the merit of collaborating with patient, family, and significant others to design, implement, and evaluate the plan of care. Answer: Collaboration and buy-in with the proposed plan of care and associated intervention is the only way to have a successful plan of care. The patient's evaluation of the effectiveness of the plan is a key part of ongoing progress toward the expected outcome.

Words of Wisdom: Endoscopic studies are considered to be scary to patients. Their fear is on several levels. First, they worry about the sedation they will receive; second, they worry about the invasiveness of the exam and if it will hurt; and, third, they worry about the results and what it will mean in the context of their lives. Giving them as much information as you can up front will go a long way to allaying their fears. So what should you tell them? Just ask yourself, if you were the one lying in the bed, what would you want to know? Then you will know what to say.

BIBLIOGRAPHY

American Cancer Society. (2014). Recommendations for colorectal cancer. Retrieved from http://www.cancer.org/cancer/colonandrectumcancer/moreinformation/colonandrectumcancerearlydetection/index

Cavanaugh, B. (2003). Nurse's manual of laboratory and diagnostic tests (4th ed.). Philadelphia, PA: F.A. Davis Company.

Cohen, L. (2007). AGA Institute review of endoscopic sedation. Retrieved from www.gastrojournal.org/article/PIIS0016508507011158/fulltext

Cystometry. (2014). Retrieved from http://www.webmd.com/urinary-incontinence-oab/cystometry-test

Graham, D., Hay, J., Clague, J., Nisar, M., & Earis, J. (1992). Comparison of three different methods used to achieve local anesthesia for fiberoptic bronchoscopy. Retrieved from http://www.researchgate.net/publication/21640112_Comparison_of_three_different_methods_used_to_achieve_local_anesthesia_for_fiberoptic_bronchoscopy

Fishbach, F., & Dunning, M. (2009). A Manual of laboratory and diagnostic tests (8th ed.). Philadelphia, PA: Lippincott Williams & Wilkins.

Heron, M. (2012). Deaths: Leading causes for 2008. Retrieved from www.cdc.gov/nchs/data/nvsr/nvsr60/nvsr60_06.pdf

Kim, J. (n.d.) Mammary ductoscopy: Current and future applications (Breast cancer and benign disease). Retrieved from cancernews.com/data/Article/236.asp

Lieberman, D. (2010). Progress and challenges in colorectal cancer screening and surveillance. Retrieved from www.gastrojournal.org/article/S0016-5085(10)00178-2/abstract

National Kidney and Urologic Diseases Information Clearinghouse. (2014). Urodynamic testing. Retrieved from http://kidney.niddk.nih.gov/kudiseases/pubs/urodynamic/

Practice guidelines for preoperative fasting and the use of pharmacologic agents to reduce the risk of pulmonary aspiration: Application to healthy patients undergoing elective procedures: An updated report by the American Society of Anesthesiologists Committee on Standards and Practice Parameters. (2011). Retrieved from http://www.asahq.org/~/media/Sites/ASAHQ/Files/Public/Resources/standards-guidelines/practice-guidelines-for-preoperative-fasting.pdf.

Rodgers, S. (2008). Medical-surgical nursing care plans (1st Ed.). Clifton Park, NY: Delmar Learning.

Saslow, D., Solomon, D., Lawson, H., Killackey, M., Kulasingam, S., Cain, J., Garcia, F., Moriarty, A., Waxman, A., Wilbur, D., Wentzensen, N., Downs, L., Spitzer, M., Moscicki, A., Franco, E., Stoler, M., Schiffman, M., Castle, P., Myers, E., & ACS-ASCCP-ASCP Cervical Cancer Guideline Committee. (2012). American Cancer Society, American Society for Colposcopy and Cervical Pathology, and American Society for Clinical Pathology screening guidelines for the prevention and early detection of cervical cancer. Retrieved from http://onlinelibrary.wiley.com/doi/10.3322/caac.21139/full

The U.S. Preventive Services Task Force on Screening for Colorectal Cancer. (2014). Retrieved from www.uspreventiveservicestaskforce.org/uspstf/uspscolo.htm

University of Maryland Medical Center. Endoscopy Overview. (2011). Retrieved from www.umm.edu/ency/article/003338.htm

Uroflowmetry. (2014). Retrieved from http://www.nlm.nih.gov/medlineplus/ency/article/003325.htm

Van Leeuwen, A., and Bladh, M. (2015). Davis's comprehensive handbook of laboratory and diagnostic testing with nursing implications (6th ed.). Philadelphia, PA: F.A. Davis Company.

Venes, D. (Ed.). (2009). Taber's cyclopedic medical dictionary (21st ed.). Philadelphia, PA: F.A. Davis Company.

Go to Section II of this book and www.davisplus.com for the Clinical Reasoning Tool and its case studies to provide you with a safe place to explore patient care situations. There are a total of 26 different case studies; 2 cases are presented for each of 13 body systems. One set of 13 cases are found in the Section II chapters, and a second set of 13 cases are available online at www.davisplus.com. Each case is designed with the specific goal of helping you to connect the dots of clinical reasoning. Cases are designed to reflect possible clinical scenarios; the outcomes may or may not be positive—you decide.

Fecal Analysis Studies

OVERVIEW

Fecal analysis includes a variety of tests performed on stool (feces) to assist with the diagnosis of conditions that affect the digestive tract, liver, and pancreas. The test results can provide evidence of irritation of the intestinal lining from a variety of sources, conditions that affect digestion or the absorption of nutrients from the digestive tract, infection from parasites or microorganisms, or evidence that can assist in the diagnosis of cancer. Laboratory analysis of stool includes both macroscopic and microscopic examination. The specimen will be observed for color, consistency, weight, shape, odor, the presence of blood streaks, and the presence of mucus. The stool may be chemically tested for pH, occult blood, fat, meat fibers, bile, white blood cells, reducing substances (carbohydrates), or enzymes. A stool culture is performed to identify bacterial infection in the digestive tract.

The information in the Part I studies is organized in a manner to help the student see how the five basic components of the nursing process (assessment, diagnosis, planning, implementation, and evaluation) can be applied to each phase of laboratory and diagnostic testing. The goal is to use nursing process to understand the integration of care (laboratory, diagnostic, nursing care) toward achieving a positive expected outcome.

- **Assessment** is the collection of information for the purpose of answering the question, "is there a problem?" Knowledge of the patient's health history, medications, complaints, and allergies as well as synonyms or alternate test names, common use for the procedure, specimen requirements, and normal ranges or interpretive comments provide the foundation for diagnosis.
- **Diagnosis** is the process of looking at the information gathered during assessment and answering the

questions, "what is the problem?" and "what do I need to do about it?" Test indications tell us why the study has been requested, and potential diagnoses tell us the value or importance of the study relative to its clinical utility.

- **Planning** is a blueprint of the nursing care before the procedure. It is the process of determining how the nurse is going to partner with the patient to fix the problem (e.g., "The patient has a study ordered and this is what I should know before I successfully carry out the plan to have the study completed"). Knowledge of interfering factors, social and cultural issues, preprocedural restrictions, the need for written and informed consent, anxiety about the procedure, and concerns regarding pain are some considerations for planning a successful partnership.
- **Implementation** is putting the plan into action with an idea of what the expected outcome should be. Collaboration with the departments where the laboratory test or diagnostic study is to be performed is essential to the success of the plan. Implementation is where the work is done within each healthcare team member's scope of practice.
- **Evaluation** answers the question, "did the plan work or not?" Was the plan completely successful, partially successful, or not successful? If the plan did not work, evaluation is the process where you determine what needs to be changed to make the plan work better. This includes a review of all expected outcomes. Nursing care after the procedure is where information is gathered to evaluate the plan. Review of results, including critical findings, in relation to patient symptoms and other tests performed provides data that form a more complete picture of health or illness.
- **Expected Outcomes** are positive outcomes related to the test. They are the outcomes the nurse should expect if all goes well.

A number of pretest, intratest, and post-test universal points are presented in this overview section because the information applies to fecal analysis studies in general.

Universal Pretest Pearls (Planning)

- Obtain a history of the patient's complaints, including a list of known allergens, especially allergies or sensitivities to medications or latex so their use can be avoided or their effects mitigated if an allergy is present. Carefully evaluate all medications currently being taken by the patient. A list of the patient's current medications, prescribed and over the counter (including anticoagulants, aspirin and other salicylates, and dietary supplements), should also be obtained. Ensure that all allergies are clearly noted in the medical record, and ensure that the patient is wearing an allergy and medical record armband. Report information that could interfere with, or delay proceeding with, the study to the health-care provider (HCP) and laboratory.
- Obtain a history of the patient's affected body system, symptoms, and results of previously performed laboratory tests and diagnostic and surgical procedures. Previous test results will provide a basis of comparison between old and new data.
- An important aspect of planning is understanding the factors that may alter study findings or cause abnormal results. Interdepartmental communication is a key factor in the planning process. The inability of a patient to cooperate or remain still during the procedure because of age, significant pain, or mental status should be among the anticipated factors. Recent or past procedures, medications, or existing medical conditions that could complicate or interfere with test results should be noted.
- Review the steps of the study with the patient or caregiver. Expect patients to be nervous about the procedure itself and the pending results. Educating the patient on his or her role during the procedure and what to expect can facilitate this. The patient's role during the procedure is to cooperate and follow instructions. The actual time required to complete each study will depend on a number of conditions including the type of equipment being used and how well a patient will cooperate.
- Address any concerns about pain and explain or describe, as appropriate, the level and type of discomfort that may be expected. Advise the patient that normally no discomfort should be experienced.
- Provide additional instructions and patient preparation regarding medication, diet, fluid intake, or activity if appropriate. Unless specified in the individual study, there are no special instructions or restrictions.
- Always be sensitive to any cultural or psychosocial issues, including a concern for modesty before, during, and after the procedure.

Universal Intratest Pearls (Implementation)

- Correct patient identification is crucial prior to any procedure. Positively identify the patient using two unique identifiers such as patient name, date of birth, Social Security number, or medical record number.
- Ensure the patient has complied with pretesting instructions, including dietary, fluid, medication, and activity restrictions as given for the procedure.
- Standard Precautions must be followed.
- Before leaving the patient's side, appropriate specimen containers should always be labeled with the corresponding patient demographics, initials of the person collecting the sample, collection date, time of collection, and applicable special notes. They should then be promptly transported to the laboratory for processing and analysis.

Universal Post Test Pearls (Evaluation)

- Note that completed test results are made available to the requesting HCP, who will discuss them with the patient.
- Answer questions and address concerns voiced by the patient or family and reinforce information given by the patient's HCP regarding further testing, treatment, or referral to another HCP. Recognize that patients will have anxiety related to test results. Provide teaching and information regarding the clinical implications of the test results on the patient's lifestyle, as appropriate.
- Note that test results should be evaluated in context with the patient's signs, symptoms, and diagnosis. Depending on the results of the procedure, additional testing may be performed to evaluate or monitor progression of the disease process and determine the need for a change in therapy.
- When a person goes through a traumatic event such as an illness or being given information that will impact his or her lifestyle, there are universal human reactions that occur. These include knowledge deficit, fear, anxiety, and coping; in some situations, grieving may occur. HCPs should always be aware of the human response and how it may affect the plan of care and expected outcomes.

DISCUSSION POINT

Regarding Post-Test Critical Findings: Timely notification of a critical finding for lab or diagnostic studies is a role expectation of the professional nurse. Notification processes will vary among facilities. Upon receipt of the critical finding, the information should be read back to the caller to verify accuracy. Most policies require immediate notification of the primary HCP, hospitalist, or on-call HCP. Reported information includes the patient's name, unique identifiers, critical finding, name of the person giving the report, and name of the person receiving the report. Documentation of notification should be made in the medical record with the name of the HCP notified, time and date of notification, and any orders received. Any delay in a timely report of a critical finding may require completion of a notification form with review by Risk Management.

STUDIES

- Culture, Bacterial, Stool
- Fecal Analysis

LEARNING OUTCOMES

Providing safe, effective nursing care (SENC) includes mastery of core competencies and standards of care. SENC is based on a judicious application of nursing knowledge in combination with scientific principles. The Art of Nursing lies in blending what you know with the ability to effectively apply your knowledge in a compassionate manner.

After reading/studying this chapter you will be able to:

Thinking

1. Examine the scope of practice related to specific aspects of care such as information management; evidence-based education; and organizational, patient, family, and ancillary communication.

Doing

1. Accept the leadership role required to meet specific clinical situations.

Caring

1. Examine how the process of personal reflection on care practices can influence patient outcomes.

Culture, Bacterial, Stool

Quick Summary

SYNONYM ACRONYM: N/A.

COMMON USE: To identify pathogenic bacterial organisms in the stool as an indicator for appropriate therapeutic interventions to treat organisms such as *Clostridium difficile* and *Escherichia coli*.

SPECIMEN: Fresh, random stool collected in a clean plastic container.

NORMAL FINDINGS: (Method: Culture on selective media for identification of pathogens usually to include *Salmonella, Shigella, Escherichia coli* O157:H7, *Yersinia enterocolitica*, and *Campylobacter*; latex agglutination or enzyme immunoassay for *Clostridium* A and B toxins). Polymerase chain reaction (PCR) may be used to identify bacterial, protozoan, or viral pathogens. Negative: No growth of pathogens. Normal fecal flora is 96% to 99% anaerobes and 1% to 4% aerobes. Normal flora present may include *Bacteroides, Candida albicans, Clostridium, Enterococcus, E. coli, Proteus, Pseudomonas*, and *Staphylococcus aureus*.

Test Explanation

Stool culture involves collecting a sample of feces so that organisms present can be isolated and identified. Certain bacteria are normally found in feces. However, when overgrowth of these organisms occurs or pathological organisms are present, diarrhea or other signs and symptoms of systemic infection occur. These symptoms are the result of damage to the intestinal tissue by the pathogenic organisms. Routine stool culture normally screens for a small number of common pathogens associated with food poisoning, such as *S. aureus, Salmonella*, and *Shigella*. Identification of other bacteria is initiated by special request or upon consultation with a microbiologist when there is knowledge of special circumstances. An example of this situation is an outbreak of *C. difficile* in a nursing home or hospital unit where the infection can spread rapidly from one person to the next. A life-threatening *C. difficile* infection of the bowel may occur in patients who are immunocompromised or are receiving broad-spectrum antibiotic therapy (e.g., clindamycin, ampicillin, cephalosporins). The bacteria release a toxin that causes necrosis of the colon tissue. The toxin can be more rapidly identified from a stool sample using an immunochemical method than from a routine culture. Appropriate interventions can be quickly initiated and might include IV replacement of fluid and electrolytes, cessation of broad-spectrum antibiotic administration, and institution of vancomycin or metronidazole antibiotic therapy. The laboratory will initiate antibiotic sensitivity testing if indicated by test results. Sensitivity testing identifies the antibiotics to which organisms are susceptible to ensure an effective treatment plan. The subspecialty of microbiology has been revolutionized by molecular diagnostics. Molecular diagnostics involves the identification of specific sequences of DNA. The application of molecular diagnostics techniques, such as PCR, has led to the development of automated instruments that can identify a single infectious agent or multiple pathogens from a small amount of stool in less than 2 hours. The instruments can detect the presence of bacteria, viruses, or protozoans commonly associated with gastrointestinal infections.

Nursing Implications

Assessment

Indications	Potential Nursing Problems
Assist in establishing a diagnosis for diarrhea of unknown etiology Identify pathogenic organisms causing gastrointestinal disease and carrier states	• Breathing • Body Image • Communication • Diarrhea • Electrolyte • Fatigue • Fluid Volume • Gas Exchange • Health Management • Human Response • Mobility • Skin • Weakness

Diagnosis: Clinical Significance of Test Results
POSITIVE FINDINGS
- Bacterial infection: Gram-negative organisms such as *Aeromonas* spp., *Campylobacter*, *E. coli* including serotype O157: H7, *Plesiomonas shigelloides*, *Salmonella*, *Shigella*, *Vibrio*, and **Yersinia**
- Bacterial infection: Gram-positive organisms such as *Bacillus cereus*, *C. difficile*, and *Listeria*. Isolation of *Staphylococcus aureus* may indicate infection or a carrier state.
- Botulism: *Clostridium botulinum* (the bacteria must also be isolated from the food or the presence of toxin confirmed in the stool specimen)
- Parasitic enterocolitis

Planning
Considerations for planning a successful partnership should include clear communication of what to expect during the test to decrease anxiety and improve cooperation. Obtain a history of the patient's travel to foreign countries, and note any medication the patient is taking that may interfere with test results, especially antibiotics. Before the procedure is performed, plan to review the steps with the patient. Inform the patient of the importance of good hand-washing techniques. Instruct the patient not to contaminate the specimen with urine, water, or toilet tissue. Address concerns about pain, and explain that there may be some discomfort during the specimen collection if the patient is constipated.

SPECIAL CONSIDERATIONS
An important aspect of planning is understanding the factors that may alter study findings or cause abnormal results. Interdepartmental communication is a key factor in the planning process. The following should be noted when planning for this study:

- A rectal swab does not provide an adequate amount of specimen for evaluating the carrier state and should be avoided in favor of a standard stool specimen.
- A rectal swab should never be submitted for *Clostridium* toxin studies as it does not provide sufficient fecal matter for evaluation; stool is the specimen of choice. A positive culture will be reflex tested for toxin identification. Specimens for *Clostridium* toxins should be refrigerated or frozen per laboratory requirements if they are not immediately transported to the laboratory because toxins degrade rapidly.
- A rectal swab is not the preferred specimen for *Campylobacter* culture. Excessive exposure of the sample to air or room temperature may damage this bacterium so that it will not grow in the culture.
- Failure to transport the culture within 1 hour of collection or urine contamination of the sample may affect results.

It is also important to understand which medications or substances the patient may be exposed to in the health care setting that can interfere with accurate testing:

- Therapy with antibiotics before specimen collection may decrease the type and the amount of bacteria.
- Barium and laxatives used less than 1 week before the test may reduce bacterial growth.

Implementation
Patient education is key to obtaining the patient's cooperation in following directions, and providing an explanation for the purpose of the procedure is an important part of this process. Inform the patient that this study can assist with identification of the organism-causing infection. Instruct the patient to collect the ordered stool specimen; place it directly into a clean, dry container; and then tightly cap the container. If the patient is not ambulatory, collect the specimen in a clean, dry bedpan. Then use a tongue blade to transfer the specimen to the container, and include any mucoid and bloody portions. Make sure that representative portions of the stool are sent for analysis: Collect a specimen sample from the first, middle, and last portion of the stool. Note the specimen appearance on the collection container label. Specimens for routine stool culture that cannot be delivered to the lab within 2 hours should be transferred from the original collection container into the appropriate transport media, an orange-capped Para-Pak enteric transport medium (Carey-Blair), and transported at room temperature.

Evaluation

Recognize anxiety related to test results, and instruct the patient to report symptoms such as pain related to tissue inflammation or irritation. Advise the patient that final test results may take up to 72 hours but that antibiotic therapy may be started immediately. Instruct the patient regarding the importance of completing the entire course of antibiotic therapy, even if no symptoms are present. Note: Antibiotic therapy is frequently contraindicated for Salmonella infection unless the infection has progressed to a systemic state. Emphasize the importance of reporting continued signs and symptoms of the infection.

✅ Critical Findings

- Bacterial pathogens: *Campylobacter, C. difficile, E. coli* including 0157:H7, *Listeria, Rotavirus* (especially in children), *Salmonella, Shigella, Vibrio, Yersinia*, or parasites *Acanthamoeba, Ascaris* (hookworm), *Cyclospora, Cryptosporidium, Entamoeba histolytica, Giardia*, and *Strongyloides* (tapeworm), parasitic ova, proglottid, and larvae.

Note and immediately report to the health-care provider (HCP) positive results for bacterial pathogens or parasites and related symptoms.

Note and immediately report to the requesting HCP any critical findings and related symptoms. A listing of these findings varies among facilities.

✅ Study Specific Complications

N/A

✅ Related Tests

- Related tests include capsule endoscopy, colonoscopy, fecal analysis, Gram stain, ova and parasites, and proctosigmoidoscopy.
- Refer to the Gastrointestinal and Immune systems tables at the end of the book for related tests by body system.

Expected Outcomes

Expected outcomes associated with Culture, Bacterial, Stool are

- Understanding the cause of diarrhea and the precautions required to prevent further exposure
- Describing proper handwashing technique and discussing the reasons for always using good hand hygiene
- Verbalizing at-risk behaviors that could cause exposure to organisms

Fecal Analysis

Quick Summary

COMMON USE: To assess for the presence of blood in the stool toward diagnosing gastrointestinal bleeding, cancer, inflammation, and infection.

SPECIMEN: Stool.

NORMAL FINDINGS: (Method: Macroscopic examination, for appearance and color; microscopic examination, for cell count and presence of meat fibers; leukocyte esterase, for leukocytes; Benedict's solution (copper sulfate) for reducing substances; guaiac, for occult blood; x-ray paper, for trypsin.)

Characteristic	Normal Result
Appearance	Solid and formed
Color	Brown
Epithelial cells	Few to moderate
Fecal fat	See "Fecal Fat" study
Leukocytes (white blood cells)	Negative
Meat fibers	Negative
Occult blood	Negative
Reducing substances	Negative
Trypsin	2+ to 4+

Test Explanation

Feces consist mainly of cellulose and other undigested foodstuffs, bacteria, and water. Other substances normally found in feces include epithelial cells shed from the gastrointestinal (GI) tract, small amounts of fats, bile pigments in the form of urobilinogen, GI and pancreatic secretions, electrolytes, and trypsin. Trypsin is a proteolytic enzyme produced in the pancreas. The average adult excretes 100 to 300 g of fecal material per day, the residue of approximately 10 L of liquid material that enters the GI tract each day. The laboratory analysis of feces includes macroscopic examination (volume, odor, shape, color, consistency, presence of mucus), microscopic examination (leukocytes, epithelial cells, meat fibers), and chemical tests for specific substances (occult blood, trypsin, estimation of carbohydrate). Detection of occult blood is the most common test performed on stool (see Fig. 10.1). The prevalence of

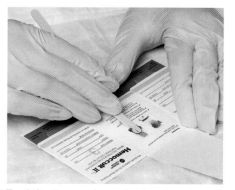

FIGURE 10.1 Fecal occult blood testing. *Used with permission, from Wilkinson, J., & Treas, L. (2010). Fundamentals of Nursing (2nd ed.). FA Davis Company.*

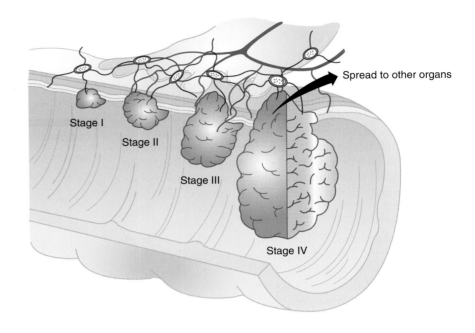

FIGURE 10.2 Stages of colon cancer. *Used with permission, from Tamparo, C., & Lewis, M. (2011). Diseases of the human body (5th ed.). FA Davis Company.*

colorectal adenoma is greater than 30% in people aged 60 and older. Progression from adenoma to carcinoma occurs over a period of 5 to 12 years; from carcinoma to metastatic disease in 2 to 3 years (see Fig. 10.2).

Nursing Implications

Assessment

Indications	Potential Nursing Problems
Assist in diagnosing disorders associated with GI bleeding or drug therapy that leads to bleeding	• Bleeding
	• Body Image
	• Electrolyte
Assist in the diagnosis of pseudomembranous enterocolitis after use of broad-spectrum antibiotic therapy	• Fluid Volume
	• Human Response
	• Infection
Assist in the diagnosis of suspected inflammatory bowel disorder	• Self-Care
Detect altered protein digestion	• Self-Esteem
Detect intestinal parasitic infestation, as indicated by diarrhea of unknown cause	• Skin
Investigate diarrhea of unknown cause	
Monitor effectiveness of therapy for intestinal malabsorption or pancreatic insufficiency	
Screen for cystic fibrosis	

Diagnosis: Clinical Significance of Test Results

UNUSUAL APPEARANCE
- Bloody: *Excessive intestinal wall irritation or malignancy*
- Bulky or frothy: *Malabsorption*
- Mucous: *Inflammation of intestinal walls*
- Slender or ribbonlike: *Obstruction*

UNUSUAL COLOR
- Black: *Bismuth (antacid) or charcoal ingestion, iron therapy, upper GI bleeding*
- Grayish white: *Barium ingestion, bile duct obstruction*
- Green: *Antibiotics, biliverdin, green vegetables*
- Red: *Beets and food coloring, lower GI bleed, phenazopyridine hydrochloride compounds, rifampin*
- Yellow: *Rhubarb*

INCREASED
- Blood: *Related to bleeding in the digestive tract*
- Carbohydrates/reducing substances: *Malabsorption syndromes, inability to digest some sugars*
- Epithelial cells: *Inflammatory bowel disorders*
- Fat: *Pancreatitis, sprue (celiac disease), cystic fibrosis related to malabsorption*
- Leukocytes: *Inflammation of the intestines related to bacterial infections of the intestinal wall, salmonellosis, shigellosis, or ulcerative colitis*
- Meat fibers: *Altered protein digestion, pancreatitis*
- Occult blood: *Anal fissure, diverticular disease, esophageal varices, esophagitis, gastritis, hemorrhoids, infectious diarrhea, inflammatory bowel disease, Mallory-Weiss tears, polyps, tumors, ulcers*
- pH: *Related to inflammation in the intestine from colitis, cancer, or antibiotic use*

DECREASED
- Carbohydrates: *Sprue, cystic fibrosis, malnutrition, medications such as colchicine (gout) or birth control pills*
- Leukocytes: *Amebic colitis, cholera, disorders resulting from toxins, parasites, viral diarrhea*

- pH: *Related to poor absorption of carbohydrate or fat*
- Trypsin: *Cystic fibrosis, malabsorption syndromes, pancreatic deficiency*

Planning

Considerations for planning a successful partnership should include clear communication of what to expect during the test to decrease anxiety and improve cooperation. Before the procedure is performed, plan to review the steps with the patient. Inform the patient of the importance of good hand-washing techniques. Instruct the patient not to contaminate the specimen with urine, water, or toilet tissue. Address concerns about pain, and explain that there should be no discomfort during the procedure. Instruct the patient to follow a normal diet unless the test is being performed to identify blood. If the test is being performed for occult blood, instruct the patient to follow a special diet that includes small amounts of chicken, turkey, and tuna (no red meats), raw and cooked vegetables and fruits, and bran cereal for several days before the test. Foods to avoid on the special diet include beets, turnips, cauliflower, broccoli, bananas, parsnips, and cantaloupe, because these foods can interfere with the occult blood test.

SPECIAL CONSIDERATIONS

An important aspect of planning is understanding the factors that may alter study findings or cause abnormal results. Interdepartmental communication is a key factor in the planning process. The following should be noted when planning for this study:

- Ingestion of a diet high in red meat, certain vegetables, and bananas can cause false-positive results for occult blood.
- Constipated stools may not indicate any trypsin activity owing to extended exposure to intestinal bacteria.

It is also important to understand which medications or substances the patient may be exposed to in the healthcare setting that can interfere with accurate testing:

- Drugs that can cause positive results for occult blood include acetylsalicylic acid, anticoagulants, colchicine, corticosteroids, iron preparations, and phenylbutazone.
- Large doses of vitamin C can cause false-negative occult blood.

Implementation

Patient education is key to obtaining the patient's cooperation in following directions, and providing an explanation for the purpose of the procedure is an important part of this process. Inform the patient that this study can assist with the diagnosis of intestinal disorders.

Ensure that the patient has complied with the ordered medication restrictions; assure that laxatives, enemas, or suppositories have been restricted for at least 3 days prior to the procedure, and note any current or recent antibiotic therapy. Instruct the patient to collect the ordered stool specimen; place it directly into a clean, dry container; and then tightly cap the container. If the patient is not ambulatory, collect the specimen in a clean, dry bedpan. Then use a tongue blade to transfer the specimen to the container, and include any mucoid and bloody portions. Make sure that representative portions of the stool are sent for analysis: Collect a specimen sample from the first, middle, and last portion of the stool. Note the specimen appearance on the collection container label. Specimens for fecal analysis should be refrigerated if they will not be transported to the laboratory within 4 hours after collection. Specimens may be collected from pediatric patients using a rectal swab; insert the swab past the anal sphincter, rotate gently, and withdraw. Place the swab in the appropriate transport container.

Evaluation

Recognize anxiety related to test results, and answer any questions or address any concerns voiced by the patient or family. Decisions regarding the need for and frequency of occult blood testing, colonoscopy, or other cancer screening procedures should be made after consultation between the patient and the health-care provider (HCP). The American Cancer Society recommends regular screening for colon cancer, beginning at age 50 years for individuals without identified risk factors; sooner for those with identified risk factors. Their recommendations for frequency of screening are to use one of the following: (1) annual for occult blood testing (fecal occult blood testing/FOBT or fecal immunochemical testing/FIT); or (2) every 5 years for flexible sigmoidoscopy, double contrast barium enema, or computed tomography (CT) colonography; or (3) every 10 years for colonoscopy; or (4) every 3 years for stool DNA testing. Abnormal findings should be followed up by colonoscopy. There are both advantages and disadvantages to the screening tests that are available today. Methods to use DNA testing of stool are being investigated and are designed to identify abnormal changes in DNA from the cells in the lining of the colon that are normally shed and excreted in stool. The DNA tests under development use multiple markers to identify colon cancers that demonstrate different, abnormal DNA changes. Unlike some of the current screening methods, the DNA tests would be able to detect precancerous polyps. The most current guidelines for colon cancer screening of the general population as well as of individuals with increased risk are available from the American Cancer Society (www.cancer.org), U.S. Preventive Services Task Force (www.uspreventiveservicestaskforce.org), and the American College of Gastroenterology (www.gi.org).

✔ Critical Findings

N/A

⊘ Study Specific Complications

N/A

⊘ Related Tests

- Related tests include α_1-antitrypsin/phenotyping, barium enema, biopsy intestine, capsule endoscopy, CEA and cancer antigens, chloride sweat, colonoscopy, CT colonoscopy, culture stool, D-xylose tolerance, fecal fat, gliadin antibody, lactose tolerance test, ova and parasites, and proctosigmoidoscopy.
- Refer to the Gastrointestinal System table at the end of the book for related tests by body system.

Expected Outcomes

Expected outcomes associated with Fecal Analysis are

- Being able to manage diarrhea and maintain baseline level of socialization
- Having skin that remains intact
- Understanding the importance of following stool specimen collection instructions to prevent inaccurate results
- Verbalizing activities that place one at risk for parasitic infection

REVIEW OF LEARNING OUTCOMES

Thinking

1. Examine the scope of practice related to specific aspects of care such as information management; evidence-based education; and organizational, patient, family, and ancillary communication. Answer: Patients need to understand the importance of specimen collection as it relates to their overall health. Without their cooperation, it is impossible to obtain the specimen needed to diagnose what is wrong with them. You need to decide how to communicate the information and education in a way that will encourage the patient to be cooperative and to follow provided instructions accurately.

Doing

1. Accept the leadership role required to meet specific clinical situations. Answer: Stool specimen collection can be very difficult for the patient, especially if the stool has a foul odor. Make a special effort to retrieve the specimen, once it has been collected, and submit it to the laboratory so it can be processed in a timely manner. This will spare the patient the embarrassment of having the specimen present when visited by others.

Caring

1. Examine how the process of personal reflection on care practices can influence patient outcomes. Answer: Think about how difficult it is for some cultures to step beyond their cultural norms and submit to specimen collection. Consideration of cultural factors will better prepare you to address the act of specimen collection in a sensitive fashion.

⟨⟩ **Words of Wisdom:** Issues related to elimination can be very embarrassing for patients. A disease process that causes the stool to have a foul odor or, in the patient's view, a funny color frightens the patient. Compassionate management of the stool is important both culturally and medically; culturally, in order to make the health-care experience less burdensome, and medically, so that the conclusions necessary for an accurate diagnosis can be reached. Part of the nursing role is to always remember the person and not just the task.

BIBLIOGRAPHY

American Cancer Society. (2014). Colorectal cancer prevention and early detection. Colorectal cancer screening tests. Retrieved from www.cancer.org/cancer/colonandrectumcancer/moreinformation/colonandrectumcancerearlydetection/colorectal-cancer-early-detection-screening-tests-used.

Stool analysis. (2010, October 13). Retrieved from www.webmd.com/digestive-disorders/stool-analysis

Stool DNA Test. (2014). Retrieved from www.ccalliance.org/screening/stool-dna.html

Van Leeuwen, A., and Bladh, M. (2015). Davis's comprehensive handbook of laboratory and diagnostic tests with nursing implications. (6th ed.). Philadelphia, PA: F.A. Davis Company.

Go to Section II of this book and www.davisplus.com for the Clinical Reasoning Tool and its case studies to provide you with a safe place to explore patient care situations. There are a total of 26 different case studies; 2 cases are presented for each of 13 body systems. One set of 13 cases are found in the Section II chapters, and a second set of 13 cases are available online at www.davisplus.com. Each case is designed with the specific goal of helping you to connect the dots of clinical reasoning. Cases are designed to reflect possible clinical scenarios; the outcomes may or may not be positive—you decide.

Manometric Studies

OVERVIEW

Manometric studies are used to assess the functionality of areas of the body that are filled with fluid or air. Types of fluids consist of blood in the arteries and veins, spinal fluid in the spinal column, food as it is digested and moves from the esophagus to the stomach, and the air volume left in the lungs at rest after exhalation. Measurements of pressure changes are made by using a transducer. Changes in pressure that are not within the normal expected findings give direction for treatment and disease management, including the integration of nursing care. The type of transducer selected is dependent upon the area of the body and the type of fluid or air pressure being measured. Some transducers may be calibrated, such as those used for measuring spinal fluid pressure. Cystometry is a urodynamic study used to assess the neuromuscular aspect of bladder function and is discussed in this chapter.

The information in the Part I studies is organized in a manner to help the student see how the five basic components of the nursing process (assessment, diagnosis, planning, implementation, and evaluation) can be applied to each phase of laboratory and diagnostic testing. The goal is to use nursing process to understand the integration of care (laboratory, diagnostic, nursing care) toward achieving a positive expected outcome.

- **Assessment** is the collection of information for the purpose of answering the question, "is there a problem?" Knowledge of the patient's health history, medications, complaints, and allergies as well as synonyms or alternate test names, common use for the procedure, specimen requirements, and normal ranges or interpretive comments provide the foundation for diagnosis.
- **Diagnosis** is the process of looking at the information gathered during assessment and answering the

questions, "what is the problem?" and "what do I need to do about it?" Test indications tell us why the study has been requested, and potential diagnoses tell us the value or importance of the study relative to its clinical utility.
- **Planning** is a blueprint of the nursing care before the procedure. It is the process of determining how the nurse is going to partner with the patient to fix the problem (e.g., "The patient has a study ordered and this is what I should know before I successfully carry out the plan to have the study completed"). Knowledge of interfering factors, social and cultural issues, preprocedural restrictions, the need for written and informed consent, anxiety about the procedure, and concerns regarding pain are some considerations for planning a successful partnership.
- **Implementation** is putting the plan into action with an idea of what the expected outcome should be. Collaboration with the departments where the laboratory test or diagnostic study is to be performed is essential to the success of the plan. Implementation is where the work is done within each healthcare team member's scope of practice.
- **Evaluation** answers the question, "did the plan work or not?" Was the plan completely successful, partially successful, or not successful? If the plan did not work, evaluation is the process where you determine what needs to be changed to make the plan work better. This includes a review of all expected outcomes. Nursing care after the procedure is where information is gathered to evaluate the plan. Review of results, including critical findings, in relation to patient symptoms and other tests performed provide data that form a more complete picture of health or illness.
- **Expected Outcomes** are positive outcomes related to the test. They are the outcomes the nurse should expect if all goes well.

A number of pretest, intratest, and post-test universal points are presented in this overview section because the information applies to manometric studies in general.

Universal Pretest Pearls (Planning)

- Obtain a history of the patient's complaints, including a list of known allergens, especially allergies or sensitivities to medications or latex so their use can be avoided or their effects mitigated if an allergy is present. Carefully evaluate all medications currently being taken by the patient. A list of the patient's current medications, prescribed and over the counter (including anticoagulants, aspirin and other salicylates, and dietary supplements), should also be obtained. Such products may be discontinued by medical direction for the appropriate number of days prior to the procedure. Ensure that all allergies are clearly noted in the medical record, and ensure that the patient is wearing an allergy and medical record armband. Report information that could interfere with, or delay proceeding with, the study to the health-care provider (HCP) and laboratory.
- Obtain a history of the patient's affected body system, symptoms, and results of previously performed laboratory tests and diagnostic and surgical procedures. Previous test results will provide a basis of comparison between old and new data.
- An important aspect of planning is understanding the factors that may alter study findings or cause abnormal results. Interdepartmental communication is a key factor in the planning process. The inability of a patient to cooperate or remain still during the procedure because of age, significant pain, or mental status should be among the anticipated factors. Recent or past procedures, medications, or existing medical conditions that could complicate or interfere with test results should be noted.
- Review the steps of the study with the patient or caregiver. Expect patients to be nervous about the procedure and the pending results. Educating the patient on his or her role during the procedure and what to expect can facilitate this. The patient's role during the procedure is to remain still. The actual time required to complete each study will depend on a number of conditions, including the type of equipment being used and how well a patient will cooperate.
- Address any concerns about pain, and explain or describe, as appropriate, the level and type of discomfort that may be expected.
- Provide additional instructions and patient preparation regarding medication, diet, fluid intake, or activity, if appropriate. Unless specified in the individual study, there are no special instructions or restrictions.
- Always be sensitive to any cultural or psychosocial issues, including a concern for modesty before, during, and after the procedure.

Reminder

Ensure that a written and informed consent has been documented in the medical record prior to the study, if required. The consent must be obtained before medication is administered.

Universal Intratest Pearls (Implementation)

- Correct patient identification is crucial prior to any procedure. Positively identify the patient using two unique identifiers such as patient name, date of birth, Social Security number, or medical record number.
- Standard Precautions must be followed.
- Children and infants may be accompanied by a parent to calm them. Keep neonates and infants covered and in a warm room and provide a pacifier or gentle touch. The testing environment should be quiet, and the patient should be instructed, as appropriate, to remain still during the test as extraneous movements can affect results.
- Ensure the patient has complied with pretesting instructions, including dietary, fluid, medication, and activity restrictions as given for the procedure. The number of days to withhold medication depends on the type of medication. Notify the HCP if pretesting instructions have not been followed (e.g., if applicable, if patient anticoagulant therapy has not been withheld).
- Baseline vital signs must be recorded and continue to be monitored throughout and after the procedure, according to organizational policy. A comparison should be made between the baseline and postprocedure vital signs and focused assessments. Protocols may vary among facilities.

Universal Post Test Pearls (Evaluation)

- Note that completed test results are made available to the requesting HCP, who will discuss them with the patient.
- Answer questions and address concerns voiced by the patient or family and reinforce information given by the patient's HCP regarding further testing, treatment, or referral to another HCP. Recognize that patients will have anxiety related to test results. Provide teaching and information regarding

the clinical implications of the test results on the patients lifestyle as appropriate.

● Note that test results should be evaluated in context with the patient's signs, symptoms, and diagnosis. Depending on the results of the procedure, additional testing may be performed to evaluate or monitor progression of the disease process and determine the need for a change in therapy.

● Be aware that when a person goes through a traumatic event such as an illness or being given information that will impact his or her lifestyle, there are universal human reactions that occur. These include knowledge deficit, fear, anxiety, and coping; in some situations, grieving may occur. HCPs should always be aware of the human response and how it may affect the plan of care and expected outcomes.

DISCUSSION POINT

Regarding Post-Test Critical Findings: Timely notification of a critical finding for lab or diagnostic studies is a role expectation of the professional nurse. Notification processes will vary among facilities. Upon receipt of the critical finding, the information should be read back to the caller to verify accuracy. Most policies require immediate notification of the primary HCP, hospitalist, or on-call HCP. Reported information includes the patient's name, unique identifiers, critical finding, name of the person giving the report, and name of the person receiving the report. Documentation of notification should be made in the medical record with the name of the HCP notified, time and date of notification, and any orders received. Any delay in a timely report of a critical finding may require completion of a notification form with review by Risk Management.

STUDIES

● Cystometry

LEARNING OUTCOMES

Providing safe, effective nursing care (SENC) includes mastery of core competencies and standards of care. SENC is based on a judicious application of nursing knowledge in combination with scientific principles. The Art of Nursing lies in blending what you know with the ability to effectively apply your knowledge in a compassionate manner.

After reading/studying this chapter, you will be able to:

Thinking

1. Recognize that as human beings we all have various strengths and weaknesses as team members.
2. Identify concerns related to diagnostic procedures and older adults.

Doing

1. Incorporate elements of care using an integrated multidisciplinary approach.
2. Identify safe nursing practices for follow-up care.
3. Develop and implement an individualized plan of care based on patient preferences and specific health-care needs.

Caring

1. Recognize that barriers to patient decision making can be resolved by providing resources that clarify misunderstanding.

Cystometry

Quick Summary

SYNONYM ACRONYM: Cystometrography (CMG), urodynamic testing of bladder function.

COMMON USE: To assess bladder function related to obstruction, neurogenic pathology, and infection including evaluation of surgical, and medical management.

AREA OF APPLICATION: Bladder, urethra.

● Amount of postvoid residual urine is less than 30–50 mL
● Normal filling pattern
● Normal sensory perception of bladder fullness, desire to void, and ability to inhibit urination; appropriate response to temperature (hot and cold)
● Normal bladder capacity: 250 to 450 mL. Bladder size and corresponding capacity vary with gender and age; in the pediatric patient the normal bladder stretches to maximum capacity without an increase in pressure
● Normal first urge to void: 175 to 250 mL; sensation of fullness and need to empty the bladder: 350 to 450 mL
● Normal functioning bladder pressure: 8 to 15 cm H_2O
● Normal bladder pressure increases 30 to 40 cm H_2O during voiding
● Normal detrusor pressure: less than 10 cm H_2O
● Urethral pressure that is higher than bladder pressure, ensuring continence

Test Explanation

Cystometry evaluates the motor and sensory function of the bladder when incontinence is present or neurological bladder dysfunction is suspected and monitors the effects of treatment for the abnormalities. This manometric study measures the bladder pressure and volume characteristics in milliliters of water (cm H_2O) during the filling and emptying phases. The test provides information about bladder structure and function that can lead to uninhibited bladder contractions, sensations of bladder fullness and need to void, and ability to inhibit voiding. These abnormalities cause incontinence and other impaired patterns of micturition. Cystometry can be performed with EEG (sleep studies for nocturnal incontinence), cystoscopy, and electromyography pelvic floor sphincter.

A postvoid residual measurement can also be done at the bedside to measure how much urine is left in the bladder after the patient voids. Completion of this test requires catheterization of the patient directly after voiding. The amount of urine remaining is measured and reported as the postvoid or residual urine. Normal postvoid residual is less than 30–50 mL of urine. This may be adjusted to less than 100 mL for those over the age of 65.

Nursing Implications

Assessment

Indications	Potential Nursing Problems
Detect congenital urinary abnormalities	• Activity
Determine cause of bladder dysfunction and pathology	• Bleeding
Determine cause of recurrent urinary tract infections (UTIs)	• Disturbed Sleep
Determine cause of urinary retention	• Human Reactions
Determine type of incontinence: *functional* (involuntary and unpredictable), *reflex* (involuntary when a specific volume is reached), *stress* (weak pelvic muscles), *total* (continuous and unpredictable), *urge* (involuntary when urgency is sensed), and *psychological* (e.g., dementia, confusion affecting awareness)	• Incontinence • Infection • Role Performance • Self-Care • Self-Perception • Sexuality • Socialization • Urination
Determine type of neurogenic bladder (motor or sensory)	
Evaluate the management of neurological bladder before surgical intervention	
Evaluate postprostatectomy incontinence	
Evaluate signs and symptoms of urinary elimination pattern dysfunction	
Evaluate urinary obstruction in male patients experiencing urinary retention	
Evaluate the usefulness of drug therapy on detrusor muscle function and tonicity and on internal and external sphincter function	
Evaluate voiding disorders associated with spinal cord injury	

Diagnosis: Clinical Significance of Test Results

ABNORMAL FINDINGS

BLADDER DYSFUNCTION RELATED TO DISORDERS OF THE NERVOUS SYSTEM

- Diabetic neuropathy
- Multiple sclerosis
- Parkinson Disease
- Spinal cord injury
- Stroke
- Tabes dorsalis

BLADDER DYSFUNCTION RELATED TO URINARY INCONTINENCE

- Emotional or psychological origin
- Hyperreflexia
- Urinary tract infection

BLADDER DYSFUNCTION RELATED TO URINARY RETENTION

- Bladder obstruction (e.g. congenital origin, tumor)
- Enlarged prostate
- Urinary tract infection

Planning

Considerations for planning a successful partnership should include clear communication of what to expect during the test to decrease anxiety and improve cooperation. Before the procedure is performed, plan to review the steps with the patient and address any concerns about pain. Explain that no discomfort should be experienced during the test, and inform the patient that the procedure is performed in a special urology room or clinic by a health-care provider (HCP) under sterile conditions, and takes approximately 30 to 45 minutes.

CONTRAINDICATIONS
- Patients with acute UTIs because the study can cause infection to spread to the kidneys
- Patients with urethral obstruction
- Inability to catheterize the patient
- Patients with cervical cord lesions because they may exhibit autonomic dysreflexia, as seen by bradycardia, flushing, hypertension, diaphoresis, and headache

SPECIAL CONSIDERATIONS
An important aspect of planning is understanding the factors that may alter study findings or cause abnormal results. Interdepartmental communication is a key factor in the planning process. The following should be noted when planning for this study:

- The inability of the patient to void in a supine position or straining to void during the study may cause abnormal results.
- A high level of patient anxiety or embarrassment, which may interfere with the study, can make it

difficult to distinguish whether the results are due to stress or organic pathology.

● The administration of drugs, such as muscle relaxants or antihistamines, can affect bladder function.

● For pediatric patients, the age of the child and the culture of the parents and child must be considered.

● Safety Tip
Make sure a written and informed consent has been signed prior to the procedure and before administering any medications.

Implementation
Patient education is an important part of this process, and providing an explanation for the purpose of the procedure is important. Inform the patient that this study can assist in assessing for disorders of the bladder. Instruct the patient not to void prior to the procedure and to change into the gown, robe, and foot coverings provided.

PEDIATRIC CONSIDERATIONS: Special care should be used when assessing the bladder function of children. Younger children may not understand the directions you provide and may not be able to follow them. Effort should be made to partner with the parents to facilitate the success of the study as appropriate. Older children who are able to understand the reason for the study will tend to be more cooperative. The use of pictures or dolls may assist with providing information more appropriate to their age level. Assessment of the urge to void will be easier to identify in older verbal versus younger nonverbal children. Nonverbal cues such as wiggling of the toes or unrest in younger children may provide clues regarding the need to void. For diagnostic purposes, in pediatric populations formulas are used to measure bladder capacity based on age.

The patient should be positioned in a supine or lithotomy position on the examination table. If spinal cord injury is present, the patient can remain on a stretcher in a supine position and can be draped appropriately.

Cystometry is performed by noting pressure changes that occur as the bladder fills and empties. Pressure readings can be taken at various times during the filling and emptying process. The information provided will identify alterations in the function of the bladder that could indicate why there is urinary difficulty. Attention will be given to the function of the bladder's detrusor muscle, which normally relaxes to store urine and contracts to facilitate urination. Bladder capacity (how much it can hold) will be evaluated along with response to thermal stimulation. Evaluation of bladder function during cystometry may be completed in four steps. In step one, ask the patient to void emptying the

bladder while the urinary stream is assessed for size, force, and stream continuity, including the presence of any dribbling. Any hesitance or straining during urination should be noted. In step two, assess how much urine is left in the bladder after voiding by inserting a catheter and measuring residual urine. In step three, assess bladder sensation by instilling first room temperature fluid (sterile water or normal saline) and then warmed fluid and ask the patient what he or she feels. In step four, attach a transducer for measuring pressure changes in the bladder (cystometer) to a urethral catheter to collect data as it is slowly filled. At some point in the process, the patient is asked to void around the catheter to measure maximum intravesical pressure (pressure directed inward by the bladder walls). Once all of the data are collected, the data are placed on a graph for visual examination and diagnostic assessment (see Fig. 11.1).

Evaluation
Recognize anxiety related to test results and be supportive of impaired activity related to bladder function loss or a perceived loss of independence. Discuss the implications of abnormal test results on the patient's lifestyle. Provide teaching and information about the clinical implications of the test results as appropriate. Urinary incontinence can have a long-range impact personally, socially, and professionally.

SPECIAL CONSIDERATIONS
Consideration needs to be given to support groups that may guide the patient toward a realistic transition toward life management with a bladder deficit. Many

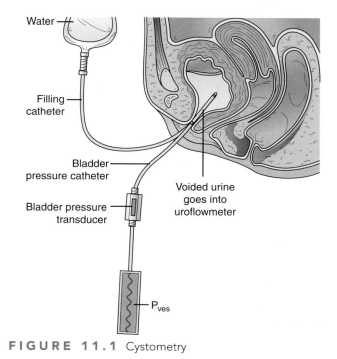

Water

Filling catheter

Bladder pressure catheter

Bladder pressure transducer

Voided urine goes into uroflowmeter

P_{ves}

FIGURE 11.1 Cystometry

people find that counseling helps them cope with their embarrassment about being incontinent. Educate the patient about access to counseling services. Provide contact information, if desired, for the Urology Care Foundation www.urologyhealth.org. When caring for a patient with altered bladder function, the forms of communication should be adapted to meet the patient's needs. Ensure him or her that special equipment and supplies are available to help manage incontinence. The process of communication chosen should be documented on the plan of care to ensure consistency and decrease frustration.

⊘ Critical Findings

N/A

⊘ Study Specific Complications

Infection and hematuria (blood in the urine) are complications that can occur post cystometry. Provide education about the signs and symptoms of infection (fever, chills, painful or difficult urination). Explain that increasing the intake of fluids, including acidic juices such as cranberry juice, can mitigate some of these symptoms. In some cases, analgesics may be needed to treat pain and antibiotics to treat infection. Sepsis and autonomic dysreflexia are rarer outcomes but can occur. Patients should be reminded to report fever, chills, and ongoing or worsening hematuria to their HCP immediately. Bladder distention is the leading cause of dysreflexia, so encourage the patient to void frequently.

⊘ Related Tests

- Related tests include bladder cancer markers, calculus kidney stone panel, Chlamydia group antibody, CBC, CBC hematocrit, CBC hemoglobin, CT pelvis, culture urine, cytology urine, IVP, MRI pelvis, PT/INR, US pelvis, and UA.
- Refer to the Genitourinary System table at the end of the book for related tests by body system.

Expected Outcomes

Expected outcomes associated with Cystometry are

- Accurate identification of any abnormalities found upon examination of the bladder
- Effective implementation of therapies for patients diagnosed with bladder damage followed by an improvement in patient status
- Sleep that remains undisturbed by urinary urgency and frequency
- Maintenance of urinary elimination of 2,000 mL per day or greater without signs of infection or obstruction

REVIEW OF LEARNING OUTCOMES

Thinking

1. Recognize that as human beings we all have various strengths and weaknesses as team members. Answer: The amount of experience you have as a nurse highly influences your self–perception of competence as a team member. The best approach is in using your personal strengths and resources to enhance your limitations while focusing on your team's goal.
2. Identify concerns related to diagnostic procedures and older adults. Answer: Age changes everything. Problems that may not occur in a younger person will be evident in older adults. Be aware of the nuances presented on assessment so that problems can be accurately identified and addressed.

Doing

1. Incorporate elements of care using an integrated multidisciplinary approach. Answer: Coordination of care includes accurate communication about individual patient preferences and any information in the medical record that would be of concern in the performance of the procedure.
2. Identify safe nursing practices in follow-up patient care. Answer: Initiate education, emotional support, and counseling for positive results. Observe the patient for possible reactions, and assure that patients understand the follow-up care needed. Be sure that parents understand all aspects of care related to their minor child. Ensure understanding with an interpreter if necessary.
3. Develop and implement an individualized plan of care based on patient preferences and specific health-care needs. Answer: Healthy decisions are interwoven with culture, personal values, and individual goals. Try to discover what is most important to your patient; this will help you frame how to meet health-care goals. Always remember that if the patient is not on board, no plan can be successful. Understanding and integrating the patient's personal preferences and expressed needs will improve compliance with obtaining diagnostic studies.

Caring

1. Recognize that barriers to patient decision making can be resolved by providing resources that clarify misunderstanding. Answer: There are many times when the patient knows the correct decision but for personal reasons is unable to commit. Your job is to figure out what

the roadblock is and provide resources that will allow the patient to come to the decision that will promote his health. However, the reality is that patients do not always make the decision we want, but they always make the decision that they believe is best for them.

Words OF Wisdom: Although the number of diagnostic tests in this section is limited, their effect on the quality of life cannot be emphasized enough. The patient will be asking him- or herself, "will I be able to continue working, spending time with my friends, and maintaining the level of intimacy I want with my life partner?" Be sensitive to the patient's emotional issues; it is not all about getting to the diagnosis. In many ways, it is more about the effect the diagnosis will have within the context of each individual's life.

BIBLIOGRAPHY

Bernstein test. (2014). Retrieved from www.nlm.nih.gov/medlineplus/ency/article/003897.htm

Cavanaugh, B. (2003). Nurse's manual of laboratory and diagnostic tests (4th Ed.). Philadelphia, PA: F.A. Davis Company.

Cystometry. (n.d.). Retrieved from www.hopkinsmedicine.org/healthlibrary/test_procedures/urology/cystometry_92,P07718/

Esophageal manometric motility study. (2014). Retrieved from http://patients.dartmouth-hitchcock.org/gi/esophageal_manometric_motility_study.html

Fishbach, F., & Dunning, M. (2009). A manual of laboratory and diagnostic tests (8th ed.). Philadelphia, PA: Lippencott Williams & Wilkins.

Gastroesophageal reflux (GER) and gastroesophageal reflux disease (GERD) in children and teens. (2013). Retrieved from http://digestive.niddk.nih.gov/ddiseases/pubs/gerinchildren/#cause

Goldani, H., Staiano, A., Borrelli, O., Thapar, N., & Lindley, K. (2010). Pediatric esophageal high resolution manometry: Utility of a standardized protocol and size-adjusted pressure topography parameters. Retrieved from www.ncbi.nlm.nih.gov/pubmed/19953088

LeMone, P., Burke, K., & Baldoff, G. (2011). Medical surgical nursing, Critical thinking in patient care (5th ed.). Upper Saddle River, NJ: Pearson.

Pagana, K., & Pagana, T. (2010), Mosby's manual of diagnostic and laboratory tests (4th ed.) St. Louis, MO: Elsevier.

Plethysmography in the evaluation of lower limb deep vein thrombosis (DVT) and occlusive peripheral arterial disease (PAD). Retrieved from www.ghc.org/all-sites/clinical/criteria/pdf/plethysmography.pdf

Richter, J., & Friedenberg, F. (2010). Gastrointestinal and liver disease (9th ed.). Philadelphia, PA: Saunders Elsevier.

Schwarz SM, MD. Pediatric Gastroesophageal Reflux Workup. Retrieved from http://emedicine.medscape.com/article/930029-workup

Van Leeuwen, A., and Bladh, M. (2015). Davis's comprehensive handbook of laboratory and diagnostic tests with nursing implications (6th ed.). Philadelphia, PA: F. A. Davis Company.

Go to Section II of this book and www.davisplus.com for the Clinical Reasoning Tool and its case studies to provide you with a safe place to explore patient care situations. There are a total of 26 different case studies; 2 cases are presented for each of 13 body systems. One set of 13 cases are found in the Section II chapters, and a second set of 13 cases are available online at www.davisplus.com. Each case is designed with the specific goal of helping you to connect the dots of clinical reasoning. Cases are designed to reflect possible clinical scenarios; the outcomes may or may not be positive—you decide.

Magnetic Resonance Imaging Studies

OVERVIEW

What can be seen when a plain image of the abdomen is placed on the viewing monitor for interpretation? Not much really because the image is gray and flat and shows little detail. If such an image is unsatisfactory, then what else can be done? Magnetic resonance imaging (MRI) uses magnets and radio waves to help us view areas of the body under diagnostic inquiry. This process is not painful and is considered to be noninvasive. MRI creates images by using the body's hydrogen ions as a point of reference, capturing how they behave when disrupted and realigned. This realignment creates images that allow us to see alterations in anatomy such as tumor and infection, and alterations of function such as blood flow. MRI images are presented as pictorial slices of the body with many images taken over a very short period of time. Images are detailed and clear without interference from the presence of fluid-filled tissue or bone. Images can be of a specific organ or a specific part of the body. Cross-sectional or multiplane views can be taken of an entire body. Transverse, coronal, or sagittal views can be taken of an area of interest. The detailed images collected are sent to the computer for storage. Stored images can be used diagnostically for initial diagnoses, review, and therapeutic evaluation. MRI units may be closed or open systems (see Fig. 12.1). Open units are more spacious and are used for pediatric patients or for those who are claustrophobic. Magnet strengths range from 0.5 to 3 Tesla, an international unit of magnetic flux density. The higher the Tesla magnetic strength, the better is the image quality. An advantage of MRI over other diagnostic tools is that it does not use ionizing radiation and can be useful for serial studies. Because magnets are the primary factor in performing this study, nurses must be vigilant in screening patients for implanted metal in

their bodies. Such a circumstance makes the patient ineligible for an MRI, and this should be communicated immediately to the health-care provider (HCP) and MRI technician.

Disadvantages of MRI use include cost and the necessity of the patient to remain immobile for extended periods of time. Ongoing technology improvements allow for MRI to be used in other specific ways. Magnetic resonance angiography (MRA) provides clear images of arterial blood flow and blockage associated with aneurysm, anatomical variants, vascular

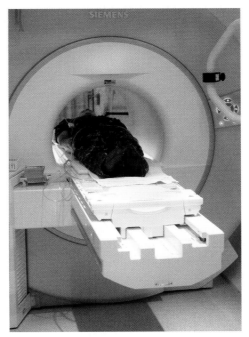

FIGURE 12.1 MRI unit. *MRI unit, released into public domain by the United States Navy. Photograph by Lance Cpl. Jonathan G. Wright. Retrieved from http://commons .wikimedia.org/wiki/File:USMC-101012-M-3392W-002.jpg*

malformations, and renal stenosis. In a similar manner, magnetic resonance venography (MRV) allows for visualization of the veins in relation to concerns such as atherosclerotic vascular disease. Magnetic resonance spectrometry (MRS) can be used to investigate body chemical distribution in multiple diseases where a more invasive procedure would place the patient at risk. Examples include HIV, Alzheimer disease, multiple sclerosis, stroke, head injury, and myocardial metabolism. Contrast in the form of a water-soluble gadolinium can be given in an oral, IV, or inhalation form and is considered safe for adult and pediatric patients. Contrast is used to gain better images of the anatomy under diagnostic inquiry. Successful pediatric imaging is dependent on the age and ability of the child to follow directions. Sedation or physical restraint may be necessary in some circumstances for body imaging. The use of sedation for extremity blood flow imaging is not recommended as it interferes with blood flow assessment. Adverse reactions to the contrast may include vomiting, respiratory distress, itching, dizziness, and headache. Some patients will complain of unusual oral sensations. Contrast can cross the placental barrier, enter the fetal circulation, and pass via the kidneys into the amniotic fluid. Although no definite adverse effects on the human fetus have been documented, the potential bio-effects of fetal exposure are not well understood. Administration should therefore be avoided during pregnancy unless no suitable alternative imaging is possible and the benefits of contrast administration outweigh the potential risk to the fetus. The value in the use of contrast is in the enhanced nature of the images.

Special Considerations

Gadolinium-based contrast agents such as Magnevist, Omniscan, OptiMark, and ProHance have been linked to the development of nephrogenic systemic fibrosis (NSF). Gadolinium-associated NSF, also known as nephrogenic fibrosing dermopathy (NFD), is a systemic disorder affecting patients with renal insufficiency who have been exposed to gadolinium-based contrast agents. Signs and symptoms resemble scleroderma with the most prominent and visible effects noted in the skin; thickening of the skin may advance to the stage where flexing of the joints becomes significantly impaired and impedes normal movement. Contrast agents containing iodine or gadolinium are primarily excreted by the kidneys. For this reason, patients over the age of 70 or with known renal insufficiency should have their renal function assessed before using contrast. This can be done simply by assessing blood urea nitrogen (BUN) and creatinine levels. Elevated creatinine and BUN levels are indicative of decreased kidney function. Creatinine and urea nitrogen are waste products that the kidneys normally remove from the blood. When the kidneys are not functioning properly, these substances may build up in the blood.

The information in the Part I studies is organized in a manner to help the student see how the five basic components of the nursing process (assessment, diagnosis, planning, implementation, and evaluation) can be applied to each phase of laboratory and diagnostic testing. The goal is to use nursing process to understand the integration of care (laboratory, diagnostic, nursing care) toward achieving a positive expected outcome.

- **Assessment** is the collection of information for the purpose of answering the question, "is there a problem?" Knowledge of the patient's health history, medications, complaints, and allergies as well as synonyms or alternate test names, common use for the procedure, specimen requirements, and normal ranges or interpretive comments provide the foundation for diagnosis.
- **Diagnosis** is the process of looking at the information gathered during assessment and answering the questions, "what is the problem?" and "what do I need to do about it?" Test indications tell us why the study has been requested, and potential diagnoses tell us the value or importance of the study relative to its clinical utility.
- **Planning** is a blueprint of the nursing care before the procedure. It is the process of determining how the nurse is going to partner with the patient to fix the problem (e.g., "The patient has a study ordered and this is what I should know before I successfully carry out the plan to have the study completed."). Knowledge of interfering factors, social and cultural issues, preprocedural restrictions, the need for written and informed consent, anxiety about the procedure, and concerns regarding pain are some considerations for planning a successful partnership.
- **Implementation** is putting the plan into action with an idea of what the expected outcome should be. Collaboration with the departments where the laboratory test or diagnostic study is to be performed is essential to the success of the plan. Implementation is where the work is done within each healthcare team member's scope of practice.
- **Evaluation** answers the question, "did the plan work or not?" Was the plan completely successful, partially successful, or not successful? If the plan did not work, evaluation is the process where you determine what needs to be changed to make the plan work better. This includes a review of all expected outcomes. Nursing care after the procedure is where information is gathered to evaluate the plan. Review of results, including critical findings, in relation to patient symptoms and other tests performed provide data that form a more complete picture of health or illness.

- **Expected Outcomes** are positive outcomes related to the test. They are the outcomes the nurse should expect if all goes well.

A number of pretest, intratest, and post-test universal points are presented in this overview section because the information applies to MRI studies in general.

Universal Pretest Pearls (Planning)

- Obtain a history of the patient's complaints, including a list of known allergens, especially allergies or sensitivities to medications or latex so their use can be avoided or their effects mitigated if an allergy is present. Carefully evaluate all medications currently being taken by the patient. A list of the patient's current medications, prescribed and over the counter (including anticoagulants, aspirin and other salicylates, and dietary supplements), should also be obtained. Such products may be discontinued by medical direction for the appropriate number of days prior to the procedure. Ensure that all allergies are clearly noted in the medical record, and ensure that the patient is wearing an allergy and medical record armband. Report information that could interfere with, or delay proceeding with, the study to the HCP and laboratory.
- Obtain a history of the patient's affected body system, symptoms, and results of previously performed laboratory tests and diagnostic and surgical procedures. Previous test results will provide a basis of comparison between old and new data.
- An important aspect of planning is understanding the factors that may alter study findings or cause abnormal results. Interdepartmental communication is a key factor in the planning process. The inability of a patient to cooperate or remain still during the procedure because of age, significant pain, or mental status should be among the anticipated factors. Recent or past procedures, medications, or existing medical conditions that could complicate or interfere with test results should be noted.
- Review the steps of the study with the patient or caregiver. Expect patients to be nervous about the procedure and the pending results. Educating the patient on his or her role during the procedure and what to expect can facilitate this. The patient's role during the procedure is to remain still. The actual time required to complete each study will depend on a number of conditions, including the type of equipment being used and how well a patient will cooperate.

- Address any concerns about pain and explain or describe, as appropriate, the level and type of discomfort that may be expected. Explain that an IV line may be inserted prior to some procedures to allow the infusion of IV fluids such as normal saline, contrast medium, or medications. Advise the patient that some discomfort may be experienced during the insertion of the IV. Make the patient aware that there may be some mild discomfort during the procedure.
- Provide additional instructions and patient preparation regarding medication, diet, fluid intake, or activity, if appropriate. Unless specified in the individual study, there are no special instructions or restrictions.
- Always be sensitive to any cultural or psychosocial issues, including a concern for modesty before, during, and after the procedure.

Reminder

Ensure that a written and informed consent has been documented in the medical record prior to the study, if required. The consent must be obtained before medication is administered.

Universal Intratest Pearls (Implementation)

- Correct patient identification is crucial prior to any procedure. Positively identify the patient using two unique identifiers such as patient name, date of birth, Social Security number, or medical record number.
- Standard Precautions must be followed.
- Children and infants may be accompanied by a parent to calm them. Keep neonates and infants covered and in a warm room, and provide a pacifier or gentle touch. The testing environment should be quiet, and the patient should be instructed, as appropriate, to remain still during the test as extraneous movements can affect results.
- Ensure the patient has complied with pretesting instructions, including dietary, fluid, medication, and activity restrictions as given for the procedure.
- The patient as appropriate, should be prepared for insertion of an IV line for infusion of IV fluids, contrast medium, antibiotics, anesthetics, analgesics, medications used in the procedure, or emergency medications. Inform the patient when prophylactic antibiotics will be administered before the procedure and assess for antibiotic allergy. Prior to administration of any fluids or medications, verify that they are accurate for the study. Bleeding or bruising can be prevented once the needle has been removed by applying direct pressure to the injection site with dry gauze for a minute or two.

The site should be observed/assessed for bleeding or hematoma formation and then covered with a gauze and adhesive bandage.

- Emergency equipment must be readily available.
- Baseline vital signs must be recorded and continuously monitored throughout and after the procedure, according to organizational policy. A comparison should be made between the baseline and postprocedure vital signs and focused assessments. Protocols may vary among facilities.

Universal Post Test Pearls (Evaluation)

- Note that completed test results are made available to the requesting HCP, who will discuss them with the patient.
- Answer questions and address concerns voiced by the patient or family, and reinforce information given by the patient's HCP regarding further testing, treatment, or referral to another HCP. Recognize that patients will have anxiety related to test results. Provide teaching and information regarding the clinical implications of the test results on the patient's lifestyle, as appropriate.
- Note that test results should be evaluated in context with the patient's signs, symptoms, and diagnosis. Depending on the results of the procedure, additional testing may be performed to evaluate or monitor progression of the disease process and determine the need for a change in therapy.
- Be aware that when a person goes through a traumatic event such as an illness or being given information that will impact his or her lifestyle, there are universal human reactions that occur. These include knowledge deficit, fear, anxiety, and coping; in some situations grieving may occur. HCPs should always be aware of the human response and how it may affect the plan of care and expected outcomes.

DISCUSSION POINT

Regarding Post-Test Critical Findings: Timely notification of a critical finding for lab or diagnostic studies is a role expectation of the professional nurse. Notification processes will vary among facilities. Upon receipt of the critical finding, the information should be read back to the caller to verify accuracy. Most policies require immediate notification of the primary HCP, hospitalist, or on-call HCP. Reported information includes the patient's name, unique identifiers, critical finding, name of the person giving the report, and name of the person receiving the report. Documentation of notification should be made in the medical record with the name

of the HCP notified, time and date of notification, and any orders received. Any delay in a timely report of a critical finding may require completion of a notification form with review by Risk Management.

STUDIES

- Magnetic Resonance Angiography
- Magnetic Resonance Imaging, Abdomen
- Magnetic Resonance Imaging, Brain
- Magnetic Resonance Imaging, Chest
- Magnetic Resonance Imaging, Musculoskeletal

LEARNING OUTCOMES

Providing safe, effective nursing care (SENC) includes mastery of core competencies and standards of care. SENC is based on a judicious application of nursing knowledge in combination with scientific principles. The Art of Nursing lies in blending what you know with the ability to effectively apply your knowledge in a compassionate manner.

After reading/studying this chapter, you will be able to:

Thinking

1. Recognize that human beings are imperfect, and failure to follow policy and standards of care or participate in work-arounds can place a patient at risk.
2. Describe the safety risks associated with MRI procedures.

Doing

1. Recognize that memory can be imperfect, and the use of assistive resources (checklists, electronic tablets, etc.) can reduce errors involving patient care.

Caring

1. Recognize the presence of both cognitive and physical personal limitations in the performance of care.
2. Recognize the merit of collaborating with patient, family, and significant others to design, implement, and evaluate the plan of care.

Magnetic Resonance Angiography

Quick Summary

SYNONYM ACRONYM: MRA.

COMMON USE: To visualize and assess blood flow in diseased and normal vessels toward diagnosis of vascular disease and to monitor and evaluate therapeutic interventions.

AREA OF APPLICATION: Vascular.

- Normal blood flow in the area being examined, including blood flow rate

Test Explanation

Magnetic resonance imaging (MRI) is very useful when the area of interest is soft tissue. The technology does not involve radiation exposure and is considered safer than other imaging methods such as radiographs and computed tomography (CT). MRI uses a magnet and radio waves to produce an energy field that can be displayed as an image of the anatomic area of interest based on the water content of the tissue. The magnetic field causes the hydrogen atoms in tissue to line up, and when radio waves are directed toward the magnetic field, the hydrogen atoms absorb the radio waves and change their position. This change in the energy field is detected by the equipment, and an image is generated by the equipment's computer system. MRI produces cross-sectional images of the vessels in multiple planes without the use of ionizing radiation or the interference of bone or surrounding tissue. Images can be obtained in two-dimensional (series of slices) or three-dimensional sequences. Standard or closed MRI equipment has the appearance of an open tube or tunnel; open MRI equipment has no sides and provides an alternative for patients who suffer from claustrophobia, pediatric patients, or patients who are obese. IV gadolinium-based contrast media may be used to better visualize the vessels and tissues in the area of interest. Clear, high-quality images of abnormalities and disease processes significantly improve the diagnostic value of the study.

Magnetic resonance angiography (MRA) is an application of MRI that provides images of blood flow and diseased and normal blood vessels. In patients who are allergic to iodinated contrast medium, MRA is used in place of angiography. MRA is particularly useful for visualizing vascular abnormalities, dissections, and other pathology. Special imaging sequences allow the visualization of moving blood within the vascular system, and two common techniques are used to obtain images of flowing blood: time-of-flight and phase-contrast MRA. In time-of-flight imaging, incoming blood makes the vessels appear bright, and surrounding tissue is suppressed. Phase-contrast images are produced by subtracting the stationary tissue surrounding the vessels where the blood is moving through vessels during the imaging, producing high-contrast images. MRA is the most accurate technique for imaging blood flowing in veins and small arteries (*laminar flow*), but it does not accurately depict blood flow in tortuous sections of vessels and distal to bifurcations and stenosis. Swirling blood may cause a signal loss and result in inadequate images, and the degree of vessel stenosis may be overestimated.

Magnetic resonance spectroscopy (MRS) is an application of MRI based on the same principles as MRI but instead of an anatomical image, the data is displayed graphically as a series of peaks. The peaks represent specific elements and compounds that provide physiological data regarding the tissue of interest. MRS can be performed using MRI equipment with software adapted for the collection and interpretation of spectral data. MRS may be used alone or in conjunction with MRI where anatomical images are first collected by MRI followed by focused MRS images that reflect specific active metabolic processes. The frequency information used in MRS identifies specific chemical compounds such as amino acids, lipids, and lactate that are commonly involved in or produced by cellular activity. The presence or absence of different metabolites in the spectral analysis can be used to identify metabolic activity associated with a suspected tumor, differentiate between tumor types, provide information about cardiac metabolism and cardiovascular dysfunction (myocardial ischemia, heart failure, peripheral vascular disease), or monitor response to therapeutic interventions. Other applications of MRS include studies of brain lesions (brain tumors, Alzheimer disease), inborn errors of metabolism (glycogen storage diseases), insulin resistance, and conditions involving skeletal muscle (muscular dystrophies).

Nursing Implications
Assessment

Indications	Potential Nursing Problems
Detect pericardial abnormalities	• Activity
Detect peripheral arterial disease (PAD)	• Bleeding
Detect thoracic and abdominal vascular diseases	• Breathing
Determine renal artery stenosis	• Cardiac Output
Differentiate aortic aneurysms from tumors near the aorta	• Confusion
Evaluate cardiac chambers and pulmonary vessels	• Fear
Evaluate postoperative angioplasty sites and bypass grafts	• Human Response
Identify congenital vascular diseases	• Infection
Monitor and evaluate the effectiveness of medical or surgical treatment	• Pain
	• Renal
	• Self-Care
	• Sexuality
	• Tissue Perfusion

Diagnosis: Clinical Significance of Test Results

ABNORMAL FINDINGS

- Aortic aneurysm
- Coarctations
- Dissections
- PAD
- Thrombosis within a vessel
- Tumor invasion of a vessel
- Vascular abnormalities
- Vessel occlusion
- Vessel stenosis

Planning

Considerations for planning a successful partnership should include clear communication of what to expect during the test to decrease anxiety and improve cooperation. Ensure the results of BUN, creatinine, and eGFR (estimated glomerular filtration rate) are obtained if GBCA is to be used. Ask if the patient has ever had any device implanted into his or her body. Obtain occupational history to determine the presence of metal in the body, such as shrapnel or flecks of ferrous metal in the eye (which can cause retinal hemorrhage). Before the procedure is performed, plan to review the steps with the patient. Explain that the procedure is usually performed in an MRI suite by an MRI technologist and takes approximately 30 to 60 minutes. Inform the patient that he or she will be lying on a flat table and placed into a cylindrical scanner for this study. Many people are fearful of pain when faced with an unknown situation. Clear communication of any potential discomfort is advised. Explain that the scanner produces a loud banging noise during the actual imaging and also that magnetophosphenes may be seen (flickering lights in the visual field); these will stop when the procedure is over. Explain that earplugs or earphones may be used to muffle the banging noise generated by the MRI machine. Explain that an IV line may be inserted to allow infusion of IV fluids such as saline, anesthetics, contrast medium, or sedatives.

CONTRAINDICATIONS

- Patients who are pregnant or suspected of being pregnant, unless the potential benefits of the MRI far outweigh the risks to the fetus and mother. *In pregnancy, gadolinium-based contrast agents (GBCAs) cross the placental barrier, enter the fetal circulation, and pass via the kidneys into the amniotic fluid. Although no definite adverse effects of GBCA administration on the human fetus have been documented, the potential bioeffects of fetal GBCA exposure are not well understood. GBCA administration should therefore be avoided during pregnancy unless no suitable alternative imaging is possible and the benefits of contrast administration outweigh the potential risk to the fetus.*
- Patients with moderate to marked renal impairment (glomerular filtration rate less than 30 mL/min/1.73 m^2); patients should be screened for renal dysfunction prior to administration. The use of GBCAs should be avoided in these patients unless the benefits of the studies outweigh the risks and if essential diagnostic information is not available using non–contrast-enhanced diagnostic studies.
- Patients with cardiac pacemakers, which can be deactivated by MRI
- Patients with metal in their body, such as dental amalgams, metallic body piercing items, tattoo inks containing iron (including tattooed eyeliners), shrapnel, bullet, ferrous metal in the eye, certain ferrous metal prosthetics, valves, aneurysm clips, intrauterine device (IUD), inner ear prostheses, or other metallic objects; these items can impair image quality. Metallic objects are also a significant safety issue for patients and health-care staff in the examination room during performance of an MRI. The MRI equipment consists of an extremely powerful magnet that can inactivate, move, or shift metallic objects inside a patient. Many metallic objects currently used in health-care procedures are made of materials that do not interfere with MRI studies; it is important for the patient to provide specific information regarding medical procedures he or she has undergone in order to identify whether the device is safe to undergo MRI. Required information includes the date of the procedure and identification of the device. Metallic objects are not allowed inside the room with the MRI equipment because items such as watches, credit cards, and car keys can become dangerous projectiles.
- Patients with transdermal patches containing metallic components; the patch's liner contains a metal that controls absorption of the substance from the patch (e.g., drugs, nicotine, steroids, hormones). The patch may cause burns to the skin *related to energy conducted through the metal, which is converted to heat during the MRI.* Other metallic objects on the skin may also cause burns.
- Patients who are claustrophobic
- Extremely obese patients whose weight cannot be supported by the table
- Patients whose physical condition is unstable, requiring the use of equipment that can be affected by the magnet

● Safety Tip

Make sure a written and informed consent has been signed prior to the procedure and before administering any medications.

Implementation

Patient education is key to obtaining the patient's cooperation in following directions, and providing an explanation for the purpose of the procedure is an important part of this process. Inform the patient that this study can assist in the detection of diseased blood vessels. Establish an IV fluid line for the injection of IV fluids such as saline, anesthetics, contrast medium, or sedatives. Ensure the patient is in compliance with pretesting instructions and that ordered premedications for allergies or anxiety have been administered. Instruct the patient to void prior to the procedure and to change into the gown, robe, and foot coverings provided. Explain to the patient that he or she will be placed on a table and remind him or her to lie very still during the procedure. Remind the patient that this study involves no radiation exposure, and supply earplugs to the patient to block out the loud, banging sounds that occur during the test. Instruct the patient to communicate with the technologist during the examination via a microphone within the scanner. If an electrocardiogram or respiratory gating is to be performed in conjunction with the scan, apply MRI-safe electrodes to the appropriate sites. Instruct the patient to take slow, deep breaths if nausea occurs during the procedure. Tell the patient that following the IV injection of 10 to 15 mL of gadolinium, the table is advanced into the scanner and imaging begins immediately. Ask the patient to inhale deeply and hold his or her breath while the images are taken, and then to exhale after the images are taken. During the imaging, monitor the patient for complications related to the procedure (e.g., allergic reaction, anaphylaxis, or bronchospasm). When the study has been completed, remove the needle or catheter and apply a pressure dressing over the puncture site. Observe/assess the needle/catheter insertion site for bleeding, inflammation, or hematoma formation.

Evaluation

Recognize anxiety related to test results and be supportive of impaired activity related to a perceived loss of independence. Observe for delayed allergic reactions, such as rash, urticaria, tachycardia, hyperpnea, hypertension, palpitations, nausea, or vomiting. Instruct the patient to immediately report symptoms such as fast heart rate, difficulty breathing, skin rash, itching, chest pain, persistent right shoulder pain, or abdominal pain. Immediately report symptoms to the appropriate health-care provider (HCP). Instruct the patient in the care and assessment of the injection site. Instruct the patient to apply cold compresses to the puncture site as needed to reduce discomfort or edema. Discuss the implications of abnormal test results on the patient's lifestyle. Provide teaching and information regarding the clinical implications of the test results as appropriate. Provide contact information, if desired, for the American Heart Association (www.americanheart.org), the National Heart, Lung, and Blood Institute (NHLBI) (www.nhlbi.nih.gov), or Legs for Life (www.legsforlife.org).

◉ Critical Findings

- Aortic aneurysm
- Aortic dissection
- Occlusion
- Tumor with significant mass effect
- Vertebral artery dissection

Note and immediately report to the requesting HCP any critical findings and related symptoms. A listing of these findings varies among facilities.

◉ Study Specific Complications

Complications are rare but do include risk for allergic reaction **related to contrast reaction.** It is important to have oxygen and endotracheal equipment in the vicinity for immediate use. In the event of an anaphylactic reaction, epinephrine, diphenhydramine, and steroids are included with resuscitative efforts.

Contrast Reactions: Signs, Symptoms and Treatment

	Minor	Intermediate	Life Threatening
Signs and Symptoms	Nausea, vomiting, urticaria, sneezing	Bronchospasms; chills and fever; chest pain, or laryngeal or tongue edema	Hypotension, cardiac dysrhythmias; seizures; lose of bowel/bladder control; laryngeal and pulmonary edema
Interventions	Antihistamines	Antihistamines, steroids, bronchodilators, IV fluids, and observation	All intermediate interventions plus intubation and ventilation, pressors, and antiseizure medications

Other complications related to the procedure may include:

- Cardiac dysrhythmias
- Acute kidney injury as a result of contrast infusion; hydration prior to the study can reduce the likelihood of this complication.
- Some patients are at risk for developing nephrogenic systemic fibrosis (NSF) as a result of the use of gadolinium-based contrast agents *related to ineffective renal clearance in patients with impaired renal function.*
- Injection of the contrast or other fluids through IV tubing into a blood vessel is an invasive procedure. There are a number of complications associated with performing a venipuncture. **Pain** is commonly associated with needles, and although the pain experienced during venipuncture is usually mild, on a rare occasion the needle may strike a nerve, causing permanent pain. Some patients experience a **vasovagal reaction** during the venipuncture procedure, evidenced by sweating, low blood pressure, fainting, or near fainting. The potential for a **fall injury** is a significant concern related to vasovagal reactions. Prolonged **bleeding** is a complication that occurs with patients who are taking blood thinners or who have coagulopathies such as hemophilia. A **hematoma** results when blood leaks into the tissue during or after a venipuncture, as evidenced by pain, bruising, and/or swelling at the venipuncture site. The swelling can cause injury by compression to surrounding nerves, which can be temporary or permanent. HCPs should watch for minor complications such as bruising and hematoma at the venipuncture site, which are fairly common. Hematomas occur more often in older adult or frail patients, or those with veins that are difficult to access. Bleeding or bruising can be prevented once the needle has been removed by applying direct pressure to the site with dry gauze for a minute or two. Some other more unusual complications of venipuncture include **cellulitis, phlebitis, inadvertent arterial puncture,** and **sepsis.** Sepsis can be caused by the introduction of bacteria from the surface of the skin into the blood as the result of improper cleansing of the venipuncture site. Immunocompromised patients are at higher risk for developing this complication. Elevated temperatures, abnormal-colored sputum, changes in breathing patterns, chills, and hypotension can all indicate infection or sepsis. Antibiotic therapy should be ordered if this occurs.

⊘ Related Tests

- Related tests include angiography of the body area of interest, BUN, CT angiography, creatinine, US arterial Doppler carotid, and US venous Doppler.
- Refer to the Cardiovascular System table at the end of the book for related tests by body system.

Expected Outcomes

Expected outcomes associated with Magnetic Resonance Angiography are:

- Maintenance of stable vital signs during the diagnostic process
- Freedom from the signs and symptoms of bleeding or rupture
- Understanding of the importance of repeat imaging to evaluate the status of the disease process
- Collaboration with the HCP to develop an effective treatment plan

Magnetic Resonance Imaging, Abdomen

Quick Summary

SYNONYM ACRONYM: Abdominal MRI.

COMMON USE: To visualize and assess abdominal and hepatic structures toward diagnosis of tumors, metastasis, aneurysm, and abscess. Also used to monitor medical and surgical therapeutic interventions.

AREA OF APPLICATION: Liver and abdominal area.

- Normal anatomic structures, soft tissue density, and biochemical constituents of body tissues, including blood flow

Test Explanation

Magnetic resonance imaging (MRI) is very useful when the area of interest is soft tissue. The technology does not involve radiation exposure and is considered safer than other imaging methods such as radiographs and computed tomography (CT). MRI uses a magnet and radio waves to produce an energy field that can be displayed as an image of the anatomic area of interest based on the water content of the tissue. The magnetic field causes the hydrogen atoms in tissue to line up, and when radio waves are directed toward the magnetic field, the hydrogen atoms absorb the radio waves and change their position; this change in the energy field is detected by the equipment, and an image is generated by the equipment's computer system. MRI produces cross-sectional images of the abdomen in multiple planes without the use of ionizing radiation or the interference of bone or surrounding tissue. Images can be obtained in two-dimensional (series of slices) or three-dimensional sequences. Standard or closed MRI equipment has the appearance of an open tube or tunnel; open MRI equipment has no sides and provides an alternative for patients who suffer from claustrophobia, pediatric patients, or patients who are obese. IV gadolinium-based contrast media may be used to better visualize the vessels and tissues in the area of interest. Clear, high-quality images of abnormalities and disease processes significantly improve the diagnostic value of the study.

Abdominal MRI is performed to assist in diagnosing abnormalities of abdominal and hepatic structures. Contrast-enhanced imaging is effective for distinguishing peritoneal metastases from primary tumors of the gastrointestinal (GI) tract. Primary tumors of the stomach, pancreas, colon, and appendix often spread by intraperitoneal tumor shedding and subsequent peritoneal carcinomatosis. MRI uses the noniodinated paramagnetic contrast medium gadopentetate dimeglumine (Magnevist), which is administered IV to enhance differences between normal and abnormal tissues.

Magnetic resonance cholangiopancreatography (MRCP) is an imaging technique used specifically to evaluate the hepatobiliary system that is comprised of the liver, gallbladder, bile ducts, pancreas, and pancreatic ducts. MRCP is a less invasive way than Endoscopic retrograde cholangiopancreatography (ERCP) to investigate abdominal pain, suspected malignancy, gall stones, or pancreatitis.

Nursing Implications

Assessment

Indications	Potential Nursing Problems
Detect abdominal aortic diseases	• Activity
Detect and stage cancer (primary or metastatic tumors of liver, pancreas, prostate, uterus, and bladder)	• Bleeding
	• Cardiac Output
	• Confusion
Detect chronic pancreatitis	• Fear
Detect renal vein thrombosis	• Grief
Detect soft tissue abnormalities	• Health Management
Determine and monitor tissue damage in renal transplant patients	• Human Response
	• Renal
Determine the presence of blood clots, cysts, fluid or fat accumulation in tissues, hemorrhage, and infarctions	• Self-Care
	• Sexuality
	• Tissue Perfusion
Determine vascular complications of pancreatitis, venous thrombosis, or pseudoaneurysm	
Differentiate aortic aneurysms from tumors near the aorta	
Differentiate liver tumors from liver abnormalities, such as cysts, cavernous hemangiomas, and hepatic amebic abscesses	
Evaluate postoperative angioplasty sites and bypass grafts	
Monitor and evaluate the effectiveness of medical or surgical interventions and the course of the disease	

Diagnosis: Clinical Significance of Test Results

ABNORMAL FINDINGS

- Acute tubular necrosis
- Aneurysm
- Cholangitis
- Glomerulonephritis
- Hydronephrosis
- Internal bleeding
- Masses, lesions, infections, or inflammations
- Renal vein thrombosis
- Vena cava obstruction

Planning

Considerations for planning a successful partnership should include clear communication of what to expect during the test to decrease anxiety and improve cooperation. Ensure the results of BUN, creatinine, and eGFR (estimated glomerular filtration rate) are obtained if GBCA is to be used. Ask if the patient has ever had any device implanted into his or her body. Obtain occupational history to determine the presence of metal in the body, such as shrapnel or flecks of ferrous metal in the eye (which can cause retinal hemorrhage). Before the procedure is performed, plan to review the steps with the patient. Explain that the procedure is usually performed in an MRI suite by an MRI technologist, and takes approximately 30 to 60 minutes. Inform the patient that he or she will be lying on a flat table and placed into a cylindrical scanner for this study. Many people are fearful of pain when faced with an unknown situation. Clear communication of any potential discomfort is advised. Explain that the scanner produces a loud banging noise during the actual imaging and also that magnetophosphenes may be seen (flickering lights in the visual field); these will stop when the procedure is over. Explain that earplugs or earphones may be used to muffle the banging noise generated by the MRI machine. Explain that an IV line may be inserted to allow the infusion of IV fluids such as saline, anesthetics, contrast medium, or sedatives.

CONTRAINDICATIONS

- Patients who are pregnant or suspected of being pregnant, unless the potential benefits of the MRI far outweigh the risks to the fetus and mother. *In pregnancy, gadolinium-based contrast agents (GBCAs) cross the placental barrier, enter the fetal circulation, and pass via the kidneys into the amniotic fluid. Although no definite adverse effects of GBCA administration on the human fetus have been documented, the potential bioeffects of fetal GBCA exposure are not well understood. GBCA administration should therefore be avoided during pregnancy unless no suitable alternative imaging is possible and the benefits of contrast administration outweigh the potential risk to the fetus.*

- Patients with moderate to marked renal impairment (glomerular filtration rate less than 30 mL/min/1.73 m²); patients should be screened for renal dysfunction prior to administration. The use of GBCAs should be avoided in these patients unless the benefits of the studies outweigh the risks and if essential diagnostic information is not available using non–contrast-enhanced diagnostic studies.
- Patients with cardiac pacemakers, which can be deactivated by MRI
- Patients with metal in their body, such as dental amalgams, metallic body piercing items, tattoo inks containing iron (including tattooed eyeliners), shrapnel, bullet, ferrous metal in the eye, certain ferrous metal prosthetics, valves, aneurysm clips, intrauterine device (IUD), inner ear prostheses, or other metallic objects; these items can impair image quality. Metallic objects are also a significant safety issue for patients and health-care staff in the examination room during performance of an MRI. The MRI equipment consists of an extremely powerful magnet that can inactivate, move, or shift metallic objects inside a patient. Many metallic objects currently used in health-care procedures are made of materials that do not interfere with MRI studies; it is important for the patient to provide specific information regarding medical procedures he or she has undergone in order to identify whether the device is safe to undergo MRI. Required information includes the date of the procedure and identification of the device. Metallic objects are not allowed inside the room with the MRI equipment because items such as watches, credit cards, and car keys can become dangerous projectiles.
- Patients with transdermal patches containing metallic components. The patch's liner contains a metal that controls absorption of the substance from the patch (e.g., drugs, nicotine, steroids, hormones). The patch may cause burns to the skin *related to energy conducted through the metal, which is converted to heat during the MRI.* Other metallic objects on the skin may also cause burns.
- Patients who are claustrophobic
- Extremely obese patients whose weight cannot be supported by the table
- Patients whose physical condition is unstable, requiring the use of equipment that can be affected by the magnet

● Safety Tip

Make sure a written and informed consent has been signed prior to the procedure and before administering any medications.

Implementation

Patient education is key to obtaining the patient's cooperation in following directions, and providing an explanation for the purpose of the procedure is an important part of this process. Inform the patient that this study can assist in the detection of abnormalities of the abdomen or liver. Establish an IV fluid line for the injection of IV fluids such as saline, anesthetics, contrast medium, or sedatives. Ensure the patient is in compliance with pretesting instructions and that ordered premedications for allergies or anxiety have been administered. Instruct the patient to void prior to the procedure and to change into the gown, robe, and foot coverings provided. Explain to the patient that he or she will be placed on a table and remind the patient to lie very still during the procedure. Remind the patient that this study involves no radiation exposure, and supply earplugs to the patient to block out the loud, banging sounds that occur during the test. Instruct the patient to communicate with the technologist during the examination via a microphone within the scanner. If an electrocardiogram or respiratory gating is to be performed in conjunction with the scan, apply MRI-safe electrodes to the appropriate sites. Instruct the patient to take slow, deep breaths if nausea occurs during the procedure. Tell the patient that following the IV injection of 10 to 15 mL of gadolinium, the table is advanced into the scanner and imaging begins immediately (see Fig. 12.2). Ask the patient to inhale deeply and hold his or her breath while the images are taken, and then to exhale after the images are taken. During the imaging, monitor the patient for complications related to the procedure (e.g., allergic reaction, anaphylaxis, or bronchospasm). When the study has been completed, remove the needle or catheter and apply a pressure dressing over the puncture site. Observe/assess the needle/catheter insertion site for bleeding, inflammation, or hematoma formation.

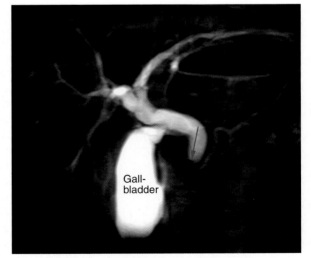

Gall-bladder

FIGURE 12.2 MRCP showing dilated biliary system secondary to calculus (arrow). *Used with permission, from Weber, E., Vilensky, J., & Fog, A. (2013). Practical radiology: a system-based approach. FA Davis Company.*

Evaluation

Recognize anxiety related to test results and be supportive of impaired activity related to a perceived loss of independence. Observe for delayed allergic reactions, such as rash, urticaria, tachycardia, hyperpnea, hypertension, palpitations, nausea, or vomiting. Instruct the patient to immediately report symptoms such as fast heart rate, difficulty breathing, skin rash, itching, chest pain, persistent right shoulder pain, or abdominal pain. Immediately report symptoms to the appropriate health-care provider (HCP). Instruct the patient in the care and assessment of the injection site. Instruct the patient to apply cold compresses to the puncture site as needed to reduce discomfort or edema. Discuss the implications of abnormal test results on the patient's lifestyle. Provide teaching and information regarding the clinical implications of the test results, as appropriate.

Critical Findings

- Acute GI bleed
- Aortic aneurysm
- Infection
- Tumor with significant mass effect

Note and immediately report to the requesting HCP any critical findings and related symptoms. A listing of these findings varies among facilities.

Study Specific Complications

Complications are rare but do include risk for allergic reaction *related to contrast reaction.* It is important to have oxygen and endotracheal equipment in the vicinity for immediate use. In the event of an anaphylactic reaction, epinephrine, diphenhydramine, and steroids are included with resuscitative efforts.

Contrast Reactions: Signs, Symptoms and Treatment

	Minor	Intermediate	Life Threatening
Signs, Symptoms	Nausea, vomiting, urticaria, sneezing	Bronchospasms; chills and fever; chest pain, or laryngeal or tongue edema	Hypotension, cardiac dysrhythmias; seizures; loss of bowel/bladder control; laryngeal and pulmonary edema
Interventions	Antihistamines	Antihistamines, steroids, bronchodilators, IV fluids, and observation	All intermediate interventions plus intubation and ventilation, pressors, and antiseizure medications

Other complications related to the procedure may include:

- Cardiac dysrhythmias
- Acute kidney injury as a result of contrast infusion; hydration prior to the study can reduce the likelihood of this complication.
- Nephrogenic systemic fibrosis (NSF) may develop in some patients as a result of the use of gadolinium-based contrast agents *related to ineffective renal clearance in patients with impaired renal function.*
- Complications associated with performing injection and venipuncture. Injection of the contrast or other fluids through IV tubing into a blood vessel is an invasive procedure. There are a number of complications associated with performing a venipuncture. **Pain** is commonly associated with needles, and although the pain experienced during venipuncture is usually mild, on a rare occasion the needle may strike a nerve causing permanent pain. Some patients experience a **vasovagal reaction** during the venipuncture procedure, evidenced by sweating, low blood pressure, fainting, or near fainting. The potential for a **fall injury** is a significant concern related to vasovagal reactions. Prolonged **bleeding** is a complication that occurs with patients who are taking blood thinners or who have coagulopathies such as hemophilia. A **hematoma** results when blood leaks into the tissue during or after a venipuncture, as evidenced by pain, bruising, and/or swelling at the venipuncture site. The swelling can cause injury by compression to surrounding nerves, which can be temporary or permanent. HCPs should watch for minor complications such as bruising and hematoma at the venipuncture site, which are fairly common. Hematomas occur more often in older adult or frail patients, or those with veins that are difficult to access. Bleeding or bruising can be prevented once the needle has been removed by applying direct pressure to the site with dry gauze for a minute or two. Some other more unusual complications of venipuncture include **cellulitis, phlebitis, inadvertent arterial puncture, and sepsis.** Sepsis can be caused by the introduction of bacteria from the surface of the skin into the blood as the result of improper cleansing of the venipuncture site. Immunocompromised patients are at higher risk for developing this complication. Elevated temperatures, abnormal-colored

sputum, changes in breathing patterns, chills, and hypotension can all indicate infection or sepsis. Antibiotic therapy should be ordered if this occurs.

✓ *Related Tests*

- Related tests include angiography abdomen, BUN, CT abdomen, creatinine, GI blood loss scan, KUB study, US abdomen, and US liver and biliary system.
- Refer to the Gastrointestinal, Genitourinary, and Hepatobiliary systems tables at the end of the book for related tests by body system.

Expected Outcomes

Expected clinical and patient-focused outcomes associated with Magnetic Resonance Imaging, Abdomen, are

- Achieving oxygenation that remains greater than 92% without an increased work of breathing
- Demonstrating coping strategies related to the diagnostic test results
- Understanding the importance of compliance with the therapeutic regime to protect transplant health
- Making positive lifestyle changes that contribute to improved overall health

Magnetic Resonance Imaging, Brain

Quick Summary

SYNONYM ACRONYM: Brain MRI.

COMMON USE: To visualize and assess intracranial abnormalities related to tumor, bleeding, lesions, and infarct such as stroke.

AREA OF APPLICATION: Brain area.
- Normal anatomic structures, soft tissue density, blood flow rate, face, nasopharynx, neck, tongue, and brain

Test Explanation

Magnetic resonance imaging (MRI) is very useful when the area of interest is soft tissue. The technology does not involve radiation exposure and is considered safer than other imaging methods such as radiographs and computed tomography (CT). MRI uses a magnet and radio waves to produce an energy field that can be displayed as an image of the anatomic area of interest based on the water content of the tissue. The magnetic field causes the hydrogen atoms in tissue to line up, and when radio waves are directed toward the magnetic field, the hydrogen atoms absorb the radio waves and change their position. This change in the energy field is detected by the equipment, and an image is generated by the equipment's computer system. MRI produces cross-sectional images of pathological lesions of the brain in multiple planes without the use of ionizing radiation or the interference of bone or surrounding tissue. Images can be obtained in two-dimensional (series of slices) or three-dimensional sequences. Standard or closed MRI equipment has the appearance of an open tube or tunnel; open MRI equipment has no sides and provides an alternative for patients who suffer from claustrophobia, pediatric patients, or patients who are obese. IV gadolinium-based contrast media may be used to better visualize the vessels and tissues in the area of interest. Clear, high-quality images of abnormalities and disease processes significantly improve the diagnostic value of the study.

Standard brain MRI can distinguish solid, cystic, and hemorrhagic components of lesions. This procedure is done to aid in the diagnosis of intracranial abnormalities, including tumors, ischemia, infection, and multiple sclerosis, and in the assessment of brain maturation in pediatric patients. Rapidly flowing blood on spin-echo MRI appears as an absence of signal or a void in the vessel's lumen. Blood flow can be evaluated in the cavernous and carotid arteries. Contrast-enhanced imaging is effective for enhancing differences between normal and abnormal tissues. Aneurysms may be diagnosed without traditional iodine-based contrast angiography, and old clotted blood in the walls of the aneurysm appear white. MRI uses the noniodinated contrast medium gadopentetate dimeglumine (Magnevist), which is administered IV.

Functional MRI (fMRI) is a neuroimaging application of MRI used to study how the brain is working. It identifies changes in blood flow, reflected by changes in the level of blood oxygenation, in response to activity. fMRI can identify metabolic changes in normal, diseased, or injured brain tissue. It is also used in research to study which parts of the brain are responsible for speech, physical movement, thought, and sensations; this type of research is also called brain mapping, and it has significant implications in understanding and managing the effects of stroke, brain tumors, and diseases like Alzheimer disease. fMRI is based on the blood oxygen level–dependent (BOLD) contrast mechanism that takes advantage of the inherent paramagnetic quality of deoxyhemoglobin. In a properly performed study, the patient is asked to perform a task; the MRI scanner detects changes in the signal strength of brain water protons produced as blood oxygen levels change, and the corresponding strength of the natural paramagnetic signal of deoxyhemoglobin changes. Magnetic resonance spectroscopy (MRS) is an application of MRI based on the same principles as MRI but instead of an anatomical image, the data is displayed graphically as a series of peaks. The peaks represent specific elements and compounds that provide physiological data regarding the tissue of interest. MRS can be performed using MRI equipment with software adapted for the collection and interpretation of spectral data. MRS may be used alone or in conjunction with MRI where anatomical images are first collected by MRI followed by focused MRS images that reflect specific active metabolic processes. The frequency information used in MRS identifies specific chemical compounds such as amino acids, lipids, and lactate that are commonly involved in or produced by cellular activity. The presence or absence of different metabolites in the spectral analysis can be used to identify metabolic activity associated with a suspected tumor, differentiate between tumor types, provide information about brain lesions (brain tumors, Alzheimer disease), or monitor response to therapeutic interventions. Other applications of MRS include studies of inborn errors of metabolism (glycogen storage diseases), insulin resistance, cardiovascular dysfunction (myocardial ischemia, heart failure, peripheral vascular disease), and conditions involving skeletal muscle (muscular dystrophies).

Nursing Implications

Assessment

Indications	Potential Nursing Problems
Detect and locate brain tumors Detect cause of cerebrovascular accident, cerebral infarct, or hemorrhage Detect cranial bone, face, throat, and neck soft tissue lesions Evaluate the cause of seizures, such as intracranial infection, edema, or increased intracranial pressure Evaluate cerebral changes associated with dementia Evaluate demyelinating disorders Evaluate intracranial infections Evaluate optic and auditory nerves Evaluate the potential causes of headache, visual loss, and vomiting Evaluate shunt placement and function in patients with hydrocephalus Evaluate the solid, cystic, and hemorrhagic components of lesions Evaluate vascularity of the brain and vascular integrity Monitor and evaluate the effectiveness of medical or surgical interventions, chemotherapy, radiation therapy, and the course of disease	• Bleeding • Communication • Confusion • Fall Risk • Fear • Health Management • Human Response • Mobility • Pain • Role Performance • Self-Care • Sensory Perception • Sexuality

Diagnosis: Clinical Significance of Test Results
ABNORMAL FINDINGS
- Abscess
- Acoustic neuroma
- Alzheimer disease
- Aneurysm
- Arteriovenous malformation
- Benign meningioma
- Cerebral aneurysm
- Cerebral infarction
- Craniopharyngioma or meningioma
- Granuloma
- Intraparenchymal hematoma or hemorrhage
- Lipoma
- Metastasis
- Multiple sclerosis
- Optic nerve tumor
- Parkinson disease
- Pituitary microadenoma
- Subdural empyema
- Ventriculitis

Planning
Considerations for planning a successful partnership should include clear communication of what to expect during the test to decrease anxiety and improve cooperation. Ensure the results of BUN, creatinine, and eGFR (estimated glomerular filtration rate) are obtained if gadolinium-based contrast agent (GBCA) is to be used. Ask if the patient has ever had any device implanted into his or her body. Obtain occupational history to determine the presence of metal in the body, such as shrapnel or flecks of ferrous metal in the eye (which can cause retinal hemorrhage). Before the procedure is performed, plan to review the steps with the patient. Explain that the procedure is usually performed in an MRI suite by an MRI technologist and takes approximately 30 to 60 minutes. Inform the patient that he or she will be lying on a flat table and placed into a cylindrical scanner for this study. Many people are fearful of pain when faced with an unknown situation. Clear communication of any potential discomfort is advised. Explain that the scanner produces a loud banging noise during the actual imaging and also that magnetophosphenes may be seen (flickering lights in the visual field); these will stop when the procedure is over. Explain that earplugs or earphones may be used to muffle the banging noise generated by the MRI machine. Explain that an IV line may be inserted to allow the infusion of IV fluids such as saline, anesthetics, contrast medium, or sedatives.

CONTRAINDICATIONS
- Patients who are pregnant or suspected of being pregnant, unless the potential benefits of the MRI far outweigh the risks to the fetus and mother.

In pregnancy, GBCAs cross the placental barrier, enter the fetal circulation, and pass via the kidneys into the amniotic fluid. Although no definite adverse effects of GBCA administration on the human fetus have been documented, the potential bioeffects of fetal GBCA exposure are not well understood. GBCA administration should therefore be avoided during pregnancy unless no suitable alternative imaging is possible and the benefits of contrast administration outweigh the potential risk to the fetus.

- Patients with moderate to marked renal impairment (glomerular filtration rate less than 30 mL/min/1.73 m²); patients should be screened for renal dysfunction prior to administration. The use of GBCAs should be avoided in these patients unless the benefits of the studies outweigh the risks and if essential diagnostic information is not available using non–contrast-enhanced diagnostic studies.
- Patients with cardiac pacemakers, which can be deactivated by MRI
- Patients with metal in their body, such as dental amalgams, metallic body piercing items, tattoo inks containing iron (including tattooed eyeliners), shrapnel, bullet, ferrous metal in the eye, certain ferrous metal prosthetics, valves, aneurysm clips, intrauterine device (IUD), inner ear prostheses, or other metallic objects; these items can impair image quality. Metallic objects are also a significant safety issue for patients and health-care staff in the examination room during performance of an MRI. The MRI equipment consists of an extremely powerful magnet that can inactivate, move, or shift metallic objects inside a patient. Many metallic objects currently used in health-care procedures are made of materials that do not interfere with MRI studies; it is important for the patient to provide specific information regarding medical procedures he or she has undergone in order to identify whether the device is safe to undergo MRI. Required information includes the date of the procedure and identification of the device. Metallic objects are not allowed inside the room with the MRI equipment because items such as watches, credit cards, and car keys can become dangerous projectiles.
- Patients with transdermal patches containing metallic components; the patch's liner contains a metal that controls absorption of the substance from the patch (e.g., drugs, nicotine, steroids, or hormones). The patch may cause burns to the skin *related to energy conducted through the metal which is converted to heat during the MRI.* Other metallic objects on the skin may also cause burns.
- Patients who are claustrophobic
- Extremely obese patients whose weight cannot be supported by the table

- Patients whose physical condition is unstable, requiring the use of equipment that can be affected by the magnet

● Safety Tip

Make sure a written and informed consent has been signed prior to the procedure and before administering any medications.

Implementation

Patient education is key to obtaining the patient's cooperation in following directions, and providing an explanation for the purpose of the procedure is an important part of this process. Inform the patient that this study can assist in the detection of intracranial abnormalities. Establish an IV fluid line for the injection of IV fluids such as saline, anesthetics, contrast medium, or sedatives. Ensure the patient is in compliance with pretesting instructions and that ordered premedications for allergies or anxiety have been administered. Instruct the patient to void prior to the procedure and to change into the gown, robe, and foot coverings provided. Explain to the patient that he or she will be placed on a table, and remind him or her to lie very still during the procedure. Remind the patient that this study involves no radiation exposure, and supply earplugs to the patient to block out the loud, banging sounds that occur during the test. Instruct the patient to communicate with the technologist during the examination via a microphone within the scanner. If an electrocardiogram or respiratory gating is to be performed in conjunction with the scan, apply MRI-safe electrodes to the appropriate sites. Instruct the patient to take slow, deep breaths if nausea occurs during the procedure. Tell the patient that following the IV injection of 10 to 15 mL of gadolinium, the table is advanced into the scanner and imaging begins immediately. Ask the patient to inhale deeply and hold his or her breath while the images are taken, and then to exhale after the images are taken (see Figs. 12.3 and 12.4). During the imaging, monitor the patient for complications related to the procedure (e.g., allergic reaction, anaphylaxis, bronchospasm). When the study has been completed, remove the needle or catheter and apply a pressure dressing over the puncture site. Observe/assess the needle/catheter insertion site for bleeding, inflammation, or hematoma formation.

Evaluation

Recognize anxiety related to test results and be supportive of impaired activity related to a perceived loss of independence. Observe for delayed allergic reactions, such as rash, urticaria, tachycardia, hyperpnea, hypertension, palpitations, nausea, or vomiting. Instruct the patient to immediately report symptoms such as

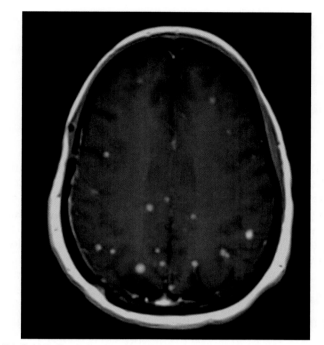

FIGURE 12.3 MRI of patient with stage 4 breast cancer showing multiple metastatic brain lesions. *Used with permission, from Weber, E., Vilensky, J., & Fog, A. (2013). Practical radiology: a system-based approach. FA Davis Company.*

fast heart rate, difficulty breathing, skin rash, itching, chest pain, persistent right shoulder pain, or abdominal pain. Immediately report symptoms to the appropriate health-care provider (HCP). Instruct the patient in the care and assessment of the injection site. Instruct the patient to apply cold compresses to the puncture site as needed to reduce discomfort or edema. Discuss the implications of abnormal test results on the patient's lifestyle. Provide teaching and information regarding the clinical implications of the test results as appropriate. Direct the family to resources that may help them understand the implications of dementia or Alzheimer disease, such as the Alzheimer's Association www.alz.org/ or the Alzheimer's Foundation of America www.alzfdn.org/.

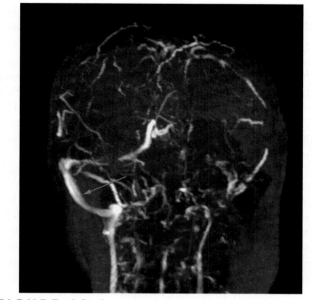

FIGURE 12.4 MR venogram with thrombosed saggital sinus. *Used with permission, from Weber, E., Vilensky, J., & Fog, A. (2013). Practical radiology: a system-based approach. FA Davis Company.*

✓ Critical Findings

- Abscess
- Cerebral aneurysm
- Cerebral infarct
- Hydrocephalus
- Skull fracture or contusion
- Tum or with significant mass effect

Note and immediately report to the HCP any critical findings and related symptoms. A listing of these findings varies among facilities.

✓ Study Specific Complications

Complications are rare but do include risk for allergic reaction *related to contrast reaction.* It is important to have oxygen and endotracheal equipment in the vicinity for immediate use. In the event of an anaphylactic reaction, epinephrine, diphenhydramine, and steroids are included with resuscitative efforts.

Contrast Reactions: Signs, Symptoms and Treatment

	Minor	Intermediate	Life Threatening
Signs, Symptoms	Nausea, vomiting, urticaria, sneezing	Bronchospasms; chills and fever; chest pain, and laryngeal or tongue edema	Hypotension, cardiac dysrhythmias; seizures; loss of bowel/bladder control; laryngeal and pulmonary edema
Interventions	Antihistamines	Antihistamines, steroids, bronchodilators, IV fluids, and observation	All intermediate interventions plus intubation and ventilation, pressors, and antiseizure medications

Other complications related to the procedure may include:

- Cardiac dysrhythmias
- Acute kidney injury as a result of contrast infusion; hydration prior to the study can reduce the likelihood of this complication.
- Nephrogenic systemic fibrosis (NSF) may develop in some patients as a result of the use of GBCAs *related to ineffective renal clearance in patients with impaired renal function.*
- Complications associated with injection and venipuncture. Injection of the contrast or other fluids through IV tubing into a blood vessel is an invasive procedure. There are a number of complications associated with performing a venipuncture. **Pain** is commonly associated with needles, and although the pain experienced during venipuncture is usually mild, on a rare occasion the needle may strike a nerve, causing permanent pain. Some patients experience a **vasovagal reaction** during the venipuncture procedure, evidenced by sweating, low blood pressure, fainting, or near fainting. The potential for a **fall injury** is a significant concern related to vasovagal reactions. Prolonged **bleeding** is a complication that occurs with patients who are taking blood thinners or who have coagulopathies such as hemophilia. A **hematoma** results when blood leaks into the tissue during or after a venipuncture, as evidenced by pain, bruising, and/or swelling at the venipuncture site. The swelling can cause injury by compression to surrounding nerves, which can be temporary or permanent. HCPs should watch for minor complications such as bruising and hematoma at the venipuncture site, which are fairly common. Hematomas occur more often in older adult or frail patients, or those with veins that are difficult to access. Bleeding or bruising can be prevented once the needle has been removed by applying direct pressure to the site with dry gauze for a minute or two. Some other more unusual complications of venipuncture include **cellulitis, phlebitis, inadvertent arterial puncture, and sepsis.** Sepsis can be caused by the introduction of bacteria from the surface of the skin into the blood as the result of improper cleansing of the venipuncture site. Immunocompromised patients are at higher risk for developing this complication. Elevated temperatures, abnormal-colored sputum, changes in breathing patterns, chills, and hypotension can all indicate infection or sepsis. Antibiotic therapy should be ordered if this occurs.

✅ *Related Tests*

- Related tests include Alzheimer disease markers, angiography of the carotids, BUN, CSF analysis, CT

brain, creatinine, EMG, evoked brain potentials, and PET brain.
- Refer to the Cardiovascular and Musculoskeletal systems tables at the end of the book for related tests by body system.

Expected Outcomes

Expected outcomes associated with Magnetic Resonance Imaging, Brain, are

- Demonstrates ability to communicate needs and wants
- Participates in activities of daily living
- Expresses fear associated with a potential tumor that may interfere with role performance
- Identifies coping strategies that will assist in dealing with devastating test results

Magnetic Resonance Imaging, Chest

Quick Summary

SYNONYM ACRONYM: Chest MRI.

COMMON USE: To visualize and assess pulmonary and cardiovascular structures toward diagnosing tumor, masses, aneurysm, infarct, air, fluid, and evaluate the effectiveness of medical, and surgical interventions.

AREA OF APPLICATION: Chest/thorax.
- Normal heart and lung structures, soft tissue, and function, including blood flow rate

Test Explanation

Magnetic resonance imaging (MRI) is very useful when the area of interest is soft tissue. The technology does not involve radiation exposure and is considered safer than other imaging methods such as radiographs and computed tomography (CT). MRI uses a magnet and radio waves to produce an energy field that can be displayed as an image of the anatomic area of interest based on the water content of the tissue. The magnetic field causes the hydrogen atoms in tissue to line up, and when radio waves are directed toward the magnetic field, the hydrogen atoms absorb the radio waves and change their position. This change in the energy field is detected by the equipment, and an image is generated by the equipment's computer system. MRI produces cross-sectional images of the chest in multiple planes without the use of ionizing radiation or the interference of bone or surrounding tissue. Images can be obtained in two-dimensional (series of slices) or three-dimensional sequences. Standard or closed MRI equipment has the appearance of an open tube or tunnel; open MRI equipment has no sides and provides an alternative for patients who suffer from claustrophobia, pediatric patients, or patients who are obese. IV gadolinium-based contrast media may be used to better visualize the vessels and tissues in the area of interest. Clear, high-quality images of abnormalities and disease processes significantly improve the diagnostic value of the study.

Chest MRI scanning is performed to assist in diagnosing abnormalities of cardiovascular and pulmonary structures. Two special techniques are available for evaluation of cardiovascular structures. One is the electrocardiograph (ECG)–gated multislice spin-echo sequence, used to diagnose anatomic abnormalities of the heart and aorta, and the other is the ECG-referenced gradient refocused sequence used to diagnose heart function and analyze blood flow patterns.

Magnetic resonance spectroscopy (MRS) is an application of MRI based on the same principles as MRI but instead of an anatomical image, the data is displayed graphically as a series of peaks. The peaks represent specific elements and compounds that provide physiological data regarding the tissue of interest. MRS can be performed using MRI equipment with software adapted for the collection and interpretation of spectral data. MRS may be used alone or in conjunction with MRI where anatomical images are first collected by MRI followed by focused MRS images that reflect specific active metabolic processes. The frequency information used in MRS identifies specific chemical compounds such as amino acids, lipids, and lactate that are commonly involved in or produced by cellular activity. The presence or absence of different metabolites in the spectral analysis can be used to identify metabolic activity associated with a suspected tumor, differentiate between tumor types, provide information about cardiac metabolism and cardiovascular dysfunction (myocardial ischemia, heart failure, peripheral vascular disease), or monitor response to therapeutic interventions. Other applications of MRS include studies of brain lesions (brain tumors, Alzheimer disease), inborn errors of metabolism (glycogen storage diseases), insulin resistance, and conditions involving skeletal muscle (muscular dystrophies).

Nursing Implications
Assessment

Indications	Potential Nursing Problems
Confirm diagnosis of cardiac and pericardiac masses	• Activity
Detect aortic aneurysms	• Airway
Detect myocardial infarction and cardiac muscle ischemia	• Breathing
Detect pericardial abnormalities	• Cardiac Output
Detect pleural effusion	• Fatigue
Detect thoracic aortic diseases	• Fear
Determine blood, fluid, or fat accumulation in tissues, pleuritic space, or vessels	• Fluid Volume
	• Gas Exchange
	• Human Response

Indications	Potential Nursing Problems
Determine cardiac ventricular function	• Pain
Differentiate aortic aneurysms from tumors near the aorta	• Self-Care
Evaluate cardiac chambers and pulmonary vessels	• Tissue Perfusion
Evaluate postoperative angioplasty sites and bypass grafts	
Identify congenital heart diseases	
Monitor and evaluate the effectiveness of medical or surgical therapeutic regimen	

Diagnosis: Clinical Significance of Test Results
ABNORMAL FINDINGS
• Aortic dissection
• Congenital heart diseases, including pulmonary atresia, aortic coarctation, agenesis of the pulmonary artery, and transposition of the great vessels
• Constrictive pericarditis
• Intramural and periaortic hematoma
• Myocardial infarction
• Pericardial hematoma or effusion
• Pleural effusion

Planning
Considerations for planning a successful partnership should include clear communication of what to expect during the test to decrease anxiety and improve cooperation. Ensure the results of BUN, creatinine, and eGFR (estimated glomerular filtration rate) are obtained if GBCA is to be used. Ask if the patient has ever had any device implanted into his or her body. Obtain occupational history to determine the presence of metal in the body, such as shrapnel or flecks of ferrous metal in the eye (which can cause retinal hemorrhage). Before the procedure is performed, plan to review the steps with the patient. Explain that the procedure is usually performed in an MRI suite by an MRI technologist, and takes approximately 30 to 60 minutes. Inform the patient that he or she will be lying on a flat table and placed into a cylindrical scanner for this study. Many people are fearful of pain when faced with an unknown situation. Clear communication of any potential discomfort is advised. Explain that the scanner produces a loud banging noise during the actual imaging and also that magnetophosphenes may be seen (flickering lights in the visual field); these will stop when the procedure is over. Explain that earplugs or earphones may be used to muffle the banging noise generated by the MRI machine. Explain that an IV line may be inserted to allow the infusion of IV fluids such as saline, anesthetics, contrast medium, or sedatives.

CONTRAINDICATIONS

- Patients who are pregnant or suspected of being pregnant, unless the potential benefits of the MRI far outweigh the risks to the fetus and mother. *In pregnancy, gadolinium-based contrast agents (GBCAs) cross the placental barrier, enter the fetal circulation, and pass via the kidneys into the amniotic fluid. Although no definite adverse effects of GBCA administration on the human fetus have been documented, the potential bioeffects of fetal GBCA exposure are not well understood. GBCA administration should therefore be avoided during pregnancy unless no suitable alternative imaging is possible and the benefits of contrast administration outweigh the potential risk to the fetus.*

- Patients with moderate to marked renal impairment (glomerular filtration rate less than 30 mL/min/1.73 m²); patients should be screened for renal dysfunction prior to administration. The use of GBCAs should be avoided in these patients unless the benefits of the studies outweigh the risks and if essential diagnostic information is not available using non–contrast-enhanced diagnostic studies.

- Patients with cardiac pacemakers, which can be deactivated by MRI

- Patients with metal in their body, such as dental amalgams, metallic body piercing items, tattoo inks containing iron (including tattooed eyeliners), shrapnel, bullet, ferrous metal in the eye, certain ferrous metal prosthetics, valves, aneurysm clips, intrauterine device (IUD), inner ear prostheses, or other metallic objects; these items can impair image quality. Metallic objects are also a significant safety issue for patients and health-care staff in the examination room during performance of an MRI. The MRI equipment consists of an extremely powerful magnet that can inactivate, move, or shift metallic objects inside a patient. Many metallic objects currently used in health-care procedures are made of materials that do not interfere with MRI studies; it is important for the patient to provide specific information regarding medical procedures he or she has undergone in order to identify whether their device is safe to undergo MRI. Required information includes the date of the procedure and identification of the device. Metallic objects are not allowed inside the room with the MRI equipment because items such as watches, credit cards, and car keys can become dangerous projectiles.

- Patients with transdermal patches containing metallic components; the patch's liner contains a metal that controls absorption of the substance from the patch (e.g., drugs, nicotine, steroids, and hormones). The patch may cause burns to the skin *related to energy conducted through the metal which is converted to heat during the MRI.* Other metallic objects on the skin may also cause burns.

- Patients who are claustrophobic

- Extremely obese patients whose weight cannot be supported by the table

- Patients whose physical condition is unstable requiring the use of equipment that can be affected by the magnet

● Safety Tip

Make sure a written and informed consent has been signed prior to the procedure and before administering any medications.

Implementation

Patient education is key to obtaining the patient's cooperation in following directions, and providing an explanation for the purpose of the procedure is an important part of this process. Inform the patient that this study can assist in the detection of abnormalities of the cardiovascular and pulmonary structures. Establish an IV fluid line for the injection IV fluids such as saline, anesthetics, contrast medium, or sedatives. Ensure the patient is in compliance with pretesting instructions and that ordered premedications for allergies or anxiety have been administered. Instruct the patient to void prior to the procedure and to change into the gown, robe, and foot coverings provided. Explain to the patient that he or she will be placed on a table and remind the patient to lie very still during the procedure. Remind the patient that this study involves no radiation exposure, and supply earplugs to the patient to block out the loud, banging sounds that occur during the test. Instruct the patient to communicate with the technologist during the examination via a microphone within the scanner. If an electrocardiogram or respiratory gating is to be performed in conjunction with the scan, apply MRI-safe electrodes to the appropriate sites. Instruct the patient to take slow, deep breaths if nausea occurs during the procedure. Tell the patient that following the IV injection of 10 to 15 mL of gadolinium, the table is advanced into the scanner and imaging begins immediately. Ask the patient to inhale deeply and hold his or her breath while the images are taken, and then to exhale after the images are taken. During the imaging, monitor the patient for complications related to the procedure (e.g., allergic reaction, anaphylaxis, bronchospasm). When the study has been completed, remove the needle or catheter and apply a pressure dressing over the puncture site. Observe/assess the needle/catheter insertion site for bleeding, inflammation, or hematoma formation.

Evaluation

Recognize anxiety related to test results and be supportive of impaired activity related to a perceived loss of independence. Observe for delayed allergic reactions, such as rash, urticaria, tachycardia, hyperpnea, hypertension, palpitations, nausea, or vomiting. Instruct the patient to immediately report symptoms such as fast heart rate, difficulty breathing, skin rash, itching, chest pain, persistent right shoulder pain, or abdominal pain. Immediately report symptoms to the appropriate health-care provider (HCP). Instruct the patient in the care and assessment of the injection site. Instruct the patient to apply cold compresses to the puncture site as needed to reduce discomfort or edema. Discuss the implications of abnormal test results on the patient's lifestyle. Provide teaching and information regarding the clinical implications of the test results as appropriate.

Critical Findings

- Aortic aneurysm
- Aortic dissection
- Tumor with significant mass effect

Note and immediately report to the requesting HCP any critical findings and related symptoms. A listing of these findings varies among facilities.

Study Specific Complications

Complications are rare but do include risk for allergic reaction *related to contrast reaction.* It is important to have oxygen and endotracheal equipment in the vicinity for immediate use. In the event of an anaphylactic reaction, epinephrine, diphenhydramine, and steroids are included with resuscitative efforts.

Contrast Reactions: Signs, Symptoms and Treatment

	Minor	Intermediate	Life Threatening
Signs, Symptoms	Nausea, vomiting, urticaria, sneezing	Bronchospasms; chills and fever; chest pain, and laryngeal or tongue edema	Hypotension, cardiac dysrhythmias; seizures; loss of bowel/bladder control; laryngeal and pulmonary edema
Interventions	Antihistamines	Antihistamines, steroids, bronchodilators, IV fluids, and observation	All intermediate interventions plus intubation and ventilation, pressors, and antiseizure medications

Other complications related to the procedure may include:

- Cardiac dysrhythmias
- Acute kidney injury as a result of contrast infusion; hydration prior to the study can reduce the likelihood of this complication.
- Nephrogenic systemic fibrosis (NSF) may develop in some patients as a result of the use of gadolinium-based contrast agents *related to ineffective renal clearance in patients with impaired renal function.*
- Complications from injection and venipuncture. Injection of the contrast or other fluids through IV tubing into a blood vessel is an invasive procedure. There are a number of complications associated with performing a venipuncture. **Pain** is commonly associated with needles and although the pain experienced during venipuncture is usually mild, on a rare occasion the needle may strike a nerve causing permanent pain. Some patients experience a **vasovagal reaction** during the venipuncture procedure, evidenced by sweating, low blood pressure, fainting, or near fainting. The potential for a **fall injury** is a significant concern related to vasovagal reactions. Prolonged **bleeding** is a complication that occurs with patients who are taking blood thinners or who have coagulopathies such as hemophilia. A **hematoma** results when blood leaks into the tissue during or after a venipuncture, as evidenced by pain, bruising, and/or swelling at the venipuncture site. The swelling can cause injury by compression to surrounding nerves, which can be temporary or permanent. HCPs should watch for minor complications such as bruising and hematoma at the venipuncture site, which are fairly common. Hematomas occur more often in older adult or frail patients, or those with veins that are difficult to access. Bleeding or bruising can be prevented once the needle has been removed by applying direct pressure to the site with dry gauze for a minute or two. Some other more unusual complications of venipuncture include **cellulitis, phlebitis, inadvertent arterial puncture, and sepsis.** Sepsis can be caused by the introduction of bacteria from the surface of the skin into the blood as the result

of improper cleansing of the venipuncture site. Immunocompromised patients are at higher risk for developing this complication. Elevated temperatures, abnormal-colored sputum, changes in breathing patterns, chills, and hypotension can all indicate infection or sepsis. Antibiotic therapy should be ordered if this occurs.

✓ Related Tests

- Related tests include AST, BNP, blood gases, blood pool imaging, BUN, chest x-ray, CT cardiac scoring, CT thorax, CRP, CK and isoenzymes, creatinine, echocardiography, exercise stress test, Holter monitor, myocardial infarct scan, myocardial perfusion heart scan, myoglobin, pleural fluid analysis, PET scan of the heart, and troponins.
- Refer to the Cardiovascular and Respiratory systems tables at the end of the book for related tests by body system.

Expected Outcomes

Expected outcomes associated with Magnetic Resonance Imaging, Chest, are

- Relieving chest pain with rest, and the use of oxygen and nitroglycerine
- Asking questions appropriate to the clinical diagnosis and accepting the education provided
- Understanding that repeat scans are performed to assess the effectiveness of treatment
- Cooperating with HCP recommendations for change that improves health

Magnetic Resonance Imaging, Musculoskeletal

Quick Summary

SYNONYM ACRONYM: Musculoskeletal (knee, shoulder, hand, wrist, foot, elbow, hip, spine) MRI.

COMMON USE: To visualize and assess bones, joints, and surrounding structures to assist in diagnosing defects, cysts, tumors, and fracture.

AREA OF APPLICATION: Bones, joints, soft tissues.

- Normal bones, joints, and surrounding tissue structures; no articular disease, bone marrow disorders, tumors, infections, or trauma to the bones, joints, or muscles

Test Explanation

Magnetic resonance imaging (MRI) is very useful when the area of interest is soft tissue. The technology does not involve radiation exposure and is considered safer than other imaging methods such as radiographs and computed tomography (CT). MRI uses a magnet and radio waves to produce an energy field that can be displayed as an image of the anatomic area of interest based on the water content of the tissue. The magnetic field causes the hydrogen atoms in tissue to line up, and when radio waves are directed toward the magnetic field, the hydrogen atoms absorb the radio waves and change their position. This change in the energy field is detected by the equipment, and an image is generated by the equipment's computer system. MRI produces cross-sectional images of bones and joints in multiple planes without the use of ionizing radiation or the interference of bone or surrounding tissue. Images can be obtained in two-dimensional (series of slices) or three-dimensional sequences. Standard or closed MRI equipment has the appearance of an open tube or tunnel; open MRI equipment has no sides and provides an alternative for patients who suffer from claustrophobia, pediatric patients, or patients who are obese. IV gadolinium-based contrast media may be used to better visualize the vessels and tissues in the area of interest. Clear, high-quality images of abnormalities and disease processes significantly improve the diagnostic value of the study.

Musculoskeletal MRI is performed to assist in diagnosing abnormalities of bones and joints and surrounding soft tissue structures, including cartilage, synovium, ligaments, and tendons. MRI eliminates the risks associated with exposure to x-rays and causes no harm to cells. Contrast-enhanced imaging is effective for evaluating scarring from previous surgery, vascular abnormalities, and differentiation of metastases from primary tumors. MRI uses the noniodinated paramagnetic contrast medium gadopentetate dimeglumine (Magnevist), which is administered IV to enhance differences between normal and abnormal tissues. Magnetic resonance spectroscopy (MRS) is an application of MRI based on the same principles as MRI but instead of an anatomical image, the data is displayed graphically as a series of peaks. The peaks represent specific elements and compounds that provide physiological data regarding the tissue of interest. MRS can be performed using MRI equipment with software adapted for the collection and interpretation of spectral data. MRS may be used alone or in conjunction with MRI where anatomical images are first collected by MRI followed by focused MRS images that reflect specific active metabolic processes. The frequency information used in MRS identifies specific chemical compounds such as amino acids, lipids, and lactate that are commonly involved in or produced by cellular activity. The presence or absence of different metabolites in the spectral analysis can be used to identify metabolic activity associated with a suspected tumor, differentiate between tumor types, provide information about skeletal muscle disease (muscular dystrophies), or monitor response to therapeutic interventions. Other applications of MRS include studies of brain lesions (brain tumors, Alzheimer disease), inborn errors of metabolism (glycogen storage diseases), insulin resistance, and cardiovascular dysfunction (myocardial ischemia, heart failure, peripheral vascular disease).

Nursing Implications
Assessment

Indications	Potential Nursing Problems
Confirm diagnosis of osteomyelitis Detect avascular necrosis of the femoral head or knee Detect benign and cancerous tumors and cysts of the bone or soft tissue Detect bone infarcts in the epiphyseal or diaphyseal sites Detect changes in bone marrow Detect tears or degeneration of ligaments, tendons, and menisci resulting from trauma or pathology Determine cause of low back pain, including herniated disk and spinal degenerative disease Differentiate between primary and secondary malignant processes of the bone marrow Differentiate between a stress fracture and a tumor Evaluate meniscal detachment of the temporomandibular joint	• Activity • Body Image • Fall Risk • Family • Fear • Human Response • Infection • Mobility • Pain • Role Performance • Self-Care • Self-Esteem

Diagnosis: Clinical Significance of Test Results
ABNORMAL FINDINGS
- Avascular necrosis of femoral head or knee, as found in Legg-Calvé-Perthes disease
- Bone marrow disease, such as Gaucher disease, aplastic anemia, sickle cell disease, or polycythemia
- Degenerative spinal disease, such as spondylosis or arthritis
- Fibrosarcoma
- Hemangioma (muscular or osseous)
- Herniated disk
- Infection
- Meniscal tears or degeneration
- Osteochondroma
- Osteogenic sarcoma
- Osteomyelitis
- Rotator cuff tears
- Spinal stenosis
- Stress fracture
- Synovitis
- Tumor

Planning
Considerations for planning a successful partnership should include clear communication of what to expect during the test to decrease anxiety and improve cooperation. Ensure the results of BUN, creatinine, and eGFR (estimated glomerular filtration rate) are obtained if gadolinium-based contrast agent (GBCA) is to be used. Ask if the patient has ever had any device implanted into his or her body. Obtain occupational history to determine the presence of metal in the body, such as shrapnel or flecks of ferrous metal in the eye (which can cause retinal hemorrhage). Before the procedure is performed, plan to review the steps with the patient. Explain that the procedure is usually performed in an MRI suite by an MRI technologist and takes approximately 30 to 60 minutes. Inform the patient that he or she will be lying on a flat table and placed into a cylindrical scanner for this study. Many people are fearful of pain when faced with an unknown situation. Clear communication of any potential discomfort is advised. Explain that the scanner produces a loud banging noise during the actual imaging and also that magnetophosphenes may be seen (flickering lights in the visual field); these will stop when the procedure is over. Explain that earplugs or earphones may be used to muffle the banging noise generated by the MRI machine. Explain that an IV line may be inserted to allow the infusion of IV fluids such as saline, anesthetics, contrast medium, or sedatives.

CONTRAINDICATIONS
- Patients who are pregnant or suspected of being pregnant, unless the potential benefits of the MRI far outweigh the risks to the fetus and mother. *In pregnancy, GBCAs cross the placental barrier, enter the fetal circulation, and pass via the kidneys into the amniotic fluid. Although no definite adverse effects of GBCA administration on the human fetus have been documented, the potential bioeffects of fetal GBCA exposure are not well understood. GBCA administration should therefore be avoided during pregnancy unless no suitable alternative imaging is possible and the benefits of contrast administration outweigh the potential risk to the fetus.*
- Patients with moderate to marked renal impairment (glomerular filtration rate less than 30 mL/min/1.73 m^2); patients should be screened for renal dysfunction prior to administration. The use of GBCAs should be avoided in these patients unless the benefits of the studies outweigh the risks and if essential diagnostic information is not available using non–contrast-enhanced diagnostic studies.

- Patients with cardiac pacemakers, which can be deactivated by MRI
- Patients with metal in their body, such as dental amalgams, metallic body piercing items, tattoo inks containing iron (including tattooed eyeliners), shrapnel, bullet, ferrous metal in the eye, certain ferrous metal prosthetics, valves, aneurysm clips, intrauterine device (IUD), inner ear prostheses, or other metallic objects; these items can impair image quality. Metallic objects are also a significant safety issue for patients and health-care staff in the examination room during the performance of an MRI. The MRI equipment consists of an extremely powerful magnet that can inactivate, move, or shift metallic objects inside a patient. Many metallic objects currently used in health-care procedures are made of materials that do not interfere with MRI studies; it is important for the patient to provide specific information regarding medical procedures he or she has undergone in order to identify whether the device is safe to undergo MRI. Required information includes the date of the procedure and identification of the device. Metallic objects are not allowed inside the room with the MRI equipment because items such as watches, credit cards, and car keys can become dangerous projectiles.
- Patients with transdermal patches containing metallic components; the patch's liner contains a metal that controls absorption of the substance from the patch (e.g., drugs, nicotine, steroids, and hormones). The patch may cause burns to the skin *related to energy conducted through the metal which is converted to heat during the MRI.* Other metallic objects on the skin may also cause burns.
- Patients who are claustrophobic
- Extremely obese patients whose weight cannot be supported by the table
- Patients whose physical condition is unstable, requiring the use of equipment that can be affected by the magnet

● Safety Tip

Make sure a written and informed consent has been signed prior to the procedure and before administering any medications.

Implementation

Patient education is key to obtaining the patient's cooperation in following directions, and providing an explanation for the purpose of the procedure is an important part of this process. Inform the patient that this study can assist in the detection of abnormalities of bones, joints, and the surrounding tissues. Establish an IV fluid line for the injection of IV fluids such as saline, anesthetics, contrast medium, or sedatives.

Ensure the patient is in compliance with pretesting instructions and that ordered premedications for allergies or anxiety have been administered. Instruct the patient to void prior to the procedure and to change into the gown, robe, and foot coverings provided. Explain to the patient that he or she will be placed on a table and remind him or her to lie very still during the procedure. Remind the patient that this study involves no radiation exposure, and supply earplugs to the patient to block out the loud, banging sounds that occur during the test. Instruct the patient to communicate with the technologist during the examination via a microphone within the scanner. If an electrocardiogram or respiratory gating is to be performed in conjunction with the scan, apply MRI-safe electrodes to the appropriate sites. Instruct the patient to take slow, deep breaths if nausea occurs during the procedure. Tell the patient that following the IV injection of 10 to 15 mL of gadolinium, the table is advanced into the scanner and imaging begins immediately (see Figs. 12.5 and 12.6). Ask the patient to inhale deeply and hold his or her breath while the images are taken, and then to exhale after the images are taken. During the imaging, monitor the patient for complications related to the procedure (e.g., allergic reaction, anaphylaxis, bronchospasm). When the study has been completed, remove the needle or catheter and apply a pressure dressing over the puncture site. Observe/assess the needle/catheter insertion site for bleeding, inflammation, or hematoma formation.

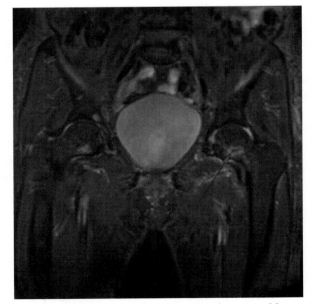

FIGURE 12.5 MRI showing stress fracture of femoral neck. *Used with permission, from Weber, E., Vilensky, J., & Fog, A. (2013). Practical radiology: a system-based approach. FA Davis Company.*

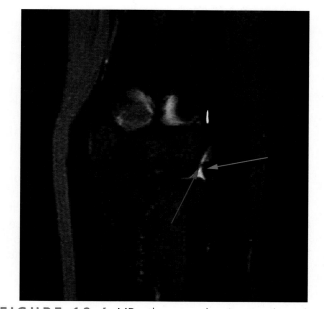

FIGURE 12.6 MR arthrogram showing tear (arrow) of the radial collateral ligament. *Used with permission, from Weber, E., Vilensky, J., & Fog, A. (2013). Practical radiology: a system-based approach. FA Davis Company.*

Evaluation

Recognize anxiety related to test results and be supportive of impaired activity related to a perceived loss of independence. Observe for delayed allergic reactions, such as rash, urticaria, tachycardia, hyperpnea, hypertension, palpitations, nausea, or vomiting. Instruct the patient to immediately report symptoms such as fast heart rate, difficulty breathing, skin rash, itching, chest pain, persistent right shoulder pain, or abdominal pain. Immediately report symptoms to the appropriate health-care provider (HCP). Instruct the patient in the care and assessment of the injection site. Instruct the patient to apply cold compresses to the puncture site as needed to reduce discomfort or edema. Discuss the implications of abnormal test results on the patient's lifestyle. Provide teaching and information regarding the clinical implications of the test results, as appropriate. Provide the contact information, if needed, for the American College of Rheumatology www.rheumatology.orgor for the Arthritis Foundation www.arthritis.org.

✓ Critical Findings

N/A

✓ Study Specific Complications

Complications are rare but do include risk for allergic reaction *related to contrast reaction.* It is important to have oxygen and endotracheal equipment in the vicinity for immediate use. In the event of an anaphylactic reaction, epinephrine, diphenhydramine, and steroids are included with resuscitative efforts.

Contrast Reactions: Signs, Symptoms and Treatment

	Minor	Intermediate	Life Threatening
Signs, Symptoms	Nausea, vomiting, urticaria, sneezing	Bronchospasms; chills and fever; chest pain, and laryngeal or tongue edema	Hypotension, cardiac dysrhythmias; seizures; loss of bowel/bladder control; laryngeal and pulmonary edema
Interventions	Antihistamines	Antihistamines, steroids, bronchodilators, IV fluids, and observation	All intermediate interventions plus intubation and ventilation, pressors, and antiseizure medications

Other complications related to the procedure may include:

- Cardiac dysrhythmias
- Acute kidney injury as a result of contrast infusion; hydration prior to the study can reduce the likelihood of this complication.
- Nephrogenic systemic fibrosis (NSF) may develop in some patients as a result of the use of gadolinium-based contrast agents *related to ineffective renal clearance in patients with impaired renal function.*

- Complications related to injection and venipuncture may occur. Injection of the contrast or other fluids through IV tubing into a blood vessel is an invasive procedure. There are a number of complications associated with performing a venipuncture. **Pain** is commonly associated with needles, and although the pain experienced during venipuncture is usually mild, on a rare occasion the needle may strike a nerve, causing permanent pain. Some patients experience a **vasovagal reaction** during the venipuncture procedure, evidenced by sweating, low blood pressure, fainting, or near fainting. The potential for a **fall injury** is a significant concern related to vasovagal reactions. Prolonged **bleeding** is a complication that occurs with patients who are taking blood thinners or who have coagulopathies such as hemophilia. A **hematoma** results when blood leaks into the tissue during or after a venipuncture, as evidenced by pain, bruising, and/or swelling at the venipuncture site. The swelling can cause injury by compression to surrounding nerves, which can be temporary or permanent. HCPs should watch for minor complications such as bruising and hematoma at the venipuncture site, which are fairly common. Hematomas occur more often in older adult or frail patients, or those with veins that are difficult to access. Bleeding or bruising can be prevented once the needle has been removed by applying direct pressure to the site with dry gauze for a minute or two. Some other more unusual complications of venipuncture include **cellulitis, phlebitis, inadvertent arterial puncture, and sepsis.** Sepsis can be caused by the introduction of bacteria from the surface of the skin into the blood as the result of improper cleansing of the venipuncture site. Immunocompromised patients are at higher risk for developing this complication. Elevated temperatures, abnormal-colored sputum, changes in breathing patterns, chills, and hypotension can all indicate infection or sepsis. Antibiotic therapy should be ordered if this occurs.

Related Tests

- Related tests include anticyclic citrullinated antibodies, ANA, arthrogram, arthroscopy, bone mineral densitometry, bone scan, BUN, CRP, CT spine, creatinine, ESR, radiography of the bone, synovial fluid analysis, RF, and vertebroplasty.
- Refer to the Musculoskeletal System table at the end of the book for related tests by body system.

Expected Outcomes

Expected outcomes associated with Magnetic Resonance Imaging, Musculoskeletal, are

- Experience decreased joint stiffness
- Have pain managed to facilitate an optimal level of activity
- Collaborate with physical therapy to use assistive devices that enhance mobility
- Agree to take necessary precautions that will prevent injury or falls

REVIEW OF LEARNING OUTCOMES

Thinking

1. Recognize that human beings are imperfect, and failure to follow policy and standards of care, or

participate in work-arounds can place a patient at risk. Answer: One of the pitfalls of nursing practice in relation to diagnostic studies such as MRI is in creating work-arounds that are perceived as making your job easier. The purpose of policy, checklists, and standardized procedures is to keep the patient safe in the potentially unsafe environment in which we work. Follow established protocols, and if you do not know what to do, ask.

2. Describe the safety risks associated with MRI procedures. Answer: Patients must be thoroughly screened for any metallic objects in the body that can cause serious effects when the patient is placed in the magnet. The magnet can move the metal object within the body, causing serious injury to the patient.

Doing

1. Recognize that memory can be imperfect and the use of assistive resources (checklists, electronic tablets, etc.) can reduce errors related to patient care. Answer: Each organization has developed some kind of checklist to assist you in making sure you have sufficiently cleared your patient for an MRI. Make sure you use the checklist, provided it will make the procedure much safer for your patient and will provide you the peace of mind that you have prevented an inadvertent error that could have devastating results.

Caring

1. Recognize the presence of both cognitive and physical personal limitations in the performance of care. Answer: Always remember that anyone can make a mistake. Following the rules set by a department such as MRI can prevent injury to the patient. This includes accurate screening prior to the performance of MRI to make sure there is no patient history of magnetic-sensitive materials that would cause injury once the procedure begins. Do not take any shortcuts.

2. Recognize the merit of collaborating with patient, family, and significant others to design, implement, and evaluate the plan of care. Answer: Depending on the age or cognitive status of the patient, it may be necessary to engage and rely more on the surrogate in the development, implementation, and evaluation of the plan of care than on the patient him- or herself. Always include the patient as much as you can, but understand that may not always be possible. Carefully assess the situation culturally and move forward cautiously when working with a large family. There may be family issues of which you are unaware.

◖ *Words* OF *Wisdom*: It is impossible to understand what an emotional tightrope a person walks when having one of these diagnostic exams. What happens if his or her greatest fear is proven to be correct? What happens if after all of the treatment nothing has worked and nothing else can be done? What if the end is near and the family is devastated, what can a nurse do? Part of the nursing role is to understand your place in each clinical situation. End of life and helping the patient to have a good death is as important a part of nursing care as making people better and sending them home. Your job when a patient is dying is to make sure the patients is as comfortable as possible, whatever that means to him or her. Then turn your attention to the family and make sure they are also as comfortable as possible, emotionally, culturally, and religiously. You are the only person who can make this happen, so make it so.

BIBLIOGRAPHY

Cavanaugh, B. (2003). Nurse's manual of laboratory and diagnostic tests (4th ed). Philadelphia, PA: F.A. Davis Company.

Fishbach, F., & Dunning, M. (2009). A manual of laboratory and diagnostic tests (8th ed.). Philadelphia, PA: Lippencott Williams & Wilkins.

Hulisz, D. (2008). Are topical patches safe during MRI or CT scans? Retrieved from www.medscape.com/viewarticle/572561

Magnetic resonance angiography (MRA). (n.d.). Retrieved from www.hopkinsmedicine.org/healthlibrary/test_procedures/cardiovascular/magnetic_resonance_angiography_mra_135,14/

Magnetic Resonance Imaging (MRI)—Chest. (2013). Retrieved from www.radiologyinfo.org/en/info.cfm?pg=chestmr

MR Safety. (2012). Retrieved from www.acr.org/Quality-Safety/Radiology-Safety/MR-Safety

Sheinfeld, A. (2014). Nephrogenic systemic fibrosis. Retrieved from http://emedicine.medscape.com/article/1097889-overview

Snopek, A. (2009). Fundamentals of special radiographic procedures (5th ed.). St. Louis, MO: Saunders Elsevier.

Van Leeuwen, A., and Bladh, M. (2015). Davis's comprehensive handbook of laboratory and diagnostic testing with nursing implications (6th ed.). Philadelphia, PA: F.A. Davis Company.

Venes, D. (Ed.). (2009). Taber's cyclopedic medical dictionary (21st ed.). Philadelphia, PA: F.A. Davis Company.

Go to Section II of this book and www.davisplus.com for the Clinical Reasoning Tool and its case studies to provide you with a safe place to explore patient care situations. There are a total of 26 different case studies; 2 cases are presented for each of 13 body systems. One set of cases for each of the 13 body systems is presented in the Section II chapters, and one set is presented online at DavisPlus. Each case is designed with the specific goal of helping you to connect the dots of clinical reasoning. Cases are designed to reflect possible clinical scenarios; the outcomes may or may not be positive—you decide.

CHAPTER

13

Nuclear Medicine Studies

OVERVIEW

Nuclear medicine diagnostic studies are used as an investigative tool in three specific ways: (1) to diagnose a disease based on the patient's presenting symptoms, (2) to evaluate the effectiveness of the therapeutic modality chosen to treat the disease, and (3) to serve as a medical research tool. Nuclear studies is a medical specialty that uses low-level radioactive materials to achieve these goals. *Radiopharmaceutical* is a term that describes the use of radioactive compounds called *tracers*. Tracers enter the body by injection through a vein, by swallow, by intrathecal pump, by intramuscular or intraperitoneal injection, or by inhalation. The method chosen should be explained to the patient. Once introduced, tracers will locate and settle in areas under diagnostic inquiry. Tracer results are used to identify a medical problem based on tissue or organ function. Each radioactive tracer is carefully selected to provide the lowest amount of radiation exposure to the patient while ensuring a satisfactory examination or therapeutic goal. A health-care team ensures that nuclear medicine scans are performed and interpreted correctly.

Nuclear medicine studies use different tracers to study different parts of the body. Tracers are chosen for their ability to settle in specific tissues or organs. Tracers, or radiopharmaceuticals, that are commonly used in nuclear medicine scanning are gallium, thallium, technetium-99m, fluorodeoxyglucose, and iodine. Radiopharmaceuticals can be classified in one of two groups: those produced in a nuclear reactor (by the process of fission in a nuclear chain reaction) or those produced in a cyclotron (a type of particle accelerator that operates within a magnetic field).

Examples of Radiopharmaceuticals

Tracer	Common Use	Method of Production
Iodine 131 [131I]	Thyroid studies: tracer is specific for thyroid tissue	Nuclear reactor
Fluorine-18 [18F]	Positron emission tomography (PET) studies	Cyclotron
Technetium-99m [99mTc]	There are 31 different isotopes of technetium-99m; each was developed to evaluate specific functions in any of the major body systems	Purified in a generator from its parent isotope, molybdenum-99, which is produced in a nuclear reactor

All radionuclides have a specific half-life that is identifiable within the tissues and is noted as a tracer dose. Units of radioactivity are measured as microcuries (μCi), millicuries (mCi), or becquerel (Bq). Radiation risks from the diagnostic use of radionuclides are very small. Radionuclides half-life is short, and the dosage used is low. Most radionuclides leave the body within 6 to 24 hours. The radiation dose patients receive is actually less than that received in most x-ray studies. The use of radionuclides for these diagnostic studies does not require that care providers or others protect themselves from the presence of radiation in the patient. However, there are instances in which this is necessary, such as when higher doses of radiation are administered as therapeutic doses. These doses can be about 1000 times greater than a diagnostic dose.

Nuclear medicine team members consist of physicians, technologists, pharmacists, and a physicist, who are all experienced in the technology of nuclear medicine. Scans may be performed by certified nuclear medicine technologists. Completed scans are interpreted by radiologists or nuclear medicine physicians. These procedures are performed in the hospital nuclear medicine department.

DISCUSSION POINT

There are many radioisotopes used in the specialty of nuclear medicine to investigate, diagnose, and provide treatment for disease. Each year there are thousands of people who are treated with radioisotopes, and millions who are diagnostically examined with tests that use radioisotopes. Imaging from nuclear studies provides real-time information regarding the physiology and metabolic processes of target organs because the tracers are developed to selectively identify an area of specific interest in the thyroid gland, long bones, liver, brain, or lungs. There are numerous other applications that include cardiology (e.g., stress testing), oncology (e.g., identification of a sentinel node biopsy site), nephrology (e.g., investigation of renal insufficiency), gastroenterology (e.g., evaluation of suspected acute cholecystitis), or the imaging required to diagnose an infection (e.g., gallium scan). It is important to remind the patient that he or she is exposed to radiation every day with the largest single source of radiation exposure in the United States coming from radon in the soil as tabulated by the National Council on Radiation Protection & Measurements (NCRP).

Imaging Equipment. Nuclear medicine scans use a specialized gamma or scintillation camera to capture images created from the emission of gamma and positron rays. Captured images interface with a computer that converts the information into a diagnostic format for use by the health-care provider (HCP). Images can be captured dynamically in multiple frames over seconds to evaluate blood flow. Static imaging captures a two-dimensional view of a particular structure, organ, or view, like taking a snapshot in time. Whole-body imaging uses a moving detector system that captures two-dimensional images of the entire body. Each view is designed to provide diagnostic information about the area of concern. Images are created from the emissions of the tracers used for each study. Changing emission levels of the administered tracer are monitored by the camera to capture images and count rate information. Information from the camera about the location and energy level of the tracer rays is sent to a computer.

In turn, the computer converts that information into a two-dimensional picture to be viewed immediately. The information captured by the camera is stored in the computer for future viewing, analysis, and comparison. The amount of time between when the radiopharmaceutical is administered and the scanning begins is dependent upon the organ being assessed. Scanning can begin immediately or start in a specified number of hours or days. Single-photon emission computed tomography (SPECT) imaging provides an additional three-dimensional view with improved viewing resolution. Computed tomography (CT) can be added to nuclear medicine scanning with this process. This will allow the nuclear medicine scan and CT scan to be completed at the same time.

Scanned images can be printed on a scale that shows varying shades of gray. Variances in the shading identify the distribution of the radionuclide in parts of the organ. This information is then interpreted by a radiologist once the study is completed. Variances in color are viewed as hot spots or cold spots. Dark spots are known as hot spots and indicate a greater concentration of the tracer in that area. Spots that do not take up the radionuclide are identified by light-shaded areas and are known as cold spots. Both can be an abnormal result depending on the disease process being imaged. Images can also be recorded in color.

DISCUSSION POINT

Ionizing radiation can be used for therapeutic reasons due to its ability to kill targeted cells by penetrating and depositing the energy within them. The energy prevents the cell from dividing and growing. An example of this type of use is in treating malignancies of the thyroid, chest, and abdomen, and in hyperthyroidism and polycythemia.

PET Scans. Positron emission tomography (PET) scan is a noninvasive nuclear imaging technique. PET scans use the administration of a positron-emitting radioactive molecule to assess tissue and organ metabolism, perfusion, function, structure, density, and body fluid volume or flow. PET scans also allow for accurate collection of data by creating clear diagnostic images for HCP use. The radioactive tracer chosen for the scan is dependent upon the tissue or organ being evaluated and its similarity to that organ's biochemical elements. Tracers gravitate to areas of higher metabolic function. Areas of higher metabolic function show up as hot spots. See Figure 13.1, which shows a PET scan of the brain. Note the areas in red, yellow, and blue. Red and yellow represent areas with significant brain activity; blue demonstrates areas with less active brain activity. Figure 13.2 shows a benign astrocytoma located in the large blue area on the right side of the image. The large growth was determined to be benign as evidenced by the blue color rather than yellow or

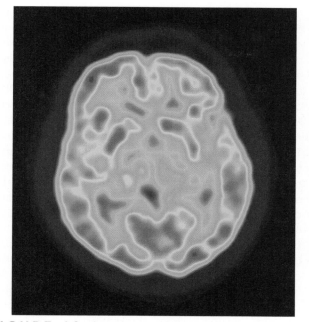

FIGURE 13.1 PET scan of the normal brain. *PET scan of the brain, released into public domain by I. Jens Langner. Accessed at www.commons.wikimedia.org/wiki/File:PET -image.jpg*

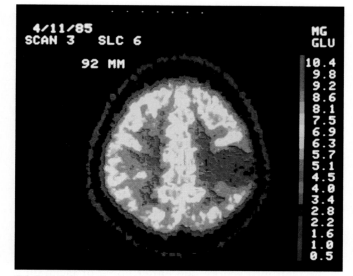

FIGURE 13.2 PET scan showing astrocytoma. *PET scan showing astrocytoma, released into public domain by the National Cancer Institute and Dr. Giovanni Di Chiro. Accessed at http://commons.wikimedia.org/wiki/File:Pet_ scan-_astrocytoma_(grade_1).jpg*

red. Red would reflect significantly increased glucose metabolism, an indication of the rapid cell multiplication associated with malignant tumors. Therapeutically, these hot spots not only identify areas of disease and its progression but provide insight into the effectiveness of chosen treatment modalities. Because only small amounts of the radiopharmaceutical are administered to the patient, the body's homeostasis is not disturbed. For example, if the radiopharmaceutical chosen is a form of sugar as a tracer, it will behave in the body like sugar normally does. The PET scanner follows the movement of the sugar tracer within the body taking computer images that measure the distribution of the radioactivity concentration as a function of time. The time study evaluation of the sugar tracer allows for identification of local tissue metabolism. PET scanning is commonly used to asses the function of disease of the heart and brain, and to identify types of cancer. Therefore, the HCPs most likely to use PET scans are cardiologists, neurologists, and oncologists. Cardiologists use a PET scan to diagnose heart diseases by evaluating cardiac blood flow while assessing the need for angioplasty or coronary artery bypass surgery. Neurologists can use the PET scan to help diagnose tumor, discover the cause of seizure, evaluate the activity of the brain during specified tasks such as memory, assess dementia, and assist in pinpointing surgical areas. Oncologists use PET scans to diagnose cancer and evaluate the effectiveness of cancer treatment modalities. Not all cancers show up with a PET scan. Those types of cancer for which the functionality of a PET is most beneficial

to the patient are brain, breast, cervical, colon, thyroid, pancreatic, esophogeal, and lung cancer, as well as lymphoma and melanoma.

The information in the Part I studies is organized in a manner to help the student see how the five basic components of the nursing process (assessment, diagnosis, planning, implementation, and evaluation) can be applied to each phase of laboratory and diagnostic testing. The goal is to use nursing process to understand the integration of care (laboratory, diagnostic, and nursing care) toward achieving a positive expected outcome.

- **Assessment** is the collection of information for the purpose of answering the question, "is there a problem?" Knowledge of the patient's health history, medications, complaints, and allergies as well as synonyms or alternate test names, common use for the procedure, specimen requirements, and normal ranges or interpretive comments provide the foundation for diagnosis.
- **Diagnosis** is the process of looking at the information gathered during assessment and answering the questions, "what is the problem?" and "what do I need to do about it?" Test indications tell us why the study has been requested, and potential diagnoses tell us the value or importance of the study relative to its clinical utility.
- **Planning** is a blueprint of the nursing care before the procedure. It is the process of determining how the nurse is going to partner with the patient to fix the problem (e.g., "The patient has a study ordered, and this is what I should know before I successfully carry out the plan to have the study

completed"). Knowledge of interfering factors, social and cultural issues, preprocedure restrictions, the need for written and informed consent, anxiety about the procedure, and concerns regarding pain are some considerations for planning a successful partnership.

- **Implementation** is putting the plan into action with an idea of what the expected outcome should be. Collaboration with the departments where the laboratory test or diagnostic study is to be performed is essential to the success of the plan. Implementation is where the work is done within each healthcare team member's scope of practice. Assessment is used to decide if there is something that needs to be addressed. Diagnosis places a name on the identified problem. The plan is what we are going to do about the identified problem. Implementation is putting the plan into action, and either doing or facilitating its completion.

- **Evaluation** answers the question, "did the plan work or not?" Was the plan completely successful, partially successful, or not successful? If the plan did not work, evaluation is the process where you determine what needs to be changed to make the plan work better. This includes a review of all expected outcomes. Nursing care after the procedure is where information is gathered to evaluate the plan. Review of results, including critical findings, in relation to patient symptoms and other tests performed provide data that form a more complete picture of health or illness.

- **Expected Outcomes** are positive outcomes related to the test. They are the outcomes the nurse should expect if all goes well.

A number of pretest, intratest, and post-test universal points are presented in this overview section because the information applies to nuclear scan studies in general.

Universal Pretest Pearls (Planning)

- Record the date of the last menstrual period and determine the possibility of pregnancy in premenopausal and perimenopausal women should be accomplished prior to scheduling all examinations using radiation. Notify the appropriate testing department if the patient may be pregnant, is breastfeeding, or is younger than 18 years of age. Children are not generally considered candidates for nuclear scanning unless the dosage is carefully calculated, although there are indications, as in cancer treatment, when frequent scanning is performed. Because of the potential effect of radiation on cell growth if a fetus is exposed to radiation, pregnant women may not be considered

candidates for some procedures unless the benefits outweigh the risk to the fetus and mother. Nuclear medicine testing may sometimes be performed in pregnant women to identify the risks of various diseases when studies utilizing no radiation, such as ultrasound and magnetic resonance imaging (MRI), cannot provide the necessary information needed. Radiopharmaceuticals can readily cross the placenta, resulting in minimal exposure to the fetus. The primary method to reduce radiation exposure to the unborn child is to strongly recommend to the mother that she drink a lot of fluid (water preferably). Increased hydration and frequent urination can reduce the radiation dose substantially. Lactating women may need to avoid nuclear scans due to the risk to the fetus. The National Council on Radiation and Protection (NCRP) Report No. 174, Preconception and Prenatal Radiation Exposure: Health Effects and Protective Guidance contains information on risks from ionizing (e.g., nuclear studies) and non-ionizing sources of radiation (e.g., MRI, US, and RF). Subsequent advances have been made in determining the potentially adverse effects of both pre- and postconception maternal irradiation, and of irradiation at various stages of pregnancy. There are no concerns to the fetus if a patient is planning on becoming pregnant soon after a diagnostic procedure using radiation. Future pregnancies should be planned for after the use of therapeutic agents in nuclear medicine. The recommendations of the International Commission on Radiation Protection (ICRP) are that women do not become pregnant until the estimated fetal dose falls below 1 mGy (1 mGy = 100 mrem).

- Obtain a history of the patient's complaints, including a list of known allergens, especially allergies or sensitivities to medications, latex, or radionuclides, so their use can be avoided or their effects mitigated if an allergy is present. Carefully evaluate all medications currently being taken by the patient. A list of the patient's current medications, prescribed and over the counter (including dietary supplements), should also be obtained. Such products should be discontinued by medical direction for the appropriate number of days prior to the procedure. **Ensure that all allergies are clearly noted in the medical record, and ensure the patient is wearing an allergy and medical record armband. Report information that could interfere with, or delay proceeding with, the scan to the HCP and nuclear medicine department.**

- Obtain a history of the patient's affected body system, symptoms, and results of previously performed laboratory tests and diagnostic and surgical procedures. Previous test results will provide a basis of comparison between old and new data.

Complete a set of preprocedure vital signs and a focused assessment prior to sending the patient for the scan. This will provide a baseline for comparison when the patient's study has been completed and postprocedure vital signs and focused assessment are conducted.

- An important aspect of planning is understanding the factors that may alter study findings or cause abnormal results. Interdepartmental communication is a key factor in the planning process. The inability of a patient to cooperate or remain still during the procedure because of age, significant pain, or mental status should be among the anticipated factors. Recent or past procedures, medications, or existing medical conditions that could complicate or interfere with test results should be noted.
- Review the steps of the study with the patient or caregiver. Expect patients to be nervous about the procedure and the pending results. Educating the patient on his or her role during the procedure and what to expect can facilitate this. The patient's role during the procedure is to remain still. The actual time for each study will depend on many conditions, including the type of imaging equipment being used, the time necessary for the chosen radiopharmaceutical to become concentrated in the tissues (which may cause a delay before imaging), the level of cooperation of the patient, the physical size of the patient, and the number of images taken based on department protocol.
- Address any concerns about pain, and explain or describe, as appropriate, the level and type of discomfort that may be expected. Explain that an IV line may be inserted prior to some procedures to allow the infusion of IV fluids such as normal saline, radionuclides, anesthetics, sedatives, radionuclides, medications used in the procedure, or emergency medications. Advise the patient that some discomfort may be experienced during insertion of the IV. Advise the patient that some mild discomfort may be experienced during the scan.
- Provide additional instructions and patient preparation regarding medication, diet, fluid intake, or activity, if appropriate. Unless specified in the individual study, there are no special instructions or restrictions.
- Always be sensitive to any cultural or psychosocial issues, including a concern for modesty before, during, and after the procedure.

Reminder

Ensure that a written and informed consent has been documented in the medical record, as appropriate, prior to a nuclear medicine scan. The consent must be obtained before medication is administered.

● *Safety Tip*

Safety in the administration of a radionuclide is a priority. This process begins with accurate patient identification to avoid administration of an incorrect radiopharmaceutical, which can be a common source of error. The identification, calculation, documentation, administration, and monitoring of the radionuclide used during an in vitro, imaging, or therapeutic procedure are required, following the facility's NRC-mandated quality management program related to patient identification and the use of therapeutic radionuclides. Radiopharmaceuticals are defined as those medications used to evoke a specific physiological or biochemical response. This includes safe handling during the preparation and administration of oral and IV contrast used in the performance of nuclear studies.

Universal Intratest Pearls (Implementation)

- Correct patient identification is crucial prior to any procedure. Positively identify the patient using two unique identifiers such as patient name, date of birth, Social Security number, or medical record number. Although the nurse will not be performing the nuclear scan, nursing is responsible to ensure that the patient understands how the study will be performed, and her or his role in ensuring its success.
- Standard Precautions must be followed.
- Children and infants may be accompanied by a parent to calm them. Keep neonates and infants covered and in a warm room, and provide a pacifier or gentle touch. The testing environment should be quiet, and the patient should be instructed, as appropriate, to remain still during the test as extraneous movements can affect results. Information on the Image Gently Campaign can be found at the Alliance for Radiation Safety in Pediatric Imaging (www.pedrad.org/associations/5364/ig/).
- Ensure the patient has complied with pretesting instructions, including dietary, fluid, medication, and activity restrictions as given for the procedure. The number of days to withhold medication depends on the type of medication. Notify the HCP if pretesting instructions have not been followed (e.g., if patient anticoagulant therapy has not been withheld).
- The patient as appropriate should be prepared for the insertion of an IV line for infusion of IV fluids, radionuclides, antibiotics, anesthetics, analgesics, or radionuclides must be made. Prior to the administration of any fluids or medications, verify that they are accurate for the study. Bleeding or bruising can be prevented, once the needle has been removed, by applying direct pressure to the injection site with dry gauze for a minute or two. The site should be observed/assessed for bleeding or hematoma formation and then covered with a gauze and adhesive bandage.

- Emergency equipment should be readily available.
- Baseline vital signs must be recorded and monitored throughout and after the procedure, according to organizational policy. A comparison should be made between the baseline and postprocedure vital signs and focused assessments. Protocols may vary among facilities.

● *Safety Tip*

Elimination of the radioisotope occurs normally in breast milk, urine, feces, and other body fluid. Mothers who are breastfeeding should not resume breastfeeding for about 3 days. Milk should be expressed to prevent cessation of milk production and then discarded until breastfeeding can be resumed.

Universal Post Test Pearls (Evaluation)

- Note that completed test results are made available to the requesting HCP, who will discuss them with the patient.
- Answer questions and address concerns voiced by the patient or family, and reinforce information given by the patient's HCP regarding further testing, treatment, or referral to another HCP. Recognize that patients will have anxiety related to test results. Provide teaching and information regarding the clinical implications of the test results on the patient's lifestyle as appropriate.
- Note that test results should be evaluated in context with the patient's signs, symptoms, and diagnosis. Depending on the results of the procedure, additional testing may be performed to evaluate or monitor progression of the disease process and determine the need for a change in therapy.
- Be aware that when a person goes through a traumatic event such as an illness or being given information that will impact his or her lifestyle, there are universal human reactions that occur. These include knowledge deficit, fear, anxiety, and coping; in some situations, grieving may occur. HCPs should always be aware of the human response and how it may affect the plan of care and expected outcomes.

Reminder

Remind the patient that no other radionuclide tests should be scheduled for 24 to 48 hours following this procedure. The radionuclide is eliminated from the body within 24 to 48 hours; unless contraindicated, advise the patient to drink increased amounts of fluids during this period to assist in elimination of the radionuclide from the body.

● *Safety Tip*

After the procedure, special care should be taken in relation to urine and stool elimination. Patients should flush the toilet numerous times immediately after use. Hands should be washed vigorously after toileting for 48 hours postprocedure. Health-care personnel assisting patients should wear gloves for handling stool or urine. Gloved hands should be vigorously washed prior to their removal. Bare hands should then be vigorously washed after glove removal.

DISCUSSION POINT

Regarding Post-Test Critical Findings: Timely notification of a critical finding for lab or diagnostic studies is a role expectation of the professional nurse. Notification processes will vary among facilities. Upon receipt of the critical finding, the information should be read back to the caller to verify accuracy. Most policies require immediate notification of the primary HCP, hospitalist, or on-call HCP. Reported information includes the patient's name, unique identifiers, critical finding, name of the person giving the report, and name of the person receiving the report. Documentation of notification should be made in the medical record with the name of the HCP notified, time and date of notification, and any orders received. Any delay in a timely report of a critical finding may require completion of a notification form with review by Risk Management.

STUDIES

- Bone Scan
- Hepatobiliary Scan
- Myocardial Infarct Scan
- Myocardial Perfusion Heart Scan
- Positron Emission Tomography, Brain
- Positron Emission Tomography, Heart

LEARNING OUTCOMES

Providing safe, effective nursing care (SENC) includes mastery of core competencies and standards of care. SENC is based on a judicious application of nursing knowledge in combination with scientific principles. The Art of Nursing lies in blending what you know with the ability to effectively apply your knowledge in a compassionate manner.

After reading/studying this chapter, you will be able to:

Thinking

1. Identify safety precautions for handling stool and urine post scan.
2. Identify the most common route of administration of radionuclides.

Doing

1. Describe the cause and appropriate intervention for treatment of an IV hematoma.
2. Discuss the postprocedure patient assessments.

Caring

1. Understand and value the patient's choice of how involved he or she wishes to be in the provision of care.

Bone Scan

Quick Summary

SYNONYM ACRONYM: Bone imaging, radionuclide bone scan, bone scintigraphy, whole-body bone scan.

COMMON USE: To assist in diagnosing bone disease such as cancer or other degenerative bone disorders.

AREA OF APPLICATION: Bone/skeleton.

NORMAL FINDINGS: No abnormalities, as indicated by homogeneous and symmetric distribution of the radionuclide throughout all skeletal structures

Test Explanation

This nuclear medicine scan assists in diagnosing and determining the extent of primary and metastatic bone disease and bone trauma and monitors the progression of degenerative disorders. Abnormalities are identified by scanning 1 to 3 hours after the IV injection of a radionuclide such as technetium-99m methylene diphosphonate. Areas of increased uptake and activity on the bone scan represent abnormalities unless they occur in normal areas of increased activity, such as the sternum, sacroiliac, clavicle, and scapular joints in adults, and growth centers and cranial sutures in children (see Figs. 13.3 and 13.4). A number of types of cancer, such as breast, lung, lymphomas, and prostate, are known to metastasize to bone. The radionuclide mimics calcium physiologically and therefore localizes in bone with an intensity proportional to the degree of metabolic activity. Gallium, magnetic resonance imaging (MRI), or white blood cell scanning may be performed after a bone scan to obtain a more sensitive study if acute inflammatory conditions such as osteomyelitis or septic arthritis are suspected. Bone scan is very sensitive; abnormalities can be identified weeks or months before they might be detected by x-ray. In addition, bone scan can detect fractures in patients who continue to have pain even though x-rays have proved negative. A gamma camera detects the radiation emitted from the injected radioactive material. Whole-body or representative images of the skeletal system can be obtained. Single-photon emission computed tomography (SPECT) has significantly improved the resolution and accuracy of bone scanning and may or may not be included as part of the examination. SPECT enables images to be recorded from multiple angles around the body and reconstructed by a computer to produce images or "slices" representing the area of interest at different levels (see Fig. 13.5).

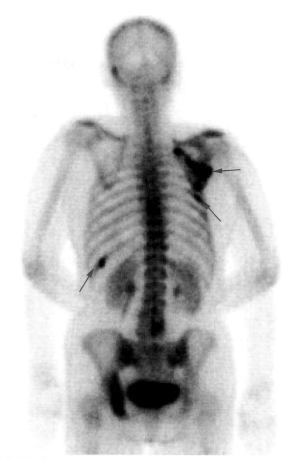

FIGURE 13.3 Bone scan showing metastases to the ribs and scapula. *Used with permission, from Weber, E., Vilensky, J., & Fog, A (2013). Practical radiology: A symptom-based approach. FA Davis Company.*

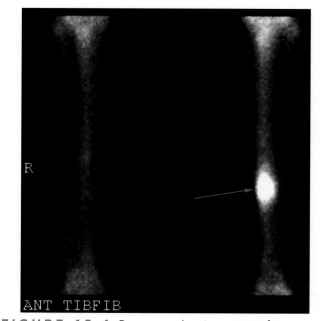

FIGURE 13.4 Bone scan showing a stress fracture of the lower leg. *Used with permission, from Weber, E., Vilensky, J., & Fog, A (2013). Practical radiology: A symptom-based approach. FA Davis Company.*

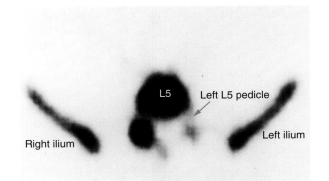

FIGURE 13.5 Cross-sectional SPECT image showing abnormal findings of the lumbar spine vertebrae at level 5 (L5). *Used with permission, from Weber, E., Vilensky, J., & Fog, A (2013). Practical radiology: A symptom-based approach. FA Davis Company.*

Nursing Implications

Assessment

Indications	Potential Nursing Problems
Aid in the diagnosis of benign tumors or cysts	• Activity
Aid in the diagnosis of metabolic bone diseases	• Body Image
Aid in the diagnosis of osteomyelitis	• Conflicted Decision Making
Aid in the diagnosis of primary malignant bone tumors (e.g., osteogenic sarcoma, chondrosarcoma, Ewing sarcoma, metastatic malignant tumors)	• Fear • Grief • Human Reactions • Infection
Aid in the detection of traumatic or stress fractures	• Injury Risk
Assess degenerative joint changes or acute septic arthritis	• Mobility • Pain
Assess suspected child abuse	• Self-esteem
Confirm temporomandibular joint derangement	• Self-care
Detect Legg-Calvé-Perthes disease	• Skin
Determine the cause of unexplained bone or joint pain	
Evaluate the healing process following fracture, especially if an underlying bone disease is present	
Evaluate prosthetic joints for infection, loosening, dislocation, or breakage	
Evaluate tumor response to radiation or chemotherapy	
Identify appropriate site for bone biopsy, lesion excision, or débridement	

Diagnosis: Clinical Significance of Test Results

ABNORMAL FINDINGS

Uneven distribution of the radionuclide, deposited in concentrated "hot spots" indicate areas where lesions, trauma, or degeneration in bone tissue are located.

- Bone necrosis
- Degenerative arthritis
- Fracture
- Legg-Calvé-Perthes disease
- Metastatic bone neoplasm
- Osteomyelitis
- Paget disease
- Primary metastatic bone tumors
- Renal osteodystrophy
- Rheumatoid arthritis

Planning

Considerations for planning a successful partnership should include clear communication of what to expect during the test to decrease anxiety and improve cooperation. Before the procedure is performed, plan to review the steps with the patient and address any concerns about pain. Explain that an IV line will be inserted to allow the infusion of IV fluids such as normal saline, anesthetics, sedatives, radionuclides, medications used in the procedure, or emergency medications, and that there may be some discomfort during the venipuncture. Reassure the patient that the radionuclide poses no radioactive hazard and rarely produces side effects. Explain that the camera takes pictures only and does not give off any radiation. Advise the patient that after initial images are taken, additional scanning will begin about 3 hours after injection with the radiopharmaceutical and takes approximately 30 to 60 minutes; also inform the patient that there may be some minimal pain or discomfort during the scan. Repeat scans may be performed for up to 24 hours after the initial radiopharmaceutical injection.

PEDIATRIC CONSIDERATIONS

Preparing a child for a bone scan depends on the age of the child. Encourage parents to be truthful about what the child may experience during the procedure (e.g., they may feel a pinch or minor discomfort when the IV needle is inserted) and to use words they know their child will understand. Toddlers and preschool-age children have a very short attention span, so the best time to talk about the test is right before the procedure. The child should be assured that she or he will be allowed to bring a favorite comfort item into the examination room and, if appropriate, that a parent will be with them during the procedure. Explain the importance of remaining still while the images are taken.

It is important to understand factors that can interfere with accurate testing. It is essential that the patient remain still during the scanning portion of the study in order to obtain clear images. Children or adult patients who are unable to lie still may need to be pre-medicated with an appropriate sedative. Foam wedges may be used during a bone scan to assist the patient in remaining immobile. Recent administration of x-ray contrast or other radionuclides may interfere with test results.

SPECIAL CONSIDERATIONS

An important aspect of planning is understanding the factors that may alter study findings or cause abnormal results. Interdepartmental communication is a key factor in the planning process. It should be noted when planning for this study that the existence of multiple myeloma or thyroid cancer can result in a false-negative scan for bone abnormalities.

● *Safety Tip*

Make sure a written and informed consent has been signed prior to the procedure and before administering any medications.

Implementation

Patient education is key to obtaining the patient's cooperation in following directions, and providing an explanation for the purpose of the procedure is an important part of this process. Inform the patient that this study can assist with assessing for disorders of the bones. A bone scan can identify areas of disease even before they show up on plain radiography, allowing for early access to treatment. Bone scans can also be used to assess the effectiveness of therapeutic interventions for diseases such as cancer and infection. Scanning is often used to assess if cancer from other areas in the body has moved to the bones.

SPECIAL CONSIDERATIONS

Patients should be encouraged to fully empty their bladder prior to the procedure as a distended bladder may obscure pelvic detail in a bone scan.

Prior to the procedure, ensure that the patient has removed all external metallic objects from the area to be examined. Establish an IV line for the administration of saline, anesthetics, sedatives, radionuclides, or emergency medications. If the patient has a history of allergic reactions to any substance or drug, administer ordered prophylactic steroids or antihistamines. Place the patient in a supine position on a flat table with foam wedges to help maintain position and immobilization. A patient may have SPECT to evaluate areas of suspicious radionuclide localization by providing a three-dimensional picture of the area of concern.

Evaluation

Recognize anxiety related to test results and answer any questions or address any concerns voiced by the patient or family. Discuss the implications of abnormal test results on the patient's lifestyle. Provide teaching and information regarding the clinical implications of the test results as appropriate. Provide contact information, if desired, for the American College of Rheumatology (www.rheumatology.org), the American Cancer Society (www.cancer.org), or the Arthritis Foundation (www.arthritis.org).

Unless contraindicated, advise the patient to drink increased amounts of fluids for 24 to 48 hours to eliminate the radionuclide from the body. Inform the patient that radionuclide is eliminated from the body within 6 to 24 hours. Follow the universal postscan recommendations as discussed in the chapter overview.

✓ *Critical Findings*

N/A

✓ *Study Specific Complications*

- Radionuclide scans are considered a fairly safe procedure. The actual scans are noninvasive and cause little patient discomfort. However, like x-rays, they expose the body to a small dose of radiation. This can damage cells and cause mutations, particularly in growing fetuses. Patients should be made aware of the potential risks to the fetus.

- Contrast reactions can be an additional complication of diagnostic studies, especially when iodinated contrast is used. **Iodinated contrast mediums may cause minor-to-severe allergic reactions in a patient.** Consideration may be given to oral administration of diphendydramine in the case of mild allergic reaction; IV or IM epinephrine or diphenhydramine may be considered in cases of moderate to severe allergic reaction; a request for resuscitation by a specially trained emergency response team may be required in the case of severe allergic reaction.

- Inaccurate injection of the radiopharmaceutical may cause the tracer to end up in subcutaneous tissue, causing infiltration, and may lead to extravasation or even entering deep into muscle tissue, resulting in false hot spots and inaccurate results.

- There are a number of complications associated with performing a venipuncture. **Pain** is commonly associated with needles, and although the pain experienced during venipuncture is usually mild, on a rare occasion the needle may strike a nerve, causing permanent pain. Some patients experience a **vasovagal reaction** during the venipuncture procedure, evidenced by sweating, low blood pressure, fainting, or near fainting. The potential for a **fall injury** is a significant concern related to vasovagal reactions. Prolonged **bleeding** is a complication that occurs in patients who are taking blood thinners or who have coagulopathies such as hemophilia. A **hematoma** results when blood leaks into the tissue during or after a venipuncture, as evidenced by pain, bruising, and/or swelling at the venipuncture site.

The swelling can cause injury by compression to surrounding nerves, which can be temporary or permanent. Health-care providers should watch for minor complications such as bruising and hematoma at the venipuncture site, which are fairly common. Hematomas occur more often in older adult or frail patients, or in those whose veins are difficult to access. Bleeding or bruising can be prevented once the needle has been removed by applying direct pressure to the site with dry gauze for a minute or two. Some other more unusual complications of venipuncture include **cellulitis, phlebitis, inadvertent arterial puncture,** and **sepsis.** Sepsis can be caused by introduction of bacteria from the surface of the skin into the blood as the result of improper cleansing of the venipuncture site. Immunocompromised patients are at a higher risk for developing this complication.

Related Tests

- Related tests include antibodies, anticyclic citrullinated peptide, ANA, arthroscopy, BMD, calcium, CRP, collagen cross-linked telopeptide, CT pelvis, CT spine, culture blood, ESR, MRI musculoskeletal, MRI pelvis, osteocalcin, radiography bone, RF, synovial fluid analysis, and white blood cell scan.
- Refer to the Musculoskeletal System table at the end of the book for related tests by body system.

Expected Outcomes

Expected outcomes associated with Bone Scans are

- Adapting to the loss of a limb and a change in body image
- Managing activity with the use of assistive devices
- Adapting to limited mobility and revised self-concept in the performance of the patient's expected role
- Expressing grief at the loss of functioning appropriately

Hepatobiliary Scan

Quick Summary

SYNONYM ACRONYM: Biliary tract radionuclide scan, cholescintigraphy, hepatobiliary imaging, hepatobiliary scintigraphy, gallbladder scan, HIDA or hepatobiliary iminodiacetic scan.

COMMON USE: To visualize and assess the cystic and common bile ducts of the gallbladder toward diagnosing obstructions, stones, inflammation, and tumor.

AREA OF APPLICATION: Bile ducts.

NORMAL FINDINGS: Normal shape, size, and function of the gallbladder with patent cystic and common bile ducts; radionuclide should pass through the biliary system and a significant amount be visualized in the gallbladder within 15–30 minutes

Test Explanation

The hepatobiliary scan is a nuclear medicine study of the hepatobiliary excretion system. It is primarily used to determine the patency of the cystic and common bile ducts, but it can also be used to determine overall hepatic function, gallbladder function, presence of gallstones (indirectly), and sphincter of Oddi dysfunction. A technetium (Tc-99m) labelled iminodiacetic acid analogue (e.g., tribromoethyl) is injected IV and excreted into the bile duct system. A gamma camera detects the radiation emitted from the injected contrast medium, and a representative image of the duct system is obtained. The results are correlated with other diagnostic studies, such as IV cholangiography, computed tomography (CT) scan of the gallbladder, and ultrasonography. Gallbladder emptying or ejection fraction can be determined by administering a fatty meal or cholecystokinin to the patient. This procedure can be used before and after surgery to determine the extent of bile reflux.

Nursing Implications
Assessment

Indications	Potential Nursing Problems
Aid in the diagnosis of acute and chronic cholecystitis	• Diarrhea
Aid in the diagnosis of suspected gallbladder disorders, such as inflammation, perforation, or calculi	• Fluid Volume
	• Gas Exchange
	• Human Reaction
Assess enterogastric reflux	• Infection
Assess obstructive jaundice when done in combination with radiography or ultrasonography	• Injury Risk
	• Jaundice
Determine common duct obstruction caused by tumors or choledocholithiasis	• Nutrition
	• Pain
Evaluate biliary enteric bypass patency	• Skin
Postoperatively evaluate gastric surgical procedures and abdominal trauma	

Diagnosis: Clinical Significance of Test Results
ABNORMAL FINDINGS

Uneven distribution of the radionuclide, deposited in concentrated "hot spots" indicate areas where lesions, trauma, abnormal anatomy, or obstructions in the biliary system are located. An extended amount of time (greater than 30–60 minutes) taken for the radionuclide to pass through the gallbladder is also abnormal.

- Cholecystitis (acalculous, acute, chronic) *evidenced by visualization of the biliary tree and lack of visualization of the gallbladder related to obstruction of the cystic duct by gallstones*

- Common bile duct obstruction secondary to gallstones, tumor, or stricture *evidenced by visualization in the bile duct but absent visualization of the tracer in the small intestine, related to bile duct obstruction*
- Congenital biliary atresia or choledochal cyst *evidenced by delayed visualization of the tracer and low ejection fracture (less than 35%)*
- Postoperative biliary leak, fistula, or obstruction
- Trauma-induced bile leak or cyst

Planning

Considerations for planning a successful partnership should include clear communication of what to expect during the test to decrease anxiety and improve cooperation. Before the procedure is performed, plan to review the steps with the patient and address any concerns about pain. Explain that an IV line will be inserted to allow infusion of IV fluids such as normal saline, anesthetics, sedatives, radionuclides, medications used in the procedure, or emergency medications, and that there may be some discomfort during the venipuncture. Reassure the patient that the radionuclide poses no radioactive hazard and rarely produces side effects. Advise the patient that initial images are taken after injection of the radionuclide. Additional scans will periodically be performed; the entire procedure takes approximately 1 to 4 hours. Imaging time depends on the patient's hepatobiliary function. Repeat scans may be performed for up to 24 hours after the initial radiopharmaceutical injection. Also inform the patient that there may be some minimal pain or discomfort during the scan. For some studies, a medication is given to cause the gallbladder to empty, and the patient may briefly experience some abdominal discomfort or nausea. Instruct the patient to fast for 4 to 6 hours before the scan. Check the patient's medication administration record for opiates. Opiate-based pain medications must not be taken for 4 to 6 hours prior to the study because they may interfere with the study. Morphine is used interventionally when the gallbladder cannot be seen because it causes the sphincter of Oddi to contract and draw the radiolabeled bile into the gallbladder, which can then be visualized.

PEDIATRIC CONSIDERATIONS

Hepatobiliary scans can be valuable in the pediatric population in differentiating between biliary atresia and neonatal hepatitis. Other uses of this scan for children and infants are to assess for liver trauma and congenital anomalies and to identify the cause of upper quadrant pain. Preparing children for a hepatobiliary scan depends on the age of the child. Encourage parents to be truthful about what the child may experience during the procedure (e.g., they may feel a pinch or minor discomfort when the IV needle is inserted) and to use words they know their child will understand. Toddlers and preschool-age children have a very short attention span, so the best time to talk about the test is right before the procedure. The child should be assured that she or he will be allowed to bring a favorite comfort item into the examination room and, if appropriate, that a parent will be with the child during the procedure. Explain the importance of remaining still while the images are taken.

SPECIAL CONSIDERATIONS

An important aspect of planning is understanding the factors that may alter study findings or cause abnormal results. Interdepartmental communication is a key factor in the planning process. The following should be noted when planning for this study:

- Scanning may be cancelled for patients who fail to comply with dietary instructions.
- Fasting for more than 24 hours before the procedure, or being on total parenteral nutrition, can interfere by preventing filling of the gallbladder, which can result in inaccurate scan results.
- The patient must remain still during the scanning portion of the study in order to obtain clear images. Children or adult patients who are unable to lie still may need to be premedicated with an appropriate sedative.
- Recent administration of x-ray contrast medium or other radionuclides may interfere with test results.
- Bilirubin levels greater than or equal to 30 mg/dL, depending on the radionuclide used, may decrease hepatic uptake.

● *Safety Tip*

Make sure a written and informed consent has been signed prior to the procedure and before administering any medications.

Implementation

Note that patient education is key to obtaining the patient's cooperation in following directions, and providing an explanation for the purpose of the procedure is an important part of this process. Inform the patient that this study can assist with assessing gallbladder, biliary tree, liver, and spleen function. Ensure that the patient has complied with dietary instructions and medication restrictions, and that morphine sulfate or opiates have been withheld. Instruct the patient to void prior to the procedure and to change into the gown, robe, and foot coverings provided.

Ensure that the patient has removed all external metallic objects from the area to be examined prior to the procedure. Establish an IV line for the administration of saline, anesthetics, sedatives, radionuclides, or emergency medications. If the patient has a history of allergic reactions to any substance or drug, administer ordered prophylactic steroids or antihistamines before the procedure. Once injected with the tracer, the patient will be asked to lie on his or her back. Scanning will occur immediately and at specified intervals. Images are taken every 5 minutes for the first 30 minutes and every 10 minutes for the next 30 minutes to an hour.

DISCUSSION POINT

Some facilities will give the patient sincalide before the study begins to stimulate the release of cholecystokinin, promoting gallbladder contraction. IV morphine sulfate may be used to elicit gallbladder contractions, forcing the radionuclide into the gallbladder as a first choice, or if the sincalide is ineffective, within 1 hour of administration. The goal is to cause the sphincter of Oddi to spasm. Scans will be repeated 20 or 50 minutes later. Additional scans may be required at 2, 4, and 24 hours later. Remind the patient who is having delayed scanning to restrict fat consumption while waiting for these additional scans. If gallbladder function or bile reflux is being assessed, the patient will be given a fatty meal or cholecystokinin 60 minutes after the radionuclide injection. During contractions of the gallbladder, the percentage of isotope being ejected is measured to determine ejection fraction.

Evaluation

Recognize anxiety related to test results and answer any questions or address any concerns voiced by the patient or family. Discuss the implications of abnormal test results on the patient's lifestyle. Provide teaching and information regarding the clinical implications of the test results as appropriate. Patients can resume eating their normal diet unless changed by the health-care provider (HCP). Postprocedure vital signs are recommended and should be completed based on organizational policy.

Unless contraindicated, advise the patient to drink increased amounts of fluids for 24 to 48 hours to eliminate the radionuclide from the body. Inform the patient that radionuclide is eliminated from the body within 6 to 24 hours. Follow the universal postscan recommendations as discussed in the chapter overview.

✔ Critical Findings

N/A

✔ Study Specific Complications

- Radionuclide scans are considered a fairly safe procedure. The actual scans are noninvasive and cause little patient discomfort. However, like x-rays, they expose the body to a small dose of radiation. This can damage cells and cause mutations, particularly in growing fetuses. Patients should be made aware of the potential risks to the fetus.
- Contrast reactions can be an additional complication of diagnostic studies, especially when iodinated contrast is used. **Iodinated contrast mediums may cause minor-to-severe allergic reactions in a patient.** Consideration may be given to the administration of oral diphenhydramine in the case of mild allergic reaction; IV or IM epinephrine or diphenhydramine may be considered in cases of moderate to severe allergic reaction; a request for resuscitation by a specially trained emergency response team may be required in the case of severe allergic reaction.
- Inaccurate injection of the radiopharmaceutical may cause the tracer to end up in subcutaneous tissue, causing infiltration, and may lead to extravasation or even entering deep into muscle tissue, resulting in false hot spots and inaccurate results.
- There are a number of complications associated with performing a venipuncture. **Pain** is commonly associated with needles, and although the pain experienced during venipuncture is usually mild, on a rare occasion the needle may strike a nerve, causing permanent pain. Some patients experience a **vasovagal reaction** during the venipuncture procedure, evidenced by sweating, low blood pressure, fainting, or near fainting. The potential for a **fall injury** is a significant concern related to vasovagal reactions. Prolonged **bleeding** is a complication that occurs with patients who are taking blood thinners or who have coagulopathies such as hemophilia. A **hematoma** results when blood leaks into the tissue during or after a venipuncture, as evidenced by pain, bruising, and/or swelling at the venipuncture site. The swelling can cause injury by compression to surrounding nerves, which can be temporary or permanent. HCPs should watch for minor complications such as bruising and hematoma at the venipuncture site, which are fairly common. Hematomas occur more often in older adult or frail patients, or those with veins that are difficult to access. Bleeding or bruising can be prevented once the needle has been removed by applying direct pressure to the site with dry gauze for a minute or two. Some other more unusual complications of venipuncture include **cellulitis, phlebitis, inadvertent arterial puncture, and sepsis.** Sepsis can be caused by introduction of bacteria from the surface of the skin into the blood as the result of improper cleansing of the venipuncture site. Immunocompromised patients are at higher risk for developing this complication.

✔ Related Tests

- Related tests include amylase, bilirubin, CT abdomen, lipase, liver and spleen scan, MRI abdomen, radiofrequency ablation liver, US abdomen, and US liver and bile ducts.

- Refer to the Hepatobiliary System table at the end of the book for related tests by body system.

Expected Outcomes

Expected outcomes associated with Hepatobiliary Scans are

- Adjusting the diet to support health in relation to diagnosis
- Offering nonpharmacological pain management that is successful in decreasing anxiety
- Managing pain so that it is at an acceptable level for the patient
- Verbalizing an understanding of the diagnostic study process and that it may be uncomfortable at times

Myocardial Infarct Scan

Quick Summary

SYNONYM ACRONYM: PYP cardiac scan, infarct scan, pyrophosphate cardiac scan, acute myocardial infarction scan.

COMMON USE: To differentiate between new and old myocardial infarcts and evaluate myocardial perfusion.

AREA OF APPLICATION: Heart, chest/thorax.

NORMAL FINDINGS: Normal coronary blood flow and tissue perfusion, with no PYP localization in the myocardium No uptake above background activity in the myocardium (*Note:* when PYP uptake is present, it is graded in relation to adjacent rib activity)

Test Explanation

Technetium-99m stannous pyrophosphate (PYP) scanning, also known as *myocardial infarct imaging,* can identify areas of infarct or necrosis due to insufficient myocardial perfusion and provide information about the extent of myocardial infarction (MI). This procedure can distinguish new from old infarcts when a patient has had abnormal electrocardiograms (ECGs) and cardiac enzymes have returned to normal.

When myocardial cells are damaged, the intracellular contents, which include calcium, are released into the circulation. PYP binds to the calcium released from the damaged myocardial cells and PYP uptake can be visualized within 24–72 hours after MI. The radionuclide remains detectable for approximately 10 to 14 days after the MI, allowing for delayed diagnosis if the patient presents with persistent chest pain over a prolonged period of time. PYP uptake is proportional to the blood flow to the affected area; with large areas of necrosis, PYP uptake may be maximal around the periphery of a necrotic area, with little uptake being detectable in the poorly perfused center. Most of the PYP is concentrated in regions that have 20% to 40% of the normal blood flow.

Single-photon emission computed tomography (SPECT) can be used to visualize the heart from multiple angles and planes, providing 3-D functional images that enable areas of MI to be viewed with greater accuracy and resolution. This technique removes overlying structures that may confuse interpretation of the results. SPECT also provides accurate, quantitative information regarding the degree of cardiac damage. Multigated (MUGA) blood pool imaging, also known as radionuclide ventriculogram (RVG), may also be performed in conjunction with a PYP scan. MUGA provides information about cardiac function such as ejection fraction, ventricular wall motion, ventricular dilation, stroke volume, and cardiac output.

Nursing Implications

Assessment

Indications	Potential Nursing Problems
Aid in the diagnosis of (or confirm and locate) acute MI when ECG and enzyme testing do not provide a diagnosis Aid in the diagnosis of perioperative MI Differentiate between a new and old infarction Evaluate possible reinfarction or extension of the infarct Obtain baseline information about infarction before cardiac surgery	• Activity • Cardiac Output • Fear • Gas Exchange • Health Management • Human Reactions • Injury Risk • Nutrition • Pain • Role Performance • Self-care • Sexuality • Tissue Perfusion

Diagnosis: Clinical Significance of Test Results
ABNORMAL FINDINGS

- MI, indicated by increased PYP uptake in the myocardium

Planning

Considerations for planning a successful partnership should include clear communication of what to expect during the test to decrease anxiety and improve cooperation. Before the procedure is performed, plan to review the steps with the patient and address any concerns about pain. Explain that an IV line will be inserted to allow the infusion of IV fluids such as normal saline, anesthetics, sedatives, radionuclides, medications used in the procedure, or emergency medications, and that there may be some discomfort during the venipuncture. Reassure the patient that the radionuclide poses no radioactive hazard and rarely produces side effects. Explain that the camera takes pictures only and does not give off any radiation. Assess the patient's cardiovascular history, including current medications, and previous laboratory and diagnostic study results. Instruct the patient to fast and refrain from smoking for 4 hours prior to the procedure. Medications should be withheld for 24 hours before the procedure, as ordered by the requesting health-care provider (HCP). Advise the patient that the scanning will begin about 3 hours after injection with the radiopharmaceutical and takes approximately 60 minutes; also inform the patient that there may be some minimal pain or discomfort during the scan. Scanning will begin 2 to 4 hours after being injected. Repeat scans may be performed for up to 24 hours after the initial radiopharmaceutical injection. Complete a preprocedural set of vital signs and focused physical assessment prior to sending the patient to nuclear medicine.

SPECIAL CONSIDERATIONS

An important aspect of planning is understanding the factors that may alter study findings or cause abnormal results. Interdepartmental communication is a key factor in the planning process. The following should be noted when planning for this study:

* It is essential that the patient remain still during the scanning portion of the study in order to obtain clear images. Patients who are unable to lie still may need to be premedicated with an appropriate sedative. Foam wedges may be used during a the scan to assist the patient in remaining immobile.
* Recent administration of x-ray contrast or other radionuclides may interfere with test results.

● Safety Tip
Make sure a written and informed consent has been signed prior to the procedure and before administering any medications.

Implementation
Note that patient education is key to obtaining the patient's cooperation in following directions, and providing an explanation for the purpose of the procedure is an important part of this process. Inform the patient that this study can assist in assessing for disorders of blood flow to the heart. Ensure that the patient has complied with dietary and medication restrictions. Instruct the patient to void prior to the procedure and to change into the gown, robe, and foot coverings provided.

Ensure that the patient has removed all external metallic objects from the area to be examined prior to the procedure. Establish an IV line for the administration of saline, anesthetics, sedatives, radionuclides, or emergency medications. If the patient has a history of allergic reactions to any substance or drug, administer ordered prophylactic steroids or antihistamines before the procedure. Once injected with the tracer, the patient will be asked to lie on his or her back. Scanning will occur immediately and at specified intervals. Images are taken every 5 minutes for the first 30 minutes and every 10 minutes for the next 30 minutes to an hour. In most circumstances, SPECT is done so that the heart can be viewed from multiple angles and planes.

Evaluation
Recognize anxiety related to test results and answer any questions or address any concerns voiced by the patient or family. Discuss the implications of abnormal test results on the patient's lifestyle. Provide teaching and information regarding the clinical implications of the test results as appropriate. Provide contact information, if desired, for the American Heart Association (AHA) (www.heart.org) or the National Heart, Lung, and Blood Institute (NHLBI) (www.nhlbi.nih.gov).

Complete a focused assessment and set of vital signs upon completion of the study. This will provide a basis of comparison to the patient's baseline assessment. Continue postscan vital signs every 15 minutes for 1 hour, then every 2 hours for 4 hours or per organizational policy. Provide patient education regarding symptoms of chest pain. Explain the importance of reporting chest pain if it should occur.

Unless contraindicated, advise the patient to drink increased amounts of fluids for 24 to 48 hours to eliminate the radionuclide from the body. Inform the patient that radionuclide is eliminated from the body within 6 to 24 hours. Complete a focused assessment and vital signs upon the patient's return from nuclear medicine. This will provide you a basis of comparison to his or her baseline assessment. Continue postscan vital signs every 15 minutes for 1 hour, then every 2 hours for 4 hours or per organizational policy. Follow the universal postscan recommendations as discussed in the chapter overview.

SPECIAL CONSIDERATIONS
Nutritional Considerations for the Diabetic Patient: Abnormal glucose levels may be associated with conditions resulting from poor glucose control. There is no "diabetic diet"; however, many meal-planning approaches with nutritional goals are endorsed by the American Diabetes Association (ADA). Patients who adhere to dietary recommendations report a better general feeling of health, better weight management, greater control of glucose and lipid values, and improved use of insulin. Instruct the patient, as appropriate, in the nutritional management of diabetes. The nutritional needs of each diabetic patient need to be determined individually (especially during pregnancy) with the appropriate HCPs, particularly professionals educated in nutrition.

NUTRITIONAL CONSIDERATIONS FOR THE CARDIAC PATIENT: An abnormal myocardial infarct scan may be associated with coronary artery disease (CAD). Nutritional therapy is recommended for patients identified to be at risk for developing CAD or for individuals who have specific risk factors and/or existing medical conditions (e.g., elevated LDL cholesterol levels, other lipid disorders, type 1 diabetes, insulin-dependent type 2 diabetes, insulin resistance, or metabolic syndrome). Other changeable risk factors that warrant patient education include strategies to encourage patients, especially those who are overweight and with high blood pressure, to safely decrease sodium intake, achieve a normal weight, ensure regular participation in moderate aerobic physical activity three to four times per week, eliminate tobacco use, and adhere to a heart-healthy diet. If triglycerides also are elevated, the patient should be advised to eliminate or reduce alcohol. A variety of dietary patterns are beneficial for people with CAD and there are many meal-planning approaches with nutritional goals endorsed by the ADA. *The Guideline on Lifestyle Management to Reduce Cardiovascular Risk,* published by the American College of Cardiology (ACC) and the American Heart Association (AHA) in conjunction with the National Heart, Lung, and Blood Institute (NHLBI), recommends a "Mediterranean"-style diet rather than a low-fat diet. The guideline emphasizes inclusion of vegetables, whole grains, fruits, low-fat dairy, nuts, legumes, and nontropical vegetable oils (e.g., olive, canola, peanut, sunflower, flaxseed) along with fish and lean poultry. A similar dietary pattern known as the Dietary Approaches to Stop Hypertension (DASH) diet makes additional recommendations for the reduction of dietary sodium. Both dietary styles emphasize a reduction in consumption of red meats, which are high in saturated fats and cholesterol, and other foods containing sugar, saturated fats, trans fats, and sodium. The ADA also includes a vegetarian diet as well as other potential weight loss diets such as Weight Watchers. The nutritional needs of each patient need to be determined individually (especially during pregnancy) with the appropriate HCPs, particularly professionals educated in nutrition.

✅ Critical Findings

N/A

✅ Study Specific Complications

- Radionuclide scans are considered a fairly safe procedure. The actual scans are noninvasive and cause little patient discomfort. However, like x-rays, they expose the body to a small dose of radiation. This can damage cells and cause mutations, particularly in growing fetuses. Patients should be made aware of the potential risks to the fetus.
- Contrast reactions can be an additional complication of diagnostic studies, especially when iodinated contrast is used. Iodinated contrast mediums may cause minor-to-severe allergic reactions in a patient. Consideration may be given to the administration of oral diphenhydramine in the case of mild allergic reaction; IV or IM epinephrine or diphenhydramine may be considered in cases of moderate to severe allergic reaction; a request for resuscitation by a specially trained emergency response team may be required in the case of severe allergic reaction.
- Inaccurate injection of the radiopharmaceutical may cause the tracer to end up in subcutaneous tissue, causing infiltration, and may lead to extravasation or even entering deep into muscle tissue, resulting in false hot spots and inaccurate results.
- There are a number of complications associated with performing a venipuncture. **Pain** is commonly associated with needles, and although the pain experienced during venipuncture is usually mild, on a rare occasion the needle may strike a nerve, causing permanent pain. Some patients experience a **vasovagal reaction** during the venipuncture procedure, evidenced by sweating, low blood pressure, fainting, or near fainting. The potential for a **fall injury** is a significant concern related to vasovagal reactions. Prolonged **bleeding** is a complication that occurs with patients who are taking blood thinners or who have coagulopathies such as hemophilia. A **hematoma** results when blood leaks into the tissue during or after a venipuncture, as evidenced by pain, bruising, and/or swelling at the venipuncture site. The swelling can cause injury by compression to surrounding nerves, which can be temporary or permanent. HCPs should watch for minor complications such as bruising and hematoma at the venipuncture site, which are fairly common. Hematomas occur more often in older adult or frail patients, or those with veins that are difficult to access. Bleeding or bruising can be prevented once the needle has been removed by applying direct pressure to the site with dry gauze for a minute or two. Some other more unusual complications of venipuncture include **cellulitis, phlebitis, inadvertent arterial puncture,** and **sepsis.** Sepsis can be caused by the introduction of bacteria from the surface of the skin into the blood as the result of improper cleansing of the venipuncture site. Immunocompromised patients are at a higher risk for developing this complication.

✅ Related Tests

- Related tests include angiography abdominal, AST, BNP, blood pool imaging, chest x-ray, CT abdominal, CT thoracic, CK and isoenzymes, culture viral, echocardiography, echocardiography transesophageal, ECG, MRA, MRI chest, myocardial perfusion scan, pericardial fluid analysis, and PET heart.
- Refer to the Cardiovascular System table at the end of the book for related tests by body system.

Expected Outcomes

Expected outcomes associated with Myocardial Infarct Scans are

- Recording EKG changes that improve and return to baseline
- Experiencing no chest pain
- Understanding that the purpose of the exam is to assess for the presence of cardiac muscle damage
- Collaborating with the HCP to design a treatment plan to improve cardiac health

Myocardial Perfusion Heart Scan

Quick Summary

SYNONYM ACRONYM: Cardiac stress scan, nuclear stress test, sestamibi scan, stress thallium, thallium scan.

COMMON USE: To assess cardiac blood flow to evaluate for and assist in diagnosing coronary artery disease and myocardial infarction.

AREA OF APPLICATION: Heart, chest/thorax.

NORMAL FINDINGS: Normal wall motion, ejection fraction (55% to 70%), coronary blood flow, tissue perfusion, and ventricular size and function. Mitochondria are responsible for generating the energy required for all cellular function; the amount of radionuclide visualization should reflect normal, active cardiac tissue.

Test Explanation

Cardiac scanning is a nuclear medicine study that reveals clinical information about coronary blood flow, ventricular size, and cardiac function. Thallium-201 chloride rest or stress studies are used to evaluate myocardial blood flow to assist in diagnosing or determining the risk for ischemic cardiac disease, coronary artery disease (CAD), and myocardial infarction (MI). This procedure is an alternative to angiography or cardiac catheterization in cases in which these procedures may pose a risk to the patient. Thallium-201 is a potassium analogue and is taken up by myocardial cells proportional to blood flow to the cell and cell viability. During stress studies, the radionuclide is injected at peak exercise, after which the patient continues to exercise for several minutes. During exercise, areas of heart muscle supplied by normal arteries increase their blood supply, as well as the supply of thallium-201 delivery to the heart muscle, to a greater extent than regions of the heart muscle supplied by stenosed coronary arteries. This discrepancy in blood flow becomes apparent and quantifiable in subsequent imaging. Comparison of early stress images with images taken after 3 to 4 hours of redistribution (delayed images) enables differentiation between normally perfused, healthy myocardium (which is normal at rest but ischemic on stress) and infarcted myocardium. In most cases the exercise stress test goal is to increase heart rate to a level just below (85%) of a person's age predicted maximum target heart rate. The target heart rate can be calculated a number of ways. One way is by subtracting the patient's age from 220 (theoretical maximum heart rate) and multiplying by 0.85 (85%). For example the study target heart rate for a patient age 50 years would be: $(220 - 50) * 0.85 = 144$

Technetium-99m agents such as sestamibi (2-methoxyisobutylisonitrile) are delivered similarly to thallium-201 during myocardial perfusion imaging, but they are extracted to a lesser degree on the first pass through the heart and are taken up by the mitochondria. Over a short period, the radionuclide concentrates in the heart to the same degree as thallium-201. The advantage to technetium-99m agents is that immediate imaging is unnecessary because the radionuclide remains fixed to the heart muscle for several hours. The examination requires two separate injections, one for the rest portion and one for the stress portion of the procedure. These injections can take place on the same day or preferably over a 2-day period. Examination quality is improved if the patient is given a light, fatty meal after the radionuclide is injected to facilitate hepatobiliary clearance of the radioactivity.

If stress testing cannot be performed by exercising a vasodilator such as dipyridamole (Persantine) or adenosine, can be administered orally or IV. A coronary vasodilator is administered before the thallium-201 or other radionuclide, and the scanning procedure is then performed. Vasodilators increase blood flow in normal coronary arteries two- to threefold without exercise, and they reveal perfusion defects when blood flow is compromised by vessel pathology. Vasodilator-mediated myocardial perfusion scanning is reserved for patients who are unable to participate in treadmill, bicycle, or handgrip exercises for stress testing because of lung disease, neurological disorders (e.g., multiple sclerosis, spinal cord injury), morbid obesity, and orthopedic disorders (e.g., arthritis, limb amputation).

Single-photon emission computed tomography (SPECT) can be used to visualize the heart from multiple angles and planes, providing 3-D functional images that enable areas of ischemia to be viewed with greater accuracy and resolution. This technique removes overlying structures that may confuse interpretation of the results. SPECT also provides accurate, quantitative information regarding the degree of cardiac damage. Based on the study findings, multigated (MUGA) blood pool imaging, also known as radionuclide ventriculogram (RVG), may also be performed in conjunction with a myocardial perfusion scan. MUGA provides information about cardiac function such as ejection fraction, ventricular wall motion, ventricular dilation, stroke volume, and cardiac output.

Nursing Implications

Assessment

Indications	Potential Nursing Problems
Adult	• Activity
Aid in the diagnosis of CAD or risk for CAD	• Cardiac Output
Determine rest defects and reperfusion with delayed imaging in unstable angina	• Fear
Evaluate the extent of CAD and determine cardiac function	• Gas Exchange
	• Health Management
Assess the function of collateral coronary arteries	• Human Reactions
Evaluate bypass graft patency and general cardiac status after surgery	• Injury Risk
	• Nutrition
	• Pain
Evaluate the site of an old MI to determine obstruction to cardiac muscle perfusion	• Role Performance
	• Self-care
Evaluate the effectiveness of medication regimen and balloon angioplasty procedure on narrow coronary arteries	• Sexuality
	• Tissue Perfusion
Pediatric	
Assess athletic potential	
Establish a baseline prior to physical rehabilitation therapy	
Evaluate for cardiac dysfunction related to diagnosed or undiagnosed congenital heart defects or other cardiac issues that manifest symptoms when engaging in physical activity or exertion	

Diagnosis: Clinical Significance of Test Results

ABNORMAL FINDINGS

Poor visualization or "cold spots" are seen in areas of poor perfusion and diminished cardiac muscle activity

• Abnormal stress and resting images, indicating previous MI
• Abnormal stress images with normal resting images, indicating transient ischemia
• Cardiac hypertrophy, indicated by increased radionuclide uptake in the myocardium
• Enlarged left ventricle
• Heart chamber disorder
• Heart failure
• Ventricular septal defects

Planning

Considerations for planning a successful partnership should include clear communication of what to expect during the test to decrease anxiety and improve cooperation. Before the procedure is performed, plan to review the steps with the patient and address any concerns about pain. Explain that an IV line will be inserted to allow the infusion of IV fluids such as normal saline, anesthetics, sedatives, radionuclides, medications used in the procedure, or emergency medications, and that there may be some discomfort during the venipuncture. Reassure the patient that the radionuclide poses no radioactive hazard and rarely produces side effects. Explain that the camera takes pictures only and does not give off any radiation. Instruct the patient to fast and refrain from consuming caffeinated beverages for 4 hours, refrain from smoking for 4 to 6 hours, and withhold medications for 24 hours before the test. Instruct the patient to avoid taking anticoagulant medication or to reduce the dosage as ordered prior to the procedure. Restrictions are as ordered by the requesting health-care provider (HCP) or institutional policy. Explain that the procedure is performed in a nuclear medicine department by a nuclear medicine technologist and will take approximately 30 minutes to 2 hours. Complete a baseline focused physical assessment and vital signs prior to sending the patient for the procedure. Instruct the patient to wear walking shoes (if treadmill exercise testing is to be performed), and emphasize the importance of reporting fatigue, pain, or shortness of breath. **Pediatric Considerations** Preparing children for a perfusion heart scan depends on the age of the child. Encourage parents to be truthful about what the child may experience during the procedure and to use words that they know their child will understand. Toddlers and preschool-age children have a very short attention span, so the best time to talk about the test is right before the procedure. The child should be assured that he or she will be allowed to bring a favorite comfort item into the examination room, and if appropriate, that a parent will be with the child during the procedure. Provide older children with information about the test, and allow them to participate in as many decisions as possible (e.g., choice of clothes to wear to the appointment) in order to reduce anxiety and encourage cooperation. If the child will be asked to perform specific movements or exercises for the test, encourage the child to practice the required activities, provide a CD that demonstrates the procedure, and teach strategies to remain calm, such as deep breathing, humming, or counting to himself or herself.

● **Safety Tip**

Explain that vital signs to monitor heart rate (ECG), oxygen level (pulse oximeter), and blood pressure (sphygmomanometer) will be measured before, during (peak), and after the study. Also explain the importance of describing any adverse symptoms that may develop during the test (e.g., chest pain, fatigue, dyspnea, dysrhythmias, or changes in blood pressure), which may require the procedure to be terminated.

It is important to understand the factors that can alter study findings. It is essential that the patient remain still during the scanning portion of the study in order to obtain clear images. Recent administration of x-ray contrast or other radionuclides may interfere with test results. Clear imaging can be impaired by some medications and certain aspects of the patient's medical history. Check the patient's medication record for the administration of digoxin and quinidine as they can affect cardiac contractility. Administration of nitrates that can affect cardiac performance should also be noted. False-positive results could be obtained in patients with a history of single vessel disease, or who engage in excessive eating or exercising between the initial scan and the repeat scan 4 hours later. Imaging can be impaired when patients have difficulty controlling their angina, or who have significant cardiac dysrhythmias or recent cardioversion. Imaging can be impaired for patients who are too exhausted to achieve maximum or have suboptimal cardiac stress. Adjustments made to the equipment to accommodate those who are very thin or very obese can cause overexposure or underexposure of the scans.

CONTRAINDICATIONS

- Mycardial perfusion scan is contraindicated for patients who have taken sildenafil (Viagra) within 48 hours of this scan because nitroglycerin may be used with this scan, and the combination of sildenafil and nitroglycerin can cause life-threatening hypotension.
- Myocardial perfusion scan is also contraindicated for patients with bleeding disorders, ventricular hypertrophy, right and left bundle branch block, and hypokalemia; in those receiving cardiotonic therapy; in those who have angina at rest or asthma; and in those with severe atherosclerotic coronary artery disease in whom dipyridamole testing cannot be performed.

● *Safety Tip*

Make sure a written and informed consent has been signed prior to the procedure and before administering any medications.

Implementation

Note that patient education is key to obtaining the patient's cooperation in following directions, and providing an explanation for the purpose of the procedure is an important part of this process. Inform the patient that this study can assist in assessing blood flow to the heart. Ensure that the patient has complied with dietary and medication restrictions. Instruct the patient to void prior to the procedure and to change into the gown, robe, and foot coverings provided.

Ensure that the patient has removed all external metallic objects from the area to be examined prior to the procedure. Establish an IV line for the administration of saline, anesthetics, sedatives, radionuclides, or emergency medications. If the patient has a history of allergic reactions to any substance or drug, administer ordered prophylactic steroids or antihistamines before the procedure. A nonionic contrast may be used if the patient has a history of allergies that would compromise the performance of the scan. Cardiac monitoring ECG electrodes should be applied and a baseline cardiac rhythm identified. The patient is placed in an upright position for 15 minutes to reduce pulmonary flow before and during the injection of the radionuclide. Once injected with the tracer, the patient is then placed on the table in a supine position. Scanning will occur immediately and at specified intervals. During the scan the patient's blood pressure, heart rate, respiratory rate, and cardiac rhythm should be monitored. Images are taken every 5 minutes for the first 30 minutes and every 10 minutes for the next 30 minutes to an hour. In most circumstances single-photon emission computed tomography (SPECT) is done so that the heart can be viewed from multiple angles and planes.

Explain to the patient that if treadmill exercising is to be performed, the patient will be assisted onto a treadmill or bicycle ergometer and asked to exercise to 80% to 85% of his or her maximum heart rate, or per the established protocol. Thallium is injected 60 to 90 seconds before exercise is stopped. The patient is immediately placed in the supine position with immediate imaging and repeat imaging in 4 hours. Those who cannot exercise will be given dipridamole 4 minutes before the thallium injection.

Evaluation

Recognize anxiety related to test results and answer any questions or address any concerns voiced by the patient or family. Discuss the implications of abnormal test results on the patient's lifestyle. Provide teaching and information regarding the clinical implications of the test results as appropriate. Provide contact information, if desired, for the American Heart Association (www.americanheart.org) or the National Heart, Lung, and Blood Institute (NHLBI) (www.nhlbi.nih.gov).

Complete a focused assessment and set of vital signs upon completion of the study. This will provide a basis of comparison to the patient's baseline assessment. Continue postscan vital signs every 15 minutes for 1 hour, then every 2 hours for 4 hours or per organizational policy. Provide patient education regarding symptoms of chest pain. Explain the importance or reporting chest pain if it should occur.

Unless contraindicated, advise the patient to drink increased amounts of fluids for 24 to 48 hours to eliminate the radionuclide from the body. Inform the patient that radionuclide is eliminated from the body within 6 to 24 hours. Follow the universal postscan recommendations as discussed in the chapter overview.

SPECIAL CONSIDERATIONS

NUTRITIONAL CONSIDERATIONS FOR THE DIABETIC PATIENT: Abnormal glucose levels may be associated with conditions resulting from poor glucose control. There is no "diabetic diet"; however, many meal-planning approaches with nutritional goals are endorsed by the American Diabetes Association (ADA). Patients who adhere to dietary recommendations report a better general feeling of health, better weight management, greater control of glucose and lipid values, and improved use of insulin. Instruct the patient, as appropriate, in the nutritional management of diabetes. The nutritional needs of each diabetic patient need to be determined individually (especially during pregnancy) with the appropriate HCPs, particularly professionals educated in nutrition.

NUTRITIONAL CONSIDERATIONS FOR THE CARDIAC PATIENT: An abnormal myocardial perfusion heart scan may be associated with coronary artery disease (CAD). Nutritional therapy is recommended for patients identified to be at risk for developing CAD or for individuals who have specific risk factors and/or existing medical conditions (e.g., elevated LDL cholesterol levels, other lipid disorders, type 1 diabetes, insulin-dependent type 2 diabetes, insulin resistance, or metabolic syndrome). Other changeable risk factors that warrant patient education include strategies to encourage patients, especially those who are overweight and with high blood pressure, to safely decrease sodium intake, achieve a normal weight, ensure regular participation in moderate aerobic physical activity three to four times per week, eliminate tobacco use, and adhere to a heart-healthy diet. If triglycerides also are elevated, the patient should be advised to eliminate or reduce alcohol. A variety of dietary patterns are beneficial for people with CAD and there are many meal-planning approaches with nutritional goals endorsed by the ADA. The Guideline on Lifestyle Management to Reduce Cardiovascular Risk published by the American College of Cardiology (ACC) and the American Heart Association (AHA) in conjunction with the National Heart, Lung, and Blood Institute (NHLBI) recommends a "Mediterranean"-style diet rather than a low-fat diet. The guideline emphasizes inclusion of vegetables, whole grains, fruits, low-fat dairy, nuts, legumes, and nontropical vegetable oils (e.g., olive, canola, peanut, sunflower, flaxseed) along with fish and lean poultry. A similar dietary pattern known as the Dietary Approaches to Stop Hypertension (DASH) diet makes additional recommendations for the reduction of dietary sodium. Both dietary styles emphasize a reduction in consumption of red meats, which are high in saturated fats and cholesterol, and other foods containing sugar, saturated fats, trans fats, and sodium. The ADA also includes a vegetarian diet as well as other potential weight loss diets such as Weight Watchers. The nutritional needs of each patient need to be determined individually (especially during pregnancy) with the appropriate HCPs, particularly professionals educated in nutrition.

SENSITIVITY TO SOCIAL AND CULTURAL ISSUES: Numerous studies point to the prevalence of excess body weight in American children and adolescents. Experts estimate that obesity is present in 25% of the population ages 6 to 11 yr. The medical, social, and emotional consequences of excess body weight are significant. Special attention should be given to instructing the child and caregiver regarding health risks and weight control education.

◆ *Critical Findings*

N/A

◆ *Study Specific Complications*

- Radionuclide scans are considered a fairly safe procedure. The actual scans are noninvasive and cause little patient discomfort. However, like x-rays, they expose the body to a small dose of radiation. This can damage cells and cause mutations, particularly in growing fetuses. Patients should be made aware of the potential risks to the fetus.

- Contrast reactions can be an additional complication of diagnostic studies, especially when iodinated contrast is used. Iodinated contrast mediums may cause minor-to-severe allergic reactions in a patient. Consideration may be given to the administration of oral diphenhydramine in the case of mild allergic reaction; IV or IM epinephrine or diphenhydramine may be considered in cases of moderate to severe allergic reaction; a request for resuscitation by a specially trained emergency response team may be required in the case of severe allergic reaction.

- Inaccurate injection of the radiopharmaceutical may cause the tracer to end up in subcutaneous tissue, causing infiltration, and may lead to extravasation or even entering deep into muscle tissue, resulting in false hot spots and inaccurate results.

- There are a number of complications associated with performing a venipuncture. **Pain** is commonly associated with needles, and although the pain experienced during venipuncture is usually mild, on a rare occasion the needle may strike a nerve causing permanent pain. Some patients experience a **vasovagal reaction** during the venipuncture procedure, evidenced by sweating, low blood pressure, fainting, or near fainting. The potential for a **fall injury** is a significant concern related to vasovagal reactions. Prolonged **bleeding** is a complication that occurs with patients who are taking blood thinners or who have coagulopathies such as hemophilia. A **hematoma** results when blood leaks into the tissue during or after a venipuncture, as evidenced by pain, bruising, and/or swelling at the venipuncture site. The swelling can cause injury by compression to surrounding nerves, which can be temporary or permanent. HCPs should watch for minor complications such as bruising and hematoma at the venipuncture site, which are fairly common. Hematomas occur more often in older adult or frail patients, or those with veins that are difficult to access. Bleeding or bruising can be prevented once the needle has been removed by applying direct pressure to the site with dry gauze for a minute or two. Some other more unusual complications of venipuncture include **cellulitis, phlebitis, inadvertent arterial puncture,** and **sepsis.** Sepsis can be caused by the introduction of bacteria from the surface of the skin into the blood as the result of improper cleansing of the venipuncture site. Immunocompromised patients are at a higher risk for developing this complication.

✅ Related Tests

- Related tests include antidysrhythmic drugs, apolipoprotein A and B, AST, atrial natriuretic peptide, BNP, calcium, cholesterol (total, HDL, LDL), CT cardiac scoring, CRP, CK and isoenzymes, echocardiography, echocardiography transesophageal, ECG, exercise stress test, glucose, glycated hemoglobin, Holter monitor, homocysteine, ketones, LDH and isos, lipoprotein electrophoresis, magnesium, MRI chest, MI infarct scan, myoglobin, PET heart, potassium, triglycerides, and troponin.
- Refer to the Cardiovascular System table at the end of the book for related tests by body system.

Expected Outcomes

Expected outcomes associated with Myocardial Perfusion Heart Scans are
- Agreeing to discuss causative factors of atherosclerotic plaque development
- Agreeing to make lifestyle adjustments necessary to promote cardiac health
- Complying with the request for re-scanning post bypass graft surgery

Positron Emission Tomography, Brain

Quick Summary

SYNONYM ACRONYM: PET scan of the brain.

COMMON USE: To assess blood flow and metabolic processes of the brain to assist in diagnosis of disorders such as ischemic or hemorrhagic stroke or cancer and to evaluate head trauma.

AREA OF APPLICATION: Brain.

NORMAL FINDINGS: Normal patterns of tissue metabolism, blood flow, and homogeneous radionuclide distribution

Test Explanation

Positron emission tomography (PET) combines the biochemical properties of nuclear medicine with the anatomic accuracy of computed tomography (CT). PET uses positron emissions from specific radionuclides. The positron radiopharmaceuticals generally have short half-lives, ranging from a few seconds to a few hours, and therefore they must be produced in a cyclotron located near where the test is being done. A radionuclide is basically composed of a measurable radioactive isotope and a biologically active molecule. The isotopes are derived from elements that are either naturally present in organic molecules (oxygen, nitrogen, and carbon) or can be substituted for naturally occurring elements (fluorine can be substituted for hydrogen). Selected molecules become biologically active radiolabelled analogs of their naturally occurring forms to create radionuclides that produce detailed functional images within the body. Radionuclides are used to evaluate many aspects of organ function including oxygen consumption and glucose metabolism; most PET studies are conducted in the areas of cardiology, neurology, and oncology. The studies are used to diagnose and stage diseases as well as to monitor the efficacy of therapeutic interventions. During the PET brain scan, the radiotracer is injected into the body where it migrates to the intended target organ, becomes involved in the physiological process of interest, and accumulates to the degree that radioactive emissions are detected by the PET scanner. The PET scanner translates the emissions from the radioactivity as the positron combines with the negative electrons from the tissues and forms gamma rays that can be detected by the scanner. This information is transmitted to the computer, which determines the location and its distribution and translates the emissions as color-coded images for viewing, quantitative measurements, activity changes in relation to time, and three-dimensional computer-aided analysis.

The brain uses oxygen and glucose almost exclusively to meet its energy needs, and therefore the brain's metabolism has been studied widely with PET. Each radionuclide tracer is designed to measure a specific body process, such as glucose metabolism, blood flow, or brain tissue perfusion. Fluorine-18, in the form of fluorodeoxyglucose (FDG), is one of the most versatile and commonly used radionuclides in PET. FDG is a glucose analogue. All cells use glucose, but diseases that involve increased metabolic activity will show a high level of radionuclide visualization while those that are hypometabolic will show little to no radionuclide visualization. There is little localization of FDG in normal tissue with minimal amounts being evenly distributed, allowing rapid detection of abnormal disease states. The radionuclide can be administered by intravenous (IV) injection or inhaled as a gas. After the radionuclide becomes concentrated in the brain, PET images of blood flow or metabolic processes at the cellular level can be obtained. Oxygen-15 is used in circumstances that warrant the evaluation of blood flow in the brain to predict or identify areas affected by a stroke. PET brain has had the greatest clinical impact in patients with epilepsy, dementia, neurodegenerative diseases, inflammation, cerebrovascular disease (indirectly), and brain tumors

The expense of the study and the limited availability of radiopharmaceuticals limit the use of PET even though it is more sensitive than traditional nuclear scanning and single-photon emission computed tomography (SPECT). Isotopes approved for use in Canada for PET studies are fairly limited in number and application. FDG is approved for some cancer scans. PET/CT and SPECT/CT are imaging applications that superimpose PET or SPECT and CT findings. The images are collected and produced by a single gantry system. The co-registered or image fusion of PET/CT or SPECT/CT findings are capable of providing a very detailed combination of anatomical and functional images. PET images can also be superimposed on MRI images.

Nursing Implications

Assessment

Indications	Potential Nursing Problems
Detect Parkinson disease and Huntington disease, as evidenced by decreased metabolism Determine the effectiveness of therapy, as evidenced by biochemical activity of normal and abnormal tissues Determine physiological changes in psychosis and schizophrenia Differentiate between tumor recurrence and radiation necrosis Evaluate Alzheimer disease and differentiate it from other causes of dementia, as evidenced by decreased cerebral flow and metabolism Evaluate cranial tumors pre- and postoperatively and determine stage and appropriate treatment or procedure Identify cerebrovascular accident or aneurysm, as evidenced by decreased blood flow and oxygen use Identify focal seizures, as evidenced by decreased metabolism between seizures	• Caregiver • Communication • Confusion • Family • Guilt • Hopelessness • Human Reactions • Infection • Nutrition • Role Performance • Self-care • Self-esteem • Sexuality • Sleep

Diagnosis: Clinical Significance of Test Results

ABNORMAL FINDINGS

• Alzheimer's disease *evidenced in later stages by areas lacking radionuclide visualization related to decreased cellular activity; cellular activity decreases as the disease progresses*
• Aneurysm *evidenced by areas lacking radionuclide visualization related to decreased cellular activity; cellular activity decreases as the disease progresses*
• Cerebral metastases *evidenced by areas of intense radionuclide visualization related to abnormally increased cellular activity*
• Cerebrovascular accident *evidenced by areas lacking radionuclide visualization related to decreased cellular activity*
• Creutzfeldt-Jakob disease
• Dementia *evidenced by areas lacking radionuclide visualization related to decreased cellular activity; cellular activity decreases as the disease progresses*
• Head trauma *evidenced by areas lacking radionuclide visualization related to decreased cellular activity*
• Huntington's disease *evidenced by focal areas of intense radionuclide visualization related to hyperactivity of the affected nerves and increased cellular metabolism; cellular activity decreases as the disease progresses*
• Migraine
• Parkinson's disease *evidenced by focal areas of intense radionuclide visualization related to hyperactivity of the affected nerves and increased cellular metabolism; cellular activity decreases as the disease progresses*
• Schizophrenia
• Seizure disorders *evidenced by focal areas of intense radionuclide visualization related to hyperactivity of the affected nerves and increased cellular metabolism*
• Tumors *evidenced by areas of intense radionuclide visualization related to abnormally increased cellular activity*

Planning

Considerations for planning a successful partnership should include clear communication of what to expect during the test to decrease anxiety and improve cooperation. Before the procedure is performed, plan to review the steps with the patient and address any concerns about pain. Explain that an IV line will be inserted to allow the infusion of IV fluids such as normal saline, anesthetics, sedatives, radionuclides, medications used in the procedure, or emergency medications, and that there may be some discomfort during the venipuncture, but there should be no discomfort during the study. Reassure the patient that the radionuclide poses no radioactive hazard and rarely produces side effects. Explain that the camera takes pictures only and does not give off any radiation. Instruct the patient to fast 4 to 6 hours before the scan; restrict alcohol, nicotine, or caffeine-containing drinks for 24 hours; and with-hold medications for 24 hours prior to the study, as directed by the requesting health-care provider (HCP). Explain that the procedure is performed in a nuclear medicine department by a nuclear medicine technologist and will take approximately 1 to 2 hours. Advise the patient that the scanning is started 30 minutes after injection of the radionuclide.

PEDIATRIC CONSIDERATIONS

Preparing a child for a PET brain scan depends on the age of the child. Encourage parents to be truthful about what the child may experience during the procedure (e.g., they may feel a pinch or minor discomfort when the IV needle is inserted) and to use words they know their child will understand. Toddlers and preschool-age children have a very short attention span, so the best time to talk about the test is right before the procedure. The child should be assured that she or he will be allowed to bring a favorite comfort item into the examination room, and if appropriate, that a parent will be with them during the procedure. Explain the importance of remaining still while the images are taken.

SPECIAL CONSIDERATIONS

An important aspect of planning is understanding the factors that may alter study findings or cause abnormal results. Interdepartmental communication is a key factor in the planning process. The following should be noted when planning for this study:

- It is essential that the patient remain still during the scanning portion of the study in order to obtain clear images.
- The effects of alcohol, caffeine, or nicotine would make it difficult to evaluate the patient's true physiological state (e.g., alcohol is a vasoconstrictor and would decrease blood flow to the target organ).
- False-positive findings may occur as a result of normal gastrointestinal tract uptake and uptake in areas of infection or inflammation.

It is also important to understand which medications or substances the patient may be exposed to in the health-care setting that can interfere with accurate testing. Drugs that alter glucose metabolism, such as tranquilizers or insulin, should be withheld because hypoglycemia can alter PET results.

● Safety Tip

Make sure a written and informed consent has been signed prior to the procedure and before administering any medications.

Implementation

Note that patient education is key to obtaining the patient's cooperation in following directions, and providing an explanation for the purpose of the procedure is an important part of this process. Inform the patient that this study can assist with assessing for disorders of brain metabolism. Instruct the patient to void prior to the procedure and to change into the gown, robe, and foot coverings provided.

Ensure that the patient has removed all external metallic objects from the area to be examined prior to the procedure. Establish an IV line for the administration of saline, anesthetics, sedatives, radionuclides, or emergency medications. If the patient has a history of allergic reactions to any substance or drug, administer ordered prophylactic steroids or antihistamines before the procedure. Once injected with the tracer, the patient will be asked to lie on his or her back on the examination table. After a wait of 30 to 45 minutes, the area of interest is scanned. The patient may be asked to perform different cognitive activities (e.g., reading) to measure changes in brain activity during reasoning or remembering. The patient may be blindfolded or asked to use earplugs to decrease auditory and visual stimuli. Each image will take 2 to 6 minutes; the actual scanning time for this exam may take up to 2 hours.

Evaluation

Recognize anxiety related to test results and be supportive of a perceived loss of independent function. Answer any questions or address any concerns voiced by the patient or family, and discuss the implications of abnormal test results on the patient's lifestyle. Provide teaching and information regarding the clinical implications of the test results as appropriate.

Complete a focused assessment and set of vital signs upon completion of the study. This will provide a basis of comparison to the baseline assessment.

Unless contraindicated, advise the patient to drink increased amounts of fluids for 24 to 48 hours to eliminate the radionuclide from the body. Inform the patient that radionuclide is eliminated from the body within 6 to 24 hours. Follow the universal postscan recommendations as discussed in the chapter overview.

✓ *Critical Findings*

- Aneurysm
- Cerebrovascular accident
- Tumor with significant mass effect

Note and immediately report to the requesting HCP any critical findings and related symptoms. A listing of these findings varies among facilities.

✓ *Study Specific Complications*

- Radionuclide scans are considered a fairly safe procedure. The actual scans are noninvasive and cause little patient discomfort. However, like x-rays, they expose the body to a small dose of radiation. This can damage cells and cause mutations, particularly in growing fetuses. Patients should be made aware of the potential risks to the fetus.

- Contrast reactions can be an additional complication of diagnostic studies, especially when iodinated contrast is used. Iodinated contrast mediums may cause minor-to-severe allergic reactions in a patient. Consideration may be given to the administration of oral diphenhydramine in the case of a mild allergic reaction; IV or IM epinephrine or diphenhydramine may be considered in cases of moderate to severe allergic reaction; a request for resuscitation by a specially trained emergency response team may be required in the case of severe allergic reaction.

- Inaccurate injection of the radiopharmaceutical may cause the tracer to end up in subcutaneous tissue, causing infiltration, and may lead to extravasation or even entering deep into muscle tissue, resulting in false hot spots and inaccurate results.

- There are a number of complications associated with performing a venipuncture. **Pain** is commonly associated with needles and although the pain experienced during venipuncture is usually mild, on a rare occasion the needle may strike a nerve, causing permanent pain. Some patients experience a **vasovagal reaction** during the venipuncture procedure, evidenced by sweating, low blood pressure, fainting, or near fainting. The potential for a **fall injury** is a significant concern related to vasovagal reactions. Prolonged **bleeding** is a complication that occurs with patients who are taking blood thinners or who have coagulopathies such as hemophilia. A **hematoma** results when blood leaks into the tissue during or after a venipuncture, as evidenced by pain, bruising, and/or swelling at the venipuncture site. The swelling can cause injury by compression to surrounding nerves, which can be temporary or permanent. HCPs should watch for minor complications such as bruising and hematoma at the venipuncture site, which are fairly common. Hematomas occur more often in older adult or frail patients, or in those whose veins are difficult to access. Bleeding or bruising can be prevented once the needle has been removed by applying direct pressure to the site with dry gauze for a minute or two. Some other more unusual complications of venipuncture include **cellulitis, phlebitis, inadvertent arterial puncture, and sepsis.** Sepsis can be caused by the introduction of bacteria from the surface of the skin into the blood as the result of improper cleansing of the venipuncture site. Immunocompromised patients are at a higher risk for developing this complication.

Related Tests

- Related tests include Alzheimer disease markers, CT brain, EEG, MRI brain, and US arterial Doppler of the carotids.
- Refer to the Musculoskeletal System table at the end of the book for related tests by body system.

Expected Outcomes

Expected outcomes associated with Positron Emission Tomography, Brain Scans, are
- Ability to navigate the home environment without injury
- Acceptance by the family of caregiver support group information
- Ability to express anxiety related to altered physical function

Positron Emission Tomography, Heart

Quick Summary

SYNONYM ACRONYM: PET scan of the heart.

COMMON USE: To assess blood flow and metabolic process of the heart to assist in diagnosis of disorders such as coronary artery disease, infarct, and aneurysm.

AREA OF APPLICATION: Heart, chest/thorax, vascular system.

NORMAL FINDINGS: Normal patterns of tissue metabolism, blood flow, and homogeneous radionuclide distribution

Test Explanation

Positron emission tomography (PET) combines the biochemical properties of nuclear medicine with the anatomic accuracy of computed tomography (CT). PET uses positron emissions from specific radionuclides. The positron radiopharmaceuticals generally have short half-lives, ranging from a few seconds to a few hours, and therefore they must be produced in a cyclotron located near where the test is being done. A radionuclide is basically composed of a measurable radioactive isotope and a biologically active molecule. The isotopes are derived from elements that are either naturally present in organic molecules (oxygen, nitrogen, and carbon) or can be substituted for naturally occurring elements (fluorine can be substituted for hydrogen). Selected molecules become biologically active radiolabelled analogs of their naturally occurring forms to create radionuclides that produce detailed functional images within the body. Radionuclides are used to evaluate many aspects of organ function including oxygen consumption and glucose metabolism; most PET studies are conducted in the areas of cardiology, neurology, and oncology. The studies are used to diagnose and stage diseases as well as to monitor the efficacy of therapeutic interventions. During the PET heart scan, the radiotracer is injected into the body where it migrates to the intended target organ, becomes involved in the physiological process of interest, and accumulates to the degree that radioactive emissions are detected by the PET scanner. The PET scanner translates the emissions from the radioactivity as the positron combines with the negative electrons from the tissues and forms gamma rays that can be detected by the scanner. This information is transmitted to the computer, which determines the location and its distribution and translates the emissions as color-coded images for viewing, quantitative measurements, activity changes in relation to time, and three-dimensional computer-aided analysis.

Cardiac muscle uses oxygen and glucose in many of its essential functions, and therefore the heart's metabolism has been studied widely with PET. Each radionuclide tracer is designed to measure a specific body process, such as glucose metabolism, blood flow, or cardiac tissue perfusion. Fluorine-18, in the form of fluorodeoxyglucose (FDG), is one of the most versatile and commonly used radionuclides in PET. FDG is a glucose analogue. All cells use glucose, but diseases that involve increased metabolic activity will show a high level of radionuclide visualization while those that are hypometabolic will show little to no radionuclide visualization. There is little localization of FDG in normal tissue with minimal amounts being evenly distributed, allowing rapid detection of abnormal disease states. The radionuclide can be administered by intravenous (IV) injection or inhaled as a gas. After the radionuclide becomes concentrated in the brain, PET images of blood flow or metabolic processes at the cellular level can be obtained. Oxygen-15 is used in circumstances that warrant the evaluation of blood flow in the brain to predict or identify areas affected by a stroke. PET brain has had the greatest clinical impact in patients with epilepsy, dementia, neurodegenerative diseases, inflammation, cerebrovascular disease (indirectly), and brain tumors.

The expense of the study and the limited availability of radiopharmaceuticals limit the use of PET even though it is more sensitive than traditional nuclear scanning and single-photon emission computed tomography (SPECT). PET/CT and SPECT/CT are imaging applications that superimpose PET or SPECT and CT findings. The images are collected and produced by a single gantry system. The co-registered or image fusion of PET/CT or SPECT/CT findings are capable of providing a very detailed combination of anatomical and functional images. PET images can also be superimposed on MRI images.

Nursing Implications
Assessment

Indications	Potential Nursing Problems
Assess tissue permeability Determine the effects of therapeutic drugs on malfunctioning or diseased tissue Determine localization of areas of heart metabolism Determine the presence of coronary artery disease (CAD), as evidenced by metabolic state during ischemia and after angina Determine the size of heart infarcts Identify cerebrovascular accident or aneurysm, as evidenced by decreasing blood flow and oxygen use	• Bleeding • Conflicted Decision Making • Death • Fatigue • Gas Exchange • Health Management • Human Reactions • Nutrition • Tissue Perfusion

Diagnosis: Clinical Significance of Test Results
ABNORMAL FINDINGS
- Chronic obstructive pulmonary disease
- Areas of tissue necrosis and scar tissue *indicated by the lack of radionuclide visualization in areas of decreased blood flow and decreased glucose concentration*
- Enlarged left ventricle
- Heart chamber disorder
- Ischemia and myocardial infarction *indicated by the lack of radionuclide visualization in areas of decreased blood flow and decreased glucose concentration*
- Pulmonary edema

Planning
Considerations for planning a successful partnership should include clear communication of what to expect during the test to decrease anxiety and improve cooperation. Before the procedure is performed, plan to review the steps with the patient and address any concerns about pain. Explain that an IV line will be inserted to allow the infusion of IV fluids such as normal saline, anesthetics, sedatives, radionuclides, medications used in the procedure, or emergency medications, and that there may be some discomfort during the venipuncture, but there should be no discomfort during the study. Reassure the patient that the radionuclide poses no radioactive hazard and rarely produces side effects. Explain that the camera takes pictures only and does not give off any radiation. Instruct the patient to fast 4 to 6 hours before the scan; restrict alcohol,

nicotine, or caffeine-containing drinks for 24 hours; and withhold medications for 24 hours prior to the study, as directed by the requesting HCP. Explain that the procedure is performed in a nuclear medicine department by a nuclear medicine technologist and will take approximately 1 to 2 hours. Advise the patient that the scanning is started 30 minutes after injection of the radionuclide.

PEDIATRIC CONSIDERATIONS

Preparing children for a PET brain scan depends on the age of the child. Encourage parents to be truthful about what the child may experience during the procedure (e.g., the child may feel a pinch or minor discomfort when the IV needle is inserted) and to use words they know their child will understand. Toddlers and preschool-age children have a very short attention span, so the best time to talk about the test is right before the procedure. The child should be assured that she or he will be allowed to bring a favorite comfort item into the examination room, and if appropriate, that a parent will be with the child during the procedure. Explain the importance of remaining still while the images are taken.

SPECIAL CONSIDERATIONS

An important aspect of planning is understanding the factors that may alter study findings or cause abnormal results. Interdepartmental communication is a key factor in the planning process. The following should be noted when planning for this study:

* It is essential that the patient remain still during the scanning portion of the study in order to obtain clear images.
* The effects of alcohol, caffeine, or nicotine would make it difficult to evaluate the patient's true physiological state.
* False-positive findings may occur as a result of normal gastrointestinal tract uptake and uptake in areas of infection or inflammation.

It is also important to understand which medications or substances the patient may be exposed to in the health-care setting that can interfere with accurate testing. Drugs that alter glucose metabolism, such as tranquilizers or insulin, should be withheld because hypoglycemia can alter PET results.

● *Safety Tip*

Make sure a written and informed consent has been signed prior to the procedure and before administering any medications.

Implementation

Note that patient education is key to obtaining the patient's cooperation in following directions, and providing an explanation for the purpose of the procedure is an important part of this process. Inform the patient that this study can assist with assessing for disorders of tissue metabolism of the heart. A high rate of glucose is needed to meet the energy needs of the heart. Nonviable myocardial tissue can be indicated by low glucose metabolism in areas of decreased blood flow. Instruct the patient to void prior to the procedure and to change into the gown, robe, and foot coverings provided.

Ensure that the patient has removed all external metallic objects from the area to be examined prior to the procedure. Establish an IV line for the administration of saline, anesthetics, sedatives, radionuclides, or emergency medications. If the patient has a history of allergic reactions to any substance or drug, administer ordered prophylactic steroids or antihistamines before the procedure. Once injected with the tracer, the patient will be asked to lie on his or her back on the examination table. After a wait of 30 to 45 minutes, the area of interest is scanned. Each image will take 2 to 6 minutes; the actual scanning time for this exam may take up to 2 hours.

Evaluation

Recognize anxiety related to test results and be supportive of a perceived loss of independent function. Answer any questions or address any concerns voiced by the patient or family, and discuss the implications of abnormal test results on the patient's lifestyle. Provide teaching and information regarding the clinical implications of the test results as appropriate.

Complete a focused assessment and set of vital signs upon completion of the study. This will provide a basis of comparison to the baseline assessment.

Unless contraindicated, advise the patient to drink increased amounts of fluids for 24 to 48 hours to eliminate the radionuclide from the body. Inform the patient that radionuclide is eliminated from the body within 6 to 24 hours. Follow the universal postscan recommendations as discussed in the chapter overview.

SPECIAL CONSIDERATIONS

NUTRITIONAL CONSIDERATIONS FOR THE DIABETIC PATIENT: Abnormal glucose levels may be associated with conditions resulting from poor glucose control. There is no "diabetic diet"; however, many meal-planning approaches with nutritional goals are endorsed by the American Diabetes Association (ADA). Patients who adhere to dietary recommendations report a better general feeling of health, better weight management, greater control of glucose and lipid values, and improved use of insulin. Instruct the patient, as appropriate, in the nutritional management of diabetes. The nutritional needs of each diabetic patient need to be determined individually (especially during pregnancy) with the appropriate health-care providers (HCPs), particularly professionals educated in nutrition.

NUTRITIONAL CONSIDERATIONS FOR THE CARDIAC PATIENT: An abnormal PET heart scan may be associated with coronary artery disease (CAD). Nutritional therapy is recommended for patients identified to be at risk for developing CAD or for individuals who have specific risk factors and/or existing medical conditions (e.g., elevated LDL cholesterol levels, other lipid disorders, type 1 diabetes, insulin-dependent type 2 diabetes, insulin resistance, or metabolic syndrome). Other changeable risk factors that warrant patient education include strategies to encourage patients, especially those who are overweight and with high blood pressure, to safely decrease sodium intake, achieve a normal weight, ensure regular participation in moderate aerobic physical activity three to four times per week, eliminate tobacco use, and adhere to a heart-healthy diet. If triglycerides also are elevated, the patient should be advised to eliminate or reduce alcohol. A variety of dietary patterns are beneficial for people with CAD and there are many meal-planning approaches with nutritional goals endorsed by the ADA. *The Guideline on Lifestyle Management to Reduce Cardiovascular Risk*, published by the American College of Cardiology (ACC) and the American Heart Association (AHA), in conjunction with the National Heart, Lung, and Blood Institute (NHLBI), recommends a "Mediterranean"-style diet rather than a low-fat diet. The guideline emphasizes inclusion of vegetables, whole grains, fruits, low-fat dairy, nuts, legumes, and nontropical vegetable oils (e.g., olive, canola, peanut, sunflower, flaxseed) along with fish and lean poultry. A similar dietary pattern known as the Dietary Approaches to Stop Hypertension (DASH) diet makes additional recommendations for the reduction of dietary sodium. Both dietary styles emphasize a reduction in consumption of red meats, which are high in saturated fats and cholesterol, and other foods containing sugar, saturated fats, trans fats, and sodium. The ADA also includes a vegetarian diet as well as other potential weight loss diets such as Weight Watchers. The nutritional needs of each patient need to be determined individually (especially during pregnancy) with the appropriate HCPs, particularly professionals educated in nutrition.

✅ *Critical Findings*

N/A

✅ *Study Specific Complications*

- Radionuclide scans are considered a fairly safe procedure. The actual scans are noninvasive and cause little patient discomfort. However, like x-rays, they expose the body to a small dose of radiation. This can damage cells and cause mutations, particularly in growing fetuses. Patients should be made aware of the potential risks to the fetus.

- Contrast reactions can be an additional complication of diagnostic studies, especially when iodinated contrast is used. Iodinated contrast mediums may cause minor-to-severe allergic reactions in a patient. Consideration may be given to the administration of oral diphenhydramine in the case of mild allergic reaction; IV or IM epinephrine or diphenhydramine may be considered in cases of moderate to severe allergic reaction; a request for resuscitation by a specially trained emergency response team may be required in the case of severe allergic reaction.

- Inaccurate injection of the radiopharmaceutical may cause the tracer to end up in subcutaneous tissue, causing infiltration, and may lead to extravasation or even entering deep into muscle tissue, resulting in false hot spots and inaccurate results.

- There are a number of complications associated with performing a venipuncture. **Pain** is commonly associated with needles, and although the pain experienced during venipuncture is usually mild, on a rare occasion the needle may strike a nerve, causing permanent pain. Some patients experience a **vasovagal reaction** during the venipuncture procedure, evidenced by sweating, low blood pressure, fainting, or near fainting. The potential for a **fall injury** is a significant concern related to vasovagal reactions. Prolonged **bleeding** is a complication that occurs with patients who are taking blood thinners or who have coagulopathies such as hemophilia. A **hematoma** results when blood leaks into the tissue during or after a venipuncture, as evidenced by pain, bruising, and/or swelling at the venipuncture site. The swelling can cause injury by compression to surrounding nerves, which can be temporary or permanent. HCPs should watch for minor complications such as bruising and hematoma at the venipuncture site, which are fairly common. Hematomas occur more often in older adult or frail patients, or in those whose veins are difficult to access. Bleeding or bruising can be prevented once the needle has been removed by applying direct pressure to the site with dry gauze for a minute or two. Some other more unusual complications of venipuncture include **cellulitis, phlebitis, inadvertent arterial puncture,** and **sepsis.** Sepsis can be caused by the introduction of bacteria from the surface of the skin into the blood as the result of improper cleansing of the venipuncture site. Immunocompromised patients are at a higher risk for developing this complication.

✅ *Related Tests*

- Related tests for cardiac indications include anion gap, antidysrhythmic drugs, apolipoprotein A and B, arterial/alveolar oxygen ratio, AST, ANP, α_1-AT, biopsy lung, blood gases, blood pool imaging, BNP, bronchoscopy, calcium, ionized calcium, carboxyhemoglobin, chest x-ray, chloride sweat, cholesterol (total, HDL, and LDL), CRP, CBC, CT cardiac scoring, CT thoracic, CK and isoenzymes, culture and smear for mycobacteria, culture bacterial sputum, culture viral, cytology sputum, echocardiography, echocardiography transesophageal, ECG, electrolytes, exercise stress test, glucose, glycated hemoglobin, gram stain, Hgb, Holter monitor, homocysteine, ketones, LDH and isoenzymes, lipoprotein electrophoresis, magnesium, MRI chest, MI infarct scan, IgE, lactic acid, lung perfusion scan, lung ventilation scan, myocardial perfusion heart scan, myoglobin, osmolality, pericardial fluid analysis, phosphorus, plethysmography, pleural fluid analysis, PET heart, PFT, potassium, pulse oximetry, TB skin test, and triglycerides. Related tests for pulmonary indications include α_1-AT, anion gap, arterial/alveolar oxygen ratio, biopsy lung, bronchoscopy, carboxyhemoglobin, chest x-ray, chloride sweat, CBC, CBC hemoglobin, CBC WBC count and differential, culture and smear for mycobacteria, culture bacterial sputum, culture viral, cytology sputum, electrolytes, gram stain, IgE, lactic acid, lung perfusion scan, lung ventilation scan, osmolality, phosphorus, plethysmography, pleural fluid analysis, and pulse oximetry.

- Refer to the Cardiovascular and Respiratory systems tables at the end of the book for related tests by body system.

Expected Outcomes

Expected outcomes associated with Positron Emission Tomography, Heart Scans, are

- Acknowledging personal cardiac risk factors and making lifestyle changes to better manage health
- Ensuring that the family accepts support in the event of patient death and considers organ donation
- Collaborating with the HCP, family, and spiritual guide to make a decision regarding ongoing healthcare choices
- Discussing end-of-life choices related to the prognosis of death

REVIEW OF LEARNING OUTCOMES

Thinking

1. Identify safety precautions for handling stool and urine post scan. Answer: Instruct the patient to flush the toilet twice and to vigorously wash his or her hands immediately after toileting. If disposing of stool or urine for the patient, wear gloves. After urine or stool disposal, flush the toilet twice.

Wash gloved hands vigorously with soap and water. Remove the gloves, and wash bare hands vigorously with soap and water. This should be done for a minimum of 48 hours.

2. Identify the most common route of administration of radionuclides. Answer: Radionuclides are most commonly administered intravenously. Other common routes of administration are oral and inhalation.

Doing

1. Describe the cause and appropriate intervention for treatment of an intravenous hematoma. Answer: Hematoma occurs when blood leaks into the surrounding tissue during or after a venipuncture. Symptoms of hematoma development are pain, bruising, and/or swelling at the venipuncture site. Swelling can cause injury by compression to surrounding nerves, which can be temporary or permanent. Hematomas occur more often in older adult or frail patients, or in those whose veins are difficult to access. Bleeding or bruising can be prevented once the needle has been removed by applying direct pressure to the site with dry gauze for a minute or two.

2. Discuss the postprocedure patient assessments. Answer: Postprocedure nursing assessment should include comparison of pre- and postprocedural vital signs and routine postprocedural vital signs as ordered until stable; comparison of pre- and postprocedure physical assessment including cognitive status; assessment of IV site; and explanation to the patient of postprocedural care related to urine and stool, increased fluid intake, follow-up scans, if any, and breastfeeding limitations if a lactating mother.

Caring

3. Understand and value the patient's choice of how involved he or she wishes to be in the provision of care. Answer: There are times when the patient and family preferences are at odds with what we would recommend. Cultural considerations are very important when conveying the results of tests exams such as nuclear studies. Western medicine values are that each person will be informed of his or her individual results. Other cultures, such as Pan Asian, feel that to provide bad news to the patient removes the patient's hope. The results may need to be conveyed to the oldest male member. Different cultures have different views and preferences. Always take this into account when engaging patients in the care process.

◖ *Words* OF *Wisdom:* Words of Wisdom: It can be challenging to have a clear understanding of the nursing role in supporting the patient through the process of being diagnosed with a devastating disease or waiting for the results of the effectiveness of therapy. When this happens, it is easy to get lost in the tasks to be performed, paying less attention to the emotional aspect of care. Stop, take a moment, and think about the patient's personal situation. Instead of the woman in room 4 with a diagnosis of cancer, you have Mari in room 4 who is a single mother with no family support and limited financial resources. An important part of the nursing role is to take a personal professional interest in your patient, thereby making sure the patient has what she or he needs most to feel supported toward a positive outcome. Know your resources, and use them wisely.

BIBLIOGRAPHY

Cavanaugh, B. (2003). Nurse's manual of laboratory and diagnostic tests (4th ed.). Philadelphia, PA: F.A. Davis Company.

Chernecky, C., & Berger, B. (2008). Laboratory and diagnostic procedures (5th ed.). St. Louis, MO: Saunders.

Fishbach, F., & Dunning, M. (2009). A manual of laboratory and diagnostic tests (8th ed.). Philadelphia, PA: Lippincott Williams & Wilkins.

Long, B.W., Rollins, J.H., and Smith, B.J. (2015). Merrill's atlas of radiographic positioning and procedures (13th ed.). St. Louis, MO: Mosby.

International Commission on Radiological Protection. (2000). Pregnancy and medical radiation. Oxford: Pergamon Press; ICRP Publication 84.

Pagana, K., & Pagana, T. (2010). Mosby's manual of diagnostic and laboratory tests (4th ed.). St. Louis, MO: Mosby.

Van Leeuwen, A., and Bladh, M. (2015). Davis's comprehensive handbook of laboratory and diagnostic testing with nursing implications (6th ed.). Philadelphia, PA: F.A. Davis.

Venes, D. (Ed.). (2009). Taber's cyclopedic medical dictionary (21st ed.). Philadelphia, PA: F.A. Davis.

Go to Section II of this book and www.davisplus.com for the Clinical Reasoning Tool and its case studies to provide you with a safe place to explore patient care situations. There are a total of 26 different case studies; 2 cases are presented for each of 13 body systems. One set of 13 cases are found in the Section II chapters, and a second set of 13 cases are available online at www.davisplus.com. Each case is designed with the specific goal of helping you to connect the dots of clinical reasoning. Cases are designed to reflect possible clinical scenarios; the outcomes may or may not be positive—you decide.

Pulmonary Function Studies

OVERVIEW

Pulmonary function tests (PFTs) are noninvasive tests used to assess respiratory abnormalities by evaluating how well a patient moves air in and out of the lungs. Respiration is controlled by the medulla of the brain in coordination with neurons to manage inspiration and expiration. Breathing is achieved through the interaction of chemoreceptors located in the medulla and lung receptors. Lung receptors found in the airways adjust breathing patterns to match respiratory changes. Multiple facets of respiration will be noted and measured during a PFT. Assessments include lung capacity and air volume and flow. Spirometry is a tool that can be used during a PFT to measure air volume and air flow rates. Information obtained by spirometry is interpreted in relation to the age, height, weight, and gender of the patient. Gas exchange will be evaluated by assessing the lungs' ability to provide oxygen to and remove carbon dioxide from body tissues and organs. Gas exchange is dependent upon three actions: (1) adequate ventilation, which is composed of inspiration and expiration; (2) diffusion, which is the ability to move gases across the alveolar capillary membrane; and (3) perfusion, which is the movement of blood through the pulmonary vasculature to the body tissues. The information provided by a PFT will assist the health-care provider (HCP) to diagnose respiratory insufficiency related to pathophysiologic abnormalities such as tumors, infections, and obstructive and restrictive disorders. PFTs in combination with other studies such as arterial blood gas (ABG) studies can be used to determine the existence and extent of pulmonary disease. Other pertinent information can be obtained from the medical history, chest radiography, CT scans of the chest, lung scans, and pulmonary angiography.

The information in the Part I studies is organized in a manner to help the student see how the five basic components of the nursing process (assessment, diagnosis, planning, implementation, and evaluation) can be applied to each phase of laboratory and diagnostic testing. The goal is to use nursing process to understand the integration of care (laboratory, diagnostic, nursing care) toward achieving a positive expected outcome.

- **Assessment** is the collection of information for the purpose of answering the question, "is there a problem?" Knowledge of the patient's health history, medications, complaints, and allergies as well as synonyms or alternate test names, common use for the procedure, specimen requirements, and normal ranges or interpretive comments provide the foundation for diagnosis.
- **Diagnosis** is the process of looking at the information gathered during assessment and answering the questions, "what is the problem?" and "what do I need to do about it?" Test indications tell us why the study has been requested, and potential diagnoses tell us the value or importance of the study relative to its clinical utility.
- **Planning** is a blueprint of the nursing care before the procedure. It is the process of determining how the nurse is going to partner with the patient to fix the problem (e.g., "The patient has a study ordered and this is what I should know before I successfully carry out the plan to have the study completed"). Knowledge of interfering factors, social and cultural issues, preprocedural restrictions, the need for written and informed consent, anxiety about the procedure, and concerns regarding pain are some considerations for planning a successful partnership.
- **Implementation** is putting the plan into action with an idea of what the expected outcome should be. Collaboration with the departments where the laboratory test or diagnostic study is to be performed is essential to the success of the plan. Implementation

is where the work is done within each health-care team member's scope of practice.

- **Evaluation** answers the question, "did the plan work or not?" Was the plan completely successful, partially successful, or not successful? If the plan did not work, evaluation is the process where you determine what needs to be changed to make the plan work better. This includes a review of all expected outcomes. Nursing care after the procedure is where information is gathered to evaluate the plan. Review of results, including critical findings, in relation to patient symptoms and other tests performed, provides data that form a more complete picture of health or illness.
- **Expected Outcomes** are positive outcomes related to the test. They are the outcomes the nurse should expect if all goes well.

A number of pretest, intratest, and post-test universal points are presented in this overview section because the information applies to pulmonary function studies in general.

Universal Pretest Pearls (Planning)

- Obtain a history of the patient's complaints, including a list of known allergens, especially allergies or sensitivities to medications or latex, so that their use can be avoided or their effects mitigated if an allergy is present. Carefully evaluate all medications currently being taken by the patient. A list of the patient's current medications, prescribed and over the counter (including anticoagulants, aspirin and other salicylates, and dietary supplements), should also be obtained. Such products may be discontinued by medical direction for the appropriate number of days prior to the procedure. Ensure that all allergies are clearly noted in the medical record, and ensure the patient is wearing an allergy and medical record armband. Report to the HCP and laboratory any information that could interfere with, or delay proceeding with, the study.
- Obtain a history of the patient's affected body system, symptoms, and results of previously performed laboratory tests and diagnostic and surgical procedures. Previous test results will provide a basis of comparison between old and new data.
- An important aspect of planning is understanding factors that may alter study findings or cause abnormal results. Interdepartmental communication is a key factor in the planning process. The inability of a patient to cooperate or remain still during the procedure because of age, significant pain, or mental status should be among the anticipated factors. Recent or past procedures, medications, or existing medical conditions that could complicate or interfere with test results should be noted.

- Review the steps of the study with the patient or caregiver. Expect patients to be nervous about the procedure itself and the pending results. Educating the patient about his or her role during the procedure and what to expect can facilitate this. The patient's role during the procedure is to remain still. The actual time required to complete each study will depend on a number of conditions, including the type of equipment being used and how well a patient will cooperate.
- Address any concerns about pain, and explain or describe, as appropriate, the level and type of discomfort that may be expected. Advise the patient that some discomfort may be experienced during the arterial puncture or venipuncture.
- Provide additional instructions and patient preparation regarding medication, diet, fluid intake, or activity if appropriate. Unless specified in the individual study, there are no special instructions or restrictions.
- Always be sensitive to any cultural or psychosocial issues, including a concern for modesty before, during, and after the procedure.

Reminder

Ensure that a written and informed consent has been documented in the medical record prior to the study, if required. The consent must be obtained before medication is administered.

Universal Intratest Pearls (Implementation)

- Correct patient identification is crucial prior to any procedure: Positively identify the patient using two unique identifiers, such as patient name, date of birth, Social Security number, or medical record number.
- Standard Precautions must be followed.
- Children and infants may be accompanied by a parent to calm them. Keep neonates and infants covered and in a warm room, and provide a pacifier or gentle touch. The testing environment should be quiet, and the patient should be instructed, as appropriate, to remain still during the test as extraneous movements can affect results.
- Ensure that the patient has complied with pretesting instructions, including dietary, fluid, medication, and activity restrictions as given for the procedure. The number of days to withhold medication depends on the type of medication. Notify the HCP if pretesting instructions have not been followed

(e.g., if applicable, if patient anticoagulant therapy has not been withheld).

- Before leaving the patient's side, appropriate specimen containers should always be labeled with the corresponding patient demographics, the initials of the person collecting the sample, collection date, time of collection, applicable special notes, especially site location and laterality, and then promptly transported to the laboratory for processing and analysis.

Universal Post Test Pearls (Evaluation)

- Note that completed test results are made available to the requesting HCP, who will discuss them with the patient.
- Answer questions and address concerns voiced by the patient or family and reinforce information given by the patient's HCP regarding further testing, treatment, or referral to another HCP. Recognize that patients will have anxiety related to test results. Provide teaching and information regarding the clinical implications of the test results on the patient's lifestyle as appropriate.
- Note that test results should be evaluated in context with the patient's signs, symptoms, and diagnosis. Depending on the results of the procedure, additional testing may be performed to evaluate or monitor progression of the disease process and determine the need for a change in therapy.
- Be aware that when a person goes through a traumatic event such as an illness or is being given information that will impact his or her lifestyle, there are universal human reactions that occur. These include knowledge deficit, fear, anxiety, and coping; in some situations, grieving may occur. Health-care providers should always be aware of the human response and how it may affect the plan of care and expected outcomes.

DISCUSSION POINT

Regarding Post-Test Critical Findings: Timely notification of a critical finding for lab or diagnostic studies is a role expectation of the professional nurse. Notification processes will vary among facilities. Upon receipt of the critical finding, the information should be read back to the caller to verify accuracy. Most policies require immediate notification of the primary HCP, hospitalist, or on-call HCP. Reported information includes the patient's name, unique identifiers, critical finding, name of the person giving the report, and name of the person receiving the report. Documentation of notification should be made in the medical record with the name of the HCP notified, time and date of notification, and any orders received. Any delay in a timely report of a critical finding may require completion of a notification form with review by Risk Management.

STUDIES

- Blood Gases
- Pulmonary Function Studies
- Pulse Oximetry

LEARNING OUTCOMES

Providing safe, effective nursing care (SENC) includes mastery of core competencies and standards of care. SENC is based on a judicious application of nursing knowledge in combination with scientific principles. The Art of Nursing lies in blending what you know with the ability to effectively apply your knowledge in a compassionate manner.

After reading/studying this chapter you will be able to:

Thinking

1. Advocate and offer emotional and physical care and support. Examine the difference between strategies that work and those that do not when providing both physical and emotional comfort and support to the patient.

Doing

1. Value the diversity of information that can be provided by other team members.

Caring

1. Recognize that the patient has personal knowledge of how to best manage his or her disease.

Blood Gases

Quick Summary

SYNONYM ACRONYM: Arterial blood gases (ABGs), venous blood gases, capillary blood gases, cord blood gases.

COMMON USE: To assess oxygenation and acid-base balance.

SPECIMEN: Whole blood. Specimen volume and collection container may vary with collection method. See Intratest section for specific collection instructions. Specimen should be tightly capped and transported in an ice slurry.

NORMAL FINDINGS: (Method: Selective electrodes for pH, Pco_2 and Po_2)

Blood Gas Value (pH)	Arterial	Venous	Capillary
Scalp	–	–	7.25–7.35
Birth, cord, full term	7.11–7.36	7.25–7.45	7.32–7.49
Adult/child	7.35–7.45	7.32–7.43	7.35–7.45

Note: SI units (conversion factor × 1).

Pco_2	Arterial	SI Units (Conventional Units × 0.133)	Venous	SI Units (Conventional Units × 0.133)	Capillary	SI Units (Conventional Units × 0.133)
Scalp	–	–	–	–	40–50 mm Hg	5.3–6.6 kPa
Birth, cord, full term	32–66 mm Hg	4.3–8.8 kPa	27–49 mm Hg	3.6–6.5 kPa	–	–
Newborn–adult	35–45 mm Hg	4.7–6 kPa	41–51 mm Hg	5.4–6.8 kPa	26–41 mm Hg	3.5–5.4 kPa

Po_2	Arterial	SI Units (Conventional Units × 0.133)	Venous	SI Units (Conventional Units × 0.133)	Capillary	SI Units (Conventional Units × 0.133)
Scalp	–	–	–	–	20–30 mm Hg	2.7–4 kPa
Birth, cord, full term	8–24 mm Hg	1.1–3.2 kPa	17–41 mm Hg	2.3–5.4 kPa	–	–
0–1 hr	33–85 mm Hg	4.4–11.3 kPa	–	–	–	–
Greater than 1 hr–adult	80–95 mm Hg	10.6–12.6 kPa	20–49 mm Hg	2.7–6.5 kPa	80–95 mm Hg	10.6–12.6 kPa

HCO_3^-	Arterial Conventional & SI Units	Venous Conventional & SI Units	Capillary Conventional & SI Units
Birth, cord, full term	17–24 mmol/L	17–24 mmol/L	N/A
2 mo–2 yr	16–23 mmol/L	24–28 mmol/L	18–23 mmol/L
Adult	22–26 mmol/L	24–28 mmol/L	18–23 mmol/L

O_2 Sat	Arterial	Venous	Capillary
Birth, cord, full term	40–90%	40–70%	–
Adult/child	95–99%	70–75%	95–98%

Values may be at the lower end of the normal range in older adults

Arterial Oxygen Content—Conventional Units	Arterial Oxygen Content—SI Units
6.6–9.7 mmol/L	15–22 volume %

Venous Oxygen Content—Conventional Units	Venous Oxygen Content—SI Units
4.9–7.1 mmol/L	11–16 volume %

Tco_2	Arterial Conventional & SI Units mmol/L	Venous Conventional & SI Units mmol/L
Birth, cord, full term	13–22 mmol/L	14–22 mmol/L
Adult/child	22–29 mmol/L	25–30 mmol/L

Base Excess Arterial	Conventional & SI Units
Birth, cord, full term	$(-10) - (-2)$ mmol/L
Adult/child	$(-2) - (+3)$ mmol/L

Test Explanation

Blood gas analysis is used to evaluate respiratory function and provide a measure for determining acid-base balance. Respiratory, renal, and cardiovascular system functions are integrated in order to maintain normal acid-base balance. Therefore, respiratory or metabolic disorders may cause abnormal blood gas findings. The blood gas measurements commonly reported are pH, partial pressure of carbon dioxide in the blood (Pco_2), partial pressure of oxygen in the blood (Po_2), bicarbonate (HCO_3^-), O_2 saturation, and base excess (BE) or base deficit (BD). pH reflects the number of free hydrogen ions (H^+) in the body. A pH less than 7.35 indicates acidosis. A pH greater than 7.45 indicates alkalosis. Changes in the ratio of free H^+ to HCO_3 will result in a compensatory response from the lungs or kidneys to restore proper acid-base balance.

Pco_2 is an important indicator of ventilation. The level of Pco_2 is controlled primarily by the lungs and is referred to as the respiratory component of acid-base balance. The main buffer system in the body is the bicarbonate–carbonic acid system. Bicarbonate is an important alkaline ion that participates along with other anions, such as hemoglobin, proteins, and phosphates, to neutralize acids. For the body to maintain proper balance, there must be a ratio of 20 parts bicarbonate to one part carbonic acid (20:1). Carbonic acid level is indirectly measured by Pco_2. Bicarbonate level is indirectly measured by the total carbon dioxide content (Tco_2). The carbonic acid level is not measured directly but can be estimated because it is 3% of the Pco_2. Bicarbonate can also be calculated from these numbers once the carbonic acid value has been obtained because of the 20:1 ratio. For example, if the Pco_2 were 40, the carbonic acid would be calculated as (3% × 40) or 1.2, and the HCO_3^- would be calculated as (20 × 1.2) or 24. The main acid in the acid-base system is carbonic acid. It is the metabolic or nonrespiratory component of the acid-base system and is controlled by the kidney. Bicarbonate levels can either be measured directly or estimated from the Tco_2 in the blood. BE/BD reflects the number of anions available in the blood to help buffer changes in pH. A BD (negative BE) indicates metabolic acidosis, whereas a positive BE indicates metabolic alkalosis.

Extremes in acidosis are generally more life threatening than alkalosis. Acidosis can develop either very quickly (e.g., cardiac arrest) or over a longer period of time (e.g., renal failure). Infants can develop acidosis very quickly if they are not kept warm and given enough calories. Children with diabetes tend to go into acidosis more quickly than do adults who have been dealing with the disease over a longer period of time. In many cases, a venous or capillary specimen is satisfactory to obtain the necessary information regarding acid-base balance without subjecting the patient to an arterial puncture with its associated risks.

As seen in the table of reference ranges, Po_2 is lower in infants than in children and adults owing to the respective level of maturation of the lungs at birth. Po_2 tends to trail off after age 30, decreasing by approximately 3 to 5 mm Hg per decade as the organs age and begin to lose elasticity. The formula used to approximate the relationship between age and Po_2 is $Po_2 = 104 - (age × 0.27)$.

The oxygen-carrying capacity of the blood indicates how much oxygen could be carried if all the hemoglobin were saturated with oxygen. Percentage of oxygen saturation is [oxyhemoglobin concentration/(oxyhemoglobin concentration + deoxyhemoglobin concentration)] × 100.

Like carbon dioxide, oxygen is carried in the body in a dissolved and combined (oxyhemoglobin) form. Most of the oxygen circulating in the body is bound to hemoglobin (98%), the rest is dissolved. One gram of hemoglobin can bind 1.34 mL of oxygen, while plasma is capable of carrying much less—0.3 mL of dissolved oxygen. Oxygen content is the sum of the dissolved and combined oxygen. Since circulating blood may contain less oxygen than it is capable of carrying it is useful to know the actual oxygen content. Oxygen content can be calculated based on measured parameters (oxygen saturation, hemoglobin, and Po_2 and a solubility factor (0.003 is the Bunsen solubility factor for dissolved oxygen in blood). The oxygen content in arterial blood is calculated: $Cao_2 = 1.34 (Sao_2 × Hgb) + 0.003 (Pao_2)$. The oxygen content of venous blood is calculated: $Cvo_2 = 1.34 (Svo_2 × Hgb) + 0.003 (Pvo_2)$.

Testing on specimens other than arterial blood is often ordered when oxygen measurements are not needed or when the information regarding oxygen can be obtained by noninvasive techniques such as pulse oximetry. Capillary blood is satisfactory for most purposes for pH and Pco_2; the use of capillary Po_2 is limited to the exclusion of hypoxia. Measurements involving oxygen are usually not useful when performed on venous samples; arterial blood is required to accurately measure Po_2 and oxygen saturation. Considerable evidence indicates that prolonged exposure to high levels of oxygen can result in injury, such as retinopathy of prematurity in infants or the drying of airways in any patient. Monitoring Po_2 from blood gases is especially appropriate under such circumstances.

Nursing Implications

Assessment

Indications	Potential Nursing Problems
This group of tests is used to assess conditions such as asthma, chronic obstructive pulmonary disease (COPD), embolism (e.g., fatty or other embolism) during coronary arterial bypass surgery, and hypoxia. It is also used to assist in the diagnosis of respiratory failure, which is defined as a Po_2 less than 50 mm Hg and Pco_2 greater than 50 mm Hg. Blood gases can be valuable in the management of patients on ventilators or being weaned from ventilators. Blood gas values are used to determine acid-base status, the type of imbalance, and the degree of compensation as summarized in the following section. Restoration of pH to near-normal values is referred to as fully compensated balance. When pH values are moving in the same direction (i.e., increasing or decreasing) as the Pco_2 or HCO_3^-, the imbalance is metabolic. When the pH values are moving in the opposite direction from the Pco_2 or HCO_3^-, the imbalance is caused by respiratory disturbances. To remember this concept, the following mnemonic can be useful: MeTRO = **Metabolic Together, Respiratory Opposite.**	• Breathing • Cardiac Output • Confusion • Dry Mouth • Fall Risk • Fatigue • Fluid Volume • Gas Exchange • Human Response • Sensory Perception • Tissue Perfusion

Acid-Base Disturbance	pH	Pco_2	Po_2	HCO_3^-
Respiratory Acidosis				
Uncompensated	Decreased	Increased	Normal	Normal
Compensated	Normal	Increased	Increased	Increased
Respiratory Alkalosis				
Uncompensated	Increased	Decreased	Normal	Normal
Compensated	Normal	Decreased	Decreased	Decreased
Uncompensated	Decreased	Normal	Decreased	Decreased
Compensated	Normal	Decreased	Decreased	Decreased
Metabolic (Nonrespiratory) Acidosis				
Uncompensated	Increased	Normal	Increased	Increased
Compensated	Normal	Increased	Increased	Increased

Diagnosis: Clinical Significance of Test Results

Acid-base imbalance is determined by evaluating pH, Pco_2, and HCO_3^- values. pH less than 7.35 reflects an acidic state, whereas pH greater than 7.45 reflects alkalosis. Pco_2 and HCO_3^- determine whether the imbalance is respiratory or nonrespiratory (metabolic). Because a patient may have more than one imbalance and may also be in the process of compensating, the interpretation of blood gas values may not always seem straightforward.

Respiratory conditions that interfere with normal breathing cause CO_2 to be retained in the blood. This results in an increase of circulating carbonic acid and a corresponding decrease in pH (respiratory acidosis). Acute respiratory acidosis can occur in acute pulmonary edema, severe respiratory infections, bronchial obstruction, pneumothorax, hemothorax, open chest wounds, opiate poisoning, respiratory depressant drug therapy, and inhalation of air with a high CO_2 content.

Chronic respiratory acidosis can be seen in patients with asthma, pulmonary fibrosis, COPD, bronchiectasis, and respiratory depressant drug therapy. Respiratory conditions that increase the breathing rate cause CO_2 to be removed from the alveoli more rapidly than it is being produced. This results in an alkaline pH. Acute respiratory alkalosis may be seen in anxiety, hysteria, hyperventilation, pulmonary embolus, and with an increase in artificial ventilation. Chronic respiratory alkalosis may be seen in high fever, administration of drugs (e.g., salicylate and sulfa) that stimulate the respiratory system, hepatic coma, hypoxia of high altitude, and central nervous system (CNS) lesions or injury that result in stimulation of the respiratory center.

Metabolic (nonrespiratory) conditions that cause the excessive formation or decreased excretion of organic or inorganic acids result in metabolic acidosis. Some of these conditions include ingestion of salicylates, ethylene glycol, and methanol, as well as uncontrolled diabetes, starvation, shock, kidney disease, and biliary or pancreatic fistula. Metabolic alkalosis results from conditions that increase pH, as can be seen in excessive intake of antacids to treat gastritis or peptic ulcer, excessive administration of HCO_3^-, loss of stomach acid caused by protracted vomiting, cystic fibrosis, or potassium and chloride deficiencies.

RESPIRATORY ACIDOSIS
- Decreased pH
- Decreased O_2 saturation
- Increased Pco_2:
  - Acute intermittent porphyria
  - Anemia (severe)
  - Anorexia
  - Anoxia
  - Asthma
  - Atelectasis
  - Bronchitis
  - Bronchoconstriction
  - Carbon monoxide poisoning
  - Cardiac disorders
  - Congenital heart defects
  - COPD
  - Cystic fibrosis
  - Depression of respiratory center
  - Drugs depressing the respiratory system
  - Electrolyte disturbances (severe)
  - Fever
  - Head injury
  - Heart failure
  - Hypercapnia
  - Hypothyroidism (severe)
  - Near drowning
  - Pleural effusion
  - Pneumonia
  - Pneumothorax
  - Poisoning
  - Poliomyelitis
  - Pulmonary edema
  - Pulmonary embolism
  - Pulmonary tuberculosis
  - Respiratory distress syndrome (adult and neonatal)
  - Respiratory failure
  - Sarcoidosis
  - Smoking
  - Tumor
- A decreased Po_2 that increases Pco_2:
  - Decreased alveolar gas exchange: cancer, compression or resection of lung, respiratory distress syndrome (newborns), sarcoidosis
  - Decreased ventilation or perfusion: asthma, bronchiectasis, bronchitis, cancer, croup, COPD, cystic fibrosis (mucoviscidosis), granulomata, pneumonia, pulmonary infarction, shock

- Hypoxemia: anesthesia, carbon monoxide exposure, cardiac disorders, high altitudes, near drowning, presence of abnormal hemoglobins
- Hypoventilation: cerebrovascular incident, drugs depressing the respiratory system, head injury
- Right-to-left shunt: congenital heart disease, intrapulmonary venoarterial shunting

COMPENSATION
- Increased Po_2:
  - Hyperbaric oxygenation
  - Hyperventilation
- Increased base excess:
  - Increased HCO_3^- to bring pH to (near) normal

RESPIRATORY ALKALOSIS
- Increased pH
- Decreased Pco_2:
  - Anxiety
  - CNS lesions or injuries that cause stimulation of the respiratory center
  - Excessive artificial ventilation
  - Fever
  - Head injury
  - Hyperthermia
  - Hyperventilation
  - Hysteria
  - Salicylate intoxication

COMPENSATION
- Decreased Po_2:
  - Rebreather mask
- Decreased base excess:
  - Decreased HCO_3^- to bring pH to (near) normal

METABOLIC ACIDOSIS
- Decreased pH
- Decreased HCO_3^-
- Decreased base excess
- Decreased Tco_2:
  - Decreased excretion of H^+: acquired (e.g., drugs, hypercalcemia), Addison disease, diabetic ketoacidosis, Fanconi syndrome, inherited (e.g., cystinosis, Wilson disease), chronic kidney disease, renal tubular acidosis
  - Increased acid intake
  - Increased formation of acids: diabetic ketoacidosis, high-fat/low-carbohydrate diets
  - Increased loss of alkaline body fluids: diarrhea, excess potassium, fistula

COMPENSATION
- Decreased Pco_2:
  - Hyperventilation

METABOLIC ALKALOSIS
- Increased pH
- Increased HCO_3^-

- Increased base excess
- Increased Tco_2:
  - Alkali ingestion (excessive)
  - Anoxia
  - Gastric suctioning
  - Hypochloremic states
  - Hypokalemic states
  - Potassium depletion: Cushing disease, diarrhea, diuresis, excessive vomiting, excessive ingestion of licorice, inadequate potassium intake, potassium-losing nephropathy, steroid administration
  - Salicylate intoxication
  - Shock
  - Vomiting

COMPENSATION

- Increased Tco_2:
  - Hypoventilation

Planning

Considerations for planning a successful partnership should include clear communication of what to expect during the test to decrease anxiety and improve cooperation. The type of oxygen, the mode of oxygen delivery, and the delivery rate should be provided as part of the test requisition process. Wait 30 minutes after a change in type or mode of oxygen delivery or rate before attempting specimen collection. Before the procedure is performed, plan to review the steps with the patient and, advise the patient rest for 30 minutes before specimen collection. Address concerns about pain, and explain that an arterial puncture may be painful. Explain that the site may be anesthetized with 1% to 2% lidocaine before the puncture. Inform the patient that specimen collection usually takes 10 to 15 minutes. The person collecting the specimen should be notified beforehand if the patient is receiving anticoagulant therapy or taking aspirin or other natural products that may prolong bleeding from the puncture site.

If the sample is to be collected by radial artery puncture, perform an Allen test before the puncture to ensure that the patient has adequate collateral circulation to the hand. The modified Allen test is performed as follows: Extend the patient's wrist over a rolled towel. Ask the patient to make a fist with the hand extended over the towel. Use your second and third fingers to locate the pulses of the ulnar and radial arteries on the palmar surface of the wrist. Your thumb should not be used to locate these arteries because it has a pulse. Compress both arteries, and ask the patient to open and close the fist several times until the palm turns pale. Release pressure on the ulnar artery only. Color should return to the palm within 5 seconds if the ulnar artery is functioning. This is a positive Allen test, and blood gases may be drawn from the radial artery site. The Allen test should then be performed on

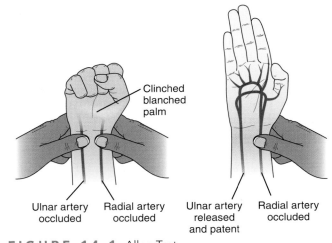

FIGURE 14.1 Allen Test.

the opposite hand. The hand to which color is restored fastest has better circulation and should be selected for specimen collection. Prepare an ice slurry in a cup or plastic bag to have ready for immediate transport of the syringe or green top tube to the laboratory (see Fig. 14.1).

CONTRAINDICATIONS

Samples for blood gases evaluation are obtained by arterial puncture, which carries a risk of bleeding, especially in patients with bleeding disorders or who are taking medications for a bleeding disorder.

SPECIAL CONSIDERATIONS

An important aspect of planning is understanding the factors that may alter study findings or cause abnormal results. Interdepartmental communication is a key factor in the planning process. The following should be noted when planning for this study:

- Values normally increase with increasing age.
- Specimens collected within 20 to 30 minutes of respiratory passage suctioning, other respiratory therapy, or the administration of antihistamines will not be accurate.
- Recent blood transfusion may produce misleading values.
- If transport to the laboratory is delayed, specimens with extremely elevated white blood cell counts will undergo misleading decreases in pH resulting from cellular metabolism.
- A falsely increased O_2 saturation may occur because of elevated levels of carbon monoxide in the blood.
- O_2 saturation is a calculated parameter based on an assumption of 100% hemoglobin A. Values may be misleading when hemoglobin variants with different oxygen dissociation curves are present. Hemoglobin S will cause a shift to the right, indicating decreased oxygen binding. Fetal hemoglobin and

methemoglobin will cause a shift to the left, indicating increased oxygen binding.

- The patient's temperature should be noted and reported to the laboratory if significantly elevated or depressed so that measured values can be corrected to the actual body temperature. Temperature affects the amount of gas in the solution. Blood gas analyzers measure samples at 37°C (98.6°F). Fever will increase actual Po_2 and Pco_2 values; therefore, the uncorrected values measured at 37°C will be falsely decreased. Hypothermia decreases actual Po_2 and Pco_2 values; therefore, the uncorrected values measured at 37°C will be falsely increased.

- *Effect of specimen collection and handling:* Exposure of the sample to room air affects the test results. Air bubbles or blood clots in the specimen are cause for rejection. Air bubbles in the specimen can falsely elevate or decrease the results, depending on the patient's blood gas status. If an evacuated tube is used for venous blood gas specimen collection, the tube must be removed from the needle before the needle is withdrawn from the arm or else the sample will be contaminated with room air.

- *Effect of anticoagulants:* Excessive amounts of heparin in the sample may falsely decrease pH, Pco_2, and Po_2. Citrates should never be used as an anticoagulant in evacuated collection tubes for venous blood gas determinations, because citrates will cause a marked analytic decrease in pH.

- *Effect of prompt and proper specimen processing, storage, and analysis:* Syringe or green-top tube specimens should be placed in ice slurry immediately after collection because blood cells continue to carry out metabolic processes in the specimen after it has been removed from the patient. These natural life processes can affect pH, Po_2, Pco_2, and the other calculated values in a short period of time. The cold temperature provided by the ice slurry will slow down, but not completely stop, metabolic changes occurring in the sample over time. Iced specimens not analyzed within 60 minutes of collection should be rejected for analysis. Electrolyte analysis from iced specimens should be carried out within 30 minutes of collection to avoid falsely elevated potassium values.

It is also important to understand which medications or substances the patient may be exposed to in the healthcare setting that can alter study findings:

- Drugs that may cause an increase in HCO_3^- include acetylsalicylic acid (initially), antacids, carbenicillin, carbenoxolone, ethacrynic acid, glycyrrhiza (licorice), laxatives, mafenide, and sodium bicarbonate. Drugs that may cause a decrease in HCO_3^- include acetazolamide, acetylsalicylic acid (long term or high doses), citrates, dimethadione, ether, ethylene glycol, fluorides, mercury compounds (laxatives),

methylenedioxyamphetamine, paraldehyde, and xylitol.

- Drugs that may cause an increase in Pco_2 include acetylsalicylic acid, aldosterone bicarbonate, carbenicillin, carbenoxolone, corticosteroids, dexamethasone, ethacrynic acid, laxatives (chronic abuse), and x-ray contrast agents. Drugs that may cause a decrease in Pco_2 include acetazolamide, acetylsalicylic acid, ethamivan, neuromuscular relaxants (secondary to postoperative hyperventilation), NSD 3004 (arterial long-acting carbonic anhydrase inhibitor), theophylline, tromethamine, and xylitol.

- Drugs that may cause an increase in Po_2 include theophylline and urokinase. Drugs that may cause a decrease in Po_2 include althesin, barbiturates, granulocyte-macrophage colony-stimulating factor, isoproterenol, and meperidine.

Implementation

Patient education is key to obtaining the patient's cooperation in following directions, and providing an explanation for the purpose of the procedure is an important part of this process. Inform the patient that this study can assist in assessing blood oxygen balance and oxygenation level. The tightly capped syringe or green-top tube should be placed in an ice slurry immediately after collection. Information on the specimen label should be protected from water in the ice slurry by first placing the specimen in a protective plastic bag. Promptly transport the specimen to the laboratory for processing and analysis.

ARTERIAL: Perform an arterial puncture and collect the specimen in an air-free heparinized syringe (see Fig. 14.2). There is no demonstrable difference in results between samples collected in plastic syringes and samples collected in glass syringes. It is very important that no room air be introduced into the collection container, because the gases in the room and in the sample will begin equilibrating immediately. The end of the

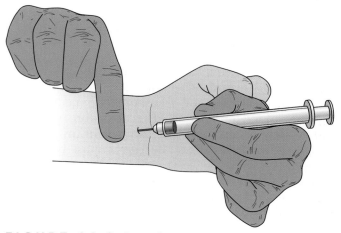

FIGURE 14.2 Arterial puncture.

syringe must be stoppered immediately after the needle is withdrawn and removed. Apply a pressure dressing over the puncture site. Samples should be mixed by gently rolling the syringe to ensure proper mixing of the heparin with the sample, which prevents the formation of small clots and rejection of the sample.

VENOUS: Central venous blood is collected in a heparinized syringe.

VENOUS: Venous blood is collected percutaneously by venipuncture in a green-top (heparin) tube (for adult patients) or a heparinized Microtainer (for pediatric patients). The vacuum collection tube must be removed from the needle before the needle is removed from the patient's arm. Apply a pressure dressing over the puncture site. Samples should be mixed by gently rolling the syringe to ensure proper mixing of the heparin with the sample, which prevents the formation of small clots and rejection of the sample.

CAPILLARY: Perform a capillary puncture and collect the specimen in two heparinized capillaries (scalp or heel for neonatal patients) or a heparinized Microtainer (for pediatric patients). Observe standard precautions. The capillary tubes should be filled as much as possible and capped on both ends. Some hospitals recommend that metal "fleas" be added to the capillary tube before the ends are capped. During transport, a magnet can be moved up and down the outside of the capillary tube to facilitate mixing and prevent the formation of clots, which would cause rejection of the sample. It is important to inform the laboratory or respiratory therapy staff of the number of fleas used so that the fleas can be accounted for and removed before the sample is introduced into the blood gas analyzers. Fleas left in the sample may damage the blood gas equipment if allowed to enter the analyzer. Microtainer samples also should be mixed by gently rolling the capillary tube to ensure proper mixing of the heparin with the sample, which prevents the formation of small clots and rejection of the sample.

CORD BLOOD: The sample may be collected immediately after delivery from the clamped cord, using a heparinized syringe.

SCALP SAMPLE: Samples for scalp pH may be collected anaerobically before delivery in special scalp-sample collection capillaries and transported immediately to the laboratory for analysis. The procedure takes approximately 5 minutes. Place the patient on her back with her feet in stirrups. The cervix must be dilated at least 3 to 4 cm. A plastic cone is placed in the vagina and fit snugly against the scalp of the fetus. The cone provides access for visualization using an endoscope and to cleanse the site. The site is pierced with a sharp blade. Containment of the blood droplet can be aided by smearing a small amount of silicone cream on the fetal skin site. The blood sample is collected in a thin, heparinized tube. Some hospitals recommend that small metal fleas be added to the scalp tube before the ends are capped. See the preceding section on capillary collection for the discussion of fleas.

Evaluation

Recognize anxiety related to test results and be supportive of impaired activity related to a perceived loss of independence. Discuss the implications of abnormal test results on the patient's lifestyle. Provide teaching and information regarding the clinical implications of the test results as appropriate. Pressure should be applied to the puncture site for at least 5 minutes in the unanticoagulated patient and for at least 15 minutes in the case of a patient receiving anticoagulant therapy. Observe/assess the puncture site for bleeding or hematoma formation and for signs or symptoms of respiratory acidosis, such as dyspnea, headache, tachycardia, pallor, diaphoresis, apprehension, drowsiness, coma, hypertension, or disorientation. Administer oxygen if appropriate. Teach the patient breathing exercises to assist with the appropriate exchange of oxygen and carbon dioxide. Teach the patient how to properly use the incentive spirometer device or mini-nebulizer if ordered. Observe/assess the patient for signs or symptoms of respiratory alkalosis, such as tachypnea, restlessness, agitation, tetany, numbness, seizures, muscle cramps, dizziness, or tingling fingertips. Instruct the patient to breathe deeply and slowly; explain that performing this type of breathing exercise into a paper bag decreases hyperventilation and quickly helps breathing return to normal. Observe/assess the patient for signs or symptoms of metabolic acidosis, such as rapid breathing, flushed skin, nausea, vomiting, dysrhythmias, coma, hypotension, hyperventilation, and restlessness. Observe/assess the patient for signs or symptoms of metabolic alkalosis, such as shallow breathing, weakness, dysrhythmias, tetany, hypokalemia, hyperactive reflexes, and excessive vomiting.

NUTRITIONAL CONSIDERATIONS: Abnormal blood gas values may be associated with diseases of the respiratory system. Malnutrition is commonly seen in patients with severe respiratory disease for reasons that include fatigue, lack of appetite, and gastrointestinal distress. Research has estimated that the daily caloric intake required for respiration in patients with COPD is 10 times higher than that of normal individuals. Inadequate nutrition can result in hypophosphatemia, especially in the respirator-dependent patient. During periods of starvation, phosphorus leaves the intracellular space and moves outside the tissue, resulting in dangerously decreased phosphorus levels. Adequate intake of vitamins A and C is also important to prevent pulmonary infection and to decrease the extent of lung tissue damage. The importance of following the prescribed diet should be stressed to the patient and/or caregiver. Water balance needs to be closely monitored in COPD patients. Fluid retention can lead to pulmonary edema.

✔ Critical Findings

Note and immediately report to the requesting health-care provider (HCP) any critical findings and related symptoms. A listing of these findings varies among facilities.

Age	Arterial Blood Gas Parameter	Less Than	Greater Than
Adult/child	pH	7.2	7.6
Adult/child	HCO_3^-	10 mmol/L	40 mmol/L
Adult/child	Pco_2	20 mm Hg (SI: 2.7 kPa)	67 mm Hg (SI: 8.9 kPa)
Adult/child	Po_2	45 mm Hg (SI: 6 kPa)	
Newborns	Po_2	37 mm Hg (SI: 4.9 kPa)	92 mm Hg (SI: 12.2 kPa)

✔ Study Specific Complications

Skin puncture is the most common invasive medical procedure performed by HCPs. There are a number of complications associated with performing an arterial puncture. **Pain** is commonly associated with needles, and although the pain experienced during arterial puncture is usually short in duration, on a rare occasion the needle may strike a nerve, causing permanent pain. Some patients experience a **vasovagal reaction** during the venipuncture procedure evidenced by sweating, low blood pressure, fainting, or near fainting. The potential for a **fall injury** is a significant concern related to vasovagal reactions. Prolonged **bleeding** is a complication that occurs with patients who are taking blood thinners or who have coagulopathies such as hemophilia. A **hematoma** results when blood leaks into the tissue during or after a skin puncture, as evidenced by pain, bruising, and/or swelling at the venipuncture site. The swelling can cause injury by compression to surrounding nerves, which can be temporary or permanent. HCPs should watch for minor complications such as bruising and hematoma at the puncture site, which are fairly common. Hematomas occur more often in older adult or frail patients, or those with blood vessels that are difficult to access. Bleeding or bruising can be prevented once the needle has been removed by applying direct pressure to the site with dry gauze for a minute or two. Some other more unusual complications of skin puncture include **cellulitis, phlebitis,**

and **sepsis.** Sepsis can be caused by the introduction of bacteria from the surface of the skin into the blood as the result of improper cleansing of the puncture site. Immunocompromised patients are at higher risk for developing this complication.

✔ Related Tests

- Related tests include α_1-AT, anion gap, arterial/alveolar oxygen ratio, biopsy lung, bronchoscopy, carboxyhemoglobin, chest x-ray, chloride sweat, CBC hemoglobin, CBC WBC and diff, culture and smear for mycobacteria, culture bacterial sputum, culture viral, cytology sputum, electrolytes, gram stain, IgE, lactic acid, lung perfusion scan, lung ventilation scan, MRI venography, osmolality, phosphorus, plethysmography, pleural fluid analysis, pulse oximetry, PFT, and TB skin tests.
- Refer to the Cardiovascular, Genitourinary, and Respiratory systems tables at the end of the book for related tests by body system.

Expected Outcomes

Expected clinical and patient-focused outcomes associated with Blood Gases are

- Maintaining normal gas exchange at rest and with activity
- Maintaining orientation to person, place, time, and purpose
- Making adjustments in lifestyle to adapt to the change in oxygenation
- Seeking assistance as needed to prevent desaturation with activity

Pulmonary Function Studies

Quick Summary

SYNONYM ACRONYM: Pulmonary function tests (PFTs).

COMMON USE: To assess respiratory function to assist in evaluating obstructive versus restrictive lung disease and to monitor and assess the effectiveness of therapeutic interventions.

AREA OF APPLICATION: Lungs, respiratory system.

NORMAL FINDINGS

- Normal respiratory volume and capacities, gas diffusion, and distribution
- No evidence of COPD or restrictive pulmonary disease

Test Explanation

Pulmonary function studies provide information about the volume, pattern, and rates of airflow involved in respiratory function. These studies may also include tests involving the diffusing capabilities of the lungs (i.e., volume of gases diffusing across a membrane). A complete pulmonary function study includes the determination of all lung volumes, spirometry, diffusing capacity, maximum voluntary ventilation, flow-volume loop, and maximum expiratory and inspiratory pressures. Other studies include small airway volumes.

The studies are conducted using a mechanical device called a *spirometer*. The amount of gas breathed in and out of the spirometer, by the patient, is measured and converted into a series of electrical signals that are displayed in a *spirogram*.

Pulmonary function studies are classified according to lung volumes and capacities, rates of flow, and gas exchange. The exception is the diffusion test, which records the movement of a gas during inspiration and expiration. Lung volumes and capacities constitute the amount of air inhaled or exhaled from the lungs; this value is compared to normal reference values specific for the patient's age, height, and gender. The following are volumes and capacities measured by spirometry that do not require timed testing.

Tidal volume	TV	Total amount of air inhaled and exhaled with one breath
Residual volume	RV	Amount of air remaining in the lungs after a maximum expiration effort; this indirect type of measurement can be done by body plethysmography (see study titled "Plethysmography")
Inspiratory reserve volume	IRV	Maximum amount of air inhaled at the point of maximum expiration
Expiratory reserve volume	ERV	Maximum amount of air exhaled after a resting expiration; can be calculated by the vital capacity (VC) minus the inspiratory capacity (IC)
Vital capacity	VC	Maximum amount of air exhaled after a maximum inspiration (can be calculated by adding the IC and the ERV)
Total lung capacity	TLC	Total amount of air that the lungs can hold after maximum inspiration; can be calculated by adding the vital capacity (VC) and the residual volume (RV)
Inspiratory capacity	IC	Maximum amount of air inspired after normal expiration; can be calculated by adding the inspiratory reserve volume (IRV) and the tidal volume (TV)
Functional residual capacity	FRC	Volume of air that remains in the lungs after normal expiration can be calculated by adding the residual volume (RV) and expiratory reserve volume (ERV)

The volumes, capacities, and rates of flow measured by spirometry that do require timed testing include the following:

Forced vital capacity in 1 sec	FEV1	Maximum amount of air that can be forcefully exhaled after a full inspiration
Forced expiratory volume	FEV	Amount of air exhaled in the first second (can also be determined at 2 or 3 sec) of forced vital capacity (FVC), which is the amount of air exhaled in seconds, expressed as a percentage
Maximal midexpiratory flow	MMEF	Also known as forced expiratory flow rate (FEF_{25-75}), or the maximal rate of airflow during a forced expiration
Forced inspiratory flow rate	FIF	Volume inspired from the RV at a point of measurement (can be expressed as a percentage to identify the corresponding volume pressure and inspired volume)
Peak inspiratory flow rate	PIFR	Maximum airflow during a forced maximal inspiration
Peak expiratory flow rate	PEFR	Maximum airflow expired during FVC
Flow-volume loops	F-V	Flows and volumes recorded during forced expiratory volume and forced inspiratory VC procedures
Maximal inspiratory-expiratory pressures		Strengths of the respiratory muscles in neuromuscular disorders
Maximal voluntary ventilation	MVV	Maximal volume of air inspired and expired in 1 min (may be done for shorter periods and multiplied to equal 1 min)

Other studies for gas-exchange capacity, small airway abnormalities, and allergic responses in hyperactive airway disorders can be performed during the conventional pulmonary function study. These include the following:

Diffusing capacity of the lungs	DL	Rate of transfer of carbon monoxide through the alveolar and capillary membrane in 1 min
Closing volume	CV	Measure of the closure of small airways in the lower alveoli by monitoring volume and percentage of alveolar nitrogen after inhalation of 100% oxygen

Isoflow volume	isoV	Flow-volume loop test followed by inhalation of a mixture of helium and oxygen to determine small airway disease
Body plethysmography		Measure of thoracic gas volume and airway resistance
Bronchial provocation		Quantification of airway response after inhalation of methacholine
Arterial blood gases	ABGs	Measure of oxygen, pH, and carbon dioxide in arterial blood

Values are expressed in units of mL, %, L, L/sec, and L/min, depending on the test performed.

Nursing Implications

Assessment

Indications	Potential Nursing Problems
Detect chronic obstructive pulmonary disease (COPD) and/or restrictive pulmonary diseases that affect the chest wall (e.g., neuromuscular disorders, kyphosis, scoliosis) and lungs, as evidenced by abnormal airflows and volumes Determine airway response to inhalants in patients with an airway-reactive disorder Determine the diffusing capacity of the lungs (DCOL) Determine the effectiveness of therapy regimens, such as bronchodilators, for pulmonary disorders Determine the presence of lung disease when other studies, such as x-rays, do not provide a definitive diagnosis, or determine the progression and severity of known COPD and restrictive pulmonary disease Evaluate the cause of dyspnea occurring with or without exercise Evaluate lung compliance to determine changes in elasticity, as evidenced by changes in lung volumes (decreased in restrictive pulmonary disease, increased in COPD and in older adult patients) Evaluate pulmonary disability for legal or insurance claims Evaluate pulmonary function after surgical pneumonectomy, lobectomy, or segmental lobectomy Evaluate the respiratory system to determine the patient's ability to tolerate procedures such as surgery or diagnostic studies Screen high-risk populations for early detection of pulmonary conditions (e.g., patients with exposure to occupational or environmental hazards, smokers, patients with a hereditary predisposition)	• Activity • Airway • Breathing • Body Image • Fear • Gas Exchange • Human Response • Role Performance • Self-care • Self-esteem • Stress

Diagnosis: Clinical Significance of Test Results

Normal adult lung volumes, capacities, and flow rates are as follows (see Fig. 14.3):

TV	500 mL at rest
RV	1,200 mL (approximate)
IRV	3,000 mL (approximate)
ERV	1,100 mL (approximate)
VC	4,600 mL (approximate)
TLC	5,800 mL (approximate)
IC	3,500 mL (approximate)
FRC	2,300 mL (approximate)
FVC	3,000–5,000 mL (approximate)
FEV_1/FVC	81%–83%
MMEF	25%–75%
FIF	25%–75%
MVV	25%–35% or 170 L/min
PIFR	300 L/min
PEFR	450 L/min
F-V loop	Normal curve
DCOL	25 mL/min per mm Hg (approximate)
CV	10%–20% of VC
V_{iso}	Based on age formula
Bronchial provocation	No change, or less than 20% reduction in FEV_1

Note: Normal values listed are estimated values for adults. Actual pediatric and adult values are based on age, height, and gender. These normal values are included on the patient's pulmonary function laboratory report. CV = closing volume; DCOL = diffusing capacity of the lungs; ERV = expiratory reserve volume; FEV_1 = forced expiratory volume in 1 sec; FIF = forced inspiratory flow rate; FRC = functional residual capacity; FVC = forced vital capacity in 1 sec; F-V loop = flow-volume loop; IC = inspiratory capacity; IRV = inspiratory reserve volume; MMEF = maximal midexpiratory flow (also known as FEF_{25-75}); MVV = maximal voluntary ventilation; PEFR = peak expiratory flow rate; PIFR = peak inspiratory flow rate; RV = residual volume; TLC = total lung capacity; TV = tidal volume; VC = vital capacity; V_{iso} = isoflow volume.

ABNORMAL FINDINGS

- Allergy
- Asbestosis
- Asthma
- Bronchiectasis
- Chest trauma
- Chronic bronchitis
- Curvature of the spine
- Emphysema
- Myasthenia gravis
- Obesity
- Pulmonary fibrosis
- Pulmonary tumors
- Respiratory infections
- Sarcoidosis

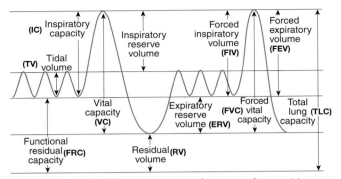

FIGURE 14.3 Respiratory volumes and capacities measured by spirometry. *Used with permission, from Van Leeuwen, A., Bladh, M., & Poelhuis-Leth, D. (2013). Davis's comprehensive handbook of laboratory and diagnostic tests with nursing implications (5th ed.). FA Davis Company.*

Planning

Considerations for planning a successful partnership should include clear communication of what to expect during the test to decrease anxiety and improve cooperation. Before the procedure is performed, plan to review the steps with the patient. Address concerns about pain, and explain that there is no discomfort during the exam. Explain that the procedure is generally performed in a specially equipped room or in a health-care provider's (HCP's) office by an HCP specializing in this procedure, and usually lasts 1 hour. Inform the patient that a nose clip may be placed over his or her nose and the spirometer's mouthpiece placed in his or her mouth during the study. Instruct the patient to refrain from smoking tobacco or eating a heavy meal for 4 to 6 hours prior to the study. The patient should avoid bronchodilators (oral or inhalant) for at least 4 hours before the study, as directed by the HCP. Prior to the study, record the patient's weight and height to assist in determining the predicted values.

CONTRAINDICATIONS

- Patients experiencing pain, which prohibits the ability to achieve deep inspiration and expiration

SPECIAL CONSIDERATIONS

An important aspect of planning is understanding the factors that may alter study findings or cause abnormal results. Interdepartmental communication is a key factor in the planning process. The following should be noted when planning for this study:

- Inadequate/poor seal around the mouthpiece affects the results.
- Lack of patient cooperation related to confusion or an inability to understand instructions may affect the results.

- The aging process can cause decreased values (FVC, DCOL) depending on the study done.
- Inability of the patient to put forth the necessary breathing effort affects the results (e.g., patients who smoke, patients who are pregnant, patients who are fatigued, patients with abdominal distention).
- Upper respiratory infections, such as a cold or acute bronchitis, in patients require consideration; abnormal test results from a transient condition may be difficult to differentiate from an underlying, more significant condition.

It is also important to understand which medications or substances the patient may be exposed to in the health-care setting that can interfere with accurate testing:

- Analgesics, bronchodilators, and sedatives can affect results.

Implementation

Patient education is key to obtaining the patient's cooperation in following directions, and providing an explanation for the purpose of the procedure is an important part of this process. Inform the patient that this study can assist in identifying the cause of poor oxygenation. Ensure that the patient has complied with dietary and medication restrictions and pretesting preparations. Obtain an inhalant bronchodilator to treat any bronchospasms that may occur with testing. Instruct the patient to void and to loosen any restrictive clothing. Place the patient in a sitting position on a chair near the spirometry equipment. If the patient wears dentures, he or she should leave them in, if necessary, for a proper mouth seal. To achieve a closed system with the spirometer, a soft nose clip is placed over the patient's nose, and the spirometer's mouthpiece is held in the mouth with the patient's lips maintaining an airtight seal. Tubing from the mouthpiece attaches to a cylinder that is connected to a computer that measures, records, and calculates the values for the tests done. The patient is instructed to breathe normally, inhale maximally, and exhale maximally. If the patient has trouble cooperating fully, a stacked vital capacity may be obtained by inserting a one-way valve. This process is repeated several times.

Evaluation

Recognize anxiety related to test results, and be supportive of impaired activity related to a perceived loss of independence. Assess the patient for dizziness or weakness and allow the patient to rest as long as necessary to recover after the test. Discuss the implications of abnormal test results on the patient's lifestyle. Provide teaching and information regarding the clinical implications of the test results as appropriate. Encourage patients who smoke to locate a smoking cessation program in their community and provide them with a Web site that may provide appropriate information, such as www.fda.gov/forconsumers/consumerupdates/ucm198176.htm.

✔ Critical Findings

N/A

✔ Study Specific Complications

N/A

✔ Related Tests

- Related tests include α_1-AT, anion gap, arterial/alveolar oxygen ratio, biopsy lung, blood gases, bronchoscopy, carboxyhemoglobin, chest x-ray, chloride sweat, CBC, CBC hemoglobin, CBC WBC count and differential, CT angiography, CT thoracic, culture and smear for mycobacteria, culture bacterial sputum, culture viral, cytology sputum, echocardiography, ECG, Gram stain, IgE, lactic acid, lung perfusion scan, lung ventilation scan, MR angiography, MRI chest, osmolality, phosphorus, plethysmography, pleural fluid analysis, potassium, PET chest, pulse oximetry, sodium, and TB skin test.
- Refer to the Cardiovascular and Respiratory systems tables at the end of the book for related tests by body system.

Expected Outcomes

Expected clinical and patient focused outcomes associated with Pulmonary Function Studies are

- Maintaining the baseline normal oxygenation level during the study
- Tolerating activity without desaturation
- Understanding the importance of using oxygen at the prescribed flow in liters per minute to support respiratory health

Pulse Oximetry

Quick Summary

SYNONYM ACRONYM: Oximetry, pulse ox.

COMMON USE: To assess arterial blood oxygenation toward evaluating respiratory status during ventilation, acute illness, activity, and sleep and to evaluate the effectiveness of therapeutic interventions.

AREA OF APPLICATION: Earlobe, fingertip; for infants, use the large toe, top or bottom of the foot, or sides of the ankle.

NORMAL FINDINGS: Greater than or equal to 95%

Test Explanation

Pulse oximetry is a noninvasive study that provides continuous readings of arterial blood oxygen saturation (SpO_2) using a sensor site (earlobe or fingertip). The SpO_2 equals the ratio of the amount of O_2 contained in the hemoglobin to the maximum amount of O_2 contained, with hemoglobin expressed as a percentage. The results obtained may compare favorably with O_2 saturation levels obtained by arterial blood gas analysis without the need to perform successive arterial punctures. The device used is a clip or probe that produces a light beam with two different wavelengths on one side. A sensor on the opposite side measures the absorption of each of the wavelengths of light to determine the O_2 saturation reading. The displayed result is a ratio, expressed as a percentage, between the actual O_2 content of the hemoglobin and the potential maximum O_2-carrying capacity of the hemoglobin.

Nursing Implications

Assessment

Indications	Potential Nursing Problems
Determine the effectiveness of pulmonary gas exchange function	• Breathing
Evaluate suspected nocturnal hypoxemia in chronic obstructive pulmonary disease	• Cardiac Output • Confusion • Fall Risk
Monitor oxygenation during testing for sleep apnea	• Fatigue • Fluid Volume
Monitor oxygenation perioperatively and during acute illnesses	• Gas Exchange • Human Response
Monitor oxygenation status in patients on a ventilator, during surgery, and during bronchoscopy	• Tissue Perfusion • Sensory Perception
Monitor O_2 saturation during activities such as pulmonary exercise stress testing or pulmonary rehabilitation exercises to determine optimal tolerance	
Monitor response to pulmonary drug regimens, especially flow and O_2 content	

Diagnosis: Clinical Significance of Test Results
ABNORMAL FINDINGS
- Abnormal gas exchange
- Hypoxemia with levels less than 95%
- Impaired cardiopulmonary function

Planning

Considerations for planning a successful partnership should include clear communication of what to expect during the test to decrease anxiety and improve cooperation. Before the procedure is performed, plan to review the steps with the patient. Explain that the procedure is usually performed bedside by a respiratory therapist, takes less than 5 minutes, and there is no pain or discomfort. If a finger probe is used, instruct the patient to remove artificial fingernails and nail polish prior to the study. Oximetry may be used to constantly monitor a patient during the perioperative period and during postanesthesia as a criteria for discharge, as well as in patients on a mechanical ventilator or under heavy sedation.

SPECIAL CONSIDERATIONS

An important aspect of planning is understanding the factors that may alter study findings or cause abnormal results. Interdepartmental communication is a key factor in the planning process. The following should be noted when planning for this study:

- Nail polish, artificial fingernails, and skin pigmentation may interrupt digital readings when a finger probe is used.
- Vasoconstriction from cool skin temperature, drugs, hypotension, or vessel obstruction causes a decrease in blood flow and can alter oximetry findings.
- Results from patients with anemic conditions are decreased, which reflects a reduction in hemoglobin, the O_2-carrying component in the blood.
- Excessive light surrounding the patient, such as from surgical lights may be detected by the meter and result in altered oximetry findings.
- Impaired cardiopulmonary function may cause variations in blood flow and result in altered oximetry findings.
- Lipid emulsion therapy and the presence of certain dyes can alter oximetry findings.
- Movement of the finger or ear or improper placement of probe or clip can alter oximetry findings.

Accuracy for most units is plus or minus 2%–3%.

Implementation

Patient education is key to obtaining the patient's cooperation in following directions, and providing an explanation for the purpose of the procedure is an important part of this process. Inform the patient that this study can assist in identifying the cause of poor oxygenation. Ensure that the patient has complied with pretesting instructions. If a finger probe is used, instruct the patient not to grip the treadmill rail or bed rail tightly; doing so restricts blood flow. Rub the area to be used, either the fingertip or the earlobe, to stimulate blood flow and clip the probe to the finger or ear. The big

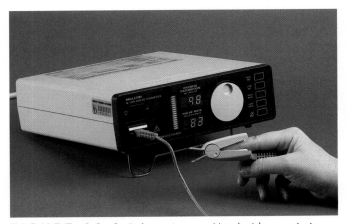

FIGURE 14.4 Pulse oximeter. *Used with permission, from Wilkinson, J., & Treas, L. (2010). Fundamentals of nursing (2nd ed.). FA Davis Company.*

toe, top or bottom of the foot, or sides of the heel may be used in infants. Place the photodetector probe over the finger in such a way that the light beams and sensors are opposite each other. Turn the power switch to the oximeter monitor, which will display information about heart rate and peripheral capillary saturation (SaO_2). The probe allows a beam of light to pass through the tissue, and the sensor measures the amount of light that the tissue absorbs (see Fig. 14.4).

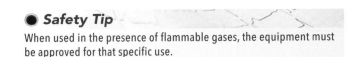

● Safety Tip

When used in the presence of flammable gases, the equipment must be approved for that specific use.

Evaluation

Recognize anxiety related to test results and be supportive of impaired activity related to a perceived loss of independence. Closely observe SpO_2, and report to the HCP if it decreases to 90%. Discuss the implications of abnormal test results on the patient's lifestyle. Provide teaching and information regarding the clinical implications of the test results as appropriate. Encourage patients who smoke to locate a smoking cessation program in their community and provide them with a Web site that may provide appropriate information, such as www.fda.gov/forconsumers/consumerupdates/ucm198176.htm.

✓ Critical Findings

Hypoxia occurs at oxygen saturation levels less than 90%. Significant hypoxia, levels less than 85%, require immediate evaluation and treatment.

Note and immediately report to the requesting HCP any critical findings and related symptoms. A listing of these findings varies among facilities.

☑ Study Specific Complications

N/A

☑ Related Tests

- Related tests include α_1-AT, anion gap, arterial/alveolar oxygen ratio, biopsy lung, blood gases, bronchoscopy, carboxyhemoglobin, chest x-ray, chloride sweat, CBC, CBC hemoglobin, CBC WBC count and differential, CT angiography, culture and smear for mycobacteria, culture bacterial sputum, culture viral, cytology sputum, ECG, Gram stain, IgE, lactic acid, lung perfusion scan, lung ventilation scan, MR angiography, MR chest, osmolality, phosphorus, plethysmography, pleural fluid analysis, potassium, pulmonary function tests, sodium, and TB skin test.
- Refer to the Cardiovascular and Respiratory systems tables at the end of the book for related tests by body system.

Expected Outcomes

Expected clinical and patient-focused outcomes associated with Pulse Oximetry are

- Maintaining oxygen saturation at level greater than 92%
- Verbalizing the importance of reporting any perceived change in the respiratory status
- Agreeing to keep the pulse oximeter on to accurately monitor oxygenation

REVIEW OF LEARNING OUTCOMES

Thinking

1. Advocate and offer emotional and physical care and support. Examine the difference between strategies that work and those that do not when providing both physical and emotional comfort and support to the patient. Answer: How do you discover what you can do to provide both physical and emotional support to your patient? Your best resources are the patient and his or her family. Find out from the patient what has worked and what has not worked in the past. Use your resources within your facility; the chaplain, social worker, and case manager can provide referrals and personal support that may be very valuable to the patient and the patient's family.

Doing

1. Value the diversity of information that can be provided by other team members. Answer:

Respiratory disease requires a team approach to meet the patient's needs and to decrease his or her shortness of breath. Team members may include the respiratory therapist to evaluate the efficacy of treatment, the pharmacist to identify medications that can decrease anxiety and work of breathing, and the physician to manage medical aspects of care.

Caring

1. Recognize that the patient has personal knowledge of how to best manage his or her disease. Answer: Most respiratory patients have devised coping strategies that will decrease the severity of their shortness of breath. Talk to your patient and, if possible, use the strategies he or she has developed to decrease the patient's shortness of breath and overcome the anxiety that difficulty breathing can elicit. You will find that the overall care runs much more smoothly.

◐ **Words OF Wisdom:** Difficulty breathing for any reason is a highly anxious event. Those patients who are experiencing difficulty breathing coupled with the fear of waiting to discover why will need "tender loving care" to cope with the situation. The terminology used to describe issues related to why one is having difficulty breathing can be confusing and add to the stress. Please make sure that in your nursing role you address the barriers that limit their understanding. Parents will be very fearful for their children, and although you may believe they understand you, the emotional aspect of the event will limit the amount of information absorbed. Always follow up to confirm their understanding in the context of the medical concern. Remember that it is your role to transfer information and provide clear communication at a level of understanding to that particular patient. Make an extra effort to individualize your care, and discover what will allow your patient to "breathe easier." This could be as simple as placing a fan on low so the patient can feel air movement or providing music and low lights. This is a your role and responsibility.

BIBLIOGRAPHY

Cavanaugh, B. (2003). Nurse's manual of laboratory and diagnostic tests (4th ed.). Philadelphia, PA: F.A. Davis Company.

Lung function tests. Retrieved from http://webmd.com/lung/lung-function-tests

Malarkey, L., & McMorrow, M. (2012). Saunders nursing guide to laboratory and diagnostic tests (2nd ed.). St. Louis, MO: Mosby Elsevier.

Pagana, K., & Pagana, T. (2010). Mosby's manual of diagnostic and laboratory tests (4th ed.). St. Louis, MO: Mosby Elsevier.

Pulmonary function test. Retrieved from http://medicalcenter.osu .edu/heart/conditions/Pages/Tests/PulmonaryFunctionTest .aspx

Pulmonary function tests. Retrieved from www.nlm.nih.gov/ medlineplus/ency/article/003853.htm

Pulmonary function tests. Retrieved from http://hopkinsmedicine .org/healthlibrary/printv.aspx?d=92,P07759

Types of lung function tests. Retrieved from http://www.nhlbi.nih .gov/health/health-topics/topics/lft/types

Van Leeuwen, A., & Bladh, M. (2015). Davis's comprehensive handbook of laboratory and diagnostic tests with nursing implications (6th ed.). Philadelphia, PA: F.A. Davis Company.

Go to Section II of this book and www.davisplus.com for the Clinical Reasoning Tool and its case studies to provide you with a safe place to explore patient care situations. There are a total of 26 different case studies; 2 cases are presented for each of 13 body systems. One set of 13 cases are found in the Section II chapters, and a second set of 13 cases are available online at www.davisplus.com. Each case is designed with the specific goal of helping you to connect the dots of clinical reasoning. Cases are designed to reflect possible clinical scenarios; the outcomes may or may not be positive—you decide.

Radiologic Studies: Contrast/Special

OVERVIEW

Radiologic studies may require the use of a contrast medium to obtain an adequate image for diagnostic inquiry. Contrast medium can be given through various routes, including IV, intra-arterial, percutaneous, oral, inhalation, rectal, or urethral catheterization. Administration of contrast medium may be invasive or noninvasive. Oral administration of barium sulfate as a contrast medium would be considered noninvasive, whereas the administration of IV iodinated dyes would be considered to be invasive. All invasive procedures require a written and informed consent. Radiologic procedures that require special contrast may be performed in a special procedure department. Precautions should be taken to prevent completing a radiologic procedure on a pregnant woman. Counting the days from the first day of the menstrual cycle to day 10, called the 10-day rule, provides a window in time when it is less likely that pregnancy has occurred. If necessary, women of childbearing years should have a pregnancy test prior to any radiologic procedure.

RADIOLOGIC PROCEDURES: There are several different types of radiologic procedures that use radiation in combination with a contrast medium to meet diagnostic needs. Special imaging procedures can cause some anxiety and discomfort, and are not without risk. Nurses and all health-care team members need to have a clear understanding of the risks, benefits, and potential complications of each type of procedure. To decrease anxiety, explain to the patient that the room where the procedure will be completed can look like an operating room. Explain also that those individuals assisting with the procedure may be masked and/or gowned, or may speak to them by microphone behind protective screens. The foreignness of the procedural area coupled with concerns about the examination results often leave the patient feeling helpless, afraid, and vulnerable. Adequate patient preparation can help decrease these feelings.

Fluoroscopy focuses on the use of contrast medium to view the function of a body part or organ in motion. A simple description of this process is to imagine that you are watching a black and white television show of a body part in motion on a digital monitor in real time. An example is the evaluation of a patient who is having trouble swallowing. The patient is given a barium solution to drink while the fluoroscope records each aspect of the swallowing process as it is happening (see Fig. 15.1).

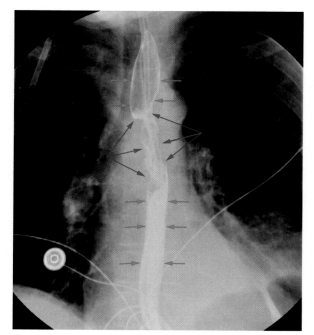

FIGURE 15.1 Esophagram showing esophageal cancer. *Used with permission, from Weber, E., Vilensky, J., & Fog, A. (2013). Practical radiology: A symptom-based approach. FA Davis Company.*

Sequences of still pictures can also be taken, and the fluoroscopic imaging can be played back as often as needed to examine areas of interest. Fluoroscopy is also frequently used to assist in various surgical procedures by providing visual guidance, for example, during insertion and placement of catheters, stents, pacemakers, or orthopedic implants (see Fig. 15.2). The use of fluoroscopy does have some risks. There can be an increase in the amount of radiation exposure, depending on the type and length of the procedure. Interventional procedures to place stents or other devices may take longer and use higher doses of radiation. Longer radiation exposure can result in short-term and long-term concerns. Short term, there may be injury to the skin and underlying tissues, and in the long term, cancers such as leukemia may occur. This is why it is important that the health-care provider (HCP) always consider the risk versus benefit to the patient when ordering radiologic procedures. To minimize the radiation risk, fluoroscopy should always be performed with the lowest acceptable exposure for the shortest time necessary.

Arteriography is used to study vascular anatomy. The focus is to study the arteries and, specifically, to assess for occlusive arterial disease. The most common arteries evaluated by arteriography are the coronary artery, the aorta and its branches, and the renal, cerebral, and adrenal arteries (see Fig. 15.3). Sites chosen for arteriography are dependent upon the diagnostic information needed. The right and left brachial arteries or femoral artery are used most often. However, other arteries can be used as appropriate to the

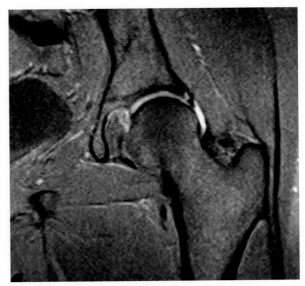

FIGURE 15.2 MR arthrogram showing torn acetabular labrum. *Used with permission, from Weber, E., Vilensky, J., & Fog, A. (2013). Practical radiology: A symptom-based approach. FA Davis Company.*

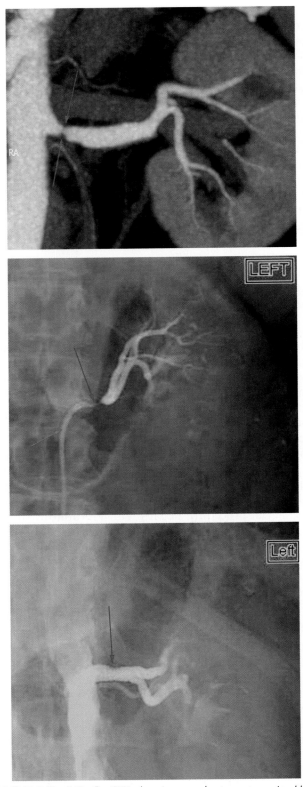

FIGURE 15.3 CTA showing renal artery stenosis. *Used with permission, from Weber, E., Vilensky, J., & Fog, A. (2013). Practical radiology: A symptom-based approach. FA Davis Company.*

situation. For example, the aortic artery may be used to evaluate circulatory problems in the lower extremities. Nurses and other HCPs should be aware of the potential complications of any procedure. Potential complications associated with arteriography are cardiac dysrhythmias, embolic stroke, allergic reactions to the contrast medium, infection and/or bleeding at the catheter insertion site, acute kidney injury, or hypertensive crisis.

Digital subtraction angiography (DSA) is an advanced digital imaging system that can allow the HCP to retrieve images within seconds of contrast injection. This process is called *digital subtraction* because the initial image taken without contrast is removed or subtracted from the rest of the images, allowing for clear visualization of arteries within dense tissues or bony areas. The digital imaging is so fast that the subtraction process appears to be almost instantaneous and can be viewed on any available picture archiving and communications system (PACS) workstation. Injection sites are the same as would be used with standard angiography.

Contrast studies include a wide variety of radiographic examinations. Because of this variety, there are different types of contrast that can be used for diagnostic inquiry. Nurses should familiarize themselves with the types of contrast used for the most commonly ordered procedures within their facility and their potential allergic reactions.

The information in the Part I studies is organized in a manner to help the student see how the five basic components of the nursing process (assessment, diagnosis, planning, implementation, and evaluation) can be applied to each phase of laboratory and diagnostic testing. The goal is to use nursing process to understand the integration of care (laboratory, diagnostic, nursing care) toward achieving a positive expected outcome.

- **Assessment** is the collection of information for the purpose of answering the question, "is there a problem?" Knowledge of the patient's health history, medications, complaints, and allergies as well as synonyms or alternate test names, common use for the procedure, specimen requirements, and normal ranges or interpretive comments provide the foundation for diagnosis.
- **Diagnosis** is the process of looking at the information gathered during assessment and answering the questions, "what is the problem?" and "what do I need to do about it?" Test indications tell us why the study has been requested, and potential diagnoses tell us the value or importance of the study relative to its clinical utility.

- **Planning** is a blueprint of nursing care before the procedure. It is the process of determining how the nurse is going to partner with the patient to fix the problem (e.g., "The patient has a study ordered, and this is what I should know before I successfully carry out the plan to have the study completed"). Knowledge of interfering factors, social and cultural issues, preprocedural restrictions, the need for written and informed consent, anxiety about the procedure, and concerns regarding pain are some considerations for planning a successful partnership.
- **Implementation** is putting the plan into action with an idea of what the expected outcome should be. Collaboration with the departments where the laboratory test or diagnostic study is to be performed is essential to the success of the plan. Implementation is where the work is done within each healthcare team member's scope of practice.
- **Evaluation** answers the question, "did the plan work or not?" Was the plan completely successful, partially successful, or not successful? If the plan did not work, evaluation is the process where you determine what needs to be changed to make the plan work better. This includes a review of all expected outcomes. Nursing care after the procedure is where information is gathered to evaluate the plan. Review of results, including critical findings, in relation to patient symptoms and other tests performed, provides data that form a more complete picture of health or illness.
- **Expected Outcomes** are positive outcomes related to the test. They are the outcomes the nurse should expect if all goes well.

A number of pretest, intratest, and post-test universal points are presented in this overview section because the information applies to contrast or special radiologic studies in general.

Universal Pretest Pearls (Planning)

- Obtain a history of the patient's complaints, including a list of known allergens, especially allergies or sensitivities to medications or latex so their use can be avoided or their effects mitigated if an allergy is present. Carefully evaluate all medications currently being taken by the patient. A list of the patient's current medications, prescribed and over the counter (including anticoagulants, aspirin and other salicylates, and dietary supplements), should also be obtained. Such products may be discontinued by medical direction for the appropriate number of days prior to the procedure. Ensure that all allergies are clearly noted in the medical record, especially allergies or sensitivities to latex, anesthetics, sedatives, or contrast medium. Patients with a known hypersensitivity to contrast medium may benefit from premedication with corticosteroids and diphenhydramine. Ensure the patient with known allergies is wearing an allergy and medical record armband. Report to the HCP and department performing the study any information that could interfere with, or delay proceeding with, the study.

- Obtain a history of the patient's affected body system, symptoms, and results of previously performed laboratory tests and diagnostic and surgical procedures. Previous test results will provide a basis of comparison between old and new data.
- An important aspect of planning is understanding the factors that may alter study findings or cause abnormal results. Interdepartmental communication is a key factor in the planning process. The inability of a patient to cooperate or remain still during the procedure because of age, significant pain, or mental status should be among the anticipated factors. Recent or past procedures, medications, or existing medical conditions that could complicate or interfere with test results should be noted.
- Review the steps of the study with the patient or caregiver. Expect patients to be nervous about the procedure itself and the pending results. Educating the patient about his or her role during the procedure and what to expect can facilitate this. The patient's role during the procedure is to remain still. The actual time required to complete each study will depend on a number of conditions, including the type of equipment being used and how well a patient will cooperate.
- Address any concerns about pain, and explain or describe, as appropriate, the level and type of discomfort that may be expected during the procedure. Explain that an IV line may be inserted prior to some procedures to allow the infusion of IV fluids such as normal saline, anesthetics, sedatives, medications used in the procedure, or emergency medications. Also explain that a separate catheter may be inserted during specific studies in order to administer contrast medium, if required. Advise the patient that some discomfort may be experienced during the insertion of the IV. Make the patient aware that there may be some mild discomfort during the procedure.
- Provide additional instructions and patient preparation regarding medication, diet, fluid intake, or activity if appropriate. Unless specified in the individual study, there are no special instructions or restrictions.
- Always be sensitive to any cultural or psychosocial issues, including a concern for modesty before, during, and after the procedure.

Reminder

Ensure that a written and informed consent has been documented in the medical record prior to the study, if required. The consent must be obtained before medication is administered.

Universal Intratest Pearls (Implementation)

- Correct patient identification is crucial prior to any procedure: Positively identify the patient using two unique identifiers, such as patient name, date of birth, Social Security number, or medical record number.
- Standard Precautions must be followed.
- Children and infants may be accompanied by a parent to calm them. Keep neonates and infants covered and in a warm room, and provide a pacifier or gentle touch. The testing environment should be quiet, and the patient should be instructed, as appropriate, to remain still during the test as extraneous movements can affect results.
- Ensure that the patient has complied with pretesting instructions, including dietary, fluid, medication, and activity restrictions as given for the procedure. The number of days to withhold medication depends on the type of medication. Notify the HCP if pretesting instructions have not been followed (e.g., if applicable, if patient anticoagulant therapy has not been withheld).
- The patient as appropriate, should be prepared for insertion of an IV line for the infusion of IV fluids, contrast medium, antibiotics, anesthetics, analgesics, medications used in the procedure, or emergency medications. Inform the patient when prophylactic antibiotics will be administered before the procedure, and assess for antibiotic allergy. Prior to administration of any fluids, contrast medium, or medications, verify that they are accurate for the study. Bleeding or bruising can be prevented, once the needle has been removed, by applying direct pressure to the injection site with dry gauze for a minute or two. The site should be observed/assessed for bleeding or hematoma formation, and then covered with a gauze and adhesive bandage.
- Emergency equipment must be readily available.

- Baseline vital signs must be recorded and continue to be monitored throughout and after the procedure, according to organizational policy. A comparison should be made between the baseline and postprocedure vital signs and focused assessments. Protocols may vary among facilities.
- After the administration of general or local anesthesia, clippers should be used to remove hair from the surgical site if appropriate, the site must be cleansed with an antiseptic solution, and the area is draped with sterile towels.
- Before leaving the patient's side, appropriate specimen containers should always be labeled, with the corresponding patient demographics, the initials of the person collecting the sample, collection date, time of collection, applicable special notes, especially site location and laterality, and then promptly transported to the laboratory for processing and analysis. Place tissue samples for standard biopsy examination in properly labeled specimen containers containing formalin solution, place tissue samples for molecular diagnostic studies in properly labeled specimen containers, and promptly transport the specimen to the laboratory for processing and analysis.

Universal Post Test Pearls (Evaluation)

- Note that completed test results are made available to the requesting HCP who will discuss them with the patient.
- Answer questions and address concerns voiced by the patient or family and reinforce information given by the patient's HCP regarding further testing, treatment, or referral to another HCP. Recognize that patients will have anxiety related to test results. Provide teaching and information regarding the clinical implications of the test results on the patients lifestyle as appropriate.
- Note that test results should be evaluated in context with the patient's signs, symptoms, and diagnosis. Depending on the results of the procedure, additional testing may be performed to evaluate or monitor progression of the disease process and determine the need for a change in therapy.
- Be aware that when a person goes through a traumatic event such as an illness or is being given information that will impact his or her lifestyle, there are universal human reactions that occur. These include knowledge deficit, fear, anxiety, and coping; in some situations, grieving may occur. HCPs should always be aware of the human response and how it may affect the plan of care and expected outcomes.

DISCUSSION POINT

Regarding Post-Test Critical Findings: Timely notification of a critical finding for lab or diagnostic studies is a role expectation of the professional nurse. Notification processes will vary among facilities. Upon receipt of the critical finding, the information should be read back to the caller to verify accuracy. Most policies require immediate notification of the primary HCP, hospitalist, or on-call HCP. Reported information includes the patient's name, unique identifiers, critical finding, name of the person giving the report, and name of the person receiving the report. Documentation of notification should be made in the medical record with the name of the HCP notified, time and date of notification, and any orders received. Any delay in a timely report of a critical finding may require completion of a notification form with review by Risk Management.

STUDIES

- Angiography, Carotid
- Angiography, Coronary
- Barium Swallow
- Cholangiography, Percutaneous Transhepatic
- Cholangiography, Postoperative
- Intravenous Pyelography
- Upper Gastrointestinal and Small Bowel Series

LEARNING OUTCOMES

Providing safe, effective nursing care (SENC) includes mastery of core competencies and standards of care. SENC is based on a judicious application of nursing knowledge in combination with scientific principles. The Art of Nursing lies in blending what you know with the ability to effectively apply your knowledge in a compassionate manner.

After reading/studying this chapter, you will be able to:

Thinking

1. Describe potential medical complications for patients undergoing arteriography.

Doing

1. Perform capably and knowledgeably within the scope of practice guidelines.

Caring

1. Value continuous improvement of your own communication and conflict resolution skills.

Angiography, Carotid

Quick Summary

SYNONYM ACRONYM: Carotid angiogram, carotid arteriography.

COMMON USE: To visualize and assess the carotid arteries and surrounding tissues for abscess, tumors, aneurysm, and evaluate for atherosclerotic disease related to stroke risk.

AREA OF APPLICATION: Neck/cervical area.

NORMAL FINDINGS:

- Normal structure, function, and patency of carotid arteries
- Contrast medium normally circulates throughout neck symmetrically and without interruption
- No evidence of obstruction, variations in number and size of vessels, malformations, cysts, or tumors

Test Explanation

This test evaluates blood vessels in the neck carrying arterial blood to the brain and is accomplished by the injection of contrast material through a catheter that has been inserted into the femoral artery. Fluoroscopy is used to guide catheter placement, and angiograms (high-speed x-ray images) provide images of the carotid artery and associated vessels in surrounding tissue which are displayed on a monitor and are recorded for future viewing and evaluation. Digital subtraction angiography (DSA) is a computerized method of removing undesired structures, like bone, from the surrounding area of interest. A digital image is taken prior to injection of the contrast and then again after the contrast has been injected. By subtracting the preinjection image from the postinjection image, a higher-quality, unobstructed image can be created. The x-ray equipment is mounted on a C-shaped arm with the x-ray device beneath the table on which the patient lies. Over the patient is an image intensifier that receives the x-rays after they pass through the patient. Patterns of circulation or changes in vessel wall appearance can be viewed to help diagnose the presence of vascular abnormalities, disease, narrowing, enlargement, blockage, trauma, or lesions. This definitive test for arterial disease may be used to evaluate chronic vascular disease, arterial or venous stenosis, and medical therapy or surgery of the vasculature. Catheter angiography still is used in patients who may undergo surgery, angioplasty, or stent placement.

Nursing Implications

Assessment

Indications	Potential Nursing Problems
Aid in angioplasty, atherectomy, or stent placement	• Cardiac Output
Allow infusion of thrombolytic drugs into an occluded artery	• Disrupted Sleep
	• Fall Risk
Detect arterial occlusion, which may be evidenced by a transection of the artery caused by trauma or penetrating injury	• Family
	• Human Response
	• Infection
	• Mobility
Detect artery stenosis, evidenced by vessel dilation, collateral vessels, or increased vascular pressure	• Pain
	• Role Performance
	• Self-esteem
Detect nonmalignant tumors before surgical resection	• Skin
Detect tumors and arterial supply, extent of venous invasion, and tumor vascularity	• Tissue Perfusion
Detect thrombosis, arteriovenous fistula, aneurysms, or emboli in vessels	
Evaluate placement of a stent	
Differentiate between tumors and cysts	
Evaluate tumor vascularity before surgery or embolization	
Evaluate the vascular system of prospective organ donors before surgery	

Diagnosis: Clinical Significance of Test Results
ABNORMAL FINDINGS

- Abscess or inflammation
- Arterial stenosis or dysplasia
- Aneurysms
- Arteriovenous fistula or other abnormalities
- Congenital anomalies
- Cysts or tumors
- Trauma causing tears or other disruption
- Vascular blockage or other disruption

Planning

Considerations for planning a successful partnership should include clear communication of what to expect during the test to decrease anxiety and improve cooperation. Before the procedure is performed, plan to review the steps with the patient. Ensure that the results of coagulation testing are obtained and recorded prior to the procedure; BUN and creatinine results are also needed if contrast medium is to be used. Note any recent procedures that can interfere with test results, including examinations using barium- or iodine-based contrast medium. Ensure that barium studies were performed more than 4 days before the CT scan. Record the date of the last menstrual period and determine the possibility of pregnancy in perimenopausal women. Explain that there may be moments of discomfort and some pain experienced during the test, and inform the patient that the procedure is usually performed in a radiology or vascular suite by a health-care provider (HCP) and takes approximately 30 to 60 minutes. Remind the patient that she or he should remain still during the procedure, and instruct the patient to remove all metal in the area to be examined. The patient should fast and restrict fluids for 2 to 4 hours prior to the procedure. Protocols may vary among facilities. Instruct the patient to avoid taking anticoagulant medication or to reduce dosage as ordered prior to the procedure. Inquire about previous allergies and contrast reactions. If iodinated contrast medium is scheduled to be used in patients receiving metformin (Glucophage) for type 2 diabetes, the drug should be discontinued on the day of the test and continue to be withheld for 48 hours after the test. Iodinated contrast can temporarily impair kidney function, and failure to withhold metformin may indirectly result in drug-induced lactic acidosis, a dangerous and sometimes fatal side effect of metformin *related to renal impairment that does not support sufficient excretion of metformin.* Patients with known pheochromocytoma should receive a beta-adrenergic blocker such as propranolol and an alpha-adrenergic blocker such as phenoxybenzamine for several days prior to the study to help prevent a malignant hypertensive episode. Explain that an IV line may be inserted to allow the infusion of IV fluids (e.g., normal saline), anesthetics, or sedatives. Explain that the contrast medium will be injected, by catheter, at a separate site from the IV line. Inform the patient that she or he may experience nausea, a feeling of warmth, a flushed sensation, a salty or metallic taste, or may notice a transient headache if contrast is used and that these reactions are considered normal.

CONTRAINDICATIONS

- Patients who are pregnant or suspected of being pregnant, unless the potential benefits of a procedure using radiation far outweigh the risk of radiation exposure to the fetus and mother
- Conditions associated with adverse reactions to the contrast medium (e.g., asthma, food allergies, or allergy to the contrast medium). Although patients are still asked specifically if they have a known allergy to iodine or shellfish, it has been well established that the reaction is not to iodine; in fact, an actual iodine allergy would be very problematic because iodine is required for the production of thyroid hormones. In the case of shellfish, the reaction is to a muscle

protein called *tropomyosin*; in the case of iodinated contrast medium, the reaction is to the noniodinated part of the contrast molecule. Patients with a known hypersensitivity to the medium may benefit from premedication with corticosteroids and diphenhydramine; the use of nonionic contrast or an alternative noncontrast imaging study, if available, may be considered for patients who have severe asthma or who have experienced moderate to severe reactions to ionic contrast medium.

- Conditions associated with preexisting renal insufficiency (e.g., chronic kidney disease, single kidney transplant, nephrectomy, diabetes, multiple myeloma, and treatment with aminoglycosides and NSAIDs) *because iodinated contrast is nephrotoxic*
- Older adult and compromised patients who are chronically dehydrated before the test *because of their risk of contrast-induced acute kidney injury*
- Patients with pheochromocytoma *because iodinated contrast may cause a hypertensive crisis*
- Patients with bleeding disorders who are receiving an arterial or venous puncture (angiography) *because the site may not stop bleeding*
- The occurrence of chest pain, severe cardiac dysrhythmias, or signs of a cerebrovascular accident, which may require terminating the procedure

SPECIAL CONSIDERATIONS

An important aspect of planning is understanding the factors that may alter study findings or cause abnormal results. Interdepartmental communication is a key factor in the planning process. The following should be noted when planning for this study:

- Large amounts of bowel gas can distort abdominal organ visualization.
- The patient's inability to cooperate or remain still during the procedure because of age, significant pain, or mental status and uncooperative patients, including children, may need sedation as motion causes artifacts on the image.
- Residual barium from previous studies blocks the transmission of x-rays.
- Metallic objects within the examination field (e.g., jewelry, body rings) may inhibit organ visualization and cause unclear images.
- Failure to follow dietary restrictions and other pretesting preparations may cause the procedure to be canceled or repeated.

● *Safety Tip*

Consultation with a HCP should occur before the procedure for radiation safety concerns regarding younger patients or patients who are lactating.

PEDIATRIC CONSIDERATIONS

Information on the Image Gently Campaign can be found at the Alliance for Radiation Safety in Pediatric Imaging (www.pedrad.org/associations/5364/ig/). Risks associated with radiation overexposure can result from frequent x-ray procedures. Personnel in the examination room with the patient should wear a protective lead apron, stand behind a shield, or leave the area while the examination is being done. Personnel working in the examination area should wear badges to record their level of radiation exposure.

Implementation

Note that patient education is key to obtaining the patient's cooperation in following directions, and providing an explanation for the purpose of the procedure is an important part of this process. Inform the patient that this study can assist in assessing for abnormalities of the carotid artery. Ensure that the patient has complied with dietary, fluid, and medication restrictions and pretesting preparations. Instruct the patient to void prior to the procedure and to change into the gown, robe, and foot coverings provided. If the patient has a history of allergic reactions to any substance or drug, administer ordered prophylactic steroids or antihistamines before the procedure. Remind the patient to remain still throughout the procedure because movement produces unreliable results. Have emergency equipment readily available. Place electrocardiographic electrodes on the patient for cardiac monitoring. Establish a baseline rhythm; determine if the patient has ventricular dysrhythmias. Using a pen, mark the site of the patient's peripheral pulses before angiography; this allows for quicker and more consistent assessment of the pulses after the procedure. Place the patient in the supine position on an examination table. Cleanse the selected area and cover with a sterile drape. A local anesthetic is injected at the site, and a small incision is made or a needle is inserted under fluoroscopy. The contrast medium is injected, and a rapid series of images is taken during and after the filling of the vessels to be examined. Delayed images may be taken to examine the vessels after a time and to monitor the venous phase of the procedure. Instruct the patient to inhale deeply and hold his or her breath while the images are taken, and then to exhale after the images are taken. Instruct the patient to take slow, deep breaths if nausea occurs during the procedure.

Monitor the patient for complications related to the procedure (e.g., allergic reaction, anaphylaxis, bronchospasm). The needle or catheter is removed, and a pressure dressing is applied over the puncture site. Observe/assess the needle/catheter insertion site for bleeding, inflammation, or hematoma formation.

Evaluation

Recognize anxiety related to test results, and be supportive of a perceived loss of independence. Instruct the patient to resume usual diet, fluids, medications, or activity as directed by the HCP. Renal function should be assessed before metformin is resumed. Monitor vital signs and neurological status every 15 minutes for 1 hour, then every 2 hours for 4 hours, and as ordered. Take the patient's temperature every 4 hours for 24 hours. Monitor intake and output at least every 8 hours. Compare all of these with baseline values. Protocols may vary from facility to facility. Observe for delayed allergic reactions, such as rash, urticaria, tachycardia, hyperpnea, hypertension, palpitations, nausea, or vomiting. Patient care after all angiographic studies is relatively uniform to prevent circulatory deficit, thrombus formation, or hemorrhage. Assess extremities for signs of ischemia or the absence of a distal pulse caused by a catheter-induced thrombus. Instruct the patient to immediately report symptoms such as a fast heart rate, difficulty breathing, skin rash, itching, chest pain, persistent right shoulder pain, or abdominal pain. Immediately report symptoms to the appropriate HCP.

Observe/assess the needle/catheter insertion site for bleeding, inflammation, or hematoma formation. Instruct the patient in the care and assessment of the site and explain that cold compresses can be applied to the puncture site as needed, to reduce discomfort or edema. Instruct the patient to maintain bedrest for 4 to 6 hours after the procedure or as ordered. Discuss the implications of abnormal test results on the patient's lifestyle. Provide teaching and information regarding the clinical implications of an abnormal study as appropriate. Instruct the patient in the use of any ordered medications. Explain the importance of adhering to the therapy regimen. As appropriate, instruct the patient about significant side effects and systemic reactions associated with the prescribed medication. Encourage him or her to review corresponding literature provided by a pharmacist. Answer any questions or address any concerns voiced by the patient or family. Educate the patient regarding access to counseling services and provide contact information, if desired. Information on carotid artery stenosis may be found at www.mayoclinic.com/health/carotid-artery-disease/DS01030.

✅ Critical Findings

N/A

✅ Study Specific Complications

Establishing an IV site and injection of contrast medium by catheter are invasive procedures. Complications are rare but do include risk for the following:

- Acute kidney injury can result from contrast infusion, *especially in dehydrated patients; hydration prior to the study can reduce the likelihood of this complication.*
- Acidosis or hypoglycemia *can occur in patients taking metformin who receive iodinated contrast; metformin should be withheld for 48 hours prior to the study.*
- Bleeding from the puncture site may occur *related to a bleeding disorder, or the effects of natural products and medications known to act as blood thinners; postprocedural bleeding from the site is rare because at the conclusion of the procedure a resorbable device, composed of non-latex-containing arterial anchor, collagen plug, and suture, is deployed to seal the puncture site.*
- Blood clots may form *related to thrombus formation on the tip of the catheter sheath surface or in the lumen of the catheter; the use of a heparinized saline flush during the procedure decreases the risk of emboli.*
- Hematoma may be seen *related to blood leakage into the tissue following needle insertion.*
- Infection *might occur if bacteria from the skin surface is introduced at the puncture site.*

- Tissue damage may occur *related to extravasation of the contrast during injection; the severity can range from a localized inflammatory reaction to more severe developments such as compartment syndrome or the formation of ulcers.*
- Nerve injury or damage to a nearby organ *might occur if the catheter strikes a nerve or perforates an organ.*

Instruct the patient to look for excessive bleeding, redness of skin, fever, or chills, and to notify her or his HCP if these symptoms occur. Antibiotic therapy should be ordered if puncture-site-related infection occurs. Elevated temperatures, abnormal-colored sputum, changes in breathing patterns, chills, and hypotension can all indicate infection or sepsis.

Injection of the contrast through a catheter into a blood vessel is an invasive procedure. Complications are rare but do include risk for allergic reaction *related to contrast reaction.* It is important to have oxygen and endotracheal equipment in the vicinity for immediate use. In the event of an anaphylactic reaction, epinephrine, diphenhydramine, and steroids are included with resuscitative efforts.

Contrast Reactions Signs, Symptoms, and Treatment

	Minor	Intermediate	Life Threatening
Signs, symptoms	Nausea, vomiting, urticaria, sneezing	Bronchospasms; chills and fever; chest pain, laryngeal or tongue edema	Hypotension, cardiac dysrhythmias; seizures; loss of bowel/bladder control; laryngeal and pulmonary edema
Interventions	Antihistamines	Antihistamines, steroids, bronchodilators, IV fluids, and observation	All intermediate interventions plus intubation and ventilation, pressors and antiseizure medications

🕒 Related Tests

- Related tests include angiography abdomen, BUN, CT angiography, CT brain, creatinine, ECG, exercise stress test, MRA, MRI brain, PT/INR, plethysmography, US arterial Doppler lower extremities, and US peripheral Doppler.
- See the Cardiovascular System table at the end of the book for related tests by body system.

Expected Outcomes

Expected outcomes associated with Angiography, Carotid, are

- No dizziness reported
- No neurological deficits noted on assessment
- An understanding verbalized of the signs and symptoms that should be reported to the HCP

Angiography, Coronary

Quick Summary

SYNONYM ACRONYM: Angiography of heart, angiocardiography, cardiac angiography, cardiac catheterization, cineangiocardiography, coronary angiography, coronary arteriography.

COMMON USE: To visualize and assess the heart and surrounding structure for abnormalities, defects, aneurysm, and tumors.

AREA OF APPLICATION: Heart.

NORMAL FINDINGS

- Normal great vessels and coronary arteries

Normal Adult Hemodynamic Pressures and Volumes Monitored During Coronary Angiography (Cardiac Catheterization)

Pressures	Description of What Measured Parameter Represents	Normal Value
Arterial blood pressure (also known as routine blood pressure)	The pressure in the brachial artery; one of the significant vital signs; reflects the pressure the heart exerts to pump blood through the circulatory system	Systolic (100–140) mm Hg/ diastolic (60–90) mm Hg
Mean arterial pressure	The average arterial pressure of one cardiac cycle; considered a better indicator of perfusion than routine blood pressure but only obtainable by direct measurement during cardiac catheterization	70–105 mm Hg
Left ventricular pressures	Peak pressure in the left ventricle during systole/peak pressure in the left ventricle at the end of diastole; indication of contractility of the heart muscle	Systolic (90–140) mm Hg/ diastolic (4–12) mm Hg
Central venous pressure (right atrial pressure)	The right-sided ventricular pressures exerted by the central veins closest to the heart (jugular, subclavian, or femoral); used to estimate blood volume and venous return	2–6 mm Hg
Pulmonary artery pressure	The pressures in the pulmonary artery	Systolic (15–30) mm Hg/ diastolic (4–12) mm Hg
Pulmonary artery wedge pressure	The pressure in the pulmonary vessels; used to provide an estimate of left atrial filling pressure, to provide an estimate of left ventricle pressure during end diastole, and a way to measure ventricular preload	4–12 mm Hg
Volumes: Cardiac output	The amount of blood pumped out by the ventricle of the heart in 1 minute	4–8 L/min
Cardiac index	The cardiac output adjusted for body surface to provide the index which is a more precise measurement; used to assess the function of the ventricle	2.5–4 L/min/m²
Arterial oxygen saturation	Concentration of oxygen in the blood	95%–100%
Stroke volume	The amount of blood pumped by each ventricle with each time it contracts in a heartbeat	60–100 mL/beat
Stroke volume index	The stroke volume adjusted for body surface to provide the index which is a more precise measurement	33–57 mL/m²
End diastolic volume (EDV)	The amount of blood in the left ventricle at the end of diastole	100–160 mL
EDV index	EDV adjusted for body surface to provide the index which is a more precise measurement	50–80 mL/m²
End systolic volume (ESV)	The amount of blood in the left ventricle at the end of systole	50–100 mL
ESV index	ESV adjusted for body surface to provide the index which is a more precise measurement	25–50 mL/m²
Ejection fraction	Stroke volume expressed as a percentage of end diastolic volume	55–70%

Test Explanation

Angiography allows x-ray visualization of the heart, aorta, inferior vena cava, pulmonary artery and vein, and coronary arteries after injection of contrast medium. Contrast medium is injected through a catheter, which has been inserted into a peripheral vein, usually the femoral or brachial vein, for a right heart catheterization or into an artery, usually the femoral or brachial artery, for a left heart catheterization; through the same catheter cardiac pressures and volumes are recorded. Fluoroscopy is used to guide catheter placement, and angiograms (high-speed x-ray images) provide images of the heart and associated vessels which are displayed on a monitor and are recorded for future viewing and evaluation. Digital subtraction angiography (DSA) is a computerized method of removing undesired structures, like bone, from the surrounding area of interest. A digital image is taken prior to injection of the contrast and then again after the contrast has been injected. By subtracting the preinjection image from the postinjection image, a higher-quality, unobstructed image can be created. Patterns of circulation, cardiac output, cardiac functions, and changes in vessel wall appearance can be viewed to help diagnose the presence of vascular abnormalities or lesions. Pulmonary artery abnormalities are seen with right heart views, and coronary artery and thoracic aorta abnormalities are seen with left heart views. Coronary angiography is useful for evaluating cardiovascular disease and various types of cardiac abnormalities.

Coronary angiography, more commonly called cardiac catheterization, is a definitive test for coronary artery disease (CAD). CAD is a condition where the blood vessels to the heart lose their elasticity and become narrowed by atherosclerotic deposits of plaque. Significant blockage is treatable using coronary artery bypass grafting (CABG) surgery. Cardiac catheterization can also be used in conjunction with less invasive interventional alternatives to CABG surgery such as percutaneous transluminal coronary angioplasty (PTCA), with or without placement of stents. PTCA is also known as balloon angioplasty because once the blockage is identified and determined to be treatable, a balloon catheter is used to help correct the problem. The balloon in the catheter is inflated to compress the plaque against the sides of the affected vessel. The balloon may be inflated multiple times and with increasing size to increase the diameter of the vessel's lumen which restores more normal blood flow. A stent, which is a small mesh tube, may be placed in the affected vessel to keep it open after the angioplasty is completed.

Carotid endarterectomy (CEA) is another procedure that can be combined with coronary angiography and may also be part of the PTCA procedure. CEA is performed to reduce stroke risk. Stroke results from severe stenosis of the carotid arteries and release of plaque emboli that travel to the brain, block circulation, and cause brain tissue death. The CEA procedure involves insertion of an additional, separate catheter to insert a device that removes plaque from the walls of the carotid arteries. The devices commonly used to perform CEA employ very small drills or rotating blades to remove the plaque. Balloon angioplasty, with or without stent placement, usually follows CEA.

Applications of Cardiac Catheterization for Infants and Pediatric Patients

Cardiac catheterization is very useful in identification of the type of heart defect, determination of the exact location of the defect, and indications regarding the severity of the defect. Some of the common operable heart defects in infants and children include repairs for ventricular septal defects, atrial septal defects, tetrology of Fallot, valve defects, and arterial switches. Cardiac catheterization can also be used as a palliative procedure prior to arterial switch repair. The catheterization, called a balloon atrial septostomy, is used to create a small hole in the inner wall of the heart between the atria that allows a greater volume of oxygenated blood to enter the circulatory system. The improved quality of circulating blood provides some time for very young patients to gain strength prior to the surgical repair. The hole is closed when the corrective surgery is completed.

Nursing Implications
Assessment

Indications	Potential Nursing Problems
Allow infusion of thrombolytic drugs into an occluded coronary	• Bleeding
Detect narrowing of coronary vessels or abnormalities of the great vessels in patients with angina, syncope, abnormal electrocardiogram, hypercholesteremia with chest pain, and persistent chest pain after revascularization	• Cardiac Output • Disrupted Sleep • Fall Risk • Family • Human Response • Infection • Mobility
Evaluate cardiac muscle function	• Nutrition
Evaluate cardiac valvular and septal defects	• Pain
Evaluate disease associated with the aortic arch	• Role Performance
Evaluate previous cardiac surgery or other interventional procedures	• Self-esteem • Skin
Evaluate peripheral arterial disease (PAD)	• Tissue Perfusion
Evaluate peripheral vascular disease (PVD)	
Evaluate ventricular aneurysms	
Monitor pulmonary pressures and cardiac output	
Perform angioplasty, perform atherectomy, or place a stent	
Quantify the severity of atherosclerotic, occlusive coronary artery disease	

Diagnosis: Clinical Significance of Test Results
ABNORMAL FINDINGS
- Aortic atherosclerosis
- Aortic dissection
- Aortitis
- Aneurysms
- Cardiomyopathy
- Congenital anomalies
- Coronary artery atherosclerosis and degree of obstruction
- Graft occlusion

- PAD
- PVD
- Pulmonary artery abnormalities
- Septal defects
- Trauma causing tears or other disruption
- Tumors
- Valvular disease

Planning

Considerations for planning a successful partnership should include clear communication of what to expect during the test to decrease anxiety and improve cooperation. Before the procedure is performed, plan to review the steps with the patient. Ensure that the results of coagulation testing are obtained and recorded prior to the procedure; BUN and creatinine results are also needed if contrast medium is used. Note any recent procedures that can interfere with test results, including examinations using barium- or iodine-based contrast medium. Ensure that barium studies were performed more than 4 days before the CT scan. Record the date of the last menstrual period, and determine the possibility of pregnancy in perimenopausal women. Explain that there may be moments of discomfort and some pain experienced during the test, and inform the patient that the procedure is usually performed in a radiology or vascular suite by a health-care provider (HCP) and takes approximately 30 to 60 minutes. Remind the patient that she or he should remain still during the procedure, and instruct the patient to remove all metal in the area to be examined. The patient should fast and restrict fluids for 2 to 4 hours prior to the procedure. Protocols may vary among facilities. Instruct the patient to avoid taking anticoagulant medication or to reduce dosage as ordered prior to the procedure. Inquire about previous allergies and contrast reactions. If iodinated contrast medium is scheduled to be used in patients receiving metformin (Glucophage) for type 2 diabetes, the drug should be discontinued on the day of the test and continue to be withheld for 48 hours after the test. Iodinated contrast can temporarily impair kidney function, and failure to withhold metformin may indirectly result in drug-induced lactic acidosis, a dangerous and sometimes fatal side effect of metformin *related to renal impairment that does not support sufficient excretion of metformin.* Patients with known pheochromocytoma should receive a beta-adrenergic blocker such as propranolol and an alpha-adrenergic blocker such as phenoxybenzamine for several days prior to the study to help prevent a malignant hypertensive episode. Explain that an IV line may be inserted to allow infusion of IV fluids (e.g., normal saline), anesthetics, or sedatives. Explain that the contrast medium will be injected, by catheter, at a separate site from the IV line. Inform the patient that she or he may experience nausea, a feeling of warmth, a flushed sensation, a salty or metallic taste, or notice a transient headache if contrast is used and that these reactions are considered normal.

CONTRAINDICATIONS

- Patients who are pregnant or suspected of being pregnant, unless the potential benefits of a procedure using radiation far outweigh the risk of radiation exposure to the fetus and mother
- Conditions associated with adverse reactions to contrast medium (e.g., asthma, food allergies, or allergy to contrast medium)

  Although patients are still asked specifically if they have a known allergy to iodine or shellfish, it has been well established that the reaction is not to iodine; in fact, an actual iodine allergy would be very problematic because iodine is required for the production of thyroid hormones. In the case of shellfish, the reaction is to a muscle protein called *tropomyosin*; in the case of iodinated contrast medium, the reaction is to the noniodinated part of the contrast molecule. Patients with a known hypersensitivity to the medium may benefit from premedication with corticosteroids and diphenhydramine; the use of nonionic contrast or an alternative noncontrast imaging study, if available, may be considered for patients who have severe asthma or who have experienced moderate to severe reactions to ionic contrast medium.
- Conditions associated with preexisting renal insufficiency (e.g., chronic kidney disease, single kidney transplant, nephrectomy, diabetes, multiple myeloma, treatment with aminoglycosides and NSAIDs) *because iodinated contrast is nephrotoxic*
- Older adult and compromised patients who are chronically dehydrated before the test *because of their risk of contrast-induced acute kidney injury*
- Patients with pheochromocytoma *because iodinated contrast may cause a hypertensive crisis*
- Patients with bleeding disorders who receive an arterial or venous puncture (angiography) *because the site may not stop bleeding*
- The occurrence of chest pain, severe cardiac dysrhythmias, or signs of a cerebrovascular accident, which may require terminating the procedure

SPECIAL CONSIDERATIONS

An important aspect of planning is understanding the factors that may alter study findings or cause abnormal results. Interdepartmental communication is a key factor in the planning process. The following should be noted when planning for this study:

- Large amounts of bowel gas can distort abdominal organ visualization.
- The patient may be unable to cooperate or remain still during the procedure because of age, significant

pain, or mental status; uncooperative patients, including children, may need sedation as motion causes artifacts on the image.

- Residual barium from previous studies blocks the transmission of x-rays.
- Metallic objects within the examination field (e.g., jewelry, body rings) may inhibit organ visualization and cause unclear images.
- Failure to follow dietary restrictions and other pretesting preparations may cause the procedure to be canceled or repeated.

● Safety Tip

Consultation with a HCP should occur before the procedure for radiation safety concerns regarding younger patients or patients who are lactating.

PEDIATRIC CONSIDERATIONS

Information on the Image Gently Campaign can be found at the Alliance for Radiation Safety in Pediatric Imaging (www.pedrad.org/associations/5364/ig/). Risks associated with radiation overexposure can result from frequent x-ray procedures. Personnel in the examination room with the patient should wear a protective lead apron, stand behind a shield, or leave the area while the examination is being done. Personnel working in the examination area should wear badges to record their level of radiation exposure.

● Safety Tip

Make sure a written and informed consent has been signed prior to the procedure if a biopsy is planned and before administering any medications.

Implementation

Patient education is an important part of this process, and providing an explanation for the purpose of the arteriogram is important. Inform the patient that this study can assist in assessing for abnormalities of the heart. Ensure that the patient has complied with dietary, fluid, and medication restrictions and pretesting preparations. Instruct the patient to void prior to the procedure and to change into the gown, robe, and foot coverings provided. If the patient has a history of allergic reactions to any substance or drug, administer ordered prophylactic steroids or antihistamines before the procedure. Remind the patient to remain still throughout the procedure because movement produces unreliable results. Have emergency equipment readily available. Place electrocardiographic electrodes on the patient for cardiac monitoring. Establish a baseline rhythm; determine if the patient has ventricular dysrhythmias. Nitroglycerin may be given to reduce or

eliminate catheter-induced spasms, or to measure its effect on the coronary arteries. Using a pen, mark the site of the patient's peripheral pulses before angiography; this allows for quicker and more consistent assessment of the pulses after the procedure. Place the patient in the supine position on an examination table. Cleanse the selected area, and cover with a sterile drape. A local anesthetic is injected at the site, and a small incision is made or a needle is inserted under fluoroscopy. The contrast medium is injected, and a rapid series of images is taken during and after the filling of the vessels to be examined (see Fig. 15.4). Delayed images may be taken to examine the vessels after a time and to monitor the venous phase of the procedure. Blood is drawn from the cardiac chambers to measure oxygen levels during the procedure. Instruct the patient to inhale deeply and hold his or her breath while the images are taken, and then to exhale after the images are taken. Instruct the patient to take slow, deep breaths if nausea occurs during the procedure.

Monitor the patient for complications related to the procedure (e.g., allergic reaction, anaphylaxis, bronchospasm). The needle or catheter is removed, and a pressure dressing is applied over the puncture site. Observe/assess the needle/catheter insertion site for bleeding, inflammation, or hematoma formation.

Evaluation

Recognize anxiety related to test results and be supportive of a perceived loss of independence. Instruct the patient to resume usual diet, fluids, medications, or activity, as directed by the HCP. Renal function should be assessed before metformin is resumed. Monitor vital signs and neurological status every 15 minutes for 1 hour, then every 2 hours for 4 hours and as ordered. Take the patient's temperature every 4 hours

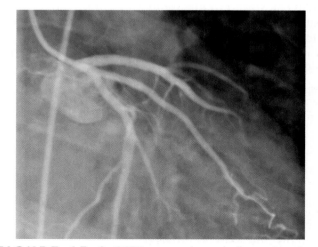

FIGURE 15.4 CCTA pre- and post balloon. *Used with permission, from Weber, E., Vilensky, J., & Fog, A. (2013). Practical radiology: A symptom-based approach. FA Davis Company.*

for 24 hours. Monitor intake and output at least every 8 hours. Compare all of these with baseline values. Protocols may vary from facility to facility. Observe for delayed allergic reactions, such as rash, urticaria, tachycardia, hyperpnea, hypertension, palpitations, nausea, or vomiting. Patient care after all angiographic studies is relatively uniform to prevent circulatory deficit, thrombus formation, or hemorrhage. Assess extremities for signs of ischemia or for the absence of a distal pulse caused by a catheter-induced thrombus. Instruct the patient to immediately report symptoms such as fast heart rate, difficulty breathing, skin rash, itching, chest pain, persistent right shoulder pain, or abdominal pain. Immediately report symptoms to the appropriate HCP.

Observe/assess the needle/catheter insertion site for bleeding, inflammation, or hematoma formation. Instruct the patient in the care and assessment of the site, and explain that cold compresses can be applied to the puncture site as needed to reduce discomfort or edema. Instruct the patient to maintain bedrest for 4 to 6 hours after the procedure or as ordered. Discuss the implications of abnormal test results on the patient's lifestyle. Provide teaching and information regarding the clinical implications of an abnormal study as appropriate. Coronary artery constriction is especially significant when greater than 70%. Common indications for surgery are narrowing of the left main coronary artery and occlusions or stenosis superiorly in the left anterior descending artery. Instruct the patient in the use of any ordered medications. Explain the importance of adhering to the therapy regimen. As appropriate, instruct the patient in significant side effects and systemic reactions associated with the prescribed medication. Encourage him or her to review corresponding literature provided by a pharmacist. Answer any questions or address any concerns voiced by the patient or family. Educate the patient regarding access to counseling services and provide contact information, if desired. Information on coronary artery disease may be found at www.nhlbi.nih.gov/health/health-topics/topics/cad/.

SPECIAL CONSIDERATIONS

Numerous studies point to the prevalence of excess body weight in American children and adolescents. Experts estimate that obesity is present in 25% of the population ages 6 to 11 years. The medical, social, and emotional consequences of excess body weight are significant. Special attention should be given to instructing the child and caregiver regarding health risks and weight-control education.

NUTRITIONAL CONSIDERATIONS FOR THE CARDIAC PATIENT: An abnormal coronary angiogram may be associated with CAD. Nutritional therapy is recommended for the patient identified to be at risk for developing CAD or for individuals who have specific risk factors and/or existing medical conditions (e.g., elevated LDL cholesterol levels, other lipid disorders, type 1 diabetes, type 2 diabetes, insulin resistance, or metabolic syndrome). Other changeable risk factors warranting patient education include strategies to encourage patients, especially those who are overweight and with high blood pressure, to safely decrease sodium intake, achieve a normal weight, ensure regular participation of moderate aerobic physical activity three to four times per week, eliminate tobacco use, and adhere to a heart-healthy diet. If triglycerides also are elevated, the patient should be advised to eliminate or reduce alcohol. A variety of dietary patterns are beneficial for people with CAD and there are many meal-planning approaches with nutritional goals endorsed by the American Diabetes Association (ADA). The Guideline on Lifestyle Management to Reduce Cardiovascular Risk published by the American College of Cardiology (ACC) and the American Heart Association (AHA) in conjunction with the National Heart, Lung, and Blood Institute (NHLBI) recommends a "Mediterranean"-style diet rather than a low-fat diet. The guideline emphasizes inclusion of vegetables, whole grains, fruits, low-fat dairy, nuts, legumes, and nontropical vegetable oils (e.g., olive, canola, peanut, sunflower, flaxseed) along with fish and lean poultry. A similar dietary pattern known as the Dietary Approaches to Stop Hypertension (DASH) diet makes additional recommendations for the reduction of dietary sodium. Both dietary styles emphasize a reduction in consumption of red meats, which are high in saturated fats and cholesterol, and other foods containing sugar, saturated fats, trans fats, and sodium. The ADA also includes a vegetarian diet as well as other potential weight loss diets such as Weight Watchers. The nutritional needs of each patient need to be determined individually (especially during pregnancy) with the appropriate health-care providers (HCPs), particularly professionals educated in nutrition.

✅ *Critical Findings*

- Aneurysm
- Aortic dissection

Note and immediately report to the requesting HCP any critical findings and related symptoms. A listing of these findings varies among facilities.

✅ *Study Specific Complications*

Establishing an IV site and the injection of contrast medium by catheter are invasive procedures. Complications are rare but do include risk for the following:

- Cardiac dysrhythmias, perforation of the myocardium of the heart, and arterial embolism from the dislodgement of arteriosclerotic plaque *may cause a stroke or an MI.*
- Acute kidney injury can result from contrast infusion, *especially in dehydrated patients; hydration prior to the study can reduce the likelihood of this complication.*
- Acidosis or hypoglycemia *can occur in patients taking metformin who receive iodinated contrast; metformin should be withheld for 48 hours prior to the study.*
- Bleeding from the puncture site may occur *related to a bleeding disorder, or the effects of natural products and medications known to act as blood thinners; postprocedural bleeding from the site is rare because at the conclusion of the procedure a resorbable device, composed of non-latex-containing arterial anchor, collagen plug, and suture, is deployed to seal the puncture site.*
- A blood clot may form *related to thrombus formation on the tip of the catheter sheath surface or in the lumen of the catheter; the use of a heparinized saline flush during the procedure decreases the risk of emboli.*
- A hematoma may form *related to blood leakage into the tissue following needle insertion.*

- Infection *might occur if bacteria from the skin surface is introduced at the puncture site.*
- Tissue damage may occur *related to extravasation of the contrast during injection; the severity can range from a localized inflammatory reaction to more severe developments such as compartment syndrome or the formation of ulcers.*
- Nerve injury or damage to a nearby organ *might occur if the catheter strikes a nerve or perforates an organ.*

Instruct the patient to look for excessive bleeding, redness of skin, fever, or chills, and to notify his or her HCP if these symptoms occur. Antibiotic therapy should be ordered if puncture-site-related infection occurs. Elevated temperatures, abnormal-colored sputum, changes in breathing patterns, chills, and hypotension can all indicate infection or sepsis.

Injection of the contrast through a catheter into a blood vessel is an invasive procedure. Complications are rare but do include risk for allergic reaction *related to contrast reaction.* It is important to have oxygen and endotracheal equipment in the vicinity for immediate use. In the event of an anaphylactic reaction, epinephrine, diphenhydramine, and steroids are included with resuscitative efforts.

Contrast Reactions Signs, Symptoms, and Treatment

	Minor	Intermediate	Life Threatening
Signs, symptoms	Nausea, vomiting, urticaria, sneezing	Bronchospasms; chills and fever; chest pain, laryngeal or tongue edema	Hypotension, cardiac dysrhythmias; seizures; loss of bowel/bladder control; laryngeal and pulmonary edema
Interventions	Antihistamines	Antihistamines, steroids, bronchodilators, IV fluids, and observation	All intermediate interventions plus intubation and ventilation, pressors, and antiseizure medications

Related Tests

- Related tests include angiography carotid, blood pool imaging, BNP, BUN, chest x-ray, cholesterol HDL and LDL, cholesterol total, CT abdomen, CT angiography, CT biliary tract and liver, CT cardiac scoring, CT spleen, CT thoracic, CK, creatinine, CRP, electrocardiography, electrocardiography transesophageal, Holter monitor, homocysteine, lipoprotein electrophoresis, MR angiography, MRI abdomen, MRI chest, myocardial perfusion heart scan, plethysmography, aPTT, PT/INR, triglycerides, troponin, and US arterial Doppler carotid.

- Refer to the Cardiovascular System table at the end of the book for related tests by body system.

Expected Outcomes

Expected outcomes associated with Angiography, Coronary, are

- Having adequate pedal pulses that are palpable bilaterally
- Understanding that the risk for infection is increased with reduced peripheral perfusion
- Adhering to the recommend diet to support cardiac health

Barium Swallow

Quick Summary

SYNONYM ACRONYM: Esophagram, video swallow, esophagus x-ray, swallowing function, esophagraphy.

COMMON USE: To assist in diagnosing disease of the esophagus such as stricture or tumor.

AREA OF APPLICATION: Esophagus.

NORMAL FINDINGS

- Normal peristalsis through the esophagus into the stomach with normal size, filling, patency, and shape of the esophagus

Test Explanation

This radiological examination of the esophagus evaluates motion and anatomic structures of the esophageal lumen by recording images of the lumen while the patient swallows a barium solution of milkshake consistency and a chalky taste. The procedure is a dynamic study and uses fluoroscopic and cineradiographic techniques. A dynamic study is one in which there is continuous monitoring of the motion being studied as opposed to a static study in which the patient and equipment are held in one position until the image has been taken. The barium swallow is often performed as part of an upper gastrointestinal (GI) series or cardiac series and is indicated for patients with a history of dysphagia and gastric reflux. The standard barium swallow study focuses on the esophageal structures of the GI tract and may identify reflux of the barium from the stomach back into the esophagus. Muscular abnormalities such as achalasia, as well as diffuse esophageal spasm, can be easily detected with this procedure. Gastroesophageal reflux disease (GERD) is a disorder of the GI system commonly seen in older adults. Because of the physiological changes associated with the aging process, numerous factors come into play that negatively impact quality of life and contribute to the development of significant complications in older adult patients as a result of GERD.

The **modified barium swallow** focuses on the oropharyngeal structures and is also used to evaluate dysphagia, or difficulty swallowing. The test may be performed and observed in the presence of a radiologist and radiology technician with or without a feeding specialist or speech pathologist depending on the reason for the examination. Nurses will encounter patients who struggle with swallowing disorders in different settings such as intensive care units, nurseries, rehabilitative units, or skilled nursing units. Situations that might indicate a modified barium swallow include the evaluation of a patient's ability to swallow food after a stroke or the inability of a child to swallow food of varying consistencies without gagging and choking during feeding.

Nursing Implications

Assessment

Indications	Potential Nursing Problems
Confirm the integrity of esophageal anastomoses in the postoperative patient	- Breathing
Detect esophageal reflux, tracheoesophageal fistulas, and varices	- Bleeding
	- Fluid Volume
	- Grief
Determine the cause of dysphagia or heartburn	- Human Response
Determine the type and location of foreign bodies within the pharynx and esophagus	- Infection
	- Nutrition
Evaluate suspected esophageal motility disorders	- Pain
Evaluate suspected polyps, strictures, Zenker diverticula, tumor, or inflammation	

Diagnosis: Clinical Significance of Test Results

ABNORMAL FINDINGS

- Achalasia
- Acute or chronic esophagitis
- Benign or malignant tumors
- Chalasia
- Congenital diaphragmatic hernia
- Diverticula
- Dysphagia with or without pain *related to constrictions, arteria lusoria, paralysis, muscle spasms, etc.*
- Esophageal motility issues *related to other conditions like scleroderma or advancing age*
- Esophageal ulcers
- Esophageal varices
- Gastroesophageal reflux disease
- Hiatal hernia
- Perforation of the esophagus
- Strictures or polyps

Planning

Considerations for planning a successful partnership should include clear communication of what to expect during the barium swallow to decrease anxiety and improve cooperation. Ensure that this procedure is performed before an upper GI study or video swallow. Before the procedure is performed, plan to review the steps with the patient. Explain that minimal discomfort may be experienced during the exam and inform the patient that the procedure is performed in a special room by a radiologist and/or a speech pathologist, and takes approximately 15 to 30 minutes. Explain that the patient will be required to drink a glass of barium used to coat the esophagus. The amount of the barium will vary depending on how rapidly it flows through the esophagus. If iodinated contrast medium (e.g., Gastrografin) is scheduled to be used in patients receiving metformin (Glucophage) for type 2 diabetes, the drug should be discontinued on the day of the test and continue to be withheld for 48 hours after the test. Iodinated contrast can temporarily impair kidney function, and failure to withhold metformin may indirectly result in drug-induced lactic acidosis, a dangerous and sometimes fatal side effect of metformin **related to renal impairment that does not support sufficient excretion of metformin.** Instruct the patient to fast and restrict fluids for 8 hours prior to the procedure. Protocols may vary among facilities.

PEDIATRIC CONSIDERATIONS

The fasting period prior to the time of the examination depends upon the child's age. General guidelines are the following: birth to 6 months: 3 hours; 7 months to 2 years: 4 hours; and 3 years and older: 6 hours.

CONTRAINDICATIONS

- Patients who are pregnant or suspected of being pregnant, unless the potential benefits of a procedure using radiation far outweigh the risk of radiation exposure to the fetus and mother
- Patients who are unable to cooperate by swallowing upon request
- Patients with an obstruction, ulcer, or suspected esophageal rupture, unless water-soluble iodinated contrast medium, such as Gastrografin, is used
- Conditions associated with adverse reactions to the contrast medium (e.g., asthma, food allergies, or allergy to the contrast medium). Although patients are still asked specifically if they have a known allergy to iodine or shellfish, it has been well established that the reaction is not to iodine' in fact, an actual iodine allergy would be very problematic because iodine is required for the production of thyroid hormones. In the case of shellfish, the reaction is to a muscle protein called *tropomyosin*; in the case of iodinated contrast medium, the reaction is to the noniodinated part of the contrast molecule. Patients with a known hypersensitivity to the medium may benefit from premedication with corticosteroids and diphenhydramine; the use of nonionic contrast or an alternative noncontrast imaging study, if available, may be considered for patients who have severe asthma or who have experienced moderate to severe reactions to ionic contrast medium.
- Patients with severe constipation or bowel obstruction as barium may make the condition worse
- Patients with a severe swallowing disorder **to the extent that aspiration might occur**
- Patients with suspected tracheoesophageal fistula, unless barium is used

SPECIAL CONSIDERATIONS

An important aspect of planning is understanding the factors that may alter study findings or cause abnormal results. Interdepartmental communication is a key factor in the planning process. The following should be noted when planning for this study:

- The procedure should be done after cholangiography and barium enema.
- The patient may be unable to cooperate or remain still during the procedure because of age, significant pain, or mental status; uncooperative patients, including children, may need sedation as motion causes artifacts on the image.
- Metallic objects within the examination field (e.g., jewelry, body rings) may inhibit organ visualization and cause unclear images.
- Failure to follow dietary restrictions and other pretesting preparations may cause the procedure to be canceled or repeated.

● *Safety Tip*

Consultation with a health-care provider (HCP) should occur before the procedure for radiation safety concerns regarding younger patients or patients who are lactating.

PEDIATRIC CONSIDERATIONS

Information on the Image Gently Campaign can be found at the Alliance for Radiation Safety in Pediatric Imaging (www.pedrad.org/associations/5364/ig/). Risks associated with radiation overexposure can result from frequent x-ray procedures. Personnel in the examination room with the patient should wear a protective lead apron, stand behind a shield, or leave the area while the examination is being done. Personnel working in the examination area should wear badges to record their level of radiation exposure.

Implementation

Patient education is an important part of this process, and providing an explanation for the purpose of the barium swallow is important. Inform the patient that this study can assist in assessing for abnormalities of the esophagus and swallowing function. Remind the patient that he or she may experience some nausea when drinking the barium, and instruct the patient to drink as instructed by the radiologist. Ensure the patient has complied with dietary and fluid restrictions for 8 hours prior to the procedure.

Place the patient erect in front of the x-ray table. The patient is provided a glass of barium with (or without) a straw and instructed to take swallows as the radiologist observes with fluoroscopy. The patient may be asked to turn his or her body in oblique and lateral positions and repeat the swallow.

If assessing for swallowing ability following a stroke, mix a small amount of barium with applesauce and ask the patient to swallow. This will be observed with fluoroscopy. If no aspiration is seen, the patient may be asked to chew and swallow some crumbled cookie mixed with barium for observation (see Fig. 15.5).

Evaluation

Recognize anxiety related to test results and be supportive of a perceived loss of independence. Instruct the patient to resume his or her usual diet, medications, and activity as directed by the HCP. Instruct the patient to increase hydration (four 8-ounce glasses) to avoid dehydration and flush the barium from the intestinal tract. Carefully monitor the patient for fatigue and fluid and electrolyte imbalance.

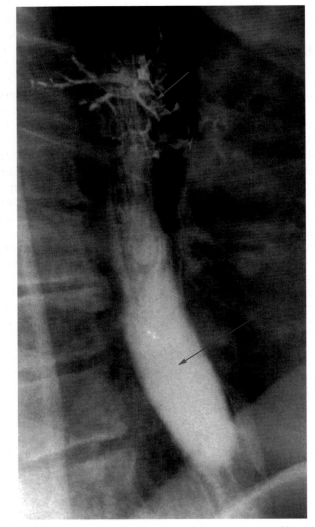

FIGURE 15.5 Esophagram showing aspirated barium. *Used with permission, from Weber, E., Vilensky, J., & Fog, A. (2013). Practical radiology: A symptom-based approach. FA Davis Company.*

PEDIATRIC CONSIDERATIONS

Instruct the parents of pediatric patients to hydrate the child with electrolyte fluid post barium swallow. Inform the patient that his or her stool will be chalky and light-colored initially but should return to normal color within 3 days.

OLDER ADULT CONSIDERATIONS

Chronic dehydration can also result in frequent bouts of constipation. Therefore, after the procedure, older adult patients should be encouraged to use a mild laxative daily until the stool is back to normal color. If the patient is unable to eliminate the barium or if stools do not return to normal color, the patient should notify the requesting HCP.

Discuss the implications of abnormal test results on the patient's lifestyle. Provide teaching and information regarding the clinical implications of an abnormal study as appropriate. Recommendations may be specific swallowing treatments (e.g., exercises to improve muscle movement, practicing positions for eating that improve the patient's ability to swallow) or specific recommendations for food and liquid textures that are easier and safer to swallow. Answer any questions or address any concerns voiced by the patient or family. Educate the patient regarding access to counseling services and provide contact information, if desired. Information on swallowing disorders (dysphagia) in adults may be found at www.asha.org/public/speech/swallowing/Swallowing-Disorders-in-Adults/.

✅ Critical Findings

N/A

✅ Study Specific Complications

While complications are rare, they may include allergic reaction **related to contrast reaction,** constipation, impaction, or bowel obstruction **related to retained barium,** and aspiration of barium **related to extreme swallowing disorders.**

✅ Related Tests

- Related tests include capsule endoscopy, chest x-ray, CT thoracic, endoscopy, esophageal manometry, gastroesophageal reflux scan, MRI chest, and thyroid scan.
- Refer to the Gastrointestinal System table at the end of the book for related tests by body system.

Expected Outcomes

Expected outcomes associated with Barium Swallow are

- Expressing concerns about the diagnosis and a possible loss of life
- Being an active partner in the decision making regarding the treatment plan

- Adapting dietary selections to the ability to swallow safely

Cholangiography, Percutaneous Transhepatic

Quick Summary

SYNONYM ACRONYM: Percutaneous cholecystogram, PTC, PTHC.

COMMON USE: To visualize and assess biliary ducts for causes of obstruction and jaundice, such as cancer or stones.

AREA OF APPLICATION: Biliary system.

NORMAL FINDINGS

- Biliary ducts are normal in diameter, with no evidence of dilation, filling defects, duct narrowing, or extravasation.
- Contrast medium fills the ducts and flows freely.
- Gallbladder appears normal in size and shape.

Test Explanation

Percutaneous transhepatic cholangiography (PTC) is a test used to visualize the biliary system in order to evaluate persistent upper abdominal pain after cholecystectomy and to determine the presence and cause of obstructive jaundice. The liver is punctured with a thin needle under fluoroscopic guidance, and contrast medium is injected as the needle is slowly withdrawn. This test visualizes the biliary ducts without depending on the gallbladder's concentrating ability. The intrahepatic and extrahepatic biliary ducts, and occasionally the gallbladder, can be visualized to determine possible obstruction. In obstruction of the extrahepatic ducts, a catheter can be placed in the duct to allow external drainage of bile. Endoscopic retrograde cholangiopancreatography (ERCP) and PTC are the only methods available to view the biliary tree in the presence of jaundice. ERCP poses less risk and is probably done more often.

Nursing Implications

Assessment

Indications	Potential Nursing Problems
Aid in the diagnosis of obstruction caused by gallstones, benign strictures, malignant tumors, congenital cysts, and anatomic variations Determine the cause, extent, and location of mechanical obstruction Determine the cause of upper abdominal pain after cholecystectomy Distinguish between obstructive and nonobstructive jaundice	• Fear • Fluid Volume • Human Response • Jaundice • Infection • Nutrition • Pain • Skin

Diagnosis: Clinical Significance of Test Results

ABNORMAL FINDINGS

- Anatomic biliary or pancreatic duct variations
- Biliary sclerosis
- Cholangiocarcinoma
- Cirrhosis
- Common bile duct cysts
- Gallbladder carcinoma
- Gallstones
- Hepatitis
- Nonobstructive jaundice
- Pancreatitis
- Sclerosing cholangitis
- Tumors, strictures, inflammation, or gallstones of the common bile duct

Planning

Considerations for planning a successful partnership should include clear communication of what to expect during the PTC to decrease anxiety and improve cooperation. Ensure that this procedure is performed before an upper GI study or barium swallow. Before the procedure is performed, plan to review the steps with the patient. The patient should fast and restrict fluids for 6 hours prior to the procedure. Instruct the patient to avoid taking anticoagulant medication or to reduce the dosage as ordered prior to the procedure. Protocols may vary among facilities. Explain that some discomfort may be experienced during the exam. Explain that an IV line may be inserted to allow the infusion of IV fluids such as normal saline, antibiotics, anesthetics, sedatives, or emergency medications. Patients who will undergo percutaneous bile drainage may have infected bile and as such should have an antibiotic administered at least 1 hour before the procedure in order to avoid spreading the infection to other parts of the body. Explain that the contrast medium will be injected, by catheter, at a separate site from the IV line. Inform the patient that the procedure is performed in a special room by a radiologist and radiographer, and takes approximately 30 to 60 minutes. Explain that a needle will be inserted into the liver and contrast will be injected through the needle. Remind the patient that she or he should remain still during the procedure and take deep breaths to relax during needle insertion. If iodinated contrast medium is scheduled to be used in patients receiving metformin (Glucophage) for type 2 diabetes, the drug should be discontinued on the day of the test and continue to be withheld for 48 hours after the test. Iodinated contrast can temporarily impair kidney function, and failure to withhold metformin may indirectly result in drug-induced lactic acidosis, a dangerous and sometimes fatal side effect of metformin ***related to renal impairment that does not support sufficient excretion of metformin.*** Type and screen the patient's blood for possible transfusion. Inform the patient that a laxative and cleansing enema may be needed the day before the procedure, with cleansing enemas on the morning of the procedure, depending on the institution's policy.

CONTRAINDICATIONS

- Patients who are pregnant or suspected of being pregnant, unless the potential benefits of a procedure using radiation far outweigh the risk of radiation exposure to the fetus and mother
- Conditions associated with adverse reactions to contrast medium (e.g., asthma, food allergies, or allergy to contrast medium). Although patients are still asked specifically if they have a known allergy to iodine or shellfish, it has been well established that the reaction is not to iodine; in fact, an actual iodine allergy would be very problematic because iodine is required for the production of thyroid hormones. In the case of shellfish, the reaction is to a muscle protein called *tropomyosin*; in the case of iodinated contrast medium, the reaction is to the noniodinated part of the contrast molecule. Patients with a known hypersensitivity to the medium may benefit from premedication with corticosteroids and diphenhydramine; the use of nonionic contrast or an alternative noncontrast imaging study, if available, may be considered for patients who have severe asthma or who have experienced moderate to severe reactions to ionic contrast medium.
- Conditions associated with preexisting renal insufficiency (e.g., chronic kidney disease, single kidney transplant, nephrectomy, diabetes, multiple myeloma, treatment with aminoglycosides and NSAIDs) because iodinated contrast is nephrotoxic
- Older adult and compromised patients who are chronically dehydrated before the test because of their risk of contrast-induced acute kidney injury
- Patients with bleeding disorders because the puncture site may not stop bleeding
- Patients with cholangitis; the injection of the contrast medium can increase biliary pressure, leading to bacteremia, septicemia, and shock

SPECIAL CONSIDERATIONS

An important aspect of planning is understanding the factors that may alter study findings or cause abnormal results. Interdepartmental communication is a key factor in the planning process. The following should be noted when planning for this study:

- Gas or feces in the gastrointestinal (GI) tract resulting from inadequate cleansing or failure to restrict food intake before the study can distort abdominal organ visualization.
- The patient may be unable to cooperate or remain still during the procedure because of age, significant pain, or mental status; uncooperative patients,

including children, may need sedation as motion causes artifacts on the image.

- Retained barium from a previous radiological procedure may inhibit organ visualization and cause unclear images.
- Metallic objects within the examination field (e.g., jewelry, body rings) may inhibit organ visualization and cause unclear images.
- Failure to follow dietary restrictions and other pretesting preparations may cause the procedure to be canceled or repeated.
- The occurrence of chest pain or severe cardiac dysrhythmias may require terminating the procedure.

● *Safety Tip*

Consultation with a health-care provider (HCP) should occur before the procedure for radiation safety concerns regarding younger patients or patients who are lactating.

PEDIATRIC CONSIDERATIONS

Information on the Image Gently Campaign can be found at the Alliance for Radiation Safety in Pediatric Imaging (www.pedrad.org/associations/5364/ig/). Risks associated with radiation overexposure can result from frequent x-ray procedures. Personnel in the examination room with the patient should wear a protective lead apron, stand behind a shield, or leave the area while the examination is being done. Personnel working in the examination area should wear badges to record their level of radiation exposure.

● *Safety Tip*

Make sure a written and informed consent has been signed prior to the procedure if a biopsy is planned and before administering any medications.

Implementation

In order to have a successful study, it is important to obtain the patient's cooperation in following directions. Patient education is an important part of this process, and providing an explanation for the purpose of the procedure is important. Inform the patient that this study can assist in assessing for disorders of the liver and bile ducts. Ensure that the patient has complied with dietary, fluid, and medication restrictions for 8 hours prior to the procedure. Assess for the completion of bowel preparation according to the institution's procedure. If the patient has a history of allergic reactions to any relevant substance or drug, administer ordered prophylactic steroids or antihistamines before the procedure. Record baseline vital signs and continue to monitor throughout the procedure. Protocols may vary among facilities. Establish an IV fluid line for the injection of saline, contrast medium, sedatives, or emergency medications.

Place the patient on the x-ray table in a supine position. A kidney, ureter, and bladder (KUB) or plain film is taken to ensure that no barium or stool will obscure visualization of the biliary system. Clean the upper abdomen on the right side over the liver and anesthetize with lidocaine. The needle is advanced through the skin into the liver under fluoroscopic guidance. When bile begins to flow freely from the needle, contrast is injected through the needle and images are taken immediately. A guide wire can be inserted into the needle and a catheter can be threaded over it if an obstruction is found. This will remain in place temporarily to establish a drainage for the biliary tract. A specimen of bile may be sent to the laboratory for culture and cytological analysis. The needle is removed, and the perforation site is bandaged.

Evaluation

Recognize anxiety related to test results and be supportive of impaired activity related to liver abnormalities and a perceived loss of independence. Maintain pressure over the needle insertion site for several hours if bleeding is persistent. Observe/assess the needle site for bleeding, inflammation, ecchymosis, leakage of bile, or hematoma formation. Advise the patient to watch for symptoms of infection, such as pain, fever, increased pulse rate, and muscle aches. Establish a closed and sterile drainage system if a catheter remains in the biliary tract. Instruct the patient to resume his or her usual diet, fluids, medications, and activity as directed by the HCP. Renal function should be assessed before metformin is restarted. Monitor vital signs and neurological status every 15 minutes for 1 hour, then every 2 hours for 4 hours, and as ordered. Take the patient's temperature every 4 hours for 24 hours. Monitor intake and output at least every 8 hours. Compare all of these with baseline values. Notify the HCP if temperature is elevated. Protocols may vary among facilities. Evaluate the patient for delayed reactions such as dyspnea, tachycardia, and urticaria following the IV injection of contrast. Antihistamines or steroids may be administered if needed. Monitor for reaction to iodinated contrast medium, including rash, urticaria, tachycardia, hyperpnea, hypertension, palpitations, nausea, or vomiting. Instruct the patient to remain on bed rest for several hours and observe for hemorrhage or bile leakage. The patient should be kept NPO for a few hours while being observed for bile extravasation or intra-abdominal bleeding, which may require surgery.

Discuss the implications of abnormal test results on the patient's lifestyle. Provide teaching and information regarding the clinical implications of the test results, as appropriate. Answer any questions or address any concerns voiced by the patient or family. Educate the patient regarding access to counseling services. Provide contact information, if desired, for the National Institutes of Health at www.nlm.nih.gov/medlineplus/liverdiseases.html.

⊘ Critical Findings

N/A

⊘ Study Specific Complications

PTC is an invasive procedure and has potential risks that include allergic reaction *related to contrast reaction,* bleeding *related to inadvertent puncture of a large hepatic blood vessel,* septicemia *related to bacteria being pushed into the bloodstream,* cholangitis *related to contrast being pushed into an obstructed bile duct,* bile peritonitis *related to bile extravasation from the liver following needle removal,* and extravasation of the contrast medium.

⊘ Related Tests

- Related tests include ALT, amylase, AMA, AST, biopsy liver, cancer antigens, cholangiography postoperative, cholangiopancreatography endoscopic retrograde, CT abdomen, GGT, hepatitis antigens and antibodies (A, B, C), hepatobiliary scan, KUB studies, laparoscopy abdominal, lipase, MRI abdomen, peritoneal fluid analysis, pleural fluid analysis, and US liver and biliary tract.
- Refer to the Gastrointestinal and Hepatobiliary systems tables at the end of the book for related tests by body system.

Expected Outcomes

Expected outcomes associated with Cholangiography, Percutaneous Transhepatic, are

- Tolerating a resumption of diet according to the dietician's recommendations
- Understanding education provided decreases the fear of potential surgery

Cholangiography, Postoperative

Quick Summary

SYNONYM ACRONYM: T-tube cholangiography.

COMMON USE: A postoperative evaluation to provide ongoing assessment of the effectiveness of bile duct or gallbladder surgery.

AREA OF APPLICATION: Gallbladder, bile ducts.

NORMAL FINDINGS
- Biliary ducts are normal in size.
- Contrast medium fills the ductal system and flows freely.

Test Explanation

After cholecystectomy, a self-retaining, T-shaped tube may be inserted into the common bile duct. Postoperative (T-tube) cholangiography is a fluoroscopic and radiographic examination of the biliary tract that involves the injection of a contrast medium through the T-tube inserted during surgery. This test may be performed during surgery and again 5 to 10 days after cholecystectomy to assess the patency of the common bile duct and to detect any remaining calculi. The procedure will also help identify areas of stenosis or the presence of fistulae (as a result of the surgery). T-tube placement may also be done after a liver transplant because biliary duct obstruction or anastomotic leakage is possible. This test should be performed before any gastrointestinal (GI) studies using barium and after any studies involving the measurement of iodinated compounds.

Nursing Implications

Assessment

Indications	Potential Nursing Problems
Determine biliary duct patency before T-tube removal Identify the cause, extent, and location of obstruction after surgery	• Activity • Breathing • Fluid Volume • Gas Exchange • Human Response • Infection • Self-care • Skin • Pain

Diagnosis: Clinical Significance of Test Results

ABNORMAL FINDINGS

• Appearance of channels of contrast medium outside of the biliary ducts, indicating a fistula
• Filling defects, dilation, or radiolucent shadows within the biliary ducts, indicating calculi or neoplasm

Planning

Considerations for planning a successful partnership should include clear communication of what to expect during the test to decrease anxiety and improve cooperation. Ensure that this procedure is performed before an upper GI study or barium swallow. Before the procedure is performed, plan to review the steps with the patient. There are no food or fluid restrictions for a postsurgical study, but the patient should follow the standard preoperative restrictions on food and fluids before an operative cholangiogram. Protocols may vary among facilities. Explain that some discomfort may be experienced during the exam. Explain that an IV line may be inserted to allow the infusion of IV fluids such as normal saline, antibiotics, anesthetics, sedatives, or emergency medications. Explain that the contrast medium will be injected through the T-tube that was left in place following surgery. Inform the patient that the procedure is performed in a special room by a

radiologist and radiographer, and takes approximately 30–60 minutes. Explain that a needle will be inserted into the liver, and contrast will be injected through the needle. Remind the patient that she or he should remain still during the procedure and take deep breaths to relax during needle insertion. If iodinated contrast medium is scheduled to be used in patients receiving metformin (Glucophage) for type 2 diabetes, the drug should be discontinued on the day of the test and continue to be withheld for 48 hours after the test. Iodinated contrast can temporarily impair kidney function, and failure to withhold metformin may indirectly result in drug-induced lactic acidosis, a dangerous and sometimes fatal side effect of metformin *related to renal impairment that does not support sufficient excretion of metformin.*

CONTRAINDICATIONS

• Patients who are pregnant or suspected of being pregnant, unless the potential benefits of a procedure using radiation far outweigh the risk of radiation exposure to the fetus and mother
• Conditions associated with adverse reactions to the contrast medium (e.g., asthma, food allergies, or allergy to the contrast medium). Although patients are still asked specifically if they have a known allergy to iodine or shellfish, it has been well established that the reaction is not to iodine; in fact, an actual iodine allergy would be very problematic because iodine is required for the production of thyroid hormones. In the case of shellfish, the reaction is to a muscle protein called *tropomyosin*; in the case of iodinated contrast medium, the reaction is to the noniodinated part of the contrast molecule. Patients with a known hypersensitivity to the medium may benefit from premedication with corticosteroids and diphenhydramine; the use of nonionic contrast or an alternative noncontrast imaging study, if available, may be considered for patients who have severe asthma or who have experienced moderate to severe reactions to ionic contrast medium.
• Conditions associated with preexisting renal insufficiency (e.g., chronic kidney disease, single kidney transplant, nephrectomy, diabetes, multiple myeloma, treatment with aminoglycosides and NSAIDs) because iodinated contrast is nephrotoxic
• Older adult and compromised patients who are chronically dehydrated before the test because of their risk of contrast-induced acute kidney injury
• Patients with bleeding disorders because the puncture site may not stop bleeding
• Patients with cholangitis; the injection of the contrast medium can increase biliary pressure, leading to bacteremia, septicemia, and shock
• Patients with acute cholecystitis or severe liver disease, as the procedure may worsen the condition

SPECIAL CONSIDERATIONS

An important aspect of planning is understanding the factors that may alter study findings or cause abnormal results. Interdepartmental communication is a key factor in the planning process. The following should be noted when planning for this study:

- Gas or feces in the GI tract resulting from inadequate cleansing or failure to restrict food intake before the study can distort abdominal organ visualization.
- The patient may be unable to cooperate or remain still during the procedure because of age, significant pain, or mental status; uncooperative patients, including children, may need sedation as motion causes artifacts on the image.
- Retained barium from a previous radiological procedure may inhibit organ visualization and cause unclear images.
- Metallic objects within the examination field (e.g., jewelry, body rings) may inhibit organ visualization and cause unclear images.
- Failure to follow dietary restrictions and other pretesting preparations may cause the procedure to be canceled or repeated.
- The occurrence of chest pain or severe cardiac dysrhythmias may require terminating the procedure.
- Air bubbles resembling calculi may be seen if there is an inadvertent injection of air.

● *Safety Tip*

Consultation with a health-care provider (HCP) should occur before the procedure for radiation safety concerns regarding younger patients or patients who are lactating.

PEDIATRIC CONSIDERATIONS

Information on the Image Gently Campaign can be found at the Alliance for Radiation Safety in Pediatric Imaging (www.pedrad.org/associations/5364/ig/). Risks associated with radiation overexposure can result from frequent x-ray procedures. Personnel in the examination room with the patient should wear a protective lead apron, stand behind a shield, or leave the area while the examination is being done. Personnel working in the examination area should wear badges to record their level of radiation exposure.

● *Safety Tip*

Make sure a written and informed consent has been signed prior to the procedure if a biopsy is planned and before administering any medications.

Implementation

Patient education is key to obtaining the patient's cooperation in following directions, and providing an explanation for the purpose of the procedure is an important part of this process. Inform the patient that this study is a diagnostic method to visualize any residual or new abnormalities of the biliary tree. Remind the patient that he or she may experience some discomfort during the insertion of the contrast medium through the T-tube, but it will only last a few seconds.

OPERATIVE CHOLANGIOGRAM: Contrast is injected directly into the common bile duct or through catheterization of the cystic duct during cholecystectomy. Images are taken while the patient is on the operating table and reviewed for residual calculi prior to closing the patient. A T-tube is left in place for follow-up study in 5 to 10 days.

T-TUBE CHOLANGIOGRAM: Position the patient supine on the table and drape the area surrounding the T-tube. The end of the T-tube is cleansed with 70% alcohol. If the T-tube site is inflamed and painful, a local anesthetic (e.g., lidocaine) may be injected around the site. A needle is inserted into the open end of the T-tube, and the clamp is removed. Contrast is administered under fluoroscopic guidance through the T-tube that is in the cystic duct, and images are taken during and after injections. The T-tube is removed if findings are normal; a dry, sterile dressing is applied to the site. If retained calculi are identified, the T-tube is left in place for 4 to 6 weeks until the tract surrounding the T-tube is healed to perform a percutaneous removal.

Evaluation

Recognize anxiety related to test results and be supportive of impaired activity related to liver abnormalities and a perceived loss of independence. After the procedure is completed, clamp the end of the T-tube or establish a sterile, closed drainage system. Observe for signs of sepsis. Monitor the T-tube site and change sterile dressing, as ordered. Instruct the patient in the care of the T-tube site. Instruct the patient to resume his or her usual diet, fluids, medications, and activity, as directed by the HCP. Monitor the patient closely for electrolyte imbalance. Renal function should be assessed before metformin is restarted. Monitor vital signs and neurological status every 15 minutes for 1 hour, then every 2 hours for 4 hours, and as ordered. Take temperature every 4 hours for 24 hours. Monitor intake and output at least every 8 hours. Compare all of these with baseline values. Notify the HCP if temperature is elevated. Protocols may vary among facilities. Evaluate the patient for delayed reactions such as dyspnea, tachycardia, and urticaria following the IV injection of contrast. Antihistamines or steroids may be administered if needed. Monitor for reaction to iodinated contrast medium, including rash, urticaria, tachycardia, hyperpnea, hypertension, palpitations, nausea, or vomiting.

Discuss the implications of abnormal test results on the patient's lifestyle. Provide teaching and information regarding the clinical implications of the test results and biliary duct abnormalities, as appropriate. Answer any questions or address any concerns voiced by the patient or family. Educate the patient regarding access to counseling services. Provide contact information, if desired, for the National Digestive Diseases Information Clearinghouse (NDDIC) at http://digestive.niddk.nih .gov/ddiseases/pubs/gallstones/.

✅ Critical Findings

N/A

✅ Study Specific Complications

Cholangiography and establishing an IV site are invasive procedures and have potential risks that include allergic reaction *related to contrast reaction,* bleeding, septicemia *related to increased pressure in the ducts caused by injection of the contrast,* bile peritonitis, and extravasation of the contrast medium.

✅ Related Tests

- Related tests include CT abdomen, hepatobiliary scan, KUB, MRI abdomen, and US liver and biliary system.
- Refer to the Gastrointestinal and Hepatobiliary systems tables at the end of the book for tests by related body systems.

Expected Outcomes

Expected outcomes associated with Cholangiography, Postoperative, are

- Remaining free of postoperative infection
- Understanding the use of postoperative incentive spirometry to prevent pneumonia
- Complying with the recommended postoperative activity schedule in order to facilitate recovery

Intravenous Pyelography

Quick Summary

SYNONYM ACRONYM: Antegrade pyelography, excretory urography (EUG), intravenous urography (IVU, IUG), IVP.

COMMON USE: To assess urinary tract dysfunction or evaluate progression of kidney disease such as stones, bleeding, and congenital anomalies.

AREA OF APPLICATION: Kidneys, ureters, bladder, and renal pelvis.

NORMAL FINDINGS

- Normal size and shape of kidneys, ureters, and bladder
- Normal bladder and absence of masses or renal calculi, with prompt visualization of contrast medium through the urinary system

Test Explanation

Intravenous pyelography (IVP) is most commonly performed to determine urinary tract dysfunction or renal disease. IVP uses IV radiopaque contrast medium to visualize the kidneys, ureters, bladder, and renal pelvis. The contrast medium concentrates in the blood and is filtered out by the glomeruli passing out through the renal tubules and concentrated in the urine. Kidney function is reflected by the length of time it takes the contrast medium to appear and to be excreted by each kidney. A series of images are taken during a 30-minute period to view passage of the contrast through the kidneys and ureters into the bladder. Tomography may be employed during the IVP to permit the examination of an individual layer or plane of the organ that may be obscured by surrounding overlying structures. Many facilities have replaced the IVP with computed tomography (CT) studies. CT provides better detail of the anatomical structures in the urinary system and therefore greater sensitivity in identification of renal pathology.

Nursing Implications

Assessment

Indications	Potential Nursing Problems
Aid in the diagnosis of renovascular hypertension	• Body Image
Evaluate the cause of blood in the urine	• Fatigue
	• Fluid Volume
Evaluate the effects of urinary system trauma	• Grief
Evaluate function of the kidneys, ureters, and bladder	• Home Management
	• Human Response
Evaluate known or suspected ureteral obstruction	• Infection
Evaluate the presence of renal, ureter, or bladder calculi	• Noncompliance
	• Nutrition
Evaluate space-occupying lesions or congenital anomalies of the urinary system	• Pain
	• Protection
	• Role Performance

Diagnosis: Clinical Significance of Test Results
ABNORMAL FINDINGS

- Absence of a kidney (congenital malformation)
- Benign and malignant kidney tumors
- Bladder tumors
- Congenital renal or urinary tract abnormalities
- Glomerulonephritis
- Hydronephrosis
- Prostatic enlargement
- Pyelonephritis
- Renal cysts
- Renal hematomas
- Renal or ureteral calculi
- Soft tissue masses
- Tumors of the collecting system

Planning

Considerations for planning a successful partnership should include clear communication of what to expect during the test to decrease anxiety and improve cooperation. Ensure that barium studies were performed more than 4 days before the IVP. Before the procedure is performed, plan to review the steps with the patient or caregiver. Explain that minimal discomfort may be experienced during contrast injection. inform the patient that the procedure is performed in a radiology room by a radiographer and takes approximately 20 to 30 minutes. Creatinine levels should be assessed prior to the procedure as abnormal renal function can worsen as a result of contrast injections. Food and fluids should be restricted for 8 hours prior to the exam or as dictated by the institution's policies. Special considerations regarding fluid restrictions may apply to patients experiencing chronic dehydration including older adult patients in whom dehydration is common; considerations may also be given to pediatric patients. Fluid restrictions for pediatric patients may be adjusted based on age and weight. A laxative is required the evening prior to the study and, in some cases, an enema or suppository is ordered the morning of the study.

> ● **Safety Tip**
>
> The combination of fluid restrictions and administration of laxatives may cause increased injury risk from falling for older adult patients, related to weakness. Additional monitoring and assistance while ambulating may be required.

If iodinated contrast medium is scheduled to be used in patients receiving metformin (Glucophage) for type 2 diabetes, the drug should be discontinued on the day of the test and continue to be withheld for 48 hours after the test. Iodinated contrast can temporarily impair kidney function, and failure to withhold metformin may indirectly result in drug-induced lactic acidosis, a dangerous and sometimes fatal side effect of metformin *related to renal impairment that does not support sufficient excretion of metformin.*

CONTRAINDICATIONS

- Patients who are pregnant or suspected of being pregnant, unless the potential benefits of a procedure using radiation far outweigh the risk of radiation exposure to the fetus and mother
- Conditions associated with adverse reactions to the contrast medium (e.g., asthma, food allergies, or allergy to the contrast medium). Although patients are still asked specifically if they have a known allergy to iodine or shellfish, it has been well established that the reaction is not to iodine; in fact, an actual iodine allergy would be very problematic because iodine is required for the production of thyroid hormones. In the case of shellfish, the reaction is to a muscle protein called *tropomyosin*; in the case of iodinated contrast medium, the reaction is to the noniodinated part of the contrast molecule. Patients with a known hypersensitivity to the medium may benefit from premedication with corticosteroids and diphenhydramine; the use of nonionic contrast or an alternative noncontrast imaging study, if available, may be considered for patients who have severe asthma or who have experienced moderate to severe reactions to ionic contrast medium.
- Conditions associated with preexisting renal insufficiency (e.g., chronic kidney disease, single kidney transplant, nephrectomy, diabetes, multiple myeloma, treatment with aminoglycocides and NSAIDs) *because iodinated contrast is nephrotoxic*
- Older adult and compromised patients who are chronically dehydrated before the test *because of their risk of contrast-induced acute kidney injury*
- Patients with bleeding disorders *because the puncture site may not stop bleeding*

SPECIAL CONSIDERATIONS

An important aspect of planning is understanding the factors that may alter study findings or cause abnormal results. Interdepartmental communication is a key factor in the planning process. The following should be noted when planning for this study:

- Gas or feces in the gastrointestinal (GI) tract resulting from inadequate cleansing or failure to restrict food intake before the study can distort abdominal organ visualization.
- The patient may be unable to cooperate or remain still during the procedure because of age, significant pain, or mental status; uncooperative patients, including children, may need sedation as motion causes artifacts on the image.
- Retained barium from a previous radiological procedure may inhibit organ visualization and cause unclear images.
- Metallic objects within the examination field (e.g., jewelry, body rings) may inhibit organ visualization and cause unclear images.
- Failure to follow dietary restrictions and other pretesting preparations may cause the procedure to be canceled or repeated.
- The occurrence of chest pain or severe cardiac dysrhythmias may require termination of the procedure.

> ● **Safety Tip**
>
> Consultation with a health-care provider (HCP) should occur before the procedure for radiation safety concerns regarding younger patients or patients who are lactating.

PEDIATRIC CONSIDERATIONS

Information on the Image Gently Campaign can be found at the Alliance for Radiation Safety in Pediatric Imaging (www.pedrad.org/associations/5364/ig/). Risks associated with radiation overexposure can result from frequent x-ray procedures. Personnel in the examination room with the patient should wear a protective lead apron, stand behind a shield, or leave the area while the examination is being done. Personnel working in the examination area should wear badges to record their level of radiation exposure.

● Safety Tip

Make sure a written and informed consent has been signed prior to the procedure if a biopsy is planned and before administering any medications.

Implementation

Patient education is key to obtaining the patient's cooperation in following directions, and providing an explanation for the purpose of the procedure is an important part of this process. Inform the patient that this study can assist in assessing for abnormalities of the kidneys. The study is performed on children to investigate vesicoureteral reflux (VUR) or the abnormal backflow of urine from the bladder to the kidneys. VUR increases the risk for bacterial infection and tissue damage in the kidneys.

PEDIATRIC CONSIDERATIONS

Preparing children for an IVP depends on the age of the child. Encourage parents to be truthful about unpleasant sensations the child may experience during the procedure and to use words that they know their child will understand. Toddlers and preschool-age children have a very short attention span, so the best time to talk about the test is right before the procedure. The child should be assured that he or she will be allowed to bring a favorite comfort item into the examination room and, if appropriate, that a parent will be with them during the procedure.

Ensure the patient has complied with dietary, fluid, and medication restrictions for 8 hours prior to the procedure. Assess for the completion of bowel preparation according to the institution's procedure. Administer enemas or suppositories on the morning of the test, as ordered. Inform the patient that he or she may experience a metallic taste in his or her mouth or a warm feeling as the contrast is injected, but that this will last only a few seconds. A kidney, ureter, and bladder (KUB) or plain film is taken to ensure that no barium or stool obscures visualization of the urinary system. Position the patient supine on the table, and clean the skin surrounding the peripheral injection site with an antiseptic solution. Following insertion of the needle or catheter into the vein, the contrast is injected. The needle or catheter remains in place for about 10 minutes to have a viable access route in the event of an allergic reaction. Once the needle is removed, the injection site is bandaged. The first image is taken 5 minutes postinjection for the nephrogram phase of the study. Images are then taken at various times to monitor the contrast as it descends the ureters and fills the bladder. The patient is monitored for any reactions to the contrast. The needle or catheter is removed, and a pressure dressing is applied over the puncture site. Instruct the patient to void if a postvoiding exposure is required to visualize the empty bladder.

Evaluation

Recognize anxiety related to test results and be supportive of a perceived loss of independence. Instruct the patient to resume his or her usual diet, medications, and activity as directed by the HCP. Renal function should be assessed before metformin is resumed if contrast was used. Instruct the patient to increase hydration to flush the contrast media from the body. Monitor urinary output as a decrease may indicate acute kidney injury. Observe for delayed reaction to the iodinated contrast medium, including rash, urticaria, tachycardia, hyperpnea, hypertension, palpitations, nausea, or vomiting. Observe/assess the needle/catheter insertion site for bleeding, inflammation, or hematoma formation. Instruct the patient in the care and assessment of the injection site. Instruct the patient to apply cold compresses to the puncture site as needed to reduce discomfort or edema.

Discuss the implications of abnormal test results on the patient's lifestyle. Provide teaching and information regarding the clinical implications of an abnormal study, as appropriate. Answer any questions or address any concerns voiced by the patient or family. Educate the patient regarding access to counseling services and provide contact information, if desired. Information on kidney disease may be found at www.nlm.nih.gov/medlineplus/ency/article/000471.htm.

✓ Critical Findings

N/A

✓ Study Specific Complications

Complications include infiltration of the contrast at the injection site, allergic reaction to contrast media, and acidosis or hypoglycemia in patients taking metformin following contrast injection.

✓ Related Tests

● Related tests include biopsy bladder, biopsy kidney, biopsy prostate, BUN, CT abdomen, CT pelvis, creatinine, cystometry, cystoscopy, gallium scan, KUB, MRI abdomen, renogram, retrograde ureteropyelography, US abdomen, US bladder, US kidney,

US prostate, urine markers of bladder cancer, urinalysis, urine cytology, and voiding cystourethrography.

- Refer to the Genitourinary System table at the end of the book for related tests by body system.

Expected Outcomes

Expected outcomes associated with Intravenous Pyelography are

- Maintaining fluid restriction as recommended to decrease fluid retention
- Returning to a normal weight without evidence of edema

Upper Gastrointestinal and Small Bowel Series

Quick Summary

SYNONYM ACRONYM: Gastric radiography, stomach series, small bowel study, upper GI series, UGI.

COMMON USE: To assess the esophagus, stomach, and small bowel for disorders related to obstruction, perforation, weight loss, swallowing, pain, cancer, reflux disease, ulcers, and structural anomalies.

AREA OF APPLICATION: Esophagus, stomach, and small intestine.

NORMAL FINDINGS

- Normal size, shape, position, and functioning of the esophagus, stomach, and small bowel

Test Explanation

The upper gastrointestinal (GI) series is a radiological examination of the esophagus, stomach, and small intestine after ingestion of barium sulfate, which is a milkshake-like, radiopaque substance. A combination of x-ray and fluoroscopy techniques are used to record the study. Air or gas may be instilled to provide double contrast and better visualization of the lumen of the esophagus, stomach, and duodenum. If perforation or obstruction is suspected, a water-soluble iodinated contrast medium is used. This test is especially useful in the evaluation of patients experiencing dysphagia, regurgitation, gastroesophageal reflux (GER), epigastric pain, hematemesis, melena, and unexplained weight loss. This test is also used to evaluate the results of gastric surgery, especially when an anastomotic leak is suspected. When a small bowel series is included, the test detects disorders of the jejunum and ileum. The patient's position is changed during the examination to allow visualization of the various structures and their function. Images of the swallowed contrast medium as it moves through the digestive system are visualized on a fluoroscopic screen, recorded, and stored electronically for review. Drugs such as glucagon may be given during an upper GI series to relax the GI tract; drugs such as metoclopramide (Reglan) may be given to accelerate the passage of the barium through the stomach and small intestine.

When the small bowel series is performed separately, the patient may be asked to drink several glasses of barium, or enteroclysis may be used to instill the barium. With enteroclysis, a catheter is passed through the nose or mouth and advanced past the pylorus and into the duodenum. Barium, followed by methylcellulose solution, is instilled via the catheter directly into the small bowel.

PEDIATRICS: An upper GI series is usually done in the pediatric population to diagnose the cause of recurrent GI signs (bleeding) and symptoms. The etiology is often related to age. In infants, recurrent symptoms such as vomiting after feeding, poor feeding, poor weight gain, and abdominal pain (evidenced by frequent crying during or after a feeding) may trigger an investigation. The most common causes of upper or lower GI bleeding in infants up to 1 month include allergies to milk proteins, anorectal fissures, bacterial enteritis, coagulopathy, esophagitis, Hirschsprung disease, intussusception, peptic ulcer, stenosis, varices, or Meckel diverticulum. Children between 2 and 23 months are most commonly diagnosed with allergies to milk proteins, anorectal fissures, esophagitis caused by GER, gastritis, intussusception, Meckel diverticulum, NSAID-induced ulcer, and ingested foreign body. Pediatric patients 24 months and older are most commonly diagnosed with esophageal varices, Mallory Weiss tears, peptic ulcer, related to Helicobacter pylori infection or peptic ulcer secondary to some other type of systemic disease (e.g., Crohn disease or inflammatory bowel disease [IBD]). Other abnormal findings in this age group include IBD, polyps, malignancy, sepsis, and Meckel diverticulum.

Nursing Implications

Assessment

Indications	Potential Nursing Problems
Determine the cause of regurgitation or epigastric pain	• Activity
	• Bleeding
Determine the presence of neoplasms, ulcers, diverticula, obstruction, foreign body, and hiatal hernia	• Cardiac Output
	• Constipation
	• Family
	• Fatigue
Evaluate suspected GER, inflammatory process, congenital anomaly, motility disorder, or structural change	• Fear
	• Fluid Volume
	• Nutrition
Evaluate unexplained weight loss or anemia	• Pain
	• Role Performance
Identify and locate the origin of hematemesis	• Self-care
	• Swallowing

Diagnosis: Clinical Significance of Test Results

ABNORMAL FINDINGS

- Achalasia
- Cancer of the esophagus
- Chalasis
- Congenital abnormalities
- Duodenal cancer, and ulcers
- Esophageal diverticula, motility disorders, ulcers, varices, and inflammation
- Foreign body
- Gastric cancer or tumors, and ulcers
- Gastritis
- Hiatal hernia
- Perforation of the esophagus, stomach, or small bowel
- Polyps
- Small bowel tumors
- Strictures

Planning

Considerations for planning a successful partnership should include clear communication of what to expect during the test to decrease anxiety and improve cooperation. Ensure that this procedure is performed before a barium swallow. Before the procedure is performed, plan to review the steps with the patient. Explain that no discomfort should be experienced during the UGI. Explain to the patient that he or she will be asked to drink a milkshake-like solution of barium sulfate that has an unpleasant chalky taste. Inform the patient that the procedure is performed in a special room by a radiologist and radiographer and takes approximately 30 minutes. Remind the patient that he or she should remain still and follow swallowing instructions during the procedure. The patient should restrict all food and fluids for 8 hours prior to the exam.

PEDIATRIC CONSIDERATIONS

The fasting period prior to the time of the examination depends the child's age. General guidelines are that the patient should not eat for the period of time between normal meals: newborns: 2 to 3 hours; infants to 4 years: 3 to 4 hours; 5 years through adolescence: 6 to 8 hours.

If iodinated contrast medium (e.g., Gastrografin) is scheduled to be used in patients receiving metformin (Glucophage) for type 2 diabetes, the drug should be discontinued on the day of the test and continue to be withheld for 48 hours after the test. Iodinated contrast can temporarily impair kidney function, and failure to withhold metformin may indirectly result in drug-induced lactic acidosis, a dangerous and sometimes fatal side effect of metformin ***related to renal impairment that does not support sufficient excretion of metformin.***

DISCUSSION POINT

PEDIATRIC CONSIDERATIONS: Preparing children for an upper GI examination depends on the age of the child. Encourage parents to be truthful about unpleasant sensations the child may experience during the procedure and to use words that they know their child will understand. Toddlers and preschool-age children have a very short attention span, so the best time to talk about the test is right before the procedure. The child should be assured that he or she will be allowed to bring a favorite comfort item into the examination room and, if appropriate, that a parent will be with them during the procedure.

CONTRAINDICATIONS

- Patients who are pregnant or suspected of being pregnant, unless the potential benefits of a procedure using radiation far outweigh the risk of radiation exposure to the fetus and mother
- Patients suspected of having upper GI perforation, unless water-soluble iodinated contrast medium, such as Gastrografin, is used
- Conditions associated with adverse reactions to contrast medium (e.g., asthma, food allergies, or allergy to contrast medium). Although patients are still asked specifically if they have a known allergy to iodine or shellfish, it has been well established that the reaction is not to iodine, in fact an actual iodine allergy would be very problematic because iodine is required for the production of thyroid hormones. In the case of shellfish the reaction is to a muscle protein called tropomyosin; in the case of iodinated contrast medium the reaction is to the noniodinated part of the contrast molecule. Patients with a known hypersensitivity to the medium may benefit from premedication with corticosteroids and diphenhydramine; the use of nonionic contrast or an alternative noncontrast imaging study, if available, may be considered for patients who have severe asthma or who have experienced moderate to severe reactions to ionic contrast medium.
- Conditions associated with preexisting renal insufficiency (e.g., chronic kidney disease, single kidney transplant, nephrectomy, diabetes, multiple myeloma, treatment with aminoglycosides and NSAIDs) ***because iodinated contrast is nephrotoxic***
- Older adult and compromised patients who are chronically dehydrated before the test, ***because of their risk of contrast-induced acute kidney injury***
- Patients with an intestinal obstruction, ***because the barium or water from the enema may make the condition worse.***

SPECIAL CONSIDERATIONS

An important aspect of planning is understanding the factors that may alter study findings or cause abnormal results. Interdepartmental communication is a key factor in the planning process. The following should be noted when planning for this study:

- Patients with swallowing problems may aspirate the barium, which could interfere with the procedure and cause patient complications.
- The patient may be unable to cooperate or remain still during the procedure because of age, significant pain, or mental status. Uncooperative patients, including children, may need sedation as motion causes artifacts on the image.
- Metallic objects within the examination field (e.g., jewelry, body rings) may inhibit organ visualization and cause unclear images.
- Failure to follow dietary restrictions and other pretesting preparations may cause the procedure to be canceled or repeated.
- Possible constipation or partial bowel obstruction caused by retained barium in the small bowel or colon may affect test results.
- This procedure should be done before a barium swallow and after a kidney x-ray (IV pyelography) or computed tomography (CT) of the abdomen or pelvis.

● *Safety Tip*

Consultation with a health-care provider (HCP) should occur before the procedure for radiation safety concerns regarding younger patients or patients who are lactating.

PEDIATRIC CONSIDERATIONS

Information on the Image Gently Campaign can be found at the Alliance for Radiation Safety in Pediatric Imaging (www.pedrad.org/associations/5364/ig/). Risks associated with radiation overexposure can result from frequent x-ray procedures. Personnel in the examination room with the patient should wear a protective lead apron, stand behind a shield, or leave the area while the examination is being done. Personnel working in the examination area should wear badges to record their level of radiation exposure.

Implementation

Patient education is key to obtaining the patient's cooperation in following directions, and providing an explanation for the purpose of the procedure is an important part of this process. Inform the patient that this study is a diagnostic method used to visualize abnormalities of the stomach and small bowel. Ensure that the patient has complied with dietary and fluid restrictions for 8 hours prior to the procedure. Remind the patient that he or she will need to swallow the barium as instructed by the radiologist.

Position the patient upright against the x-ray table and provide him or her with a cup of barium sulfate. Instruct the patient to take several swallows of the barium mixture through a straw while images are taken of the pharyngeal motion. An effervescent carbonated powder may also be administered after the barium to introduce air into the stomach if an air contrast upper GI is ordered. The air helps to further outline the gastric mucosa.

PEDIATRIC CONSIDERATIONS

For infants, barium contrast may be mixed with a small amount of the infant's feeding to take in a bottle.

If the patient is unable to drink the barium, a thin flexible tube may be placed through his or her nose to get the barium into the esophagus. The barium is observed with fluoroscopy as it flows through the esophagus and begins to fill the stomach. As soon as the patient finishes drinking the barium, the table and patient are moved into a recumbent position, and images are taken as the patient rolls in different positions (see Fig. 15.6).

If the small bowel is to be examined after the upper GI series, instruct the patient to drink an additional glass of barium while the small intestine is observed for passage of barium. Images are taken at 30- to 60-minute intervals until the barium reaches the ileocecal valve, the terminal ileum of the small intestines (see Fig. 15.7). This process can last up to 5 hours, with follow-up images taken at 24 hours.

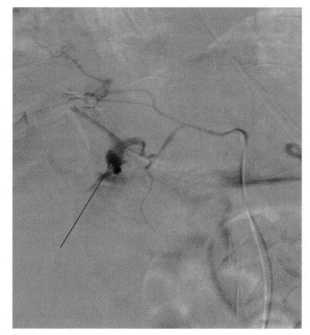

FIGURE 15.6 CTA showing GI bleeding. *Used with permission, from Weber, E., Vilensky, J., & Fog, A. (2013). Practical radiology: A symptom-based approach. FA Davis Company.*

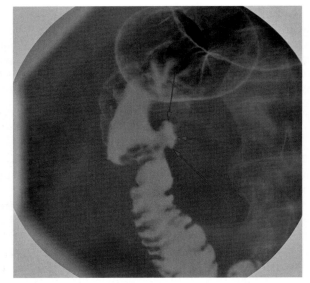

FIGURE 15.7 Duodenal ulcer. *Used with permission, from Weber, E., Vilensky, J., & Fog, A. (2013). Practical radiology: A symptom-based approach. FA Davis Company.*

Evaluation

Recognize anxiety related to test results and be supportive of a perceived loss of independence. Instruct the patient to resume usual diet as directed by the HCP. Instruct the patient to increase fluid intake (four glasses) to aid in the elimination of barium unless contraindicated. Monitor for reaction to iodinated contrast medium, including rash, urticaria, tachycardia, hyperpnea, hypertension, palpitations, nausea, or vomiting, if iodine is used. Instruct the patient to immediately report symptoms such as fast heart rate, difficulty breathing, skin rash, itching, chest pain, persistent right shoulder pain, or abdominal pain. Immediately report symptoms to the appropriate HCP. If a water-soluble contrast was used for the study, inform the patient that he or she may experience diarrhea after the procedure. Inform the patient that his or her stool will be a chalky color and should resume the normal color within 2 days. Instruct the patient to take a mild laxative and increase fluid intake (four glasses) to aid in the elimination of barium unless contraindicated.

PEDIATRIC CONSIDERATIONS

Instruct the parents of pediatric patients to hydrate the child with electrolyte fluid post barium enema.

OLDER ADULT CONSIDERATIONS

Chronic dehydration can also result in frequent bouts of constipation. Therefore, after the procedure, older adult patients should be encouraged to hydrate with fluids containing electrolytes (e.g., Gatorade, Gatorade low calorie for diabetics, or Pedialyte) and to use a mild laxative daily until the stool is back to normal color. If the patient is unable to eliminate the barium, or if the stool does not return to normal color, the patient should notify the HCP.

Discuss the implications of abnormal test results on the patient's lifestyle. Provide teaching and information regarding the clinical implications of stomach and intestinal abnormalities, as appropriate. Answer any questions or address any concerns voiced by the patient or family. Educate the patient regarding access to counseling services, and provide contact information, if desired, for the National Digestive Diseases Information Clearinghouse (NDDIC) at http://digestive.niddk.nih .gov/ddiseases/topics/stomach.aspx.

Ⓢ Critical Findings

- Foreign body
- Perforated bowel
- Tumor with significant mass effect

Note and immediately report to the requesting HCP any critical findings and related symptoms. A listing of these findings varies among facilities.

Ⓢ Study Specific Complications

Complications include allergic reaction to the contrast medium, aspiration of the barium, significant diarrhea *related to use of Gastrografin,* and partial bowel obstruction caused by thickened or congealed barium.

Ⓢ Related Tests

- Related tests include barium enema, barium swallow, capsule endoscopy, CT abdomen, endoscopic retrograde cholangiopancreatography, esophageal manometry, fecal analysis, gastric acid stimulation test, gastric emptying scan, gastrin stimulation test, gastroesophageal reflux scan, H. pylori antibody, KUB study, Meckel diverticulum scan, MRI abdomen, and US pelvis.
- Refer to the Gastrointestinal System table at the end of the book for related tests by body system.

Expected Outcomes

Expected outcomes associated with Upper Gastrointestinal and Small Bowel Series are

- Finding that white blood count remains within normal limits
- Asking appropriate questions regarding the diagnosis and therapeutic treatment
- Tolerating the diet without pain or regurgitation

REVIEW OF LEARNING OUTCOMES

Thinking

1. Describe potential medical complications for patients undergoing arteriography. Answer: Complications related to allergies to a contrast medium, the perforation of a vessel, or the possible displacement of a plaque within an artery are the greatest concerns when performing a arteriogram. Constant monitoring of the patient during the study is an important aspect of patient care.

Doing

1. Perform capably and knowledgeably within scope of practice guidelines. Answer: These types of radiology studies require the proactive participation of the nurse in collaboration with radiology department staff to prepare and, in some instances recover, individuals. Understanding the roles of nursing and radiology in this process is necessary to patient safety and the ability of the team to function successfully.

Caring

1. Recognize the usefulness of reflection in improving communication and conflict resolution skills. Answer: Nursing is a study in the application of growing clinical competence that moves from novice to expert. Becoming an expert in any part of nursing requires time and patience. Clear communication and growth of your conflict resolution skills is a part of the growing process. Value your individual growth in learning the ways of communicating specific information regarding radiology studies to your patients and assisting them to overcome conflict within themselves and their families in relation to those exams. Take every opportunity to learn from others, and ask a lot of questions.

((*Words* OF *Wisdom:* When some patients hear the word "radiology," they immediately think about radiation exposure. There is an inherent fear factor with that thought. "How many times can I do this before I get radiation poisoning?" This unfounded concern can prevent a patient from making a decision to go ahead with a radiographic study that may identify a disease in the early stages and save his or her life. Patients always have the right to refuse. Our job is to ensure that the refusal is based on a patient's having all of the information he or she needs to make an informed decision. This includes the truth about the risk of exposure to radiation.

BIBLIOGRAPHY

Alamria, H., Almoghairia, A., Alghamdib, A., Almasooda, A., Alotaibya, M., Kazima, H., Almutairia, M., & Alanazia, A. (2011). Efficacy of a single dose intravenous heparin in reducing sheath-thrombus formation during diagnostic angiography: A randomized controlled trial. Retrieved from www.sciencedirect.com/science/article/pii/S1016731511002065

American College of Obstetricians and Gynecologists. (2011). Hysterosalpingography. Retrieved from www.acog.org/For_Patients/Search_FAQs?Keyword=FAQ143

American College of Radiology. (2014). About imaging agents or tracers. Retrieved from www.acrin.org/PATIENTS/ABOUTIMAGINGEXAMSANDAGENTS/ABOUTIMAGINGAGENTSORTRACERS.aspx

American Heart Association. (2014). Patent ductus arteriosis (PDA). Retrieved from www.heart.org/HEARTORG/Conditions/CongenitalHeartDefects/AboutCongenitalHeartDefects/Patent-Ductus-Arteriosis-PDA_UCM_307032_Article.jsp

American Society of Anesthesiologists Committee. (2011). Practice guidelines for preoperative fasting and the use of pharmacologic agents to reduce the risk of pulmonary aspiration: Application to healthy patients undergoing elective procedures Retrieved from http://www.asahq.org/~/media/Sites/ASAHQ/Files/Public/Resources/standards-guidelines/practice-guidelines-for-preoperative-fasting.pdf.

Carotid endarterectomy. (2014). Retrieved from http://surgery.ucsf.edu/conditions--procedures/carotid-endarterectomy.aspx

Cleveland Clinic. (2013, November). Carotid angiography and stenting. (2010, January 22). Retrieved from http://my.clevelandclinic.org/heart/services/procedures/carotidstent.aspx.

Conditions which may contraindicate the use of IV iodinated contrast. (n.d.). Retrieved from www.fda.gov/MedicalDevices/ProductsandMedicalProcedures/InVitroDiagnostics/ucm301431.htm

Fischbach, F., & Dunning, M. (2009). A laboratory manual of laboratory and diagnostic tests (8th ed.). Philadelphia, PA: Lippincott Williams & Wilkins.

Frank, E., Long, B., & Smith, B. (2012). Merrill's atlas of radiographic positioning and procedures (12th ed.). St. Louis, MO: Elsevier.

Gandelman, G. (2012, December 9). Percutaneous transluminal coronary angioplasty (PTCA). Retrieved from www.nlm.nih.gov/medlineplus/ency/anatomyvideos/000096.htm

Goergen, S., Revell, A., & Walker, C. (2009). Iodine-containing contrast medium (ICCM). Retrieved from www.insideradiology.com.au/pages/view.php?T_id=21

Horwitch, P., & Lin, E. (2013). Adrenal adenoma imaging. Retrieved from http://emedicine.medscape.com/article/376240-overview

Johns Hopkins Medicine. (2014). Fluoroscopy procedures. Retrieved from www.hopkinsmedicine.org/healthlibrary/test_procedures/orthopaedic/fluoroscopy_procedure_92,P07662/

LeMone, P., Burke, K., & Baldoff, G. (2011). Medical surgical nursing, critical thinking in patient care. (5th ed.). Upper Saddle River, NJ: Pearson.

Maddox, T. (2002). Adverse reactions to contrast material: Recognition, prevention, and treatment. Retrieved from www.aafp.org/afp/2002/1001/p1229.html

Mayo Clinic. (2011). Carotid artery disease. Retrieved from www.mayoclinic.com/health/carotid-artery-disease/DS01030

National Institutes of Health. (2014). Salivary gland disorders. Retrieved from www.nlm.nih.gov/medlineplus/salivaryglanddisorders.html

National Institutes of Health. (2012). What is coronary artery disease? Retrieved from www.nhlbi.nih.gov/health/health-topics/topics/cad/

National Institutes of Health. (2011). What is pulmonary embolism? Retrieved from www.nhlbi.nih.gov/health/health-topics/topics/pe/

Normal hemodynamic parameters and laboratory values. (n.d.). Retrieved from http://ht.edwards.com/scin/edwards/sitecollectionimages/products/mininvasive/ar10523-normal_card_1lr.pdf

Patel, K. (2013). Deep venous thrombosis treatment and management. Retrieved from http://emedicine.medscape.com/article/1911303-treatment

RadiologyInfo. (2014). Retrieved from www.radiologyinfo.org/

Rothrock, S. (2013). Myth of shellfish, iodine, and CT contrast allergy link debunked. Retrieved from www.compactmedicalguides.com/blog/post/myth-of-shellfish-iodine-and-ct-contrast-allergy-link-debunked

Tang, Q., Liu, M., Ma, Z. Guo, X, Kuang, T., & Yang, Y. (2013, September 12). Non-invasive evaluation of hemodynamics in pulmonary hypertension by a Septal angle measured by computed tomography pulmonary angiography: Comparison with right-heart catheterization and association with N-terminal pro-B-type natriuretic peptide. Experimental and Therapeutic Medicine, 6, 1350–1358.

U.S. Food and Drug Administration. (2013). Fluoroscopy. Retrieved from www.fda.gov/radiation-emittingproducts/radiationemittingproductsandprocedures/medicalimaging/medicalx-rays/ucm115354.htm

Uterine fibroid embolization (UFE). (2013). Retrieved from www.radiologyinfo.org/en/info.cfm?pg=ufe

Van Leeuwen, A., & Bladh, M. (2015). Davis's comprehensive handbook of laboratory and diagnostic testing with nursing implications (6th ed.). Philadelphia, PA: F.A. Davis Company.

Vidalink. (2007). The IV contrast/iodine allergy myth. Retrieved from www.ct-scan-info.com/ctcontrast.html

Wu, H. (2014). Radiographic evaluation of the pediatric urinary tract. Retrieved from http://emedicine.medscape.com/article/1016549-overview#aw2aab6b5

Go to Section II of this book and www.davisplus.com for the Clinical Reasoning Tool and its case studies to provide you with a safe place to explore patient care situations. There are a total of 26 different case studies; 2 cases are presented for each of 13 body systems. One set of 13 cases are found in the Section II chapters, and a second set of 13 cases are available online at www.davisplus.com. Each case is designed with the specific goal of helping you to connect the dots of clinical reasoning. Cases are designed to reflect possible clinical scenarios; the outcomes may or may not be positive—you decide.

Radiologic Studies: Plain

OVERVIEW

Plain x-rays are used for a basic evaluation of a specific body area such as the head, chest, extremities, and abdomen. Plain x-rays do not use contrast medium or any other method to augment the image obtained and are often used as a first step in evaluation before moving on to a more invasion method of inquiry. An x-ray beam passes from one side of the body to the other, capturing an image for study. The type of image captured depends on how much radiation reaches the image receptor. Images that are obtained during x-ray look like a black-and-white photograph. Variances in the density of the image being x-rayed and the amount of energy absorbed determine how black or white the images appear. Areas that are less dense, such as those filled with fluid or air, will appear almost black because very little of the radiation is absorbed. Solid areas that are denser, such as bone, will absorb more radiation and will appear as white. Tissues and masses that absorb different amounts of radiation will appear in various shades of gray. Captured images will be displayed digitally on an imaging plate and saved onto a CD or other device.

Different views of the body can be taken for comparison and as a more accurate diagnostic tool. An example is a chest x-ray of which the health-care provider (HCP) requests an anterior view and a lateral view. The anterior view will allow the HCP to look at anatomical structures from the front to the back, and the lateral view will allow side-to-side viewing. Posteroranterior views work the same way and take the x-ray from the back to the front. The type of view chosen is dependent on the goal of the x-ray and the direction of diagnostic inquiry. Images are often taken at various angles to provide a better view of the body part to evaluate fractures, foreign bodies, tumors, and other abnormalities in different body planes. This approach allows the radiologist to locate foreign bodies, evaluate the anterior/posterior displacements of fractures, and pinpoint more exactly the location of a tumor or mass in the body. Oblique projections are required for many body parts, which is done by rotating either the patient or the x-ray in different angles.

RADIATION EXPOSURE RISKS: Risks associated with radiation exposure during x-ray are generally outweighed by the diagnostic benefit to the patient. Patients are protected as much as possible from unnecessary radiation exposure. This is achieved by using the lowest amount of radiation necessary to complete the x-ray and by providing the patient with a lead apron shield when it does not interfere with the part of the body being examined. The goal is to reduce radiation exposure to what is medically necessary. However, even with the best radiation safety practices in place, there is still a risk of damage to the cells of the body. Because of this, x-rays should not be completed unless needed. Protection from radiation exposure for both the patient and the radiology technician is always a consideration in radiology departments. The conceptual approach to safe radiography is to image gently, wisely, and at the lowest exposure to reasonably achieve the desired results. The general rule in most radiography departments is to provide shielding for all children and women of childbearing age if possible. Regardless of all of our efforts, there is still the possibility of damage to the body. The following are some types of damage:

- *Somatic effects*—These effects may occur to the individual who had been exposed to x-ray radiation. Effects can be short term or long term, as may be seen in some cases of leukemia or cancer.
- *Genetic effects*—These are effects that occur in the child instead of the individual who was exposed.

The mutation occurs in the sperm and egg cells, resulting in the infant having mild to severe effects, including mental retardation.

- *Fetal effects*—These effects occur when the fetus is exposed during the embryonic or fetal stage of development. The result of the exposure in utero will depend on the stage of fetal development at the time of exposure.

Radiation Effects in Utero

Weeks After Conception	Effect
0–1 (pre-implantation)	Intrauterine death
2–7 (organogenesis)	Developmental abnormalities/ growth retardation/cancer
8–40 (fetal stage)	Same as above with lower risk plus functional abnormalities

To prevent accidental fetal exposure, x-rays on child-bearing women should be performed using the 10-day rule. This rule recommends that x-rays should only be performed from the first day of the menstrual cycle until day 10. Generally, ovulation has not occurred during this period and there is a better chance that a viable pregnancy is not present. Women receiving an x-ray that is outside of this time frame should have a pregnancy test before being x-rayed to decrease the risk of fetal exposure.

PEDIATRIC IMAGING: Radiation risk is higher in the pediatric population because their cells divide more rapidly than adults. The younger the patient, the more radiation sensitive they are. The Image Gently Campaign was launched in 2008 to raise awareness of safety concerns related to radiation exposure from diagnostic procedures. It has grown into a national coalition of more than 40 organizations whose goal is to provide education to individuals and institutions, promoting awareness of safe pediatric imaging practices. Information for patients, parents, and HCPs, about the Image Gently Campaign, can be found at www.imagegently.org.

● Safety Tip

It is essential to follow pediatric x-ray precautions because of the effects of radiation exposure on children who weigh less than 100 pounds. Some of the reasons for these precautions include

- Epidemiologic studies show that children run a higher risk from exposure than adults.
- Because exposed children have a longer life expectancy than exposed adults, children are more likely to show radiation damage.
- Children, because of their size, are more likely to receive a higher radiation dose than necessary.

DISCUSSION POINT

Pediatric/Adolescent Preparation: Decreasing anxiety and encouraging cooperation will be necessary when working with children and adolescents. Early preparation can assist in the development of coping skills. Generally, the older the child, the earlier the preparation should begin. Using a doll to show children how they will be positioned or having them practice positioning can decrease anxiety. Encouraging the participation of adolescents in the decision-making process as much as possible can reduce their anxiety. Adolescents may benefit from watching a digital explanation of the study through a multimedia network connection via tablet, smartphone, or other application. Suggesting ways to remain calm, such as counting, deep breathing, singing, and relaxation, are good coping methods for adolescents and school-age children.

Nurses need to understand that anxiety management is a normal part of study preparation in the pediatric population. Acceptance of this as a norm can help the nurse to manage the situation when the child begins to cry as the time for the study approaches. Nurses should provide assurance that the study is not a punishment for anything the child did wrong. Giving children permission to cry, yell, or in some way express their discomfort can also decrease their anxiety.

RADIOLOGIC PROCEDURES: There are many types of procedures performed in a diagnostic imaging department. While all of them use radiation, there are many different categories. Routine, plain examinations, such as a chest x-ray, abdominal x-ray, or bone x-ray use no contrast material and are considered noninvasive procedures.

The information in the Part I studies is organized in a manner to help the student see how the five basic components of the nursing process (assessment, diagnosis, planning, implementation, and evaluation) can be applied to each phase of laboratory and diagnostic testing. The goal is to use nursing process to understand the integration of care (laboratory, diagnostic, nursing care) toward achieving a positive expected outcome.

- **Assessment** is the collection of information for the purpose of answering the question, "is there a problem?" Knowledge of the patient's health history, medications, complaints, and allergies as well as synonyms or alternate test names, common use for the procedure, specimen requirements, and normal ranges or interpretive comments provide the foundation for diagnosis.
- **Diagnosis** is the process of looking at the information gathered during assessment and answering the questions, "what is the problem?" and "what do I need to do about it?" Test indications tell us why the study has been requested, and potential

diagnoses tell us the value or importance of the study relative to its clinical utility.

- **Planning** is a blueprint of the nursing care before the procedure. It is the process of determining how the nurse is going to partner with the patient to fix the problem (e.g., "The patient has a study ordered and this is what I should know before I successfully carry out the plan to have the study completed"). Knowledge of interfering factors, social and cultural issues, preprocedural restrictions, the need for written and informed consent, anxiety about the procedure, and concerns regarding pain are some considerations for planning a successful partnership.

- **Implementation** is putting the plan into action with an idea of what the expected outcome should be. Collaboration with the departments where the laboratory test or diagnostic study is to be performed is essential to the success of the plan. Implementation is where the work is done within each healthcare team member's scope of practice.

- **Evaluation** answers the question, "did the plan work or not?" Was the plan completely successful, partially successful, or not successful? If the plan did not work, evaluation is the process where you determine what needs to be changed to make the plan work better. This includes a review of all expected outcomes. Nursing care after the procedure is where information is gathered to evaluate the plan. Review of results, including critical findings, in relation to patient symptoms and other tests performed, provides data that form a more complete picture of health or illness.

- **Expected Outcomes** are positive outcomes related to the test. They are the outcomes the nurse should expect if all goes well.

A number of pretest, intratest, and post-test universal points are presented in this overview section because the information applies to plain radiologic studies in general.

Universal Pretest Pearls (Planning)

- Obtain a history of the patient's complaints, including a list of known allergens, especially allergies or sensitivities to medications or latex so that their use can be avoided or their effects mitigated if an allergy is present. Carefully evaluate all medications currently being taken by the patient. A list of the patient's current medications, prescribed and over the counter (including anticoagulants, aspirin and other salicylates, and dietary supplements), should also be obtained. Such products

may be discontinued by medical direction for the appropriate number of days prior to the procedure. Ensure that all allergies are clearly noted in the medical record, especially allergies or sensitivities to latex, anesthetics, or sedatives. Ensure that the patient with known allergies is wearing an allergy and medical record armband. Report to the HCP and department performing the study any information that could interfere with, or delay proceeding with, the study.

- Obtain a history of the patient's affected body system, symptoms, and results of previously performed laboratory tests and diagnostic and surgical procedures. Previous test results will provide a basis of comparison between old and new data.

- An important aspect of planning is understanding the factors that may alter study findings or cause abnormal results. Interdepartmental communication is a key factor in the planning process. The inability of a patient to cooperate or remain still during the procedure because of age, significant pain, or mental status should be among the anticipated factors. Recent or past procedures, medications, or existing medical conditions that could complicate or interfere with test results should be noted.

- Review the steps of the study with the patient or caregiver. Expect patients to be nervous about the procedure itself and the pending results. Educating the patient about his or her role during the procedure and what to expect can facilitate this. The patient's role during the procedure is to remain still. The actual time required to complete each study will depend on a number of conditions, including the type of equipment being used and how well a patient will cooperate.

- Address any concerns about pain, and explain or describe, as appropriate, the level and type of discomfort that may be expected during the procedure. Make the patient aware that there may be some mild discomfort during the procedure.

- Provide additional instructions and patient preparation regarding medication, diet, fluid intake, or activity, if appropriate. Unless specified in the individual study, there are no special instructions or restrictions.

- Address any concerns about pain and explain or describe, as appropriate, the level and type of discomfort that may be expected during the procedure. Explain that an IV line or catheter may be inserted prior to some procedures to allow infusion of IV fluids such as normal saline, antibiotics, contrast medium, anesthetics, sedatives, medications used in the procedure, or emergency medications. Advise the patient that some discomfort may be experienced during the insertion of the IV. Make the patient aware that there may be some mild discomfort during the procedure.

- Always be sensitive to any cultural or psychosocial issues, including a concern for modesty before, during, and after the procedure.

Reminder

Ensure that a written and informed consent has been documented in the medical record prior to the study, if required. The consent must be obtained before medication is administered.

Universal Intratest Pearls (Implementation)

- Correct patient identification is crucial prior to any procedure: Positively identify the patient using two unique identifiers, such as patient name, date of birth, Social Security number, or medical record number.
- Standard Precautions must be followed.
- Children and infants may be accompanied by a parent to calm them. Keep neonates and infants covered and in a warm room, and provide a pacifier or gentle touch. The testing environment should be quiet, and the patient should be instructed, as appropriate, to remain still during the test as extraneous movements can affect results.
- Ensure that the patient has complied with pretesting instructions, including dietary, fluid, medication, and activity restrictions as given for the procedure. The number of days to withhold medication depends on the type of medication. Notify the HCP if pretesting instructions have not been followed (e.g., if applicable, if patient anticoagulant therapy has not been withheld).
- Enemas must be administered if ordered.
- As appropriate, preparation must be made for the insertion of an IV line for the infusion of IV fluids, antibiotics, contrast medium, anesthetics, analgesics, medications used in the procedure, or emergency medications. Inform the patient when prophylactic antibiotics will be administered before the procedure and assess for antibiotic allergy. Prior to administration of any fluids or medications, verify that they are accurate for the study. Bleeding or bruising can be prevented, once the needle has been removed, by applying direct pressure to the injection site with dry gauze for a minute or two. The site should be observed/assessed for bleeding or hematoma formation, and then covered with a gauze and adhesive bandage.
- Emergency equipment must be readily available.

- Baseline vital signs should be recorded and continue to be monitored throughout and after the procedure, according to organizational policy. A comparison should be made between the baseline and postprocedure vital signs and focused assessments. Protocols may vary among facilities.

Universal Post Test Pearls (Evaluation)

- Note that completed test results are made available to the requesting HCP, who will discuss them with the patient.
- Answer questions and address concerns voiced by the patient or family and reinforce information given by the patient's HCP regarding further testing, treatment, or referral to another HCP. Recognize that patients will have anxiety related to test results. Provide teaching and information regarding the clinical implications of the test results on the patient's lifestyle as appropriate.
- Note that test results should be evaluated in context with the patient's signs, symptoms, and diagnosis. Depending on the results of the procedure, additional testing may be performed to evaluate or monitor progression of the disease process and determine the need for a change in therapy.
- Be aware that when a person goes through a traumatic event such as an illness or is being given information that will impact his or her lifestyle, there are universal human reactions that occur. These include knowledge deficit, fear, anxiety, and coping; in some situations grieving may occur. HCPs should always be aware of the human response and how it may affect the plan of care and expected outcomes.

DISCUSSION POINT

Regarding Post-Test Critical Findings: Timely notification of a critical finding for lab or diagnostic studies is a role expectation of the professional nurse. Notification processes will vary among facilities. Upon receipt of the critical finding, the information should be read back to the caller to verify accuracy. Most policies require immediate notification of the primary HCP, hospitalist, or on-call HCP. Reported information includes the patient's name, unique identifiers, critical finding, name of the person giving the report, and name of the person receiving the report. Documentation of notification should be made in the medical record with the name of the HCP notified, time and date of notification, and any orders received. Any delay in a timely report of a critical finding may require completion of a notification form with review by Risk Management.

STUDIES

- Bone Mineral Densitometry
- Chest X-Ray
- Kidney, Ureter, and Bladder Study
- Radiography, Bone
- Vertebroplasty

LEARNING OUTCOMES

Providing safe, effective nursing care (SENC) includes mastery of core competencies and standards of care. SENC is based on a judicious application of nursing knowledge in combination with scientific principles. The Art of Nursing lies in blending what you know with the ability to effectively apply your knowledge in a compassionate manner.

Thinking

1. Recognize patient concerns as a result of age in the procedure preparation.

Doing

1. Develop and implement an individualized plan of care based on patient preferences and specific health-care needs.

Caring

1. Acknowledge the value of cultural diversity in the provision of care.

Bone Mineral Densitometry

Quick Summary

SYNONYM ACRONYM: DEXA, DXA, SXA, QCT, RA, ultrasound densitometry.

Dual-energy x-ray absorptiometry (DEXA, DXA): Two x-rays of different energy levels measure bone mineral density and predict risk of fracture.

Single-energy x-ray absorptiometry (SXA): A single-energy x-ray measures bone density at peripheral sites.

Quantitative computed tomography (QCT): QCT is used to examine the lumbar vertebrae. It measures trabecular and cortical bone density. Results are compared to a known standard. This test is the most expensive and involves the highest radiation dose of all techniques.

Radiographic absorptiometry (RA): A standard x-ray of the hand. Results are compared to a known standard.

Ultrasound densitometry: Studies bone mineral content in peripheral densitometry sites such as the heel or wrist. It is not as precise as x-ray techniques but is less expensive than other techniques.

COMMON USE: To evaluate bone density related to osteoporosis.

AREA OF APPLICATION: Lumbar spine, heel, hip, wrist, whole body.

NORMAL FINDINGS

- Normal bone mass with T-score value not less than −1.

Test Explanation

Bone mineral density (BMD) can be measured at any of several body sites, including the spine, hip, wrist, and heel. Equipment used to measure BMD include computed tomography (CT), radiographic absorptiometry, ultrasound, SXA, and most commonly, DEXA. The radiation exposure from SXA and DEXA machines is approximately one-tenth that of a standard chest x-ray.

Osteoporosis is a condition characterized by low BMD, which results in increased risk of fracture. The National Osteoporosis Foundation estimates that 4 to 6 million postmenopausal women in the United States have osteoporosis, and an additional 13 to 17 million (30% to 50%) have low bone density at the hip. It is estimated that one of every two women will experience a fracture as a result of low bone mineral content in her lifetime. The measurement of BMD gives the best indication of risk for a fracture. The lower the BMD, the greater is the risk of fracture. The most common fractures are those of the hip, vertebrae, and distal forearm. Bone mineral loss is a disease of the entire skeleton and is not restricted to the areas listed. The effect of the fractures has a wide range, from complete recovery to chronic pain, disability, and possible death.

The BMD values measured by the various techniques cannot be directly compared. Therefore, they are stated in terms of standard deviation (SD) units. The patient's T-score is the number of SD units above or below the average BMD in young adults. A Z-score is the number of SD units above or below the average value for a person of the same age as the measured patient. Since bone loss occurs naturally as part of the aging process, using a patient's Z-score in comparison to a person of the same age could be misleading, especially in the early development of osteoporosis. The World Health Organization has defined normal bone density as being within (above or below) 1 SD of the mean for young adults. Low bone density is defined as density below 1 SD and 2.5 SD the mean for young adults, bone density 2.5 SD or more below the mean for young adults is indicative of osteoporosis (osteopenia), and bone density more than 2.5 SD below the mean for young adults is defined as severe (established) osteoporosis. The baseline age for young adults is approximately 30 years of age. For most BMD readings, 1 SD is equivalent to 10% to 12% of the average young-normal BMD value. A T-score of −2.5 is therefore equivalent to a bone mineral loss of 30% when compared to a young adult.

Nursing Implications

Assessment

Indications	Potential Nursing Problems
Determine the mineral content of bone Determine a possible cause of amenorrhea Establish a diagnosis of osteoporosis Estimate the actual fracture risk compared to young adults Evaluate bone demineralization associated with chronic conditions (e.g., chronic kidney disease) or long-term use of corticosteroids Evaluate bone demineralization associated with immobilization Evaluate secondary causes of bone demineralization associated with endocrine disorders (e.g., Cushing syndrome, diabetes, eating disorders, hyperparathyroidism, hyperprolactemia) Monitor changes in BMD due to medical problems (e.g., multiple myeloma, malabsorption) or therapeutic intervention Predict future fracture risk	• Activity • Breathing • Body Image • Constipation • Fall Risk • Human Response • Injury Risk • Mobility • Nutrition • Pain • Self-care • Sexuality • Socialization

Diagnosis: Clinical Significance of Test Results

ABNORMAL FINDINGS

- Osteoporosis is defined as T-score value less than −2.5.
- Low bone mass or osteopenia has T-scores from −1 to −2.5.
- Fracture risk increases as BMD declines from young-normal levels (low T-scores).
- Low Z-scores in older adults can be misleading because low BMD is common.
- Z-scores estimate fracture risk compared to others of the same age (versus young-normal adults).

Planning

Considerations for planning a successful partnership should include clear communication of what to expect during the test to decrease anxiety and improve cooperation. Before the procedure is performed, plan to review the steps with the patient. Address concerns about pain related to the procedure, and explain that some pain may be experienced during the test or that there may be moments of discomfort. Inform the patient that the procedure is usually performed in a radiology department by a health-care provider (HCP) and staff specializing in this procedure and takes approximately 60 minutes.

CONTRAINDICATIONS

- Patients who are pregnant or suspected of being pregnant, unless the potential benefits of a procedure using radiation far outweigh the risks to the fetus and mother

SPECIAL CONSIDERATIONS

An important aspect of planning is understanding the factors that may alter study findings or cause abnormal results. Interdepartmental communication is a key factor in the planning process. The following should be noted when planning for this study:

- The use of anticonvulsant drugs, cytotoxic drugs, tamoxifen, glucocorticoids, lithium, or heparin, as well as increased alcohol intake, increased aluminum levels, excessive thyroxin, kidney dialysis, or smoking may affect the test results by either increasing or decreasing the bone mineral content.
- The patient may be unable to cooperate or remain still during the procedure because of age, significant pain, or mental status; uncooperative patients, including children, may need sedation as motion causes artifacts on the image.
- Metallic objects within the examination field (e.g., jewelry, body rings) may inhibit organ visualization and cause unclear images.

● *Safety Tip*

Consultation with a HCP should occur before the procedure for radiation safety concerns regarding younger patients or patients who are lactating.

PEDIATRIC CONSIDERATIONS

Information on the Image Gently Campaign can be found at the Alliance for Radiation Safety in Pediatric Imaging (www.pedrad.org/associations/5364/ig/). Risks associated with radiation overexposure can result from frequent x-ray procedures. Personnel in the examination room with the patient should wear a protective lead apron, stand behind a shield, or leave the area while the examination is being done. Personnel working in the examination area should wear badges to record their level of radiation exposure.

Implementation

Patient education is key to obtaining the patient's cooperation in following directions, and providing an explanation for the purpose of the procedure is an important part of this process. Inform the patient that this study can assist in assessing for mineral content of the bones.

Position the patient in a supine position on the imaging table with the patient's arms above her or his head. Foam wedges may be used to help maintain position and immobilization. The radiation source and detectors move over the area being scanned. The images are reviewed by the technologist on a special viewing

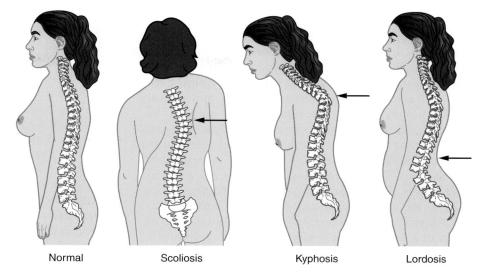

FIGURE 16.1 Spinal curvatures. *Used with permission, from Tamparo, C., & Lewis, M. (2011). Diseases of the human body (5th ed.). FA Davis Company.*

Normal   Scoliosis   Kyphosis   Lordosis

monitor in the scanning room and then recorded digitally for radiologist interpretation (see Fig. 16.1).

Evaluation

Recognize anxiety related to test results and be supportive of a perceived loss of independence. Discuss the implications of abnormal test results on the patient's lifestyle. Provide teaching and information regarding the clinical implications of bone loss as appropriate. Assure the patient that although there is no cure for osteoporosis, there are steps she or he can take to prevent, slow, or stop its progress. Answer any questions or address any concerns voiced by the patient or family. Educate the patient with vitamin D deficiency, as appropriate, that foods high in calcium and vitamin D should be included in the diet. Examples of foods rich in calcium and vitamin D are yogurt, cheese, cottage cheese, canned sardines with bones, flounder, salmon, dried figs, and dark green leafy vegetables such as spinach and broccoli. Processed foods with added calcium, such as breads and cereals, can also be included. Avoiding red meat and high-fat foods that bind calcium in the intestine can reduce loss. The excess use of alcohol, salt, or caffeine can also decrease absorption. Explain to the patient that vitamin D is also synthesized by the body, in the skin, and is activated by sunlight. Daily recommendations for calcium and vitamin D intake are based on age. Calcium and vitamin D supplements may be used if dietary intake is insufficient. Provide contact information, if desired, for the Institute of Medicine of the National Academies (www.iom.edu) or the USDA's resource for nutrition (http://www.choosemyplate.gov/). Educate the patient regarding access to counseling services, and provide contact information, if desired, for the National Osteoporosis Foundation at http://nof.org/.

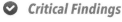 **Critical Findings**

N/A

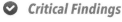 **Study Specific Complications**

N/A

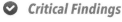 **Related Tests**

- Related tests include ALP, antibodies anticyclic citrullinated peptide, ANA, arthrogram, arthroscopy, biopsy bone, bone scan, calcium, CRP, collagen cross-linked telopeptides, CT pelvis, CT spine, ESR, MRI musculoskeletal, MRI pelvis, osteocalcin, PTH, phosphorus, radiography bone, RF, synovial fluid analysis, and vitamin D.
- Refer to the Musculoskeletal System table at the end of the book for related tests by body system.

Expected Outcomes

Expected outcomes associated with Bone Mineral Densitometry are

- Understanding that sexual dysfunction is due to pain and spinal deformity
- Proactively seeking information regarding current treatment modalities
- Adapting the home environment to prevent falls and injury

Chest X-Ray

Quick Summary

SYNONYM ACRONYM: Chest radiography, CXR, lung radiography.

COMMON USE: To assist in the evaluation of cardiac, respiratory, and skeletal structure within the lung cavity and diagnose multiple diseases such as pneumonia and heart failure.

AREA OF APPLICATION: Heart, mediastinum, lungs.

NORMAL FINDINGS
- Normal lung fields, cardiac size, mediastinal structures, thoracic spine, ribs, and diaphragm

Test Explanation

Chest radiography, commonly called chest x-ray, is one of the most frequently performed radiological diagnostic studies. This study yields information about the pulmonary, cardiac, and skeletal systems. The lungs, filled with air, are easily penetrated by x-rays and appear black on chest images. A routine chest x-ray includes a posteroanterior (PA) projection, in which x-rays pass from the posterior to the anterior, and a left lateral projection. Additional projections that may be requested are obliques, lateral decubitus, or lordotic views. Portable x-rays, done in acute or critical situations, can be done at the bedside and usually include only the anteroposterior (AP) projection with additional images taken in a lateral decubitus position if the presence of free pleural fluid or air is in question. Chest images should be taken on full inspiration and erect when possible to minimize heart magnification and demonstrate fluid levels. Expiration images may be added to detect a pneumothorax or locate foreign bodies. Rib detail images may be taken to delineate bone pathology, useful when chest radiographs suggest fractures or metastatic lesions. Fluoroscopic studies of the chest can also be done to evaluate lung and diaphragm movement. In the beginning of the disease process of tuberculosis, asthma, and chronic obstructive pulmonary disease, the results of a chest x-ray may not correlate with the clinical status of the patient and may even be normal.

Nursing Implications

Assessment

Indications	Potential Nursing Problems
Aid in the diagnosis of diaphragmatic hernia, lung tumors, IV devices, and metastasis	• Activity
	• Breathing
Evaluate known or suspected pulmonary disorders, chest trauma, cardiovascular disorders, and skeletal disorders	• Cardiac Output
	• Fall Risk
	• Family
	• Fear
Evaluate placement and position of an endotracheal tube, tracheostomy tube, nasogastric feeding tube, pacemaker wires, central venous catheters, Swan-Ganz catheters, chest tubes, and intra-aortic balloon pump	• Fluid Volume
	• Gas Exchange
	• Human Response
	• Injury Risk
	• Pain
	• Role Performance
Evaluate positive purified protein derivative (PPD) or Mantoux tests	• Self-care
	• Sexuality
Monitor resolution, progression, or maintenance of disease	• Tissue Perfusion
Monitor effectiveness of the treatment regimen	

Diagnosis: Clinical Significance of Test Results

ABNORMAL FINDINGS
- Atelectasis
- Bronchitis
- Curvature of the spinal column (scoliosis)
- Enlarged heart
- Enlarged lymph nodes
- Flattened diaphragm
- Foreign bodies lodged in the pulmonary system as seen by a radiopaque object
- Fractures of the sternum, ribs, and spine
- Lung pathology, including tumors
- Malposition of tubes or wires
- Mediastinal tumor and pathology
- Pericardial effusion
- Pericarditis
- Pleural effusion
- Pneumonia
- Pneumothorax
- Pulmonary bases, fibrosis, infiltrates
- Tuberculosis
- Vascular abnormalities

Planning

Considerations for planning a successful partnership should include clear communication of what to expect during the test to decrease anxiety and improve cooperation. Before the procedure is performed, plan to review the steps with the patient. Address concerns about pain, and explain that no pain will be experienced during the test. Inform the patient that the procedure is performed in the radiology department or at the bedside by a registered radiological technologist and takes approximately 5 to 15 minutes.

PEDIATRIC CONSIDERATIONS

Preparing children for a chest x-ray depends on the age of the child. Encourage parents to be truthful about what the child may experience during the procedure and to use words that they know their child will understand. Toddlers and preschool-age children have a very short attention span, so the best time to talk about the test is right before the procedure. The child should be assured that he or she will be allowed to bring a favorite comfort item into the examination room and, if appropriate, that a parent will be with the child during the procedure. Provide older children with information about the test and allow them to participate in as many decisions as possible (e.g., the choice of clothes to wear to the appointment) in order to reduce anxiety and encourage cooperation. If the child will be asked to maintain a certain position for the test, encourage the child to practice the required position, provide a CD that demonstrates the procedure, and teach strategies to remain calm, such as deep breathing, humming, or counting to him- or herself.

CONTRAINDICATIONS

- Patients who are pregnant or who are suspected of being pregnant, unless the potential benefits of a procedure using radiation far outweigh the risks to the fetus and mother

SPECIAL CONSIDERATIONS

An important aspect of planning is understanding the factors that may alter study findings or cause abnormal results. Interdepartmental communication is a key factor in the planning process. The following should be noted when planning for this study:

- The radiographic equipment must be properly adjusted to accommodate obese or thin patients to avoid causing underexposure or overexposure.
- The patient may be unable to cooperate or remain still during the procedure because of age, significant pain, or mental status; uncooperative patients, including children, may need sedation as motion causes artifacts on the image.
- Metallic objects within the examination field (e.g., jewelry, body rings) may inhibit organ visualization and cause unclear images.
- The occurrence of chest pain or severe cardiac dysrhythmias may require termination of the procedure

● *Safety Tip*

Consultation with a health-care provider (HCP) should occur before the procedure for radiation safety concerns regarding younger patients or patients who are lactating.

PEDIATRIC CONSIDERATIONS

Information on the Image Gently Campaign can be found at the Alliance for Radiation Safety in Pediatric Imaging (www.pedrad.org/associations/5364/ig/). Risks associated with radiation overexposure can result from frequent x-ray procedures. Personnel in the examination room with the patient should wear a protective lead apron, stand behind a shield, or leave the area while the examination is being done. Personnel working in the examination area should wear badges to record their level of radiation exposure.

Implementation

Patient education is key to obtaining the patient's cooperation in following directions, and providing an explanation for the purpose of the procedure is an important part of this process. Inform the patient that this study can assist in assessing for abnormalities of the lungs and surrounding structures.

Position the patient in an upright position with his or her anterior chest against the cassette or image detector, with hands on hips, neck extended, and shoulders rolled forward for the PA view. Instruct the patient to take in a deep breath and hold it, and then to exhale

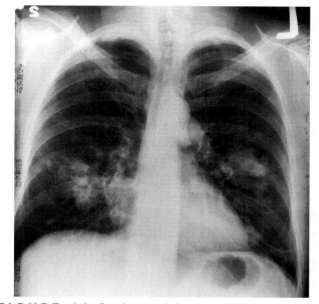

FIGURE 16.2 Abnormal chest x-ray. *Abnormal chest x-ray, released into public domain by the National Cancer Institute. Accessed at https://visualsonline.cancer.gov/details .cfm?imageid=2343*

after the images are taken. Turn the patient with his or her left side against the image board for a lateral view (this places the patient's heart closest to the image receptor for less magnification) and repeat the exposure. For portable examinations, elevate the head of the bed to the high Fowler position. The images are reviewed by the technologist on a special viewing monitor in the scanning room and then recorded digitally for radiologist interpretation (see Fig. 16.2).

Evaluation

Recognize anxiety related to test results and be supportive of a perceived loss of independence. Discuss the implications of abnormal test results on the patient's lifestyle. Provide teaching and information regarding the clinical implications of abnormal lung functions as appropriate. Answer any questions or address any concerns voiced by the patient or family.

✔ *Critical Findings*

- Foreign body
- Malposition of tube, line, or postoperative device (pacemaker)
- Pneumonia
- Pneumoperitoneum
- Pneumothorax
- Spine fracture

Note and immediately report to the requesting HCP any critical findings and related symptoms. A listing of these findings varies among facilities.

✅ Study Specific Complications

N/A

✅ Related Tests

- Related tests include biopsy lung, blood gases, bronchoscopy, CT thoracic, CBC, culture mycobacteria, culture sputum, culture viral, electrocardiogram, Gram stain, lung perfusion scan, MRI chest, pulmonary function study, pulse oximetry, and TB tests.
- Refer to the Cardiovascular and Respiratory systems tables at the end of the book for related tests by body system.

Expected Outcomes

Expected outcomes associated with Chest X-Ray are

- Adapting to an altered ability to function in the designated family role
- Understanding fall prevention education with the absence of a fall event
- Describing symptoms that may indicate a pneumothorax

Kidney, Ureter, and Bladder Study

Quick Summary

SYNONYM ACRONYM: Flat plate of the abdomen, KUB, plain film of the abdomen.

COMMON USE: To visualize and assess the abdominal organs for obstruction or abnormality related to mass, trauma, bleeding, stones, or congenital anomaly.

AREA OF APPLICATION: Kidneys, ureters, bladder, and abdomen.

NORMAL FINDINGS

- Normal size and shape of kidneys
- Normal bladder, absence of masses and renal calculi, and no abnormal accumulation of air or fluid

Test Explanation

A kidney, ureter, and bladder (KUB) x-ray examination provides information regarding the structure, size, and position of the abdominal organs; it also indicates whether there is any obstruction or abnormality of the abdomen caused by disease or congenital malformation. Calcifications of the renal calyces, renal pelvis, and any radiopaque calculi present in the urinary tract or surrounding organs may be visualized in addition to normal air and gas patterns within the intestinal tract. Perforation of the intestinal tract or an intestinal obstruction can be visualized on erect KUB images. KUB x-rays are among the first examinations done to diagnose intra-abdominal diseases such as intestinal obstruction, masses, tumors, ruptured organs, abnormal gas accumulation, and ascites.

Nursing Implications

Assessment

Indications	Potential Nursing Problems
Determine the cause of acute abdominal pain or palpable mass	• Bleeding
Evaluate the effects of lower abdominal trauma, such as internal hemorrhage	• Breathing
Evaluate known or suspected intestinal obstructions	• Constipation
Evaluate the presence of renal, ureter, or other organ calculi	• Fluid Volume
Evaluate the size, shape, and position of the liver, kidneys, and spleen	• Gastrointestinal
Evaluate suspected abnormal fluid, air, or metallic objects in the abdomen	• Human Response
	• Nutrition
	• Pain

Diagnosis: Clinical Significance of Test Results

ABNORMAL FINDINGS

- Abnormal accumulation of bowel gas
- Ascites
- Bladder distention
- Congenital renal anomaly
- Foreign body
- Hydronephrosis
- Intestinal obstruction
- Organomegaly
- Renal calculi
- Renal hematomas
- Ruptured viscus
- Soft tissue masses
- Trauma to liver, spleen, kidneys, and bladder
- Vascular calcification

Planning

Other considerations for planning a successful partnership should include clear communication of what to expect during the test to decrease anxiety and improve cooperation. Before the procedure is performed, plan to review the steps with the patient. Address concerns about pain, and explain that little to no pain is expected during the test, but that there may be moments of discomfort. Inform the patient that the procedure is performed in the radiology department or at the bedside by a registered radiologic technologist and takes approximately 5 to 15 minutes to complete.

CONTRAINDICATIONS

- Patients who are pregnant or suspected of being pregnant, unless the potential benefits of a procedure using radiation far outweigh the risks to the fetus and mother

SPECIAL CONSIDERATIONS

An important aspect of planning is understanding the factors that may alter study findings or cause abnormal results. Interdepartmental communication is a key factor in the planning process. The following should be noted when planning for this study:

- The radiographic equipment must be properly adjusted to accommodate obese or thin patients to avoid underexposure or overexposure.
- The patient may be unable to cooperate or remain still during the procedure because of age, significant pain, or mental status; uncooperative patients, including children, may need sedation as motion causes artifacts on the image.
- Metallic objects within the examination field (e.g., jewelry, body rings) may inhibit organ visualization and cause unclear images.
- Retained barium from a previous radiological procedure may cause unclear images.
- Incorrect positioning of the patient may produce poor visualization of the area to be examined, for images done by portable equipment.

● Safety Tip

Consultation with a health-care provider (HCP) should occur before the procedure for radiation safety concerns regarding younger patients or patients who are lactating.

PEDIATRIC CONSIDERATIONS

Information on the Image Gently Campaign can be found at the Alliance for Radiation Safety in Pediatric Imaging (www.pedrad.org/associations/5364/ig/). Risks associated with radiation overexposure can result from frequent x-ray procedures. Personnel in the examination room with the patient should wear a protective lead apron, stand behind a shield, or leave the area while the examination is being done. Personnel working in the examination area should wear badges to record their level of radiation exposure.

Implementation

Patient education is key to obtaining the patient's cooperation in following directions, and providing an explanation for the purpose of the procedure is an important part of this process. Inform the patient that this study can assist in assessing for abnormalities of the abdominal and pelvic structures.

Position the patient in a supine position on the x-ray table with hands relaxed at the side. Instruct the patient to take in a deep breath and hold it during the exposure. Turn the patient with his or her left side against the table if looking for an abdominal aortic aneurysm or have the patient stand for an erect KUB if looking for free abdominal air. The images are reviewed by the

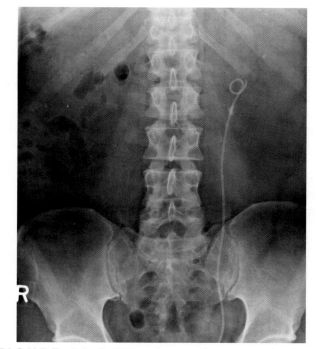

FIGURE 16.3 KUB with ureteral stent. *Used with permission, from Weber, E., Vilensky, J., & Fog, A. (2013). Practical radiology: A symptom-based approach. FA Davis Company.*

technologist on a special viewing monitor in the x-ray room and then recorded digitally for radiologist interpretation (see Fig. 16.3).

Evaluation

Recognize anxiety related to test results and be supportive of a perceived loss of independence. Discuss the implications of abnormal test results on the patient's lifestyle. Provide teaching and information regarding the clinical implications of bowel or visceral abnormalities, as appropriate. Answer any questions or address any concerns voiced by the patient or family. Educate the patient regarding access to counseling services and provide contact information, if desired, for the American Gastroenterological Association (www.gastro.org).

◉ Critical Findings

- Bowel obstruction
- Ischemic bowel
- Visceral injury

Note and immediately report to the requesting HCP any critical findings and related symptoms. A listing of these findings varies among facilities.

◉ Study Specific Complications

N/A

✅ *Related Tests*

- Related tests include angiography renal, calculus kidney stone panel, CT abdomen, CT pelvis, CT renal, IVP, and MRI abdomen, retrograde ureteropyelography, US abdomen, US kidney, US pelvis, and UA.
- Refer to the Gastrointestinal and Genitourinary systems tables at the end of the book for related tests by body system.

Expected Outcomes

Expected outcomes associated with Kidney, Ureter, and Bladder Study are

- Regain normal bowel function, evidenced by active bowel sounds with the passage of flatus and a soft-formed stool
- Have no stones or blood in the urine

Radiography, Bone

Quick Summary

SYNONYM ACRONYM: Arm x-rays, bone x-rays, leg x-rays, orthopedic x-rays, rib x-rays, spine x-rays.

COMMON USE: To assist in evaluating bone pain, trauma, and abnormalities related to disorders or events such as dislocation, fracture, abuse, and degenerative disease.

AREA OF APPLICATION: Skeleton.

NORMAL FINDINGS

- *Infants and children:* Thin plate of cartilage, known as growth plate or epiphyseal plate, between the shaft and both ends
- *Adolescents and adults:* By age 17, calcification of cartilage plate; no evidence of fracture, congenital abnormalities, tumors, or infection

Test Explanation

Skeletal x-rays are noninvasive studies used to evaluate extremity pain or discomfort due to trauma, bone and spine abnormalities, or fluid within a joint. Serial skeletal x-rays are used to evaluate growth pattern. Radiation emitted from the x-ray machine passes through the patient onto an image receptor. X-rays pass through air freely and are absorbed by the anatomical structures of the body in varying degrees based on density. Bones are very dense and therefore absorb or attenuate most of the x-rays passing into the body and appear white; organs and muscles are denser than air but not as dense as bone, so they appear in various shades of gray. Metals absorb x-rays and appear white and thus facilitate the search for foreign bodies in the patient.

Nursing Implications

Assessment

Indications	Potential Nursing Problems
Assist in detecting bone fracture, dislocation, deformity, and degeneration	• Activity
	• Body Image
	• Breathing
Evaluate for child or older adult abuse	• Caregiver
Evaluate growth pattern	• Constipation
Identify abnormalities of bones, joints, and surrounding tissues	• Fall Risk
	• Family
	• Human Response
Monitor fracture healing process	• Infection
	• Injury Risk
	• Mobility
	• Nutrition
	• Pain
	• Role Performance
	• Self-care
	• Skin
	• Sexuality

Diagnosis: Clinical Significance of Test Results

ABNORMAL FINDINGS

- Arthritis
- Bone degeneration
- Bone spurs
- Foreign bodies
- Fracture
- Genetic disturbance (achondroplasia, dysplasia, dyostosis)
- Hormonal disturbance
- Infection, including osteomyelitis
- Injury
- Joint dislocation or effusion
- Nutritional or metabolic disturbances
- Osteoporosis or osteopenia
- Soft tissue abnormalities
- Tumor or neoplastic disease (osteogenic sarcoma, Paget disease, myeloma)

Planning

Considerations for planning a successful partnership should include clear communication of what to expect during the test to decrease anxiety and improve cooperation. Before the procedure is performed, plan to review the steps with the patient. Address concerns about pain, and explain that there may be moments of discomfort and some pain experienced during the test. Inform the patient that the procedure is usually performed in the radiology department by a health-care provider (HCP), with support staff, and takes approximately 10 to 30 minutes.

CONTRAINDICATIONS

- Patients who are pregnant or suspected of being pregnant, unless the potential benefits of a procedure using radiation far outweigh the risks to the fetus and mother

SPECIAL CONSIDERATIONS

An important aspect of planning is understanding the factors that may alter study findings or cause abnormal results. Interdepartmental communication is a key factor in the planning process. The following should be noted when planning for this study:

- The patient may be unable to cooperate or remain still during the procedure because of age, significant pain, or mental status; uncooperative patients, including children, may need sedation as motion causes artifacts on the image.
- Metallic objects within the examination field (e.g., jewelry, body rings) may inhibit organ visualization and cause unclear images.
- Retained barium from a previous radiological procedure may cause unclear images.

● *Safety Tip*

Consultation with a HCP should occur before the procedure for radiation safety concerns regarding younger patients or patients who are lactating.

PEDIATRIC CONSIDERATIONS

Information on the Image Gently Campaign can be found at the Alliance for Radiation Safety in Pediatric Imaging (www.pedrad.org/associations/5364/ig/). Risks associated with radiation overexposure can result from frequent x-ray procedures. Personnel in the examination room with the patient should wear a protective lead apron, stand behind a shield, or leave the area while the examination is being done. Personnel working in the examination area should wear badges to record their level of radiation exposure.

Implementation

Patient education is key to obtaining the patient's cooperation in following directions, and providing an explanation for the purpose of the procedure is an important part of this process. Inform the patient that this study can assist in assessing for abnormalities of the bone and joint structures. The patient may be required to place the body part of interest in several different positions to obtain the proper radiographic images. They may also be asked to inhale deeply or hold their breath while images are being obtained. Explain the importance of remaining still during imaging (see Fig. 16.4).

Evaluation

Recognize anxiety related to test results and be supportive of a perceived loss of independence. Discuss the implications of abnormal test results on the patient's lifestyle. Provide teaching and information regarding

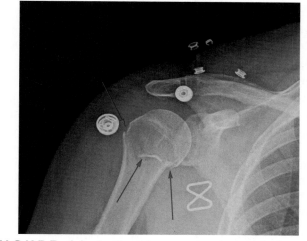

FIGURE 16.4 Shoulder x-ray showing surgical neck fracture of the humerus. *Used with permission, from Weber, E., Vilensky, J., & Fog, A (2013). Practical radiology: A symptom-based approach. FA Davis Company.*

the clinical implications of bone abnormalities and joint functions, as appropriate. Answer any questions or address any concerns voiced by the patient or family.

● *Critical Findings*

N/A

● *Study Specific Complications*

N/A

● *Related Tests*

- Related tests include antibodies anti-cyclic citrullinated peptide, ANA, arthrogram, arthroscopy, biopsy bone, BMD, bone scan, calcium, CBC, CRP, collagen cross-linked telopeptides, CT spine, ESR, MRI musculoskeletal, osteocalcin, phosphorus, synovial fluid analysis, RF, vitamin D, and WBC scan.
- Refer to the Musculoskeletal System table at the end of the book for related tests by body system.

Expected Outcomes

Expected outcomes associated with Radiography, Bone, are

- Being able to make postural changes that do not interfere with respiratory effort
- Agreeing to participate in therapy that will assist in maintaining optimal physical ability

Vertebroplasty

Quick Summary

SYNONYM ACRONYM: None.

COMMON USE: A minimally invasive procedure to treat the spine for disorders such as tumor, lesions, osteoporosis, vertebral compression, and pain.

AREA OF APPLICATION: Spine.

NORMAL FINDINGS
- Improvement in the ability to ambulate without pain
- Relief of back pain

Test Explanation

Vertebroplasty is a minimally invasive, nonsurgical therapy used to repair a broken vertebra and to provide relief of pain related to vertebral compression in the spine that has been weakened by osteoporosis or tumoral lesions. Osteoporosis affects over 10 million women in the United States and accounts for over 700,000 vertebral fractures per year. This procedure is usually successful at alleviating the pain caused by a compression fracture less than 6 months in duration with pain directly referable to the location of the fracture. Secondary benefits may include vertebra stabilization and reduction of the risk of further compression. Vertebroplasty involves the injection of an orthopedic cement mixture through a needle into a fracture site. The cement hardens, stabilizes the bone preventing further collapse, and reduces the pain caused by bone rubbing against bone. The injection is visualized with guidance from radiological imaging or fluoroscopy; a small amount of contrast (with or without iodine) may be used to provide imaged guidance for the injection of the cement. Vertebroplasty may be the preferred procedure when patients are older adults or too frail to tolerate open spinal surgery or if bones are too weak for surgical repair. Patients with a malignant tumor may benefit from vertebroplasty. Other possible applications include in younger patients whose osteoporosis is caused by long-term steroid use or a metabolic disorder. This procedure is recommended after basic treatments such as bedrest and orthopedic braces have failed or when pain medication has been ineffective or caused the patient medical problems, including stomach ulcers.

Nursing Implications

Assessment

Indications	Potential Nursing Problems
Assistance in the detection of nonmalignant tumors before surgical resection Repair of compression spinal fractures of varying ages. Fractures older than 6 months will respond but at a slower rate. Fractures less than 4 weeks old should be given a chance to heal without intervention unless they are associated with disabling pain or hospitalization Repair of spinal problems due to tumors	• Activity • Body Image • Breathing • Constipation • Fall Risk • Human Response • Injury Risk • Mobility • Nutrition • Pain • Self-care • Sexuality • Socialization

Diagnosis: Clinical Significance of Test Results

ABNORMAL FINDINGS
- Failure to reduce the patient's pain
- Failure to improve the patient's mobility

Planning

Considerations for planning a successful partnership should include clear communication of what to expect during the test to decrease anxiety and improve cooperation. Before the procedure is performed, plan to review the steps with the patient. Food and fluids should be restricted for 8 hours prior to the exam. Explain that an IV line may be inserted to allow infusion of IV fluids such as normal saline, anesthetics, sedatives, contrast medium (if a CT study is requested to verify the placement of the vertebroplasty cement), or emergency medications; the vertebroplasty cement will be injected at a separate site, in the spinal fractures. Explain that some discomfort may be experienced during the exam, but IV sedation and/or anesthetics will be administered to ease pain. Inform the patient that the procedure is performed in an interventional radiology room by a radiologist and takes approximately 60 to 90 minutes.

CONTRAINDICATIONS
- Patients who are pregnant or suspected of being pregnant, unless the potential benefits of a procedure using radiation far outweigh the risks to the fetus and mother
- Conditions associated with adverse reactions to vertebroplasty cement
- Conditions associated with adverse reactions to the contrast medium (e.g., asthma, food allergies, or allergy to the contrast medium). Although patients are still asked specifically if they have a known allergy to iodine or shellfish, it has been well established that the reaction is not to iodine; in fact, an actual iodine allergy would be very problematic because iodine is required for the production of thyroid hormones. In the case of shellfish, the reaction is to a muscle protein called *tropomyosin*; in the case of iodinated contrast medium, the reaction is to the noniodinated part of the contrast molecule. Patients with a known hypersensitivity to the medium may benefit from premedication with corticosteroids and diphenhydramine; the use of nonionic contrast or an alternative noncontrast imaging study, if available, may be considered for patients who have severe asthma or who have experienced moderate to severe reactions to ionic contrast medium.
- Conditions associated with preexisting renal insufficiency (e.g., chronic kidney disease, single kidney transplant, nephrectomy, diabetes, multiple myeloma, treatment with aminoglycosides and NSAIDs) because iodinated contrast is nephrotoxic
- Older adult and compromised patients who are chronically dehydrated before the test because of their risk of contrast-induced acute kidney injury

- Patients with bleeding disorders receiving an arterial or venous puncture because the site may not stop bleeding
- Pain that is primarily radicular in nature
- Pain that is improving or that has been present and unchanged for years
- Imaging procedures that suggest no fracture is present or that the fracture is remote from the patient's pain

SPECIAL CONSIDERATIONS

An important aspect of planning is understanding the factors that may alter study findings or cause abnormal results. Interdepartmental communication is a key factor in the planning process. The following should be noted when planning for this study:

- The patient may be unable to cooperate or remain still during the procedure because of age, significant pain, or mental status; uncooperative patients, including children, may need sedation as motion causes artifacts on the image.
- Metallic objects within the examination field (e.g., jewelry, body rings) may inhibit organ visualization and cause unclear images.
- Retained barium from a previous radiological procedure may cause unclear images.
- Gas or feces in the gastrointestinal tract resulting from inadequate cleansing or failure to restrict food intake before the study may cause unclear images.
- The occurrence of chest pain or severe cardiac dysrhythmias may require termination of the procedure.
- Failure to follow dietary restrictions before the procedure may cause the procedure to be canceled or repeated.

● *Safety Tip*

Consultation with a health-care provider (HCP) should occur before the procedure for radiation safety concerns regarding younger patients or patients who are lactating.

PEDIATRIC CONSIDERATIONS

Information on the Image Gently Campaign can be found at the Alliance for Radiation Safety in Pediatric Imaging (www.pedrad.org/associations/5364/ig/). Risks associated with radiation overexposure can result from frequent x-ray procedures. Personnel in the examination room with the patient should wear a protective lead apron, stand behind a shield, or leave the area while the examination is being done. Personnel working in the examination area should wear badges to record their level of radiation exposure.

● *Safety Tip*

Make sure a written and informed consent has been signed prior to the procedure if a biopsy is planned and before administering any medications.

Implementation

Patient education is key to obtaining the patient's cooperation in following directions, and providing an explanation for the purpose of the procedure is an important part of this process. Inform the patient this procedure can assist in repairing fractures of the vertebra. If the patient has a history of allergic reactions to any substance or drug, administer ordered prophylactic steroids or antihistamines before the procedure. Instruct the patient to void prior to the procedure and to change into the gown, robe, and foot coverings provided.

OLDER ADULT CONSIDERATIONS

Older adult patients present with a variety of concerns when undergoing diagnostic procedures. The level of cooperation and fall risk may be complicated by underlying problems such as visual and hearing impairment, joint and muscle stiffness, physical weakness, mental confusion, and the effects of medications. A fall injury can be avoided by providing assistance getting on and off the x-ray table. Older adult patients are often chronically dehydrated; anticipating the effects of hypovolemia and orthostasis can also help prevent falls. Record baseline vital signs and continue to monitor throughout the procedure. Establish an IV fluid line for injection of a anti-anxiety agent or a sedative and place ECG electrodes on the patient. Establish a baseline rhythm. Place the patient in a prone position, cleanse the selected area of the vertebra, and cover with a sterile drape. A local anesthetic is injected at the site, a small incision is made or a needle inserted, and orthopedic cement is injected under flouroscopic guidance. The needle is removed, and a pressure dressing is applied over the puncture site. Observe/assess the needle/catheter insertion site for bleeding, inflammation, or hematoma formation.

Evaluation

Recognize anxiety related to test results and be supportive of a perceived loss of independence. Instruct the patient to resume diet, fluids, and medications, as directed by the health-care providers (HCPs). Renal function should be assessed before metformin is resumed. Monitor vital signs and neurological status every 15 minutes for 1 hour, then every 2 hours for 4 hours, and then as ordered by the HCP. Take temperature every 4 hours for 24 hours. Monitor intake and output at least every 8 hours. Compare all of these with baseline values. Notify the HCP if temperature is elevated. Protocols may vary among facilities. Observe for delayed allergic reactions such as rash, urticaria, tachycardia, hyperpnea, hypertension, palpitations, nausea, or vomiting. Instruct the patient to immediately report symptoms such as fast heart rate, difficulty breathing, skin rash, itching, chest pain, persistent right shoulder pain, or abdominal pain. Immediately report symptoms to the appropriate HCP. Assess extremities for signs of ischemia or absence of distal pulse caused by a catheter-induced thrombus. Instruct the patient to remain in a supine position for about 1 hour to allow for hardening of the cement. Instruct the patient to maintain bedrest for 4 to 6 hours after the procedure or as ordered. Inform the patient that he or she may experience pain relief almost immediately after the procedure, but for some people it may take up to 72 hours. Monitor vital signs as well as intake and output for 2 to 4 hours. Antibiotics for infection and pain medication for discomfort may be prescribed following the procedure. Instruct the patient in the care and assessment of the site. Instruct the patient to apply cold compresses to the puncture site as needed to reduce discomfort or edema. Instruct the patient to avoid strenuous activity, including bending, pushing, stretching, or pulling movements for the first several weeks following the procedure. Active outpatient physical therapy (if appropriate) will begin 3 to 4 weeks after the procedure.

Discuss the implications of abnormal results on the patient's lifestyle. Provide teaching and information regarding the clinical implications of bone abnormalities and joint functions as appropriate. Answer any questions or address any concerns voiced by the patient or family.

✔ Critical Findings

N/A

✔ Study Specific Complications

Injection of the contrast through IV tubing into a blood vessel is an invasive procedure. Complications are rare but do include risk for the following: allergic reaction related to cement or contrast reaction, cardiac dysrhythmias, hematoma related to blood leakage into the tissue following insertion of the IV needle, or infection which might occur if bacteria from the skin surface is introduced at the IV needle insertion site. Other complications related to the use of the cement include soft-tissue damage and nerve impingement related to extravasation of cement, embolism to the lungs related to a blood clot or cement leakage, and respiratory and cardiac failure; risk for complications increases when more than one vertebra is treated at the same time.

✔ Related Tests

- Related tests include bone mineral densitometry, bone scan, CT spine, EMG, and MRI musculoskeletal.
- Refer to the Musculoskeletal System table at the end of the book for related tests by body system.

Expected Outcomes

Expected outcomes associated with Vertebroplasty are

- Understanding the importance of adequate dietary calcium and supplement intake
- Not having constipation as evidenced by a soft bowel movement

REVIEW OF LEARNING OUTCOMES

Thinking

1. Recognize patient concerns as a result of age in the procedure preparation. Answer: Understanding child and adolescent development will help in reducing anxiety and encouraging cooperation during a study. Try to help the child/adolescent with coping skills by suggesting age-appropriate methods.

Doing

1. Develop and implement an individualized plan of care based on patient preferences and specific health-care needs. Answer: Talk to your patient and her or his family. Explore the patient's feelings about the health issues she or he is facing. Try to identify what is most important to the patient. Once you know that, it will help you to frame your information in a way that is acceptable to her or his point of view.

Caring

1. Acknowledge the value of cultural diversity in the provision of care. Answer: Nursing school provides an abstract view of patient care. Student clinical rotations do not provide the same up-close and personal experience that the day-by-day unit assignment does. Human nature is never more evident than when in an emotionally charged clinical situation. Observing how your patients of varying cultures, ages, and ethnicities meet health-care challenges will provide a wonderful palate for your future nursing care.

◖ **Words OF Wisdom:** When some patients hear the word "radiology," they immediately think about radiation exposure. There is an inherent fear factor with that thought. "How many times can I do this before I get radiation poisoning?" This unfounded concern can prevent a patient from making a decision to go ahead with a radiographic study that may identify a disease in the early stages and save her or his life. Patients always have the right to refuse. Our job is to ensure that the refusal is based on the patient's having all of the information she or he needs to make an informed decision. This includes the truth about risk of exposure to radiation.

BIBLIOGRAPHY

ACR Practice guideline for the performance of screening and diagnostic mammography (2013). Retrieved from www.acr.org/~/media/3484ca30845348359bad4684779d492d.pdf

Chest x-ray. (2014). Why it's done. Retrieved from www.mayoclinic.com/health/chest-x-rays/MY00297/DSECTION=why-its-done

Fischbach, F., & Dunning, M. (2009). A laboratory manual of laboratory and diagnostic tests (8th ed.). Philadelphia, PA: Lippincott Williams & Wilkins.

Frank, E., Long, B., & Smith, B. (2012). Merrill's atlas of radiographic positioning and procedures (12th ed.). St. Louis, MO: Elsevier.

Hilhorst, J. (2008). GI bleeds. Retrieved from http://learnpediatrics .com/body-systems/gastrointestinal/gi-bleeds/

LeMone, P., Burke, K., & Baldoff, G. (2011). Medical surgical nursing. Critical thinking in patient care (5th ed.). Upper Saddle River, NJ: Pearson.

Locklin, J., & Wood, B. (2005). Radiofrequency ablation: A nursing perspective. Retrieved from www.ncbi.nlm.nih.gov/pmc/articles/PMC2376767/

National Institutes of Health. (2012). Bone mass measurement: What the numbers mean. Retrieved from www.niams.nih.gov/Health_Info/Bone/Bone_Health/bone_mass_measure.asp

Osteoporosis. (n.d.). Retrieved from www.stritch.luc.edu/lumen/MedEd/hmps/Family%20Medicine-Osteoporosis.htm

Pagana, K., & Pagana, T. (2010). Mosby's manual of diagnostic and laboratory tests (4th ed.). St. Louis, MO: Elsevier.

Radiofrequency ablation of liver tumors. (2013). Retrieved from http://www.radiologyinfo.org/en/info.cfm?pg=rfaliver

Society of Interventional Radiology. (2009). Nonsurgical vertebroplasty is effective pain treatment for spinal fractures caused by osteoporosis or bone tumors. Retrieved from www.sirweb.org/patients/vertebroplasty-osteoporosis/

Sohns, C., Angic, B., Sossalla, S., Konietschke, F., & Obenauer, S. (2010). Computer-assisted diagnosis in full-field digital mammography—Results in dependence of readers experiences. The Breast Journal, 16(5): 490–497. doi:10.1111/j.1524-4741.2010.00963.x

The American College of Radiology Mammography Accreditation Program: Mammography sample written mammography report. (2013). Retrieved from www.acr.org/Quality-Safety/Accreditation/Mammography/Lay-Letters

Van Leeuwen, A., & Bladh, M. (2015). Davis's comprehensive handbook of laboratory and diagnostic testing with nursing implications (6th ed.). Philadelphia, PA: F.A. Davis Company.

Venes, D. (Ed.). (2009). Taber's cyclopedic medical dictionary (21st ed.). Philadelphia, PA: F.A. Davis Company.

Vertebroplasty. (n.d.). Retrieved from www.hopkinsmedicine.org/healthlibrary/printv.aspx?d=135,37

Go to Section II of this book and www.davisplus.com for the Clinical Reasoning Tool and its case studies to provide you with a safe place to explore patient care situations. There are a total of 26 different case studies; 2 cases are presented for each of 13 body systems. One set of 13 cases are found in the Section II chapters, and a second set of 13 cases are available online at www.davisplus.com. Each case is designed with the specific goal of helping you to connect the dots of clinical reasoning. Cases are designed to reflect possible clinical scenarios; the outcomes may or may not be positive—you decide.

Sensory Studies: Auditory

OVERVIEW

Hearing is one of the five basic senses. The ear is considered to be the sensory organ of hearing. The ear is also responsible for equilibrium. Auditory evaluation assesses the ability of a person to hear sound. Sound is measured in intensity (decibels) and tone (Hertz), along with an assessment of air conduction and bone conduction. The ear is composed of an external ear, middle ear, and inner ear that transmit sound to the brain via nerve impulses from the acoustovestibular nerve (also called cranial nerve VIII) (see Fig. 17.1).

The external ear is composed of the outer ear (pinna), the external auditory canal, and the tympanic membrane (eardrum). The pinna is commonly described as the outer ear with one ear located on each side of the head. The way the outer ear (pinna) collects sound helps to identify the direction the sound is coming from. It is the outer ear's role to capture sound waves and funnel them through the external auditory canal toward the tympanic membrane (eardrum). Captured sound waves cause the tympanic membrane (eardrum) to vibrate. The way the tympanic membrane (eardrum) vibrates will determine the type of sound sensed by the individual. Fast vibrations would be sensed as a high-pitched sound.

The middle ear is another part of the ear responsible for hearing. Sound vibrations travel through three ossicles: the malleus (hammer), incus (anvil), and stapes (stirrup). The stapes connects to the oval window, a membrane that lies between the middle and inner ear. The ossicles and oval window are designed to amplify and transmit sound information from the middle to the inner ear. This information is collected by the inner ear and sent to the brain to be understood as a sound.

The inner ear has two functions, to assist hearing and regulate balance. The cochlea is a snail-shaped sensory part of the inner ear that assists with hearing. The cochlea has three fluid-filled canals that transmit information in the form of electrical impulses that the brain can recognize as sound. The first is the cochlear canal, which is filled with endolymph fluid similar in composition to intracelluar fluid. The other two are the vestibular and tympanic canals, which are filled with perilymph fluid similar in composition to cerebrospinal fluid. The different fluids in the canals relate to their role in regulating electrochemical stimulation of the hairs on the organ of Corti. The organ of Corti is found within the cochlea and has thousands of cell hairs that act as hearing receptors. Sound is received through the movement of fluids within the canals through the interaction of the bones of the middle ear and the oval window located in the cochlea. The specific hair cells within the organ of Corti that are stimulated is determined by sound pitch. Sound information is sent to the brain by way of the auditory nerve to the auditory cortex. The inner ear also regulates balance. Balance is based on the movement of fluid in the vestibular canals. Changes in movement of the fluid within these canals sends a message through the vestibular nerve to the cerebellum. This information is transformed into knowledge related to the real-time orientation of the head.

Simply stated, hearing works when sound that enters the ear causes the eardrum to vibrate, resulting in movement of the ossicles and oval window. This movement causes the fluids in the tympanic and vestibular canals of the inner ear to also move. The pressure of the fluid movement within the cochlear canal causes the basilar membrane and hair cells of the organ of Corti to move. Then nerve impulses are sent from the hair cells to the brain by way of the acoustovestibular nerve to be understood as sound.

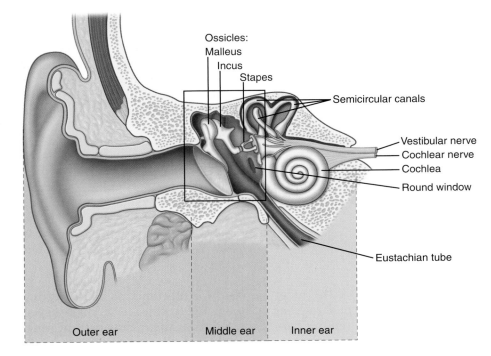

FIGURE 17.1 Anatomy of the ear. *Used with permission, from Thompson, G. (2013). Understanding anatomy & physiology. FA Davis Company.*

DISCUSSION POINT

Hearing screening is completed in every state and territory in the United States. It is the nurse's role to ensure that all newborns have appropriate hearing screens completed and to facilitate interventions. The Centers for Disease Control and Prevention has a program called CDC Hearing Loss Early Hearing Detection and Intervention (EHDI). This is a countrywide effort to facilitate hearing screens for newborns. The purpose of the newborn screening program is early hearing loss detection and intervention. The website at www.cdc.gov/ncbddd/hearingloss/ehdi-programs.html provides information for hearing screens and interventional recommendations for each state. Early hearing loss detection is a team effort that begins with the birth facility within defined protocols. Protocols may change depending on the infant's condition. For example, infants in the neonatal intensive care unit (NICU) with an admission longer than 5 days require automated auditory brainstem response testing in addition to the well-baby otoacoustic emission screen. Testing should be performed prior to discharge or transfer. Technology supports electronic submission of results and referral enrollment data to state public health departments for tracking and inquiry purposes. Facilities are also obligated to develop mechanisms for compliance review. Public health nurses, staff nurses, and others working in medical home/pediatric offices should continue the process of developmental assessment during well visits. Formal screens should be completed at 9, 18, and 24 or 30 months of age or if parents or caregivers express a concern. Objective tests should be performed at 4, 6, 8, and 10 years of age. Follow-up evaluation should be completed for newborns who fail screening. Early referral is essential once a diagnosis of hearing loss has been made.

The goal of early screening is to ensure that all infants are initially screened by 1 month of age. Infants who fail hearing screens should have an evaluation by an audiologist by age 3 months. Appropriate and timely interventions should be provided before 6 months of age. Families of infants with hearing loss should receive culturally competent support. Data management and tracking systems for newborns with hearing loss are linked with other relevant public health information systems. For more information regarding state-sponsored newborn screening, visit the EHDI recommendations for your state.

SPECIAL CONSIDERATIONS

Recognizing infants and children at risk of hearing loss is an important aspect of early detection. There are many conditions that place infants and children at risk for hearing loss. Some of these conditions are Alport, Branchio-Oto-Renal, Charcot-Marie-Tooth, Down, Hunter, Jervell and Lange-Nielsen, Pendred, Stickler, Usher, or Waardenburg craniofacial abnormalities. Family history should be evaluated for others with childhood hearing loss. The infant's mother should be evaluated for a history of infection that could contribute to hearing loss. Some possible infections are cytomegalovirus, rubella virus, syphilis treponeme, herpes virus, or toxoplasma parasite during pregnancy. Other possible causes of infant hearing loss are a history of hyperbilirubinemia that requires transfusion, pulmonary hypertension associated with mechanical ventilation, the use of extracorporeal membrane oxygenation, exposure to ototoxic medication (directly or while in utero), significant postnatal infection such as bacterial meningitis, recurrent or persistent otitis media, and head trauma. Children should be assessed for delayed speech development and any hearing loss. Some loss of hearing due to aging is normal. The degree of hearing loss is dependent on health and environmental factors. Safety precautions will be necessary to protect older adults from injury associated with failure to hear alarms, others' speech, and warnings. For more information on hearing loss in older adults, please visit www.nidcd.nih.gov/health/hearing/pages/older.aspx

The information in the Part I studies is organized in a manner to help the student see how the five basic components of the nursing process (assessment, diagnosis, planning, implementation, and evaluation) can be applied to each phase of laboratory and diagnostic testing. The goal is to use nursing process to understand the integration of care (laboratory, diagnostic, nursing care) toward achieving a positive expected outcome.

- **Assessment** is the collection of information for the purpose of answering the question, "is there a problem?" Knowledge of the patient's health history, medications, complaints, and allergies as well as synonyms or alternate test names, common use for the procedure, specimen requirements, and normal ranges or interpretive comments provide the foundation for diagnosis.
- **Diagnosis** is the process of looking at the information gathered during assessment and answering the questions, "what is the problem?" and "what do I need to do about it?" Test indications tell us why the study has been requested, and potential diagnoses tell us the value or importance of the study relative to its clinical utility.
- **Planning** is a blueprint of the nursing care before the procedure. It is the process of determining how the nurse is going to partner with the patient to fix the problem (e.g., "The patient has a study ordered and this is what I should know before I successfully carry out the plan to have the study completed"). Knowledge of interfering factors, social and cultural issues, preprocedural restrictions, the need for written and informed consent, anxiety about the procedure, and concerns regarding pain are some considerations for planning a successful partnership.
- **Implementation** is putting the plan into action with an idea of what the expected outcome should be. Collaboration with the departments where the laboratory test or diagnostic study is to be performed is essential to the success of the plan. Implementation

is where the work is done within each health-care team member's scope of practice.

- **Evaluation** answers the question, "did the plan work or not?" Was the plan completely successful, partially successful, or not successful? If the plan did not work, evaluation is the process where you determine what needs to be changed to make the plan work better. This includes a review of all expected outcomes. Nursing care after the procedure is where information is gathered to evaluate the plan. Review of results, including critical findings, in relation to patient symptoms and other tests performed provides data that form a more complete picture of health or illness.
- **Expected Outcomes** are positive outcomes related to the test. They are the outcomes the nurse should expect if all goes well.

A number of pretest, intratest, and post-test universal points are presented in this overview section because the information applies to sensory auditory studies in general.

Universal Pretest Pearls (Planning)

- Obtain a history of the patient's complaints, including a list of known allergens, especially allergies or sensitivities to medications or latex so their use can be avoided or their effects mitigated if an allergy is present. Carefully evaluate all medications currently being taken by the patient. A list of the patient's current medications, prescribed and over the counter (including anticoagulants, aspirin and other salicylates, and dietary supplements), should also be obtained. Ensure that all allergies are clearly noted in the medical record, and ensure the patient is wearing an allergy and medical record armband. Report to the health-care provider (HCP) any information that could interfere with, or delay proceeding with, the study.
- Obtain a history of the patient's affected body system, symptoms, and results of previously performed laboratory tests and diagnostic and surgical procedures. Previous test results will provide a basis of comparison between old and new data.
- An important aspect of planning is understanding the factors that may alter study findings or cause abnormal results. Interdepartmental communication is a key factor in the planning process. The inability of a patient to cooperate or remain still during the procedure because of age, significant pain, or mental status should be among the anticipated factors. Recent or past procedures, medications, or existing medical conditions that could complicate or interfere with test results should be noted.

- Review the steps of the study with the patient or caregiver. Expect patients to be nervous about the procedure itself and the pending results. Educating the patient on his or her role during the procedure and what to expect can facilitate this. The patient's role during the procedure is to remain still. The actual time required to complete each study will depend on a number of conditions, including the type of equipment being used and how well a patient will cooperate.
- Address any concerns about pain, and explain or describe, as appropriate, the level and type of discomfort that may be expected.
- Provide additional instructions and patient preparation regarding medication, diet, fluid intake, or activity, if appropriate. Unless specified in the individual study, there are no special instructions or restrictions.
- Always be sensitive to any cultural or psychosocial issues, including concern for modesty before, during, and after the procedure.

Reminder

Ensure that a written and informed consent has been documented in the medical record prior to the study, if required. The consent must be obtained before medication is administered.

Universal Intratest Pearls (Implementation)

- Correct patient identification is crucial prior to any procedure. Positively identify the patient using two unique identifiers, such as patient name, date of birth, Social Security number, or medical record number.
- Standard Precautions must be followed.
- The testing environment should be quiet and the patient or caregiver, as appropriate, should be instructed, as appropriate, to remain still during the test as extraneous movements can affect results. Children and infants may be accompanied by a parent to calm them. Keep neonates and infants covered and in a warm room, and provide a pacifier or gentle touch.
- Ensure that the patient has complied with pretesting instructions.

Universal Post Test Pearls (Evaluation)

- Completed test results are made available to the requesting HCP, who will discuss them with the patient.

- Answer questions and address concerns voiced by the patient or family and reinforce information given by the patient's HCP regarding further testing, treatment, or referral to another HCP. Recognize that patients will have anxiety related to test results. Provide teaching and information regarding the clinical implications of the test results on the patients lifestyle as appropriate.
- Note that test results should be evaluated in context with the patient's signs, symptoms, and diagnosis. Depending on the results of the procedure, additional testing may be performed to evaluate or monitor progression of the disease process and determine the need for a change in therapy.
- When a person goes through a traumatic event such as an illness or being given information that will impact his or her lifestyle, there are universal human reactions that occur. These include knowledge deficit, fear, anxiety, and coping; in some situations, grieving may occur. HCPs should always be aware of the human response and how it may affect the plan of care and expected outcomes.

DISCUSSION POINT

Regarding Post-Test Critical Findings: Timely notification of a critical finding for lab or diagnostic studies is a role expectation of the professional nurse. Notification processes will vary among facilities. Upon receipt of the critical finding, the information should be read back to the caller to verify accuracy. Most policies require immediate notification of the primary HCP, hospitalist, or on-call HCP. Reported information includes the patient's name, unique identifiers, critical finding, name of the person giving the report, and name of the person receiving the report. Documentation of notification should be made in the medical record with the name of the HCP notified, time and date of notification, and any orders received. Any delay in a timely report of a critical finding may require completion of a notification form with review by Risk Management.

STUDIES

- Audiometry, Hearing Loss

LEARNING OUTCOMES

Providing safe, effective nursing care (SENC) includes mastery of core competencies and standards of care. SENC is based on a judicious application of nursing knowledge in combination with scientific principles. The Art of Nursing lies in blending what you know with the ability to effectively apply your knowledge in a compassionate manner.

After reading/studying this chapter you will be able to:

Thinking

1. List some of the common reasons hearing test results may be misleading if pretesting interferences are not investigated, made known, or eliminated prior to the start of the hearing test.
2. List five types of medications known to be ototoxic and discuss why the nurse would need to be aware of the relationship between blood levels of these drugs and the patient's sense of hearing.

Doing

1. Discuss the role of the nurse in the EDHI program.
2. Describe the method to check for canal closure and the corrective measure that can be taken to ensure the ear canal does not close due to compression from the headphones used in the pediatric or adult audiometry hearing test.
3. Describe the safety risks associated with altered auditory perception.

Caring

1. Describe the impact of one's own communication style on others.
2. Acknowledge that there are limitations to the nurse–patient relationship.

Audiometry, Hearing Loss

Quick Summary

COMMON USE: To evaluate hearing loss in newborns and school-age children but can be used for all ages.

AREA OF APPLICATION: Ears.

NORMAL FINDINGS: Normal pure tone average of –10 to 15 dB for infants, children, or adults

Test Explanation

Tests to estimate hearing ability can be performed on patients of any age (e.g., at birth before discharge from a hospital or birthing center, as part of a school screening program, or as adults if indicated). Hearing loss audiometry includes quantitative testing for a hearing deficit. An audiometer is used to measure and record thresholds of hearing by air conduction and bone conduction tests. The test results determine if hearing loss is conductive, sensorineural, or a combination of both. An elevated air-conduction threshold with a normal bone-conduction threshold indicates a conductive hearing loss. An equally elevated threshold for both air and bone conduction indicates a sensorineural hearing loss. An elevated threshold of air conduction that is greater than an elevated threshold of bone conduction indicates a composite of both types of hearing loss. A conductive hearing loss is caused by an abnormality in the external auditory canal or middle ear, and a sensorineural hearing loss by an abnormality in the inner ear or of the VIII (auditory) nerve. Sensorineural hearing loss can be further differentiated clinically by sensory (cochlear) or neural (VIII nerve) lesions. Sensorineural hearing loss is permanent. Additional information for comparing and differentiating between conductive and sensorineural hearing loss can be obtained from hearing loss tuning fork tests. Every state and territory in the United States has a newborn screening program that includes early hearing loss detection and intervention (EHDI). The goal of EHDI is to assure that permanent hearing loss is identified before 3 months of age, appropriate and timely intervention services are provided before 6 months of age, families of infants with hearing loss receive culturally competent support, and tracking and data management systems for newborn hearing screens are linked with other relevant public health information systems.

Nursing Implications

Assessment

Indications	Potential Nursing Problems
Determine the need for a type of hearing aid and evaluate its effectiveness	• Communication
	• Fall Risk
Determine the type and extent of hearing loss and if further radiological, audiological, or vestibular procedures are needed to identify the cause	• Human Reaction
	• Infection
	• Pain
Evaluate communication disabilities and plan for rehabilitation interventions	• Self-esteem
	• Self-image
Evaluate degree and extent of preoperative and postoperative hearing loss following stapedectomy in patients with otosclerosis	• Sensory Perception
	• Socialization
Screen for hearing loss in infants and children and determine the need for a referral to an audiologist	

Diagnosis: Clinical Significance of Test Results

If findings are normal, the patient should have normal hearing. The test is conducted using earphones and/or a device placed behind the ear to deliver sounds of varying intensities. Results are categorized using ranges of pure tone recorded in decibels.

ASHA Category	Pure Tone Averages
Normal range or no impairment	−10–15 dB
Slight loss	16–25 dB
Mild loss	26–40 dB
Moderate loss	41–55 dB
Moderately severe loss	56–70 dB
Severe loss	71–90 dB
Profound loss	Greater than 91 dB

dB = decibel.

ABNORMAL FINDINGS

Causes of conductive hearing loss

- Impacted cerumen
- Hole in eardrum
- Malformed outer ear, ear canal, or middle ear
- Obstruction of external ear canal (related to presence of a foreign body)
- Otitis externa (related to infection in ear canal)
- Otitis media (related to poor eustachian tube function or infection)
- Otitis media serous (related to fluid in middle ear due to allergies or a cold)
- Otosclerosis

Causes of sensorineural hearing loss

- Congenital damage or malformations of the inner ear
- Ménire disease
- Ototoxic drugs administered orally, topically, as otic drops, by IV, or passed to the fetus in utero (aminoglycoside antibiotics, e.g., gentamicin or tobramycin, and chemotherapeutic drugs, e.g., cisplatin and carboplatin, are known to cause permanent hearing loss; quinine, loop diuretics, and salicylates, e.g., aspirin are known to cause temporary hearing loss; other categories of drugs known to be ototoxic include anesthetics, cardiac medications, mood-altering medications, and glucocorticosteroids, e.g., cortisone, steroids)
- Presbycusis (gradual hearing loss experienced in advancing age related to degeneration of the cochlea)
- Serious infections (meningitis, measles, mumps, other viral, syphilis)
- Trauma to the inner ear (related to exposure to noise in excess of 90 dB or as a result of physical trauma)
- Tumor (e.g., acoustic neuroma, cerebellopontine angle tumor, meningioma)
- Vascular disorders

Planning

Considerations for planning a successful partnership should include clear communication of what to expect during the test to decrease anxiety and improve cooperation. Before the procedure is performed, plan to review the steps with the patient. Explain that an otoscopy will be performed before an audiologist or health-care provider (HCP) performs the hearing test in a quiet, soundproof room, and that the test can take up 20 minutes to evaluate both ears. Explain that each ear will be tested separately by using earphones and/or a device placed behind the ear to deliver sounds of varying intensities. Explain and demonstrate to the patient how to communicate with the audiologist and how to exit from the room. Many people are fearful of pain when faced with an unknown situation. Clear communication of any potential discomfort is advised. An example may be to explain the earphones may feel tight when placed over the ears.

SPECIAL CONSIDERATIONS

An important aspect of planning is understanding the factors that may alter study findings or cause abnormal results. Interdepartmental communication is a key factor in the planning process. The following should be noted when planning for this study:

- Attention to testing equipment is essential because improper earphone fit or erroneous audiometer calibration can significantly affect results.
- Tinnitus or other sensations can also cause abnormal responses.

It is also important to understand which medications or substances the patient may be exposed to in the health-care setting that can interfere with accurate testing:

- The effects of ototoxic medications can cause temporary, intermittent, or permanent hearing loss. Patients should be made aware of the potential side effects of ototoxic drugs and should be instructed to report any change in hearing. Vigilance should be used to assess hearing during and after drug use.

Implementation
DISCUSSION POINT

Prior to the start of the test, an otoscopy examination should be performed to ensure that the external ear canal is free from any obstruction (see Fig. 17.2). Test for closure of the canal from the pressure of the earphones by compressing the tragus. Tendency for the canal to close (often the case in children and older adult patients) can be corrected by the careful insertion of a small stiff plastic tube into the anterior canal.

● *Safety Tip*

Address concerns about claustrophobia, as appropriate. Ensure informed and written consent has been obtained before the administration of any medications for claustrophobia, as appropriate.

Patient education is key to obtaining the patient's cooperation in following directions, and providing an explanation for the purpose of the procedure is an important

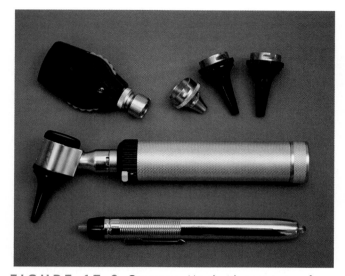

FIGURE 17.2 Otoscope. *Used with permission, from Burton, M. (2011). Fundamentals of nursing care: Concepts, Connections, & Skills. FA Davis Company.*

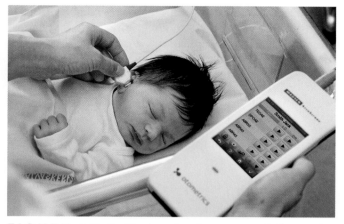

FIGURE 17.3 Newborn hearing screen. *© Otometrics, used with permission.*

part of this process. Inform the patient that this study can assist in the detection of hearing loss. The patient should be placed in a sitting position in close proximity to the audiometer in a soundproof room. The ear not being tested should be masked to prevent crossover of test tones, and the earphones should be positioned on the head and over the ear canals. Age-appropriate equipment, such as insert earphones or ear muffins, may be used to test infants and children unless contraindicated. The auditory response for air conduction is measured through electrodes placed on the infant's scalp. If bone conduction testing is to be performed as part of the hearing assessment, an oscillating probe may be placed on the forehead or over the mastoid process behind the ear (Fig. 17.3).

The test is started by providing a trial tone at 15 to 20 dB above the expected threshold for 1 to 2 seconds in order to familiarize the patient with the type of sounds used during the test. The patient should be instructed to press the button each time a tone is heard, no matter how loudly or faintly it is perceived. If there is no response made by the patient to the trial tone, the HCP conducting the test will increase the level until a response is obtained. The test is continued by increasing the level in 10-dB increments or until the audiometer's limit is reached for the test frequency.

Testing is repeated until the same response is achieved at a 50% response rate at the same hertz level. The threshold is derived from the lowest decibel level at which the patient correctly identifies three out of six responses to a tone at that hertz level. The test is continued for each ear with tones delivered at 1,000 Hz, 2,000 Hz, 4,000 Hz, and 8,000 Hz, and then again at 1,000 Hz, 500 Hz, and 250 Hz to determine a second threshold. Averaging the thresholds at the 500-Hz, 1,000-Hz, and 2,000-Hz levels reveals the degree of hearing loss and is called the pure tone average (PTA).

Results are recorded on a graph called an audiogram. An analysis of thresholds for air and bone conduction tones is done to determine the type of hearing loss (conductive, sensorineural, or mixed).

There are alternative approaches to assist in the assessment of hearing loss in pediatric patients. Minimal response levels in children between 6 months and 2 years of age can be determined by behavioral responses to test tones; playing audiometry that requires the child to perform a task or raise a hand in response to a specific tone is useful in testing children 2 years and older. Children 12 years and older can be asked to follow directions in identifying objects, and their response to speech of specific intensities can be used to evaluate hearing loss that is affected by speech frequencies.

Evaluation

Recognize anxiety related to test results and be supportive of impaired activity related to hearing loss or a perceived loss of independence. Discuss the implications of abnormal test results on the patient's lifestyle. As appropriate, instruct the patient in the use, cleaning, and storage of a hearing aid. Provide teaching and information regarding the clinical implications of the test results as appropriate. Profound hearing loss can have a long-range impact personally, socially, and professionally. Consideration needs to be given to support groups that may guide the patient toward a realistic transition toward life management with an auditory deficit. Educate the patient regarding access to counseling services. Provide contact information, if desired, for the National Center for Hearing Assessment and Management (http://infanthearing.org) or for the American Speech-Language-Hearing Association (www.asha.org) or for assistive technology at ABLEDATA (sponsored by the National Institute on Disability and Rehabilitation Research, www.abledata.com). When caring for a patient with altered auditory function, forms of communication should be adapted to meet the patient's needs. The process of communication chosen should be documented on the plan of care to ensure consistency and decrease frustration.

✅ Critical Findings

N/A

✅ Study Specific Complications

N/A

✅ Related Tests

- Related tests include analgesic and antipyretic drugs, antimicrobial drugs, cultures bacterial (ear), evoked brain potential studies for hearing loss, gram stain, newborn screening, otoscopy, spondee speech reception threshold, and tuning fork tests (Webber, Rinne).
- Refer to the table of tests associated with the Auditory System at the end of the book.

Expected Outcomes

Expected clinical and patient-focused outcomes associated with Audiometry, Hearing Loss, testing are

- Accurate measurement and classification of the patient's hearing level
- Effective implementation of rehabilitative therapies for patients diagnosed with hearing loss followed by an improvement in patient status
- Demonstrated ability to communicate needs with a minimum of frustration
- Commitment to learn and utilize alternate methods of communication

REVIEW OF LEARNING OUTCOMES

Thinking

1. List some of the common reasons hearing test results may be misleading if pretesting interferences are not investigated, made known, or eliminated prior to the start of the hearing test. Answer: There are a number of factors that can affect the outcome of hearing studies. Medical conditions such as tinnitus, obstruction of the auditory canal with cerumen, dried drainage, foreign bodies, or the effects of ototoxic medications can cause temporary, intermittent, or permanent hearing loss. Test results can be affected by the following: problems with equipment, such as improper earphone fit or audiometer calibration; inappropriate testing conditions, such as a noisy test environment; an inability of the patient to understand how to identify responses; or an unwillingness of the patient to cooperate during the test because of age, language barriers, significant pain, or mental status.

2. List five types of medications known to be ototoxic, and discuss why the nurse would need to be aware of the relationship between blood levels of these drugs and the patient's sense of hearing. Answer: The degree of hearing loss associated with ototoxic drug use is dependent upon the drug prescribed. Aminoglycoside antibiotics such as gentamicin, tobramycin, neomycin, kanomycin, and streptomycin, as well as chemotherapeutic drugs such as cisplatin and carboplatin are known to cause permanent hearing loss. Temporary hearing loss can be caused by quinine, salicylates such as aspirin and loop diuretics such asethacrynic acid, furosemide, and bumetanide. It is important to consider the possibility that the patient may be receiving different types of ototoxic medications at the same time. Sedated or bed-bound patients may not be aware of problems with balance, which increases fall risk. Careful attention to blood levels for antibiotics and frequent symptom assessments could make the difference in preventing permanent hearing loss in the patient.

Doing

1. Discuss the role of the nurse in the EDHI program. Answer: EDHI is a team effort that begins with the nurse in the birth facility. Generally, there are separate protocols for NICU and well-infant nursery hearing screens; for example, NICU admissions longer than 5 days require automated auditory brainstem response in addition to the otoacoustic emission screen performed on well infants. Testing should be performed prior to discharge or transfer and technology is available for facilities to electronically submit results and referral enrollment data to state public health departments for tracking and inquiry purposes. Recognizing infants and children at risk of hearing loss is an important aspect of early detection. Patient and a family history of current or past conditions and their treatments, as well as direct observation, provide important information. Public health departments, nurses in public health services, and nurses and other staff in the medical home/pediatric offices continue the process of developmental assessment during well visits, follow up on evaluations for failed newborn screens, and make referrals for early intervention services once a diagnosis of hearing loss has been established.

2. Describe the method to check for canal closure and the corrective measures that can be taken to ensure the ear canal does not close due to compression from the headphones used in the pediatric or adult audiometry hearing test. Answer: Test for closure of the canal from the pressure of the earphones by

compressing the tragus. Tendency for the canal to close (often the case in children and older adult patients) can be corrected by the careful insertion of a small, stiff plastic tube into the anterior canal.

3. Describe the safety risks associated with altered auditory perception. Answer: An increased fall risk exists due to equilibrium issues, misunderstanding, or not receiving important directions.

Caring

1. Describe the impact of one's own communication style on others. Answer: Acknowledging one's personal communication style allows for making adjustments to better meet patient needs. Remember that the best method of communication is whatever works best for them and allows for accurate communication of information, needs, and wants.

2. Acknowledge that there are limitations to the nurse–patient relationship. Answer: Collaborate with the patient to meet care needs. Some patients want you to do everything for them, both simple and small tasks. Some patients want to be independent to the point of injury risk. Your job is to discover what works and does not work and then to use what works to encourage the patient to engage in activities that will provide the best outcome with the least risk.

Words OF Wisdom: Accurate communication is clearly a nursing role. How can you collaborate with your patients in planning their care if you cannot communicate with them? You cannot. To be successful in meeting your patient's needs, you will have to discover what works and what does not work as an alternate means of communication. Hand gestures can be a way to communicate, but the problem is that some hand gestures are culturally inappropriate. Remember that to lose one of your senses is terrifying, especially your hearing. Work with your patient to discover the answer to the question, "How can we talk to each other in a way that causes the least amount of frustration, with the best level of understanding?" You will find this to be one of the biggest challenges throughout your nursing career.

BIBLIOGRAPHY

American Academy of Pediatrics. (2007). Year 2007 Position statement: Principles and guidelines for early hearing detection and intervention programs. Retrieved from http://pediatrics.aap-publications.org/content/120/4/898.full?ijkey=oj9BAleq21OlA&keytype=ref&siteid=aapjournals

Cavanaugh, B. (2003). Nurse's manual of laboratory and diagnostic tests (4th ed.). Philadelphia, PA: F.A. Davis Company.

CDC Hearing Loss Early Hearing Detection and Intervention (EHDI). Retrieved from www.cdc.gov/ncbddd/hearingloss/ehdi-programs.html

Cone, B., Dorn, P., Konrad-Martin, D., Lister, J., Ortiz, C., & Schairer, K. (2012). Ototoxic medications. Retrieved from www.asha.org/public/hearing/Ototoxic-Medications/

How Hearing Works. Retrieved from http://healthhowstuffworks.com/mental-health/human-nature/perception/hearing1.html

How the ear works. (n.d.). Retrieved from www.hearingcentral.com/howtheearworks.asp

Janssen, R. (2009). Syndromes commonly associated with hearing loss in children. Retrieved from http://libguides.lib.umanitoba.ca/content.php?pid=264188&sid=2181101

Kaufman, O. (2000). Ototoxic medications. Retrieved from http://www.nvrc.org/wp-content/uploads/2010/12/Drugs-that-Cause-HL.pdf

Mudd, P. (2012). Ototoxicity. Retrieved from http://emedicine.medscape.com/article/857679-overview

Smith, R., Shearer, A.E., Hildebrand, M., and Van Camp, G. (2014). Deafness and hereditary hearing loss overview. Retrieved from http://www.ncbi.nlm.nih.gov/books/NBK1434/

Van Leeuwen, A., & Bladh, M. (2015). Davis's comprehensive handbook of laboratory and diagnostic testing with nursing implications (6th ed.). Philadelphia, PA: F.A. Davis Company.

Venes, D. (Ed.). (2009). Taber's cyclopedic medical dictionary (21st ed.). Philadelphia, PA: F.A. Davis Company.

Go to Section II of this book and www.davisplus.com for the Clinical Reasoning Tool and its case studies to provide you with a safe place to explore patient care situations. There are a total of 26 different case studies; 2 cases are presented for each of 13 body systems. One set of 13 cases are found in the Section II chapters, and a second set of 13 cases are available online at www.davisplus.com. Each case is designed with the specific goal of helping you to connect the dots of clinical reasoning. Cases are designed to reflect possible clinical scenarios; the outcomes may or may not be positive—you decide.

Sensory Studies: Ocular

OVERVIEW

People have five senses: touch, taste, smell, sight, and hearing. This chapter covers studies that evaluate sight. The eye is the sensory organ of vision. The eye is very small and complex and is composed of the cornea, pupil, iris, lens, retina, and optic nerve. Vision can be altered if any of these components is compromised. The sclera is the outermost layer of the eye and helps the eye keep its shape. The cornea is found at the front of the sclera and is a protective transparent covering for the iris, pupil, and anterior portion of the eye. The cornea bends light waves that pass the iris and enter the pupil. The iris is the colored part of the eye; it may be blue, green, brown, hazel, or a combination of colors. The color of the iris is distinctive to each individual. The iris has two muscles, a dilator and a sphincter, which control the amount of light that enters the pupil. The dilator muscle will make the pupil larger, allowing more light in, and the sphincter muscle will make the pupil smaller, allowing less light in. The result is that the pupil becomes smaller in bright light and larger in dimmer light. The lens is located inside of the eye and acts as a barrier between two different fluids. The vitreous humor is a clear gel fluid located behind the lens, and the aqueous humor is located in front of the lens. Once light passes through the pupil, it travels through the lens to the retina, which is located at the back of the eye. The retina is responsible for providing central vision, color vision, peripheral vision, night vision, and fine detail in overall visual acuity. The retina contains two types of photoreceptor cells called *rods* and *cones*. The cones are found in the center of the retina, in an area called the *macula*. Together the macula and cones provide finely detailed central vision in color. Rods are distributed throughout the periphery of the retina. The purpose of the rods is to detect motion and support both night vision and peripheral vision. Light is converted by these cells into electrical impulses that are sent to the brain by the optic nerve and are transformed into images (see Fig. 18.1).

The optic system is fully developed by 20 years of age and remains fairly stable until the age of 40. The exception to this is pregnancy, when changes from fluid retention, hormones, blood pressure, and the development of gestational diabetes can alter sight. As people age, the lens of the eye becomes more rigid, causing presbyopia or farsightedness. This change in vision occurs between 40 and 60 years of age and can be improved with corrective eyewear. The development of cataracts is another age-related change in vision. It should be noted that cataracts can develop at any age as the result of an eye injury due to trauma, illness, or chronic exposure to certain medications. A cataract occurs when the lens becomes cloudy, affecting vision. Cataract surgery is a common way to improve sight and restore vision.

Nurses should collect historical information about each patient's eye health. Appropriate questions include asking about the presence of any known or suspected vision loss; changes in visual acuity, including the type and cause; the use of glasses or contact lenses; eye conditions with treatment regimens; and complaints such as pain, itching, drainage, and flashers or floaters.

DISCUSSION POINT

An accurate eye examination may require the pupils to be dilated to better examine eye structures. Education should be provided to patients to ensure they understand that since they are having their pupils dilated, it will be about 4 hours before their eyes return to normal. Because of this, they will need to arrange to have someone available to take them home once the examination is completed. Mydriatic drops will be ordered to

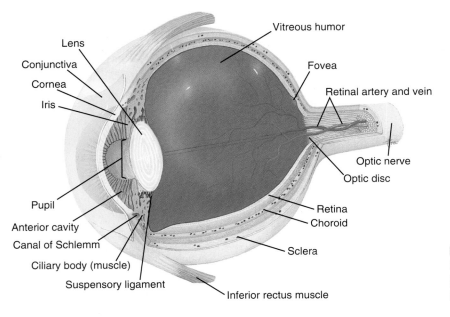

FIGURE 18.1 Anatomy of the eye. *Used with permission from Venes, D. (Ed.). (2009). Taber's cyclopedic medical dictionary (21st ed.). FA Davis Company.*

be instilled in each eye for dilation. When administering drops, have the patient look up. Drops should be instilled in the white of the eye near to where the cornea and sclera meet. Neither the dropper nor the bottle should touch the eyelashes (see Fig. 18.2). The patient may be asked to sit in a darkened waiting area for 10 to 15 minutes while the eyes dilate. Pupil dilation tends to occur faster and to last longer in people with light-colored eyes.

Explain to the patient that during the eye examination, she or he will be asked to fix her or his sight on a specific point in the room and not move his or her gaze away from that spot until asked to do so. Patients will also be asked to keep their eyes completely open during the study. Those who wear contacts or glasses may be asked to remove them during the eye examination.

DISCUSSION POINT

Assess the patient for any allergy to mydriatics before placing the drops in the patient's eyes. Patients should

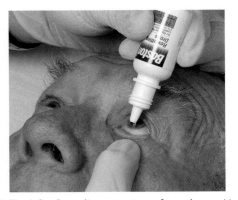

FIGURE 18.2 Administration of eyedrops. *Used with permission from Burton, M. (2011). Fundamentals of nursing care: Concepts, connections, & skills. FA Davis Company.*

be screened for current eyedrop use. Those who are currently using eyedrops may be asked to refrain from use for a minimum of 1 day before the eye examination. For example, the patient may be asked to refrain from using miotic eyedrops prescribed to treat glaucoma, because the drops cause pupil constriction and would obstruct the view of the fundus during examination.

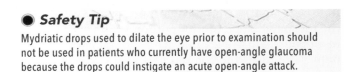

● *Safety Tip*

Mydriatic drops used to dilate the eye prior to examination should not be used in patients who currently have open-angle glaucoma because the drops could instigate an acute open-angle attack.

The information in the Part I studies is organized in a manner to help the student see how the five basic components of the nursing process (assessment, diagnosis, planning, implementation, and evaluation) can be applied to each phase of laboratory and diagnostic testing. The goal is to use nursing process to understand the integration of care (laboratory, diagnostic, nursing care) toward achieving a positive expected outcome.

- **Assessment** is the collection of information for the purpose of answering the question, "is there a problem?" Knowledge of the patient's health history, medications, complaints, and allergies as well as synonyms or alternate test names, common use for the procedure, specimen requirements, and normal ranges or interpretive comments provide the foundation for diagnosis.
- **Diagnosis** is the process of looking at the information gathered during assessment and answering the questions, "what is the problem?" and "what do I need to do about it?" Test indications tell us why the study has been requested, and potential

diagnoses tell us the value or importance of the study relative to its clinical utility.

- **Planning** is a blueprint of the nursing care before the procedure. It is the process of determining how the nurse is going to partner with the patient to fix the problem (e.g., "The patient has a study ordered and this is what I should know before I successfully carry out the plan to have the study completed"). Knowledge of interfering factors, social and cultural issues, preprocedural restrictions, the need for written and informed consent, anxiety about the procedure, and concerns regarding pain are some considerations for planning a successful partnership.

- **Implementation** is putting the plan into action with an idea of what the expected outcome should be. Collaboration with the departments where the laboratory test or diagnostic study is to be performed is essential to the success of the plan. Implementation is where the work is done within each health-care team member's scope of practice.

- **Evaluation** answers the question, "did the plan work or not?" Was the plan completely successful, partially successful, or not successful? If the plan did not work, evaluation is the process where you determine what needs to be changed to make the plan work better. This includes a review of all expected outcomes. Nursing care after the procedure is where information is gathered to evaluate the plan. Review of results, including critical findings, in relation to patient symptoms and other tests performed provides data that form a more complete picture of health or illness.

- **Expected Outcomes** are positive outcomes related to the test. They are the outcomes the nurse should expect if all goes well.

A number of pretest, intratest, and post-test universal points are presented in this overview section because the information applies to sensory ocular studies in general.

Universal Pretest Pearls (Planning)

- Obtain a history of the patient's complaints, including a list of known allergens, especially allergies or sensitivities to medications or latex so their use can be avoided or their effects mitigated if an allergy is present. Carefully evaluate all medications currently being taken by the patient. A list of the patient's current medications, prescribed and over the counter (including anticoagulants, aspirin and other salicylates, and dietary supplements), should also be obtained. Such products may be discontinued by medical direction for the appropriate number of days prior to the procedure. Ensure that all allergies are clearly noted in the medical record, and ensure the patient is wearing an allergy and medical record armband. Report to the health-care provider (HCP) information that could interfere with, or delay proceeding with, the study.

- Obtain a history of the patient's affected body system, symptoms, and results of previously performed laboratory tests and diagnostic and surgical procedures. Previous test results will provide a basis of comparison between old and new data.

- An important aspect of planning is understanding the factors that may alter study findings or cause abnormal results. Interdepartmental communication is a key factor in the planning process. The inability of a patient to cooperate or remain still during the procedure because of age, significant pain, or mental status should be among the anticipated factors. Recent or past procedures, medications, or existing medical conditions that could complicate or interfere with test results should be noted.

- Review the steps of the study with the patient or caregiver. Expect patients to be nervous about the procedure itself and the pending results. Educating the patient on his or her role during the procedure and what to expect can facilitate this. The patient's role during the procedure is to remain still. The actual time required to complete each study will depend on a number of conditions, including the type of equipment being used and how well a patient will cooperate.

- Address any concerns about pain, and explain or describe, as appropriate, the level and type of discomfort that may be expected.

- Provide additional instructions and patient preparation regarding medication, diet, fluid intake, or activity, if appropriate. Unless specified in the individual study, there are no special instructions or restrictions.

- Always be sensitive to any cultural or psychosocial issues, including a concern for modesty before, during, and after the procedure.

Universal Intratest Pearls (Implementation)

- Correct patient identification is crucial prior to any procedure. Positively identify the patient using two unique identifiers such as patient name, date of birth, Social Security number, or medical record number.

- Standard Precautions must be followed.

- Ensure that the patient has complied with pretesting instructions, including dietary, fluid, medication, and activity restrictions as given for the procedure.

- Children and infants may be accompanied by a parent to calm them. Keep neonates and infants covered and in a warm room, and provide a pacifier or gentle touch. The testing environment should be quiet, and the patient should be instructed, as appropriate, to remain still during the test as extraneous movements can affect results.

Universal Post Test Pearls (Evaluation)

- Note that completed test results are made available to the requesting HCP, who will discuss them with the patient.
- Answer questions and address concerns voiced by the patient or family and reinforce information given by the patient's HCP regarding further testing, treatment, or referral to another HCP. Recognize that patients will have anxiety related to test results. Provide teaching and information regarding the clinical implications of the test results on the patient's lifestyle, as appropriate.
- Note that test results should be evaluated in context with the patient's signs, symptoms, and diagnosis. Depending on the results of the procedure, additional testing may be performed to evaluate or monitor progression of the disease process and determine the need for a change in therapy.
- Be aware that when a person goes through a traumatic event such as an illness or being given information that will impact his or her lifestyle, there are universal human reactions that occur. These include knowledge deficit, fear, anxiety, and coping; in some situations, grieving may occur. HCPs should always be aware of the human response and how it may affect the plan of care and expected outcomes.

DISCUSSION POINT

Regarding Post-Test Critical Findings: Timely notification of a critical finding for lab or diagnostic studies is a role expectation of the professional nurse. Notification processes will vary among facilities. Upon receipt of the critical finding, the information should be read back to the caller to verify accuracy. Most policies require immediate notification of the primary HCP, hospitalist, or on-call HCP. Reported information includes the patient's name, unique identifiers, critical finding, name of the person giving the report, and name of the person receiving the report. Documentation of notification should be made in the medical record with the name of the HCP notified, time and date of notification, and any orders received. Any delay in a timely report of a critical finding may require completion of a notification form with review by Risk Management.

STUDIES

- Fundus Photography
- Gonioscopy
- Intraocular Pressure
- Pachymetry
- Refraction
- Slit-Lamp Biomicroscopy
- Visual Fields Test

LEARNING OUTCOMES

Providing safe, effective nursing care (SENC) includes mastery of core competencies and standards of care. SENC is based on a judicious application of nursing knowledge in combination with scientific principles. The Art of Nursing lies in blending what you know with the ability to effectively apply your knowledge in a compassionate manner.

After reading/studying this chapter you will be able to:

Thinking

1. List three tests commonly used to indicate whether diabetes has affected a patient's eyesight.
2. Select and discuss potential nursing diagnoses commonly encountered when interacting with adult and older patients undergoing ocular studies.
3. Identify an important instruction that should be given prior to having a study that includes dilation of the pupils.

Doing

1. Review the visual acuity (VA) findings from the patient's slit-lamp results, previous VA findings (20/80), and current VA findings (20/20), and interpret whether the patient's vision is improved, has stayed the same, or is worse.
2. Identify two important contraindications for the use of mydriatic drugs prior to a dilated eye examination.

Caring

1. Acknowledge how patient's hopes affect the outcome of designed care strategies to control identified pain and distress.
2. Recognize that there can be instances where the patient's choices conflict with organizational policy and ethical standards of care.

Fundus Photography

Quick Summary

COMMON USE: To evaluate vascular and structural changes in the eye in assessing the progression of diseases such as glaucoma, diabetic retinopathy, and macular degeneration.

AREA OF APPLICATION: Eyes.

NORMAL FINDINGS
- Normal optic nerve and vessels
- No evidence of other ocular abnormalities

Test Explanation

Fundoscopy is performed as part of a routine eye examination. This test involves the examination of the structures of the eye to document the condition of the eye, detect abnormalities, and assist in following the progress of treatment. The fundus is the inner lining of the eye. The retina, optic disc, and macula can be visualized directly or indirectly by fundoscopic examination. Photographic images may be taken through dilated pupils to document findings for review and comparison. The Amsler grid is an additional test that may be included in the eye examination, especially if macular degeneration is suspected. This simple test for central vision can be performed using a grid with instructions printed from a home computer (see Figs. 18.3 and 18.4).

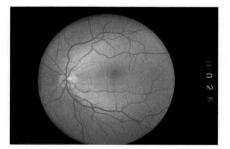

FIGURE 18.3 Normal fundus. *Used with permission, from Dillon, P. (2006). Nursing health assessment: A critical thinking, case studies approach (2nd ed.). FA Davis Company.*

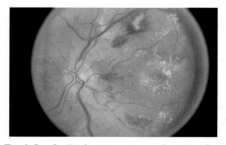

FIGURE 18.4 Diabetic retinopathy. *Used with permission, from Dillon, P. (2006). Nursing health assessment: A critical thinking, case studies approach (2nd ed.). FA Davis Company.*

Nursing Implications

Assessment

Indications	Potential Nursing Problems
Detect the presence of choroidal nevus Detect various types and stages of glaucoma Document the presence of diabetic retinopathy Document the presence of macular degeneration and any other degeneration and any associated hemorrhaging Observe ocular effects resulting from the long-term use of high-risk medications	• Human Reaction • Injury Risk • Pain • Tissue Perfusion • Self-care • Sensory Perception

Diagnosis: Clinical Significance of Test Results

ABNORMAL FINDINGS
- Aneurysm
- Atrial hypertension
- Benign intracranial hypertension from brain tumor
- Choroidal nevus
- Color vision deficiencies
- Diabetic retinopathy
- Disorders of the optic nerve
- Glaucoma
- Histoplasmosis
- Macular degeneration
- Obstructive disorders of the arteries or veins that lead to collateral circulation
- Papilledema
- Raised intracranial pressure associated with hydrocephalus
- Retinal detachment or tear
- Sickle cell anemia
- Stroke

Planning

Considerations for planning a successful partnership should include clear communication of what to expect during the test to decrease anxiety and improve cooperation. Before the procedure is performed, plan to review the steps with the patient. Address concerns about pain and explain that mydriatics, if used, may cause blurred vision and sensitivity to light. There may also be a brief stinging sensation when the drop is put in the eye, but no discomfort will be experienced during the examination. Inform the patient that a health-care provider (HCP) performs the test in a quiet, darkened room, and that to dilate and evaluate both eyes, the test can take up to 60 minutes.

SPECIAL CONSIDERATIONS

An important aspect of planning is understanding the factors that may alter study findings or cause abnormal results. Interdepartmental communication is a key factor in the planning process. The following should be noted when planning for this study:

- Clinical conditions such as the presence of cataracts may interfere with the fundal view.
- Ineffective dilation of the pupils and rubbing or squeezing the eyes during the study may impair clear imaging.

Implementation

Patient education is key to obtaining the patient's cooperation in following directions, and providing an explanation for the purpose of the procedure is an important part of this process. Inform the patient that this study can assist in detecting changes in the eye that affect vision.

> ● **Safety Tip**
>
> Ensure that the patient has complied with medication restrictions; ensure that eye medications, especially miotics and mydriatics, have been withheld, as ordered, for at least 1 day prior to the test.

Seat the patient in a chair that faces the camera. Instruct the patient to place the chin in the chin rest and gently press the forehead against the support bar. Instruct the patient to open his or her eyes wide and look at desired target while the HCP examines the fundus, with or without dilation. The examination is performed at a variety of prescribed levels of gaze. The patient should be encouraged to maintain a constant gaze but told they can blink as needed. The direct examination is performed using an instrument called an ophthalmoscope. The instrument is about the size of penlight through which a beam of light is directed into the pupil while the HCP uses magnifying lenses to visualize the interior of the fundus. The indirect examination is carried out using either a binocular indirect ophthalmoscope, a slit lamp microscope and hand lens, or a hand lens with the light source affixed to the HCP's head. When the examination is completed instruct the patient to open his or her eyes wide and look at the desired target while a sequence of photographs are taken.

Evaluation

Recognize anxiety related to test results, and be supportive of impaired activity related to vision loss or an anticipated loss of driving privileges. Discuss the implications of abnormal test results on the patient's lifestyle. Provide teaching and information regarding the clinical implications of the test results, as appropriate. Emphasize, as appropriate, that good glycemic control delays the onset of and slows the progression of diabetic retinopathy, nephropathy, and neuropathy. Provide education regarding smoking cessation as appropriate. Instruct the patient to resume usual medications, as directed by the HCP. Instruct the patient, as ordered, to avoid strenuous physical activities, such as lifting heavy objects, that may increase pressure in the eye. Provide contact information regarding vision aids, if desired, for ABLEDATA (sponsored by the National Institute on Disability and Rehabilitation Research [NIDRR], available at www.abledata.com). The American Optometric Association provides recommendations for the frequency of eye examinations at their Web site (www.aoa.org). Information can also be obtained from the American Macular Degeneration Foundation (www.macular.org), the American Diabetes Association (www.diabetes.org), or the American Heart Association (www.americanheart.org). Inform the patient that visual acuity and responses to light may change. Suggest that the patient wear dark glasses until the pupils return to normal size.

✔ *Critical Findings*

- Detached retina

Flashers, floaters, or a veil that moves across the field of vision may indicate detached retina or retinal tear. This condition requires immediate examination by an ophthalmologist. Untreated, full retinal detachment can result in irreversible and complete loss of vision in the affected eye.

Note and immediately report to the requesting HCP any critical findings and related symptoms. A listing of these findings varies among facilities.

✔ *Study Specific Complications*

Dilation can initiate a severe and sight-threatening open-angle attack in patients with narrow-angle glaucoma.

✔ *Related Tests*

- Related tests include fluorescein angiography, fructosamine, glucagon, glucose, glycated hemoglobin, gonioscopy, insulin, intraocular pressure, microalbumin, plethysmography, refraction, slit-lamp biomicroscopy, and visual field testing.
- Refer to the Ocular System table at the end of the book for related tests by body system.

Expected Outcomes

Expected clinical and patient-focused outcomes associated with Fundus Photography are

- Obtaining acceptable images for proper diagnosis
- Seeking healthy behaviors to decrease the loss of visual acuity
- Understanding how health management decisions affect eyesight

Gonioscopy

Quick Summary

COMMON USE: To detect abnormalities in the structure of the anterior chamber of the eye such as in glaucoma.

AREA OF APPLICATION: Eyes.

NORMAL FINDINGS: Normal appearance of anterior chamber structures and wide, unblocked, normal angle

Test Explanation

Gonioscopy is a technique used for examination of the anterior chamber structures of the eye (i.e., the trabecular meshwork and the anatomical relationship of the trabecular meshwork to the iris). The trabecular meshwork is the drainage system of the eye, and gonioscopy is performed to determine if the drainage angle is damaged, blocked, or clogged. Gonioscopy in combination with biomicroscopy is considered to be the most thorough basis to confirm a diagnosis of glaucoma and to differentiate between open-angle and angle-closure glaucoma. The angle structures of the anterior chamber are normally not visible because light entering the eye through the cornea is reflected back into the anterior chamber. Placement of a special contact lens (goniolens) over the cornea allows reflected light to pass back through the cornea and onto a reflective mirror in the contact lens. It is in this way that the angle structures can be visualized. There are two types of gonioscopy: indirect and direct. The more commonly used indirect technique employs a mirrored goniolens and biomicroscope. Direct gonioscopy is performed with a gonioscope containing a dome-shaped contact lens known as a gonioprism. The gonioprism eliminates internally reflected light, allowing direct visualization of the angle. Interpretation of visual examination is usually documented in a colored hand-drawn diagram. Scheie's classification is used to standardize definition of angles based on appearance by gonioscopy. Shaffer's classification is based on the angular width of the angle recess.

Nursing Implications

Assessment

Indications	Potential Nursing Problems
Assessment of peripheral anterior synechiae (PAS) Conditions affecting the ciliary body Degenerative conditions of the anterior chamber Evaluation of glaucoma (confirmation of normal structures and estimation of angle width) Growth or tumor in the angle Hyperpigmentation Post-trauma evaluation for angle recession Suspected neovascularization of the angle Uveitis	• Human Reaction • Injury Risk • Pain • Tissue Perfusion • Self-care • Sensory Perception

Diagnosis: Clinical Significance of Test Results

Scheie Classification Based on Visible Angle Structures

Classification	Appearance
Wide open	All angle structures seen
Grade I narrow	Difficult to see over the iris root
Grade II narrow	Ciliary band obscured
Grade III narrow	Posterior trabeculum hazy
Grade IV narrow	Only Schwalbe line visible

Shaffer Classification Based on Angle Width

Classification	Appearance
Wide open (20°–45°)	Closure improbable
Moderately narrow (10°–20°)	Closure possible
Extremely narrow (less than 10°)	Closure possible
Partially/totally closed	Closure present

ABNORMAL FINDINGS

- Corneal endothelial disorders (Fuchs endothelial dystrophy, iridocorneal endothelial syndrome)
- Glaucoma
- Lens disorders (cataract, displaced lens)
- Malignant ocular neoplasm in angle
- Neovascularization in angle
- Ocular hemorrhage
- PAS
- Schwartz syndrome
- Trauma
- Tumors
- Uveitis

Planning

Considerations for planning a successful partnership should include clear communication of what to expect during the test to decrease anxiety and improve cooperation. Before the procedure is performed, plan to review the steps with the patient. Instruct the patient to remove contact lenses or glasses, as appropriate. Address concerns about pain, and explain that no pain will be experienced during the test, and that some discomfort may be experienced after the test, when the numbness wears off from anesthetic drops administered before the test. Explain the importance of keeping the eyes open and fixated during the procedure. Inform the patient that the test is performed by a health-care provider (HCP) or optometrist specially trained to perform this procedure and takes about 5 minutes to complete.

SPECIAL CONSIDERATIONS

An important aspect of planning is understanding the factors that may alter study findings or cause abnormal results. Interdepartmental communication is a key factor in the planning process. It should be noted when preparing for this study that rubbing or squeezing the eyes may affect results.

Implementation

Patient education is key to obtaining the patient's cooperation in following directions, and providing an explanation for the purpose of the procedure is an important part of this process. Inform the patient that this study can assist in evaluating the eye for disease.

Seat the patient comfortably. Instill topical anesthetic in each eye, as ordered, and allow time for it to work. Topical anesthetic drops are placed in the eye with the patient looking up and the solution directed at the six o'clock position of the sclera (the white of the eye) near the limbus (the gray, semitransparent area of the eyeball where the cornea and sclera meet). Neither the dropper nor the bottle should touch the eyelashes. Ask the patient to place the chin in the chin rest and gently press the forehead against the support bar. Ask the patient to open his or her eyes wide and look at desired target. Explain that the HCP will place a lens on the eye while a narrow beam of light is focused on the eye.

Evaluation

Recognize anxiety related to test results, and be supportive of impaired activity related to vision loss or an anticipated loss of driving privileges. Discuss the implications of abnormal test results on the patient's lifestyle. Provide teaching and information regarding the clinical implications of the test results as appropriate.

✔ *Critical Findings*

N/A

✔ *Study Specific Complications*

N/A

✔ *Related Tests*

- Related tests include fundus photography, pachymetry, slit-lamp biomicroscopy, and visual field testing.
- Refer to the Ocular System table at the end of the book for related tests by body system.

Expected Outcomes

Expected clinical and patient-focused outcomes associated with Gonioscopy are

- Agreeing to use visual aids to increase one's ability to provide self-care
- Collaborating with family members to create a clutter-free home environment to decrease fall risk

Intraocular Pressure

Quick Summary

SYNONYM ACRONYM: IOP.

COMMON USE: To evaluate changes in ocular pressure to assist in diagnosis of disorders such as glaucoma.

AREA OF APPLICATION: Eyes.

NORMAL FINDINGS: Normal IOP is between 10 and 20 mm Hg

Test Explanation

The intraocular pressure (IOP) of the eye depends on a number of factors. The two most significant are the amount of aqueous humor present in the eye and the circumstances by which it leaves the eye. Other physiological variables that affect IOP include respiration, pulse, and the degree of hydration of the body. Individual eyes respond to IOP differently. Some can tolerate high pressures (20 to 30 mm Hg), and some will incur optic nerve damage at lower pressures. With respiration, variations of up to 4 mm Hg in IOP can occur, and changes of 1 to 2 mm Hg occur with every pulsation of the central retinal artery. IOP is measured with a tonometer; normal values indicate the pressure at which no damage is done to the intraocular contents. The rate of fluid leaving the eye, or its ability to leave the eye unimpeded, is the most important factor regulating IOP. There are three primary conditions that result in occlusion of the outflow channels for fluid. The most common condition is open-angle glaucoma, in which the diameters of the openings of the trabecular meshwork become narrowed, resulting in an increased IOP due to an increased resistance of fluid moving out of the eye. In secondary or angle-closure glaucoma, the trabecular meshwork becomes occluded by tumor cells, pigment, red blood cells in hyphema, or other material. Additionally, the obstructing material may cover parts of the meshwork itself, as with scar tissue or other types of adhesions that form after severe iritis, an angle-closure glaucoma attack, or a central retinal vein occlusion. The third condition impeding fluid outflow in the trabecular channels occurs with pupillary block, most commonly associated with primary angle-closure glaucoma. In eyes predisposed to this condition, dilation of the pupil causes the iris to fold up like an accordion against the narrow-angle structures of the eye. Fluid in the posterior chamber has difficulty circulating into the anterior chamber; therefore, pressure in the posterior chamber increases, causing the iris to bow forward and obstruct the outflow channels even more. Angle-closure attacks occur quite suddenly and do not give the eye a chance to adjust itself to the sudden increase in pressure. The eye becomes very red, the cornea edematous (patient may report seeing halos), and the pupil fixed and dilated, accompanied by a complaint of moderate pain. Pupil dilation can be initiated by emotional arousal or fear, conditions in which the eye must adapt to darkness (movie theaters), or mydriatics. Acute angle-closure glaucoma is an ocular emergency usually resolved by a peripheral iridotomy to allow movement of fluid between the anterior and posterior chambers. Iridotomy uses a laser to create a hole in the iris and is the preferred method of treatment. An iridectomy is another more invasive and less often used procedure that constitutes removal of a portion of the peripheral iris either by traditional surgery or by laser. Laser iridotomy is facilitated by the neodymium yttrium-aluminum-garnet laser, also known as the Nd:YAG laser. In some cases an argon laser may may be used alone or in combination with the YAG laser.

Nursing Implications
Assessment

Indications	Potential Nursing Problems
Diagnosis or ongoing monitoring of glaucoma Screening test included in a routine eye examination	• Fall • Home Maintenance • Human Reaction • Injury Risk • Role Performance • Safety • Self-care • Self-esteem • Sensory Perception • Socialization

Diagnosis: Clinical Significance of Test Results
ABNORMAL FINDINGS
• Open-angle glaucoma
• Primary angle-closure glaucoma
• Secondary glaucoma

Planning
Considerations for planning a successful partnership should include clear communication of what to expect during the test to decrease anxiety and improve cooperation. Before the procedure is performed, plan to review the steps with the patient. Address concerns about pain, and explain that the patient will be requested to fixate the eyes during the procedure. Explain that the patient may feel coldness or a slight sting when the anesthetic drops are instilled at the beginning of the procedure, but that no discomfort will be experienced during the test. Instruct the patient about what should be expected with the use of the tonometer. The patient will experience less anxiety if he or she understands that the tonometer tip will touch the tear film and not the eye directly.

Inform the patient that a health-care provider (HCP) performs the test in a quiet, darkened room, and that to evaluate both eyes, the test can take 1 to 3 minutes.

SPECIAL CONSIDERATIONS
An important aspect of planning is understanding the factors that may alter study findings or cause abnormal results. Interdepartmental communication is a key factor in the planning process. It should be noted when planning for this study that rubbing or squeezing the eyes may affect results.

Implementation
Note that patient education is key to obtaining the patient's cooperation in following directions, and providing an explanation for the purpose of the procedure is an important part of this process. Inform the patient that this study can assist in measuring eye pressure.

Seat the patient comfortably. Instill topical anesthetic/fluorescein dye in each eye, as ordered, and allow time for it to work. A number of techniques are used to measure IOP. It can be measured at the slit lamp or with a miniaturized, handheld applanation tonometer or an airpuff tonometer. When the applanation tonometer is positioned on the patient's cornea, the instrument's headrest is placed against the patient's forehead. The tonometer should be held at an angle with the handle slanted away from the patient's nose. The tonometer tip should not touch the eyelids. When the tip is properly aligned and in contact with the fluorescein-stained tear film, force is applied to the tip using an adjustment control to the desired endpoint. The tonometer is removed from the eye. The reading is taken a second time, and if the pressure is elevated, a third reading is taken. The procedure is repeated on the other eye. With the airpuff tonometer, an air pump blows air onto the cornea, and the time it takes for the air puff to flatten the cornea is detected by infrared light and photoelectric cells. This time is directly related to the IOP.

Evaluation
Recognize anxiety related to test results and be supportive of impaired activity related to vision loss or an anticipated loss of driving privileges. Discuss the implications of abnormal test results on the patient's lifestyle. Provide teaching and information regarding the clinical implications of the test results, as appropriate. Provide contact information, if desired, for the Glaucoma Research Foundation (www.glaucoma.org). Instruct the patient in the use of any ordered medications, usually eyedrops, that are intended to decrease IOP. Explain the importance of adhering to the therapy regimen, especially because increased IOP does not present symptoms. Instruct the patient in both the ocular side effects and systemic reactions associated with the prescribed medication. Encourage him or her to review corresponding literature provided by a pharmacist.

✅ Critical Findings

Increased IOP in the presence of sudden pain, sudden change in vision, a partially dilated and nonreactive pupil, and firm globe implies acute angle closure glaucoma (AACG), which is an ocular emergency requiring immediate attention to avoid permanent vision loss.

Note and immediately report to the requesting HCP any critical findings and related symptoms. A listing of these findings varies among facilities.

AACG requires immediate examination by an ophthalmologist. Iridotomy is the most likely intervention.

✅ Study Specific Complications

N/A

✅ Related Tests

- Related tests include fundus photography, gonioscopy, nerve fiber analysis, pachymetry, slit-lamp biomicroscopy, and visual field testing.
- Refer to the Ocular System table at the end of the book for related tests by body system.

Expected Outcomes

Expected clinical and patient-focused outcomes associated with Intraocular Pressure are

- Obtaining an accurate measurement of the patient's IOP
- Recommending therapeutic interventions, if appropriate, followed by improving or stabilizing the patient's vision
- Verbalizing an understanding of the pathophysiology of glaucoma
- Recognizing the importance of following medical recommendations to preserve eyesight

Pachymetry

Quick Summary

COMMON USE: To assess the thickness of the cornea prior to LASIK surgery and evaluate glaucoma risk.

AREA OF APPLICATION: Eyes.

NORMAL FINDINGS: Normal corneal thickness of 535 to 555 micron

Test Explanation

Pachymetry is the measurement of the thickness of the cornea using an ultrasound device called a pachymeter. Refractive surgery procedures such as LASIK (laser-assisted in situ keratomileusis) remove tissue from the cornea. Pachymetry is used to ensure that enough central corneal tissue remains after surgery to prevent ectasia, or abnormal bowing, of thin corneas. Also, studies point to a correlation between increased risk of glaucoma and decreased corneal thickness. This correlation has influenced some health-care providers (HCPs) to include pachymetry as a part of a regular eye health examination for patients who have a family history of glaucoma or who are part of a high-risk population. African Americans have a higher incidence of glaucoma than any other ethnic group.

Nursing Implications

Assessment

Indications	Potential Nursing Problems
Assist in the diagnosis of glaucoma (*Note*: the intraocular pressure in glaucoma patients with a thin cornea, 530 micron or less, may be higher than in patients whose corneal thickness is within normal limits) Determine corneal thickness in potential refractive surgery candidates Monitor the effects of various therapies using eyedrops, laser, or filtering surgery	• Fall Risk • Health Maintenance • Human Reaction • Injury Risk • Role Performance • Self-care • Self-esteem • Sensory Perception

The intraocular pressure in glaucoma patients with a thin cornea, 530 micron or less, may be higher than in patients whose corneal thickness is within normal limits.

Diagnosis: Clinical Significance of Test Results

ABNORMAL FINDINGS

- Bullous keratopathy
- Corneal rejection after penetrating keratoplasty
- Fuchs endothelial dystrophy
- Glaucoma

Planning

Considerations for planning a successful partnership should include clear communication of what to expect during the test to decrease anxiety and improve cooperation. Before the procedure is performed, plan to review the steps with the patient. Address concerns about pain, and explain and explain that no discomfort should be experienced during the test, but there may be some discomfort experienced after the test, when the numbness from anesthetic drops administered before the test wears off. Explain that during the test a probe tip will gently touch the surface of the cornea. Inform the patient that an HCP performs the test and that, to evaluate both eyes, the test can take 3 to 5 minutes.

SPECIAL CONSIDERATIONS

An important aspect of planning is understanding the factors that may alter study findings or cause abnormal results. Interdepartmental communication is a key factor in the planning process. It should be noted when planning for this study that improper technique during application of the probe tip to the cornea may affect results.

Implementation

Patient education is key to obtaining the patient's cooperation in following directions, and providing an explanation for the purpose of the procedure is an important part of this process. Inform the patient that this study can assist in measuring the thickness of the cornea in the eye.

Seat the patient comfortably. Instill topical anesthetic in each eye, as ordered, and allow time for it to work. Request that the patient look straight ahead while the probe of the pachymeter is applied directly on the cornea of the eye. The average of three readings for each eye is taken. Individual readings should be within 10 microns. Results on both eyes should be similar.

Evaluation

Recognize anxiety related to test results. Encourage the family to recognize and be supportive of impaired activity related to vision loss, the anticipated loss of driving privileges, or the possibility of requiring corrective lenses (self-image). Discuss the implications of test results on the patient's lifestyle. Reassure the patient regarding concerns related to impending cataract surgery. Provide teaching and information regarding the clinical implications of the test results as appropriate. Provide contact information, if desired, for the Glaucoma Research Foundation (www.glaucoma.org).

✔ Critical Findings

N/A

✔ Study Specific Complications

N/A

✔ Related Tests

- Related tests include fundus photography, gonioscopy, intraocular pressure, and visual field testing.
- Refer to the Ocular System table at the end of the book for related tests by body system.

Expected Outcomes

Expected clinical and patient-focused outcomes associated with Pachymetry are

- Accurate measurement of the patient's corneal thickness
- Successful surgical outcome
- Adjustment of the home environment to decrease fall and injury risk

Refraction

Quick Summary

COMMON USE: To assess the visual acuity of the eyes in patients of all ages, to evaluate visual acuity as required by driver licensing laws, and to assist in evaluating the eyes prior to therapeutic interventions such as eyeglasses, contact lenses, low vision aids, cataract surgery, or LASIK surgery.

AREA OF APPLICATION: Eyes.

NORMAL FINDINGS: Normal visual acuity; 20/20 (with corrective lenses if appropriate).

Test Explanation

This noninvasive procedure tests the visual acuity (VA) of the eyes and determines abnormalities or refractive errors that need correction. Refractions are performed using a combination of different pieces of equipment. Refractive error can be quickly and accurately measured using computerized automatic refractors or manually with a viewing system consisting of an entire set of trial lenses mounted on a circular wheel (phoropter). A projector may also be used to display test letters and characters from Snellen eye charts for use in assessing VA (see Fig. 18.5). If the VA is worse than 20/20, the pinhole test may be used to quickly assess the best corrected vision. Refractive errors of the peripheral cornea and lens can be reduced or eliminated by having the patient look through a pinhole at the vision test. Patients with cataracts or visual field defects will not show improved results using the pinhole test. The retinoscope is probably the most valuable instrument that can be used to objectively assess VA (see Fig. 18.6). It is

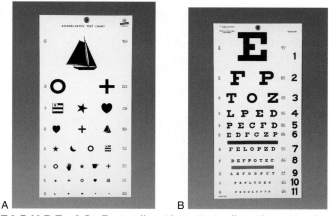

FIGURE 18.5 A. Allen Chart. B. Snellen Chart. *Used with permission, from Ward, S. (2009). Maternal-child nursing care: Optimizing outcomes for mothers, children, and families. FA Davis Company.*

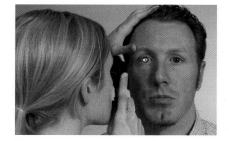

FIGURE 18.6 Examining internal structures of the eye with a retinoscope. *Used with permission, from Wilkinson, J., & Treas, L. (2010). Fundamentals of nursing (2nd ed.). FA Davis Company.*

also the only objective means of assessing refractive error in pediatric patients and patients who are unable to cooperate with other techniques of assessing refractive error due to illiteracy, senility, or inability to speak the same language as the examiner. Visual defects identified through refraction, such as hyperopia (farsightedness), in which the point of focus lies behind the retina; myopia (nearsightedness), in which the point of focus lies in front of the retina; and astigmatism, in which the refraction is unequal in different curvatures of the eyeball, can be corrected by glasses, contact lenses, or refractive surgery.

Nursing Implications

Assessment

Indications	Potential Nursing Problems
Determine if an optical defect is present and if light rays entering the eye focus correctly on the retina	• Fall Risk
	• Human Reaction
	• Infection
Determine the refractive error prior to refractive surgery such as radial keratotomy (RK), photorefractive keratotomy (PRK), laser-assisted in situ keratomileusis (LASIK), intracorneal rings (Intacs), limbal relaxing incisions (LRI), implantable contact lens (phakic intraocular lens [IOL]), clear lens replacement	• Injury Risk
	• Pain
	• Self-esteem
	• Sensory Perception
Determine the type of corrective lenses (e.g., biconvex or plus lenses for hyperopia, biconcave or minus lenses for myopia, compensatory lenses for astigmatism) needed for refractive errors	
Diagnose refractive errors in vision	

Diagnosis: Clinical Significance of Test Results

Visual Acuity Scale

Foot	Meter	Decimal
20/200	6/60	0.1
20/160	6/48	0.13
20/120	6/36	0.17
20/100	6/30	0.2
20/80	6/24	0.25
20/60	6/18	0.33
20/50	6/15	0.4

Foot	Meter	Decimal
20/40	6/12	0.5
20/30	6/9	0.67
20/25	6/7.5	0.8
20/20	6/6	1
20/16	6/4.8	1.25
20/12	6/3.6	1.67
20/10	6/3	2

VA can be expressed fractionally in feet, fractionally in meters, or as a decimal where perfect vision of 20/20 feet or 6/6 meters is equal to 1. Comparing the fraction in feet or meters to the decimal helps demonstrate that acuity less than 20/20, or less than 1, is "worse" vision, and acuity greater than 20/20, or greater than 1, is "better." A patient who cannot achieve best corrected VA of 20/200 or above (greater than 0.1) in his or her better eye is considered legally blind in the United States.

Uncorrected Visual Acuity	Foot	Meter	Decimal
Mild vision loss	20/30–20/70	6/9–6/21	0.67–0.29
Moderate vision loss	20/80–20/160	6/24–6/48	0.25–0.13
Severe vision loss	20/200–20/400	6/60–6/120	0.1–0.05
Profound vision loss	20/500–20/1,000	6/150–6/300	0.04–0.02

ABNORMAL FINDINGS
• Refractive errors such as anisometropia, astigmatism, hyperopia, myopia and presbyopia.

Planning

Considerations for planning a successful partnership should include clear communication of what to expect during the test to decrease anxiety and improve cooperation. Before the procedure is performed, plan to review the steps with the patient. Address concerns about pain, and explain that mydriatics, if used, may cause blurred vision and sensitivity to light. There may also be a brief stinging sensation when the drop is put in the eye. Inform the patient that a health-care provider (HCP) performs the test in a quiet, darkened room, and that to evaluate both eyes, the test can take up to 30 minutes (including time for the pupils to dilate before the test is actually performed).

SPECIAL CONSIDERATIONS
An important aspect of planning is understanding the factors that may impair the procedure or cause abnormal results. Interdepartmental communication is a

key factor in the planning process. It should be noted when planning for this study that improper pupil dilation may prevent adequate examination for refractive error.

Implementation

Patient education is key to obtaining the patient's cooperation in following directions, and providing an explanation for the purpose of the procedure is an important part of this process. Inform the patient that this study can assist in assessing visual acuity.

If dilation is to be performed, administer the ordered mydriatic to each eye, and repeat in 5 to 15 minutes. Ask the patient to place the chin in the chin rest and gently press the forehead against the support bar. Request that the patient look straight ahead while the eyes are examined with the instrument. The examiner will sit about 2 feet away at eye level with the patient. The retinoscope light is held in front of the eyes and directed through the pupil. Each eye is also examined for the characteristics of the red reflex, the reflection of the light from the retinoscope, which normally moves in the same direction as the light. After the examination, different lenses are tried to provide the best corrective lenses to be prescribed. When optimal VA is obtained with the trial lenses in each eye, a prescription for corrective lenses is written.

Evaluation

Recognize anxiety related to test results, and be supportive of impaired activity related to vision loss, the anticipated loss of driving privileges, or the possibility of requiring corrective lenses (self-image). Discuss the implications of abnormal test results on the patient's lifestyle. Provide teaching and information regarding the clinical implications of the test results, as appropriate. Provide contact information, if desired, for a general patient education Web site on the topic of eye care (e.g., www.allaboutvision.com). Inform the patient that visual acuity and responses to light may change. Suggest that the patient wear dark glasses after the test until the pupils return to normal size.

✔ Critical Findings

N/A

✔ Study Specific Complications

Dilation can initiate a severe and sight-threatening open-angle attack in patients with narrow-angle glaucoma.

✔ Related Tests

- Related tests include color perception test, intraocular muscle function, intraocular pressure, Schirmer tear test, and slit-lamp biomicroscopy.

- Refer to the Ocular System table at the end of the book for related tests by body system.

Expected Outcomes

Expected clinical and patient-focused outcomes associated with Refraction are

- Obtaining accurate measurement of the patient's refractive error
- Making recommendations for corrective therapy, if appropriate, followed by noting improvement in the patient's vision
- Understanding the importance of wearing corrective lenses to prevent injury
- Agreeing to routine eye examinations to maintain adequate visual acuity

Slit-Lamp Biomicroscopy

Quick Summary

SYNONYM ACRONYM: Slit-lamp examination.

COMMON USE: To detect abnormalities in the external and anterior eye structures to assist in diagnosing disorders such as corneal injury, hemorrhage, ulcers, and abrasion.

AREA OF APPLICATION: Eyes.

NORMAL FINDINGS: Normal anterior tissues and structures of the eyes

Test Explanation

This noninvasive procedure is used to visualize the anterior portion of the eye and its parts, including the eyelids and eyelashes, sclera, conjunctiva, cornea, iris, lens, and anterior chamber, and to detect pathology of any of these areas of the eyes. The slit lamp has a binocular microscope and light source that can be adjusted to examine the fluid, tissues, and structures of the eyes. For example, slit lamp ophthalmoscopy can be performed using the microscope part of the slit lamp and a special lens placed close to the eye to examine the retina, optic disc, choroid, and blood vessels in the back or fundus of the eye. Ophthalmoscopy is helpful in the identification of retinal detachment, diseases such as glaucoma that affect the movement of eye fluid, or diseases that affect the blood vessels in the eyes such as hypertension and diabetes. Special attachments to the slit lamp are used for special studies and more detailed views of specific areas. Dilating drops or mydriatics may be used to enlarge the pupil in order to allow the examiner to see the eye in greater detail. Mydriatics work either by temporarily paralyzing the muscle that makes the pupil smaller or by stimulating the iris dilator muscle. Blue or hazel eyes dilate faster than brown eyes (see Fig. 18.7).

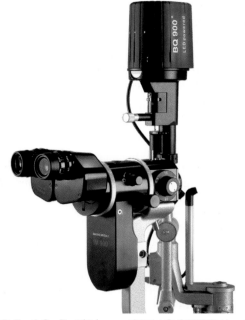

FIGURE 18.7 Slit lamp. *©HAAG-STREIT. Used with permission.*

Nursing Implications

Assessment

Indications	Potential Nursing Problems
Detect conjunctival and corneal injuries by foreign bodies and determine if ocular penetration or anterior chamber hemorrhage is present Detect corneal abrasions, ulcers, or abnormal curvatures (keratoconus) Detect deficiency in tear formation indicative of lacrimal dysfunction causing dry eye disease that can lead to corneal erosions or infection Detect lens opacities indicative of cataract formation Determine the presence of blepharitis, conjunctivitis, hordeolum, entropion, ectropion, trachoma, scleritis, and iritis Evaluate the fit of contact lenses	• Human Reaction • Infection • Inflammation • Injury Risk • Noncompliance • Pain • Sensory Perception

Diagnosis: Clinical Significance of Test Results

ABNORMAL FINDINGS
- Blepharitis
- Conjunctivitis
- Corneal abrasions
- Corneal foreign bodies
- Corneal ulcers
- Diabetes

- Ectropion
- Entropion
- Glaucoma
- Hordeolum
- Iritis
- Keratoconus (abnormal curvatures)
- Lens opacities
- Scleritis
- Trachoma

Planning

Considerations for planning a successful partnership should include clear communication of what to expect during the test to decrease anxiety and improve cooperation. Before the procedure is performed, plan to review the steps with the patient. Address concerns about pain, and explain that mydriatics, if used, may cause blurred vision and sensitivity to light. There may also be a brief stinging sensation when the drop is put in the eye. Inform the patient that a health-care provider (HCP) performs the test in a quiet, darkened room, and that to evaluate both eyes, the test can take up to 30 minutes (including time for the pupils to dilate before the test is actually performed).

SPECIAL CONSIDERATIONS

An important aspect of planning is understanding the factors that may alter study findings or cause abnormal results. Interdepartmental communication is a key factor in the planning process. It should be noted when planning for this study that rubbing or squeezing the eyes can affect the results.

Implementation

Note that patient education is key to obtaining the patient's cooperation in following directions, and providing an explanation for the purpose of the procedure is an important part of this process. Inform the patient that this study can assist in evaluating the structures of the eye.

Seat the patient comfortably. If dilation is to be performed, administer the ordered mydriatic to each eye and repeat in 5 to 15 minutes. Ask the patient to place the chin in the chin rest and gently press the forehead against the support bar. The slit lamp is placed in front of the patient's eyes in line with the examiner's eyes. The external structures of the eyes are inspected with the special bright light and microscope of the slit lamp. The light is then directed into the patient's eyes to inspect the anterior fluids and structures and is adjusted for the shape, intensity, and depth needed to visualize these areas. Magnification of the microscope is also adjusted to optimize visualization of the eye structures.

Note that special attachments and procedures can also be used to obtain further diagnostic information about the eyes. These may include, for example, a camera to photograph specific parts, gonioscopy to determine anterior chamber closure, and a cobalt-blue filter to detect minute corneal scratches, breaks, and abrasions with corneal staining.

Evaluation

Recognize anxiety related to test results, and encourage the family to recognize and be supportive of impaired activity related to vision loss, the anticipated loss of driving privileges, or the possibility of requiring corrective lenses (self-image). Discuss the implications of the abnormal test results on the patient's lifestyle. Provide contact information, if desired, for a general patient education Web site on the topic of eye care (e.g., www.allaboutvision.com). Instruct the patient to resume usual medications, as directed by the HCP. Inform the patient that visual acuity and responses to light may change. Suggest that the patient wear dark glasses after the test until the pupils return to normal size.

✅ Critical Findings

N/A

✅ Study Specific Complications

Dilation can initiate a severe and sight-threatening open-angle attack in patients with narrow-angle glaucoma.

✅ Related Tests

- Related tests include color perception test, fluorescein angiography, gonioscopy, intraocular muscle function, intraocular pressure, nerve fiber analysis, refraction, Schirmer tear test, and visual field testing.
- Refer to the Ocular System table at the end of the book for related tests by body system.

Expected Outcomes

Expected clinical and patient-focused outcomes associated with Slit-Lamp Biomicroscopy are

- Obtaining acceptable images for proper diagnosis
- Understanding the importance of keeping eye examination appointments
- Managing eye pain at a level acceptable to the patient

Visual Fields Test

Quick Summary

SYNONYM ACRONYM: Perimetry, VF.

COMMON USE: To assess visual field function related to the retina, optic nerve, and optic pathways to assist in diagnosing visual loss disorders such as brain tumors, macular degeneration, and diabetes.

AREA OF APPLICATION: Eyes.

NORMAL FINDINGS: Normal central vision field extends in a circle approximately 25° to 30° on all sides of central fixation and out 60° superiorly (upward), 60° nasally (medially), 75° inferiorly (downward), and 90° temporally (laterally). There is a normal physiological blind spot, 12° to 15° temporal to the central fixation point, and approximately 1.5° below the horizontal meridian which is approximately 7.5° high and 5.5° wide. The patient should be able to see the test object throughout the entire central vision field except within the physiological blind spot.

Test Explanation

The visual field (VF) is the area within which objects can be seen by the eye as it fixes on a central point. The central field is an area extending 25° surrounding the fixation point. The peripheral field is the remainder of the area within which objects can be viewed. This test evaluates the central VF, except within the physiological blind spot, through systematic movement of the test object across a tangent screen. It tests the function of the retina, optic nerve, and optic pathways. VF testing may be performed manually by the examiner (confrontation VF examination) or by using partially or fully automated equipment (tangent screen, Goldman, Humphrey VF examination). In the manual VF test, the patient is asked to cover one eye and fix his or her gaze on the examiner. The examiner moves his or her hand out of the patient's VF and then gradually brings it back into the patient's VF. The patient signals the examiner when the hand comes back into view. The test is repeated on the other eye. The manual test is frequently used for screening because it is quick and simple. Tangent screen or Goldman testing is an automated method commonly used to create a map of the patient's VF.

Nursing Implications

Assessment

Indications	Potential Nursing Problems
Detect field vision loss and evaluate its progression or regression	- Fall Risk - Human Reaction - Injury Risk - Role Performance - Safety - Self-care - Self Image - Sensory Perception - Socialization

Diagnosis: Clinical Significance of Test Results

ABNORMAL FINDINGS

- Amblyopia
- Blepharochalasis
- Blurred vision

- Brain injury
- Brain tumors
- Cerebrovascular accidents
- Choroidal nevus
- Diabetes with ophthalmic manifestations
- Glaucoma
- Headache
- Macular degeneration
- Macular drusen
- Nystagmus
- Optic neuritis or neuropathy
- Ptosis of eyelid
- Retinal detachment, hole, or tear
- Retinal exudates or hemorrhage
- Retinal occlusion of the artery or vein
- Retinitis pigmentosa
- Rheumatoid arthritis
- Stroke
- Subjective visual disturbance
- Use of high-risk medications
- VF defect
- Vitreous traction syndrome

Planning

Considerations for planning a successful partnership should include clear communication of what to expect during the test to decrease anxiety and improve cooperation. Instruct the patient to wear corrective lenses if appropriate and if they are needed for distance vision. Instruct the patient regarding the importance of keeping the eyes open for the test. Before the procedure is performed, plan to review the steps with the patient. Address concerns about pain, and explain that no discomfort should be experienced during the test. Inform the patient that a health-care provider (HCP) performs the test in a quiet, darkened room and that to evaluate both eyes, the test can take up to 30 minutes.

SPECIAL CONSIDERATIONS

An important aspect of planning is understanding the factors that may alter study findings or cause abnormal results. Interdepartmental communication is a key factor in the planning process. The following should be noted when planning for this study:

- Measuring visual acuity with and without corrective lenses prior to testing is highly recommended.
- Assessing and noting the patient's cooperation and reliability as good, fair, or poor because it is difficult to evaluate factors such as general health, fatigue, or reaction time, all of which affect test performance. An uncooperative patient or a patient with severe vision loss who has difficulty seeing even a large vision screen may have test results that are invalid.

Implementation

Patient education is key to obtaining the patient's cooperation in following directions, and providing an explanation for the purpose of the procedure is an important part of this process. Inform the patient that this study can assist in assessing visual field function and vision loss.

The patient should be seated 3 feet away from the tangent screen with the eye being tested directly in line with the central fixation tangent, usually a white disk, on the screen. The eye not being tested should be covered. Ask the patient to place the chin in the chin rest and gently press the forehead against the support bar. Reposition the patient as appropriate to ensure that the eye to be tested is properly aligned in front of the VF testing equipment. While the patient stares at the disk on the screen, the examiner moves an object toward the patient's visual field. The patient signals the examiner when the object enters his or her visual field. The patient's responses are recorded, and a map of the patient's VF, including areas of visual defect, can be drawn on paper manually or by a computer.

Evaluation

Recognize anxiety related to test results and be supportive of impaired activity related to vision loss, a perceived loss of driving privileges, or the possibility of requiring corrective lenses. Discuss the implications of the test results on the patient's lifestyle. Provide contact information, if desired, for a general patient education Web site on the topic of eye care (e.g., www.allaboutvision.com). Provide contact information regarding vision aids, if desired, for ABLEDATA (sponsored by the National Institute on Disability and Rehabilitation Research [NIDRR], available at www.abledata.com). Information can also be obtained from the American Macular Degeneration Foundation (www.macular.org), the Glaucoma Research Foundation (www.glaucoma.org), and the American Diabetes Association (www.diabetes.org). Instruct the patient in the use of any ordered medications. Explain the importance of adhering to the therapy regimen. As appropriate, instruct the patient in significant side effects and systemic reactions associated with the prescribed medication. Encourage him or her to review the corresponding literature provided by a pharmacist.

✓ Critical Findings

N/A

✓ Study Specific Complications

N/A

✓ Related Tests

- Related tests include CT brain, EEG, evoked brain potentials, fluorescein angiography, fructosamine, fundus photography, glucagon, glucose, glycated hemoglobin, gonioscopy, insulin, intraocular pressure, microalbumin, plethysmography, PET brain, and slit-lamp biomicroscopy.

- Refer to the Ocular System table at the end of the book for related tests by body system.

Expected Outcomes

Expected clinical and patient-focused outcomes associated with Visual Fields Test are

- Obtaining acceptable mapping of the patient's visual field for proper diagnosis
- Adapting activities to the level of the visual field loss in order to prevent injury
- Demonstrating the ability to express feelings about the progressive loss of vision

REVIEW OF LEARNING OUTCOMES

Thinking

1. List three tests commonly used to indicate whether diabetes has affected a patient's eyesight. Answer: All sight involves the retina; therefore, anything that affects the blood vessels of the retina has the potential to affect eyesight. With diabetes, the vessels weaken as the disease progresses, allowing fluid and proteins to leak from the vessels. The fluid accumulates, causing the retina to swell, which, in turn, distorts vision. Pictures of the structures of the eye taken during fundus photography studies are very useful to document changes in the eye during the progression of diabetes. Fluorescein angiography is a type of fundus photography in which a fluorescent dye is used to document patterns of blood flow in a series of photographs taken after the dye has been administered by an IV site in the patient's arm. The retina is responsible for peripheral or side vision that can be evaluated using visual fields studies.

2. Select and discuss potential nursing diagnoses commonly encountered when interacting with adult and older patients undergoing sensory studies. Answer: Risk for fall or injury, alterations in sensory perception, anxiety, impaired home maintenance, fear, and ineffective coping/family coping, self care, communication, self-esteem.

3. Identify an important instruction that should be given prior to having a study that includes dilation of the pupils. Answer: Inform the patient that visual acuity and responses to light may change as a result of pupil dilation. Suggest that the patient wear dark glasses until the pupils return to normal size. Ensure that a patient having a study that includes dilation of the pupils understands that he or she must refrain from driving until the pupils return to normal after the test (about 4 hours) and has made arrangements to have someone else be responsible for transportation after the study.

Doing

1. Review the visual acuity (VA) findings from the patient's slit-lamp results, previous VA findings (20/80), and current VA findings (20/20), and interpret whether the patient's vision improved, has stayed the same, or is worse. Answer: Review of the Snelling visual acuity chart shows the patient's vision improved.

2. Identify two important contraindications for the use of mydriatic drugs prior to a dilated eye examination. Answer: Dilation of the pupils is contraindicated for patients with allergies to mydriatic drugs and for patients with narrow-angle glaucoma, as dilation can initiate a severe and sight-threatening attack.

Caring

1. Acknowledge how patient's hopes affect the outcome of designed care strategies to control identified pain and distress. Answer: After receiving test results that indicate failing vision, the patient may be despondent. Attitude matters. One way to assist the patient to view the situation in a more positive light is to provide information to better understand the medical issue. A second way is to have the patient talk to someone who has been in the same situation in order to provide emotional support. Which should you use? That depends on the emotional needs of your patient.

2. Recognize that there can be instances where the patient's choices conflict with organizational policy and ethical standards of care. Answer: Sometimes a patient may make a decision about his or her health that you know is not in the patient's best interests. Refusal of care is common. Why they are refusing is what you need to discover. The answer to that question is the key to assisting the patient to achieve a positive outcome. However, you must accept that you cannot make the decisions for your patient, and sometimes you cannot change his or her mind.

Words OF Wisdom: Imagine that you have spent your life as an artist, a pianist, or a computer software developer and your physician tells you that you are losing your vision. Now you are in the hospital and you are angry and afraid that, in a very basic sense, who you are is about to change forever. As the nurse, what can you do? The place to begin is understanding your nursing role and who you are in relation to this situation. You are the person who will try to discover why your patient is angry, sad, and withdrawn. You are the person who will then select the resources that will allow your patient to begin to cope with this change in her or his life. By virtue of the amount of time you spend with the patient, you are the only person who can create a workable plan that will make the sensory loss transition less traumatic. Why? Because it is the nurse's role to identify problems, create a plan, and coordinate care toward a positive outcome. Know your resources and know how to use them.

BIBLIOGRAPHY

About color vision defects. (n.d.). Retrieved from http://www.opticaldiagnostics.com/info/color_vision_defects.html

Beers, M., Porter, R., Jones, T., Kaplan, J., & Berkwits, M. (Eds.). (2006). Approach to the ophthalmologic patient. The MERCK Manual (18th ed., pp. 869-885). Whitehouse Station; NJ: Merck Research Laboratories.

Bennett, T. (2012). Fundamentals of fluorescein angiography. Retrieved from http://www.opsweb.org/?page=FA

Bianco, C. (2000). How vision works. Retrieved from http://health.howstuffworks.com/mental-health/human-nature/perception/eye.htm

Cavanaugh, B. (2003). Nurse's manual of laboratory and diagnostic tests (4th ed.). Philadelphia, PA: F.A. Davis Company.

Color vision deficiency. (n.d.). Retrieved from http://www.aoa.org/patients-and-public/eye-and-vision-problems/glossary-of-eye-and-vision-conditions/color-deficiency?sso=y

Hancock, S. (2008). Clinical decision making I: Visual field interpretation. Retrieved from http://www.apcthai.com/webboard/uploads/Visual_Field_Interpretation.pdf

Iserson, K. (2001). Color blindness and health care personnel. Retrieved from http://archinte.jamanetwork.com/article.aspx?volume=161&issue=18&page=2265

Understanding nerve fiber analysis. (2002). Retrieved from http://cms.revoptom.com/handbook/oct02_sec4_p.htm

Van Leeuwen, A., & Bladh, M. (2015). Davis's comprehensive handbook of laboratory and diagnostic testing with nursing implications (6th ed.). Philadelphia, PA: F.A. Davis Company.

Venes, D., Fenton, B., Patwell, J., & Enright, A. (2009). Tabers cyclopedic medical dictionary (21st ed.). Philadelphia: PA: F.A. Davis.

Sheppard, J. (2012). Visual field testing: Vision tests to detect glaucoma and other eye disorders. Retrieved from www.medicinenet.com/visual_field_test/article.htm

Waggoner, T. Sr., & Waggoner, T. Jr. (n.d.). The truth about color vision in healthcare. Retrieved from http://www.testing colorvision.com/tcvuploads/cvdh.pdf

Walker, H., Hall, W., & Hurst, J. (Eds.). (1990). Clinical methods: The history, physical, and laboratory examinations (3rd ed.). Retrieved from http://www.ncbi.nlm.nih.gov/books/NBK220/

Web MD. (2011). Diabetic retinopathy: What happens. Retrieved from http://diabetes.webmd.com/tc/diabetic-retinopathy-what-happens

Go to Section II of this book and www.davisplus.com for the Clinical Reasoning Tool and its case studies to provide you with a safe place to explore patient care situations. There are a total of 26 different case studies; 2 cases are presented for each of 13 body systems. One set of 13 cases are found in the Section II chapters, and a second set of 13 cases are available online at www.davisplus.com. Each case is designed with the specific goal of helping you to connect the dots of clinical reasoning. Cases are designed to reflect possible clinical scenarios; the outcomes may or may not be positive—you decide.

Skin Tests

OVERVIEW

Skin tests are done to provide diagnostic information related to the body's immunity to infectious disease. There are a wide variety of skin tests available as diagnostic tools. Culture is covered in this section (see Fig. 19.1).

Skin culture is used to identify a bacterial, fungal, or viral infection and provide direction as to the treatment that will kill the organism, thereby curing the infection. Intact skin is a natural barrier that protects us from invading microorganisms. Once a break in the skin occurs, the door opens, allowing microorganisms to walk right in. Treatment for infection should begin with obtaining ordered samples from the infected sites for testing. Types of samples include skin cells, pus, or other fluids. Samples should be obtained with sterile technique using either a sterile swab or container. It is the nurse's responsibility to make sure that collected samples go to the laboratory in a timely manner, with the correct patient identification and test label. Most samples will be tested for gram stain, culture, and possibly antibiotic sensitivity. Because there are some types of bacteria that normally live on the skin, the laboratory may report those results as normal flora. Results that return as abnormal may identify the predominant organism, how much of the organism is present, and may the known pathogen.

The information in the Part I studies is organized in a manner to help the student see how the five basic components of the nursing process (assessment, diagnosis, planning, implementation, and evaluation) can be applied to each phase of laboratory and diagnostic testing. The goal is to use nursing process to understand the integration of care (laboratory, diagnostic, nursing care) toward achieving a positive expected outcome.

- **Assessment** is the collection of information for the purpose of answering the question, "is there a problem?" Knowledge of the patient's health history, medications, complaints, and allergies as well as synonyms or alternate test names, common use for the procedure, specimen requirements, and normal ranges or interpretive comments provide the foundation for diagnosis.
- **Diagnosis** is the process of looking at the information gathered during assessment and answering the questions, "what is the problem?" and "what do I need to do about it?" Test indications tell us why the study has been requested, and potential diagnoses tell us the value or importance of the study relative to its clinical utility.
- **Planning** is a blueprint of the nursing care before the procedure. It is the process of determining how the nurse is going to partner with the patient to fix the problem (e.g., "The patient has a study ordered and this is what I should know before I successfully carry out the plan to have the study completed"). Knowledge of interfering factors, social and cultural issues, preprocedural restrictions, the need for written and informed consent, anxiety about the procedure, and concerns regarding pain are some considerations for planning a successful partnership.
- **Implementation** is putting the plan into action with an idea of what the expected outcome should be. Collaboration with the departments where the laboratory test or diagnostic study is to be performed is essential to the success of the plan. Implementation

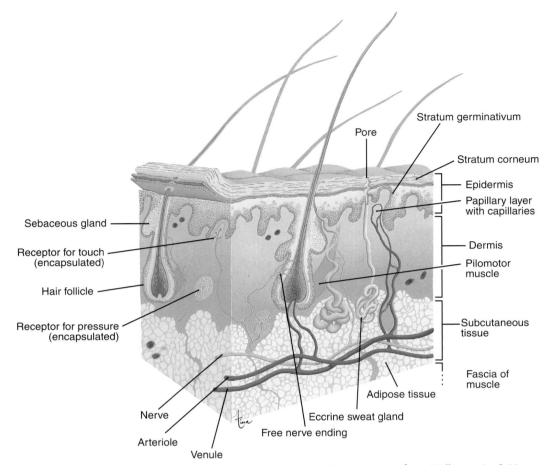

FIGURE 19.1 Structure of skin and subcutaneous tissue. *Used with permission, from Williams, L., & Hopper, P. (2010). Understanding medical surgical nursing (4th ed.). FA Davis Company.*

is where the work is done within each health-care team member's scope of practice.

- **Evaluation** answers the question, "did the plan work or not?" Was the plan completely successful, partially successful, or not successful? If the plan did not work, evaluation is the process where you determine what needs to be changed to make the plan work better. This includes a review of all expected outcomes. Nursing care after the procedure is where information is gathered to evaluate the plan. Review of results, including critical findings, in relation to patient symptoms and other tests performed, provides data that form a more complete picture of health or illness.

- **Expected Outcomes** are positive outcomes related to the test. They are the outcomes the nurse should expect if all goes well.

A number of pretest, intratest, and post-test universal points are presented in this overview section, because the information applies to skin tests in general.

Universal Pretest Pearls (Planning)

- Obtain a history of the patient's complaints, including a list of known allergens, especially allergies or sensitivities to medications or latex, so their use can be avoided or their effects mitigated if an allergy is present. Carefully evaluate all medications currently being taken by the patient. A list of the patient's current medications, prescribed and over the counter (including anticoagulants, aspirin and other salicylates, and dietary supplements) should also be obtained. Ensure that all allergies are clearly noted in the medical record, and ensure the patient is wearing an allergy and medical record armband. Report to the healthcare provider (HCP) any information that could interfere with, or delay proceeding with the study.

- Obtain a history of the patient's affected body system, symptoms, and results of previously performed laboratory tests and diagnostic and surgical procedures. Previous test results will provide a basis of comparison between old and new data.

- An important aspect of planning is understanding the factors that may alter study findings or cause abnormal results. Interdepartmental communication is a key factor in the planning process. The inability of a patient to cooperate or remain still during the procedure because of age, significant pain, or mental status should be among the anticipated factors. Recent or past procedures, medications, or existing medical conditions that could complicate or interfere with test results should be noted.
- Review the steps of the study with the patient or caregiver. Expect patients to be nervous about the procedure and the pending results. Educating the patient on his or her role during the procedure and what to expect can facilitate this. The patient's role during the procedure itself is to remain still. The actual time required to complete each study will depend on a number of conditions, including the type of equipment being used and how well a patient will cooperate.
- Address any concerns about pain, and explain or describe, as appropriate, the level and type of discomfort that may be expected.
- Provide additional instructions and patient preparation regarding medication, diet, fluid intake, or activity, if appropriate. Unless specified in the individual study, there are no special instructions or restrictions.
- Always be sensitive to any cultural or psychosocial issues, including concern for modesty before, during, and after the procedure.

Reminder

Ensure that a written and informed consent has been documented in the medical record prior to the study, if required. The consent must be obtained before medication is administered.

Universal Intratest Pearls (Implementation)

- Correct patient identification is crucial prior to any procedure. Positively identify the patient using two unique identifiers, such as patient name, date of birth, Social Security number, or medical record number.
- Standard Precautions must be followed.
- Children and infants may be accompanied by a parent to calm them. Keep neonates and infants covered and in a warm room, and provide a pacifier

or gentle touch. The testing environment should be quiet, and the patient should be instructed, as appropriate, to remain still during the test as extraneous movements can affect results.
- Ensure that the patient has complied with pretesting instructions.

Universal Post Test Pearls (Evaluation)

- Note that completed test results are made available to the requesting HCP, who will discuss them with the patient.
- Answer questions and address concerns voiced by the patient or family, and reinforce information given by the patient's HCP regarding further testing, treatment, or referral to another HCP. Recognize that patients will have anxiety related to test results. Provide teaching and information regarding the clinical implications of the test results on the patients lifestyle, as appropriate.
- Note that test results should be evaluated in context with the patient's signs, symptoms, and diagnosis. Depending on the results of the procedure, additional testing may be performed to evaluate or monitor progression of the disease process and determine the need for a change in therapy.
- Be aware that when a person goes through a traumatic event such as an illness or being given information that will impact his or her lifestyle, there are universal human reactions that occur. These include knowledge deficit, fear, anxiety, and coping; in some situations, grieving may occur. HCPs should always be aware of the human response and how it may affect the plan of care and expected outcomes.

DISCUSSION POINT

Regarding Post-Test Critical Findings: Timely notification of a critical finding for lab or diagnostic studies is a role expectation of the professional nurse. Notification processes will vary among facilities. Upon receipt of the critical finding, the information should be read back to the caller to verify accuracy. Most policies require immediate notification of the primary HCP, hospitalist, or on-call HCP. Reported information includes the patient's name, unique identifiers, critical finding, name of the person giving the report, and name of the person receiving the report. Documentation of notification should be made in the medical record with the name of the HCP notified, time and date of notification, and any orders received. Any delay in a timely report of a critical finding may require completion of a notification form with review by Risk Management.

STUDIES

- Culture, Bacterial, Anal/Genital, Ear, Eye, Skin, and Wound

LEARNING OUTCOMES

Providing safe, effective nursing care (SENC) includes mastery of core competencies and standards of care. SENC is based on a judicious application of nursing knowledge in combination with scientific principles. The Art of Nursing lies in blending what you know with the ability to effectively apply your knowledge in a compassionate manner.

After reading/studying this chapter, you will be able to:

Thinking

1. Explain the importance of collecting a specimen using sterile technique.

Doing

1. Describe three necessary actions to ensure a sample is correctly obtained and sent to the laboratory.

Caring

1. Recognize the value of working as a health-care team in meeting clinical objectives.

Culture, Bacterial, Anal/Genital, Ear, Eye, Skin, and Wound

Quick Summary

COMMON USE: To identify pathogenic bacterial organisms as an indicator for appropriate therapeutic interventions for multiple sites of infection.

SPECIMEN: Sterile fluid or swab from affected area placed in transport media tube provided by laboratory.

NORMAL FINDINGS: (Method: Culture aerobic and/or anaerobic on selected media; cell culture followed by use of direct immunofluorescence, nucleic acid amplification, Polymerase Chain Reaction, and DNA probe assays [e.g., Gen-Probe] are available for identification of Neisseria gonorrhoeae, Streptococcus agalactiae (Group B Streptococcus), and Chlamydia trachomatis.) Culture, Negative: no growth of pathogens. Culture Enhanced PCR or other DNA assays, Negative: None detected.

Test Explanation

When indicated by patient history, anal and genital cultures may be performed to isolate the organism responsible for sexually transmitted infections. Chlamydia, gonorrhea, and syphilis are reportable sexually transmitted infections. Anal and genital cultures may also be performed on pregnant women in order to identify the presence of Group B streptococcus (GBS), a significant and serious neonatal infection transmitted as the newborn passes through the birth canal of colonized mothers. Neonatal GBS is the most common cause of sepsis, pneumonia, or meningitis in newborns. The disease is classified as either early onset (first week of life) and late onset (after the first week of life). The Centers for Disease Control and Prevention (CDC), American Academy of Family Physicians (AAFP), American Academy of Pediatrics (AAP), American College of Nurse-Midwives (ACNM), and American College of Obstetricians and Gynecologists (ACOG) recommend universal screening for all pregnant women at 35 to 37 wk gestation. Pregnant patients with positive results for a GBS urinary tract infection at any time during pregnancy should receive appropriate medical treatment at the time of diagnosis and also receive intrapartum antibiotic prophylaxis in order to offer continued protection in the absence of complete eradication of the infection at the time of delivery. Rapid GBS test kits can provide results within minutes on vaginal or rectal fluid swab specimens submitted in a sterile red-top tube. Negative rapid test findings should be followed up with culture and gram stain or culture enhanced molecular methods.

Ear and eye cultures are performed to isolate the organism responsible for chronic or acute infectious disease of the ear and eye.

Skin and soft tissue samples from infected sites must be collected carefully to avoid contamination from the surrounding normal skin flora. Skin and tissue infections may be caused by both aerobic and anaerobic organisms. Therefore, a portion of the sample should be placed in aerobic and a portion in anaerobic transport media. Care must be taken to use transport media that are approved by the laboratory performing the testing.

Sterile fluids can be collected from the affected site. Refer to related body fluid studies (i.e., amniotic fluid, cerebrospinal fluid, pericardial fluid, peritoneal fluid, pleural fluid, and synovial fluid) for specimen collection.

A wound culture involves collecting a specimen of exudates, drainage, or tissue so that the causative organism can be isolated and pathogens identified. Specimens can be obtained from superficial and deep wounds (see Fig. 19.2).

Optimally, specimens should be obtained before antibiotic use. The method used to culture and grow the organism depends on the suspected infectious organism. There are transport media specifically for bacterial agents. The laboratory will select the appropriate media for suspect organisms and will initiate antibiotic sensitivity testing if indicated by test results. Sensitivity

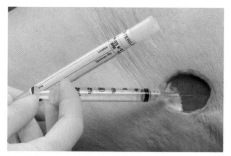

FIGURE 19.2 Wound culture. *Used with permission, from Wilkinson, J., & Treas, L. (2010). Fundamentals of nursing (2nd ed.). FA Davis Company.*

testing identifies the antibiotics to which organisms are susceptible to ensure an effective treatment plan (see Fig. 19.3).

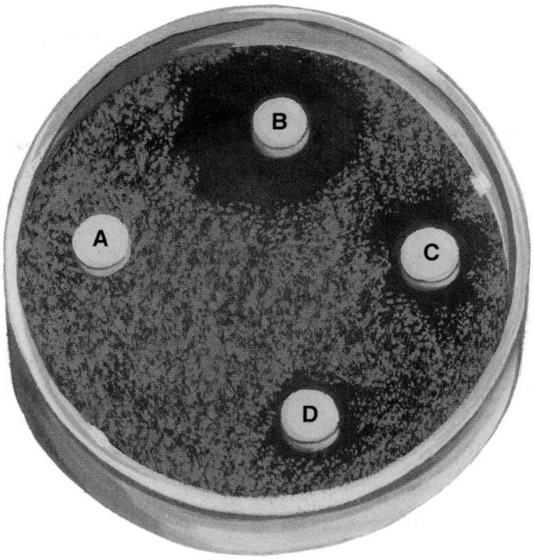

Nursing Implications
Assessment

FIGURE 19.3 Bacterial culture. *Used with permission, from Scanlon, V., & Sanders, T. (2010). Essentials of anatomy and physiology (6th ed.). FA Davis Company.*

Indications	Potential Nursing Problems
Anal/Genital Assist in the diagnosis of sexually transmitted infections. Determine the cause of genital itching or purulent drainage. Determine effective antimicrobial therapy specific to the identified pathogen. Conduct routine prenatal screening for vaginal and rectal GBS colonization. **Ear** Isolate and identify organisms responsible for ear pain, drainage, or changes in hearing. Isolate and identify organisms responsible for outer-, middle-, or inner-ear infection. Determine effective antimicrobial therapy specific to the identified pathogen. **Eye** Isolate and identify pathogenic microorganisms responsible for infection of the eye. Determine effective antimicrobial therapy specific to identified pathogen. **Skin** Isolate and identify organisms responsible for skin eruptions, drainage, or other evidence of infection. Determine effective antimicrobial therapy specific to the identified pathogen.	• Activity • Fear • Human Reactions • Infection • Mobility • Nutrition • Pain • Self-esteem • Sensory Perception **(related to a loss of visual and auditory acuity)** • Sexuality • Skin

Indications

Sterile Fluids
Isolate and identify organisms before surrounding tissue becomes infected.
Determine effective antimicrobial therapy specific to the identified pathogen.

Wound
Detect abscess or deep-wound infectious process.
Determine if an infectious agent is the cause of wound redness, warmth, or edema with drainage at a site.
Determine the presence of infectious agents in stage 3 and stage 4 decubitus ulcers.
Isolate and identify organisms responsible for the presence of pus or other exudate in an open wound.
Determine effective antimicrobial therapy specific to the identified pathogen.

Diagnosis: Clinical Significance of Test Results
POSITIVE FINDINGS IN

ANAL/ENDOCERVICAL/GENITAL

Infections or carrier states are caused by the following organisms: Chlamydia trachomatis, obligate intracellular bacteria without a cell wall, gram-variable Gardnerella vaginalis, gram negative Neisseria gonorrhoeae, Treponema pallidum, and toxin-producing strains of gram-positive Staphylococcus aureus, and gram-positive GBS.

EAR

Commonly identified gram-negative organisms include Escherichia coli, Proteus spp., Pseudomonas aeruginosa, gram-positive S. aureus, and β-hemolytic streptococci.

EYE

Commonly identified organisms include C. trachomatis (transmitted to newborns from infected mothers), gram-negative Haemophilus influenzae (transmitted to newborns from infected mothers), H. aegyptius, N. gonorrhoeae (transmitted to newborns from infected mothers), P. aeruginosa, gram-positive S. aureus, and Streptococcus pneumoniae.

SKIN

Commonly identified gram-negative organisms include Bacteroides, Pseudomonas, gram-positive Clostridium, Corynebacterium, staphylococci, and group A streptococci.

STERILE FLUIDS

Commonly identified pathogens include gram-negative Bacteroides, E. coli, P. aeruginosa, gram-positive Enterococcus spp., and Peptostreptococcus spp.

WOUND

Aerobic and anaerobic microorganisms can be identified in wound culture specimens. Commonly identified gram-negative organisms include Klebsiella, Proteus, Pseudomonas, gram-positive Clostridium perfringens, S. aureus, and group A streptococci.

Planning

Considerations for planning a successful partnership should include clear communication of what to expect during the test to decrease anxiety and improve cooperation. Note any recent medications that can interfere with test results, such as antibiotics. Pretest antimicrobial therapy will delay or inhibit the growth of pathogens. Instruct female patients not to douche for 24 hours before a cervical or vaginal specimen is to be obtained. Before the procedure is performed, plan to review the steps with the patient. Address concerns about pain, and explain that there may be some discomfort during the specimen collection.

SPECIAL CONSIDERATIONS

An important aspect of planning is understanding the factors that may alter study findings or cause abnormal results. Interdepartmental communication is a key factor in the planning process. The following should be noted when planning for this study:

- Failure to collect an adequate specimen, improper collection or storage technique, and failure to transport the specimen in a timely fashion are causes for specimen rejection.

- Testing specimens more than 1 hour after collection may result in decreased growth or no growth of organisms.
- The specimen should not be frozen or allowed to dry.

Implementation

Patient education is key to obtaining the patient's cooperation in following directions, and providing an explanation for the purpose of the procedure is an important part of this process. Inform the patient that this study can assist in identifying the organism-causing infection. Ensure that the patient has complied with medication restrictions prior to the procedure. Specify the exact specimen source/origin (e.g., vaginal lesion).

DISCUSSION POINT

Chlamydia is an intracellular obligate pathogen. Culture of infected epithelial cells is considered the gold standard for the identification of chlamydia because of the higher sensitivity of nucleic acid amplification or DNA probe assays relative to antibody assays. Therefore, culture should always be the test of choice in cases of suspected or known child abuse.

There are a number of other commonly used ways to diagnose chlamydial infection from samples containing a sufficient number of infected epithelial cells, including:

1. Specimens collected in liquid-based PAP test kits that can be "split" specifically for detection of Chlamydia trachomatis.
2. Specimens collected by cervical or urethral culture for females and urethral culture for males, followed by direct immunofluorescence, nucleic acid amplification, or DNA probe assays (e.g., Gen-Probe APTIMA)
   A. *Cervix or urethra (female)* Position the patient on the gynecological examination table with her feet in stirrups. Drape the patient's legs to provide privacy and reduce chilling. Remove mucus and pus with a swab, discard, and use gentle, rotating pressure for 10 to 30 seconds with another swab to obtain the specimen for culture. Carefully withdraw the swab to avoid contact with the vaginal mucosa. Place the swab specimen in the transport tube, and break the swab shaft at the scoreline. Tightly recap the swab specimen. The cervical swab may be combined with a urethral swab in the same transport medium tube.
   B. *Urethra (male)* Explain that there may be some burning and pressure as the culture is being taken but that it will dissipate after a few minutes. The patient should not have urinated for at least 1 hour prior to specimen collection. Insert the specimen collection swab at least 2 cm and up to 4 cm into the urethra. Gently rotate the swab for 2 to 3 seconds and then carefully withdraw the swab and place it into the specimen transport

tube. Place the swab specimen in the transport tube, and break the swab shaft at the scoreline. Tightly recap the swab specimen.

3. First-void urine specimens followed by nucleic acid amplification or DNA probe assays (e.g., Gen-Probe APTIMA®). The patient should not have urinated for at least 1 hour prior to specimen collection, and female patients should not cleanse the labial area prior to providing the specimen. Instruct the patient to provide 20 to 30 mL of a first-catch urine into a sterile urine collection cup. The required volume can be indicated by making a mark on the urine collection cup. Specimen volume is an important consideration because larger volumes may result in specimen dilution and smaller volumes may not provide an adequate amount of organisms into the specimen of urine. The specimen must be transferred into the APTIMA specimen transport within 24 hours of collection and before being assayed. Add 2 mL of urine from the well-mixed first-catch urine to the APTIMA collection device.

4. Specimens collected by swab from other sites:
   A. *Conjunctiva* Remove mucus and exudate. Use a swab and firm pressure to scrape away epithelial cells from upper and lower lids.
   B. *Posterior nasopharynx or throat* Collect epithelial cells by using a swab.
   C. *Rectum* Collect epithelial cells from anal crypts by using a swab. Avoid contamination with fecal material.

ANAL: Place the patient in a lithotomy or side-lying position and drape for privacy. Insert the swab 1 in. into the anal canal and rotate it, moving it from side to side to allow it to come into contact with the microorganisms. Remove the swab. Place the swab in the Culturette tube, and squeeze the bottom of the tube to release the transport medium. Ensure that the end of the swab is immersed in the medium. Repeat with a clean swab if the swab is pushed into feces.

EAR: Cleanse the area surrounding the site with a swab that contains cleaning solution to remove any contaminating material or flora that have collected in the ear canal. If needed, assist the appropriate HCP in removing any cerumen that has collected. Insert a Culturette swab approximately 1/4 in. into the external ear canal. Rotate the swab in the area that contains the exudate. Carefully remove the swab, ensuring that it does not touch the side or opening of the ear canal. Place the swab in the Culturette tube, and squeeze the bottom of the tube to release the transport medium. Ensure that the end of the swab is immersed in the medium.

EYE: Pass a moistened swab over the appropriate site, avoiding the eyelid and eyelashes unless those areas are selected for study. Collect any visible pus or other exudate. Place the swab in the Culturette or Gen-Probe transport tube, and squeeze the bottom of the tube to release the transport medium. Ensure that the end of the swab is immersed in the medium. An appropriate HCP should perform procedures requiring eye culture.

GENITAL
1. *Female* Position the patient on the gynecological examination table with her feet in stirrups. Drape the patient's legs to provide privacy and reduce chilling. Cleanse the external genitalia and perineum from front to back with towelettes provided in the culture kit. Using a Culturette swab, obtain a sample of the lesion or discharge from the urethra or vulva. Place the swab in the Culturette tube, and squeeze the bottom of the tube to release the transport medium. Ensure that the end of the swab is immersed in the medium. To obtain a vaginal and endocervical culture, insert a water-lubricated vaginal speculum. Insert the swab into the cervical orifice, and rotate the swab to collect the secretions containing the microorganisms. Remove and place it in the appropriate culture medium or Gen-Probe transport tube. Material from the vagina can be collected by moving a swab along the sides of the vaginal mucosa. The swab is removed and then placed in a tube of saline medium.
2. *Male* To obtain a urethral culture, cleanse the penis (retracting the foreskin) and have the patient milk the penis to express discharge from the urethra. Insert a swab into the urethral orifice, and rotate the swab to obtain a sample of the discharge. Place the swab in the Culturette or Gen-Probe transport tube, and squeeze the bottom of the tube to release the transport medium. Ensure that the end of the swab is immersed in the medium.

SKIN: Assist the appropriate HCP in obtaining a skin sample from several areas of the affected site. If indicated, the dark, moist areas of the folds of the skin and outer growing edges of the infection where microorganisms are most likely to flourish should be selected. Place the scrapings in a collection container or spread on a slide. Aspirate any fluid from a pustule or vesicle using a sterile needle and tuberculin syringe. The exudate will be flushed into a sterile collection tube. If the lesion is not fluid filled, open the lesion with a scalpel, and swab the area with a sterile cotton-tipped swab. Place the swab in the Culturette tube, and squeeze the bottom of the tube to release the transport medium. Ensure that the end of the swab is immersed in the medium.

STERILE FLUID: Refer to related body fluid studies (i.e., amniotic fluid, cerebrospinal fluid, pericardial fluid, peritoneal fluid, pleural fluid, synovial fluid) for specimen collection instructions.

WOUND: Place the patient in a comfortable position, and drape the site to be cultured. Cleanse the area around the wound to remove flora indigenous to the skin. Place a Culturette swab in a superficial wound where the exudate is the most excessive without touching the wound edges. Place the swab in the Culturette tube, and squeeze the bottom of the tube to release the transport medium. Ensure that the end of the swab is immersed in the medium. Use more than one swab and Culturette tube to obtain specimens from other areas of the wound. To obtain a deep wound specimen, insert a sterile syringe and needle into the wound and aspirate the drainage. Following aspiration, inject the material into a tube containing an anaerobic culture medium.

Evaluation

Recognize anxiety related to test results, and instruct the patient to report symptoms such as pain related to tissue inflammation or irritation. Instruct the patient to resume taking usual medication as directed by the HCP or to begin antibiotic therapy as prescribed. Discuss the importance of completing the entire course of antibiotic therapy even if no symptoms are present. Advise the patient that final test results may take 24 to 72 hours, depending on the organism suspected, but that antibiotic therapy may be started immediately. Inform the patient that a repeat culture may be needed 1 week after completion of the antimicrobial regimen. Instruct the patient in wound care and nutritional requirements (e.g., protein, vitamin C) to promote wound healing.

Emphasize the importance of reporting continued signs and symptoms of the infection. Provide information regarding vaccine-preventable diseases where indicated (e.g., cervical cancer, hepatitis A and B, human papillomavirus). Provide contact information, if desired, for the CDC (www.cdc.gov/vaccines/vpd-vac). Instruct the patient in the use of any ordered medications (oral, topical, drops). Instruct the patient in the proper use of sterile technique for cleansing the affected site and applying dressings as directed. Explain the importance of adhering to the therapy regimen. As appropriate, instruct the patient in significant side effects and systemic reactions associated with the prescribed medication. Encourage him or her to review corresponding literature provided by a pharmacist.

Inform the patient awaiting results of anal, endocervical, or genital cultures that final results may take from 24 to 72 hr depending on the method used and organism suspected. Advise the patient to avoid sexual contact until test results are available. Instruct the female patient in vaginal suppository and medicated cream installation as well as the administration of topical medication to treat specific conditions as indicated. Inform infected patients that all sexual partners must be tested for the microorganism. Inform the patient that positive culture findings for certain organisms must be reported to a local health department official who will question him or her regarding sexual partners. Offer support, as appropriate, to patients who may be the victims of rape or sexual assault. Educate the patient regarding access to counseling services. Provide a nonjudgmental, nonthreatening atmosphere for discussing the risks of sexually transmitted infections. It is also important to address problems the patient may experience (e.g., guilt, depression, and anger).

✔ Critical Findings

- Listeria in genital cultures: Listeriosis in pregnant women may result in premature birth, miscarriage, or stillbirth. The earlier in pregnancy the infection occurs, the more likely that it will lead to miscarriage or fetal death. After 20 weeks' gestation, listeriosis is more likely to cause premature labor and birth.
- Methicillin-resistant S. aureus (MRSA) in skin or wound cultures
- GBS in urine or anal/genital cultures

Note and immediately report to the requesting healthcare provider (HCP) any critical findings and related symptoms. A listing of these findings may vary among facilities; specific organisms are required to be reported to local, state, and national departments of health.

✔ Study Specific Complications

N/A

✔ Related Tests

- Related tests include relevant amniotic fluid analysis, antimicrobial drugs, audiometry hearing loss, biopsy site, cerebrospinal fluid (CSF) analysis, culture viral, Gram stain, otoscopy, pericardial fluid analysis, Pap smear, peritoneal fluid analysis, pleural fluid analysis, procalcitonin, spondee speech reception threshold, synovial fluid analysis, syphilis serology, tuning fork tests, vitamin C, and zinc.
- Refer to the Immune System table at the end of the book for related tests by body system.

Expected Outcomes

Expected clinical and patient-focused outcomes associated with Culture, Bacterial, Anal/Genital, Ear, Eye, Skin, and Wound are

- Collecting and transporting specimens to the laboratory without contamination
- Exhibiting sensitivity related to specimen collection in cases of rape
- Complying with specimen collection techniques and following instructions correctly
- Verbalizing that the purpose of specimen collection is to identify infecting organism
- Complying with the recommended treatment designed by the HCP
- Understanding that surgery may be necessary to treat infection related to the decubitus ulcer

REVIEW OF LEARNING OUTCOMES

Thinking

1. Explain the importance of collecting a specimen using sterile technique. Answer: The purpose of collecting a specimen and sending it to the laboratory for testing is to identify infecting organisms. Using sterile technique to collect a specimen will decrease the risk of contaminating the specimen with other organisms that could interfere with the validity of treatment decisions made by the HCP.

Doing

1. Describe three necessary actions to ensure a sample is correctly obtained and sent to the laboratory. Answer; Three basic steps of accurate specimen collection include making sure you have the correct patient, making sure you have the correct specimen container, and making sure you complete all of the required specimen collection information prior to sending it to the laboratory to prevent it from being discarded.

Caring

1. Recognize the value of working as a health-care team in meeting clinical objectives. Answer: Specimen collection is very much a team effort. Collaboration is required between the nurse, patient, family, and laboratory technician. The mutual goal is to find out what the infecting organism is so that it can be treated. The nurse convinces the patient that the specimen is needed and explains how to collect it. The patient partners with us by agreeing to collect and report the specimen to be picked up. The laboratory technician or technologist follows specific procedures to culture the specimen, identifying the infecting organism and which drugs can kill it. The HCP orders treatment based on the laboratory results. Any break in this chain of teamwork can cause error and delay treatment. We need to remember that we do not work alone but as part of a health-care team—we need each other to achieve a successful outcome.

Words OF Wisdom: Patients are very sensitive to the suggestion that they may have brought harm to their loved ones. With a diagnosis such as tuberculosis, there are societal and cultural connotations that are not positive. Be cognizant of what kind of emotional impact your words have. Use care in phrasing cause and effect. Use your resources, case management, social services, and the chaplain to assist your patient over the emotional hurtles.

BIBLIOGRAPHY

Aplisol (tuberculin-purified protein derivative) injection. (2009). Retrieved from http://dailymed.nlm.nih.gov/dailymed/lookup.cfm?setid=1e91a67c-1694-4523-9548-58f7a8871134

Centers for Disease Control and Prevention. (2012). Mantoux Tuberculin Skin Test DVD Facilitator Guide. Retrieved from www.cdc.gov/tb/education/mantoux/guide.htm

Centers for Disease Control and Prevention. (2013). Testing for TB infection. Retrieved from www.cdc.gov/tb/topic/testing/default.htm

Ryan, K., Ray, C., Ahmad, N., Drew, W., & Plorde, J. (2010). Sherris medical microbiology (5th ed.). Columbus, OH: McGraw-Hill.

Selekman, J. (2006). Changes in the screening for tuberculosis in children. Retrieved from http://medscape.com/viewarticle/525640

Targeted tuberculin skin testing and treatment and treatment of latent tuberculosis infection in children and adolescents. (2004). Pediatrics, 114, 1175. doi: 10.1542/peds.2004–0809

Thompson, G. (2013). Understanding anatomy & physiology: A visual, auditory, interactive approach. Philadelphia: F.A. Davis Company.

Van Leeuwen, A., & Bladh, M. (2015). Davis's comprehensive handbook of laboratory and diagnostic testing with nursing implications (6th ed.). Philadelphia, PA: F.A. Davis Company.

Go to Section II of this book and www.davisplus.com for the Clinical Reasoning Tool and its case studies to provide you with a safe place to explore patient care situations. There are a total of 26 different case studies; 2 cases are presented for each of 13 body systems. One set of 13 cases are found in the Section II chapters, and a second set of 13 cases are available online at www.davisplus.com. Each case is designed with the specific goal of helping you to connect the dots of clinical reasoning. Cases are designed to reflect possible clinical scenarios; the outcomes may or may not be positive—you decide.

Tissue and Cell Microscopy Studies: Histology/Cytology

OVERVIEW

Tissue and cell microscopy studies can be used as an investigative tool for suspected disease. Cancer is an example of the type of diagnosis that may be made from a tissue or cell study. The body's different organs and tissues have unique cell types with specific functions. These differences are apparent under microscopic examination. Pathology is a medical subspecialty that studies the difference between healthy tissue and diseased tissue. Histology is the study of tissue structure and organization. Cytology is the study of cellular structure.

Tissue samples are usually obtained by biopsy. Biopsies can be collected using a fine needle or core needle technique. The collection technique is dependent upon the health-care provider's (HCP) clinical plan and the size of the sample required to make a definitive diagnosis. Fine needle biopsy uses a thin needle to aspirate a small tissue specimen. Guided imagery can be used to assist the HCP to locate and collect tissue specimens. The drawback with fine needle aspiration is the risk that there will not be enough tissue collected to make a diagnosis. Larger tissue specimens can be obtained by using a core or punch needle. Core needles have a larger bore, which allows the HCP to remove a larger cylinder of tissue. Core needle biopsies also provide information regarding the degree of tumor penetration. Biopsy is an important tool that assists the HCP to develop the best therapeutic treatment modality for the patient.

The *frozen section* is a special procedure performed at the time of surgery. Once a tissue specimen has been obtained, it is visually examined, and then preserved by rapidly freezing it in a special medium. The frozen specimen is thinly sliced and placed on glass slides. The slides are rapidly processed and stained to be read by a pathologist. This procedure takes about 20 minutes and can be completed while a patient is under anesthesia. The value

of a frozen section to a surgeon is in obtaining quick information related to tumor removal. Tumors that are confirmed as nonmalignant can be removed during surgery. Other tumors confirmed as malignant may require the surgeon to rethink the decision to go forward with the surgery as planned or to complete a more extensive procedure. Frozen sections are also used to ensure that all of the cancer has been removed by verifying that the tumor margins are clear. Biopsy results are essential in helping the HCP decide which therapy or therapies—radiation, chemotherapy, or a combination of both—will have the best chance of eradicating the cancer.

When a routine specimen for pathology is obtained, it should be placed in a container with a preservative such as formalin and labeled with the correct information. The pathology requisition should include information that identifies the patient, the name of the person who submitted the specimen, the date and time the specimen was collected, the clinical history, and the preoperative diagnosis. Once received by the pathologist, the specimen will be given a gross visual examination. The sample will be weighed, measured, and described based on characteristics such as color and consistency. Gross examination helps a pathologist see how disease has changed the sample and helps to direct him or her where to begin a microscopic review. Tissue samples will be prepared for microscopic review by processing them in various chemicals and then placing them in hot wax molds. Once the wax molds cool, the samples are cut into very thin slices that are fixed on glass slides and stained. Hematoxylin and eosin are the most common stains used for tissue evaluation. The stained slides allow the pathologist to evaluate the samples for the anatomical cell structure, and the organization of the cells into the tissue. There are many other microscopic, enzymatic, and antibody techniques that can enhance different cell features. Histological examination of a specimen provides information about a tumor and the involved tissue's basement membrane. A histological examination can differentiate carcinoma, connective tissue, and blood vessels. If additional samples are needed, they can be stained for further review at any point after collection.

Cytology can be used to screen for disease or to render a diagnosis. Cytology focuses on examining single cells or clusters of cells. The type of specimen obtained will determine how the specimen is prepared for examination. Specimens can be obtained for examination by aspirating, scraping, or brushing cells from tissue surfaces, collecting secretions, or removing fluids that contain cells. Some samples, such as body fluids, may need to be concentrated before there are enough cells to examine. The cells are fixed on a glass slide and stained for microscopic review. During microscopic examination, a cytologist will use a special pen to mark abnormal cells. Marked samples will be sent to a pathologist, who will evaluate the appearance of the marked cells and their nuclei. The advantages of cytology are that it is fast, inexpensive, convenient, and less painful with fewer complications.

The information in the Part I studies is organized in a manner to help the student see how the five basic components of the nursing process (assessment, diagnosis, planning, implementation, and evaluation) can be applied to each phase of laboratory and diagnostic testing. The goal is to use nursing process to understand the integration of care (laboratory, diagnostic, nursing care) toward achieving a positive expected outcome.

- **Assessment** is the collection of information for the purpose of answering the question, "is there a problem?" Knowledge of the patient's health history, medications, complaints, and allergies as well as synonyms or alternate test names, common use for the procedure, specimen requirements, and normal ranges or interpretive comments provide the foundation for diagnosis.
- **Diagnosis** is the process of looking at the information gathered during assessment and answering the questions, "what is the problem" and "what do I need to do about it?" Test indications tell us why the study has been requested, and potential diagnoses tell us the value or importance of the study relative to its clinical utility.
- **Planning** is a blueprint of the nursing care before the procedure. It is the process of determining how the nurse is going to partner with the patient to fix the problem (e.g.,"The patient has a study ordered and this is what I should know before I successfully carry out the plan to have the study completed"). Knowledge of interfering factors, social and cultural issues, preprocedural restrictions, the need for written and informed consent, anxiety

about the procedure, and concerns regarding pain are some considerations for planning a successful partnership.

- **Implementation** is putting the plan into action with an idea of what the expected outcome should be. Collaboration with the departments where the laboratory test or diagnostic study is to be performed is essential to the success of the plan. Implementation is where the work is done within each healthcare team member's scope of practice.
- **Evaluation** answers the question, "did the plan work or not?" Was the plan completely successful, partially successful, or not successful? If the plan did not work, evaluation is the process where you determine what needs to be changed to make the plan work better. This includes a review of all expected outcomes. Nursing care after the procedure is where information is gathered to evaluate the plan. Review of results, including critical findings, in relation to patient symptoms and other tests performed, provides data that form a more complete picture of health or illness.
- **Expected Outcomes** are positive outcomes related to the test. They are the outcomes the nurse should expect if all goes well.

A number of pretest, intratest, and post-test universal points are presented in this overview section, because the information applies to tissue and cell microscopy (histology/cytology) studies in general.

Universal Pretest Pearls (Planning)

- Obtain a history of the patient's complaints, including a list of known allergens, especially allergies or sensitivities to medications or latex, so their use can be avoided or their effects mitigated if an allergy is present. Carefully evaluate all medications currently being taken by the patient. A list of the patient's current medications, prescribed and over the counter (including anticoagulants, aspirin and other salicylates, and dietary supplements) should also be obtained. Such products may be discontinued by medical direction for the appropriate number of days prior to the procedure. Ensure that all allergies are clearly noted in the medical record, and ensure the patient is wearing an allergy and medical record armband. Report to the HCP and laboratory any information that could interfere with, or delay proceeding with, the study
- Obtain a history of the patient's affected body system, symptoms, and results of previously performed laboratory tests and diagnostic and surgical procedures. Previous test results will provide a basis of comparison between old and new data.

- An important aspect of planning is understanding factors that may alter study findings or cause abnormal results. Interdepartmental communication is a key factor in the planning process. The inability of a patient to cooperate or remain still during the procedure because of age, significant pain, or mental status should be among the anticipated factors. Recent or past procedures, medications, or existing medical conditions that could complicate or interfere with test results should be noted.
- Review the steps of the study with the patient or caregiver. Expect patients to be nervous about the procedure and the pending results. Educating the patient on his or her role during the procedure and what to expect can facilitate this. The patient's role during the procedure itself is to remain still. The actual time required to complete each study will depend on a number of conditions, including the type of equipment being used and how well a patient will cooperate.
- Address any concerns about pain, and explain or describe, as appropriate, the level and type of discomfort that may be expected during the procedure. Explain that an IV line may be inserted prior to some procedures to allow the infusion of IV fluids such as normal saline, anesthetics, sedatives, medications used in the procedure, or emergency medications. Advise the patient that some discomfort may be experienced during the insertion of the IV. Make the patient aware that there may be some mild discomfort during the procedure.
- Provide additional instructions and patient preparation regarding medication, diet, fluid intake, or activity, if appropriate. Unless specified in the individual study, there are no special instructions or restrictions.
- Always be sensitive to any cultural or psychosocial issues, including a concern for modesty before, during, and after the procedure.

Reminder

Ensure that a written and informed consent has been documented in the medical record prior to the study, if required. The consent must be obtained before medication is administered.

Universal Intratest Pearls (Implementation)

- Correct patient identification is crucial prior to any procedure. Positively identify the patient using two unique identifiers such as patient name, date of birth, Social Security number, or medical record number.
- Standard Precautions must be followed.

- Ensure that the patient has complied with pretesting instructions, including dietary, fluid, medication, and activity restrictions as given for the procedure. The number of days to withhold medication depends on the type of medication. Notify the HCP if pretesting instructions have not been followed, for example, if applicable, if patient anticoagulant therapy has not been withheld.
- The patient as appropriate, should be prepared for insertion of an IV line for infusion of IV fluids, antibiotics, anesthetics, or analgesics. Inform the patient when prophylactic antibiotics will be administered before the procedure, and assess for antibiotic allergy. Prior to administration of any fluids or medications, verify that they are accurate for the study. Bleeding or bruising can be prevented, once the needle has been removed, by applying direct pressure to the injection site with dry gauze for a minute or two. The site should be observed/assessed for bleeding or hematoma formation, and then covered with a gauze and an adhesive bandage.
- Emergency equipment should be readily available.
- Baseline vital signs must be recorded and continuously monitored throughout and after the procedure, according to organizational policy. A comparison should be made between the baseline and postprocedure vital signs and focused assessments. Protocols may vary among facilities.
- Before leaving the patient's side, appropriate specimen containers should always be labeled with the corresponding patient demographics, initials of the person collecting the sample, collection date, time of collection, applicable special notes, especially site location and laterality, and then be promptly transported to the laboratory for processing and analysis. Place tissue samples for standard biopsy examination in properly labeled specimen containers containing formalin solution; place tissue samples for molecular diagnostic studies in properly labeled specimen containers. Promptly transport the specimen to the laboratory for processing and analysis.

Universal Post Test Pearls (Evaluation)

- Note that completed test results are made available to the requesting HCP, who will discuss them with the patient.
- Answer questions and address concerns voiced by the patient or family and reinforce information given by the patient's HCP regarding further testing, treatment, or referral to another HCP. Recognize that patients will have anxiety related to test results. Provide teaching and information regarding

the clinical implications of the test results on the patient's lifestyle, as appropriate.

- Note that test results should be evaluated in context with the patient's signs, symptoms, and diagnosis. Depending on the results of the procedure, additional testing may be performed to evaluate or monitor progression of the disease process and determine the need for a change in therapy.
- Be aware that when a person goes through a traumatic event such as an illness or being given information that will impact his or her lifestyle, there are universal human reactions that occur. These include knowledge deficit, fear, anxiety, and coping; in some situations, grieving may occur. Health-care providers should always be aware of the human response and how it may affect the plan of care and expected outcomes.

DISCUSSION POINT

Regarding Post-Test Critical Findings: Timely notification of a critical finding for lab or diagnostic studies is a role expectation of the professional nurse. Notification processes will vary among facilities. Upon receipt of the critical finding, the information should be read back to the caller to verify accuracy. Most policies require immediate notification of the primary HCP, hospitalist, or on-call HCP. Reported information includes the patient's name, unique identifiers, critical finding, name of the person giving the report, and name of the person receiving the report. Documentation of notification should be made in the medical record with the name of the HCP notified, time and date of notification, and any orders received. Any delay in a timely report of a critical finding may require completion of a notification form with review by Risk Management.

STUDIES

- Biopsy, Chorionic Villus
- Papanicolaou Smear

LEARNING OUTCOMES

Providing safe, effective nursing care (SENC) includes mastery of core competencies and standards of care. SENC is based on a judicious application of nursing knowledge in combination with scientific principles. The Art of Nursing lies in blending what you know with the ability to effectively apply your knowledge in a compassionate manner.

Thinking

1. Recognize that as human beings, we all have various strengths and weaknesses as team members.

Doing

1. Recognize that barriers to patient decision making can be resolved by providing resources that clarify misunderstanding.

Caring

1. Recognize that there is value in collaborating with other disciplines to provide patient care.

Biopsy, Chorionic Villus

Quick Summary

COMMON USE: To assist in diagnosing genetic fetal abnormalities such as Down syndrome.

SPECIMEN: Chorionic villus tissue.

NORMAL FINDINGS: (Method: Tissue culture) Normal karyotype.

Test Explanation

This test is used to detect fetal abnormalities caused by numerous genetic disorders. Examples of genetic defects that are commonly tested for and can be identified from a chorionic villus sampling include sickle cell anemia and cystic fibrosis. The advantage over amniocentesis is that it can be performed as early as the eighth week of pregnancy, permitting earlier decisions regarding termination of pregnancy. However, unlike amniocentesis, this test will not detect neural tube defects (see Fig. 20.1).

Nursing Implications

Assessment

Indications	Potential Nursing Problems
Assist in the diagnosis of in utero metabolic disorders such as cystic fibrosis or other errors of lipid, carbohydrate, or amino acid metabolism	• Family
	• Grief
	• Human Reactions
	• Self-esteem
Detect abnormalities in the fetus of women of advanced maternal age	• Spirituality
	• Role Performance
Determine fetal gender when the mother is a known carrier of a sex-linked abnormal gene that could be transmitted to male offspring, such as hemophilia or Duchenne muscular dystrophy	
Evaluate fetus in families with a history of genetic disorders, such as Down syndrome, Tay-Sachs disease, chromosome or enzyme anomalies, or inherited hemoglobinopathies	

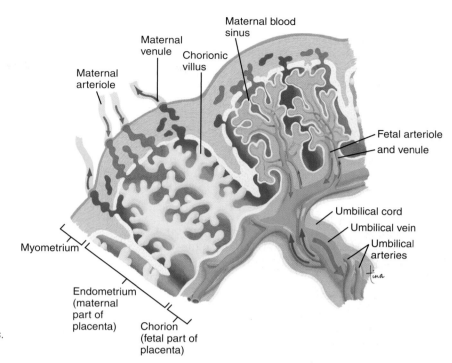

FIGURE 20.1 Diagram of the placenta showing the chorionic villus. *Used with permission, from Ward, S. (2009). Maternal-child nursing care: Optimizing outcomes for mothers, children, and families. FA Davis Company.*

Diagnosis: Clinical Significance of Test Results

ABNORMAL KARYOTYPE

Numerous genetic disorders. Generally, the laboratory provides detailed interpretive information regarding the specific chromosome abnormality detected.

Planning

Considerations for planning a successful partnership should include clear communication of what to expect during the test to decrease anxiety and improve cooperation. Include any family history of genetic disorders such as cystic fibrosis, Duchenne muscular dystrophy, hemophilia, sickle cell anemia, Tay-Sachs disease, thalassemia, and trisomy 21. Obtain maternal Rh type, and if the patient is Rh-negative, check for prior sensitization by obtaining a history of previous pregnancy. Record the date of the last menstrual period and determine that the pregnancy is in the first trimester between the 10th and 12th weeks. Obtain a history of IV drug use, high-risk sexual activity, or occupational exposure. Before the procedure is performed, plan to review the steps with the patient. Address concerns about pain, and provide information about the administration of pain medication appropriate for the procedure to be performed, an explanation about the need for establishing IV access, and other pretest preparation instructions. Warn the patient that normal results do not guarantee a normal fetus. Assure the patient that precautions to avoid injury to the fetus will be taken by locating the fetus with ultrasound. Explain that during the transabdominal procedure, any discomfort with a needle biopsy will be minimized with local anesthetics. Explain that during the transvaginal procedure, some cramping may be experienced as the catheter is guided through the cervix. Encourage relaxation and controlled breathing during the procedure to aid in reducing any mild discomfort. Inform the patient that specimen collection is performed by health-care provider (HCP) specializing in this procedure and usually takes approximately 10 to 15 minutes to complete. Instruct the patient to drink a glass of water about 30 minutes prior to testing so that the bladder is full. This elevates the uterus higher in the pelvis.

CONTRAINDICATIONS

The test is contraindicated in the patient with a history of or in the presence of incompetent cervix, vaginal infection, or Rh sensitization.

SPECIAL CONSIDERATIONS

An important aspect of planning is understanding the factors that may alter study findings or cause abnormal results. Interdepartmental communication is a key factor in the planning process. It should be noted when planning for this study that the patient should not void before the procedure. Failure to follow the instructions given before the procedure may cause the procedure to be canceled or repeated.

● Safety Tip

Make sure a written and informed consent has been signed prior to the procedure and before administering any medications.

Implementation

Note that patient education is key to obtaining the patient's cooperation in following directions, and providing an explanation for the purpose of the procedure is an important part of this process. Inform the patient that this study can assist in establishing a diagnosis of in utero genetic disorders.

Ensure that the patient has a full bladder before the procedure. Have emergency equipment readily available. Have the patient remove her clothes below the waist. Record maternal and fetal baseline vital signs, and continue to monitor throughout the procedure. Monitor for uterine contractions. Monitor fetal vital signs using ultrasound. Protocols may vary among facilities.

TRANSABDOMINAL BIOPSY

Assist the patient into a supine position on the examination table with her abdomen exposed. Drape the patient's legs, leaving the abdomen exposed. Assess the position of the amniotic fluid, fetus, and placenta using ultrasound. A needle is inserted through the abdomen into the uterus, avoiding contact with the fetus. A syringe is connected to the needle and the specimen of chorionic villus cells is withdrawn from the uteroplacental area. Pressure is applied to the site for 3 to 5 minutes, and then a sterile pressure dressing is applied.

TRANSVAGINAL BIOPSY

Assist the patient into a lithotomy position on a gynecologic examination table (with her feet in stirrups). Drape the patient's legs. Assess the position of the fetus and placenta using ultrasound. A speculum is inserted into the vagina and is opened to gently spread apart the vagina for inspection of the cervix. The cervix is cleansed with a swab of antiseptic solution. A catheter is inserted through the cervix into the uterus, avoiding contact with the fetus. A syringe is connected to the catheter, and the specimen of chorionic villus cells is withdrawn from the uteroplacental area.

Evaluation

Recognize anxiety related to test results, and monitor vital signs (both maternal and fetal) and neurological status, complete an assessment for postprocedural complications, provide instructions regarding diet, and administer ordered medications. Monitor for premature labor. Assess for nausea and pain. Administer antiemetic and analgesic medications as needed and as directed by the HCP. Instruct the patient in the care and assessment of the site. Instruct the patient to immediately report chills or fever, bleeding, or pain at the biopsy site. Advise the patient to expect mild cramping, leakage of small amount of amniotic fluid, and vaginal spotting for up to 2 days following the procedure but to report moderate to severe abdominal pain or cramps, increased or prolonged leaking of amniotic fluid from vagina or abdominal needle site, and vaginal bleeding that is heavier than spotting. Administer antibiotic therapy if ordered. Remind the patient of the importance of completing the entire course of antibiotic therapy, even if signs and symptoms disappear before the completion of therapy. Administer Rh o (D) immune globulin (RhoGAM IM or Rhophylac IM or IV) to maternal Rh-negative patients to prevent maternal Rh sensitization should the fetus be Rh-positive. Discuss the implications of abnormal test results on the patient's lifestyle. Provide teaching and information regarding the clinical implications of the test results, as appropriate. There are numerous tests for fetal genetic testing associated with inherited diseases and congenital abnormalities. The tests can be performed from chorionic villus sampling or amniotic fluid by methods that include polymerase chain reaction, microarray, and cell culture with karyotyping comparison. Educate the patient regarding access to counseling services. Encourage family to seek counseling if concerned with pregnancy termination or to seek genetic counseling if chromosomal abnormality is determined. Decisions regarding elective abortion should take place in the presence of both parents. Provide a nonjudgmental, nonthreatening atmosphere for a discussion during which the risks of delivering a developmentally challenged infant are discussed with options (termination of pregnancy or adoption). It is also important to discuss problems the mother and father may experience (guilt, depression, anger) if fetal abnormalities are detected.

✓ Critical Findings

- Identification of abnormalities in chorionic villus tissue.

Note and immediately report to the requesting HCP any critical findings and related symptoms. A listing of these findings varies among facilities.

✓ Study Specific Complications

Women at risk for or with known cervical abnormalities should be aware of the risks of miscarriage due to an incompetent (loose) cervix *related to passing a catheter or other instrument through the cervix, weakening the cervix*. Rh-negative women risk mixing of the maternal and fetal blood supply *related to the invasive nature of the procedure, potentially resulting in development of maternal antibodies directed against fetal blood cells which is a situation that can develop into hemolytic disease of the newborn*

✓ Related Tests

- Related tests include amniotic fluid analysis, and L/S ratio, chromosome analysis, α_1 fetoprotein, HCG, hexosaminidase A and B, newborn screening, US biophysical profile, and US obstetric.
- Refer to the Reproductive System table at the end of the book for related tests by body system.

Expected Outcomes

Expected outcomes associated with Biopsy, Chorionic Villus, are

- Consulting with the significant other or a spiritual leader regarding the potential termination of pregnancy related to lack of fetal viability
- Agreeing to seek genetic counseling related to the advisability of a future pregnancy
- Expressing concerns related to the ability to provide care to a special needs child

Papanicolaou Smear

Quick Summary

SYNONYM ACRONYM: Pap smear, cervical smear.

COMMON USE: To establish a cytological diagnosis of cervical and vaginal disease and identify the presence of genital infections, such as human papillomavirus, herpes, and cytomegalovirus.

SPECIMEN: Cervical and endocervical cells.

NORMAL FINDINGS: Method: (Microscopic examination of fixed and stained smear) Reporting of Pap smear findings may follow one of several formats and may vary by laboratory. Simplified content of the two most common formats for interpretation are listed in the table.

Bethesda System

Specimen type
- Smear, liquid-based, or other.

Specimen adequacy
- *Satisfactory* for evaluation—endocervical transformation zone component is described as present or absent, along with other quality indicators (e.g., partially obscuring blood, inflammation).
- *Unsatisfactory* for evaluation—either the specimen is rejected and the reason given, or the specimen is processed and examined but not evaluated for epithelial abnormalities and the reason is given.

General categorization
- *Negative for intraepithelial lesion or malignancy.*
- *Epithelial cell abnormality* (abnormality is specified in the interpretation section of the report).
- *Other comments.*

Interpretation/result
1. Negative for intraepithelial lesion or malignancy
   A. *List organisms causing infection:*
      - *Trichomonas vaginalis;* fungal organisms consistent with *Candida* spp.; shift in flora suggestive of bacterial vaginosis; bacteria morphologically consistent with *Actinomyces* spp.; cellular changes consistent with herpes simplex virus
   B. *Other nonneoplastic findings:*
      - Reactive cellular changes associated with inflammation, radiation, intrauterine device; glandular cell status post-hysterectomy; atrophy.

3. Epithelial cell abnormalities
   A. *Squamous cell abnormalities*
      - ASC of undetermined significance (ASC-US) cannot exclude HSIL (ASC-H)
      - LSIL encompassing HPV, mild dysplasia, CIN 1
      - HSIL encompassing moderate and severe dysplasia, CIS/CIN 2 and CIN 3 with features suspicious for invasion (if invasion is suspected)
      - Squamous cell carcinoma
   B. *Glandular cell*
      - Atypical glandular cells (NOS or specify otherwise)
      - Atypical glandular cells, favor neoplastic (NOS or specify otherwise)
      - Endocervical adenocarcinoma *in situ*
      - Adenocarcinoma
3. Other
   A. Endometrial cells (in a woman of 40 years or greater)

Automated review
- *Indicates the case was examined by an automated device and the results are listed along with the name of the device.*

Ancillary testing
- *Describes the test method and result.*

Educational notes and suggestions
- *Should be consistent with clinical follow-up guidelines published by professional organizations with references included.*

ASC = atypical squamous cells; ASC-H = high-grade atypical squamous cells; ASC-US = atypical squamous cells undetermined significance; CIN = cervical intraepithelial neoplasia; CIS = carcinoma in situ; HSIL = high-grade squamous intraepithelial lesion; LSIL = low-grade squamous intraepithelial lesion.

Test Explanation

The Papanicolaou (Pap) smear is primarily used for the early detection of cervical cancer. The interpretation of Pap smears is as heavily dependent on the collection and fixation technique as it is on the completeness and accuracy of the clinical information provided with the specimen. The patient's age, date of last menstrual period, parity, surgical status, postmenopausal status, use of hormone therapy (including use of oral contraceptives), history of radiation or chemotherapy, history of abnormal vaginal bleeding, and history of previous Pap smears are essential for proper interpretation. Human papillomavirus (HPV) is the most common sexually transmitted virus and primary causal factor in the development of cervical cancer. Therefore, specimens for HPV are often collected simultaneously with the PAP smear. The laboratory should be consulted about the availability of this option prior to specimen collection because specific test kits are required to allow for simultaneous sample collection. HPV infection can be successfully treated once it has been identified. There are three HPV vaccines (Cervarix, Gardasil, and Gardasil 9), usually given as a series of three shots, at 2 and 6 months after the initial injection. Vaccination is recommended in the preteen years because the vaccine's protection is most effective if the immune response to HPV develops prior to sexual activity. All three vaccines protect against the HPV strains that carry the highest infection risk (strains 16 and 18) and are associated with approximately 65–70% of cervical cancers and the majority of other HPV related anal/genital cancers. Cervarix is a 2-valent vaccine that targets HPV types 16 and 18; Gardasil is a 4-valent vaccine that targets HPV types 6, 11, 16, and 18; and Gardasil 9 is a 9-valent vaccine that targets HPV types 6, 11, 16, 18, 31, 33, 45, 52, and 58. Gardasil and Gardasil 9 are effective against HPV types that account for another 15–20% of cervical cancers; they are also effective against HPV types 6 and 11, the types that cause genital warts. The Centers for Disease Control and Prevention recommends vaccination for males (4–v HPV or 9–v HPV) ages 11 or 12 years through 21 years if not already vaccinated or who have not completed the entire 3 dose series; vaccination of males through 26 years (4–v HPV or 9–v HPV) for immunocompromised men or men who have oral or anal intercourse with other men; and females (2–v HPV, 4–v HPV, or 9–v HPV) ages 11 or 12 years through 26 years if not already vaccinated or who have not completed the entire 3 dose series. NOTE: Vaccination can begin at age 9 years for either males or females. FDA approval was recently received for administration of Gardasil 9 for females ages 9–25 and males ages 9–15 years. Additional FDA approval has been requested for males ages 16–26 years. The Advisory Committee on Immunization Practices has reviewed the preliminary data and recommended off-label use for males ages 16–26 years.

A wet prep can be prepared simultaneously from a cervical or vaginal sample. The swab is touched to a microscope slide, and a small amount of saline is dropped on the slide. The slide is examined by microscope to determine the presence of harmful bacteria or Trichomonas.

A Schiller test entails applying an iodine solution to the cervix. Normal cells pick up the iodine and stain brown. Abnormal cells do not pick up any color.

Improvements in specimen preparation have added to the increased quality of screening procedures. Liquid-based Pap tests have largely replaced the traditional Pap smear. Cervical cells collected in the liquid media are applied in a very thin layer onto slides, using a method that clears away contaminants such as blood or vaginal discharge. Samples can be "split" so that questionable findings by cytological screening can be followed up with more specific molecular methods like nucleic acid hybridization probes, polymerase chain reaction, intracellular microRNA quantification, or immunocytochemistry to detect the presence of high-risk HPV, Chlamydia trachomatis,

and Neisseria gonorrhoeae. Computerized scanning systems are also being used to reduce the number of smears that require manual review by a cytotechnologist or pathologist.

There are some alternatives to cone biopsy and cryosurgery for the treatment of cervical dysplasia. Patients with abnormal Pap smear results may have a cervical loop electrosurgical excision procedure (LEEP) performed to remove or destroy abnormal cervical tissue. In the LEEP procedure, a speculum is inserted into the vagina, the cervix is numbed, and a special electrically charged wire loop is used to painlessly remove the suspicious area. Postprocedure cramping and bleeding can occur. Laser ablation is another technique that can be employed for the precise removal of abnormal cervical tissue.

Nursing Implications

Assessment

Indications	Potential Nursing Problems
Assist in the diagnosis of cervical dysplasia	• Bleeding
Assist in the diagnosis of endometriosis, condyloma, and vaginal adenosis	• Human Reactions
Assist in the diagnosis of genital infections (herpes, *Candida* spp., *Trichomonas vaginalis*, cytomegalovirus, *Chlamydia*, lymphogranuloma venereum, HPV, and *Actinomyces* spp.)	• Pain • Self-esteem • Sexuality
Assist in the diagnosis of primary and metastatic neoplasms	
Evaluate hormonal function	

Diagnosis: Clinical Significance of Test Results
POSITIVE FINDINGS IN
(See table [Bethesda system])

DECREASED IN
N/A

Planning
Considerations for planning a successful partnership should include clear communication of what to expect during the test to decrease anxiety and improve cooperation. Before the procedure is performed, plan to review the steps with the patient. Address concerns about pain, and explain that there may be some discomfort during the procedure. Instruct the patient to avoid douching or sexual intercourse for 24 hours before specimen collection. Verify that the patient is not menstruating. Inform the patient that the specimen collection is performed by an HCP specializing in this procedure and takes approximately 5 to 10 minutes.

SPECIAL CONSIDERATIONS

An important aspect of planning is understanding the factors that may impair the procedure or cause abnormal results. Interdepartmental communication is a key factor in the planning process. The following should be noted when planning for this study:

- The smear should not be allowed to air dry before fixation as the cells may become distorted and may become unable to be properly evaluated.
- Lubricating jelly should not be used on the speculum as it may interfere with the readability of the smear.
- Use of an improper collection site may result in specimen rejection. Samples for cancer screening are obtained from the posterior vaginal fornix and from the cervix. Samples for hormonal evaluation are obtained from the vagina.
- Douching, sexual intercourse, using tampons, or using vaginal medication within 24 hours prior to specimen collection can interfere with the specimen's results.
- Collection of other specimens prior to the collection of the Papanicolaou (Pap) smear may be cause for specimen rejection.
- Contamination with blood from samples collected during the patient's menstrual period may be cause for specimen rejection.

It is also important to understand which medications or substances the patient may be exposed to in the healthcare setting that can interfere with accurate testing.

- If the patient is taking vaginal antibiotic medication, testing should be delayed for 1 month after the treatment has been completed.

Implementation

Patient education is key to obtaining the patient's cooperation in following directions, and providing an explanation for the purpose of the procedure is an important part of this process. Inform the patient that this study can assist in diagnosing disease of the reproductive system.

Have the patient remove her clothes below the waist. Assist the patient into a lithotomy position on a gynecological examination table (with feet in stirrups). Drape the patient's legs. A plastic or metal speculum is inserted into the vagina and is opened to gently spread apart the vagina for inspection of the cervix. The speculum may be dipped in warm water to aid in comfortable insertion. After the speculum is properly positioned, the cervical and vaginal specimens are obtained. A synthetic fiber brush is inserted deep enough into the cervix to reach the endocervical canal. The brush is then rotated one turn and removed. A plastic or wooden spatula is used to lightly scrape the cervix and vaginal wall (see Fig. 20.2).

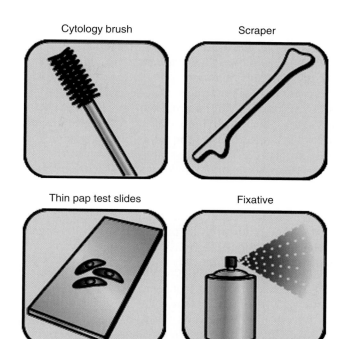

FIGURE 20.2 Equipment used for pelvic exam. *Used with permission, from Dillon, P. (2006). Nursing health assessment: A critical thinking, case studies approach (2nd ed.). FA Davis Company.*

CONVENTIONAL COLLECTION

Specimens from both the brush and the spatula are plated on the glass slide. The brush specimen is plated using a gentle rolling motion, whereas the spatula specimen is plated using a light gliding motion across the slide. The specimens are immediately fixed to the slide with a liquid or spray containing 95% ethanol. The speculum is removed from the vagina. A pelvic and/or rectal examination is usually performed after specimen collection is completed. Provide a sanitary pad if cervical bleeding occurs.

THINPREP COLLECTION

The ThinPrep bottle lid is opened and removed, exposing the solution. The brush and spatula specimens are then gently swished in the ThinPrep solution to remove the adhering cells. The brush and spatula are then removed from the ThinPrep solution, and the bottle lid is replaced and secured. Cleanse or allow the patient to cleanse secretions or excess lubricant (if a pelvic and/or rectal examination is also performed) from the perineal area. Provide a sanitary pad if cervical bleeding occurs.

CHLAMYDIA VAGINAL SWAB COLLECTION FOLLOWED BY NAA

- *Care provider specimen:* Collect vaginal fluid sample using the Gen-Probe® APTIMA® Vaginal Swab Kit by contacting the swab to the lower third of the vaginal wall, rotating the swab for 10 to 30 seconds to absorb the fluid. Immediately place the swab into the transport tube, and carefully break the swab shaft against the side of the tube. Tightly screw on the cap.

- *Patient self-collection instructions:* Partially open the package. Do not touch the soft tip or lay the swab down. If the soft tip is touched, the swab is laid down, or the swab is dropped, use a new APTIMA® Vaginal Swab Specimen Collection Kit. Remove the swab. Carefully insert the swab into the vagina about 2 in. past the introitus, and gently rotate the swab for 10 to 30 seconds, making sure the swab touches the walls of the vagina so that moisture is absorbed by the swab. Withdraw the swab without touching the skin. Immediately place the swab into the transport tube, and carefully break the swab shaft against the side of the tube. Tightly screw on the cap.

FOR CHLAMYDIA ENDOCERVICAL SWAB

Remove excess mucus from the cervical os and surrounding mucosa using the cleaning swab (the white shaft swab in the package with red printing). Discard this swab. Insert the specimen collection swab (the blue shaft swab in the package with green printing) into the endocervical canal. Gently rotate the swab clockwise for 10 to 30 seconds in the endocervical canal to ensure adequate sampling. Withdraw the swab carefully; avoid contact with the vaginal mucosa. Remove the cap from the swab specimen transport tube, and immediately place the specimen collection swab into the transport tube. Carefully break the swab shaft at the scoreline, using care to avoid splashing the contents. Recap the swab specimen transport tube tightly.

CHLAMYDIA MALE URETHRAL SWAB

The patient should not have urinated for at least 1 hour prior to specimen collection. Insert the specimen collection swab (the blue shaft swab in the package with the green printing) 2 to 4 cm into the urethra. Gently rotate the swab clockwise for 2 to 3 seconds in the urethra to ensure adequate sampling. Withdraw the swab carefully. Remove the cap from the swab specimen transport tube, and immediately place the specimen collection swab into the specimen transport tube. Carefully break the swab shaft at the scoreline using care to avoid splashing the contents. Recap the swab specimen transport tube tightly.

URINE SPECIMEN

The patient should not have urinated for at least 1 hour prior to specimen collection. Direct the patient to provide a first-catch urine (approximately 20 to 30 mL of the initial urine stream) into a urine collection cup free of any preservatives. The collection of larger volumes of urine may result in specimen dilution that may reduce

test sensitivity; lesser volumes may not adequately rinse organisms into the specimen. Female patients should not cleanse the labial area prior to providing the specimen. Add urine to the APTIMA® COMBO 2 urine collection device. The final volume must be between the two black lines on the device (about 2 mL).

Evaluation

Recognize anxiety related to test results and offer support. Discuss the implications of abnormal test results on the patient's lifestyle. Provide teaching and information regarding the clinical implications of the test results, as appropriate. Decisions regarding the need for and frequency of conventional or liquid-based Pap tests or other cancer screening procedures should be made after consultation between the patient and the HCP. The most current guidelines for cervical cancer screening of the general population as well as of individuals with increased risk are available from the American Cancer Society (www.cancer.org) and the American College of Obstetricians and Gynecologists (ACOG) (www.acog.org). Educate the patient regarding access to counseling services. Provide information regarding vaccine preventable diseases where indicated (e.g., cervical cancer, human papillomavirus). Provide contact information, if desired, for the Centers for Disease Control and Prevention (www.cdc.gov/vaccines/vpd-vac).

✔ *Critical Findings*

N/A

✔ *Study Specific Complications*

N/A

✔ *Related Tests*

- Related tests include biopsy cervical, cancer antigens, Chlamydia group antibody, colposcopy, culture anal/genital, culture throat, culture urine, culture viral, CMV, cytology urine, laparoscopy gynecologic, US pelvis, and UA.
- Refer to the Immune and Reproductive systems tables at the end of the book for related tests by body system.

Expected Outcomes

Expected outcomes associated with Papanicolaou (PAP) Smear are

- Verbalizing an understanding that intercourse may be painful and that abstinence may be required while the disease is treated in order to prevent injury to one's self or others
- Decreasing vaginal bleeding and discharge

REVIEW OF LEARNING OUTCOMES

Thinking

1. Recognize that as human beings we all have various strengths and weaknesses as team members. Answer: It is important to know your own strengths and limitations so that you know when to ask for help. Each patient is unique in her or his needs and wants. Each situation will require an approach to fit the unique situation. Understanding yourself will better allow you to access the resources that will best fit the situation with the least amount of frustration for you and your patient in high-stress situations such as diagnosing cancer.

Doing

1. Recognize that barriers to patient decision making can be resolved by providing resources that clarify misunderstanding. Answer: What are you thinking when your biopsy comes back positive and your HCP recommends breast removal or amputation? Does this give you pause; do you hesitate to say yes? Decisional conflict is a real possibility for your patients. How do you know which choice is best? An informed decision requires that all of the patient's questions be answered to his or her satisfaction. Your role is to find out what the questions are and use your resources to provide the answers so that the conflict is resolved and a decision is made.

Caring

1. Recognize that there is value in collaborating with other disciplines to provide patient care. Answer: Providing care for a patient in the current health-care environment is very much a team effort. Consider the patient who has had a biopsy with devastating results. How can you help her or him cope with the situation? Design the interaction to meet the patient's needs by collaborating with others. You can provide the patient with information about her or his interventional options. Ask the Chaplain for spiritual support based on the patient's religious affiliation. Include social services for support groups, financial assistance, and someone to talk to. Consider all of the other ancillary departments at your disposal, and assess what they can do to meet the patient's needs.

Words of Wisdom: The term "biopsy" is very difficult for patients to hear. Having a biopsy will put your patient on an emotional roller coaster, riding high with the hope that nothing is wrong and going low to the depths of despair when the patient's worst fears are confirmed. Responses will range from denial to anger and back again. Concern will not just be for him- or herself but also for the patient's loved ones, especially in the case in which small children may be left without a parent. How can you help? Tell the patient the truth. Provide him or her with the facts, including all the options that are recommended by the HCP. Help the patient find what coping strategies work for him or her and recommend using them. Finally, provide resources that can be used outside of the hospital or physician's office. Speaking with those in similar circumstances can help to work through the grief and fear in a way that nothing else can.

BIBLIOGRAPHY

Bladder cancer. Retrieved August 12, 2013, from www.medicinenet.com/bladder_cancer/article.htm

Can Hodgkin disease be found early. Retrieved August 11, 2013, from www.cancer.org/cancer/hodgkindisease/detailedguide/hodgkin-disease-detection

Chapin, J. Malignant Hyperthermia. (February 11, 2014). Retrieved from http://emedicine.medscape.com/article/1445509-overview#a11

Cleveland Clinic. (2014). Vital signs (body temperature, pulse rate, respiration rate, blood pressure). Retrieved from http://my.clevelandclinic.org/health/healthy_living/hic_Pre-participation_Evaluations/hic_Vital_Signs

Kidney cancer. Retrieved August 11, 2013, from www.mayoclinic.com/health/kidney-cancer/DS00360

Lung cancer signs and symptoms . Retrieved August 10, 2013, from www.cancer.org/cancer/lungcancer-non-smallcell/detailedguide/non-small-cell-lung-cancer-diagnosis

Liver biopsy. (July 22, 2010). Retrieved from www.webmd.com/hepatitis/percutaneous-liver-biopsy

Lorenz, J., & Blum, M. (2006). Complications of percutaneous chest biopsy. Retrieved from www.ncbi.nlm.nih.gov/pmc/articles/PMC3036363/

Melanoma skin cancer. Retrieved August 11, 2013, from http://www.cancer.org/cancer/skincancer-melanoma/detailedguide/melanoma-skin-cancer-detection

Mescher, A. (2009). Junqueira's basic histology: Text and atlas (12th ed.). New York, NY: McGraw-Hill.

Myopathy information page. Retrieved August 13, 2013, from http://ninds.nih.gov/disorders/myopathy/myopathy.htm

Overview of biopsy types. (March 7, 2013). Retrieved from www.cancer.org/treatment/understandingyourdiagnosis/examsandtestdescriptions/testingbiopsyandcytologyspecimensforcancer/testing-biopsy-and-cytology-specimens-for-cancer-biopsy-types

Polyzos, S., & Anastasilakis, A. (2011). Rare potential complications of thyroid fine needle biopsy. Retrieved from www.ncbi.nlm.nih.gov/pmc/articles/PMC3209672/

Practice guidelines for preoperative fasting and the use of pharmacologic agents to reduce the risk of pulmonary aspiration: Application to healthy patients undergoing elective procedures: An updated report by the American Society of Anesthesiologists Committee on Standards and Practice Parameters. (2011). Retrieved from http://www.asahq.org/~/media/Sites/ASAHQ/Files/Public/Resources/standards-guidelines/practice-guidelines-for-preoperative-fasting.pdf

Protocol and procedures for allergic reactions, including anaphylaxis in adults, infants, and children. (n.d.). Retrieved from https://dph.georgia.gov/sites/dph.georgia.gov/files/related_files/site_page/Emergency%20Protocols%20and%20Procedures.pdf

Rosenberg, H., Sambuughin, N., Riazi, S., & Dirksen, R. Malignant hyperthermia susceptibility. (January 31, 2013). Retrieved from www.ncbi.nlm.nih.gov/books/NBK1146/

Ross, M., & Pawlina, W. (2010). Histology: A text and atlas (6th ed.). Philadelphia, PA: Lippincott Williams & Wilkins.

Saslow, D., Solomon, D., Lawson, H., Killackey, M., Kulasingam, S., Cain, J., Garcia, F., Moriarty, A., Waxman, A., Wilbur, D., ... ACS-ASCCP-ASCP Cervical Cancer Guideline Committee. (2012). American Cancer Society, American Society for Colposcopy and Cervical Pathology, and American Society for Clinical Pathology screening guidelines for the prevention and early detection of cervical cancer. Retrieved from http://onlinelibrary.wiley.com/doi/10.3322/caac.21139/full

Symptoms of cervical cancer. (n.d.). Retrieved from http://www.cdc.gov/cancer/cervical/basic_info/symptoms.htm

Thyroid cancer. Retrieved August 12, 2013, from http://www.mayoclinic.com/health/thyroid-cancer/DS00492/DESCETION=symptoms

Van Leeuwen, A., & Bladh, M. (2015). Davis's comprehensive handbook of laboratory and diagnostic testing with nursing implications (6th ed.). Philadelphia, PA: F.A. Davis Company.

Vital signs. (n.d.). Retrieved from www.rnpedia.com/home/notes/fundamentals-of-nursing-notes/vital-signs

Go to Section II of this book and www.davisplus.com for the Clinical Reasoning Tool and its case studies to provide you with a safe place to explore patient care situations. There are a total of 26 different case studies; 2 cases are presented for each of 13 body systems. One set of 13 cases are found in the Section II chapters, and a second set of 13 cases are available online at www.davisplus.com. Each case is designed with the specific goal of helping you to connect the dots of clinical reasoning. Cases are designed to reflect possible clinical scenarios; the outcomes may or may not be positive—you decide.

Ultrasound Studies

OVERVIEW

Ultrasound began in the late 1940s with patients sitting in water-filled gun turrets. The diagnostic use of ultrasound has advanced from the 1950s, when it was used in obstetrics and for the evaluation of the heart and abdomen, to the 1970s, when the introduction of grayscale imaging allowed the health-care provider (HCP) to see a cross section of their patients' anatomy. With the advent of computer technology in the 1980s and color Doppler in the 1990s, ultrasound technology entered the modern age to become a widely used diagnostic tool that provides high-quality, detailed images of the human body in real time.

Ultrasound technology creates viewable images of the body by using a transducer in combination with high-frequency sound waves. The transducer can be placed against the skin or in a probe which is inserted into a body cavity. The transducer contains peizo-electric crystals that are activated, when an electric current is applied, to emit harmless, high-frequency sound waves into the body. Images are created by sound waves that bounce between the transducer and the tissues, body fluids, or organs being evaluated. Organ density will affect the way sound waves "bounce," allowing for differentiation between healthy and diseased tissue. Computers can then provide visual three-dimensional diagnostic information to be used by the HCP. Common uses of ultrasound as a diagnostic tool are in evaluating heart disease, the brain with stroke, and to assess for abdominal or reproductive changes. Because ultrasound does not use ionizing radiation like conventional radiography, it is a good choice as a diagnostic tool for pregnant women and children. The benefits of ultrasound include that it is safe for multiple use, noninvasive, portable, and accessible in multiple types of settings with all kinds of patients. Ultrasound is portable with different sizes of transducer, which make it very useful when working with the neonate, pediatric, and geriatric populations. Examples of some ways ultrasound can be beneficial to diagnose conditions in these populations include in diagnosing spina bifida, hydrocephalus, intracranial hemorrhage, appendicitis, foreign body detection, osteoporosis, or cardiac conditions (see Figs. 21.1 through 21.3).

Ultrasound transducers placed inside a patient can be used to examine areas such as the prostate and heart to diagnose and monitor disease progression. Cardiac evaluation can be completed with ultrasound by doing a transesophageal echocardiography (TEE). During a TEE, a fiberoptic endoscope is placed into the esophagus to evaluate the heart. This close-up view of the heart is not obstructed by the thorax or lungs and allows the HCP to obtain a clearer image for diagnostic review.

Doppler ultrasound is another way to use this technology as a diagnostic tool. Dopplers can assess blood flow through the body's veins and arteries. Areas of investigation include the abdomen, arms, legs, and neck.

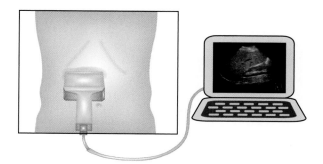

FIGURE 21.1 Ultrasound imaging. *Used with permission, from Weber, E., Vilensky, J., & Fog, A. (2013). Practical radiology: A symptom-based approach. FA Davis Company.*

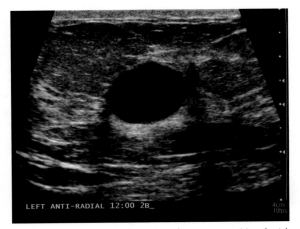

FIGURE 21.2 US showing a breast cyst. *Used with permission, from Weber, E., Vilensky, J., & Fog, A. (2013). Practical radiology: A symptom-based approach. FA Davis Company.*

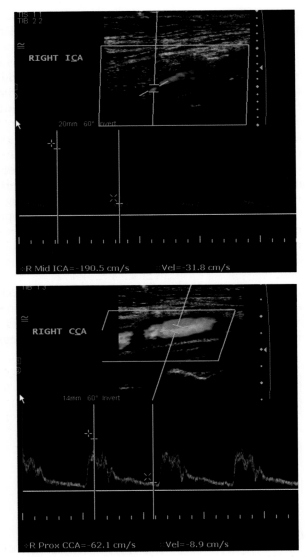

FIGURE 21.3 Carotid US showing stenosis. *Used with permission, from Weber, E., Vilensky, J., & Fog, A. (2013). Practical radiology: A symptom-based approach. FA Davis Company.*

Ultrasound can also be used to assess the blood flow to a mass in the breast, or to assess for deep vein thrombosis (DVT). Color Doppler ultrasound can be used to assess peripheral arteries in patients with peripheral vascular disease. Overall, ultrasound is a good complementary tool to other types of diagnostic studies designed to identify disease processes and evaluate the effectiveness of therapeutic interventions. The table below reviews types of ultrasound scanning techniques.

Ultrasound Scanning Techniques

Real-time imaging	Rapid sequence of data instantly converted into images
Doppler imaging	Used to assess blood flow through the conversion of sound waves into audible sounds or graphs. This technique is used to assess fetal heart rate and blood flow to organs.
Color flow Doppler	Used to evaluate blood flow in the chambers of the heart by determining the velocity (shades of flow) and direction (recorded as colors) of the blood flow
Duplex scanning	Used to demonstrate aneurysms, detect arterial plaque, or assess transplants for rejection
B-scan	Produces two-dimensional images from a series of single echoes
M-mode scan	Used to show the motion (M) of the heart over time, referred to as M-mode cardiography

The information in the Part I studies is organized in a manner to help the student see how the five basic components of the nursing process (assessment, diagnosis, planning, implementation, and evaluation) can be applied to each phase of laboratory and diagnostic testing. The goal is to use nursing process to understand the integration of care (laboratory, diagnostic, nursing care) toward achieving a positive expected outcome.

- **Assessment** is the collection of information for the purpose of answering the question, "is there a problem?" Knowledge of the patient's health history, medications, complaints, and allergies as well as synonyms or alternate test names, common use for the procedure, specimen requirements, and normal ranges or interpretive comments provide the foundation for diagnosis.

- **Diagnosis** is the process of looking at the information gathered during assessment and answering the questions, "what is the problem," and "what do I need to do about it?" Test indications tell us why the study has been requested, and potential diagnoses tell us the value or importance of the study relative to its clinical utility.

- **Planning** is a blueprint of the nursing care before the procedure. It is the process of determining how the nurse is going to partner with the patient to fix the problem (e.g., "The patient has a study ordered, and this is what I should know before I successfully carry out the plan to have the study completed"). Knowledge of interfering factors, social and cultural issues, preprocedural restrictions, the need for written and informed consent, anxiety about the procedure, and concerns regarding pain are some considerations for planning a successful partnership.
- **Implementation** is putting the plan into action with an idea of what the expected outcome should be. Collaboration with the departments where the laboratory test or diagnostic study is to be performed is essential to the success of the plan. Implementation is where the work is done within each health-care team member's scope of practice.
- **Evaluation** answers the question, "did the plan work or not?" Was the plan completely successful, partially successful, or not successful? If the plan did not work, evaluation is the process where you determine what needs to be changed to make the plan work better. This includes a review of all expected outcomes. Nursing care after the procedure is where information is gathered to evaluate the plan. Review of results, including critical findings, in relation to patient symptoms and other tests performed, provides data that form a more complete picture of health or illness.
- **Expected Outcomes** are positive outcomes related to the test. They are the outcomes the nurse should expect if all goes well.

A number of pretest, intratest, and post-test universal points are presented in this overview section, because the information applies to ultrasound studies in general.

Universal Pretest Pearls (Planning)

- Obtain a history of the patient's complaints, including a list of known allergens, especially allergies or sensitivities to medications or latex so their use can be avoided or their effects mitigated if an allergy is present. Carefully evaluate all medications currently being taken by the patient. A list of the patient's current medications, prescribed and over the counter (including anticoagulants, aspirin and other salicylates, and dietary supplements) should also be obtained. Such products may be discontinued by medical direction for the appropriate number of days prior to the procedure. Ensure that all allergies are clearly noted in the medical record, and ensure that the patient is wearing an allergy and medical record armband. Report information that could interfere with, or delay proceeding with, the study to the HCP and laboratory.
- Obtain a history of the patient's affected body system, symptoms, and results of previously performed laboratory tests and diagnostic and surgical procedures. Previous test results will provide a basis of comparison between old and new data.
- An important aspect of planning is understanding the factors that may alter study findings or cause abnormal results. Interdepartmental communication is a key factor in the planning process. The inability of a patient to cooperate or remain still during the procedure because of age, significant pain, or mental status should be among the anticipated factors. Recent or past procedures, medications, or existing medical conditions that could complicate or interfere with test results should be noted.
- Review the steps of the study with the patient or caregiver. Expect patients to be nervous about the procedure and the pending results. Educating the patient on his or her role during the procedure and what to expect can facilitate this. The patient's role during the procedure is to remain still. The actual time required to complete each study will depend on a number of conditions, including the type of equipment being used and how well a patient will cooperate.
- Address any concerns about pain and explain or describe, as appropriate, the level and type of discomfort that may be expected. Explain that an IV line may be inserted prior to some procedures to allow the infusion of fluids such as saline, contrast medium, or medications. Advise the patient that some discomfort may be experienced during insertion of an IV or collection of biopsy specimens, if ordered. Make the patient aware there may be some mild discomfort during the procedure.
- Provide additional instructions and patient preparation regarding medication, diet, fluid intake, or activity, if appropriate. Unless specified in the individual study, there are no special instructions or restrictions.
- Always be sensitive to any cultural or psychosocial issues, including a concern for modesty before, during, and after the procedure.

Reminder

Ensure that a written and informed consent has been documented in the medical record prior to the study, if required. The consent must be obtained before medication is administered.

Universal Intratest Pearls (Implementation)

- Correct patient identification is crucial prior to any procedure. Positively identify the patient using two unique identifiers such as patient name, date of birth, Social Security number, or medical record number.
- Standard Precautions must be followed.
- Children and infants may be accompanied by a parent to calm them. Keep neonates and infants covered and in a warm room, and provide a pacifier or gentle touch. The testing environment should be quiet, and the patient should be instructed, as appropriate, to remain still during the test as extraneous movements can affect results.
- Ensure the patient has complied with pretesting instructions, including dietary, fluid, medication, and activity restrictions as given for the procedure.
- The patient as appropriate, should be prepared for insertion of an IV line for infusion of IV fluids, antibiotics, contrast medium, anesthetics, analgesics, or medications used in the procedure or emergency medications. Inform the patient when prophylactic antibiotics will be administered before the procedure, and assess for antibiotic allergy. Prior to administration of any fluids or medications, verify that they are accurate for the study. Bleeding or bruising can be prevented, once the needle has been removed, by applying direct pressure to the injection site with dry gauze for a minute or two. The site should be observed/assessed for bleeding or hematoma formation, and then covered with a gauze and an adhesive bandage.
- Emergency equipment must be readily available.
- Baseline vital signs should be recorded and continuously monitored throughout and after the procedure, according to organizational policy. A comparison should be made between the baseline and postprocedure vital signs and focused assessments. Protocols may vary among facilities.
- Before leaving the patient's side, appropriate specimen containers should always be labeled, with the corresponding patient demographics, initials of the person collecting the sample, collection date, time of collection, and applicable special notes, especially site location and laterality, and then promptly transported to the laboratory for processing and analysis. Place tissue samples for standard biopsy examination in properly labeled specimen containers containing formalin solution, place tissue samples for molecular diagnostic studies in properly labeled specimen containers, and promptly transport the specimen to the laboratory for processing and analysis.

Universal Post Test Pearls (Evaluation)

- Note that completed test results are made available to the requesting HCP, who will discuss them with the patient.
- Answer questions and address concerns voiced by the patient or family and reinforce information given by the patient's HCP regarding further testing, treatment, or referral to another HCP. Recognize that patients will have anxiety related to test results. Provide teaching and information regarding the clinical implications of the test results on the patient's lifestyle as appropriate.
- Note that test results should be evaluated in context with the patient's signs, symptoms, and diagnosis. Depending on the results of the procedure, additional testing may be performed to evaluate or monitor progression of the disease process and determine the need for a change in therapy.
- Be aware that when a person goes through a traumatic event such as an illness or being given information that will impact his or her lifestyle, there are universal human reactions that occur. These include knowledge deficit, fear, anxiety, and coping; in some situations, grieving may occur. HCPs should always be aware of the human response and how it may affect the plan of care and expected outcomes.

DISCUSSION POINT

Regarding Post-Test Critical Findings: Timely notification of a critical finding for lab or diagnostic studies is a role expectation of the professional nurse. Notification processes will vary among facilities. Upon receipt of the critical finding, the information should be read back to the caller to verify accuracy. Most policies require immediate notification of the primary HCP, hospitalist, or on-call HCP. Reported information includes the patient's name, unique identifiers, critical finding, name of the person giving the report, and name of the person receiving the report. Documentation of notification should be made in the medical record with the name of the HCP notified, time and date of notification, and any orders received. Any delay in a timely report of a critical finding may require completion of a notification form with review by Risk Management.

STUDIES

- Echocardiography
- Echocardiography, Transesophageal
- Ultrasound, Abdomen
- Ultrasound, Arterial Doppler, Carotid Studies
- Ultrasound, Bladder

- Ultrasound, Liver and Biliary System
- Ultrasound, Pancreas
- Ultrasound, Pelvis (Gynecologic, Nonobstetric)
- Ultrasound, Prostate (Transrectal)

LEARNING OUTCOMES

Providing safe, effective nursing care (SENC) includes mastery of core competencies and standards of care. SENC is based on a judicious application of nursing knowledge in combination with scientific principles. The Art of Nursing lies in blending what you know with the ability to effectively apply your knowledge in a compassionate manner.

After reading/studying this chapter you will be able to:

Thinking

1. State how ultrasound is integrated into the process of disease diagnosis and therapeutic treatment.

Doing

1. Quantify quality care with data collection to validate best practice in health care.
2. Coordinate the integration of care regarding general planning guidelines for ultrasound studies.

Caring

1. Value how failure to follow standards of practice affects care outcomes.

Echocardiography

Quick Summary

SYNONYM ACRONYM: Doppler echo, Doppler ultrasound of the heart, echo, Sonogram of the heart, Transthoracic echocardiogram (TTE).

COMMON USE: To assist in diagnosing cardiovascular disorders such as defect, heart failure, tumor, infection, and bleeding.

AREA OF APPLICATION: Chest/thorax.

NORMAL FINDINGS

- Normal appearance in the size, position, structure, and movements of the heart valves visualized and recorded in a combination of ultrasound modes; and normal heart muscle walls of both ventricles and left atrium, with adequate blood filling. Established values for the measurement of heart activities obtained by the study may vary by health-care provider (HCP) and institution.

Test Explanation

Echocardiography, a noninvasive ultrasound (US) procedure, uses high-frequency sound waves of various intensities to assist in diagnosing cardiovascular disorders. The procedure records the echoes created by the deflection of an ultrasonic beam off the cardiac structures and allows visualization of the size, shape, position, thickness, and movement of all four valves, atria, ventricular and atria septa, papillary muscles, chordae tendineae, and ventricles. This study can also determine blood-flow velocity and the direction and presence of pericardial effusion during the movement of the transducer over areas of the chest. Electrocardiography and phonocardiography can be done simultaneously to correlate the findings with the cardiac cycle. These procedures can be done at the bedside or in a specialized department, HCP's office, or clinic.

Included in the study are the M-mode method, which produces a linear tracing of timed motions of the heart, its structures, and associated measurements over time; and the two-dimensional gray scale method, or two dimensional real-time Doppler color-flow imaging with pulsed and continuous-wave Doppler spectral tracings, which produces a cross section of the structures of the heart and their relationship to one another, including changes in the coronary vasculature, velocity and direction of blood flow, and areas of eccentric blood flow. Red and blue colors are assigned to represent the direction of blood flow while the intensity of the color is an indication of velocity. Doppler color-flow imaging may also be helpful in depicting the function of biological and prosthetic valves.

Echocardiography has become the method of choice for cardiac stress testing and evaluation of chest pain. Congenital heart disease such as atrial or ventricular septal defects are frequently evaluated with echocardiography. Cardiac contrast medium, composed of noniodinated lipid microspheres, such as DEFINITY or Optison may be used to improve the visualization of the heart.

Nursing Implications

Assessment

Indications	Potential Nursing Problems
Detect atrial tumors (myxomas) Detect subaortic stenosis ***as evidenced either by displacement of the anterior atrial leaflet or by a reduction in aortic valve flow, depending on the obstruction*** Detect ventricular or atrial mural thrombi and evaluate cardiac wall motion after myocardial infarction	• Activity • Bleeding • Cardiac Output • Fluid Volume • Gas Exchange • Human Response • Nutrition • Role Performance • Skin • Tissue Perfusion

Continued

Table Continued

Determine the presence
of pericardial effusion,
tamponade, and
pericarditis

Determine the severity of
valvular abnormalities such
as stenosis, prolapse, and
regurgitation

Evaluate congenital heart
disorders

Evaluate endocarditis

Evaluate or monitor
prosthetic valve
function

Evaluate the presence of
shunt flow and continuity
of the aorta and pulmonary
artery

Evaluate unexplained chest
pain, electrocardiographic
changes, and abnormal
chest x-ray *(evidenced
by an enlarged cardiac
silhouette)*

Evaluate ventricular
aneurysms and/or
thrombus

Measure the size of the
heart's chambers and
determine if hypertrophic
cardiomyopathy or heart
failure is present

Diagnosis: Clinical Significance of Test Results

ABNORMAL FINDINGS

- Aortic aneurysm
- Aortic valve abnormalities
- Cardiac neoplasm
- Cardiomyopathy
- Congenital heart defect
- Coronary artery disease (CAD)
- Endocarditis
- Heart failure
- Mitral valve abnormalities
- Myxoma
- Pericardial effusion, tamponade, and pericarditis
- Pulmonary hypertension
- Pulmonary valve abnormalities
- Septal defects
- Ventricular hypertrophy
- Ventricular or atrial mural thrombi

Planning

Considerations for planning a successful partnership should include clear communication of what to expect during the test to decrease anxiety and improve cooperation. Before the procedure is performed, plan to review the steps with the patient. Explain that an IV line may be inserted to allow the infusion of IV fluids such as normal saline, anesthetics, sedatives, dye, or emergency medications. Address concerns about pain related to the procedure and explain that there should be no discomfort during the procedure but there may be some discomfort during insertion of the IV needle. Inform the patient that the procedure is performed in a special room or at the bedside by an ultrasound technologist, and takes approximately 30 to 45 minutes. Explain that echocardiography does not use radiation and is considered safe.

SPECIAL CONSIDERATIONS

An important aspect of planning is understanding the factors that may alter study findings or cause abnormal results. Interdepartmental communication is a key factor in the planning process. The following should be noted when planning for this study:

- Dehydration may result in failure to demonstrate the boundaries between organs and tissue structures.
- Incorrect placement of the transducer over the desired test site may affect the quality of the study; the quality of the ultrasound study is very dependent upon the skill of the ultrasonographer.
- Bandages and dressings on postoperative patients may prohibit the required direct contact of the transducer on the skin.
- Fatty tissue in obese patients may affect results, because sound waves are distorted by fatty tissue.
- Metallic objects (e.g., jewelry, body rings) within the examination field may inhibit organ visualization and cause unclear images.
- The inability of the patient to cooperate or remain still during the procedure because of age, significant pain, or mental status may affect results; motion may cause artifacts
- An inadequate amount of gel or lubricant applied to the body to ensure the proper transmission of sound waves to and from the body may affect results.
- The presence of chronic obstructive pulmonary disease or the use of mechanical ventilation increases the air between the heart and chest wall (hyperinflation) and can attenuate the ultrasound waves.
- The enlarged space between the transducer and the heart in obese patients may affect results.
- The presence of dysrhythmias may cause unclear images.

● *Safety Tip*

Make sure a written and informed consent has been signed prior to the procedure if a biopsy is planned and before administering any medications.

Implementation

Note that patient education is key to obtaining the patient's cooperation in following directions, and providing an explanation for the purpose of the procedure is an important part of this process. Inform the patient that this study can assist in assessing for disorders of the heart.

Position the patient in a supine position on the examination table with foam wedges to help maintain position and immobilization and drape appropriately. Place electrocardiographic leads (EKG) on the chest, and apply a conductive gel on the patient's skin to improve the transmission and reception of the sound waves. Place the transducer on the chest surface along the left sternal border, the subxiphoid area, the suprasternal notch, and the supraclavicular areas to obtain views and tracings of the portions of the heart. Scan the areas by systematically moving the probe in a perpendicular position to direct the ultrasound waves to each part of the heart. To obtain different views or information about heart function, position the patient on the left side and/or sitting up, or request that the patient breathe slowly or hold the breath during the procedure. To evaluate heart function changes, the patient may be asked to inhale amyl nitrate (a vasodilator). Tracings are recorded from the reflected sound waves received. Administer dye, if ordered, and obtain a second series of images. Following the completion of securing the images, wipe the gel from the patient's chest.

Evaluation

Recognize anxiety related to test results, and be supportive of impaired activity related to cardiac insufficiency. Discuss the implications of abnormal test results on the patient's lifestyle. Provide teaching and information regarding the clinical implications of the test results as appropriate. Provide contact information, if desired, for the American Heart Association (www.americanheart.org) or the National Heart, Lung, and Blood Institute (NHLBI) (www.nhlbi.nih.gov).

SPECIAL CONSIDERATIONS

Numerous studies point to the prevalence of excess body weight in American children and adolescents. Experts estimate that obesity is present in 25% of the population ages 6 years to 11 years. The medical, social, and emotional consequences of excess body weight are significant. Special attention should be given to instructing the child and caregiver regarding health risks and weight-control education.

NUTRITIONAL CONSIDERATIONS FOR THE CARDIAC PATIENT: An abnormal myocardial infarct scan may be associated with coronary artery disease (CAD). Nutritional therapy is recommended for the patient identified to be at risk for developing CAD or for individuals who have specific risk factors and/or existing medical conditions (e.g., elevated LDL cholesterol levels, other lipid disorders, type 1 diabetes, type 2 diabetes, insulin resistance, or metabolic syndrome). Other changeable risk factors warranting patient education include strategies

to encourage patients, especially those who are overweight and with high blood pressure, to safely decrease sodium intake, achieve a normal weight, ensure regular participation of moderate aerobic physical activity three to four times per week, eliminate tobacco use, and adhere to a heart-healthy diet. If triglycerides also are elevated, the patient should be advised to eliminate or reduce alcohol. A variety of dietary patterns are beneficial for people with CAD and there are many meal-planning approaches with nutritional goals endorsed by the American Diabetes Association (ADA). The Guideline on Lifestyle Management to Reduce Cardiovascular Risk published by the American College of Cardiology (ACC) and the American Heart Association (AHA) in conjunction with the National Heart, Lung, and Blood Institute (NHLBI) recommends a "Mediterranean"-style diet rather than a low-fat diet. The guideline emphasizes inclusion of vegetables, whole grains, fruits, low-fat dairy, nuts, legumes, and nontropical vegetable oils (e.g., olive, canola, peanut, sunflower, flaxseed) along with fish and lean poultry. A similar dietary pattern known as the Dietary Approaches to Stop Hypertension (DASH) diet makes additional recommendations for the reduction of dietary sodium. Both dietary styles emphasize a reduction in consumption of red meats, which are high in saturated fats and cholesterol, and other foods containing sugar, saturated fats, trans fats, and sodium. The ADA also includes a vegetarian diet as well as other potential weight loss diets such as Weight Watchers. The nutritional needs of each patient need to be determined individually (especially during pregnancy) with the appropriate HCPs, particularly professionals educated in nutrition.

✅ Critical Findings

- Aortic aneurysm
- Infection
- Obstruction
- Tumor with significant mass effect (rare)

Note and immediately report to the requesting HCP any critical findings and related symptoms. A listing of these findings varies among facilities.

✅ Study Specific Complications

N/A

✅ Related Tests

- Related tests include antidysrhythmic drugs, apolipoprotein A and B, AST, atrial natriuretic peptide, BNP, blood gases, blood pool imaging, calcium, chest x-ray, cholesterol (total, HDL, LDL), CT cardiac scoring, CT thorax, CRP, CK and isoenzymes, echocardiography, echocardiography transesophageal, electrocardiogram, exercise stress test, glucose, glycated hemoglobin, Holter monitor, homocysteine, ketones, LDH and isos, lipoprotein electrophoresis, lung perfusion scan, magnesium, MRI chest, MI infarct scan, myocardial perfusion heart scan, myoglobin, PET heart, potassium, pulse oximetry, sodium, triglycerides, and troponin.

- Refer to the Cardiovascular System table at the end of the book for related tests by body system.

Expected Outcomes

Expected outcomes associated with Echocardiography are

- Decreasing fluid retention evidenced by decreasing weight and less edema
- Improved activity tolerance

Echocardiography, Transesophageal

Quick Summary

SYNONYM ACRONYM: Echo, TEE.

COMMON USE: To assess and visualize cardiovascular structures toward diagnosing disorders such as tumors, congenital defects, valve disorders, chamber disorders, and bleeding.

AREA OF APPLICATION: Chest/thorax.

NORMAL FINDINGS

- Normal appearance of the size, position, structure, movements of the heart valves and heart muscle walls, and chamber blood filling; no evidence of valvular stenosis or insufficiency, cardiac tumor, foreign bodies, or CAD. The established values for the measurement of heart activities obtained by the study may vary by health-care provider (HCP) and institution.

Test Explanation

Transesophageal echocardiography (TEE) is performed to assist in the diagnosis of cardiovascular disorders when noninvasive echocardiography is contraindicated or does not reveal enough information to confirm a diagnosis. Noninvasive echocardiography may be an inadequate procedure for patients who are obese, have chest wall structure abnormalities, or have chronic obstructive pulmonary disease (COPD). TEE provides a better view of the posterior aspect of the heart, including the atrium and aorta. It is done with a transducer attached to a gastroscope that is inserted into the esophagus. The transducer and the ultrasound (US) instrument allow the beam to be directed to the back of the heart. The echoes are amplified and recorded on a screen for visualization and recorded on graph paper or videotape. The depth of the endoscope and movement of the transducer are controlled to obtain various images of the heart structures. TEE is usually performed during surgery; it is also used on patients who are in the intensive care unit, in whom the transmission of waves

to and from the chest has been compromised and more definitive information is needed. The images obtained by TEE have better resolution than those obtained by routine transthoracic echocardiography because TEE uses higher-frequency sound waves and offers closer proximity of the transducer to the cardiac structures. Cardiac contrast medium, composed of nonionated lipid microspheres, such as DEFINITY or Optison, is used to improve the visualization of viable myocardial tissue within the heart.

Nursing Implications

Assessment

Indications	Potential Nursing Problems
Confirm diagnosis if conventional echocardiography does not correlate with other findings.	• Bleeding
Detect and evaluate congenital heart disorders.	• Cardiac Output
Detect atrial tumors (myxomas).	• Fluid Volume
Detect or determine the severity of valvular abnormalities and regurgitation.	• Human Response
Detect subaortic stenosis as evidenced by displacement of the anterior atrial leaflet and reduction in aortic valve flow, depending on the obstruction.	• Infection
Detect thoracic aortic dissection and coronary artery disease (CAD).	• Injury Risk
Detect ventricular or atrial mural thrombi and evaluate cardiac wall motion after myocardial infarction.	• Noncompliance
Determine the presence of pericardial effusion.	• Protection
Evaluate aneurysms and ventricular thrombus.	• Sleep
Evaluate or monitor biological and prosthetic valve function.	• Tissue Perfusion
Evaluate septal defects.	
Measure the size of the heart's chambers and determine if hypertrophic cardiomyopathy or congestive heart failure is present.	
Monitor cardiac function during open heart surgery (most sensitive method for monitoring ischemia).	
Reevaluate after inadequate visualization with conventional echocardiography as a result of obesity, trauma to or deformity of the chest wall, or lung hyperinflation associated with COPD.	

Diagnosis: Clinical Significance of Test Results

ABNORMAL FINDINGS

- Aortic aneurysm
- Aortic valve abnormalities
- CAD

- Cardiomyopathy
- Congenital heart defects
- Heart failure
- Mitral valve abnormalities
- Myocardial infarction
- Myxoma
- Pericardial effusion
- Pulmonary hypertension
- Pulmonary valve abnormalities
- Septal defects
- Shunting of blood flow
- Thrombus
- Ventricular hypertrophy
- Ventricular or atrial mural thrombi

Planning

Considerations for planning a successful partnership should include clear communication of what to expect during the test to decrease anxiety and improve cooperation. Before the procedure is performed, plan to review the steps with the patient. Address concerns about pain related to the procedure. Explain that some pain may be experienced during the test, and there may be moments of discomfort during insertion of the scope. Lidocaine is sprayed in the patient's throat to reduce discomfort caused by the presence of the endoscope. Inform the patient that the procedure is performed in an endoscopy suite or at the bedside by a gastroenterologist or a cardiologist, and takes approximately 20 to 30 minutes. Explain that echocardiography does not use radiation and is considered safe. Inform the patient that a light sedation will be used and will be given through an IV. Explain that he or she will need to remove any dentures or partials prior to the procedure. Remind the patient that he or she should have no food, fluid, or medication for 6 hours unless by medical direction.

CONTRAINDICATIONS

This procedure is contraindicated under a variety of circumstances that may be considered absolute or relative depending on the facility's providers:

- Barrett esophagus
- Bleeding disorders
- Esophageal obstruction (e.g., spasm, stricture, tumor)
- Esophageal trauma (e.g., laceration, perforation)
- Esophageal varices
- Known upper esophagus disease
- Tracheoesophageal fistula
- Recent esophageal surgery (e.g., esophagectomy or esophagogastrectomy)
- Unstable cardiac or respiratory status
- Zenker diverticulum

SPECIAL CONSIDERATIONS

An important aspect of planning is understanding the factors that may alter study findings or cause abnormal results. Interdepartmental communication is a key factor in the planning process. The following should be noted when planning for this study:

- Incorrect placement of the transducer over the desired test site may affect test results; the quality of the US study is very dependent upon the skill of the ultrasonographer.
- Bandages and dressings of postoperative patients prohibit the required direct contact of the transducer on the skin, which may affect results.
- Fatty tissue of obese patients may affect clarity of images, because sound waves are distorted by fatty tissue.
- The inability of the patient to cooperate or remain still during the procedure because of age, significant pain, or mental status may affect results; motion may cause artifacts.
- An inadequate amount of gel or lubricant applied to the body to ensure the proper transmission of sound waves to and from the body may affect results.
- The presence of chronic obstructive pulmonary disease or the use of mechanical ventilation increases the air between the heart and chest wall (hyperinflation) and can attenuate the ultrasound waves.
- Due to the enlarged space between the transducer and the heart in obese patients, the quality of the images may be affected.
- The presence of dysrhythmias may affect the results.
- Dehydration results in failure to demonstrate the boundaries between organs and tissue structures.
- Metallic objects (e.g., jewelry, body rings) within the examination field may inhibit organ visualization and cause unclear images.
- A large diaphragmatic hernia may affect imaging.
- An unknown upper esophageal pathology may affect imaging.
- Conditions such as esophageal dysphagia and irradiation of the mediastinum *related to difficulty manipulating the US probe once it has been inserted in the esophagus* may affect imaging.
- Failure to follow dietary restrictions before the procedure may cause the procedure to be canceled or repeated.

● *Safety Tip*

Make sure a written and informed consent has been signed prior to the procedure and before administering any medications.

Implementation

Note that patient education is key to obtaining the patient's cooperation in following directions, and providing an explanation for the purpose of the procedure is an important part of this process. Inform the patient that this study can assist in assessing for disorders of the heart muscles and valves. Ensure that the patient has complied with dietary and fluid restriction for at least 6 hours prior to the procedure. Ask the patient, as appropriate, to remove his or her dentures. Establish an IV fluid line for the injection of saline, sedatives, or emergency medications.

Place the patient in a left side-lying position on a flat table with foam wedges to help maintain position and immobilization, and drape appropriately. Insert an IV and administer a short-acting sedation as prescribed. Place electrocardiograph leads (EKG) on the chest, and continually monitor the patient's heart rhythm. Secure a blood pressure cuff and pulse oximeter, and take baseline readings and monitor vital signs throughout the procedure. Anesthetize the pharynx with a locally applied topical agent to depress the gag reflex. The endoscope is inserted into the mouth and into the upper portion of the esophagus. Ask the patient to swallow while the transducer is advanced through the endoscope and is located behind the heart. Dim the lights in the room to display the images on the monitor and obtain printouts, if requested. Administer dye, if ordered, and obtain a second series of images. The endoscope and transducer are withdrawn following the procedure, and a dressing is placed on skin following removal of the IV. Remove the EKG leads and clean off the skin.

Evaluation

Recognize anxiety related to test results, and be supportive of impaired activity related to cardiac abnormalities. Observe the patient for 30 to 60 minutes after the procedure to monitor the effects of the sedation and assess the patient's swallowing function. Monitor vital signs and neurological status every 15 minutes for 1 hour, then every 2 hours for 4 hours, and as ordered. Take the temperature every 4 hours for 24 hours. Monitor intake and output at least every 8 hours. Compare with baseline values. Notify the HCP if temperature is elevated. Protocols may vary among facilities. Instruct the patient to treat throat discomfort with lozenges and warm gargles when the gag reflex returns. Instruct the patient to resume the usual diet and activity 4 to 6 hours after the test, as directed by the HCP. Discuss the implications of abnormal test results on the patient's lifestyle, and provide teaching and information regarding the clinical implications of the test results as appropriate.

SPECIAL CONSIDERATIONS

Numerous studies point to the prevalence of excess body weight in American children and adolescents. Experts estimate that obesity is present in 25% of the population ages 6 years to 11 years. The medical, social, and emotional consequences of excess body weight are significant. Special attention should be given to instructing the child and caregiver regarding health risks and weight-control education.

NUTRITIONAL CONSIDERATIONS FOR THE CARDIAC PATIENT: An abnormal myocardial infarct scan may be associated with CAD. Nutritional therapy is recommended for the patient identified to be at risk for developing CAD or for individuals who have specific risk factors and/or existing medical conditions (e.g., elevated LDL cholesterol levels, other lipid disorders, type 1 diabetes, type 2 diabetes, insulin resistance, or metabolic syndrome). Other changeable risk factors warranting patient education include strategies to encourage patients, especially those who are overweight and with high blood pressure, to safely decrease sodium intake, achieve a normal weight, ensure regular participation of moderate aerobic physical activity three to four times per week, eliminate tobacco use, and adhere to a heart-healthy diet. If triglycerides also are elevated, the patient should be advised to eliminate or reduce alcohol. A variety of dietary patterns are beneficial for people with CAD and there are many meal-planning approaches with nutritional goals endorsed by the American Diabetes Association (ADA). The Guideline on Lifestyle Management to Reduce Cardiovascular Risk published by the American College of Cardiology (ACC) and the American Heart Association (AHA) in conjunction with the National Heart, Lung, and Blood Institute (NHLBI) recommends a "Mediterranean"-style diet rather than a low-fat diet. The guideline emphasizes inclusion of vegetables, whole grains, fruits, low-fat dairy, nuts, legumes, and nontropical vegetable oils (e.g., olive, canola, peanut, sunflower, flaxseed) along with fish and lean poultry. A similar dietary pattern known as the Dietary Approaches to Stop Hypertension (DASH) diet makes additional recommendations for the reduction of dietary sodium. Both dietary styles emphasize a reduction in consumption of red meats, which are high in saturated fats and cholesterol, and other foods containing sugar, saturated fats, trans fats, and sodium. The ADA also includes a vegetarian diet as well as other potential weight loss diets such as Weight Watchers. The nutritional needs of each patient need to be determined individually (especially during pregnancy) with the appropriate HCPs, particularly professionals educated in nutrition.

✅ Critical Findings

- Aortic aneurysm
- Aortic dissection

Note and immediately report to the requesting HCP any critical findings and related symptoms. A listing of these findings varies among facilities.

✅ Study Specific Complications

While complications are rare, trauma to the upper GI tract (e.g., esophageal bleeding, perforation, or rupture) may occur. Other potential complications include undiagnosed esophageal pathology, laryngospasm, or bronchospasm.

Related Tests

- Related tests include antidysrhythmic drugs, apolipoprotein A and B, AST, atrial natriuretic peptide, BNP, blood gases, blood pool imaging, calcium, chest x-ray, cholesterol (total, HDL, LDL), CT cardiac scoring, CT thorax, CRP, CK and isoenzymes, echocardiography, electrocardiogram, exercise stress test, glucose, glycated hemoglobin, Holter monitor, homocysteine, ketones, LDH and isos, lipoprotein electrophoresis, lung perfusion scan, magnesium, MRI chest, MI infarct scan, myocardial perfusion heart scan, myoglobin, PET heart, potassium, pulse oximetry, sodium, triglycerides, and troponin.
- Refer to the Cardiovascular System table at the end of the book for related tests by body system.

Expected Outcomes

Expected outcomes associated with Echocardiography, Transesophageal, are

- Understanding that those with valve prolapse can live normal lives with therapeutic management
- Acknowledging the importance of altering one's lifestyle to better manage health

Ultrasound, Abdomen

Quick Summary

SYNONYM ACRONYM: Abdominal ultrasound, abdomen sonography.

COMMON USE: To visualize and assess the solid organs of the abdomen, including the aorta, bile ducts, gallbladder, kidneys, pancreas, spleen, and other large abdominal blood vessels. This study is used to perform biopsies and assist in diagnosing disorders such as aortic aneurysm, infections, fluid collections, masses, and obstructions. This procedure can also be used to evaluate therapeutic interventions such as organ transplants.

AREA OF APPLICATION: Abdomen from the xiphoid process to the umbilicus.

NORMAL FINDINGS
- Absence of ascites, aortic aneurysm, cysts, obstruction, or tumors
- Normal size, position, and shape of intra-abdominal organs and associated structures

Test Explanation

Ultrasound (US) procedures are diagnostic, noninvasive, and relatively inexpensive. They take a short time to complete, do not use radiation, and cause no harm to the patient. High-frequency sound waves of various intensities are delivered by a transducer, a flashlight-shaped device, pressed against the skin. The waves are bounced back off internal anatomical structures and fluids, converted to electrical energy, amplified by the transducer, and displayed as images on a monitor. US is often used as a diagnostic and therapeutic tool for guiding minimally invasive procedures such as needle biopsies and fluid aspiration (paracentesis). The contraindications and complications for biopsy and fluid aspiration are discussed in detail in the individual studies.

Abdominal US is valuable in determining aortic aneurysms, in determining the internal components of organ masses (solid versus cystic), and for evaluating other abdominal diseases, ascites, and abdominal obstruction. Abdominal US can be performed on the same day as a radionuclide scan or other radiological procedure and is especially valuable in patients who have hypersensitivity to contrast medium or are pregnant. US is also widely used for pediatric patients to help diagnose appendicitis and for infants to assign cause for recurrent vomiting.

Nursing Implications
Assessment

Indications	Potential Nursing Problems
Determine the patency and function of abdominal blood vessels, including the abdominal aorta; vena cava; and portal, splenic, renal, and superior and inferior mesenteric veins. Detect and measure an abdominal aortic aneurysm. Monitor abdominal aortic aneurysm expansion to prevent rupture. Determine changes within small aortic aneurysms pre- and postsurgery. Evaluate abdominal ascites. Evaluate size, shape, and pathology of intra-abdominal organs.	• Breathing • Body Image • Cardiac Output • Confusion • Electrolytes • Fall Risk • Fluid Volume • Grief • Hopelessness • Human Response • Infection • Nutrition • Pain • Powerlessness • Sexuality • Tissue Perfusion • Urination

Diagnosis: Clinical Significance of Test Results
ABNORMAL FINDINGS
- Abdominal abscess, ascitic fluid, or hematoma
- Aortic aneurysm greater than 4 cm
- Congenital absence or malplacement of organs
- Gallbladder or renal calculi
- Tumor, liver, spleen, or retroperitoneal space

Planning

Considerations for planning a successful partnership should include clear communication of what to expect during the test to decrease anxiety and improve cooperation. Retained air, barium, or gas from a previous radiological procedure may block the transmission of sound waves; there should be 24 hours between potentially interfering procedures and this test. Alternatively, endoscopic retrograde cholangiopancreatography, colonoscopy, or procedures involving barium, if ordered, should be scheduled after this procedure. Before the procedure is performed, plan to review the steps with the patient. There are no food or fluid restrictions for most US studies; however, restrictions for US studies such as liver, pancreas, biliary tree, and gallbladder may require fasting for 8 hours by medical direction. Address concerns about pain related to the procedure. Explain to the patient that there may be moments of discomfort experienced during the test. Inform the patient that the procedure is performed in a special room or at the bedside by an ultrasound technologist, and takes approximately 20 to 30 minutes. Explain that ultrasound does not use radiation and is considered safe.

SPECIAL CONSIDERATIONS

An important aspect of planning is understanding the factors that may alter study findings or cause abnormal results. Interdepartmental communication is a key factor in the planning process. The following should be noted when planning for this study:

- Incorrect placement of the transducer over the desired test site may affect results; the quality of the US study is very dependent upon the skill of the ultrasonographer.
- Bandages and dressings of the postoperative patient may prohibit the required direct contact of the transducer on the skin.
- The fatty tissue of obese patients may affect results, because sound waves are distorted by fatty tissue.
- The inability of the patient to cooperate or remain still during the procedure because of age, significant pain, or mental status may affect the quality of the images, as motion may cause artifacts.
- An inadequate amount of gel or lubricant applied to the body may affect the proper transmission of sound waves to and from the body.
- The presence of chronic obstructive pulmonary disease or the use of mechanical ventilation increases the air between the heart and chest wall (hyperinflation) and can attenuate the ultrasound waves.
- Attenuation of the sound waves by the ribs can impair clear imaging of the upper abdominal structures.
- Retained air, barium, or gas from a previous radiological procedure may block the transmission of sound waves.
- Large amounts of bowel gas may distort abdominal organ visualization.
- Dehydration may result in failure to demonstrate the boundaries between organs and tissue structures.
- Failure to follow dietary restrictions before the procedure may cause the procedure to be canceled or repeated.

- Metallic objects (e.g., jewelry, body rings) within the examination field may inhibit organ visualization and cause unclear images.

● *Safety Tip*

Make sure a written and informed consent has been signed prior to the procedure if a biopsy is planned and before administering any medications.

Implementation

Note that patient education is key to obtaining the patient's cooperation in following directions, and providing an explanation for the purpose of the procedure is an important part of this process. Inform the patient that this study can assist in assessing for disorders of the abdominal organs. Ensure that food and fluids have been restricted, if required, prior to the procedure.

Position the patient in a supine position on the examination table and drape appropriately. The right- or left-side-up positions may be used to allow gravity to reposition the liver, gas, and fluid to facilitate better organ visualization. A conductive gel is applied on the patient's skin to improve the transmission and reception of the sound waves. The ultrasound transducer is moved across the abdomen in specific directions over the area of interest and images are recorded from the reflected sound waves received. Following completion of the images, wipe the gel from the patient's abdomen. If a biopsy was performed, cover the puncture site with a sterile dressing and promptly transport the specimen to the laboratory for processing and analysis (see Figs. 21.4 and 21.5).

Evaluation

Recognize anxiety related to test results and be supportive of impaired activity related to a perceived loss of independence. Discuss the implications of abnormal test

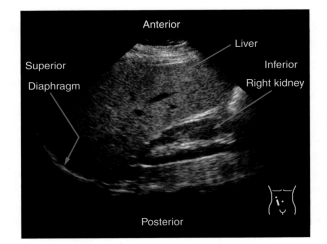

FIGURE 21.4 US of right upper abdomen. *Used with permission, from Weber, E., Vilensky, J., & Fog, A. (2013). Practical radiology: A symptom-based approach. FA Davis Company.*

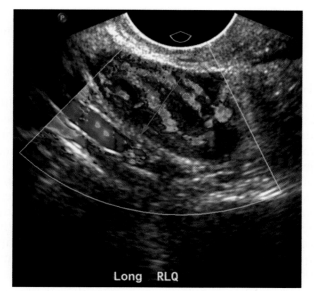

FIGURE 21.5 Color flow US of right lower abdomen; thickened and distended appendix (arrow). *Used with permission, from Weber, E., Vilensky, J., & Fog, A. (2013). Practical radiology: A symptom-based approach. FA Davis Company.*

results on the patient's lifestyle. Provide teaching and information regarding the clinical implications of the test results as appropriate. If a biopsy was completed, monitor the puncture site and instruct the patient to contact his or her health-care provider (HCP) if the puncture site shows indications of redness or inflammation, or if the patient experiences a fever that persists.

NUTRITIONAL CONSIDERATIONS:
A low-fat, low-cholesterol, and low-sodium diet should be consumed to reduce current disease processes and/or decrease the risk of hypertension and coronary artery disease.

✓ Critical Findings

- Aortic aneurysm measuring 5 cm or more in diameter.

Note and immediately report to the requesting HCP any critical findings and related symptoms. A listing of these findings varies among facilities.

✓ Study Specific Complications

Complications following an ultrasound-guided biopsy include hemorrhage from highly vascular tissue or infection. Instruct the patient to look for excessive bleeding, redness of skin, or fever or chills, and to notify his or her HCP if these symptoms occur.

✓ Related Tests

- Related tests include ACTH and challenge tests, albumin, ALKP, ALT, amylase, angiography abdomen, AST, biopsy intestinal, biopsy liver, bilirubin and fractions, BUN, calcium, calculus kidney stone panel, cancer antigens, carbon dioxide, CBC, CBC hematocrit, CBC hemoglobin, CBC WBC and differential, chloride, cortisol and challenge tests, creatinine, CT abdomen, GGT, HCG, hepatobiliary scan, infectious mononucleosis, IVP, KUB, LDH, lipase, magnesium, MRI abdomen, peritoneal fluid analysis, phosphorus, potassium, PT/INR, renogram, sodium, US kidney, US liver and biliary, US pancreas, US spleen, uric acid, urinalysis, and WBC scan.
- Refer to the Cardiovascular, Gastrointestinal, Genitourinary, and Hepatobiliary systems tables at the end of the book for related tests by body system.

Expected Outcomes

Expected outcomes associated with Ultrasound, Abdomen, are
- Understanding that ultrasound can locate and remove fluid to improve breathing
- Recognizing the importance of using ultrasound to pinpoint tumor location

Ultrasound, Arterial Doppler, Carotid Studies

Quick Summary

SYNONYM ACRONYM: Carotid Doppler, carotid ultrasound, arterial ultrasound, cerebrovascular ultrasound.

COMMON USE: To visualize and assess blood flow through the carotid arteries toward evaluating risk for stroke related to atherosclerosis.

AREA OF APPLICATION: Arteries.

NORMAL FINDINGS
- Normal blood flow through the carotid arteries with no evidence of occlusion or narrowing

Test Explanation

Ultrasound (US) procedures are diagnostic, noninvasive, and relatively inexpensive. They take a short time to complete, do not use radiation, and cause no harm to the patient. High-frequency sound waves of various intensities are delivered by a transducer, a flashlight-shaped device, pressed against the skin. The waves are bounced back off internal anatomical structures and fluids, converted to electrical energy, amplified by the transducer, and displayed as images on a monitor.

Using the duplex scanning method, carotid US records sound waves to obtain information about the carotid arteries. The amplitude and waveform of the carotid pulse are measured, resulting in a two-dimensional image of the artery. Carotid arterial sites used for the studies include the common carotid, external carotid, and internal carotid. Blood flow direction, velocity, and the presence of flow disturbances can be readily assessed. The sound waves that hit the moving red blood cells and are reflected back to the transducer correspond to the velocity of the blood flow through the vessel. Color doppler US can be used with the duplex method where red and blue are assigned to represent the direction of blood flow while the intensity of the color is an indication of velocity. The result is the visualization of the artery to assist in the diagnosis (i.e., presence, amount, location) of plaque causing vessel stenosis or atherosclerotic occlusion affecting the flow of blood to the brain. Depending on the degree of stenosis causing a reduction in vessel diameter, additional testing can be performed to determine the effect of stenosis on the hemodynamic status of the artery.

The combined information obtained from carotid US and ankle-brachial index (ABI) provides significant support for predicting coronary artery disease. ABI is a noninvasive, simple comparison of blood pressure measurements in the arms and legs and can be used to detect peripheral arterial disease (PAD). A Doppler stethoscope is used to obtain the systolic pressure in either the dorsalis pedis or the posterior tibial artery. This ankle pressure is then divided by the highest brachial systolic pressure acquired after taking the blood pressure in both of the patient's arms. This index should be greater than 1 with a range of 0.85 to 1.4. When the index falls below 0.5, blood flow impairment is considered significant. Patients should be scheduled for a vascular consult for an abnormal ABI. Patients with diabetes or kidney disease, and some older adult patients, may have a falsely elevated ABI due to calcifications of the vessels in the ankle causing an increased systolic pressure. The ABI test approaches 95% accuracy in detecting PAD. However, a normal ABI value does not absolutely rule out the possibility of PAD for some individuals, and additional tests should be done to evaluate symptoms.

Nursing Implications

Assessment

Indications	Potential Nursing Problems
Assist in the diagnosis of carotid artery occlusive disease, as evidenced by visualization of blood flow disruption. Detect irregularities in the structure of the carotid arteries. Detect plaque or stenosis of the carotid artery, as evidenced by turbulent blood flow or changes in Doppler signals indicating occlusion.	• Caregiver • Communication • Family • Fear • Human Response • Mobility • Nutrition • Powerlessness • Self-care • Sensory Perception • Swallowing

Diagnosis: Clinical Significance of Test Results
ABNORMAL FINDINGS
- Arterial aneurysm
- Carotid artery occlusive disease (atherosclerosis)

- Plaque or stenosis of carotid artery
- Reduction in vessel diameter of more than 16%, indicating stenosis
- Tumor

Planning
Considerations for planning a successful partnership should include clear communication of what to expect during the test to decrease anxiety and improve cooperation. Before the procedure is performed, plan to review the steps with the patient. Address concerns about pain related to the procedure, and explain that some pain may be experienced during the test, and there may be moments of discomfort. Inform the patient that the procedure is performed in a special room or at the bedside by an ultrasound technologist, and takes approximately 15 to 30 minutes. Explain that ultrasound does not use radiation and is considered safe.

SPECIAL CONSIDERATIONS
An important aspect of planning is understanding the factors that may alter study findings or cause abnormal results. Interdepartmental communication is a key factor in the planning process. The following should be noted when planning for this study:

- Incorrect placement of the transducer over the desired test site may affect results; the quality of the US study is very dependent upon the skill of the ultrasonographer.
- Bandages and dressings of postoperative patients prohibit the required direct contact of the transducer on the skin.
- Fatty tissue of obese patients may affect results, because sound waves are distorted by fatty tissue
- The inability of the patient to cooperate or remain still during the procedure because of age, significant pain, or mental status may affect the quality of the images; motion may cause artifacts.
- An inadequate amount of gel or lubricant applied to the body to ensure the proper transmission of sound waves to and from the body may affect the quality of the images.
- Attenuation of the sound waves by bony structures can impair clear imaging of the vessels.
- Dehydration may result in failure to demonstrate the boundaries between organs and tissue structures.
- Metallic objects (e.g., jewelry, body rings) within the examination field may inhibit organ visualization and cause unclear images.

Implementation
Note that patient education is key to obtaining the patient's cooperation in following directions, and providing an explanation for the purpose of the procedure is an important part of this process. Inform the patient that this study can assist in assessing for disorders of the carotid arteries.

Position the patient in a supine position on the examination table and support the head to prevent the patient from turning it laterally. A conductive gel is applied on the patient's neck to improve the transmission and reception of the sound waves. The ultrasound transducer is moved across the skin in specific directions, and images of the carotid artery and blood flow are recorded from the reflected sound waves received. Vertebral artery blood flow can also be visualized during a carotid Doppler. Following completion of the images, wipe the gel from the patient's neck.

Evaluation

Recognize anxiety related to test results, and be supportive of impaired activity related to carotid artery function or a perceived loss of independence. Discuss the implications of abnormal test results on the patient's lifestyle. Provide teaching and information regarding the clinical implications of the test results as appropriate. Provide contact information, if desired, for the American Heart Association (AHA) (www.americanheart.org), the National Heart, Lung, and Blood Institute (NHLBI) (www.nhlbi.nih.gov), or the Legs for Life (www.legsforlife.org).

SPECIAL CONSIDERATIONS

Numerous studies point to the prevalence of excess body weight in American children and adolescents. Experts estimate that obesity is present in 25% of the population ages 6 years to 11 years. The medical, social, and emotional consequences of excess body weight are significant. Special attention should be given to instructing the child and caregiver regarding health risks and weight-control education.

NUTRITIONAL CONSIDERATIONS FOR THE CARDIAC PATIENT:

An abnormal myocardial infarct scan may be associated with CAD. Nutritional therapy is recommended for the patient identified to be at risk for developing CAD or for individuals who have specific risk factors and/or existing medical conditions (e.g., elevated LDL cholesterol levels, other lipid disorders, type 1 diabetes, type 2 diabetes, insulin resistance, or metabolic syndrome). Other changeable risk factors warranting patient education include strategies to encourage patients, especially those who are overweight and with high blood pressure, to safely decrease sodium intake, achieve a normal weight, ensure regular participation of moderate aerobic physical activity three to four times per week, eliminate tobacco use, and adhere to a heart-healthy diet. If triglycerides also are elevated, the patient should be advised to eliminate or reduce alcohol. A variety of dietary patterns are beneficial for people with CAD and there are many meal-planning approaches with nutritional goals endorsed by the American Diabetes Association (ADA). The Guideline on Lifestyle Management to Reduce Cardiovascular Risk published by the American College of Cardiology (ACC) and the American Heart Association (AHA) in conjunction with the National Heart, Lung, and Blood Institute (NHLBI) recommends a "Mediterranean"-style diet rather than a low-fat diet. The guideline emphasizes inclusion of vegetables, whole grains, fruits, low-fat dairy, nuts, legumes, and nontropical vegetable oils (e.g., olive, canola, peanut, sunflower, flaxseed) along with fish and lean poultry. A similar dietary pattern known as the Dietary Approaches to Stop Hypertension (DASH) diet makes additional recommendations for the reduction of dietary sodium. Both dietary styles emphasize a reduction in consumption of red meats, which are high in saturated fats and cholesterol, and other foods containing sugar, saturated fats, trans fats, and sodium. The ADA also includes a vegetarian diet as well as other potential weight loss diets such as Weight Watchers. The nutritional needs of each patient need to be determined individually (especially during pregnancy) with the appropriate health-care providers (HCPs), particularly professionals educated in nutrition.

✓ Critical Findings

N/A

✓ Study Specific Complications

N/A

✓ Related Tests

- Related tests include angiography carotid, angiography coronary, antidysrhythmic drugs, apolipoprotein A & B, AST, blood gases, calcium, cholesterol (total, HDL, LDL), CT angiography, CT cardiac scoring, echocardiography, CRP, CK and isoenzymes, glucose, glycated hemoglobin, Holter monitor, homocysteine, ketones, LDH and isoenzymes, lipoprotein electrophoresis, magnesium, MRI angiography, MRI chest, MRI venography, myocardial infarction scan, myocardial perfusion heart scan, myoglobin, PET heart, triglycerides, troponin, US arterial Doppler upper and lower extremities, and US venous Doppler extremity.
- Refer to the Cardiovascular System table at the end of the book for related tests by body system.

Expected Outcomes

Expected outcomes associated with Ultrasound, Arterial Doppler, Carotid Studies, are

- Being able to interact with the environment on the affected side
- Understanding that an endarterctomy or stent placement may be necessary based on study results

Ultrasound, Bladder

Quick Summary

SYNONYM ACRONYM: Bladder sonography.

COMMON USE: To visualize and assess the bladder toward diagnosing disorders such as retention, obstruction, distention, cancer, infection, bleeding, and inflammation.

AREA OF APPLICATION: Bladder.

NORMAL FINDINGS
- Normal size, position, and contour of the bladder

Test Explanation

Ultrasound (US) procedures are diagnostic, noninvasive, and relatively inexpensive. They take a short time to complete, do not use radiation, and cause no harm to the patient. High-frequency sound waves of various intensities are delivered by a transducer, a flashlight-shaped device, pressed against the skin. The waves are bounced back off internal anatomical structures and fluids, converted to electrical energy, amplified by the transducer, and displayed as images on a monitor. US is often used as a diagnostic and therapeutic tool for guiding minimally invasive procedures such as needle biopsies and fluid aspiration. The contraindications and complications for biopsy and fluid aspiration are discussed in detail in the individual studies.

Bladder US evaluates the structure and position of the contents of the bladder and identifies disorders of the bladder, such as masses or lesions. The methods for imaging may include the transrectal, transurethral, and transvaginal approaches. The examination is helpful for monitoring a patient's response to therapy for bladder disease. Bladder images can be included in other US studies such as the kidneys, ureters, bladder, urethra, and gonads in diagnosing renal/neurological disorders.

The bladder scan is another noninvasive US study commonly used to assess postvoid residual. Advantages of the bladder scan over other studies, such as cystometry, is that the study can be performed at the bedside and does not require the patient to be catheterized, thereby eliminating the possibility of the patient developing a catheter-related UTI. The patient's gynecological history should be obtained prior to using the scanner in order to select the proper setting. The scanners have settings for male, female, and child, but scanning a female patient who has had a hysterectomy and is without a uterus should be performed using the settings for a male patient. This test is not usually performed on pregnant women. Normal findings are less than 30–50 mL. Report a residual urine that is greater than 100 mL or as directed by the requesting healthcare provider (HCP).

Nursing Implications

Assessment

Indications	Potential Nursing Problems
Assess residual urine after voiding to diagnose urinary tract obstruction causing overdistention.	• Bleeding
Detect tumor of the bladder wall or pelvis, as evidenced by distorted position or changes in bladder contour.	• Fear • Hopelessness • Human Response
Determine end-stage malignancy of the bladder caused by extension of a primary tumor of the ovary or other pelvic organ.	• Infection • Nutrition • Pain • Spirituality
Evaluate the cause of urinary tract infection, urine retention, and flank pain.	• Urination
Evaluate hematuria, urinary frequency, dysuria, and suprapubic pain.	
Measure urinary bladder volume by transurethral or transvaginal approach.	

Diagnosis: Clinical Significance of Test Results
ABNORMAL FINDINGS
- Bladder diverticulum
- Cyst
- Cystitis
- Malignancy of the bladder
- Tumor
- Ureterocele
- Urinary tract obstruction

Planning

Considerations for planning a successful partnership should include clear communication of what to expect during the test to decrease anxiety and improve cooperation. Retained air, barium, or gas from a previous radiological procedure may block the transmission of sound waves; there should be 24 hours between potentially interfering procedures and this test. Alternatively, endoscopic retrograde cholangiopancreatography, colonoscopy, or procedures involving barium, if ordered, should be scheduled after this procedure. Before the procedure is performed, plan to review the steps with the patient. Instruct the patient receiving transabdominal US to drink three to four glasses of fluid 90 minutes before the procedure and not to void because the procedure requires a full bladder. Patients receiving transvaginal US only do not need to have a full bladder. Inform the patient that, for the transvaginal approach, a sterile latex- or sheath-covered probe will be inserted into the vagina. Address concerns about pain related to the procedure. Explain to the patient that some pain may be experienced during the test, and there may be moments of discomfort. Inform the patient that the procedure is performed in an ultrasound room by a sonographer, and takes approximately 15 to 30 minutes. If a fine-needle aspiration is to be performed, a radiologist will be present to do the procedure and there may be minimal discomfort. Explain that ultrasonography does not use radiation and is considered safe.

SPECIAL CONSIDERATIONS

An important aspect of planning is understanding the factors that may alter study findings or cause abnormal results. Interdepartmental communication is a key factor in the planning process. The following should be noted when planning for this study:

- Incorrect placement of the transducer over the desired test site may affect results; the quality of the US study is very dependent upon the skill of the ultrasonographer.
- Bandages and dressings of postoperative patients may prohibit the required direct contact of the transducer on the skin.
- Fatty tissue of obese patients may affect results, because sound waves are distorted by fatty tissue.
- The inability of the patient to cooperate or remain still during the procedure because of age, significant pain, or mental status may affect the quality of the images; motion may cause artifacts.
- An inadequate amount of gel or lubricant applied to the body to ensure the proper transmission of sound waves to and from the body may affect image quality.
- Retained air, barium, or gas from a previous radiological procedure may block the transmission of sound waves.
- Large amounts of bowel gas may distort abdominal organ visualization.
- Dehydration may result in failure to demonstrate the boundaries between organs and tissue structures.
- Metallic objects (e.g., jewelry, body rings) within the examination field may inhibit organ visualization and cause unclear images.

● *Safety Tip*

Make sure a written and informed consent has been signed prior to the procedure if a biopsy is planned and before administering any medications.

Implementation

Note that patient education is key to obtaining the patient's cooperation in following directions, and providing an explanation for the purpose of the procedure is an important part of this process. Inform the patient that this study can assist in assessing for disorders of the bladder and pelvis. Ensure that the patient receiving transabdominal US drank five to six glasses of fluid and has not voided unless directed by the sonographer prior to the procedure.

Position the patient in a supine position on the examination table and drape appropriately. ***Transabdominal approach:*** Conductive gel is applied to the skin, and a transducer is moved over the skin while the bladder is distended to obtain images of the area of interest. ***Transvaginal approach:*** A covered and lubricated probe is inserted into the vagina and moved to different levels during scanning. When the full bladder images are completed, instruct the patient to void and return to the table. Additional scans are taken to check for residual urine volume and, following completion of the images, the gel is removed from the patient's pelvis (see Fig. 21.6).

If a direct percutaneous biopsy is to be performed, the area of concern is located with the ultrasound transducer. The skin is wiped with a cleansing solution, a local anesthesia is given subcutaneously at the puncture site, and the needle is guided into the area of concern for a small tissue sample or to drain a cyst. Following removal of the needle, cover the puncture site with a sterile dressing, and promptly transport the specimen to the laboratory for processing and analysis.

Evaluation

Recognize anxiety related to test results, and discuss the implications of abnormal test results on the patient's lifestyle. If a needle biopsy was performed, instruct the patient to contact his or her HCP if the puncture site shows indications of redness or inflammation, or

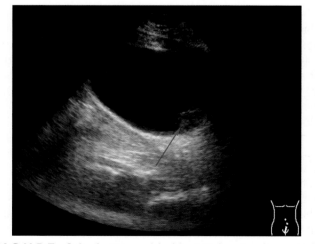

FIGURE 21.6 Urinary bladder US showing a mucosal polyp (arrow). *Used with permission, from Weber, E., Vilensky, J., & Fog, A. (2013). Practical radiology: A symptom-based approach. FA Davis Company.*

if the patient experiences a fever that persists. Inform the patient that he or she may experience mild soreness following this procedure. Provide teaching and information regarding the clinical implications of the test results as appropriate. Refer the patient to appropriate counseling resources if needed and provide contact information, if desired, for the American Cancer Society at www.cancer.org.

✅ Critical Findings

N/A

✅ Study Specific Complications

Complications following an ultrasound-guided biopsy include hemorrhage from highly vascular tissue or infection. Instruct the patient to look for excessive bleeding, redness of skin, or fever or chills, and to notify his or her HCP if these symptoms occur.

✅ Related Tests

- Related tests include bladder cancer markers urine, CT pelvis, cystoscopy, IVP, KUB study, and MRI pelvis.
- Refer to the Genitourinary System table in the end of the book for related tests by body system.

Expected Outcomes

Expected outcomes associated with Ultrasound, Bladder, are
- Maintaining urinary output in excess of 2,000 mL per day without signs of obstruction
- Verbalizing the importance of appropriate diet and fluid intake to prevent future stone formation

Ultrasound, Liver and Biliary System

Quick Summary

SYNONYM ACRONYM: Gallbladder ultrasound, liver ultrasound, hepatobiliary sonography.

COMMON USE: To visualize and assess liver and gallbladder structure and function, assist in obtaining a biopsy, and diagnose disorders such as gallstones, cancer, tumors, cysts, and bleeding. Also used to evaluate the effectiveness of therapeutic interventions

AREA OF APPLICATION: Liver, gallbladder, bile ducts

NORMAL FINDINGS
- Normal size, position, and shape of the liver and gallbladder as well as patency of the cystic and common bile ducts

Test Explanation

Ultrasound (US) procedures are diagnostic, noninvasive, and relatively inexpensive. They take a short time to complete, do not use radiation, and cause no harm to the patient. High-frequency sound waves of various intensities are delivered by a transducer, a flashlight-shaped device, pressed against the skin. The waves are bounced back off internal anatomical structures and fluids, converted to electrical energy, amplified by the transducer, and displayed as images on a monitor. US is often used as a diagnostic and therapeutic tool for guiding minimally invasive procedures such as needle biopsies, tube placement, and fluid aspiration. The contraindications and complications for biopsy and fluid aspiration are discussed in detail in the individual studies.

Hepatobiliary US is used to evaluate the structure, size, and position of the liver and gallbladder in the right upper quadrant (RUQ) of the abdomen. The gallbladder and biliary system collect, store, concentrate, and transport bile to the intestines to aid in digestion. This procedure allows visualization of the gallbladder and bile ducts when the patient may have impaired liver function, and it is especially helpful when done on patients in whom gallstones cannot be visualized with oral or IV radiological studies. Liver US can be done in combination with a nuclear scan to obtain information about liver function and density differences in the liver.

Nursing Implications

Assessment

Indications	Potential Nursing Problems
Detect cysts, polyps, hematoma, abscesses, hemangioma, adenoma, metastatic disease, hepatitis, or solid tumor of the liver or gallbladder, as evidenced by echoes specific to tissue density and sharply or poorly defined masses.	• Bleeding • Breathing • Fluid Volume • Health Management • Human Response • Infection • Jaundice • Nutrition • Pain • Skin • Urination
Detect gallstones or inflammation when oral cholecystography is inconclusive.	
Detect hepatic lesions, as evidenced by density differences and echo-pattern changes.	
Determine the cause of unexplained hepatomegaly and abnormal liver function tests.	
Determine cause of unexplained RUQ pain.	
Determine patency and diameter of the hepatic duct for dilation or obstruction.	
Differentiate between obstructive and nonobstructive jaundice by determining the cause.	
Evaluate response to therapy for tumor, as evidenced by a decrease in size of the organ.	
Guide biopsy or tube placement.	
Guide catheter placement into the gallbladder for stone dissolution and gallbladder fragmentation.	

Diagnosis: Clinical Significance of Test Results
ABNORMAL FINDINGS
- Biliary or hepatic duct obstruction/dilation
- Cirrhosis
- Gallbladder inflammation, stones, carcinoma, polyps
- Hematoma or trauma
- Hepatic tumors, metastasis, cysts, hemangioma, hepatitis
- Hepatocellular disease, adenoma
- Hepatomegaly
- Intrahepatic abscess
- Subphrenic abscesses

Planning
Considerations for planning a successful partnership should include clear communication of what to expect during the test to decrease anxiety and improve cooperation. Retained air, barium, or gas from a previous radiological procedure may block the transmission of sound waves; there should be 24 hours between potentially interfering procedures and this test. Alternatively, endoscopic retrograde cholangiopancreatography, colonoscopy, or procedures involving barium, if ordered, should be scheduled after this procedure. Before the procedure is performed, plan to review the steps with the patient. The patient should fast and restrict fluids for 8 hours prior to the procedure in order to reduce the presence of bowel gas; the patient may be asked to eat a low- or fat-free diet the night before the procedure. Protocols may vary among facilities. Address concerns about pain related to the procedure and explain that some pain may be experienced during the test, and there may be moments of discomfort. Inform the patient that the procedure is performed in a special room or at the bedside by an ultrasound technologist, and takes approximately 20 to 30 minutes. Explain that ultrasound does not use radiation and is considered safe.

SPECIAL CONSIDERATIONS
An important aspect of planning is understanding the factors that may alter study findings or cause abnormal results. Interdepartmental communication is a key factor in the planning process. The following should be noted when planning for this study:

- Incorrect placement of the transducer over the desired test site may affect results; the quality of the US study is very dependent upon the skill of the ultrasonographer.
- Bandages and dressings of postoperative patients may prohibit the required direct contact of the transducer on the skin.
- Fatty tissue of obese patients may affect the quality of images, because sound waves are distorted by fatty tissue.
- The inability of the patient to cooperate or remain still during the procedure because of age, significant

pain, or mental status may affect image quality; motion may cause artifacts.
- An inadequate amount of gel or lubricant applied to the body to ensure the proper transmission of sound waves to and from the body may affect results.
- Retained air, barium, or gas from a previous radiological procedure may block the transmission of sound waves.
- Large amounts of bowel gas may distort abdominal organ visualization.
- Attenuation of the sound waves by bony structures may impair clear imaging of the right lobe of the liver.
- Dehydration may result in failure to demonstrate the boundaries between organs and tissue structures.
- Metallic objects (e.g., jewelry, body rings) within the examination field may inhibit organ visualization and cause unclear images.
- Failure to follow dietary restrictions may cause the procedure to be canceled or repeated.

● Safety Tip
Make sure a written and informed consent has been signed prior to the procedure if a biopsy is planned and before administering any medications.

Implementation
Patient education is key to obtaining the patient's cooperation in following directions, and providing an explanation for the purpose of the procedure is an important part of this process. Inform the patient that this study can assist in assessing for disorders of the liver and biliary tree. Ensure that food and fluids have been restricted for at least 8 hours prior to the procedure.

Position the patient in a supine position on the examination table and drape appropriately. The right- or left-side-up positions may be used to allow gravity to reposition the liver, gas, and fluid to facilitate better organ visualization. A conductive gel is applied on the patient's skin to improve the transmission and reception of the sound waves. The ultrasound transducer is moved across the upper right quadrant of the abdomen in specific directions over the area of interest, and images are recorded from the reflected sound waves received. Following completion of the images, wipe the gel from the patient's abdomen (see Figs. 21.7 through 21.9). If a biopsy was performed, cover the puncture site with a sterile dressing, and promptly transport the specimen to the laboratory for processing and analysis.

Evaluation
Recognize anxiety related to test results, and be supportive of impaired activity related to a perceived loss of independence. Instruct the patient to resume usual diet and fluids, as directed by the health-care provider (HCP). Discuss the implications of abnormal test results

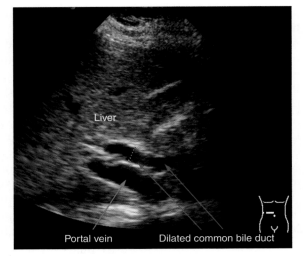

FIGURE 21.7 US image showing a dilated common bile duct. *Used with permission, from Weber, E., Vilensky, J., & Fog, A. (2013). Practical radiology: A symptom-based approach. FA Davis Company.*

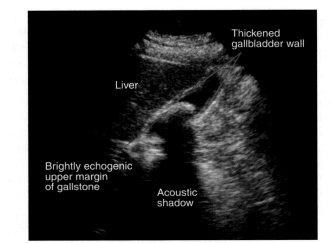

FIGURE 21.8 US of upper right abdomen demonstrating cholelithiasis. *Used with permission, from Weber, E., Vilensky, J., & Fog, A. (2013). Practical radiology: A symptom-based approach. FA Davis Company.*

on the patient's lifestyle. Provide teaching and information regarding the clinical implications of the test results as appropriate. If a biopsy was completed, monitor the puncture site and instruct the patient to contact her or his HCP if the puncture site shows indications of redness or inflammation, or if she or he experiences a fever that persists.

✔ Critical Findings

N/A

✔ Study Specific Complications

Complications following an ultrasound-guided biopsy include hemorrhage from highly vascular tissue or infection. Instruct the patient to look for excessive

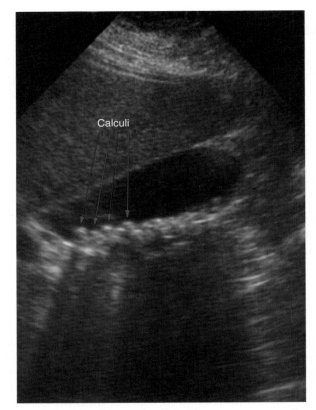

FIGURE 21.9 US of gallbladder containing small stones. *Used with permission, from Weber, E., Vilensky, J., & Fog, A. (2013). Practical radiology: A symptom-based approach. FA Davis Company.*

bleeding, redness of skin, or fever or chills, and to notify her or his HCP if these symptoms occur.

✔ Related Tests

- Related tests include ALP, ALT, AST, bilirubin, biopsy liver, cholangiography, colonoscopy, CT abdomen, endoscopy, ERCP, GGT, haptoglobin, hepatitis (A, B, C antigens and/or antibodies), hepatobiliary scan, laparoscopy abdominal, MRI abdomen, radiofrequency ablation liver, and US abdomen.
- Refer to the Hepatobiliary System table at the end of the book for related tests by body system.

Expected Outcomes

Expected outcomes associated with Ultrasound, Liver and Biliary System, are
- Confirming that pain does not occur after eating
- Having breath sounds that are clear bilaterally

Ultrasound, Pancreas

Quick Summary

SYNONYM ACRONYM: Pancreatic ultrasonography.

COMMON USE: To visualize and assess the pancreas toward diagnosing disorders such as tumor, cancer, obstruction, and cysts. Also used as a tool for biopsy and to evaluate the effectiveness of therapeutic interventions.

AREA OF APPLICATION: Pancreas and upper abdomen

NORMAL FINDINGS

- Normal size, position, contour, and texture of the pancreas

Test Explanation

Ultrasound (US) procedures are diagnostic, noninvasive, and relatively inexpensive. They take a short time to complete, do not use radiation, and cause no harm to the patient. High-frequency sound waves of various intensities are delivered by a transducer, a flashlight-shaped device, pressed against the skin. The waves are bounced back off internal anatomical structures and fluids, converted to electrical energy, amplified by the transducer, and displayed as images on a monitor. US is often used as a diagnostic and therapeutic tool for guiding minimally invasive procedures such as needle biopsies and fluid aspiration. The contraindications and complications for biopsy and fluid aspiration are discussed in detail in the individual studies.

Pancreatic US is used to determine the size, shape, and position of the pancreas; determine the presence of masses or other abnormalities of the pancreas; and examine the surrounding viscera. Pancreatic US is usually done in combination with computed tomography (CT) or magnetic resonance imaging (MRI) of the pancreas.

Nursing Implications

Assessment

Indications	Potential Nursing Problems
Detect anatomic abnormalities as a consequence of pancreatitis. Detect pancreatic cancer, as evidenced by a poorly defined mass or a mass in the head of the pancreas that obstructs the pancreatic duct. Detect pancreatitis, as evidenced by pancreatic enlargement with increased echoes. Detect pseudocysts, as evidenced by a well-defined mass with absence of echoes from the interior. Monitor therapeutic response to tumor treatment. Provide guidance for percutaneous aspiration and fine-needle biopsy of the pancreas.	• Breathing • Gas Exchange • Health Management • Human Response • Infection • Nutrition • Pain • Protection

Diagnosis: Clinical Significance of Test Results

ABNORMAL FINDINGS

- Acute pancreatitis
- Calculi
- Pancreatic duct obstruction
- Pancreatic tumor
- Pseudocysts

Planning

Considerations for planning a successful partnership should include clear communication of what to expect during the test to decrease anxiety and improve cooperation. Retained air, barium, or gas from a previous radiological procedure may block the transmission of sound waves; there should be 24 hours between potentially interfering procedures and this test. Alternatively, endoscopic retrograde cholangiopancreatography, colonoscopy, or procedures involving barium, should be scheduled after this procedure. Before the procedure is performed, plan to review the steps with the patient. The patient should fast and restrict fluids for 8 hours prior to the procedure in order to reduce the presence of bowel gas; the patient may be asked to eat a low- or fat-free diet the night before the procedure. Protocols may vary among facilities. Address concerns about pain related to the procedure and explain that some pain may be experienced during the test, and there may be moments of discomfort. Inform the patient that the procedure is performed in a special room or at the bedside by an ultrasound technologist, and takes approximately 20 to 30 minutes. Explain that ultrasound does not use radiation and is considered safe.

SPECIAL CONSIDERATIONS

An important aspect of planning is understanding the factors that may alter study findings or cause abnormal results. Interdepartmental communication is a key factor in the planning process. The following should be noted when planning for this study:

- Incorrect placement of the transducer over the desired test site may affect results; the quality of the US study is very dependent upon the skill of the ultrasonographer.
- Bandages and dressing of postoperative patients may prohibit the required direct contact of the transducer on the skin.
- Fatty tissue of obese patients may affect the quality of the images, because sound waves are distorted by fatty tissue.
- The inability of the patient to cooperate or remain still during the procedure because of age, significant pain, or mental status may affect results; motion may cause artifacts.
- An inadequate amount of gel or lubricant applied to the body to ensure the proper transmission of sound waves to and from the body may affect image quality.
- Retained air, barium, or gas from a previous radiological procedure may block the transmission of sound waves.
- Large amounts of bowel gas may distort abdominal organ visualization.

- Dehydration may result in failure to demonstrate the boundaries between organs and tissue structures.
- Metallic objects (e.g., jewelry, body rings) within the examination field may inhibit organ visualization and cause unclear images.

Implementation

Patient education is key to obtaining the patient's cooperation in following directions, and providing an explanation for the purpose of the procedure is an important part of this process. Inform the patient that this study can assist in assessing for disorders of the pancreas. Ensure that food and fluids have been restricted for at least 8 hours prior to the procedure.

Place the patient in the supine position on an examination table. The right- or left-side-up position may be used to allow gravity to reposition the liver, gas, and fluid to facilitate better organ visualization. Expose the abdominal area and drape the patient. Conductive gel is applied to the skin, and a transducer is moved over the skin to obtain images of the area of interest.

Evaluation

Recognize anxiety related to test results and be supportive of impaired activity related to a perceived loss of independence. Discuss the implications of abnormal test results on the patient's lifestyle. Provide teaching and information regarding the clinical implications of the test results as appropriate. If a biopsy was completed, monitor the puncture site and instruct the patient to contact his or her health-care provider (HCP) if the puncture site shows indications of redness or inflammation, or if he or she experiences a fever that persists.

✔ Critical Findings

N/A

✔ Study Specific Complications

Complications following an ultrasound-guided biopsy include hemorrhage from highly vascular tissue or infection. Instruct the patient to look for excessive bleeding, redness of skin, or fever or chills, and to notify his or her HCP if these symptoms occur.

✔ Related Tests

- Related tests include amylase, cancer antigens, CT abdomen, CT pancreas, C peptide, ERCP, KUB study, laparoscopy abdominal, lipase, MRI abdomen, MRI pancreas, peritoneal fluid analysis, and US abdomen.
- Refer to the Gastrointestinal System table at the end of the book for related tests by body system.

Expected Outcomes

Expected outcomes associated with Ultrasound, Pancreas, are

- Recognizing the importance of refraining from alcohol consumption toward preventing stone formation

- Understanding that smoking should be avoided to prevent placing stress on the pancreas

Ultrasound, Pelvis (Gynecologic, Nonobstetric)

Quick Summary

SYNONYM ACRONYM: Lower abdominal ultrasound, pelvic gynecologic (GYN) sonogram, pelvic sonography.

COMMON USE: To visualize and assess the pelvis for disorders such as uterine mass, tumor, cancer, cyst, and fibroids. This procedure can also be useful in evaluating ovulation and fallopian tube function related to fertility issues.

AREA OF APPLICATION: Pelvis and appendix region

NORMAL FINDINGS

- Normal size, position, location, and structure of pelvic organs (e.g., uterus, ovaries, fallopian tubes, vagina); intrauterine contraceptive device (IUD) properly positioned within the uterine cavity

Test Explanation

Ultrasound (US) procedures are diagnostic, noninvasive, and relatively inexpensive. They take a short time to complete, do not use radiation, and cause no harm to the patient. High-frequency sound waves of various intensities are delivered by a transducer, a flashlight-shaped device, pressed against the skin. The waves are bounced back off internal anatomical structures and fluids, converted to electrical energy, amplified by the transducer, and displayed as images on a monitor. US is often used as a diagnostic and therapeutic tool for guiding minimally invasive procedures such as needle biopsies and fluid aspiration. The contraindications and complications for biopsy and fluid aspiration are discussed in detail in the individual studies.

Gynecologic US is used to determine the presence, size, and structure of masses and cysts and determine the position of an IUD; evaluate postmenopausal bleeding; and examine other abnormalities of the uterus, ovaries, fallopian tubes, and vagina. This procedure is done by a transabdominal or transvaginal approach. The transabdominal approach provides a view of the pelvic organs posterior to the bladder. It requires a full bladder, thereby allowing a window for transmission of the US waves, pushing the uterus away from the pubic symphysis, pushing the bowel out of the pelvis, and acting as a reference for comparison in the evaluation of the internal structures of a mass or cyst being examined. The transvaginal approach focuses on the female reproductive organs and is often used to monitor ovulation over a period of days in patients undergoing fertility assessment. This approach is also used in obese patients or in patients with retroversion of the uterus because the sound waves are better able to reach the organ from the vaginal site. Transvaginal images are significantly more accurate compared to anterior transabdominal images in identifying paracervical, endometrial, and ovarian pathology, and the transvaginal approach does not require a full bladder.

Nursing Implications
Assessment

Indications	Potential Nursing Problems
Detect and monitor the treatment of pelvic inflammatory disease (PID) when done in combination with other laboratory tests.	• Family
	• Fear
Detect bleeding into the pelvis resulting from trauma to the area or ascites associated with tumor metastasis.	• Hopelessness
	• Human Response
	• Infection
Detect masses in the pelvis and differentiate them from cysts or solid tumors, as evidenced by differences in sound-wave patterns.	• Pain
	• Role Performance
	• Self-esteem
	• Sexuality
Detect pelvic abscess or peritonitis caused by a ruptured appendix or diverticulitis.	
Detect the presence of ovarian cysts and malignancy and determine the type, if possible, as evidenced by size, outline, and change in position of other pelvic organs.	
Evaluate the effectiveness of tumor therapy, as evidenced by a reduction in mass size.	
Evaluate suspected fibroid tumor or bladder tumor.	
Evaluate the thickness of the uterine wall.	
Monitor placement and location of an IUD.	
Monitor follicular size associated with fertility studies or remove follicles for in vitro transplantation.	

Diagnosis: Clinical Significance of Test Results
ABNORMAL FINDINGS
- Abscess
- Adnexal torsion
- Appendicitis
- Endometrioma
- Fibroids (leiomyoma)
- Infection
- Nonovarian cyst
- Ovarian cysts
- Ovarian tumor
- Peritonitis

- PID
- Uterine tumor or adnexal tumor

Planning
Considerations for planning a successful partnership should include clear communication of what to expect during the test to decrease anxiety and improve cooperation. Retained air, barium, or gas from a previous radiological procedure may block the transmission of sound waves; there should be 24 hours between potentially interfering procedures and this test. Alternatively, endoscopic retrograde cholangiopancreatography, colonoscopy, or procedures involving barium, if ordered, should be scheduled after this procedure. Before the procedure is performed, plan to review the steps with the patient. Address concerns about pain related to the procedure and explain that some pain may be experienced during the test, and there may be moments of discomfort. Explain that a latex or sterile sheath-covered probe will be inserted into the vagina for the transvaginal approach. Instruct the patient receiving transabdominal US to drink three to four glasses of fluid 90 minutes before the examination and not to void, because the procedure requires a full bladder. Patients receiving transvaginal US only do not need to have a full bladder. Inform the patient that the procedure is performed in a special room or at the bedside by an ultrasound technologist, and takes approximately 20 to 30 minutes.

CONTRAINDICATIONS
Patients with latex allergy; use of the vaginal probe requires the probe to be covered with a condom-like sac, usually made from latex. Latex-free covers are available.

SPECIAL CONSIDERATIONS
An important aspect of planning is understanding the factors that may alter study findings or cause abnormal results. Interdepartmental communication is a key factor in the planning process. The following should be noted when planning for this study:

- Incorrect placement of the transducer over the desired test site may affect results; the quality of the US study is very dependent upon the skill of the ultrasonographer.
- Bandages and dressings of postoperative patients may prohibit the required direct contact of the transducer on the skin.
- Fatty tissue of obese patients may affect the quality of the images, because sound waves are distorted by fatty tissue.
- The inability of the patient to cooperate or remain still during the procedure because of age, significant pain, or mental status may affect image quality; motion may cause artifacts.
- An inadequate amount of gel or lubricant applied to the body to ensure the proper transmission of sound waves to and from the body may affect results.

- Retained air, barium, or gas from a previous radiological procedure may block the transmission of sound waves.
- Large amounts of bowel gas may distort abdominal organ visualization.
- Dehydration may result in failure to demonstrate the boundaries between organs and tissue structures.
- An insufficiently full bladder may fail to push the bowel from the pelvis and the uterus from the symphysis pubis, thereby prohibiting clear imaging of the pelvic organs in transabdominal imaging.
- Metallic objects (e.g., jewelry, body rings) within the examination field may inhibit organ visualization and cause unclear images.

● Safety Tip

Make sure a written and informed consent has been signed prior to the procedure if a biopsy is planned and before administering any medications.

Implementation

Patient education is key to obtaining the patient's cooperation in following directions, and providing an explanation for the purpose of the procedure is an important part of this process. Inform the patient that this study can assist in assessing for disorders of the pelvis or fetus. Verify that she has complied with fluid instructions and has not voided.

Position the patient in a supine position on the examination table and drape appropriately. ***Transabdominal approach:*** Conductive gel is applied to the skin, and a transducer is moved over the skin while the bladder is distended to obtain images of the area of interest. ***Transvaginal approach:*** A covered and lubricated probe is inserted into the vagina and moved to different levels. For transvaginal scanning, place a pillow under the buttocks and have the patient bend her knees. A lithotomy position may be used as an alternative. Place a small amount of gel on the transducer face before covering it with a condom or transducer cover. The transducer is manipulated to take images in the saggital, coronal, and transverse sections of the uterus and adnexa. Following completion of the exam, remove the transducer and provide the patient with a warm cloth to clean herself. Allow the patient to void, as needed (see Fig. 21.10).

Evaluation

Recognize anxiety related to test results, and be supportive of impaired activity related to a perceived loss of independence. Discuss the implications of abnormal test results on the patient's lifestyle. Provide teaching and information regarding the clinical implications of the test results as appropriate. If a biopsy

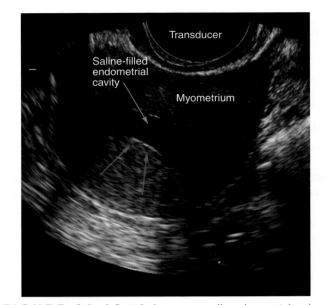

FIGURE 21.10 US showing small endometrial polyp. *Used with permission, from Weber, E., Vilensky, J., & Fog, A. (2013). Practical radiology: A symptom-based approach. FA Davis Company.*

was completed, monitor the puncture site, and instruct the patient to contact her health-care provider (HCP) if the puncture site shows indications of redness or inflammation, or if she experiences a fever that persists.

✓ Critical Findings

- Abscess
- Adnexal torsion
- Appendicitis
- Infection
- Tumor with significant mass effect

Note and immediately report to the requesting HCP any critical findings and related symptoms. A listing of these findings varies among facilities.

✓ Study Specific Complications

Complications following an ultrasound-guided biopsy include hemorrhage from highly vascular tissue or infection. Instruct the patient to look for excessive bleeding, redness of skin, or fever or chills, and to notify her HCP if these symptoms occur.

✓ Related Tests

- Related tests include cancer antigens, colposcopy, CT abdomen, hysterosalpingography, KUB study, laparoscopy gynecologic, MRI abdomen, Pap smear, and PET pelvis.
- Refer to the Reproductive System table at the end of the book for related tests by body system.

Expected Outcomes

Expected outcomes associated with Ultrasound, Pelvis (Gynecologic, Nonobstetric), are

- Expressing fear about the inability to conceive
- Being afebrile with an absence of vaginal discharge

Ultrasound, Prostate (Transrectal)

Quick Summary

SYNONYM ACRONYM: Prostate sonography, TRUS.

COMMON USE: To visualize and assess the prostate gland as an adjunct of prostate-specific antigen (PSA) blood testing and examination to assist in diagnosing disorders such as tumor and cancer. Also used to assist in guiding biopsy of the prostate.

AREA OF APPLICATION: Prostate, seminal vesicles

NORMAL FINDINGS
- Normal size, consistency, and contour of the prostate gland

Test Explanation

Ultrasound (US) procedures are diagnostic, noninvasive, and relatively inexpensive. They take a short time to complete, do not use radiation, and cause no harm to the patient. High-frequency sound waves of various intensities are delivered by a transducer, a candle-shaped device, which is lubricated, sheathed with a condom, and inserted a few inches into the rectum. The waves are bounced back off internal anatomical structures and fluids, converted to electrical energy, amplified by the transducer, and displayed as images on a monitor. US is often used as a diagnostic and therapeutic tool for guiding minimally invasive procedures such as needle biopsies and fluid aspiration. The contraindications and complications for biopsy and fluid aspiration are discussed in detail in the individual studies.

Prostate US is used to evaluate the structure, size, and position of the contents of the prostate (e.g., masses). This procedure can evaluate abnormal pathology in prostate tissue, the seminal vesicles, and surrounding perirectal tissue. Prostate US aids in the diagnosis of prostatic cancer by evaluating palpable nodules as a complement to a digital rectal examination (DRE) or in response to an elevated PSA level. The DRE is a simple procedure used to examine, by palpation, the lower rectum and prostate gland. It is performed by the health-care provider (HCP) who inserts a lubricated, gloved finger into the rectum while the patient is properly positioned. Prostate US can also be used to stage carcinoma and to assist in radiation seed placement. Micturition disorders can also be evaluated by this procedure. The examination is helpful in monitoring patient response to therapy for prostatic disease.

Nursing Implications

Assessment

Indications	Potential Nursing Problems
Aid in the diagnosis of micturition disorders. Aid in prostate cancer diagnosis. Assess prostatic calcifications. Assist in guided needle biopsy of a suspected tumor. Assist in radiation seed placement. Determine prostatic cancer staging. Detect prostatitis.	• Human Response • Pain • Self-esteem • Sexuality • Urination

Diagnosis: Clinical Significance of Test Results

ABNORMAL FINDINGS
- Benign prostatic hyperplasia
- Micturition disorders
- Perirectal abscess
- Perirectal tumor
- Prostate abscess
- Prostate cancer
- Prostatitis
- Rectal tumor
- Seminal vesicle tumor

Planning

Considerations for planning a successful partnership should include clear communication of what to expect during the test to decrease anxiety and improve cooperation. Retained air, barium, or gas from a previous radiological procedure may block the transmission of sound waves; there should be 24 hours between potentially interfering procedures and this test. Alternatively, colonoscopy or procedures involving barium, if ordered, should be scheduled after this procedure. The patient may be asked to restrict anticoagulants, aspirin, and other salicylates by medical direction for the appropriate number of days prior to the procedure. Before the procedure is performed, plan to review the steps with the patient. Explain that an enema will be given prior to the study to remove any residual fecal material that could interfere with the rectal probe. Address concerns about pain related to the procedure, and explain that some pain may be experienced during the test, and there may be moments of discomfort. If a biopsy is to be performed, antibiotics may be administered prior to the procedure. Inform the patient that the procedure is performed in a special room or a urologist's office by an ultrasound technologist, and takes approximately 20 to

30 minutes. Explain that ultrasound does not use radiation and is considered safe.

CONTRAINDICATIONS

This study is contraindicated for patients with latex allergy because the rectal probe is covered with a latex condom-like sac.

An important aspect of planning is understanding the factors that may alter study findings or cause abnormal results. Interdepartmental communication is a key factor in the planning process. The following should be noted when planning for this study:

- Incorrect placement of the transducer over the desired test site may affect results; the quality of the US study is very dependent upon the skill of the ultrasonographer.
- Fatty tissue of obese patients may affect the quality of the images, because sound waves are distorted by fatty tissue.
- Attenuation of the sound waves by pelvic bones can impair clear imaging of the prostate.
- The inability of the patient to cooperate or remain still during the procedure because of age, significant pain, or mental status may affect image quality; motion may cause artifacts.
- An inadequate amount of gel or lubricant applied to the body to ensure the proper transmission of sound waves to and from the body may affect image quality.
- Retained air, barium, or gas from a previous radiological procedure may block the transmission of sound waves.
- Dehydration may result in failure to demonstrate the boundaries between organs and tissue structures.
- Metallic objects (e.g., jewelry, body rings) within the examination field may inhibit organ visualization and cause unclear images.

● Safety Tip

Make sure a written and informed consent has been signed prior to the procedure if a biopsy is planned and before administering any medications.

Implementation

Note that patient education is key to obtaining the patient's cooperation in following directions, and providing an explanation for the purpose of the procedure is an important part of this process. Inform the patient that this study can assist in assessing for disorders of the prostate. Instruct the patient not to void prior to the procedure. Verify that he has complied with fluid instructions and has not voided.

Position the patient in a left lateral position on the examination table and drape appropriately. A conductive gel is applied on the rectal transducer to improve the transmission and reception of the sound waves. The ultrasound transducer is covered with a lubricated condom, placed inside the rectum, and scans are obtained in various planes. Following completion of the images, remove the transducer and offer the patient a warm cloth to clean the perianal area. If a biopsy was performed, cover the puncture site with a sterile dressing and promptly transport the specimen to the laboratory for processing and analysis.

Evaluation

Recognize anxiety related to test results, and be supportive of impaired activity related to a perceived loss of independence. Discuss the implications of abnormal test results on the patient's lifestyle. Provide teaching and information regarding the clinical implications of the test results as appropriate. If a biopsy was completed, monitor the puncture site and instruct the patient to contact his HCP if the puncture site shows indications of redness or inflammation, or if he experiences a fever that persists. Provide contact information, if desired, for the National Cancer Institute (www.cancer.gov) or the Prostate Cancer Foundation (www.prostatecancerfoundation.org). Recommendations made by various medical associations and national health organizations regarding prostate cancer screening are moving away from routine PSA screening and toward informed decision making. The American Cancer Society's guidelines recommend that discussions about screening should begin at age 50 years for men at average risk, 45 years for men at high risk, and 40 years for men at the highest risk of developing prostate cancer. The most current guidelines for prostate cancer screening of the general population as well as of individuals with increased risk are available from the American Cancer Society (www.cancer.org) and the American Urological Association (www.aua.org).

NUTRITIONAL CONSIDERATIONS: There is growing evidence that inflammation and oxidation play key roles in the development of numerous diseases, including prostate cancer. Research also indicates that diets containing dried beans, fresh fruits and vegetables, nuts, spices, whole grains, and smaller amounts of red meats can increase the amount of protective antioxidants. Regular exercise, especially in combination with a healthy diet, can bring about changes in the body's metabolism that decrease inflammation and oxidation.

● *Critical Findings*

N/A

● *Study Specific Complications*

Complications following an ultrasound-guided biopsy include hemorrhage from highly vascular tissue or infection. Instruct the patient to look for excessive bleeding, redness of skin, or fever or chills, and to notify his HCP if these symptoms occur.

⊘ *Related Tests*

- Related tests include biopsy prostate, CT pelvis, cystoscopy, cystourethrography voiding, IVP, KUB study, MRI pelvis, proctosigmoidoscopy, PSA, renogram, retrograde ureteropyelography, and semen analysis.
- Refer to the Genitourinary System table at the end of the book for related tests by body system.

Expected Outcomes

Expected outcomes associated with Ultrasound, Prostate (Transrectal), are

- Absence of bladder distention or urinary retention
- Absence of bladder spasms

REVIEW OF LEARNING OUTCOMES

Thinking

1. State how ultrasound is integrated into the process of disease diagnosis and therapeutic treatment. Answer: Ultrasound imaging is diagnostic tool that can be used to assess a fetus or multiple body areas such as the kidneys, ovaries, abdomen, heart, pancreas, spleen, uterus, and more. Ultrasound is painless and portable and can be used for all age levels without exposure to radiation. This makes follow-up ultrasounds that are completed to evaluate the effectiveness of therapeutic management a good alternative to other choices.

Doing

1. Quantify quality care with data collection to validate best practice in health care. Answer: Nursing has something we call *standards of practice*. Standards of practice are based on evidence that indicates which interventions will provide the best outcome for our patients. This is a cultural shift from "doing it this way because that is the way we have always done it." Always ask yourself if there is a better way to approach a task. If necessary, research it and share your findings with those who can support your efforts. One person can make a difference—let that be you.
2. Coordinate the integration of care regarding general planning guidelines for ultrasound studies. Answer: It is the nurse's responsibility to prepare the patient for ultrasound. An integral part of that preparation is to assess the patient's condition and communicate that information to the ultrasound department. This will ensure that the patient completes the study safely without incident. All protocols related to handing the patient off and receiving the patient back from ultrasound are within the nurse's purview. Patient concerns regarding the procedure should be addressed by the nurse and discussed with the physician and ultrasound department as appropriate.

Caring

1. Value how failure to follow standards of practice affects care outcomes. Answer: Sometimes alterations in care occur regardless of our best efforts. Mistakes happen. One day you will make a mistake. No one goes to work thinking, "today I hope to make a mistake that may cause injury to my patient." Overall, nursing is chosen as a profession by those who want to serve others. Pay attention to any mistake you make, any mistake you observe, and think about the lesson learned that will allow you to make more careful choices in the future. This is one of the best ways to do no harm.

○ **Words OF Wisdom:** Ultrasound is used most often to look for cancer, tumor, obstruction, and cysts. Ultrasound is also used to gauge whether or not the diagnosed disease is getting better or worse. Ultrasound can become invasive if used as a tool for guided biopsy. In all cases, this is a very anxiety-producing event. That's not because it is painful but because the patient knows that there is a possibility of a poor result. On the other hand, ultrasound can be a fairly inexpensive way to give the patient peace of mind that the treatment is working and his or her health is improving.

BIBLIOGRAPHY

AIUM Practice guideline for the performance of peripheral arterial ultrasound examinations using color and spectral Doppler imaging. (2014). Retrieved from www.aium.org/resources/guidelines/peripheralArterial.pdf

Contraindications to Transesophageal Echocardiography. (2014). Retrieved from http://www.scahq.org/files/Conference_2014_Annual_Syllabi_Sessions/Advanced_TEE_SCA_2014%5B1%5D.docx.

LeMone, P., Burke, K., & Baldoff, G. (2011). Medical surgical nursing, Critical thinking in patient care (5th ed.). Upper Saddle River, NJ: Pearson.

Facts about Peripheral Artery Disease. (2006). Retrieved from www.nhlbi.nih.gov/health/public/heart/pad/docs/pad_extfctsht_general_508.pdf

Fishbach, F., & Dunning, M. (2009). A manual of laboratory and diagnostic tests (8th ed.). Philadelphia, PA: Lippincott Williams & Wilkins.

Gray-Scale and color Doppler sonography of scrotal disorders in children: An update. (2005). Retrieved from http://radiographics.rsna.org/content/25/5/1197.full#content-block

Kawamura, D., & Lunsford, B. (2012). Abdomen and superficial structures (3rd ed.). Philadelphia, PA: Lippincott Williams & Wilkins.

Practice guidelines for perioperative transesophageal echocardiography. An updated report by the American Society of

Anesthesiologists and the Society of Cardiovascular Anesthesiologists Task Force on Transesophageal Echocardiography. (2010). Retrieved from www.guideline.gov/content.aspx?id=23846

Sanders, R., & Winter, T. (2007). Clinical sonography: A practical guide. Baltimore, MD: Lippincott Williams & Wilkins.

Snopek, A. (2009). Fundamentals of special radiographic procedures (5th ed.). St. Louis, MO: Saunders Elsevier.

Sound medicine: Understanding ultrasound and its benefits. (2014). Retrieved from www.sdms.org/public/soundmedicine.asp

Stephenson, S. (2012). Obstetrics and gynecology (3rd ed.). Philadelphia, PA: Lippincott Williams & Wilkins.

Stone, M., Price, D., & Anderson, B. (2006). Ultrasonographic investigation of the effect of reverse Trendelenburg on the cross-sectional area of the femoral vein. Journal of Emergency Medicine, 30, 211–213.

Ultrasound—Breast. (2013). Retrieved from www.radiologyinfo.org/en/info.cfm?pg=breastus

Van Leeuwen, A., & Bladh, M. (2015). Davis's comprehensive handbook of laboratory and diagnostic testing with nursing implications (6th ed.). Philadelphia, PA: F.A. Davis Company.

Venes, D. (Ed.). (2009). Taber's cyclopedic medical dictionary (21st ed.). Philadelphia, PA: F.A. Davis Company.

Go to Section II of this book and www.davisplus.com for the Clinical Reasoning Tool and its case studies to provide you with a safe place to explore patient care situations. There are a total of 26 different case studies; 2 cases are presented for each of 13 body systems. One set of 13 cases are found in the Section II chapters, and a second set of 13 cases are available online at www.davisplus.com. Each case is designed with the specific goal of helping you to connect the dots of clinical reasoning. Cases are designed to reflect possible clinical scenarios; the outcomes may or may not be positive—you decide.

Urine Studies

OVERVIEW

The importance of urine studies to assess health or illness has been recognized for more than 6,000 years. Evidence of the interest in urine studies to evaluate health has been found in artifacts from the earliest civilizations known; the cave man, the Babylonians, the Egyptians, the Greeks, the Romans, the Vikings, through the Middle Ages, and into more modern times urinalysis is still being performed today. As science progressed through the ages, a greater understanding of anatomy and physiology, coupled with the invention and refinement of microscopy, has led to the development of valuable and important technology that has greatly benefited the area of urinalysis. Simple, rapid, cost-effective urinalysis results can be obtained from manual dipstick and microscopic evaluations or from automated instruments in a variety of settings such as physician offices, health clinics, hospitals, and private laboratories. Other more complex and quantitative urine studies are performed by laboratory technicians and technologists using a variety of instruments in a clinical or reference laboratory setting. Urine studies are frequently included in routine health examinations for a number of reasons. They are easily and painlessly collected and can reveal diseases that would have otherwise gone undetected. Diseases like type 2 diabetes or chronic urinary tract infections typically do not demonstrate characteristic signs and symptoms but rather produce vague and general complaints.

Urine is evaluated by its physical appearance, chemical composition, and microscopic components. Specimen collection and handling are important factors that contribute to the accuracy of test results. Changes to the composition of a urine specimen begin to take place as soon as it is collected. As such, appropriate patient preparation, specimen collection technique, the interval of time between collection and analysis, storage temperature, as well as the handling and use of indicated preservatives are important issues in maintaining the integrity of the specimen.

Urine is formed by the kidneys from the filtration of circulating blood. Approximately 20% to 25% of the blood circulated by the heart is filtered by the kidneys each day at a rate of about 1,200 mL/min or 600 mL/min/kidney. As such, many of the substances from blood are also present in urine, and in general, with normal kidney function, the concentrations of substances found in the urine will reflect plasma levels. Which is to say that if the plasma concentration of a substance is elevated, more of it will be present in the urine than normal. Conversely, if the plasma concentration of a substance is lower than normal, less will be present in the urine. This is because urine is an ultrafiltrate of plasma, which retains substances essential to the body through the process of reabsorption, and which eliminates substances that are not needed through the process of excretion. The substances most readily reabsorbed include water, glucose, amino acids, and electrolytes (sodium, chloride, potassium). Substances commonly excreted from the body include urea, electrolytes (sodium, chloride, potassium), uric acid, creatinine, ammonia, pigments (medications, the breakdown of heme, digested foods), enzymes, hormones and their metabolites, vitamins, minerals, and drugs. Proteins and substances bound to plasma proteins are not normally found in the ultrafiltrate. Factors that affect blood levels also affect urine levels, such as dietary intake (deficient versus sufficient versus excessive), body metabolism (hyper versus hypo), endocrine function (complex interaction of feedback mechanisms), physical activity (active versus at rest), body position (supine versus recumbent), and the time of day (circadian versus diurnal variation).

The kidneys are responsible for multiple, essential functions of the body as described in other chapters of this book and include:

1. Regulation of body fluids *(by controlling the movement of water and sodium ions)*
2. Regulation of acid–base balance *(by excreting H⁺ ions when there is excess acid, HCO_3^- ions when there is excess base, and synthesizing ammonia)*
3. Regulation of electrolyte balance including Na^+, K^+, Ca^{2+}, Mg^{2+}, Cl^-, bicarbonate (HCO_3^-), phosphate, and sulfate ions
4. Regulation of blood pressure *(by controlling the movement of sodium ions via stimulation/suppression of the renin-angiotensin-aldosterone system)*
5. Production of erythropoietin *(for the formation of RBCs)*
6. Production of vitamin D
7. Excretion of waste products from the body, including urea (a nitrogen-containing waste product created from the breakdown of protein), uric acid (a waste product created from purine metabolism), and creatinine (a breakdown product of muscle metabolism)

The kidneys react to changes brought about by the function of the body's other organs and are influenced by changes in blood volume, blood pressure, and hormone levels.

Normally, the kidneys are paired organs located in the small of the back on each side of the spine, underneath the 12th rib. Each adult kidney measures about 4 inches (10 cm) long, by 2 inches (5 cm) wide, by 1 inch (2.5 cm) thick, is about the size of a closed fist, and weighs about 150 g. The structure of the kidney is composed of two main portions: the outer renal cortex where urine production occurs, and the interior renal medulla where urine collection occurs, surrounded by a thick fibrous capsule. Blood vessels, nerves, lymphatic vessels, and ureters enter and exit the kidney through a structure called the hilum, a slit located in the concave notch on the medial side of each organ. Blood enters the kidney through the renal artery and leaves from the renal vein (see Fig. 22.1).

The kidney is a very vascular, innervated organ supplied by multitudes of tiny afferent arterioles that carry blood to the nephrons and smaller efferent arterioles that carry blood away from the nephrons. The basic functional filtration unit of the kidney is the nephron, and there are over one million nephrons in each kidney (see Fig. 22.2). The nephron has two main functions: filtrating blood from the heart and forming urine for excretion. Each nephron has a rich supply of capillaries that are organized into a network called the glomerulus. The filtration function of the nephron is accomplished by the renal corpuscle,

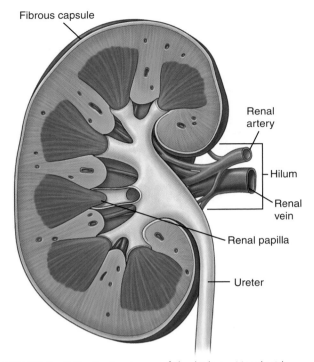

FIGURE 22.1 Anatomy of the kidney. *Used with permission, from Thompson, G. (2013). Understanding anatomy & physiology. FA Davis Company.*

which is composed of a glomerulus and a Bowman or glomerular capsule. Each nephron contains a structure called the juxtaglomerular apparatus, which is formed by the distal convoluted tubule and the glomerular afferent arteriole. The apparatus is a region of specialized cells that produce and release renin, making its main function regulating blood pressure and assuring a steady filtration rate from the glomerulus. Ultrafiltrate from the glomerulus enters a series of renal tubules where the urine is formed. The renal tubule is a very long structure divided into four distinct areas that each performs a specific function: the proximal convoluted tubule lined with thousands of microvilli to enhance reabsorption and secretion, the nephron loop (the descending and ascending limb are collectively referred to as the loop of Henle), the distal convoluted tubule, and the collecting duct. The glomerulus and convoluted tubules (proximal and distal) are located in the cortex of the kidney, while the loop of Henle dips slightly down toward the medulla in most of the cortical nephrons, where substances then exit the efferent arterioles into the peritubular capillaries and ultimately return to be circulated to where they are needed. Juxtamedullary nephrons, a different type of nephron that composes about 15% of all nephrons, have a very long loop of Henle that extends deep into the medulla, has different permeability and transport properties, and has two types of postglomerular

Detailed structure of a nephron

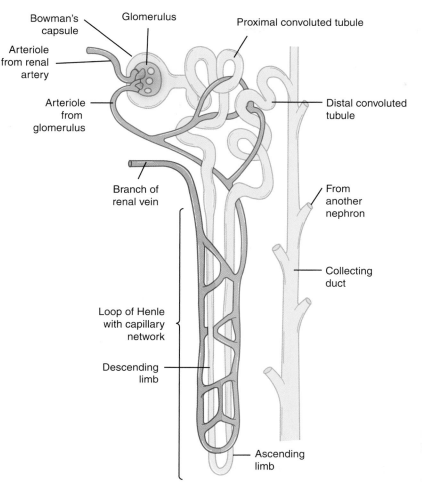

FIGURE 22.2 Nephron with associated blood vessels. *Used with permission, from Tamparo, C., & Lewis, M. (2011). Diseases of the human body (5th ed.). FA Davis Company.*

capillaries (the peritubular capillaries and vasa recta). The collecting ducts of all nephrons pass into one of 8 to 10 lobes that contain cone-shaped structures called renal pyramids. The collecting ducts eventually merge to transport the urine away from the cortex toward the point of the pyramid, called the renal papilla, which faces the hilum. The renal papilla funnel urine into cup-shaped structures called minor calyxes, which merge to form a major calyx. The major calyces merge to form the renal pelvis, which channels the urine to the bladder via the ureters for excretion through the urethra.

The amount of fluid filtered by the glomeruli of both kidneys is about 180 L a day, of which 90% to 99% is reabsorbed, leaving 1 to 2 L to be excreted as urine. Filtration occurs in the kidney by benefit of different pressure gradients. Water and other substances move through the tubules by both active and passive transport. The afferent arterioles are larger than the efferent arterioles, allowing blood to flow in faster than it exits, increasing pressure within the glomerular

vessels, forcing water and dissolved low molecular weight substances into the space between the glomerulus and the Bowman capsule, and from there into the proximal renal tubule. As the filtrate passes through the proximal tubule, water and other substances are carried from the glomerulus by the efferent arterioles into a second capillary network entwined around the renal tubules called the peritubular capillaries. Substances eventually reabsorbed into the circulating fluids include:

- Larger substances such as plasma proteins, blood cells, protein-bound hormones, minerals, and other high molecular weight materials
- Low molecular weight substances such as water, amino acids, important ions (sodium, chloride, bicarbonate, potassium, calcium, magnesium, phosphate), glucose, and other threshold substances needed by the body

As the filtrate moves through the proximal tubules, sulfates, glucuronides, hippurates, hydrogen ions, and

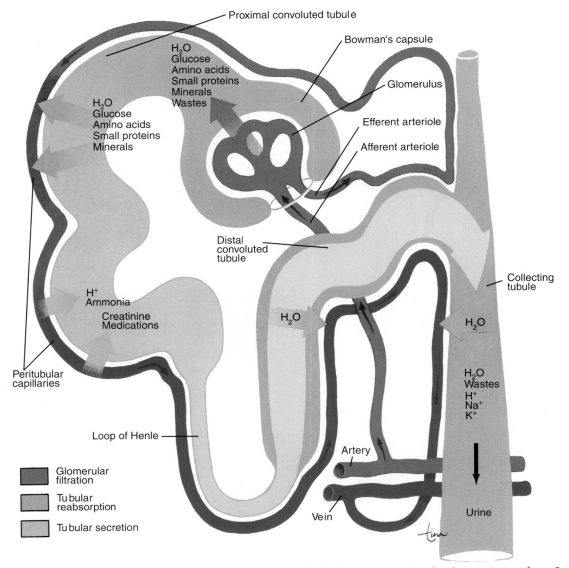

FIGURE 22.3 Glomerular filtration, tubular reabsorption, and tubular secretion. *Used with permission, from Scanlon, V., & Sanders, T. (2010). Essentials of anatomy and physiology (6th ed.). FA Davis Company.*

drugs such as penicillin are added to it by the process of secretion. Like the proximal tubule, the descending limb of the loop of Henle is very permeable to water, and water readily diffuses out of the descending loop, further concentrating the filtrate that remains in the tubules. Some sodium and chloride is actively pumped out of the ascending limb of the loop of Henle and is re-absorbed into the interstitial fluid. Water does not follow the sodium ions into the interstitial fluid due to the selective properties of the cells in the membrane of the ascending limb. As a result of the loss of sodium chloride and retained water, the fluid that leaves the loop of Henle has a lower osmolality than plasma. Water, potassium, sodium, and chloride are reabsorbed from

the distal tubules and hydrogen ions are secreted into the distal tubule. The main function of the distal and collecting tubules is to adjust the pH, osmolality, and the electrolyte content of the formed urine before it is excreted (see Fig. 22.3).

Polyuria is an abnormal increase in the volume of urine, as is commonly associated with diabetes, the overuse of diuretics, and excessive IV fluid administration. Oliguria is a decrease in urinary volume such as occurs in preeclampsia, eclampsia, shock, and acute nephritis. Anuria, which is the inability to pass urine, is a rare finding and may be associated with extreme blockage of the kidney or with blocked or crimped urinary catheter tubing.

Normal Urine Volume per 24 Hours

The ranges below are very general averages and were not calculated based on normal average body weights. Literature also shows that the expected urinary output can be estimated by formula where the expected output is: Infants—1 to 2 mL/kg/hr, Children and Adolescents—0.5 to 1 mL/kg/hr, and Adults and Older Adults—1 mL/kg/hr.

Newborns	15–60 mL
Infants	
3–10 days	100–300 mL
11–59 days	250–450 mL
2–12 months	400–500 mL
Children and Adolescents	
13 months–4 years	500–700 mL
5–7 years	650–1,000 mL
8–14 years	800–1,400 mL
Adults and Older Adults	800–2,500 mL (average 1,200 mL)

Normally, more urine is produced during the day than at night. With advancing age, the reverse will often occur. The total expected outcome for adults appears to remain the same regardless of age.

The information in the Part I studies is organized in a manner to help the student see how the five basic components of the nursing process (assessment, diagnosis, planning, implementation, and evaluation) can be applied to each phase of laboratory and diagnostic testing. The goal is to use nursing process to understand the integration of care (laboratory, diagnostic, nursing care) toward achieving a positive expected outcome.

- **Assessment** is the collection of information for the purpose of answering the question, "is there a problem?" Knowledge of the patient's health history, medications, complaints, and allergies as well as synonyms or alternate test names, common use for the procedure, specimen requirements, and normal ranges or interpretive comments provide the foundation for diagnosis.
- **Diagnosis** is the process of looking at the information gathered during assessment and answering the questions, "what is the problem" and "what do I need to do about it?" Test indications tell us why the study has been requested and potential diagnoses tell us the value or importance of the study relative to its clinical utility.
- **Planning** is a blueprint of the nursing care before the procedure. It is the process of determining how the nurse is going to partner with the patient to fix the problem (e.g., "the patient has a study ordered and this is what I should know before I successfully carry out the plan to have the study completed"). Knowledge of interfering factors, social and cultural issues, preprocedure restrictions, the need for written and informed consent, anxiety about the procedure, and concerns regarding pain are some considerations for planning a successful partnership.
- **Implementation** is putting the plan into action with an idea of what the expected outcome should be. Collaboration with the departments where the laboratory test or diagnostic study is to be performed is essential to the success of the plan. Implementation is where the work is done within each health-care team member's scope of practice.
- **Evaluation** answers the question, "did the plan work or not?" Was the plan completely successful, partially successful, or not successful? If the plan did not work, evaluation is the process where you determine what needs to be changed to make the plan work better. This includes a review of all expected outcomes. Nursing care after the procedure is where information is gathered to evaluate the plan. Review of results, including critical findings, in relation to patient symptoms and other tests performed, provides data that form a more complete picture of health or illness.
- **Expected Outcomes** are positive outcomes related to the test. They are the outcomes the nurse should expect if all goes well.

A number of pretest, intratest, and post-test universal points are presented in this overview section because the information applies to urine studies in general.

Universal Pretest Pearls (Planning)

- Obtain a history of the patient's complaints, including a list of known allergens, especially allergies or sensitivities to medications or latex so their use can be avoided or their effects mitigated if an allergy is present. Carefully evaluate all medications currently being taken by the patient. A list of the patient's current medications, prescribed and over the counter (including anticoagulants, aspirin and other salicylates, and dietary supplements) should also be obtained. Such products may be discontinued by medical direction for the appropriate number of days prior to the procedure. Ensure that all allergies are clearly noted in the medical record, and ensure that the patient is wearing an allergy and medical record armband. Report information that could interfere with, or delay proceeding with, the study to the health-care provider (HCP) and laboratory.

- Obtain a history of the patient's affected body system, symptoms, and results of previously performed laboratory tests and diagnostic and surgical procedures. Previous test results will provide a basis of comparison between old and new data.
- An important aspect of planning is understanding factors that may alter study findings or cause abnormal results. Interdepartmental communication is a key factor in the planning process. The inability of a patient to cooperate or remain still during the procedure because of age, significant pain, or mental status should be among the anticipated factors. Recent or past procedures, medications, or existing medical conditions that could complicate or interfere with test results should be noted.
- Review the steps of the study with the patient or caregiver. Expect patients to be nervous about the procedure and the pending results. Educating the patient on his or her role during the procedure and what to expect can facilitate this. The actual time required to complete each study will depend on a number of conditions, including the type of equipment being used and how well a patient will cooperate.
- Address any concerns about pain and explain or describe, as appropriate, the level and type of discomfort that may be expected.
- Provide additional instructions and patient preparation regarding medication, diet, fluid intake, or activity if appropriate. Unless specified in the individual study, there are no special instructions or restrictions.
- Always be sensitive to any cultural or psychosocial issues, including a concern for modesty before, during, and after the procedure.

Reminder

Ensure that a written and informed consent has been documented in the medical record prior to the study, if required. The consent must be obtained before medication is administered.

Universal Intratest Pearls (Implementation)

- Correct patient identification is crucial prior to any procedure. Positively identify the patient using two unique identifiers such as patient name, date of birth, Social Security number, or medical record number.
- Standard Precautions must be followed.
- Children and infants may be accompanied by a parent to calm them. Keep neonates and infants covered and in a warm room and provide a pacifier or gentle touch. The testing environment should be quiet, and the patient should be instructed, as appropriate, to remain still during the test as extraneous movements can affect results.
- Ensure that the patient has complied with pretesting instructions, including dietary, fluid, medication, and activity restrictions as given for the procedure.
- Appropriate specimen containers should always be labeled, before leaving the patient's side, with the corresponding patient demographics, initials of the person collecting the sample, collection date, time of collection, applicable special notes, and then they should be promptly transported to the laboratory for processing and analysis.

Universal Post Test Pearls (Evaluation)

- Note that test results are made available to the requesting HCP, who will discuss them with the patient.
- Answer questions and address concerns voiced by the patient or family and reinforce information given by the patient's HCP regarding further testing, treatment, or referral to another HCP. Recognize that patients will have anxiety related to test results. Provide teaching and information regarding the clinical implications of the test results on the patient's lifestyle as appropriate.
- Note that test results should be evaluated in context with the patient's signs, symptoms, and diagnosis. Depending on the results of the procedure, additional testing may be performed to evaluate or monitor progression of the disease process and determine the need for a change in therapy.
- Be aware that when a person goes through a traumatic event such as an illness or being given information that will impact his or her lifestyle, there are universal human reactions that occur. These include knowledge deficit, fear, anxiety, and coping; in some situations, grieving may occur. HCPs should always be aware of the human response and how it may affect the plan of care and expected outcomes.

DISCUSSION POINT
Regarding Post-Test Critical Findings: Timely notification of a critical finding for lab or diagnostic studies is a role expectation of the professional nurse. Notification processes will vary among facilities. Upon receipt of the critical finding, the information should be read back to the caller to verify accuracy. Most policies require immediate notification of the primary HCP, hospitalist,

or on-call HCP. Reported information includes the patient's name, unique identifiers, critical finding, name of the person giving the report, and name of the person receiving the report. Documentation of notification should be made in the medical record with the name of the HCP notified, time and date of notification, and any orders received. Any delay in a timely report of a critical finding may require completion of a notification form with review by Risk Management.

STUDIES

- Creatinine, Urine, and Creatinine Clearance, Urine
- Drugs of Abuse
- Protein, Urine: Total Quantitative and Fractions
- Urinalysis

LEARNING OUTCOMES

Providing safe, effective nursing care (SENC) includes mastery of core competencies and standards of care. SENC is based on a judicious application of nursing knowledge in combination with scientific principles. The Art of Nursing lies in blending what you know with the ability to effectively apply your knowledge in a compassionate manner.

After reading/studying this chapter you will be able to:

Thinking

1. Describe the basic anatomy of the kidney.
2. List the seven major functions of the kidneys.
3. Identify four things that influence kidney function.

Doing

1. Discuss the four main types of urine specimen collection.
2. Ensure clear communication of patient preferences to ancillaries who are providing care.

Caring

1. Voluntarily collaborate with others who may have a different point of view on how to provide care.

Creatinine, Urine, and Creatinine Clearance, Urine

Quick Summary

COMMON USE: To assess and monitor kidney function related to acute or chronic nephritis.

SPECIMEN: Urine from an unpreserved random or timed specimen collected in a clean plastic collection container.

NORMAL FINDINGS: (Method: Spectrophotometry)

Age	Conventional Units	SI Units
		Urine Creatinine (Conventional Units × 8.84)
2–3 yr	6–22 mg/kg/ 24 hr	53–194 micromol/ kg/24 hr
4–18 yr	12–30 mg/kg/ 24 hr	106–265 micromol/ kg/24 hr
Adult male	14–26 mg/kg/ 24 hr	124–230 micromol/ kg/24 hr
Adult female	11–20 mg/kg/ 24 hr	97–177 micromol/ kg/24 hr
		Creatinine Clearance (Conventional Units × 0.0167)
Children	70–140 mL/ min/1.73 m^2	1.17–2.33 mL/s/ 1.73 m^2
Adult male	85–125 mL/ min/1.73 m^2	1.42–2.08 mL/s/ 1.73 m^2
Adult female	75–115 mL/ min/1.73 m^2	1.25–1.92 mL/s/ 1.73 m^2
For each decade after 40 yr	Decrease of 6–7 mL/min/ 1.73 m^2	Decrease of 0.06–0.07 mL/s/1.73 m^2

Test Explanation

Creatinine is the end product of creatine metabolism. Creatine resides almost exclusively in skeletal muscle, where it participates in energy-requiring metabolic reactions. In these processes, a small amount of creatine is irreversibly converted to creatinine, which then circulates to the kidneys and is excreted. The amount of creatinine generated in an individual is proportional to the mass of skeletal muscle present and remains fairly constant, unless there is massive muscle damage resulting from crushing injury or degenerative muscle disease. Creatinine values decrease with advancing age owing to diminishing muscle mass. Although the measurement of urine creatinine is an effective indicator of renal function, the creatinine clearance test is more precise. The creatinine clearance test measures a blood sample and a urine sample to determine the rate at which the kidneys are clearing creatinine from the blood; this reflects the glomerular filtration rate (GFR) and is based on an estimate of body surface.

Chronic kidney disease (CKD) is a significant health concern worldwide. International studies have been undertaken to evaluate the risk factors common to cardiovascular disease, diabetes, and hypertension; these three diseases are all associated with CKD. Albuminuria can be the result of increased glomerular permeability to proteins is considered an independent risk factor predictive of kidney or cardiovascular disease. There has also been an international effort to standardize methods to identify and monitor CKD undertaken by the National Kidney Disease Education Program (NKDEP), the International Confederation of Clinical Chemistry and Laboratory Medicine, and the European Communities Confederation of Clinical Chemistry (since renamed the European Federation of Clinical Chemistry and Laboratory Medicine). International efforts have resulted in development of an isotope dilution mass spectrometry (IDMS) reference method for standardized measurement of creatinine and use of equations to estimate glomerular filtration rate (eGFR) for both adults and children under the age of 18 years. The equation for adults is based on factors identified in either the NKF Modification of Diet in Renal Disease (MDRD) study or the Chronic Kidney Disease Epidemiology Collaboration (CKD-EPI) equation using creatinine results from a method that has calibration traceable to IDMS. The equation includes four factors: serum or plasma creatinine value, age in years, gender, and race. The equation for adults is valid only for patients between the ages of 18 and 70. A correction factor is incorporated in the equation if the patient is African American because CKD is more prevalent in African Americans; results are approximately 20% higher. An IDMS-traceable equation using serum creatinine results from a method that has a calibration traceable to the IDMS and referred to as the "bedside" Schwartz equation is recommended for estimating GFR for patients less 18 years of age. The formula uses the patient's height in centimeters and the serum creatinine value where the GFR (mL/min/1.73 m²) = (0.41 × height cm)/serum creatinine mg/dL (SI Units: GFR (mL/min/1.73 m²) = (36.2 × height cm)/serum creatinine micromol/L. It is very important to know whether the creatinine has been measured using an IDMS traceable test method because the values will differ; results are lower. The equations have not been validated for pregnant women (GFR is significantly increased in pregnancy); patients older than 70; patients with serious comorbidities; or patients with extremes in body size, muscle mass, or nutritional status. eGFR calculators can be found at the NKDEP (www.nkdep.nih.gov/professionals/gfr_calculators/index.htm).

- Creatinine clearance can be estimated from a blood creatinine level: Creatinine clearance = [1.2 × (140 − age in years) × (weight in kg)]/blood creatinine level.

The result is multiplied by 0.85 if the patient is female; the result is multiplied by 1.18 if the patient is African American.

Nursing Implications

Assessment

Indications	Potential Nursing Problems
Determine the extent of nephron damage in known kidney disease (at least 50% of functioning nephrons must be lost before values are decreased).	• Airway
	• Cardiac Output
	• Fluid Volume
Determine kidney function before administering nephrotoxic drugs.	• Infection
	• Injury Risk
Evaluate accuracy of a 24-hr urine collection based on the constant level of creatinine excretion.	• Human Response
	• Pain
Evaluate glomerular function.	
Monitor effectiveness of treatment in kidney disease.	

Diagnosis: Clinical Significance of Test Results

INCREASED IN

- Acromegaly *(related to increased muscle mass)*
- Carnivorous diets *(related to increased intake of creatine, which is metabolized to creatinine and excreted by the kidneys)*
- Exercise *(related to muscle damage; increased renal blood flow)*
- Gigantism *(related to increased muscle mass)*

DECREASED IN

Conditions that decrease GFR, impair kidney function, or reduce renal blood flow will decrease renal excretion of creatinine

- Acute or chronic glomerulonephritis
- Chronic bilateral pyelonephritis
- Leukemia
- Muscle wasting diseases *(related to abnormal creatinine production; decreased production reflected in decreased excretion)*
- Paralysis *(related to abnormal creatinine production; decreased production reflected in decreased excretion)*
- Polycystic kidney disease
- Pregnancy-induced hypertension *(related to reduced GFR)*
- Shock
- Urinary tract obstruction (e.g., from calculi)
- Vegetarian diets *(evidenced by diets that exclude intake of animal muscle, the creatine source metabolized to creatinine and excreted by the kidneys)*

Planning

Considerations for planning a successful partnership should include clear communication of what to expect during the test to decrease anxiety and improve cooperation. Before the procedure is performed, plan to review the steps with the patient. Consumption of large amounts of meat, excessive exercise, and stress should be avoided for 24 hours before the test. Protocols may vary among facilities. Provide an appropriate collection container. Address concerns about pain, and explain that there should be no discomfort during the urine collection procedure. Inform the patient that a blood sample for creatinine will be required on the day urine collection begins or at some point during the 24-hour collection period.

SPECIAL CONSIDERATIONS

An important aspect of planning is understanding the factors that may alter study findings or cause abnormal results. Interdepartmental communication is a key factor in the planning process. The following should be noted when planning for this study:

- Excessive ketones in urine may cause falsely decreased values.
- Specimen handling during collection is essential. Failure to refrigerate the specimen throughout the urine collection period allows the decomposition of creatinine, causing falsely decreased values. Failure to follow proper technique in collecting a 24-hour specimen may invalidate test results.
- Failure to follow dietary restrictions before the procedure may cause the procedure to be canceled or repeated.

It is also important to understand which medications or substances the patient may be exposed to in the healthcare setting that can interfere with accurate testing:

- Drugs that may increase urine creatinine levels include ascorbic acid, cefoxitin, cephalothin, corticosteroids, fluoxymesterone, levodopa, methandrostenolone, methotrexate, methyldopa, nitrofurans (including nitrofurazone), oxymetholone, phenolphthalein, and prednisone.
- Drugs that may increase urine creatinine clearance include enalapril, oral contraceptives, prednisone, and ramipril.
- Drugs that may decrease urine creatinine levels include anabolic steroids, androgens, captopril, and thiazides.
- Drugs that may decrease the urine creatinine clearance include acetylsalicylic acid, amphotericin B, carbenoxolone, chlorthalidone, cimetidine, cisplatin, cyclosporine, guancidine, ibuprofen, indomethacin, mitomycin, oxyphenbutazone, probenecid (coadministered with digoxin), puromycin, and thiazides.

Implementation

Patient education is key to obtaining the patient's cooperation in following directions, and providing an explanation for the purpose of the procedure is an important part of this process. Inform the patient that this study can assist in assessing kidney function.

SPECIMEN COLLECTION TYPES AND INSTRUCTIONS

- *Random Clean-Catch Specimen (Specimens collected first thing in the morning, before the ingestion of any food or fluids, provide the most useful information because the likelihood of identifying abnormalities is greater in a more concentrated specimen. The first morning clean-catch specimen is normally hypertonic due to decreased fluid intake, usually occurring overnight, with a specific gravity greater than 1.022. A specific gravity less than 1.022 is an indication that the kidneys are unable to concentrate urine during the natural period of dehydration, while a healthy patient sleeps.*
  - *Infant/Pediatric Patient:* Put on gloves. Clean and dry the genital area, remove the covering over the adhesive strips on the collector bag, and apply securely over the genital area. Diaper the child and observe for voiding. When the specimen is obtained, place the entire collection bag in a sterile urine container. Remove the collection device carefully from the skin to prevent irritation. Transfer the urine into a specimen container. For the dipstick method, place the dipstick or reagent pad into the urine specimen or on the diaper saturated with urine. Remove, compare with the color chart, and record the results.
  - *Male Patient:* Instruct the patient to do the following: (1) thoroughly wash his hands, (2) cleanse the meatus, (3) void a small amount into the toilet to flush the epithelial cells or bacteria from the outer urethra, and then (4) void directly into the specimen container.
  - *Female Patient:* Instruct the patient to do the following: (1) thoroughly wash her hands; (2) cleanse the labia from front to back; (3) while keeping the labia separated, void a small amount into the toilet to flush epithelial cells or bacteria from the outer urethra; and (4) without interrupting the urine stream, void directly into the specimen container.
- *Urinary Catheterization:* Place female patients in the lithotomy position and male patients in the supine position. Using sterile technique, open the straight urinary catheterization kit and perform urinary catheterization. Place the retained urine in a sterile specimen container. Urinary catheterization is a common procedure with potentially significant complications. Improper catheter insertion, improper catheter care, or excessive movement of the catheter for any reason may cause trauma to the urethra or bladder. Aside from the physical damage caused to the urinary organs, iatrogenic hematuria from the tissue trauma may cause abnormal and misleading results that could negatively affect patient care. Insertion and maintenance of urinary catheters also carries a significant risk for causing a hospital-acquired infection (HAI) or catheter-associated urinary tract infection (CAUTI). The Centers for Disease Control and Prevention (CDC) and other national

health organizations have published recommendations regarding the standard of care for prevention of CAUTI.

- *Indwelling Catheter:* Put on gloves. Empty the drainage tube of urine. It may be necessary to clamp off the catheter for 15 to 30 minutes before specimen collection. Cleanse the specimen port with an antiseptic swab and then aspirate 5 mL of urine with a 21- to 25-gauge needle and syringe. Transfer the urine to a sterile container.
- *Suprapubic Aspiration:* Place the patient in a supine position. Cleanse the area with antiseptic and drape with sterile drapes. A needle is inserted through the skin into the bladder. A syringe attached to the needle is used to aspirate the urine sample. The needle is then removed, and a sterile dressing is applied to the site. Place the sterile sample in a sterile specimen container. Do not collect urine from the pouch from the patient with a urinary diversion (e.g., ileal conduit). Instead, perform catheterization through the stoma.
- *Timed Specimen:* Obtain a clean 3-L urine specimen container, a toilet-mounted collection device, and a plastic bag (for transport of the specimen container). The specimen must be refrigerated or kept on ice throughout the entire collection period. If an indwelling urinary catheter is in place, replace the tubing and container system at the start of the collection time and keep the drainage bag on ice. Begin the test between 6 a.m. and 8 a.m. if possible. Collect first voiding and discard. Record the time the specimen was discarded as the beginning of the timed collection period. The next morning, ask the patient to void at the same time the collection was started and add this last voiding to the container. Urinary output should be recorded throughout the collection time. At the conclusion of the test, compare the quantity of urine with the urinary output record for the collection; if the specimen contains less than what was recorded as output, some urine may have been discarded, invalidating the test. Include on the collection container's label the total volume of urine collected, test start and stop times, and the ingestion of any foods or medications that can affect test results.

Usually a 24-hour time frame for urine collection is ordered. Inform the patient that all urine must be saved during that 24-hour period. A sign can be placed in the bathroom to remind the patient to save all urine. Instruct the patient not to void directly into the laboratory 24-hour collection container, but instead to void all urine into the collection device, and then to pour the urine into the laboratory collection container. Caution the patient to avoid defecating in the collection device and to prevent toilet tissue from getting into the collection device.

Evaluation

Recognize anxiety related to test results, and be supportive of impaired activity related to fear of a shortened life expectancy. Discuss the implications of abnormal test results on the patient's lifestyle. Help the patient to cope with long-term implications. Provide teaching and information regarding the clinical implications of the test results as appropriate. Educate the patient regarding access to counseling services. Recognize that anticipatory anxiety and grief related to potential lifestyle changes may be expressed when someone is faced with a chronic disorder. Provide contact information, if desired, for the NKF (www.kidney.org) or the NKDEP (www.nkdep.nih.gov).

✓ Critical Findings

- Degree of impairment:
- Borderline: 62.5–80 mL/min/1.73 m² (SI: 1–1.3 mL/s/1.73 m²)
- Slight: 52–62.5 mL/min/1.73 m² (SI: 0.9–1 mL/s/1.73 m²)
- Mild: 42–52 mL/min/1.73 m² (SI: 0.7–0.9 mL/s/1.73 m²)
- Moderate: 28–42 mL/min/1.73 m² (SI: 0.5–0.7 mL/s/1.73 m²)
- Marked: Less than 28 mL/min/1.73 m² (SI: Less than 0.5 mL/s/1.73 m²)

Note and immediately report to the requesting healthcare provider (HCP) any critical findings and related symptoms. A listing of these findings varies among facilities.

✓ Study Specific Complications

N/A

✓ Related Tests

- Related tests include anion gap, antimicrobial drugs, antibodies antiglomerular basement membrane, ANF, biopsy kidney, biopsy muscle, blood gases, BNP, BUN, calcium, calculus kidney stone analysis, C4, CT abdomen, CT renal, CK and isoenzymes, creatinine, culture urine, cytology urine, cystoscopy, echocardiography, echocardiography transesophageal, electrolytes, EMG, ENG, EPO, gallium scan, glucagon, glucose, haptoglobin, insulin, IVP, KUB studies, lung perfusion scan, microalbumin, osmolality, phosphorus, renogram, retrograde ureteropyelography, TSH, thyroxine, US kidney, uric acid, and UA.
- Refer to the Genitourinary System table at the end of the book for related tests by body system.

Expected Outcomes

Expected outcomes associated with Creatinine and Creatinine Clearance, Urine, are

- Maintaining normal fluid volume with an absence of edema
- Not having any seizure activity
- Verbalizing the importance of collecting all of the urine voided within the designated 24-hour period
- Nursing provision of clear direction about when to begin and end the urine collection

Drugs of Abuse

Quick Summary

- Amphetamines
- Ethanol (Alcohol)
- Cannabinoids
- Opiates
- Cocaine
- Phencyclidine

SYNONYM ACRONYM: Amphetamines, cannabinoids (THC), cocaine, ethanol (alcohol, ethyl alcohol, ETOH), phencyclidine (PCP), opiates (heroin)

COMMON USE: To assist in rapid identification of commonly abused drugs in suspected drug overdose or for workplace drug screening

NORMAL FINDINGS: (Method: Spectrophotometry for ethanol; immunoassay for drugs of abuse)

Ethanol: None detected
Drug screen: None detected

Test Explanation

Drug abuse continues to be a significant social and economic problem in the workforce. The Substance Abuse and Mental Health Services Administration (SAMHSA) has identified opiates, cocaine, cannabinoids, amphetamines, and phencyclidines (PCPs) as the most commonly abused illicit drugs. Alcohol is the most commonly encountered legal substance of abuse. Chronic alcohol abuse can lead to liver disease, high blood pressure, cardiac disease, and birth defects. Regulations relating to workplace drug and alcohol testing are defined at the federal level by the Drug-Free Workplace Act (DFWA), Americans with Disabilities Act (ADA), Family and Medical Leave Act (FMLA), and Fair Credit Reporting Act (FRCA). The DFWA pertains to some Federal contractors and all Federal grantees who receive a contract or grant from a Federal source. The U.S. Department of Transportation (DOT) also has stipulations regarding which of its agencies must participate in a workplace screening program, and at defined levels of employee participation. Employers not covered by FDWA or DOT regulations may be covered by the laws of their particular state(s) and by their individual company's Human Resource policies. When applicable federal and state laws coexist, employers need to follow the legislation that best benefits their employees.

Nursing Implications

Assessment

Indications	Potential Nursing Problems
Differentiate alcohol intoxication from diabetic coma, cerebral trauma, or drug overdose. Investigate suspected drug abuse. Investigate suspected drug overdose. Investigate suspected noncompliance with drug or alcohol treatment program. Monitor ethanol levels when administered to treat methanol intoxication. Conduct routine workplace screenings.	• Conflicted Decision-making • Family • Human Response • Morality • Role Performance • Sleep • Socialization

	Screening Cutoff Concentrations for Drugs of Abuse Recommended by SAMHSA	Confirmatory Cutoff Concentrations for Drugs of Abuse Recommended by SAMHSA	Detectable Duration After Last Single-Use Dose	Detectable Duration After Last Dose: Prolonged Use
Hallucinogens				
Cannabinoids	50 ng/mL	15 ng/mL	2–7 days	1–2 mo
Phencyclidine	25 ng/mL	25 ng/mL	1 wk	2–4 wk
Opiates	2,000 ng/mL	2,000 ng/mL	1–3 days	1–3 days
6–Acetylmorphine	10 ng/mL	10 ng/mL	20 hr	1–7 days
Stimulants				
Amphetamines (either amphetamine or methamphetamine)[a]	500 ng/mL	250 ng/mL	48 hr	7–10 days
Cocaine	150 ng/mL	100 ng/mL	3 days	4 days
MDMA (either methylenedioxymethamphetamine, methylenedioxyamphetamine, or methylenedioxyethylamphetamine)	500 ng/mL	250 ng/mL	24 hr	24 hr

[a] To be reported as positive for methamphetamine, the specimen must also contain amphetamine at a concentration of 100 ng/mL or greater.

Diagnosis: Clinical Significance of Test Results

A urine screen merely identifies the presence of these substances in urine; it does not indicate time of exposure, amount used, quality of the source used, or level of impairment. Positive screens should be considered presumptive. Drug-specific confirmatory methods should be used to investigate questionable results of a positive urine screen.

Planning

Considerations for planning a successful partnership should include clear communication of what to expect during the test to decrease anxiety and improve cooperation. Before the procedure is performed, plan to review the steps with the patient, especially if the circumstances require the collection of urine and blood specimens using a chain-of-custody protocol. Inform the patient that specimen collection takes approximately 5 to 10 minutes but may vary depending on the level of patient cooperation. Provide an appropriate collection container. Address concerns about pain and explain that there may be some discomfort during the venipuncture, but there should be no discomfort during urine specimen collection.

SPECIAL CONSIDERATIONS

An important aspect of planning is understanding the factors that may alter study findings or cause abnormal results. Interdepartmental communication is a key factor in the planning process. The following should be noted when planning for this study:

- Adulterants such as bleach or other strong oxidizers can produce erroneous urine drug screen results.
- Alcohol is a volatile substance, and specimens should be stored in a tightly stoppered containers to avoid falsely decreased values. It is equally important to avoid using an alcohol prep to cleanse the venipuncture site as blood alcohol level may be falsely increased; an alcohol-free prep should be used.

It is also important to understand which medications or substances the patient may be exposed to in the healthcare setting that can interfere with accurate testing:

- Codeine-containing cough medicines and antidiarrheal preparations, as well as the ingestion of large amounts of poppy seeds, may produce a false-positive opiate result.

DISCUSSION POINT

Make sure a written and informed consent has been signed prior to the procedure.

Implementation

Patient education is key to obtaining the patient's cooperation in following directions, and providing an explanation for the purpose of the procedure is an important part of this process. Inform the patient that this study can assist with the identification of drugs in the body.

For alcohol level, use a non-alcohol-containing solution to cleanse the venipuncture site before specimen collection. Perform a venipuncture as appropriate.

RANDOM CLEAN-CATCH SPECIMEN COLLECTION INSTRUCTIONS

- *Infant/Pediatric Patient:* Put on gloves. Clean and dry the genital area, remove the covering over the adhesive strips on the collector bag, and apply securely over the genital area. Diaper the child and observe for voiding. When the specimen is obtained, place the entire collection bag in a sterile urine container. Remove the collection device carefully from the skin to prevent irritation. Transfer the urine into a specimen container. For the dipstick method, place the dipstick or reagent pad into the urine specimen or on the diaper saturated with urine. Remove, compare with the color chart, and record the results.
- *Male Patient:* Instruct the patient to do the following: (1) thoroughly wash his hands, (2) cleanse the meatus, (3) void a small amount into the toilet to flush the epithelial cells or bacteria from the outer urethra, and then (4) void directly into the specimen container.
- *Female Patient:* Instruct the patient to do the following: (1) thoroughly wash her hands; (2) cleanse the labia from front to back; (3) while keeping the labia separated, void a small amount into the toilet to flush epithelial cells or bacteria from the outer urethra; and (4) without interrupting the urine stream, void directly into the specimen container.

Follow the chain-of-custody protocol, if required. Monitor specimen collection, labeling, and packaging to prevent tampering. This protocol may vary by institution.

Evaluation

Recognize anxiety related to test results, and ensure that results are communicated to the proper individual, as indicated in the chain-of-custody protocol. Educate the patient regarding access to counseling services. Provide support and information regarding detoxification programs, as appropriate. Provide contact information, if desired, for the National Institute on Drug Abuse (www.nida.nih.gov).

⊘ Critical Findings

Note and immediately report to the requesting healthcare provider (HCP) any critical findings and related symptoms. A listing of these findings varies among facilities.

The legal limit for ethanol intoxication varies by state, but in most states, greater than 80 mg/dL (0.08%) is considered impaired for driving. Levels greater than 300 mg/dL are associated with amnesia, vomiting, double vision, and hypothermia. Levels of 400 to 700 mg/dL are associated with coma and may be fatal. Possible interventions for ethanol toxicity include administration of tap water or 3% sodium bicarbonate lavage, breathing support, and hemodialysis (usually indicated only if levels exceed 300 mg/dL).

Amphetamine intoxication (greater than 1 mcg/mL) causes psychoses, tremors, convulsions, insomnia, tachycardia, dysrhythmias, impotence, cerebrovascular accident, and respiratory failure. Possible interventions include emesis (if orally ingested and if the patient has a gag reflex and normal central nervous system [CNS] function), administration of activated charcoal followed by magnesium citrate cathartic, acidification of the urine to promote excretion, and administration of liquids to promote urinary output.

Cocaine intoxication (greater than 1 mcg/mL) causes short-term symptoms of CNS stimulation, hypertension, tachypnea, mydriasis, and tachycardia. Possible interventions include emesis (if orally ingested and if the patient has a gag reflex and normal CNS function), gastric lavage (if orally ingested), whole-bowel irrigation (if packs of the drug were ingested), airway protection, cardiac support, and administration of diazepam or phenobarbital for convulsions. The use of beta blockers is contraindicated.

Heroin and morphine are opiates that at toxic levels (greater than 200 ng/mL) cause bradycardia, flushing, itching, hypotension, hypothermia, and respiratory depression. Possible interventions include airway protection and the administration of naloxone (Narcan).

PCP intoxication (greater than 1 mg/mL) causes a variety of symptoms depending on the stage of intoxication. Stage I includes psychiatric signs, muscle spasms, fever, tachycardia, flushing, small pupils, salivation, nausea, and vomiting. Stage II includes stupor, convulsions, hallucinations, increased heart rate, and increased blood pressure. Stage III includes further increases of heart rate and blood pressure that may culminate in cardiac and respiratory failure. Possible interventions may include providing respiratory support, administering activated charcoal with a cathartic such as sorbitol, gastric lavage and suction, administering IV nutrition and electrolytes, and acidifying urine to promote PCP excretion.

⊘ Study Specific Complications

N/A

⊘ Related Tests

- Refer to the Therapeutic/Toxicology table at the end of the book for related tests.

Expected Outcomes

Expected outcomes associated with Drugs of Abuse are
- Expressing an interest in seeking assistance for drug rehabilitation
- Accepting the support of outside resources to make a positive, drug-free lifestyle change
- Nursing following the protocol to assure that a urine specimen obtained is from the patient

Protein, Urine: Total Quantitative and Fractions

Quick Summary

SYNONYM ACRONYM: None.

COMMON USE: To assess for the presence of protein in the urine toward diagnosing disorders affecting the kidneys and urinary tract, such as cancer, infection, and pre-eclampsia.

SPECIMEN: Urine from an unpreserved random or timed specimen collected in a clean plastic collection container.

NORMAL FINDINGS: (Method: Spectrophotometry for total protein, electrophoresis for protein fractions)

	Conventional Units	SI Units (Conventional Units × 0.001)
Total protein	30–150 mg/24 hr	0.03–0.15 g/24 hr
2nd & 3rd trimester of pregnancy	45–185 mg/24 hr	0.045–0.185 g/24 hr

The 24 hr urine volume is recorded and provided with the results of the protein measurement. Electrophoresis for fractionation is qualitative: No monoclonal gammopathy detected. (Urine protein electrophoresis should be ordered along with serum protein electrophoresis.)

Test Explanation

Most proteins, with the exception of the immunoglobulins, are synthesized and catabolized in the liver, where they are broken down into amino acids. The amino acids are converted to ammonia and ketoacids. Ammonia is converted to urea via the urea cycle. Urea is excreted in the urine. Normally, proteins do not pass from the blood through the kidneys' filtration process into the urine. The presence of protein in the urine is a significant indication of kidney disease. Chronic conditions such as diabetes, hypertension, and sickle cell anemia cause incremental and potentially irreversible kidney damage. Acute conditions such as urinary tract infections and kidney stones can also damage the kidneys.

Nursing Implications

Assessment

Indications	Potential Nursing Problems
Assist in the detection of Bence Jones proteins (light chains). Assist in the diagnosis of myeloma, Waldenström macroglobulinemia, lymphoma, and amyloidosis. Evaluate kidney function.	• Body Image • Confusion • Fear • Fluid Volume • Human Response • Infection • Injury Risk • Noncompliance • Nutrition • Pain • Self-care

Diagnosis: Clinical Significance of Test Results

INCREASED IN

- Diabetic nephropathy *(related to disease involving renal glomeruli, which increases permeability of protein)*
- Fanconi syndrome *(related to abnormal protein deposits in the kidney, which can cause Fanconi syndrome)*
- Heavy metal poisoning *(related to disease involving renal glomeruli, which increases permeability of protein)*
- Malignancies of the urinary tract *(tumors secrete protein into the urine)*
- Monoclonal gammopathies *(evidenced by large amounts of Bence Jones protein light chains excreted in the urine)*
- Multiple myeloma *(evidenced by large amounts of Bence Jones protein light chains excreted in the urine)*
- Nephrotic syndrome *(related to disease involving renal glomeruli, which increases permeability of protein)*
- Postexercise period *(related to muscle exertion)*
- Pre-eclampsia *(numerous factors contribute to increased permeability of the kidneys to protein)*
- Sickle cell disease *(related to increased destruction of red blood cells and excretion of hemoglobin protein)*
- Urinary tract infections *(related to disease involving renal glomeruli, which increases permeability of protein)*

DECREASED IN

N/A

Planning

Considerations for planning a successful partnership should include clear communication of what to expect during the test to decrease anxiety and improve cooperation. Before the procedure is performed, plan to review the steps with the patient. Provide an appropriate collection container. Address concerns about pain, and explain that there should be no discomfort during the procedure.

SPECIAL CONSIDERATIONS

An important aspect of planning is understanding the factors that may impair the procedure or cause abnormal results. Interdepartmental communication is a key factor in the planning process. It should be noted when planning for this study that all urine voided for the timed collection period must be included in the collection or else falsely decreased values may be obtained. Compare output records with the volume collected to verify that all voids were included in the collection.

It is also important to understand which medications or substances the patient may be exposed to in the health-care setting that can interfere with accurate testing:

- Drugs and substances that may increase urine protein levels include acetaminophen, aminosalicylic acid, amphotericin B, ampicillin, antimony compounds, antipyrine, arsenicals, ascorbic acid, bacitracin, bismuth subsalicylate, bromate, capreomycin, captopril, carbamazepine, carbarsone, carbenoxolone, carbutamide, cephaloglycin, cephaloridine, chlorpromazine, chlorpropamide, chlorthalidone, chrysarobin, colistimethate, colistin, corticosteroids, cyclosporine, demeclocycline, 1,2-diaminopropane, diatrizoic acid, dihydrotachysterol, doxycycline, enalapril, gentamicin, gold, hydrogen sulfide, iodoalphionic acid, iodopyracet, iopanoic acid, iophenoxic acid, ipodate, kanamycin, corn oil (Lipomul), lithium, mefenamic acid, melarsonyl, melarsoprol, mercury compounds, methicillin, methylbromide, mezlocillin, mitomycin, nafcillin, naphthalene, neomycin, NSAIDs, oxacillin, paraldehyde, penicillamine, penicillin, phenolphthalein, phenols, phensuximide, phosphorus, picric acid, piperacillin, plicamycin, polymyxin, probenecid, promazine, pyrazolones, quaternary ammonium compounds, radiographic agents, rifampin, sodium bicarbonate, streptokinase, sulfisoxazole, suramin, tetracyclines, thallium, thiosemicarbazones, tolbutamide, tolmetin, triethylenemelamine, and vitamin D.
- Drugs that may decrease urine protein levels include benazepril, captopril, cyclosporine, diltiazem, enalapril, fosinopril, interferon, lisinopril, losartan, lovastatin, prednisolone, prednisone, and quinapril.

Implementation

Patient education is key to obtaining the patient's cooperation in following directions, and providing an explanation for the purpose of the procedure is an important part of this process. Inform the patient that this study can assist in assessing the cause of protein in the urine.

SPECIMEN COLLECTION TYPES AND INSTRUCTIONS

- *Random Clean-Catch Specimen (Specimens collected first thing in the morning, before the ingestion of any food or fluids, provide the most useful information because the likelihood of identifying abnormalities is greater in a more concentrated specimen. The first morning clean-catch specimen is normally hypertonic due to decreased fluid intake, usually occurring overnight, with a specific gravity greater than 1.022. A specific gravity less than 1.022 is an indication that the kidneys are unable to concentrate urine during the natural period of dehydration, while a healthy patient sleeps.*
- *Infant/Pediatric Patient:* Put on gloves. Clean and dry the genital area, remove the covering over the adhesive strips on the collector bag, and apply securely over the genital area. Diaper the child and observe for voiding. When the specimen is obtained, place the entire collection bag in a

sterile urine container. Remove the collection device carefully from the skin to prevent irritation. Transfer the urine into a specimen container. For the dipstick method, place the dipstick or reagent pad into the urine specimen or on the diaper saturated with urine. Remove, compare with the color chart, and record the results.

- *Male Patient:* Instruct the patient to do the following: (1) thoroughly wash his hands, (2) cleanse the meatus, (3) void a small amount into the toilet to flush the epithelial cells or bacteria from the outer urethra, and then (4) void directly into the specimen container.
- *Female Patient:* Instruct the patient to do the following: (1) thoroughly wash her hands; (2) cleanse the labia from front to back; (3) while keeping the labia separated, void a small amount into the toilet to flush epithelial cells or bacteria from the outer urethra; and (4) without interrupting the urine stream, void directly into the specimen container.

- *Urinary Catheterization:* Place female patients in the lithotomy position and male patients in the supine position. Using sterile technique, open the straight urinary catheterization kit and perform urinary catheterization. Place the retained urine in a sterile specimen container. Urinary catheterization is a common procedure with potentially significant complications. Improper catheter insertion, improper catheter care, or excessive movement of the catheter for any reason may cause trauma to the urethra or bladder. Aside from the physical damage caused to the urinary organs, iatrogenic hematuria from the tissue trauma may cause abnormal and misleading results that could negatively affect patient care. Insertion and maintenance of urinary catheters also carries a significant risk for causing a hospital-acquired infection (HAI) or a catheter-associated urinary tract infection (CAUTI). The Centers for Disease Control and Prevention (CDC) and other national health organizations have published recommendations regarding the standard of care for prevention of CAUTI.
- *Indwelling Catheter:* Put on gloves. Empty the drainage tube of urine. It may be necessary to clamp off the catheter for 15 to 30 minutes before specimen collection. Cleanse the specimen port with an antiseptic swab and then aspirate 5 mL of urine with a 21- to 25-gauge needle and syringe. Transfer the urine to a sterile container.
- *Suprapubic Aspiration:* Place the patient in a supine position. Cleanse the area with antiseptic, and drape with sterile drapes. A needle is inserted through the skin into the bladder. A syringe attached to the needle is used to aspirate the urine sample. The needle is then removed, and a sterile dressing is applied to the site. Place the sterile sample in a sterile specimen container. Do not collect urine from the pouch from the patient with a urinary diversion (e.g., ileal conduit). Instead, perform catheterization through the stoma.
- *Timed Specimen:* Obtain a clean 3-L urine specimen container, a toilet-mounted collection device, and a plastic bag (for transport of the specimen container). The specimen must be refrigerated or kept on ice throughout the entire collection period. If an indwelling urinary catheter is in place, replace the tubing and container system at the start of the collection time and keep the drainage bag on ice. Begin the test between 6 a.m. and 8 a.m. if possible. Collect first voiding and discard. Record the time the specimen was discarded as the beginning of the timed collection period. The next morning, ask the patient to void at the same time the collection was started, and add this last voiding to the container. Urinary output should be recorded throughout the collection time. At the conclusion of the test, compare the quantity of urine with the urinary output record for the collection; if the specimen contains less than what was recorded as output, some urine may have been discarded, invalidating the test. Include on the collection container's label the total volume of urine collected, test start and stop times, and the ingestion of any foods or medications that can affect test results.

Usually a 24-hour time frame for urine collection is ordered. Inform the patient that all urine must be saved during that 24-hour period. A sign can be placed in the bathroom to remind the patient to save all urine. Instruct the patient not to void directly into the laboratory 24-hour collection container, but instead to void all urine into the collection device, and then to pour the urine into the laboratory collection container. Caution the patient to avoid defecating in the collection device and to prevent toilet tissue from getting into the collection device.

Evaluation
Recognize anxiety related to test results and answer any questions or address any concerns voiced by the patient or family.

✅ Critical Findings
N/A

✅ Study Specific Complications
N/A

✅ Related Tests
- Related tests include amino acid screen, ACE, β_2-microglobulin, biopsy bladder, biopsy bone marrow, bladder cancer markers, BUN, calcium, CBC, CT pelvis, CT renal, creatinine, cryoglobulin, culture urine, cytology urine, cystometry, cystoscopy,

glucose, glycated hemoglobin, Hgb electrophoresis, IgA, IgG, IgM, IFE, IVP, lead, LAP, MRI musculoskeletal, microalbumin, osmolality, porphyrins, protein blood total and fractions, renogram, sickle cell screen, US bladder, US spleen, UA, and voiding cystourethrography.

- Refer to the Genitourinary and Immune systems tables at the end of the book for related tests by body system.

Expected Outcomes

Expected outcomes associated with Protein, Urine: Total Quantitative and Fractions, are

- Understanding the importance of maintaining an adequate fluid volume
- Noting no alteration in sensorium
- Verbalizing an understanding that abnormal results increase the health risk to one's self and one's fetus

Urinalysis

Quick Summary

SYNONYM ACRONYM: UA.

COMMON USE: To screen urine for multiple substances such as infection, blood, sugar, bilirubin, urobilinogen, nitrates, and protein to assist in diagnosing disorders such as kidney and liver disease as well as to assess hydration status.

SPECIMEN: Urine from an unpreserved, random specimen collected in a clean plastic collection container.

NORMAL FINDINGS: (Method: Macroscopic evaluation by dipstick and microscopic examination) Urinalysis composes a battery of tests including a description of the color and appearance of urine; measurement of specific gravity and pH; and semiquantitative measurement of protein, glucose, ketones, urobilinogen, bilirubin, hemoglobin, nitrites, and leukocyte esterase. Urine sediment may also be examined for the presence of crystals, casts, renal epithelial cells, transitional epithelial cells, squamous epithelial cells, white blood cells (WBCs), red blood cells (RBCs), bacteria, yeast, sperm, and any other substances excreted in the urine that may have clinical significance. Examination of urine sediment is performed microscopically under high power, and results are reported as the number seen per high-power field (hpf). The color of normal urine ranges from light yellow to deep amber. The color depends on the patient's state of hydration (more concentrated samples are darker in color), diet, medication regimen, and exposure to other substances that may contribute to unusual color or odor. The appearance of normal urine is clear. Cloudiness is sometimes attributable to the presence of amorphous phosphates or urates as well as blood, WBCs, fat, or bacteria.

Dipstick

pH	4.5–8
Protein	Less than 20 mg/dL
Glucose	Negative
Ketones	Negative
Hemoglobin	Negative
Bilirubin	Negative
Urobilinogen	Up to 1 mg/dL
Nitrite	Negative
Leukocyte esterase	Negative
Specific gravity	1.005–1.03

Microscopic Examination

Red blood cells	Less than 5/hpf
White blood cells	Less than 5/hpf
Renal cells	None seen
Transitional cells	None seen
Squamous cells	Rare; usually no clinical significance
Casts	Rare hyaline; otherwise, none seen
Crystals in acid urine	Uric acid, calcium oxalate, amorphous urates
Crystals in alkaline urine	Triple phosphate, calcium phosphate, ammonium biurate, calcium carbonate, amorphous phosphates
Bacteria, yeast, parasites	None seen

Test Explanation

Routine urinalysis, one of the most widely ordered laboratory procedures, is used for basic screening purposes. It is a group of tests that evaluate the kidneys' ability to selectively excrete and reabsorb substances while maintaining proper water balance. The results can provide valuable information regarding the overall health of the patient and the patient's response to disease and treatment. The urine dipstick has a number of pads on it to indicate various biochemical markers (see Fig. 22.4). Urine pH is an indication of the kidneys' ability to help maintain balanced hydrogen ion concentration in the blood. Specific gravity is a reflection of the concentration ability of the kidneys. Urine protein is the most common indicator of kidney disease, although there are conditions that can

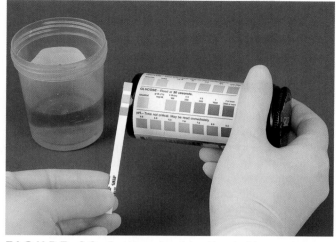

FIGURE 22.4 Urine dipsticks. *Used with permission, from Ward, S. (2009). Maternal-child nursing care: Optimizing outcomes for mothers, children, and families. FA Davis Company.*

cause benign proteinuria. Glucose is used as an indicator of diabetes. The presence of ketones indicates impaired carbohydrate metabolism. Hemoglobin indicates the presence of blood, which is associated with kidney disease. Bilirubin is used to assist in the detection of liver disorders. Urobilinogen indicates hepatic or hematopoietic conditions. Nitrites and leukocytes are used to test for bacteriuria and other sources of urinary tract infections (UTIs). Most laboratories have established criteria for the microscopic examination of urine based on patient population (e.g., pediatric, oncology, urology), unusual appearance, and biochemical reactions.

Nursing Implications
Assessment

Indications	Potential Nursing Problems
Determine the presence of a genitourinary infection or abnormality. Monitor the effects of physical or emotional stress. Monitor fluid imbalances or treatment for fluid imbalances. Monitor the response to drug therapy and evaluate undesired reactions to drugs that may impair kidney function. Provide screening as part of a general physical examination, especially on admission to a health-care facility or before surgery.	• Activity • Bleeding • Blood Glucose • Confusion • Electrolytes • Fluid Volume • Human Response • Infection • Self-care • Skin • Urination

Diagnosis: Clinical Significance of Test Results

Unusual Color

Color	Presence of
Deep yellow	Riboflavin
Orange	Bilirubin, chrysophanic acid, phenazopiridine, santonin
Pink	Beet pigment, hemoglobin, myoglobin, porphyrin, rhubarb
Red	Beet pigment, hemoglobin, myoglobin, porphyrin, uroerythrin
Green	Oxidized bilirubin, Clorets (breath mint)
Blue	Diagnex, indican, methylene blue
Brown	Bilirubin, hematin, methemoglobin, metronidazole, nitrofurantoin, metabolites of rhubarb, senna
Black	Homogentisic acid, melanin
Smoky	Red blood cells

Test	Increased in	Decreased in
pH	Ingestion of citrus fruits Vegetarian diets Metabolic and respiratory alkalosis	Ingestion of cranberries High-protein diets Metabolic or respiratory acidosis
Protein	Benign proteinuria owing to stress, physical exercise, exposure to cold, or standing Diabetic nephropathy Glomerulonephritis Nephrosis Toxemia of pregnancy	N/A
Glucose	Diabetes	N/A
Ketones	Diabetes Fasting Fever High-protein diets Isopropanol intoxication Postanesthesia period Starvation Vomiting	N/A
Hemoglobin	Diseases of the bladder Exercise (march hemoglobinuria) Glomerulonephritis Hemolytic anemia or other causes of hemolysis (e.g., drugs, parasites, transfusion reaction)	N/A

Continued

Table Continued

Test	Increased in	Decreased in
Hemoglobin (continued)	Malignancy Menstruation Paroxysmal cold hemoglobinuria Paroxysmal nocturnal hemoglobinuria Pyelonephritis Snake or spider bites Trauma Tuberculosis Urinary tract infections Urolithiasis	
Urobilinogen	Cirrhosis Heart failure Hemolytic anemia Hepatitis Infectious mononucleosis Malaria Pernicious anemia	Antibiotic therapy (suppresses normal intestinal flora) Obstruction of the bile duct
Bilirubin	Cirrhosis Hepatic tumor Hepatitis	N/A
Nitrites	Presence of nitrite-forming bacteria (e.g., **Citrobacter, Enterobacter, Escherichia coli, Klebsiella, Proteus, Pseudomonas, Salmonella**, and some species of **Staphylococcus**)	N/A
Leukocyte esterase	Bacterial infection Calculus formation Fungal or parasitic infection Glomerulonephritis Interstitial nephritis Tumor	N/A
Specific gravity	Adrenal insufficiency Dehydration Diabetes Diarrhea Fever Heart failure Proteinuria Sweating Vomiting Water restriction X-ray dyes	Diuresis Excess IV fluids Excess hydration Hypothermia Impaired renal concentrating ability

FORMED ELEMENTS IN URINE SEDIMENT
CELLULAR ELEMENTS

- Clue cells (cell wall of the bacteria causes adhesion to epithelial cells) are present in nonspecific vaginitis caused by Gardnerella vaginitis, Mobiluncus cortisii, and M. mulieris.
- RBCs are present in glomerulonephritis, lupus nephritis, focal glomerulonephritis, calculus, malignancy, infection, tuberculosis, infarction, renal vein thrombosis, trauma, hydronephrosis, polycystic kidney, urinary tract disease, prostatitis, pyelonephritis, appendicitis, salpingitis, diverticulitis, gout, scurvy, subacute bacterial endocarditis, infectious mononucleosis, hemoglobinopathies, coagulation disorders, heart failure, and malaria (see Fig. 22.5).
- Renal cells that have absorbed cholesterol and triglycerides are also known as oval fat bodies.
- Renal cells come from the lining of the collecting ducts, and increased numbers indicate acute tubular damage as seen in acute tubular necrosis, pyelonephritis, malignant nephrosclerosis, acute glomerulonephritis, acute drug or substance (salicylate, lead, or ethylene glycol) intoxication, or chemotherapy, resulting in desquamation, urolithiasis, and kidney transplant rejection.
- Squamous cells line the vagina and distal portion of the urethra. The presence of normal squamous epithelial cells in female urine is generally of no clinical significance. Abnormal cells with enlarged nuclei indicate the need for cytological studies to rule out malignancy (see Fig. 22.6).
- Transitional cells line the renal pelvis, ureter, bladder, and proximal portion of the urethra. Increased numbers are seen with infection, trauma, and malignancy.
- WBCs are present in acute UTI, tubulointerstitial nephritis, lupus nephritis, pyelonephritis, kidney transplant rejection, fever, and strenuous exercise (see Fig. 22.7).

CASTS

- Granular casts are formed from protein or by the decomposition of cellular elements. They may be seen in kidney disease, viral infections, or lead intoxication.
- Large numbers of hyaline casts may be seen in renal diseases, hypertension, congestive heart failure, or nephrotic syndrome and in more benign conditions

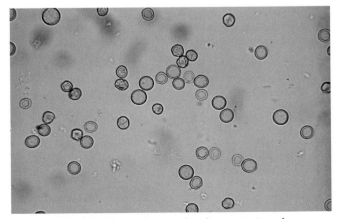

FIGURE 22.5 RBCs. *Used with permission, from Strasinger, S. (1994). Urinalysis and body fluids (3rd ed.). FA Davis Company.*

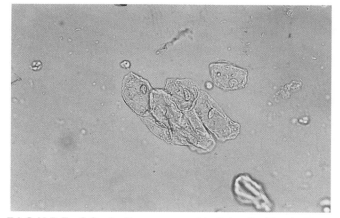

FIGURE 22.6 Squamous epithelial cells. *Used with permission, from Strasinger, S. (1994). Urinalysis and body fluids (3rd ed.). FA Davis Company.*

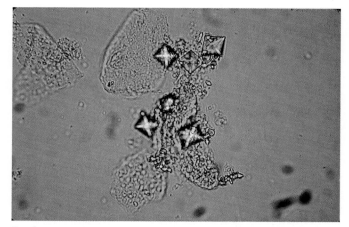

FIGURE 22.8 Calcium oxalate crystals. *Used with permission, from Strasinger, S. (1994). Urinalysis and body fluids (3rd ed.). FA Davis Company.*

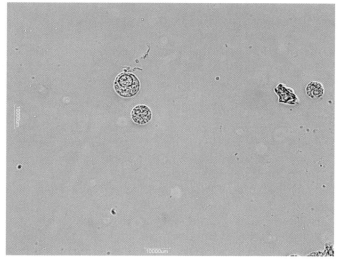

FIGURE 22.7 WBCs. *Used with permission, from Strasinger, S. (1994). Urinalysis and body fluids (3rd ed.). FA Davis Company.*

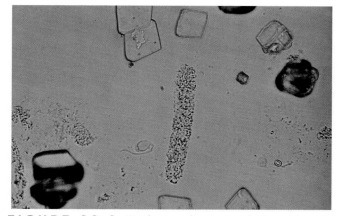

FIGURE 22.9 Finely granular cast and uric acid crystals. *Used with permission, from Strasinger, S. (1994). Urinalysis and body fluids (3rd ed.). FA Davis Company.*

such as fever, exposure to cold temperatures, exercise, or diuretic use.

- RBC casts may be found in acute glomerulonephritis, lupus nephritis, and subacute bacterial endocarditis.
- Waxy casts are seen in chronic kidney disease or conditions such as kidney transplant rejection, in which there is renal stasis.
- WBC casts may be seen in lupus nephritis, acute glomerulonephritis, interstitial nephritis, and acute pyelonephritis.

CRYSTALS

- Crystals found in freshly voided urine have more clinical significance than crystals seen in a urine sample that has been standing for more than 2 to 4 hours.
- Calcium oxalate crystals are found in ethylene glycol poisoning, urolithiasis, high dietary intake of oxalates, and Crohn disease (see Fig. 22.8).

- Cystine crystals are seen in patients with cystinosis or cystinuria.
- Leucine or tyrosine crystals may be seen in patients with severe liver disease.
- Large numbers of uric acid crystals are seen in patients with urolithiasis, gout, high dietary intake of foods rich in purines, or who are receiving chemotherapy (see study titled "Uric Acid, Urine")(see Fig. 22.9).

YEAST

- Yeast cells, usually Candida albicans, may be seen in diabetes and vaginal moniliasis (see Fig. 22.10).

Planning

Considerations for planning a successful partnership should include clear communication of what to expect during the test to decrease anxiety and improve cooperation. Before the procedure is performed, plan to review the steps with the patient. Provide an appropriate collection container. Address concerns about pain, and

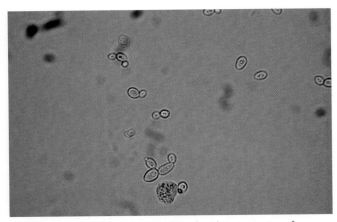

FIGURE 22.10 Yeast. *Used with permission, from Strasinger, S. (1994). Urinalysis and body fluids (3rd ed.). FA Davis Company.*

explain that there should be no discomfort during the procedure.

SPECIAL CONSIDERATIONS

An important aspect of planning is understanding the factors that may alter study findings or cause abnormal results. Interdepartmental communication is a key factor in the planning process. It is also important to understand which medications or substances the patient may be exposed to in the health-care setting that can interfere with accurate testing. The following should be noted when planning for this study:

ODOR

- Certain foods, such as onion, garlic, and asparagus, contain substances that may give urine an unusual odor. An ammonia-like odor may be produced by the presence of bacteria. Urine with a maple syrup–like odor may indicate a congenital metabolic defect (maple syrup urine disease).

PROTEIN

- The various biochemical strips are subject to interference that may produce false-positive or false-negative results. The dipstick method for protein detection is mostly sensitive to the presence of albumin; light-chain or Bence Jones proteins may not be detected by this method. Alkaline pH may produce false-positive protein results.

GLUCOSE

- Large amounts of ketones or ascorbic acid may produce false-negative or decreased color development on the glucose pad. Contamination of the collection container or a specimen with chlorine, sodium hypochlorite, or peroxide may cause false-positive glucose results.

KETONES

- False-positive ketone results may be produced in the presence of ascorbic acid, levodopa metabolites, valproic acid, phenazopyridine, phenylketones, or phthaleins.

HEMOGLOBIN

- The hemoglobin pad may detect myoglobin, intact RBCs, and free hemoglobin. Contamination of the collection container or the specimen with sodium hypochlorite or iodine may cause false-positive hemoglobin results. Negative or decreased hemoglobin results may occur in the presence of formalin, elevated protein, nitrite, ascorbic acid, or high specific gravity.

NITRITE

- False-negative nitrite results are common. Negative or decreased results may be seen in the presence of ascorbic acid and high specific gravity. Other causes of false-negative values relate to the amount of time the urine was in the bladder before voiding or the presence of pathogenic organisms that do not reduce nitrates to nitrites.

LEUKOCYTE ESTERASE

- False-positive leukocyte esterase reactions result from specimens contaminated by vaginal secretions. The presence of high glucose, protein, or ascorbic acid concentrations may cause false-negative results. Specimens with high specific gravity may also produce false-negative results. Patients with neutropenia (e.g., oncology patients) may also have false-negative results because they do not produce enough WBCs to exceed the sensitivity of the biochemical reaction.

OTHER

- Specimens that cannot be delivered to the laboratory or tested within 1 hour should be refrigerated or should have a preservative added that is recommended by the laboratory. Specimens collected more than 2 hours before submission may be rejected for analysis.
- Because changes in the urine specimen occur over time, prompt and proper specimen processing, storage, and analysis are important to achieve accurate results. Changes that may occur over time include the following: Production of a stronger odor and an increase in pH (bacteria in the urine break urea down to ammonia); a decrease in clarity (as bacterial growth proceeds or precipitates form); a decrease in bilirubin and urobilinogen (oxidation to biliverdin and urobilin); a decrease in ketones (lost through volatilization); decreased glucose (consumed by

bacteria); an increase in bacteria (growth over time); disintegration of casts, WBCs, and RBCs; and an increase in nitrite (overgrowth of bacteria).

Implementation

Patient education is key to obtaining the patient's cooperation in following directions, and providing an explanation for the purpose of the procedure is an important part of this process. Inform the patient that this study can assist in assessing for disease, infection, and inflammation, and evaluate for dehydration.

SPECIMEN COLLECTION TYPES AND INSTRUCTIONS

- *Random Clean-Catch Specimen (Specimens collected first thing in the morning, before the ingestion of any food or fluids, provide the most useful information because the likelihood of identifying abnormalities is greater in a more concentrated specimen. The first morning clean-catch specimen is normally hypertonic due to decreased fluid intake, usually occurring overnight, with a specific gravity greater than 1.022. A specific gravity less than 1.022 is an indication that the kidneys are unable to concentrate urine during the natural period of dehydration, while a healthy patient sleeps.*

  - *Infant/Pediatric Patient:* Put on gloves. Clean and dry the genital area, remove the covering over the adhesive strips on the collector bag, and apply securely over the genital area. Diaper the child and observe for voiding. When the specimen is obtained, place the entire collection bag in a sterile urine container. Remove the collection device carefully from the skin to prevent irritation. Transfer the urine into a specimen container. For the dipstick method, place the dipstick or reagent pad into the urine specimen or on the diaper saturated with urine. Remove, compare with the color chart, and record the results.

  - *Male Patient:* Instruct the patient to do the following: (1) thoroughly wash his hands, (2) cleanse the meatus, (3) void a small amount into the toilet to flush the epithelial cells or bacteria from the outer urethra, and then (4) void directly into the specimen container.

  - *Female Patient:* Instruct the patient to do the following: (1) thoroughly wash her hands; (2) cleanse the labia from front to back; (3) while keeping the labia separated, void a small amount into the toilet to flush epithelial cells or bacteria from the outer urethra; and (4) without interrupting the urine stream, void directly into the specimen container.

- *Urinary Catheterization:* Place female patients in the lithotomy position and male patients in the supine position. Using sterile technique, open the straight urinary catheterization kit and perform urinary catheterization. Place the retained urine in a sterile specimen container. Urinary catheterization is a common procedure with potentially significant complications. Improper catheter insertion, improper catheter care, or excessive movement of the catheter for any reason may cause trauma to the urethra or bladder. Aside from the physical damage caused to the urinary organs, iatrogenic hematuria from the tissue trauma may cause abnormal and misleading results that could negatively affect patient care. Insertion and maintenance of urinary catheters also carries a significant risk for causing a hospital-acquired infection (HAI) or catheter-associated urinary tract infection (CAUTI). The Centers for Disease Control and Prevention (CDC) and other national health organizations have published recommendations regarding the standard of care for prevention of CAUTI.

- *Indwelling Catheter:* Put on gloves. Empty the drainage tube of urine. It may be necessary to clamp off the catheter for 15 to 30 minutes before specimen collection. Cleanse the specimen port with an antiseptic swab, and then aspirate 5 mL of urine with a 21- to 25-gauge needle and syringe. Transfer the urine to a sterile container.

- *Suprapubic Aspiration:* Place the patient in a supine position. Cleanse the area with antiseptic, and drape with sterile drapes. A needle is inserted through the skin into the bladder. A syringe attached to the needle is used to aspirate the urine sample. The needle is then removed and a sterile dressing is applied to the site. Place the sterile sample in a sterile specimen container. Do not collect urine from the pouch from the patient with a urinary diversion (e.g., ileal conduit). Instead, perform catheterization through the stoma.

Evaluation

Recognize anxiety related to test results, and instruct the patient to report symptoms such as pain related to tissue inflammation, pain or irritation during void, bladder spasms, or alterations in urinary elimination. Observe/assess for signs of inflammation if the specimen is obtained by suprapubic aspiration. Instruct the patient with a UTI, as appropriate, about the proper technique for wiping the perineal area (front to back) after a bowel movement. UTIs are more common in women who use diaphragm/spermicide contraception. These patients can be educated, as appropriate, in the proper insertion and removal of the contraceptive device to avoid recurrent UTIs. Instruct the patient to begin antibiotic therapy, as prescribed, and instruct the patient in the importance of completing the entire course of antibiotic therapy, even if symptoms are no longer present.

✓ Critical Findings

Possible critical values are the presence of uric acid, cystine, leucine, or tyrosine crystals.

The combination of grossly elevated urine glucose and ketones is also considered significant.

Note and immediately report to the requesting health-care provider (HCP) any critical findings and related symptoms. A listing of these findings varies among facilities.

✓ Study Specific Complications

N/A

✓ Related Tests

- Related tests include amino acids, angiography renal, antibodies, anti-glomerular basement membrane, biopsy bladder, biopsy kidney, bladder cancer marker, BUN, calcium, calculus kidney stone panel, CBC, creatinine, culture urine, cystometry, cystoscopy, cystourethrography voiding, cytology urine, electrolytes, glucose, glycated hemoglobin, IFE, IVP, ketones, KUB study, microalbumin, osmolality, oxalate, protein total, phosphorus, renogram, retrograde ureteropyelography, urea nitrogen urine, uric acid (blood and urine), and US abdomen.
- Refer to the Endocrine, Genitourinary, Immune, Hematopoietic, and Hepatobiliary systems tables at the end of the book for related tests by body system.

Expected Outcomes

Expected outcomes associated with Urinalysis are

- Agreeing to save urine for visual inspection
- Having urine characteristics that do not indicate infection
- Verbalizing symptoms that would indicate an infection

REVIEW OF LEARNING OUTCOMES

Thinking

1. Describe the basic anatomy of the kidney. Answer: The structure of the kidney is surrounded by a thick fibrous capsule and is composed of two main portions: the outer renal cortex, where urine production occurs, and the interior renal medulla, where urine collection occurs. Blood vessels, nerves, lymphatic vessels, and ureters enter and exit the kidney through a structure called the hilium, a slit located in the concave notch on the medial side of each organ. Blood enters the kidney through the renal artery and leaves from the renal vein. The basic functional filtration unit of the kidney is the nephron, which is supplied by capillaries organized into a network called the glomerulus. The filtration function of the nephron is accomplished by the renal corpuscle, which is composed of a glomerulus and a Bowman's or glomerular capsule. Ultrafiltrate from the glomerulus enters a series of renal tubules where the urine is formed. The renal tubule is a very long structure divided into four distinct areas that each performs a specific function: (1) the proximal convoluted tubule lined with thousands of microvilli to enhance reabsorption and secretion, (2) the nephron loop (the descending and ascending limbs are collectively referred to as the loop of Henle), (3) the distal convoluted tubule, and (4) the collecting duct. The collecting ducts of all nephrons pass into cone-shaped structures called renal pyramids and eventually merge into the renal papilla, which faces the hilium. The renal papilla funnel urine into cup-shaped structures called minor calyxes, which merge to form a major calyx. The major calyces merge to form the renal pelvis, which channels the urine to the bladder via the ureters for excretion through the urethra.

2. List the seven major functions of the kidneys. Answer: The regulation of body fluids, the regulation of acid-base balance, the regulation of electrolyte balance, the regulation of blood pressure, the production of erythropoeitin to facilitate RBC formation, the production of vitamin D, and the excretion of waste products.

3. Identify four things that influence kidney function. Answer: The kidneys react to changes brought about by the function of the body's other organs and are influenced by changes in blood volume, blood pressure, and hormone levels.

Doing

1. Discuss the four main types of urine specimen collection. Answer: Clean catch, catheter, suprapubic, and timed.

2. Ensure clear communication of patient preferences to ancillaries who are providing care. Answer: Understanding and integrating patients' personal preferences and expressed needs will improve compliance with obtaining diagnostic studies.

Caring

1. Voluntarily collaborate with others who may have a different point of view on how to provide care. Answer: Healthy decisions are interwoven with culture, personal values, and individual goals. Try to discover what is most important to your patient; this will help you frame how to meet health-care goals. Always remember that if the patient is not on board, no plan can be successful.

((*Words* OF *Wisdom:* There is a large variety of urine studies used for a multitude of reasons. One of the barriers to accurate urine studies is the way in which the sample is handled. As the nurse, you are required to clearly understand how to collect and transport the specimen to meet diagnostic standards. This can be confusing to some. If you have questions, call the laboratory and ask. It is the nurse's role to seek information from reliable resources to meet both nursing and medical goals. From the patient perspective, it can be embarrassing to save urine specimens for study. Be culturally sensitive and age sensitive. How you approach the patient matters. Older generations tend to be more modest regarding body functions than those of a younger generation. Some cultures may not ever openly discuss them.

BIBLIOGRAPHY

Cavanaugh, B. (2003). Nurse's manual of laboratory and diagnostic tests (4th ed.). Philadelphia, PA: F.A. Davis Company.

Echeverry, G., Hortin, G., & Rai, A. (2010). Introduction to urinalysis: historical perspectives and clinical application. Methods Molecular Biology, 641:1–12. doi: 10.1007/978-1-60761-711-2_1

Estridge, B., Reynolds, A., & Walters, N. (2000). Basic medical laboratory techniques. Albany, NY: Delmar.

Graff, L. (1983). A handbook of routine urinalysis. Philadelphia, PA: Lippincott Williams & Wilkins.

Haber, M. (1988, September 8). Pisse prophecy: a brief history of urinalysis. Clinical Laboratory Medicine, 8(3):415–430.

Methodist Children's Hospital and Women's Services, San Antonio, Texas. (April, 2012). Pediatric reference guide. Retrieved from www.methodistaircare.com/pdfGuides/revised/Neonatal%20and%20Pediatric/AirCare_Pediatric_Reference_Guide.pdf

Nguyen, T., & Abilez, O. (2009). Practical guide to the care of the surgical patient. The pocket scalpel. Retrieved from www.us.elsevierhealth.com/media/us/samplechapters/9780323039772/Chapter%2002.pdf

Tanner, G. (n.d.). Renal physiology and body fluids. Retrieved from http://downloads.lww.com/wolterskluwer_vitalstream_com/sample-content/9780781768528_Rhoades/samples/Rhoades_PT6-CH22.pdf

The Postnatal. (2011). Urine output at different ages. Retrieved from www.thepostnatal.com/2011/06/urine-output-at-different-ages/

The routine urinalysis. (n.d.). Retrieved from www.austincc.edu/kotrla/UALect3RoutineUA.pdf

Thompson, G. (2013). Understanding anatomy and physiology. A visual, auditory, interactive approach. Philadelphia, PA: F.A. Davis Company.

Urinalysis. (n.d.). Retrieved from www.nlm.nih.gov/medlineplus/ency/article/003579.htm

Urinalysis. (n.d.). Retrieved from http://library.med.utah.edu/WebPath/TUTORIAL/URINE/URINE.html

Van Leeuwen, A., & Bladh, M. (2015). Davis's comprehensive handbook of laboratory and diagnostic tests with nursing implications (6th ed.). Philadelphia, PA: F.A. Davis Company.

Yoquinto, L. (2011, August 15). The fascinating history of urine tests. Retrieved from www.livescience.com/35819-history-urine-tests.html

Wu, A. (Ed.). (2006). Tietz clinical guide to laboratory tests (4th ed.). St. Louis, MO: W.B. Saunders Company.

Go to Section II of this book and www.davisplus.com for the Clinical Reasoning Tool and its case studies to provide you with a safe place to explore patient care situations. There are a total of 26 different case studies; 2 cases are presented for each of 13 body systems. One set of 13 cases are found in the Section II chapters, and a second set of 13 cases are available online at www.davisplus.com. Each case is designed with the specific goal of helping you to connect the dots of clinical reasoning. Cases are designed to reflect possible clinical scenarios; the outcomes may or may not be positive—you decide.

Clinical Reasoning Tool Case Studies: Applying Laboratory and Diagnostic Testing Clinically

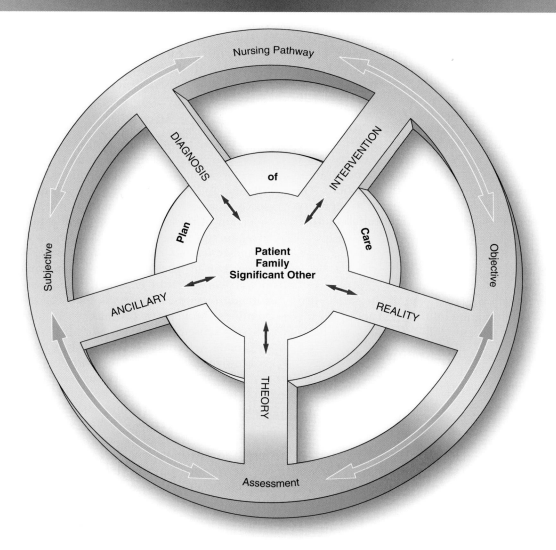

Clinical Reasoning Tool and Case Study User Guide

Introduction

Critical thinking is the essence of what a nurse does. It is a dynamic integration of science and art. Critical thinking is taking scientific evidence-based concepts and molding them to fit that specific situation with the patient, family, or significant other toward a positive expected outcome. The Clinical Reasoning Tool was developed through years of bedside nursing practice and working with nursing students and is designed to assist in achieving that goal.

Purpose of the Clinical Reasoning Tool

The purpose of the Clinical Reasoning Tool is to guide you into "thinking like a nurse." It is designed to take you by the hand and help you see the possibilities within a patient care situation. The tool is a visual representation of nursing process and is represented visually by a wheel consisting of an outer rim, a central hub, and corridors that connect the two. The outer rim is the Nursing Pathway, which represents deliberate nursing action and movement. The Hub of the wheel represents the point of care and a focus centered on the patient, family, and significant other. The Nursing Pathway and Hub are connected by five corridors: Diagnosis, Interventions, Reality Check, Theory, and Ancillary. Each corridor provides a link between nurse and patient and represents nursing activities, thoughts, and actions. The hope is that you, as the learner, will begin to see nursing process as an integrative artistic application of nursing principles. Let's take a closer look.

Nursing Pathway

The Nursing Pathway is where you, as the nurse, proactively collect and integrate information about the disease process and the patient. Ask yourself,

- What do I know about this disease process?
- Do I understand the pathophysiology?
- Do I know which lab tests or diagnostic studies would apply?
- What type of medical management would I expect to see used?
- How does this relate to my patient?

Collected information (data) will begin to provide the palate for an artistic application of nursing process.

Data collected will be *subjective* (i.e., what the patient tells you about her or his symptoms and feelings). Any information expressed by the patient that is pertinent to the clinical situation should be considered. Encouraging general nonthreatening conversation with the patient is a good way to begin the data collection process.

Collected data will also be *objective*. Sources of information pertinent to the care of the patient will be found in a review of labs, diagnostic studies, medical history, and physician notes. Objective data can also be obtained from other nurses, health-care providers (HCPs) such as physical therapists, and family members or significant others. Head-to-toe assessment is another part of objective data collection because you, as the nurse, learn about the patient through your own evaluation. Assessment data are updated continuously, providing the foundation for clinical reasoning and decision making for all of your interactions.

Once all of the data have been collected and assessed, the nurse can decide on a diagnosis and move forward with the provision of care. Care decisions are ongoing and revised as new information is received.

Clinical Corridors

The clinical corridors are where applications that can assist you in providing care to your patient reside. The corridors—Diagnosis, Interventions, Reality Check, Theory, and Ancillary—connect you to the patient and serve as conduits for purposeful nursing action. Your selection of these applications is dependent upon your assessment of the situation. *It is for you to choose the applications that best fit a specific patient scenario and artistically apply them at the point of care.* Movement from corridor to corridor can be orderly, such as first choosing nursing diagnoses and then choosing associated interventions. Movement can also be intuitive, using that nursing sense of what will work best to enter corridors and make selections as needed. It is expected that you will move in and out of the corridors at will while selecting and refining your choices.

A realistic and artistic application of scientific principles occurs by framing diagnoses, interventions, and expected outcomes to fit a specific set of facts individualized for that patient. The corridors of ancillary and nursing theory are visual reminders for you of the resources available for use in the planning and implementation of care. Reality Check is a corridor that reminds you to consider each patient's circumstances in devising and implementing his or her plan. If the plan does not work for the patient, then the plan *does not work*. Throughout the case studies, information will be provided to you from each of these corridors. In the step-by-step guide for using the Clinical Reasoning Tool, each corridor will be more fully discussed.

Plan of Care

The Plan of Care encircles the patient who resides at the hub of the wheel. Everything that you decide to do in collaboration with your patient and interdisciplinary team needs to be documented in a central location. The plan of care serves as a road map by giving direction for care to others; this is the reason why you must have a plan of care. As the nurse, you are responsible for co-ordinating care, and you cannot do that if you do not know what is going on. The plan of care is refined and redesigned on an ongoing basis according to assessment findings and the needs of the patient. Completion of a "reality check" is necessary for any plan of care to be successful.

Care Hub

The hub of the wheel represents the patient as the center of nursing care. Along with the patient in the hub of the wheel are the family and significant others. All care activities occur at the hub of the wheel. Care may need to be provided to or in collaboration with family and significant others as well as provided to the patient. Life issues such as culture, religion, and age can influence how care is approached. It is your role as the nurse to coordinate the management of care among the health-care team members.

Evaluation of a plan's success is made within the hub of the wheel at the patient's bedside and point of care. Each goal of the plan is evaluated as *met* (the plan was a success and the goal achieved), *partially met* (the goal was partially achieved, but some revisions in the plan will need to be made), or *not met* (the plan was not successful, and the goal was not achieved). All goals must be measurable and realistic for the patient situation. We may wish for a paraplegic to walk, but it is an unrealistic goal that cannot be achieved.

Clinical Reasoning Tool: Step-By-Step Case Study Application

The purpose of using case studies is not to give you the answers on how to perform patient care but to assist you to mentally explore the possibilities—essentially, using science to point your mind in the *direction of*

thinking like a nurse. The steps in each case study are the following:

Step 1:   Data Collection
Step 2:   Potential Problem/Diagnoses
Step 3:   Potential Interventions and Expected Outcome
              Putting It All Together: Application of the Nursing Process
Step 4:   Assessment
Step 5:   Reality Check: Detour Ahead
              Critical Thinking Moment
Step 6:   Actual Problems/Diagnoses
Step 7:   Planning: Actual Interventions
              Critical Thinking Moment
Step 8:   Implementation
              Nursing Theory: How Do I Do It?
              Ancillary Support: Who Will Help Me?
Step 9:   Plan of Care
Step 10:   Evaluation

Step 1: Data Collection

As the learner, you enter the Nursing Pathway and begin to collect information (data) about the specific case. Pathophysiology, signs and symptoms, labs, diagnostics, and medical management for each illness are provided for you to read. This opens the case study and begins your journey.

Step 2: Potential Problems/Diagnoses

What are my patient's problems? Now that you have had a chance to explore the disease process and associated concepts, what nursing diagnoses would apply? Visually, the Clinical Reasoning Tool contains selections in the Diagnosis corridor. Here you choose those nursing problems that may apply to this specific clinical scenario. For every medical diagnosis presented, there are potential nursing diagnoses based upon the pathophysiology of the disease process and associated symptoms. The first question a nurse should ask is, "What are the possible patient problems/nursing diagnoses that could be connected with this particular disease process?" The answer is the beginning of clinical reasoning and sets the stage for thinking like a nurse by framing nursing process as a commonsense approach to patient care.

There are "universal diagnoses" that hold true for every patient regardless of the disease process or assessment data. Universal diagnoses are those human responses common to all people when placed in situations in which we feel at risk. The four most common human responses are

- *Knowledge,* because there is always something a patient can learn

- *Anxiety* and *coping*, because, regardless of what a patient tells you, he or she is always stressed
- *Fear*, if the patient's life or lifestyle are threatened

Many times the human response is integrated into other problems and addressed in the overall picture. However, if there is a defined need, it should be evaluated as an individual problem. For example, a patient may be admitted for cellulitis where education (knowledge) about infection and treatment may be imbedded with the discussion of medication and skin. In contrast, a newly diagnosed diabetic will require a deliberate series of educational offerings (knowledge) and emotional support (coping/anxiety) prior to discharge. This requires the human response to be addressed as specific issues rather than integrated into the whole.

The choice of how to proceed is up to your artistic sense of the individual and the situation at hand. The nursing role is to understand and consider the science of the disease process and consider the possibilities prior to applying that knowledge to a patient situation.

Step 3: Potential Interventions and Expected Outcome

What should I do about the diagnoses/problems I have identified? What are my options? Now we brainstorm once again and think about what possible *potential interventions* could be used to address each of the identified *potential problems*. Intervention selections should include three categories: assessment (what you need to evaluate or monitor), therapeutic (what you are going to do), and teaching (what you are going to tell the patient/family/significant other). Always think about the expected outcomes of the interventions that are considered. This answers the question, what do I expect to see happen?

In the Clinical Reasoning Tool, these aspects of care are represented visually by the Interventions corridor. This corridor represents possible interventions to be used in patient care. All selections are based upon best-practice guidelines. Linking the potential diagnoses with the corresponding potential interventions is the first step in connecting the dots and thinking like a nurse. After this has been done, you now have a potential nursing plan. Always remember that an essential part of clinical reasoning is using common sense in conjunction with scientific principles in addressing a patient care situation.

Putting It All Together: Application of the Nursing Process

Putting It All Together is where the art and science of nursing meet to provide the best patient outcomes. We take the *potential diagnoses and interventions* and place them into the context of the patient situation.

To accomplish this, we use nursing process and nursing theory to provide the palate for patient care.

Step 4: Assessment

As the learner, you are now introduced to your patient. Provided information includes demographics, chief complaint, history of the present illness, past medical history, and family history.

From there the focus is on the application of nursing process, beginning with assessment. Each case provides narrative information for both subjective and objective assessment.

- Subjective assessment is information you get from the patient about how the patient perceives his or her health, or how the patient is feeling. Findings could be a physical and/or an emotional response to illness. Assessment data are provided in a narrative format in each case, challenging you to draw your own conclusions.
- Objective assessment encompasses any reliable source of information. Sources of information may include shift report, chart information, the physician, other nurses, and other HCPs. Objective assessment also includes your findings from the head-to-toe assessment (general appearance and physical assessment), lab values, diagnostic studies, and medications. This includes an overall impression of the patient's health.

Step 5: Reality Check: Detour Ahead

It is critical to consider the "reality" of the patient's life and integrate that information into all aspects of the nursing process. In this part of the case study, you are challenged to identify *real-life issues* from the information provided and apply them in meaningful, artistic, and realistic ways. *It is essential that the chosen interventions fit within the reality of the patient situation for the outcomes to be successful.* A reality check must be done before a plan is developed and implemented. Consideration needs to be given to factors such as culture, religion, socioeconomic status, level of education, developmental level, marital status, employment, age, and gender. Reality for any individual is ever changing, and you must be flexible and adaptable to change for your plan to be successful. Reality Check is a corridor in the Clinical Reasoning Tool that must be visited often to ensure that the chosen plan is congruent with patient expectations as a collaborative process.

Critical Thinking Moment

After you have completed the subjective and objective assessments, you will need to make a decision about the patient's *actual* problems and nursing diagnoses based upon the data you have collected and the potential problems you identified. Outcomes must be realistic and measurable.

Step 6: Actual Problems/Diagnoses

It is only after consideration of the *possible* diagnoses and associated interventions that you can select *actual* diagnoses and interventions. Choices are made based upon your consideration of collected data and life issues. For each case you will need to revisit your list of *potential diagnoses* and choose from among those the *actual diagnoses* identified based upon your evaluation of the case study information provided. A problem statement must be completed for each identified problem/diagnosis. The goal is to choose the "best fit" for a specific patient. Information to consider in making this decision comes from the objective and subjective data collected during assessment.

Step 7: Planning; Actual Interventions

Once *actual* nursing diagnoses have been chosen, it is time to decide which of your *potential interventions* will "fit" the clinical situation. These then become your *actual interventions* to be used within the patient's reality in hopes of meeting your expected outcomes. Interventions need to be identified in three categories: Assessment, Therapeutic, and Education. It is necessary to indicate a rationale (reason) for each intervention choice. Ask yourself: why have I chosen that particular intervention? Each problem statement must have an expected outcome. What is the overall goal for the chosen problem? Remember that expected outcomes must be reasonable and measurable. An intervention should never be chosen without a full understanding of what the expected outcome should be. If you do not understand what should happen, then how can you tell if your chosen intervention worked? Consider this simple example: You have a patient who is having trouble breathing. You recommend to the HCP the application of oxygen as your chosen intervention. Your expectation is that once the oxygen is applied, your patient's breathing will improve.

Step 8: Implementation

Implementation is simply putting the plan in motion and seeing what happens. There are multiple factors that need to be considered in the implementation of a plan. The two biggest questions are (1) *how do I do it?* and (2) *who can help?* Both of those questions need to be answered.

Nursing Theory: How Do I Do It?

Believe it or not, nursing theorists provide guidance on the best way to approach care. Most nursing programs choose a nursing theory around which they explain their approach to care. Thinking that one single theory will work in every clinical situation is unrealistic. A better plan is to use multiple theories to approach different aspects of care and specific situations. The practical application of nursing theory prevents this "one size fits all" approach. For example, imagine that you are caring for a first-generation Asian immigrant admitted for an appendectomy and postoperative care. Based on what you know about this surgical procedure, you identify two possible nursing diagnoses, pain and infection. Your expectation is that in providing care you will have to consider the patient's Asian culture. Yet it is important to manage the pain, prevent infection, and assess the patient's understanding. To meet your goal, you choose three theorists for this single clinical situation: (1) Madeleine Leninger's theory of transcultural nursing is used to ensure culturally competent pain management; (2) Florence Nightingale's theory on environment is used to address hygiene, the environment of care, and infection prevention; and (3) Dorothea Orem's theory of self-care management is used to assess the patient's ability to participate in wound care. Inclusion of these theories at the bedside is a key component in the application of evidenced-based and relationship-based care. Understanding the place of nursing theory in practice provides a professional and scientific foundation for practice.

Ancillary Support: Who Will Help Me?

Patient care does not occur in a vacuum. As the nurse, you are responsible for coordinating the care of the patient with other departments. You must make recommendations to the physician and act as the patient advocate. Support from other HCPs is often interwoven into your plan of care. Communication and collaboration with other teams such as respiratory therapy, physical therapy, occupational therapy, case management, social services, chaplain, and more are necessary for positive outcomes. Viewing the HCP as a team member in the process is integral to its success. Nurses spend up to 12 hours a day with the patient. This makes you the best arbiter of how that individual is progressing day by day. Although it is out of your scope of practice to order medications and treatments, it is not out of your scope of practice to make informed recommendations to the physician as part of the health-care team.

Step 9: Plan of Care

The nursing plan of care is a road map and an interdisciplinary communication tool to coordinate patient care among disciplines. The plan is refined and redesigned collaboratively and on an ongoing basis according to the needs of the patient. Expected entries would include identified problems, corresponding interventions, and expected outcomes. Individual preferences must be noted. Consider the 5-year-old who sleeps with a teddy bear for comfort.

Step 10: Evaluation

Evaluation is an active process in which you "connect the dots" to decide if the expected outcomes (goals) that were established have been met, partially met, or not met. The question you should ask is, how successful was I in meeting the goals that were set for this patient? Was the plan successful and all of the goals met? Was it partially successful with some of the goals met and some revisions needed? Or were the goals not met or not achieved? The case evaluation includes an evaluation of both the problem and the outcome.

The evaluation of success does not always lie solely with the nurse but is an integrative conversation with the patient, family, significant other, and other health-care team members. For example, if the goal is to have your patient verbalize an understanding of wound care, then evaluation of the success of this teaching goal will depend on your assessment of the patient's response along with the input from the wound care nurse and the son who will be assisting with home care. Evaluation can be simple or complex depending upon the situation. Eventually you have to decide if care is going in the right direction. Is the patient the same, getting better, or getting worse? This overarching consideration will also provide direction for care. Each case provides a narrative summary that challenges your conclusions.

Good luck!

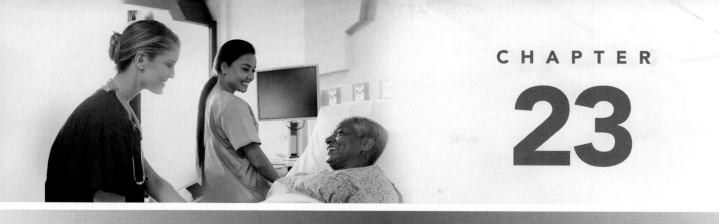

Cardiovascular System

Case Study: Myocardial Infarction

Common Nursing Study Name	Section 1 Study	Section 1 Chapter Number
Chest x-ray (CXR)	Chest x-ray	Chapter 16
CK-MB (creatine kinase-MB isoenzyme)	Creatine kinase and isoenzymes	Chapter 1
Computed tomography (CT) of the head	Computed tomography, brain	Chapter 7
Coronary angiography	Angiography, coronary	Chapter 15
C-Reactive protein (CRP)	C-Reactive protein	Chapter 1
Echocardiogram	Echocardiography	Chapter 21
	Echocardiography, transesophageal	Chapter 21
Electrocardiogram (ECG)	Electrocardiogram	Chapter 8
Electrolytes	Carbon dioxide	Chapter 1
	Chloride, blood	Chapter 1
	Potassium, blood	Chapter 1
	Sodium, blood	Chapter 1
Electroencephalogram (EEG)	Electroencephalography	Chapter 8
Hemogram and platelet count	Complete blood count, hematocrit	Chapter 2
	Complete blood count, hemoglobin	Chapter 2
	Complete blood count, platelet count	Chapter 3
	Complete blood count, RBC count	Chapter 2
	Complete blood count, RBC indices	Chapter 2
	Complete blood count, WBC count	Chapter 2
Magnetic resonance imaging (MRI) Angiography and MRI of the chest	Magnetic resonance angiography	Chapter 12
	Magnetic resonance imaging, chest	Chapter 12
Myocardial radionuclide imaging	Myocardial infarct scan	Chapter 13
	Myocardial perfusion heart scan	Chapter 13
Myoglobin	Myoglobin	Chapter 1
Oxygen saturation (pulse oximetry)	Pulse oximetry	Chapter 14
Partial thromboplastin time (aPTT)	Partial thromboplastin time, activated	Chapter 3
Prothrombin time (PT) with international normalized ratio (INR)	Prothrombin time and international normalized ratio	Chapter 3
Positron emission tomography (PET), heart	Positron emission tomography, heart	Chapter 13
Transesophogeal echocardiogram (TEE)	Echocardiography, transesophageal	Chapter 21
Troponin I	Troponins I and II	Chapter 1

STEP 1: DATA COLLECTION

Pathophysiology

Heart attack, the most common name for myocardial infarction (MI), remains the leading cause of death in the United States. A heart attack occurs when a part of the heart has a sudden or progressive deprivation of oxygen causing the heart muscle to die.

Risk Factors

General risk factors for MI are

- Age (men greater than 45 years and women greater than 55 years, without estrogen replacement)
- Family history
- Hypertension
- Diabetes
- Smoking
- Elevated high-density lipoproteins

Classification

The universal definition of MI is an alteration in cardiac-sensitive biomarkers such as troponin plus at least one of the following five diagnostic criteria: (1) symptoms of ischemia; (2) new and significant ST/T wave changes or left bundle branch block; (3) electrocardiogram (ECG) notation of pathological Q wave changes; (4) imaging verification of recent loss of viable myocardium or motion abnormality; and (5) verification of an intracoronary thrombus during angiography or autopsy. MI can be classified by type. Type 1 MI is spontaneous related to plaque, rupture, dissection, or ulceration with underlying coronary artery disease (CAD). Type 2 is a MI related to ischemia and injury with necrosis caused by oxygen imbalance from an event other than CAD such as arterial spasm, rupture, embolism, anemia, or a respiratory event. Type 3 is a MI that causes death before diagnostic studies such as cardiac biomarkers can be performed. Type 4 is a MI associated with either percutaneous coronary intervention or stent placement with resulting thrombus. Type 5 is a MI associated with a coronary artery bypass graft.

Another way to classify MI is as a ST-elevated MI (STEMI) with cardiac biomarkers, or as a non-ST-elevated MI (NSTEMI) with cardiac biomarkers. Both a STEMI and a NSTEMI are housed under the designation of acute coronary syndrome (ACS), along with unstable angina. Unstable angina is defined as chest pain in which there is no ST-segment elevation and no cardiac markers. A further MI differentiation is as a Q-wave MI or non-Q-wave MI based on the presence or absence of Q waves on the ECG.

Non-ST-Elevated MI (NSTEMI)

An NSTEMI is characterized by a decrease in oxygen to the heart through a disruption of coronary blood flow causing an imbalance between myocardial oxygen supply and demand. This imbalance is usually due to a narrowing of the coronary artery from a nonocclusive thrombus associated with a disruption of atherosclerotic plaque. The concern with NSTEMI is the possibility that it may progress to a STEMI if the artery becomes occluded. Careful monitoring of a NSTEMI is essential. Other events that could cause cardiac oxygen deprivation are coronary artery spasm, coronary artery embolism, infectious disease, arterial inflammation, hypoxia, anemia, stress, and surgical procedures.

ST-Elevated MI (STEMI)

A STEMI occurs when a clot or thrombus blocks a coronary artery. Thrombus is a common cause of MI in individuals whose coronary artery has narrowed 70% or more. Clots form from progressive damage of the coronary vessel as a result of hypertension, smoking, diabetes, high cholesterol, or a combination of these factors. The body tries to fix vessel damage by creating a plaque Band-Aid made of platelets and white blood cells (WBC). Over time the plaque grows, causing the lumen of the coronary artery to narrow. Unstable plaque is supported by increasing numbers of platelets. Increasing support is provided by the activation of collagen and thrombin to produce glycoprotein IIb and IIIa which bind fibrinogen. The repetitive process of platelet aggregation and fibrinogen binding creates larger and larger thrombi until coronary artery vessel blockage occurs.

Disrupted oxygenation causes layers of cardiac muscle damage to spread from the point of infarct outward. It is at the point of infarction that cardiac muscle cell death and irreversible necrosis occurs. Surrounding the area of necrosis is a layer of injury where the heart muscle is inflamed but can be saved if oxygenation is restored. The area of injury is surrounded by a layer of ischemia where the heart muscle is hurt but not damaged. Ischemia is reversible if coronary blood flow is restored before there is permanent damage. The area of the myocardial infarction is dependent upon the coronary artery involved and how the blood supply is affected.

- *Left Main Coronary Artery and Left Anterior Descending Coronary Artery:* Anterior or anteroseptal infarcts occur when the left anterior descending coronary artery or one of its branches occludes. These arteries supply blood to bundle branches, the anterior wall of the left ventricle, and part of the interventricular septum.
- *Right Coronary Artery:* Infarcts of the right ventricle (most often inferior wall) occur when the right coronary artery or one of its branches occludes. This artery supplies blood to the atrioventricular node, right ventricle, and the inferior and posterior left ventricular walls.
- *Left Circumflex Artery:* This supplies blood to the lateral left ventricular wall.
- *Posterior Descending Coronary Artery:* This supplies blood to the posterior wall of the left ventricle.

Reinfarction, infarct extension, or recurrent ischemia in the first 24 hours after the initial cardiac event is a concern. Other potential complications of MI include

- Dysrhythmias
- Sudden death
- Bundle branch block
- Heart failure
- Cardiogenic shock
- Cardiomyopathy
- Cardiac or papillary muscle rupture
- Ventricular aneurysm
- Pericarditis
- Dissection of coronary arteries
- Psychiatric problems

Signs and Symptoms

The cardinal symptom of MI is chest pain lasting 15 to 20 minutes or longer, caused by a lack of blood flow beyond the occlusion, resulting in cell death. Pain can vary with gender and associated medical conditions such as diabetes. Generally, chest pain is described as substernal, severe, crushing, squeezing, heaviness, tightness, burning, knife-like, dull, or diffuse. Chest pain can radiate to the left arm, shoulders, neck, back, or jaw. Radiating pain may be intermittent or continuous depending on activity. Chest pain causes fear and anxiety which, in turn, will increase heart rate, blood pressure (BP), and respiratory rate. Other classic symptoms of MI are provided in Box 23-1.

Box 23-1 Classic Symptoms of Myocardial Infarction

- Feeling of impending doom
- Diaphoresis, cool clammy skin, pallor
- Shortness of breath
- Blood pressure changes (high or low)
- Heart rate changes (high or low)
- Palpitations
- Sensorium changes (confusion, disorientation, restlessness)
- Nausea and vomiting
- Weakness and dizziness

Sometimes patients will not have any symptoms; this is called a silent MI. Women, older adults, diabetics, and dialysis patients often have vague symptoms that they attribute to noncardiac causes. Patients will describe feeling bad, or having fatigue, epigastric pain, gas, right-sided chest pain or tightness, and chest discomfort. The older adult in particular may present with hypotension, hypothermia, syncope, vague discomfort, mild perspiration, or stroke-like symptoms.

Laboratory Studies

Laboratory values are especially important in evaluating the presence of MI because of the cardiac markers left in the presence of cardiac muscle injury. All muscle cells have protein enzymes that leak into the bloodstream when the cells are damaged. Laboratory studies that capture these changes are categorized as specific biomarkers and nonspecific biomarkers for MI. Specific MI biomarkers may be diagnostic with a single draw, whereas nonspecific biomarkers may be drawn as a series of tests every 6 hours for the first 24 hours to confirm diagnosis. Typically, elevation of laboratory values will be seen over several hours. The goal is to obtain biomarker results in the first 30 to 60 minutes after a cardiac event.

Specific Biomarkers

- **Troponin I** is a cardiac-specific contractile protein that leaks out of cells in the presence of cardiac muscle damage. Troponin I is a very sensitive test in that it can identify small amounts of cardiac muscle damage. A Troponin I that is elevated above the normal range in the first 24 hours after a suspected cardiac event is considered to be diagnostic for MI. Troponin I usually rises within 3 hours of an MI and peaks within 15 to 20 hours.

Nonspecific Biomarkers

- **CK-MB** is an isoenzyme specifically found in heart muscle and is often performed in conjunction with Troponin I in diagnosis of MI. CK-MB rises within 4 to 6 hours of an MI and peaks within the first 24 hours. Rapid CK-MB mass assays have largely replaced CK-MB isoenzyme measurement by electrophoresis.
- **Myoglobin** is rapidly released from necrotic tissue and is detected 1 to 3 hours after an MI. Myoglobin is a sensitive indicator of early MI, but it lacks specificity because myoglobin levels can be affected by skeletal muscle damage. While an increase in myoglobin can help support a diagnosis of MI, the absence of an increase in myoglobin is more effective in ruling out MI.
- **C-reactive protein (CRP) and WBC** count can both be elevated due to inflammation in the presence of an MI.

Diagnostic Studies

- **Electrocardiogram (ECG)** detects changes in heart function as early as 2 hours from the occurrence of an MI and as late as 96 hours after. An ECG is valuable in differentiating STEMI from NSTEMI. If there is ST-segment elevation on the ECG the patient is having a STEMI, typically associated with coronary thrombus. If there is no ST-segment elevation on the ECG the patient is having an NSTEMI, typically associated with a transient thrombus or incomplete coronary artery occlusion. An ECG can also indicate patterns of necrosis, injury, or ischemia of myocardial tissue.

An abnormal Q wave indicates necrosis, ST elevation indicates injury, and ST depression with T-wave inversion indicates ischemia. Identification of infarct location is associated with lead placement and noted ischemic changes. It is important to note that a normal ECG does not rule out MI since changes may be evidenced over time. Only about half of patients experiencing MI have an initial diagnostic ECG. Therefore, serial ECGs completed at 15- or 30-minute intervals may be a helpful diagnostic tool in evaluating evolving myocardial injury.

- **Coronary angiography** is considered by many to be the gold standard for the evaluation of the coronary arteries. The performance of angiography requires cardiac catheterization, which is an invasive procedure that will also evaluate cardiac pressures, ejection fraction, ventricular function, and the patency of coronary arteries. Angiography allows for visualization of the coronary vasculature to check for narrowing or obstruction. Arterial narrowing greater than 50% is considered to be significant.
- **Myocardial radionuclide imaging** studies such as a myocardial infarct scan and myocardial perfusion heart scan are useful in checking for areas of decreased coronary perfusion and reduced ejection fraction.
- **Positron emission tomography (PET)** scan can check for the presence of irreversible heart muscle damage and evaluate response to treatment.
- **Magnetic resonance imaging (MRI) of the chest** can evaluate for cardiac muscle dysfunction. **Magnetic resonance angiography (MRA)** can assess cardiac perfusion through high-resolution imaging. MRI detects small areas of MI and differentiate between MI and diseases that may mimic an MI such as myocarditis.
- **Echocardiogram** can be used to check for cardiac muscle, thickness, dysfunction, or structural defects. Its strength is in visualization of the heart with assessment of cardiac perfusion and the ability to locate obstruction.
- **Chest x-ray (CXR)** can help to assess for heart failure and other diagnoses such as dissecting aneurysm and pneumothorax. However, CXR cannot determine the age of an infarct and may miss small infarcts.

General/Medical Management

Early Treatment: MONA

Management is focused on early diagnosis and early treatment. The goal of early treatment is to reverse ischemia as soon as possible in order to preserve cardiac muscle function, reduce infarct size, and decrease mortality. Oxygen supply and demand must be addressed first to prevent additional dysrhythmias and progression of the coronary event. Therefore, accomplishing immediate reperfusion is essential by whatever means is available. Common reperfusion strategies are thrombolytics/fibrinolytics or percutaneous coronary intervention (PCI). When a patient presents with a suspected cardiac event, an acronym that is commonly used in the early stages of diagnosis and treatment is MONA:

- **M = Morphine** is used to treat chest pain (2 to 4 mg every 5 minutes until pain is relieved). If hypotension occurs it should be treated with fluid boluses. Morphine decreases myocardial workload and preload.
- **O = Oxygen** is essential to reduce hypoxia (keep saturation greater than 90%). This is a standard treatment for all MI patients especially during the first 3 hours. Oxygen should be titrated to maintain adequate saturation. Oxygen administration supports cardiac function by treating hypoxia.
- **N = Nitrates** are used to improve peripheral, coronary, and venous vasodilation and decrease preload. Nitroglycerin is used to dilate peripheral vessels, relax vascular smooth muscle, and decrease preload. Nitrates are recommended for use during the first 24 hours unless there is hypotension and systolic BP is less than 90 mm Hg, or there is persistent severe bradycardia. Hypotension can be treated by elevating the legs and administering fluids. The administered dose of nitroglycerin (NTG) is usually 0.4 mg SL every 5 minutes for three doses. If IV NTG is used, a recommended dose is 10 to 20 mcg/min, titrated up by 5 mcg to 10 mcg every 5 to 10 minutes to assist in controlling ischemia. Vigilant BP monitoring will be necessary when IV NTG is being administered.
- **A = Aspirin** (ASA) is used for platelet aggregation. A dose of 160 to 325 mg chewed has been shown to reduce mortality rates. If the patient is nauseated and unable to take ASA orally, a suppository may be used.

Thrombolytic and Fibrinolytic Therapies

Thrombolytic/fibrinolytic agents are used to assist in reestablishing blood flow to coronary vessels by dissolving clots. Recommended drugs to accomplish this are tissue plasma activators (tPAs) such as streptokinase, reteplase, and alteplase. Criteria for administration of a thrombolytic is ST elevation greater than 0.1 mV in two or more contiguous leads, bundle branch block, and acute coronary syndrome in patients seen less than 12 hours after the initial onset of symptoms. Ideally, thrombolytic should be administered with a door-to-drug time of 30 minutes. Hypertension should be controlled before thrombolytic use to prevent hemorrhagic stroke risk. Screening of contraindications is necessary and includes sinus bradycardia, second- or third-degree heart block, and accelerated idioventricular rhythm, stroke within the previous year, active bleeding, suspected aortic dissection, streptokinase within the previous 2 years, current anticoagulant use, or severe uncontrolled hypertension (greater than 180/110 mm Hg).

Anticoagulants such as unfractionated heparin or low molecular weight heparin prevent conversion of fibrinogen to fibrin and can be used in patients who are not receiving thrombolytic therapy. Anticoagulants have been shown to decrease the death rates. Laboratory tests to be monitored are activated partial thromboplastin time (aPTT), hemogram for hemoglobin (Hgb) and hematocrit (Hct), and platelet count. One recommendation for initial IV heparin is a bolus of 60 units/kg, followed by a continuous infusion of 12 units/kg/hr adjusted to keep the patient's aPTT between 1.5 and 2 times the patient's baseline.

Platelet glycoprotein IIb and IIIa inhibitors (abciximab, eptifibatide, and tirofiban) are used to prevent platelet aggregation and fibrinogen binding. Note that with this class of medications there is a chance of bleeding risk, so Hgb, Hct, and platelet count should be monitored daily. Glycoprotein IIb and IIIa can decrease risk of death but are contraindicated for concurrent use with thrombolytics.

Beta Blockers

Beta-adrenergic blockers are used (atenolol, metoprolol) to reduce cardiac contractility, cardiac output, and heart rate. This drug may decrease the rate of reocclusion in patients taking a thrombolytic and may reduce the size of the infarct in patients who are not taking thrombolytic if started within the first few hours after a coronary event.

ACE Inhibitors

Angiotensin-converting enzyme (ACE) inhibitors such as captopril are used to decrease endothelial dysfunction and prevent angiotensin conversion. The general recommendation is to start ACE inhibitors within 24 hours after thrombolytic therapy is completed and hypertension is managed.

Calcium Channel Blockers

Calcium channel blockers are used if beta blockers are ineffective or contraindicated. Some literature states this class of drugs is routinely recommended.

Magnesium and Lidocaine

Magnesium may be used for replacement of low magnesium starting within 6 hours of onset of symptoms, but magnesium use is not routinely recommended. Lidocaine is useful in treating ventricular dysrhythmia and amiodarone can be used to decrease ventricular irritability.

Coronary Interventions

PERCUTANEOUS CORONARY INTERVENTIONS (PCIs): These procedures are used to attempt to open up occluded coronary arteries and restore blood flow and oxygenation. Typically, the results are best if these procedures are completed within 12 hours of initial symptoms or 90 minutes after arrival in the emergency department (ED).

PERCUTANEOUS TRANSLUMINAL CORONARY ANGIOPLASTY (PTCA): There are invasive procedures available to improve coronary perfusion. PTCA is an alternative for reperfusion when thrombolytics are contraindicated, for patients who are high risk, or if the ECG does not show ST-segment elevation. Recommended door-to-needle time for PTCA is 90 minutes. The goal of PTCA is to widen a narrowed coronary artery so that blood flow and oxygenation are improved. This is accomplished by inflating a balloon that is inserted and removed to widen the arterial lumen. This process may need to be completed one or more times to widen the arterial lumen enough to improve blood flow and provide space for possible stent placement.

CORONARY STENTS: These are tubes used in conjunction with PTCA to essentially prop open the arterial wall and keep it open after the balloon is deflated and removed. The goal is to maintain blood flow and oxygenation. Laser angioplasty uses pulsating laser energy to vaporize plaque, thereby reopening occluded arteries.

CORONARY ATHERECTOMY: This technique reopens narrowed arteries by using a directional atherectomy catheter to cut away layers of plaque, restoring blood flow and oxygen.

CORONARY ARTERY BYPASS GRAFT (CABG): This procedure should be performed within 6 hours of MI. CABG is a surgical revascularization that is used to bypass (go around) an occluded coronary artery to supply blood and oxygen to the ischemic part of the heart. Most surgeons use the internal mammary artery or saphenous leg vein for bypass grafts. Daily lab draws may include cardiac markers, electrolytes, and coagulation studies.

Patient Education

Patient education is a very important part of general management of MI. Patients will need information on lifestyle changes such as reducing their cholesterol levels, adhering to a diet low in saturated fats, and strictly managing diabetes, hypertension, and heart failure. Clear explanations of treatment guidelines and the expected results should be provided. Comprehensive education about cardiac disease, when to report signs and symptoms, when to seek treatment, how to take medications, and how to incorporate activity into their lives will be necessary. Treatment for depression should be provided if appropriate.

STEP 2: POTENTIAL PROBLEMS/ DIAGNOSES

It is important that nurses understand and consider the science of the disease process and the possibilities prior to applying that knowledge to a patient situation. We begin that process with questioning.

💬 *Question:* Based upon your review of the content presented, what possible *potential problems* would you expect for a patient with these diagnoses?

💬 *Answer:* Pain, anxiety, fear, bleeding risk, tissue perfusion, activity tolerance, and hemodynamic instability

STEP 3: POTENTIAL INTERVENTIONS AND EXPECTED OUTCOMES

💬 *Question:* Based upon your identification of patient problems, what possible interventions would you recommend for these diagnoses, and what would you expect to happen? This would be considered your "grocery list" of the possible actions you could use to assist your patient.

💬 *Answer:* See the following problems, interventions, and expected outcomes:

Problem	Interventions	Expected Outcome
Fear	• Encourage the patient's verbalization of fears. • Assess coping mechanisms. • Assess the patient's level of fear. • Explain in simple terms the purpose of interventions. • Assist the patient to understand that emotions and feelings are normal. • Provide access to spiritual assistance.	The patient demonstrates situational coping.
Decreased Cardiac Output	• Monitor the patient's heart rate and rhythm. • Monitor ECG changes. • Monitor oxygenation. • Assess for a change in the level of consciousness. • Prepare with a standby pacemaker. • Administer medications as appropriate to the rhythm. • Monitor for changes in blood pressure. • Administer IV fluids as ordered. • Administer diuretics as appropriate. • Educate the patient and family about the purpose of interventions.	The patient maintains adequate coronary output.
Tissue Perfusion	• Monitor for recurrent chest pain. • Monitor for recurrent ischemia. • Administer oxygen. • Explain to the patient possible emergency procedures. • Monitor the patient's extremities for temperature. • Monitor for pallor. • Assess for capillary refill. • Assess for sensorium changes. • Monitor electrolytes. • Prepare for temporary pacing. • Administer antidysrhythmic drugs per protocol. • Provide continuous ECG monitoring.	Tissue perfusion is adequate.
Bleeding	• Monitor for bruising or hematomas. • Monitor for any complaints of back pain related to retroperitoneal bleeding. • Monitor for blood in stool, emesis, or urine. • Coordinate lab draws to minimize punctures. • Monitor INR, PT, and Hgb. • Monitor for changes in mental status.	Bleeding is absent.

Problem	Interventions	Expected Outcome
Activity	<ul><li>Provide a comfortable room temperature.</li><li>Pace activities to include rest periods.</li><li>Explain the importance of limiting activities to help the heart heal.</li><li>Assist with activities.</li><li>Monitor for orthostatic hypotension.</li><li>Encourage restful activities.</li><li>Increase activity gradually while monitoring tolerance.</li><li>Elevate the patient's feet when out of bed to promote venous return.</li><li>Explain how to evaluate the body's response to activity.</li><li>Collaborate to create an individualized activity program.</li></ul>	The patient can tolerate progressive activity.
Hemodynamic Instability	<ul><li>Monitor for hypertension every 2 hours as it increases afterload and oxygen demands.</li><li>Monitor respirations every 2 hours.</li><li>Auscultate the patient's lungs to check for crackles.</li><li>Monitor for dyspnea.</li><li>Check the patient's heart rate every 2 hours.</li><li>Monitor for jugular venous distention.</li><li>Take the patient's temperature every 4 hours.</li><li>Monitor the patient's skin for warmth and color.</li><li>Monitor urine output greater than or equal to 30 mL/hr.</li><li>Monitor for dysrhythmias.</li><li>Monitor laboratory values.</li></ul>	Vital signs are stable, there is adequate urine output, there is no dyspnea, and dysrhythmias are absent.
Anxiety	<ul><li>Assess for hypoperfusion.</li><li>Administer oxygen.</li><li>Administer sedatives if appropriate and explain the reason.</li><li>Assess for side effects from sedative administration.</li><li>Assist in the identification of and use of relaxation techniques that work.</li><li>Consistency of care (same nurse) can assist in decreasing anxiety.</li><li>Explain the reason for admission.</li><li>Explain the reason for equipment and its use.</li><li>Discuss the anticipated plan of care with the patient.</li><li>Discuss visiting hours with the patient.</li><li>Assess for signs of anxiety.</li></ul>	The patient is coping with anxiety.
Pain	<ul><li>Assess for pain intensity, location, and duration.</li><li>Administer oxygen.</li><li>Teach the patient to take deep breaths.</li><li>Administer morphine.</li><li>Provide reassurance.</li><li>Administer nitroglycerin.</li><li>Monitor vital signs.</li><li>Monitor oxygen saturation.</li></ul>	Pain is at a level acceptable to the patient.

PUTTING IT ALL TOGETHER: APPLICATION OF THE NURSING PROCESS

Putting it all together is where the art and science of nursing meet to provide the best patient outcomes. We take the possibilities and place them into the context of the patient situation. To accomplish this we use nursing diagnosis, nursing interventions, nursing outcomes, and nursing theory to provide the palate for nursing care.

STEP 4: ASSESSMENT

PATIENT INFORMATION: Steven Lewis, a 57-year-old Caucasian male

CHIEF COMPLAINT: Chest pain 10/10 described as crushing with shortness of breath

HISTORY OF THE PRESENT ILLNESS: Patient thought he had indigestion after a dinner. When there was no improvement and he started to have some trouble breathing, he had his live-in girlfriend drive him to the ED. Upon arrival at the ED, he started having chest pain and shortness of breath and became anxious and diaphoretic.

PAST MEDICAL HISTORY: Smoker for 40 years, with hypertension and high cholesterol

FAMILY HISTORY: Married, separated from his wife, in a long-term relationship with a live-in girlfriend; has two children with the live-in girlfriend, ages 6 and 8; parents are deceased: father from a heart attack and mother from pneumonia

CHART REVIEW AND REPORT: Arvin James (AJ) receives the following report from the off-going nurse. Steve Lewis arrived in ED about 6 hours ago with crushing chest pain described as a 10/10, shortness of breath, anxiety, and diaphoresis. An ECG was completed in the first 10 minutes on arrival to ED and showed ST-segment elevation. Steve was treated in ED using the MONA acronym. He received morphine 4 mg IVP for pain relief, oxygen 3L NC with an oxygen saturation of 94%, nitroglycerin 0.4 mg times three doses for vasodilatation, and chewable aspirin 325 mg. Cardiac biomarkers, troponin I and CK-MB, were drawn with normal results.

Within 60 minutes of arrival to the ED, Steve was seen by a cardiologist and taken to interventional radiology for a coronary angiogram as a diagnostic tool to assess appropriate reperfusion therapy. During the coronary angiogram the cardiologist found that Steve's left main artery was 90% occluded. The cardiologist decided to insert an intra-aortic balloon pump as a temporary measure to improve coronary perfusion

until Steve could go to surgery. Anticoagulant therapy of a continuous heparin infusion was started, along with a continuous nitroglycerin infusion to promote vasodilation.

After the cardiac catheterization and balloon placement, Steve was transferred to critical care to wait for the CABG scheduled for the morning. Steve arrived post cardiac catheterization with an augmented pressure of 150 mm Hg, a pulse of 58 beats per minute, and a reported ejection fraction of 45%.

Three hours after arrival in critical care Steve became hemodynamically unstable. He complained of crushing, stabbing, chest pain 10/10, became short of breath, and his oxygen saturation dropped to 76% on 3 L NC. As a result, Steve's oxygen delivery is changed to a 100% nonrebreather mask with an improved oxygen saturation of 90%. Steve also became hypotensive with an augmented pressure of 90 mm Hg. His hourly urine dropped from 100 mL/hr to 60 mL/hr of amber urine. As a result of ongoing hemodynamic instability, Steve was taken for an emergency CABG and has just returned.

AJ enters Steve's room and tells the recovery room nurse that she can give you her report. Steve had a four-vessel CABG using the left internal mammary and saphenous vein of the left leg. His heparin infusion was discontinued. He remains on a nitroglycerin drip. His urine output during surgery was less than 30 mL/hr of dark amber urine. A transesophageal echocardiogram (TEE) was completed in surgery with a reported change in ejection fraction to between 35% and 40%. When the anesthesiologist attempted to bring Steve out of the anesthesia, he had a grand mal seizure and as a result was resedated. Computed tomography (CT) of the head was completed in surgery, and it appears that Steve had a stroke on the table during surgery. The cardiologist believes the stroke is related to an air embolism.

SUBJECTIVE ASSESSMENT: Lori, Steve's live-in girlfriend, is at the bedside. AJ was told by the off-going nurse that Steve introduced Lori as the wife of his heart even though they are not legally married. AJ is aware that Lori has been at Steve's bedside since his arrival to the hospital and that prior to surgery Steve and Lori spoke about his wishes if the surgery should "go badly." Steve said that he did not want to live on a machine like a "vegetable." Lori is at the bedside, appearing tearful but stoic. She says, "He knew he wasn't going to make it, he doesn't want to live on a machine, we both told the last nurse what we want." AJ replies, *"Sara, your last nurse, told me that she was in the room with you both before Steve went for surgery and that he was clear about his wishes."* "Yes," Lori continues, "we agreed years ago that we would protect each other from living a hopeless vegetative life, and from what I just have been told it sounds pretty hopeless."

OBJECTIVE ASSESSMENT: Steve's general appearance is pale and nonresponsive due to sedation. He does not appear to be in any pain. Airway is supported by mechanical ventilation with 100% oxygen, and a saturation of 92%. There are two chest tubes in place, one mid-sternum and one left lateral chest with a total of 250 mL of bloody drainage. Foley catheter is in place with 45 mL of dark amber urine. Vital signs are BP 90/50 mm Hg, heart rate 56 beats per minute, skin is cool to touch, peripheral pulses are weak with the Doppler bilaterally, and capillary refill is less than 3 seconds. Breath sounds are coarse, and bowel sounds are absent.

- *Preoperative Laboratory Studies:*
  - CK-MB is 64 ng/mL
  - Troponin I is 12.6 ng/mL
- *Diagnostic Studies:*
  - CT scan of the head shows extensive damage possibly from an air embolism.
  - EEG confirms minimal electrical brain activity.
- *Medications:*
  - Nitroglycerin IV infusion of 20 mcg/min
  - Dopamine 5 mc/kg/min to support blood pressure
  - Midazolam 3 mg/hr titrated to keep sedated

STEP 5: REALITY CHECK: DETOUR AHEAD

Reality Check occurs when the nurse takes a moment to think about individualized patient information that needs to be considered in framing diagnoses and interventions. This information is retrievable from any legitimate source (e.g., family, case management, other nurses, any ancillary, a doctor, etc.). These are the "wrenches" that create challenging situations, such as culture, religion, socioeconomic status, level of education, developmental level, marital status, employment, age, and gender.

Psychosocial History

Steve has been working as a Web-based pastry chef. His plan was to eventually open his own bakery. Currently he has been earning about $50,000 a year. He is a high school graduate who is self-taught in pastry arts since he was unable to afford culinary school.

Steve has been legally married for 30 years. He has been separated from his wife Jennifer for the last 15 years due to irreconcilable differences. Steve has been living with his girlfriend Lori as husband and wife for the past 10 years even though they are not legally married. The separation between Steve and Jennifer was bitter, and there were no children from the marriage. Steve felt that Jennifer was not really interested in marriage, instead putting all of her energy into getting ahead in her career and refusing to have children. Steve and Lori have two children

ages 6 and 8 years and are active in their local Christian church. Steve often donates pastry goods for fundraisers.

Jennifer resents Lori for taking her place in Steve's life. Steve and Lori have been talking lately about finally getting a divorce so that they can be legally married. Jennifer has always blocked any divorce attempts in the hope that she and Steve can reconcile. Steve has had no intention of reconciling with Jennifer but has not pursued a divorce because of the cost of a lengthy court battle. Coincidentally, Lori and Steve had a recent discussion about what the other would want in the event of a catastrophic occurrence and decided that neither would seek life support measures if there was medical agreement that those measures would only prolong death. In accordance with this conversation and the results of the CT scan of the head, EEG results, and neurology consult, a do not resuscitate (DNR) order is created for Steve.

Steve's estranged wife Jennifer arrived at the hospital this morning after hearing from a friend that Steve had suffered a heart attack. Jennifer insisted on speaking with the attending physician and told him that she wants Steve to be made a full "code" (that is, resuscitation efforts should be performed, as compared with an order not to resuscitate). The physicians explain Steve's poor prognosis, but Jennifer refuses to listen. She tells the physician that she loves her husband even though they have been separated for the last 15 years and does not want him to die before they have a chance to reconcile their differences. Jennifer also threatens to sue both the hospital and physicians if they do not do as she has requested. Lori is devastated by this turn of events and requests the physicians do something to honor Steve's request. The physicians made Steve a full "code."

Critical Thinking Moment

You just completed the assessment of Steve Lewis and need to make a decision about the patient's *actual* problems and nursing diagnoses based upon the data you collected and the potential problems you identified. Outcomes must be realistic and measurable.

STEP 6: ACTUAL PROBLEMS/DIAGNOSES

The *first step* in problem identification is to revisit the list of *potential diagnoses* and choose *actual diagnoses* based upon the learner's evaluation of the case study information provided. A problem statement must be completed for each identified problem/diagnosis. The actual problems for this case study are cardiac output, tissue perfusion, and a dysfunctional family.

STEP 7: PLANNING: ACTUAL INTERVENTIONS

After actual diagnoses have been chosen, it is necessary to evaluate the list of *potential interventions* and choose *actual interventions* that will fit within the patient's reality and meet expected outcomes. Each intervention requires a rationale. Interventions are identified in three categories: (1) assessment, (2) therapeutic, and (3) education.

Diagnostic Statement

Decreased cardiac output related to electrical instability secondary to ischemia and cardiac muscle necrosis as evidenced by hypotension, an irregular heart rate of 46 beats per minute, and an ejection fraction of 35%.

Assessment

- Assess for hypotension. *Rationale: This allows you to check for hemodynamic stability.*
- Assess for oxygenation. *Rationale: Hypoxia may become evident with altered cardiac output.*
- Assess and monitor the heart rate and rhythm. *Rationale: This allows you to evaluate for changes in cardiac stability.*

Therapeutic Interventions

- Assess vital signs every 15 minutes. *Rationale: This allows you to note hemodynamic trends.*
- Auscultate breath sounds every 4 hours. *Rationale: This allows you to evaluate early symptoms of heart failure, such as crackles in the bases.*
- Monitor and record the chest tube output hourly. *Rationale: This allows you to evaluate Hgb and Hct in relation to blood loss.*

Education

- For the family, to understand the purpose of hemodynamic monitoring. *Rationale: Understanding of the purpose can decrease anxiety.*
- For the family, to understand the purpose of keeping a temporary pacemaker kit at the bedside. *Rationale: This provides for cardiac support, if needed.*
- For the family, to recognize the symptoms of poor cardiac perfusion. *Rationale: This allows the family to act as partners in recognizing and reporting concerns.*

Expected Outcome

- The best possible cardiac rhythm and ejection fraction is maintained or improved.

Diagnostic Statement

Insufficient tissue perfusion related to impaired cardiac function as evidenced by cool skin, pallor, weak peripheral pulses, and capillary refill greater than 3 seconds.

Assessment

- Assess capillary refill. *Rationale: This allows you to evaluate for adequate perfusion.*
- Assess peripheral pulses. *Rationale: This allows you to evaluate for adequate perfusion.*
- Assess for trends in vital signs. *Rationale: This may show an indication of altered cardiac status.*

Therapeutic Interventions

- Continuous ECG monitoring: Monitor cardiac rhythms and treat. *Rationale: This allows for the timely identification and treatment of dysrhythmias.*
- Administer antidysrhythmic drugs per critical care protocol. *Rationale: Protocols allow for immediate interventions that can improve perfusion outcomes.*
- Administer oxygen to keep saturation greater than 93%. *Rationale: Oxygen administration can support improved perfusion by decreasing the cardiac workload.*

Education

- For the family, to understand the purpose of oxygen administration. *Rationale: Understanding the purpose can decrease anxiety and promote cooperation.*
- For the family, to understand the pathophysiology behind poor perfusion. *Rationale: Understanding can improve cooperation with the plan of care.*
- For the family, to understand signs and symptoms to report to the nurse. *Rationale: Understanding will allow for recognition and reporting of future events.*

Expected Outcome

- Improved tissue perfusion

Diagnostic Statement

Impaired family function related to the denial of clinical events as evidenced by refusal of the estranged wife to accept a DNR status, unresolved conflict between the patient and his estranged wife, and conflict between the estranged wife and the live-in girlfriend secondary to clinical decision making.

Assessment

- Assess for areas of conflict. *Rationale: This allows you to better understand the situation and create an effective plan of care.*
- Assess for spiritual support. *Rationale: This assists with end-of-life issues.*
- Assess for coping mechanisms. *Rationale: This assists Lori in supporting the patient's health-care decisions.*

Therapeutic Interventions

- Arrange a family conference to discuss patient prognosis. *Rationale: This provides family members with information for appropriate decision making.*

- Arrange for social services to meet with family members. *Rationale: This assists in the identification and resolution of conflict.*
- Facilitate spiritual support. *Rationale: This provides a framework for making end-of-life decisions.*

Education

- Patient prognosis. *Rationale: This assists Jennifer and Lori in understanding the clinical picture.*
- Options in relation to prognosis. *Rationale: This helps the family support Steve's health-care decisions.*
- Palliative care options. *Rationale: This assists Steve to have a good death.*

Expected Outcome

- Lori and Jennifer will agree on a plan of care for Steve in line with clinical realities.

STEP 8: IMPLEMENTATION

Nursing Theory

Steve had a stroke during the CABG that left him in a persistent vegetative state. This is a devastating outcome for his family. In addition, Lori and Jennifer are at odds on how to proceed from this point. Nursing theory needs to support the reality of the medical prognosis that Steve's life is at risk and that whatever happens, he will never fully recover. Although Steve will be given all of the medical support available, he cannot interact on an interpersonal level. The focus now shifts from Steve to the family and how to support them while advocating for Steve regarding his end-of-life wishes. In their theory of caring, Anne Boykin and Savina Schoenhofer explain that to influence outcomes, nurses need to make a personal connection with the patient or family. This caring connection can allow the nurse and family to discover the best way of helping and nurturing. Each caring connection will be unique and beneficial to those involved. Focus is on the patient, not on the task, in an artistic application of nursing. Although in this case Steve is not able to participate in creating this relationship, AJ will have the challenge of attempting to do so with both Lori and Jennifer. The level of caring and appropriateness will need to be integrated with the situation's ethical issues.

Ancillary Support

Case management and social services should be contacted, and a family meeting should be arranged with the physicians to discuss prognoses in relation to code status. The meeting would include both Lori, Jennifer, and the nurses who have cared for Steve and been party to the end-of-life discussions. Respiratory therapy will support oxygenation and ventilation until some decision is made.

STEP 9: PLAN OF CARE

The plan of care is a road map for patient care and should be used as a communication tool between disciplines. Expected entries on the plan of care would be each identified problem, intervention, and expected outcome, including any information from ancillary support. Individualized care for Steve should focus on what keeps him comfortable during the dying process. This may include pain management, supportive oxygenation, or music. A discussion with Lori regarding what he likes would be helpful.

STEP 10: EVALUATION

Evaluation is an active process in which the nurse "connects the dots" to decide if the expected outcomes (goals) that were established have been met, partially met, or not met. If the goals are met, we continue with the plan as outlined. If the goal was partially met, we revise the parts of the plan that did not work. If the goals were not met, we start all over with a new plan.

End-of-Shift Narrative

Lori remained at Steve's bedside; Jennifer was there sporadically. Lori attempted to approach Jennifer regarding Steve's wishes about end-of-life matters; Jennifer simply walked out of the room. Steve's perfusion status has worsened; he did not awaken when attempting to wean him off of the midazolam. He occasionally has runs of tachycardia. Currently his extremities are cold bilaterally, nail beds are dusky, and legs are mottled to mid-calf. Steve is very pale and his oxygen saturation dropped to 86% on 100% oxygen. There has been no urinary output for the last 2 hours. An hour ago Steve coded, and full resuscitation efforts were made. Steve remains on full ventilator support with medications to assist in maintaining hemodynamic stability. When Steve coded, Jennifer became hysterical and started screaming at the nurses to "fix him!" Jennifer initially refused to leave the room during the code but was escorted out by the chaplain. Lori attempted to talk to Jennifer again, but she refuses to speak with anyone.

The family conference was held with both Jennifer and Lori in attendance. The nurse who was in the room for the conversation between Lori and Steve regarding his wish to not be resuscitated (DNR) was present and relayed what Steve said to Jennifer. The cardiologist and neurologist explained in simple terms that Steve's cardiac status was unstable and that he was in a persistent vegetative state due to the significant brain damage from the stroke. Lori asked Jennifer to remove her objection to making Steve a DNR. Jennifer continued adamantly to refuse. After much discussion among all parties, clinical leadership decided to take this case to the Ethics Committee for discussion and review. Currently Steve is on ventilator support and remains in a persistent vegetative state.

Problem Evaluation

PROBLEM 1: Cardiac Output. The expected outcome is that sinus rhythm is maintained. The goal is not met: Steve has been having runs of tachycardia with poor perfusion. Revised plan: Continue to discuss revised code status with family, and encourage palliative care.

PROBLEM 2: Tissue Perfusion. The expected outcome is improved tissue perfusion. The goal is not met: Steve has mottling of the lower extremities, all extremities are cold, his nail beds are dusky, oxygenation has decreased to 86%, peripheral pulses are absent, and capillary refill remains greater than 3 seconds. Revised plan: Continue to discuss revised code status with the family, and encourage palliative care.

PROBLEM 3: Family Dysfunction. The expected outcome is that the family will agree on a plan of care in line with clinical realities. The goal is not met: Lori wants to honor Steve's wishes; Jennifer does not and is threatening to sue anyone who tries to make him a DNR. Revised plan: DNR to be discussed in the Ethics Committee. The neurologist has recommended a cerebral angiogram to confirm brain dysfunction.

Overall Evaluation

In comparing Steve's current overall health status against his morning assessment, Steve is declining.

REFERENCES

Alcola, N., & Shapiro, S. (2000, September). Less than common acute MI symptoms. American Journal of Nursing, 100(9), 5–7.

Beers, M., Porter, R., Jones, T., Kaplan, J., & Berkwits, M. (Eds.). (2006). Cardiovascular tests and procedures. The MERCK Manual (18th ed., pp. 589–604). Whitehouse Station, NJ: Merck Research Laboratories.

Corona, G. (2005). Is my patient having an acute MI. Nursing 2005, 35(6), 32–35.

George, J. (2011). Nursing theories. The base for professional nursing practice (6th ed.). Upper Saddle River, NJ: Pearson Education.

Goldrich, G. (2005, September). Myocardial infarction: Getting in line with the new guidelines. Nursing 2005, 35(9), 32–39.

Gulanick, M., & Meyers J., (2013). Nursing care plans nursing diagnosis and intervention (8th ed.). St. Louis, MO: Mosby.

Holloway, N. (2004). Medical surgical nursing care planning (4th ed.). Springhouse, PA: Lippincott, Williams & Wilkins.

Kirwar, M. (2009, January/February). An eye for MI. Nursing Made Incredibly Easy, 7(1), 5–10.

LeMone, P., Burke, K., & Baldoff, G. (2011). Medical surgical nursing, Critical thinking in patient care (5th ed.). Upper Saddle River, NJ: Pearson.

Moore, J., & Wilson, M. (2010, September). Treatment of acute MI emergencies in a community hospital setting. American Journal of Nursing, 110(9), 15–19.

Nagle, B., & Nee, C. (2002). Recognizing and responding to acute myocardial infarction. Nursing 2002 , 32(10), 50–54.

Overbaugh, K. (2009, May). Acute coronary syndrome. American Journal of Nursing, 109(5), 42–52.

Pagana, K., & Pagana, T. (2010). Mosby's manual of diagnostic and laboratory tests (4th ed.). St Louis, MO: Elsevier.

Parker, M.E. (2006). Nursing theories and nursing practice (2nd ed.). Philadelphia, PA: F.A. Davis.

Rodgers, S. (2008). Medical surgical nursing care plans. Clifton Park, NY: Thomson Delmar.

Thygesen, K., Alpert, J.S., Jaffe, A.S., Simoons, M.L., Chaitman, B.R., & White, H.D. (2012). Third universal definition of myocardial infarction. Retrieved from http://circ.ahajournals.org/content/126/16/2020.full

Van Leeuwen, A., & Bladh, M. (2015). Davis's comprehensive handbook of laboratory and diagnostic testing with nursing implications (6th ed.). Philadelphia, PA: F.A. Davis Company.

Wilansky, S., Moreno, C., & Lester, S. (2007). Complications of MI. Critical Care Medicine, 35(8), 348–354.

Wilkinson, J., & Ahern, N. (2009). In Nursing Diagnosis Handbook (9th ed.). Upper Saddle River, NJ: Prentice Hall.

Wilson, B., Shannon, M., & Stang, C. (2006). Nurses drug guide. Upper Saddle River, NJ: Prentice Hall.

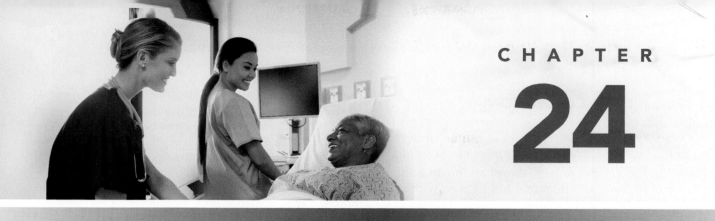

Endocrine System

Case Study: Osteoporosis

Common Nursing Study Name	Section 1 Study	Section 1 Chapter Number
Alkaline phosphatase	Alkaline phosphatase and isoenzymes	Chapter 1
Bone mineral densitometry (BMD)	Bone mineral densitometry	Chapter 16
Calcium	Calcium, blood	Chapter 1
Chest x-ray	Chest x-ray	Chapter 16
Complete blood count (CBC)	Complete blood count, hematocrit	Chapter 2
	Complete blood count, hemoglobin	Chapter 2
	Complete blood count, platelet count	Chapter 3
	Complete blood count, RBC count	Chapter 2
	Complete blood count, RBC indices	Chapter 2
	Complete blood count, RBC morphology and inclusions	Chapter 2
	Complete blood count, WBC count and differential	Chapter 2
Electrolytes	Carbon dioxide	Chapter 1
	Chloride, blood	Chapter 1
	Potassium, blood	Chapter 1
	Sodium, blood	Chapter 1
Free thyroxine (FT4)	Thyroxine, free	Chapter 1
Parathyroid hormone	Parathyroid hormone	Chapter 1
Testosterone	Testosterone, total	Chapter 1
Thyroid-stimulating hormone (TSH)	Thyroid-stimulating hormone	Chapter 1
Vertebroplasty	Vertebroplasty	Chapter 16
Vitamin D	Vitamin D	Chapter 1

STEP 1: DATA COLLECTION

Pathophysiology

Bones are the structural foundation of the body, supporting and protecting organs. Bones are made from a mixture of collagen and minerals, interwoven with calcium, phosphorus, and glycosaminoglycan to hold everything together.

There are two types of bone tissue: trabecular and cortical bone. Trabecular bone is the spongy porous inside found mostly at the ends of long bones. Cortical bone is the hard compact outer part of the bone. Bone is made out of osteoprogenitor cells called osteoblasts, osteocytes, and osteoclasts. Each bone cell has a different function.

Osteoblasts secrete osteocalcin, osteonectin, and thrombospondin collagen proteins that create both trabecular and cortical bone tissue. Bone health is regulated through a process of osteoblast bone formation and osteoclast bone resorption. During growth, new bone forms faster than old bone is broken down and reabsorbed. This continues until peak bone mass is reached. Eventually, the rate of bone replacement occurs almost concurrently with bone resorption.

Calcium balance is maintained by hormones secreted by the thyroid and parathyroid. Parathyroid hormone speeds up bone breakdown when calcium is needed. In contrast, the thyroid gland secretes calcitonin to block parathyroid hormone and conserve calcium in the bones. Calcium absorbed from the digestive system is deposited in the bones. This is a normal process used to replace weaker bone with stronger bone while balancing calcium levels in the blood.

New bone is created by cells called *osteocytes*. Osteocytes are mature osteoblasts that live inside the bone matrix. Their function is to control the level of calcium and phosphorus embedded in the bone's collagen fibers.

Osteoclasts are cells that control bone resorption and are thought to come from stem cells in the bone marrow. These cells eat old bone, releasing calcium and phosphorus into the blood as part of the remodeling process.

Osteoporosis occurs when bone resorption occurs faster than bone formation, creating porous bones with less mass. Osteoclast activity in women is increased from estrogen loss due to menopause. Men lose bone at a lesser degree with a decrease in testosterone levels. These gender-related hormone losses are why osteoporosis is associated with estrogen loss in postmenopausal women and testosterone loss in men. Osteoporosis is also associated with the natural aging that results in reduced bone production. Initially, as aging begins, women and men lose a similar amount of cortical bone.

Menopause changes everything. With the loss of estrogen, women begin to lose cortical bone twice as fast as men. Women also lose more than half of their trabecular bone by the age of 80.

Osteoporosis literally means "porous bones" and is called the *silent thief* because until damage occurs, symptoms are either absent or so vague as to be indiscernible. A way to visualize how osteoporosis changes bone structure is to imagine a solid outer layer of bone filled with a honeycomb design. This is the design of a strong bone. Osteoporosis thins the outer bone and makes the holes in the honeycomb larger. Porous bones are more fragile, have a lower bone mass, and are more susceptible to fractures that occur from nontraumatic causes such as sneezing. Fractures from estrogen loss happen more in the trabecular bone of the vertebrae, forearm, or wrist. Those fractures from normal aging are seen in trabecular or cortical bone like the femur.

Risk Factors

Gender is the biggest risk factor. Women have the highest risk from less overall bone mass and increased bone loss after menopause. Men have a greater bone mass than women, placing them less at risk. Other risk factors include being small-boned, thin, or of white or Asian ethnicity; an immediate family history of osteoporosis; menopause or ovary removal prior to the age of 45; smoking; two or more alcoholic drinks a day; a lack of exercise; prior fracture; steroid use for more than 3 months; low calcium intake; vitamin D deficiency; high caffeine intake; smoking; immobility; and a low testosterone level.

The greater the number of risk factors, the greater the risk of fracture associated with osteoporosis. Some medications can increase osteoporosis risk. Steroids cause the greatest amount of damage. Other medications that may increase risk are protease inhibitors, aromatase inhibitors, some serotonin uptake inhibitors, prolactin-raising antiepileptic inhibitors, heparin, warfarin, thyroid hormone, cyclosporine, glucocorticoids, and some chemotherapy drugs.

Osteoporosis can also be attributed to other disease process. Some of these contributing diseases include idiopathic hypercalciuria, cystic fibrosis, calcium and vitamin D malabsorption, anorexia nervosa, estrogen or testosterone deficiency, excess thyroid hormone, Cushing syndrome, celiac disease, Crohn disease, ulcerative colitis, cirrhosis, hepatitis, lupus, rheumatoid arthritis, and aseptic necrosis.

Signs and Symptoms

Osteoporosis can occur without symptoms, making it difficult to know if the bones are becoming weaker. Symptoms do not appear until a significant amount of bone mass has been lost. Indicators of osteoporosis are a gradual shortening of height and bone fracture with pain.

Kyphosis

Kyphosis, which is the development of a stooped back, is a visual indicator of osteoporosis. Kyphosis is caused from the loss of trabecular bone in the spine. The result is vertebral collapse with shortening stature, which causes the spine to bend forward. Kyphosis can become so extreme that patients become bent over, with the lower ribs resting on the pelvis. Severe curvature can decrease lung expansion, interfere with oxygenation, cause difficulty breathing, contribute to lung infections, and result in a protruding abdomen with gastrointestinal problems. The awkwardness of the spine's position can cause pain that interferes with activities of daily living.

Fracture

Fracture can be the first nonvisual indicator of osteoporosis. Fracture risk increases after the age of 65. Some fractures will occur from falls associated with muscle weakness, imbalance, visual deficits, and agitation. Home environmental factors such as loose rugs, poor light, slippery surfaces, obstacles, or a lack of assistive devices can also increase the fall risk.

Vertebral fractures in the mid-thoracic or thoracic area can occur without injury. Many vertebral fractures are asymptomatic and are often misdiagnosed as back strain with chronic pain.

Hip fractures from osteoporosis are serious because of the inactivity associated with healing. Inactivity can lead to pneumonia, embolism, decubitus ulcers, depression, malnutrition, and urinary tract infections. Functional loss has severe psychosocial ramifications for the elderly in relation to independent living. Affected areas are mobility associated with activities such as grocery shopping, and housekeeping. A fear of falling and sustaining another serious injury is a concern for this age group.

Depression

Depression associated with physical limitations is a possibility. Altered body images cause people to feel like strangers to their own skin. Shrunken height, or chronic or acute pain associated with fracture, and deficits in activities of daily living can lead to social isolation and depression.

Laboratory Studies

Laboratory studies are not used to diagnose osteoporosis. However, there are studies that can act as indicators of risk. Calcium is normally 8.2 to 10.2 mg/dL.

Calcium levels are usually normal with osteoporosis but may be elevated with other bone diseases. Vitamin D 25-hydroxy and vitamin D 1,25-dihydroxy are laboratory studies that are used to check vitamin D levels. The vitamin D 25-hydroxy level is considered deficient when less than 20 ng/mL, insufficient when between 20 and 30 ng/mL, and optimal when between 30 and 100 ng/mL. The normal range for vitamin D 1,25-dihydroxy is 18 to 72 pg/mL. Vitamin D 25-hydroxy is the major circulating form of vitamin D, while vitamin D 1,25-dihydroxy is the more biologically active form. Vitamin D is necessary to absorb calcium. Some recommend repeat testing every 3 months to assess the effectiveness of supplement therapy.

Thyroid tests are used to rule out hypothyroidism which can increase bone resorption. The sensitive or third-generation thyroid-stimulating hormone (TSH) test is useful in the evaluation of hypothyroidism. A normal TSH varies by age. For adults ages 20 years and older, a normal TSH is 0.4 to 4.2 micro-international units/mL. The free thyroxine (FT4) test is used to follow up on an abnormal or borderline TSH level. A normal FT4 for adults is 0.8 to 1.5 ng/dL. Parathyroid hormone is used to check for hyperparathyroidism as the parathyroid hormone regulates calcium resorption. A normal result is 10 to 65 pg/mL. Testosterone, total levels that are low can contribute to osteoporosis in men. A normal result for an adult female is 15 to 70 ng/dL. An alkaline phosphatase level that is elevated can indicate a problem with the bones. A normal level for women 21 years and older is 25 to 125 units/L.

Diagnostic Studies

Unlike laboratory studies, there are diagnostic studies that can be used to identify and assess osteoporosis. Bone mineral densitometry (BMD) is a painless, noninvasive examination that uses low-level radiation and is considered to be the gold standard for diagnosis of osteoporosis. BMD evaluates the amount of bone mineral content and density in a specific area of bone. Bone strength is dependent upon bone mineral density. Women over the age of 65 and men over the age of 70 should have a bone density evaluation. Postmenopausal women with a history of fracture, any disease that may cause bone loss such as rheumatoid arthritis, or individuals taking medication related to bone loss such as steroids, should have a BMD evaluation. Bone density results are reported in terms of standard deviation and associated T-score. A normal bone mass finding would be a T-score value not less than −1. A T-score value of −2.5 is indicative of osteoporosis. The most common type of BMD test is called the dual-energy x-ray absorptiometry (DEXA). DEXA uses two x-rays of different energies to measure bone mineral density. DEXA is valuable as a tool to identify bone density prior to a fracture, predict fracture risk, confirm a diagnosis of osteoporosis once a fracture occurs, and evaluate the effectiveness of osteoporosis treatment. The lower the bone density, the greater is the risk for fracture. Densitometry of the heel or wrist can also be evaluated by ultrasound. This is less expensive than DEXA, but the quality of the results may not be as precise. Chest x-ray is a valuable tool for visualization of fractures or kyphosis related to osteoporosis but is not a tool that is useful in diagnosing osteoporosis because bone mineral density depletion is not picked up until there has been about a 30% loss.

General/Medical Management

The management of osteoporosis begins with a good assessment with history and physical. Postmenopausal women should be assessed for fall risk with an evaluation of balance, gait, and muscle strength. Fall risk factors that should be evaluated are the home environment and participation in high-risk activities.

In individuals with osteoporosis, the early detection of vertebral fractures can help to prevent further disability. The measurement of height is an easy way to screen for fracture risk. During office visits, height should be measured to catch shrinking. Women who have lost more than 2.5 inches in height should have BMD testing to rule out fracture. Once 3 inches in height has been lost, the risk of fracture can increase to more than 150%.

Prevention: Dietary Support

Prevention is the best treatment for osteoporosis. Once a fracture has occurred, it is too late to implement the best strategies. Stopping or slowing bone loss is the focus of osteoporosis management. Calcium and vitamin D supplements can assist in preventing osteoporosis.

Dietary calcium is the only source of natural calcium outside of the body. Calcium intake can decrease osteoporosis risk by maximizing bone strength. The recommended dietary intake of calcium is based on age. For men and women ages 31 to 50 years, the recommended intake is 800 mg/day, for men and women ages 51 to 70, the recommended daily intake is 1000 mg/day. The body will regulate calcium levels by increasing intestinal absorption when levels are too low and excreting excess calcium through the kidneys when levels are too high. When calcium is needed but is not available, the body will take calcium from the bones. Vitamin D is necessary for the absorption of calcium.

Foods high in calcium and vitamin D should be included in the diet. Examples of foods rich in calcium and vitamin D are yogurt, cheese, cottage cheese, canned sardines with bones, flounder, salmon, dried figs, and dark green leafy vegetables such as spinach. Processed foods with added calcium, such as breads and cereals, can also be included. Avoiding red meat and high-fat foods that bind calcium in the intestine can reduce loss. The excess use of alcohol, salt, or caffeine can also decrease absorption.

Calcium and vitamin D supplements may be used if dietary intake is insufficient. The recommended calcium supplement dose is based on age and gender. Women ages 51 to 70 years of age should take 1,200 mg daily and men of the same age range should take 1,000 mg daily. Men and women older than age 71 should take 1,200 mg daily. The types of calcium supplements are calcium carbonate and calcium citrate. Calcium carbonate is best taken with food to help prevent gas or constipation. Calcium citrate can be taken with or without food. Calcium should be taken in divided doses because the body will only absorb 500 mg at a time. Calcium supplements should be used to make up the difference between the consumption of calcium-rich foods and the body's calcium needs. Adequate calcium consumption can retard bone loss and improve bone mass in women with low estrogen. Iron or other medications that need to be taken on an empty stomach can interfere with absorption.

The recommended dietary intake allowance of vitamin D is 600 international units for men and women ages 51 to 70, and 800 international units for men and women 71 years of age and older. A recommendation for vitamin D supplementation is 1,000 international units daily. Vitamin D is necessary to assist in the absorption of calcium. Good dietary sources of vitamin D are oily fish, such as mackerel, and fortified products such as milk, yogurt, orange juice, and breakfast cereals. Exposure to sunlight is necessary for vitamin D production, but the quality of that exposure is limited by weather and other factors. Exposure to sunlight for 5 to 30 minutes twice a week between late morning and early afternoon hours without the use of sunscreen on the face, arms, and back is thought to be sufficient to meet vitamin D synthesis requirements.

Prevention: Medications

In addition to supplemental calcium and vitamin D, there are medications that can be prescribed to assist in treating osteoporosis. Generally, these medications are designed to decrease fracture risk and increase bone density. Bisphosphonates such as risedronate, ibandronate, and alendronate sodium can be used to slow bone remodeling, increase bone density, decrease fracture rates, and suppress osteoclast activity. Side effects of bisphosphonates include heartburn, nausea, stomach and esophageal irritation; bone, joint, or muscle pain; difficulty swallowing; fever; chest pain;

or headache. Antiresorptive medications such as calcitonin salmon can reduce vertebral fracture risk and be used as an off-label analgesic for the reduction of bone pain.

Estrogen and progesterone hormone therapy can reduce bone loss and increase bone density. The lowest effective dose of hormone therapy may be used for women who have moderate-to-severe menopause. Benefits of hormone therapy may fail when the medication is discontinued. The use of hormone therapy does have some risk, including stroke, uterine cancer, heart attack, blood clots, breast cancer, endometrial cancer, vaginal bleeding, breast tenderness, and gallbladder disease. Estrogen agonists or an estrogen receptor modulator such as raloxifene hydrochloride can also decrease vertebral fractures and increase bone mineral density in the hips and spine. Side effects may include hot flashes, leg cramps, blood clots, flu-like symptoms, and ovarian and uterine disease.

Bone-forming medications such as teriparatide can increase the rate of bone formation, reduce fractures, and assist in building bones. Possible side effects include leg cramps, dizziness, and increased urine and serum calcium.

Prevention: Lifestyle Choices

There are lifestyle choices that can decrease osteoporosis risk. Regular exercise is a choice that can strengthen both bones and muscles. Exercise works by increasing cortical thickness, bone strength, and bone mineral density. The types of exercise that are thought to have an impact on osteoporosis are weight-bearing exercises such as running, walking, and weightlifting. Weight-bearing resistance exercise is most beneficial if done three to four times a week. Exercise can also improve balance, which decreases fall risk. Structured physical therapy programs may be beneficial in understanding proper body mechanics and safe lifting practices.

Smoking is a lifestyle choice that has been found to decrease estrogen levels, may be associated with early menopause, and may increase bone loss and fracture risk. Alcohol consumption has been linked with fracture risk, so the recommendation is to limit its use. Alcohol does have a negative effect on the liver, which helps convert vitamin D to a usable form. Caffeine from soft drinks, coffee, and tea has been linked with wasting calcium in the body.

Environment modification can decrease fall risk, thereby decreasing fracture risk. Strategies include keeping the room temperature at 65°F to prevent drowsiness, getting up slowly to prevent orthostatic hypotension, strategically placing lights to prevent tripping, keeping walking spaces free of clutter, avoiding throw rugs, and installing hand rails in bathrooms and hallways.

Pain Relief

The primary treatment for vertebral fractures is pain relief. Acute pain can be treated with opioids and chronic pain with nonsteroidal anti-inflammatory drugs (NSAIDs). Physiotherapy and calcitonin may also be beneficial. Surgery is rarely used unless the back pain is intractable.

Surgery

Surgical options are vertebroplasty or kyphoplasty, in which cement is injected into the fractured vertebra. Kyphoplasty has the added benefit of restoring height and decreasing kyphosis by inflating a balloon to expand the vertebral space prior to cement injection. Both have been able to decrease pain and improve functionality.

Hip fractures contribute to early death more than any other kind of fracture. Hip fracture occurs most often from a sideways fall. The preferred treatment of hip fracture is surgical repair. The type of surgical approach is dependent on the severity of fracture and physician preference. Rehabilitation after surgery is necessary.

Patient Education

Independent living is the cornerstone of a person's self-concept. The loss of independence due to a chronic debilitating disease such as osteoporosis can be devastating. The emotional impact regarding a change in independent living may cause education challenges. As the educator, the goal is to provide information clearly and consistently in a manner that is appropriate to age and culture. It is difficult to do that when the patient is in denial about the existence of her or his limitations. Try to begin by asking the patient what is most important to her or him. Then take that information and frame the education on how you and the patient will work together to help to adapt her or his current reality to keep what is most important to the patient in whatever form is possible with what assistance is needed.

STEP 2: POTENTIAL PROBLEM/ DIAGNOSES

It is important that nurses understand and consider the science of the disease process and the possibilities prior to applying that knowledge to a patient situation. We begin that process with questioning.

Question: Based upon your review of the content about asthma, what *possible problems* would you expect for a patient with this diagnosis?

Answer: Knowledge, mobility, nutrition, pain, body image, and injury

STEP 3: POTENTIAL INTERVENTIONS AND EXPECTED OUTCOMES

💬 *Question:* Based upon your identification of patient problems, what possible interventions would you recommend for these diagnoses, and what would you expect to happen? This would be considered your "grocery list" of the possible actions you could use to assist your patient.

💬 *Answer:* See the following problems, interventions, and expected outcomes:

Problem	Interventions	Expected Outcome
Knowledge	• Teach the importance of taking calcium and vitamin D supplements. • Teach the value of engaging in weight-bearing exercises to build and maintain strong bones. • Assess the patient's eating habits to determine if calcium- and vitamin D–rich foods are being eaten. • Assess the patient's willingness to adhere to osteoporosis treatment modalities. • Explain how changes in diet can assist in lessening the severity of osteoporosis. • Explain how estrogen therapy can assist in decreasing the bone fracture risk associated with osteoporosis. • Encourage smoking cessation as smoking has been associated with the early onset of menopause. • Encourage limiting caffeine intake as it can increase diuresis and calcium loss; encourage limiting alcohol intake as it is associated with altering intestinal calcium resorption. • Assess if any medications are being taken that can interfere with calcium absorption.	Verbalize how factors such as smoking, caffeine use, alcohol use, and inadequate diet can contribute to osteoporosis severity.
Mobility	• Exercise a minimum of three times a week for 30 minutes each day to promote bone growth. • Use assistive devices as necessary to participate in activities of daily living since any activity will promote bone growth. • Teach about fall precautions; assess the home environment for fall risks. • Evaluate medications for contributory causes related to recent falls. • Access physical therapy to facilitate moderate exercise. • Ask what types of activity cause pain and if there is any interference with lifestyle activities. • Observe the patient's ability to move and ambulate. • Reinforce mobility techniques, such as active or passive range of motion. • Assist with ambulation as needed. • Teach that low, comfortable walking shoes can promote safe ambulation. • Teach to avoid activities that could result in fracture.	Maintain optimal physical activity.
Nutrition	• The patient should eat food that will maintain a calcium intake of 1,200 mg a day minimally. • Collaborate with the dietician to design an acceptable high-calcium diet. • Discuss foods that can interfere with calcium maintenance. • Teach the purpose of recommended vitamin D and calcium intake. • Assess the patient's ability to make high-calcium food choices. • Provide sample menus to assist in making beneficial dietary choices. • Teach the importance of sunlight exposure as related to vitamin D deficiency. • Administer calcium and vitamin D supplements.	Verbalize the importance of an appropriate diet in osteoporosis prevention.
Pain	• Suggest modifications in activity that may reduce pain. • Administer anti-inflammatory medications to reduce pain. • Assess pain intensity and characteristics, and assess the patient's response to the administration of pain medication.	Pain should be at a level acceptable to the individual.

Body Image	• Assess the patient's perception of body changes. • Assess the perceived impact of change on social activities, work, and interpersonal relationships. • Acknowledge feelings about physical changes. • Encourage self-care to become comfortable with physical changes. • Reinforce self-care techniques suggested by the occupational therapist. • Encourage participation in support groups.	Decreased anxiety about postural changes.
Injury	• Assess environmental factors that could contribute to fall risks. • Encourage adequate calcium and vitamin D intake (diet and supplement). • Encourage the patient to begin an exercise program to strengthen upper and lower body strength, which decreases fall risks. • Teach the patient to avoid lifting objects heavier than 10 pounds to decrease vertebral fracture risk.	Verbalize safety factors that can decrease fracture risk.

PUTTING IT ALL TOGETHER: APPLICATION OF THE NURSING PROCESS

Putting it all together is where the art and science of nursing meet to provide the best patient outcomes. We take the possibilities and place them into the context of the patient situation. To accomplish this, we use nursing diagnosis, nursing interventions, nursing outcomes, and nursing theory to provide the palette for nursing care.

STEP 4: ASSESSMENT

PATIENT INFORMATION: 56-year-old female Celesta Blade

CHIEF COMPLAINT: Severe low back pain

HISTORY OF THE PRESENT ILLNESS: Sudden onset of severe low back pain without injury.

PAST MEDICAL HISTORY: Early menopause at the age of 38; has never taken hormone replacement therapy. Smokes one pack of cigarettes a day for the past 25 years, and has a couple glasses of wine each evening before bed.

FAMILY HISTORY: Mother died at the age of 76 from complications after a fall that resulted in a hip fracture. Celesta has a sister age 60 who was recently diagnosed with osteoporosis. Mother was a single parent and father is unknown.

CHART REVIEW AND REPORT: Celesta came to the emergency department (ED) for severe low back pain. She states she did not do anything to injure her back. Visually there is a small curvature of the upper spine. Celesta reports her height as 5'8" but measures at 5'6½". Radiographic x-ray of the spine shows a curvature of the spine indicative of kyphosis but no fracture is seen. Laboratory studies consisting of a complete blood count and electrolytes are within normal limits. A bone mineral density study, dual-energy x-ray absorptiometry (DEXA), has been ordered. Celesta has been told by the HCP that based on her family history coupled with the suddenness of the back pain and evidence of beginning spinal curvature with height loss, he suspects osteoporosis. Celesta rated the back pain at a 10/10 in the ED for which she was given morphine sulfate 2 mg IV push with the pain decreasing to a 2/10. Celesta currently has hydrocodone with acetaminophen, one tablet every 6 hours ordered for moderate pain rated a 4/10 to 6/10 in intensity with morphine 2 mg IVP for severe pain rated 7/10 in intensity. Celesta was given the hydrocodone with acetaminophen for pain rated at a 5/10 one hour earlier. Vital signs are within normal limits except for BP, which was elevated to 186/90 mm Hg due to pain. After receiving pain medication, the BP reading changed to 126/82 mm Hg. Celesta is starting on ibuprofen 800 mg every 8 hours per her request, indicating that she prefers not to take narcotics. Celesta is also started on calcium with vitamin D 500 mg twice a day.

SUBJECTIVE ASSESSMENT: Arvin James (AJ) enters the room and sees Celesta sitting in a chair by the window watching the rain. AJ introduces himself, *"good morning my name is AJ, and I will be your nurse today. How are you feeling this morning?"* Celesta replies, "I'm OK, I guess. Actually I was just thinking that I am pretty lucky." *"How so?"* "Well, it looks like I have osteoporosis, like my mom and my sister. I should have known something was wrong when I had trouble finding blouses to fit me; they just seemed tight across the back. You know, my aunt was bent over like a pretzel before she died. It was horrible. The doctor says that the curvature I have right now is small, and with treatment we can keep it from getting worse. I can live with that. I think we caught it soon enough to prevent any real damage. The DEXA will let me know where I stand with that." *"It's been about an hour since you took the hydrocodone with acetaminophen, how's the pain now?"* "Pretty good, it just feels like a dull ache, maybe a 1/10. Nothing close to what it was before. The doctor says I can probably go home today after the DEXA. I don't know a lot about this disease, can you get me some information?" *"Of course,"* AJ responds.

OBJECTIVE ASSESSMENT: Celesta appears to have a slight curvature of the upper back that is noticeable when looking at her profile while she is sitting in the chair. When asked to lay in the bed for a morning assessment, it is noted that she has a steady gait and does not appear to be a fall risk. When asked to point to the area that was painful, Celesta indicated the lower third of her back. Vital signs are within normal limits, and BP is 124/80 mm Hg. Radiology comes to pick Celesta up for the DEXA just as the assessment is completed.

- *Laboratory Studies:*
  - CBC: Normal results: Hgb 13 g/dL, Hct 39%, WBC 6.8×10^3/microL
  - Electrolytes: Normal results: Na^+ 137 mEq/L, K^+ 3.8 mEq/L, Cl^- 100 mEq/L
- *Diagnostic Studies:*
  - DEXA indicates there is bone mineral density loss, indicating osteopenia.

STEP 5: REALITY CHECK: DETOUR AHEAD

Reality Check occurs when the nurse takes a moment to think about individualized patient information that needs to be considered in framing diagnoses and interventions. This information is retrievable from any legitimate source (e.g., family, case management, other nurses, any ancillary, a physician, etc.). These are the "wrenches" that create challenging situations, such as culture, religion, socioeconomic status, level of education, developmental level, marital status, employment, age, and gender.

Psychosocial History

Celesta comes from a financially well off family. Although she did not know her father, her mother went to live with her parents after she was born. Her mother's parents gave them an entire wing of their estate that included a small kitchen. Celesta's grandfather paid for private schooling for both her and her sister and financed both of their college educations. When her grandparents died their estate was divided between their mother and aunt. When their mother died, it was passed on to them. Celesta is financially independent and does not need to work.

Celesta volunteers at a homeless shelter working long hours and is often so busy that she eats whatever is handy. Celesta confesses that she lives on coffee and donuts. This type of diet has been going on for 20 plus years. Celesta considers herself to be a wine connoisseur. She likes to go to vineyards and do wine tasting and enjoys drinking two to three glasses of wine every evening before bed. Celesta does smoke and has no intention of quitting. Celesta never married and has no children. She currently lives on the family estate with her sister where she grew up.

Critical Thinking Moment

You have just completed the assessment of Celesta and need to make a decision about the patient's actual problems and nursing diagnoses based upon the data you have collected and the potential problems you identified. Outcomes must be realistic and measurable.

STEP 6: ACTUAL PROBLEMS/DIAGNOSES

The *first step* in problem identification is to revisit the list of *potential diagnoses* and choose *actual diagnoses* based upon the learner's evaluation of the case study information provided. A problem statement must be completed for each identified problem/diagnosis. The actual problems for this case study are pain, knowledge, and nutrition.

STEP 7: PLANNING: ACTUAL INTERVENTIONS

After actual diagnoses have been chosen, it is necessary to evaluate the list of *potential interventions* and choose *actual interventions* that will fit within the patient's reality and meet expected outcomes. Each intervention requires a rationale. Interventions are identified in three categories: (1) assessment, (2) therapeutic, and (3) education.

Diagnostic Statement

A **lack of knowledge** related to osteoporosis prevention and treatment is evidenced by Celesta's request for information.

Assessment

- Assess Celesta's understanding of osteoporosis as a disease. *Rationale: This allows for establishing a baseline for discussion.*
- Assess Celesta's willingness to adhere to osteoporosis treatment modalities. *Rationale: The nurse-patient collaboration with the plan of care is necessary for success.*

- Assess Celesta's eating habits. *Rationale: Evaluate if calcium-rich foods are being eaten.*

Therapeutic Interventions

- Encourage limiting alcohol use (wine). *Rationale: Alcohol use is associated with altered intestinal calcium resorption.*
- Explain how estrogen therapy can decrease bone fracture risk. *Rationale: This will help Celesta understand how prescribed medication can help to prevent bone fracture.*
- Encourage Celesta to limit caffeine intake. *Rationale: Caffeine can increase diuresis and calcium loss.*

Education

- Teach the importance of taking calcium and vitamin D supplements as prescribed. *Rationale: This is necessary to support bone health when dietary intake is insufficient. Taking too much calcium can result in hypercalcemia.*
- Explain how changes in diet can assist in decreasing the severity of osteoporosis. *Rationale: Inclusion of foods rich in calcium and vitamin D can assist in meeting recommended daily requirements that support bone health.*
- Teach the value of engaging in weight-bearing exercises. *Rationale: This assists in maintaining strong bones and decreases fracture risk.*

Expected Outcome

- Verbalize how lifestyle choices can contribute to osteoporosis severity.

Diagnostic Statement

Pain related to osteoporosis is evidenced by a self-report of back pain with an intensity rating of 10/10 prior to medication.

Assessment

- Assess the patient's pain intensity and characteristics. *Rationale: This allows you to adequately create a plan to treat pain.*
- Assess the patient's response to pain medication in order to evaluate the need for a pain management plan.
- Assess what makes the patient's pain better or worse. *Rationale: This allows you to identify what influences the pain.*

Therapeutic Interventions

- Suggest modifications in activity that may reduce pain. *Rationale: This reduces the patient's pain.*
- Administer ibuprofen 800 mg. *Rationale: This reduces the patient's pain and inflammation.*
- Administer hydrocodone with acetaminophen 2 tablets as needed. *Rationale: This reduces the patient's pain.*

Education

- Teach Celesta to report changes in pain. *Rationale: Increased pain can indicate a worsening condition.*
- Teach Celesta to call for medication before her pain becomes uncontrollable. *Rationale: Adequate pain management is more challenging and less effective when the severity is high.*
- Instruct Celesta to take ibuprofen with food. *Rationale: This prevents gastrointestinal upset.*

Expected Outcome

- Pain at a level acceptable to the patient

Diagnostic Statement

Nutrition related to poor diet as evidenced by history of eating "on the fly"

Assessment

- Assess Celesta's ability to make high-calcium food choices. *Rationale: The adequate dietary supplement of calcium can support bone health.*
- Assess Celesta's willingness to make dietary changes. *Rationale: Collaboration with the patient is necessary for the success of the plan of care.*
- Assess Celesta's understanding of the risks associated with eating "on the fly" (e.g., coffee, donuts). *Rationale: Long-standing eating habits are hard to change unless the patient understand the risks to her or his health and agrees to change.*

Therapeutic Interventions

- Administer calcium and vitamin D supplements 500 mg twice a day. *Rationale: This supports the patient's calcium intake.*
- Discuss foods that can interfere with calcium maintenance. *Rationale: This assists the patient in making beneficial dietary choices.*
- Provide sample menus. *Rationale: This may improve the patient's dietary choices.*

Education

- Assist Celesta to collaborate with the dietician to design an acceptable high-calcium diet. *Rationale: This will provide Celesta with information to make wise food choices.*
- Teach Celesta the importance of sunlight exposure as related to vitamin D deficiency. *Rationale: This encourages the minimum sun exposure to support vitamin D synthesis and calcium utilization.*
- Teach Celesta the purpose of the recommended vitamin D and calcium intake. *Rationale: This supports bone health.*

Expected Outcome

- The patient verbalizes the importance of an appropriate diet in osteoporosis prevention.

STEP 8: IMPLEMENTATION

Nursing Theory

Celesta is accepting of her diagnosis of osteoporosis and wants to do what is necessary to improve her health. Lydia Hall suggests that we assist Celesta to think about what she can do to improve her perform health. To achieve a positive outcome, we will need to carry out physician orders either independently or with the assistance of ancillaries.

Ancillary Support

Dietary information can help by providing dietary direction to Celesta about foods rich in calcium and vitamin D. Sample menus can be explored, as well as foods to avoid.

STEP 9: PLAN OF CARE

The plan of care is a road map for patient care and should be used as a communication tool between disciplines. Expected entries on the plan of care would be each identified problem, intervention, and expected outcome. Other information that should be added to the plan of care is how Celesta likes to learn (e.g., video, written material, computer access). The types of educational material provided, such as information about diet, medication, and activity, should be coordinated to allow the team to move forward as a group without frustrating repetition.

STEP 10: EVALUATION

Evaluation is an active process in which the nurse "connects the dots" to decide if the expected outcomes (goals) that were established have been met, partially met, or not met. If the goals are met, we continue with the plan as outlined. If the goal was partially met, we revise the parts of the plan that did not work. If the goals were not met, we start all over with a new plan.

End-of-Shift Narrative

Celesta has accessed the hospital's online library to read about osteoporosis and the best treatments. At her request, the physician has placed her on alendronic acid 5 mg daily. Celesta tells AJ she is very interested in joining an exercise club to begin weight-bearing exercises and strengthen her bones, preventing fracture. After speaking with the dietician, Celesta agrees that she needs to limit alcohol use and plans to cut down to one small glass of wine each night before bed. Celesta has spent the afternoon creating several simple menus that she feels will work well with her lifestyle. She plans to continue her work at the homeless shelter but says she will drink less coffee and eat fewer donuts. When asked about the pain, Celesta says that the hydrocodone with acetaminophen tablets she has been taking keep her pain minimal at a 2/10. She is very comfortable and does not require any other medication. Celesta insists that she has no interest in quitting smoking.

Problem Evaluation

PROBLEM 1: **Lack of Knowledge.** The expected outcome is that Celesta verbalizes how factors such as high caffeine use, alcohol use, and an inadequate diet can contribute to osteoporosis severity. The goal is met: Celesta has been proactive about searching out information related to osteoporosis, has been engaged with the dietician in meal planning, and is ready to make changes to improve her health.

PROBLEM 2: **Pain.** The expected outcome is pain at a level acceptable to the patient. The goal is met: Celesta reports that the hydrocodone with acetaminophen has kept her pain at a level of 2/10, which is acceptable to her.

PROBLEM 3: **Nutrition.** The expected outcome is that the patient verbalizes the importance of an appropriate diet in osteoporosis. The goal is met: Celesta has embraced making healthier menu plans with plans to drink less wine and coffee.

Overall Evaluation

Based on the end-of-shift assessment and comparison of Celesta's progress during this shift, Celesta is found to be improving.

REFERENCES

Dietary Reference Intakes (DRIs): Estimated Average Requirements, Food and Nutrition Board, Institute of Medicine, National Academies. Retrieved from http://www.iom.edu/Activities/Nutrition/SummaryDRIs/~/media/Files/Activity%20Files/Nutrition/DRIs/5_Summary%20Table%20Tables%201-4.pdf

Doheny, M., Sedlak, C., Estok, P., & Zeller, R. (2011, July/August). Bone density, health beliefs, and osteoporosis preventing behaviors in men. Orthopaedic Nursing, 30(4), 266–272.

Drugs.com. Actonel. Official FDA information. Retrieved from http://www.drugs.com/pro/actonel.html

Drugs.com. Boniva. Official FDA information. Retrieved from http://www.drugs.com/pro/boniva.html

Drugs.com. Fosamax. Official FDA information. Retrieved from http://www.drugs.com/pro/fosamax.html

Gatullo, B., Cichminski, L., Kumar, C., & Giachetta, D. (2011, November/December). Fine-tuning osteoporosis. Nursing Made Incredibly Easy, 26–37.

George, J. (2011). Nursing theories: The base for professional nursing practice (6th ed.). Upper Saddle River, NJ: Pearson Education.

Grossman, J. (2011). Osteoporosis prevention. Current Opinion in Rheumatology, 23, 203–210.

Gulanick, M., & Meyers J. (2013). Nursing care plans: Nursing diagnosis and intervention (8th ed.). St Louis, MO: Mosby.

Halcomb, S. (2006). Osteoporosis. Nursing 2006, 36(4), 48–49.

Holloway, N. (2004). Medical surgical nursing care planning (4th ed.). Springhouse, PA: Lippincott, Williams & Wilkins.

Kamienski, M., Tate, D., & Vega, M. (2011, May/June). The silent thief diagnosis and management of osteoporosis. Orthopaedic Nursing, 30(3), 162–171.

LeMone, P., Burke, K., & Baldoff, G. (2011). Medical surgical nursing, Critical thinking in patient care (5th ed.). Upper Saddle River, NJ: Pearson.

Mayo Clinic. Vitamin D. Retrieved from http://www.mayoclinic.com/health/vitamin-d/NS_patient-vitamind/DSECTION= dosing

Medscape. Updated Position Statement for Calcium Intake in Postmenopausal Women. Retrieved from http://www.medscape.org/viewarticle/548054

National Center for Biotechnology Information (NCBI). Bone Health and Osteoporosis: A Report of the Surgeon General. Retrieved from http://www.ncbi.nlm.nih.gov/books/NBK45506/

National Institutes of Health, Office of Dietary Supplements. Dietary Supplement Fact Sheet: Calcium Retrieved from http://ods.od.nih.gov/factsheets/Calcium-HealthProfessional/

National Institutes of Health, Office of Dietary Supplements. Dietary Supplement Fact Sheet: Vitamin D. Retrieved from http://ods.od.nih.gov/factsheets/VitaminD-HealthProfessional/

Parker, M. (2006). Nursing theories and nursing practice (2nd ed.). Philadelphia, PA: FA Davis.

Rodgers, S. (2008). Medical surgical nursing care plans. Clifton Park, NY: Thomson Delmar.

Roush, K. (2011, August). Prevention and treatment of osteoporosis in postmenopausal women: A review. American Journal of Nursing, 111(8), 26–31.

Simmons, S. (2005, March/April). Boning up on osteoporosis. Nursing Made Incredibly Easy, 6–15.

Swearingen, P. (2008). All in one care planning resource (2nd ed.). St Louis, MO: Mosby.

Van Leeuwen, A., & Bladh, M. (2015). Davis's comprehensive handbook of laboratory and diagnostic testing with nursing implications (6th ed.). Philadelphia, PA: F.A. Davis Company.

Wilkinson, J., & Ahern, N. (2009). In Nursing Diagnosis Handbook (9th ed.). Saddle River, NJ: Prentice Hall.

Wilson, B., Shannon, M., & Stang, C. (2006). Nurses drug guide. Upper Saddle River, NJ: Prentice Hall.

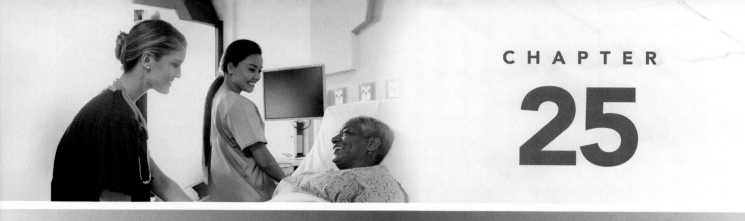

25

Gastrointestinal System

Case Study: Pancreatitis

Common Nursing Study Name	Section 1 Study	Section 1, Chapter Number
Abdominal X-Rays, Plain (KUB)	Kidney, Ureter, and Bladder Study	Chapter 16
Amylase	Amylase	Chapter 1
Arterial Blood Gas (ABG)	Blood Gases	Chapter 14
Blood Culture	Culture, Bacterial, Blood	Chapter 5
Blood Sugar	Glucose	Chapter 1
Calcium	Calcium, Blood	Chapter 1
Computed Tomography (CT) of the Pancreas	Computed Tomography, Pancreas	Chapter 7
Endoscopic Retrograde Cholangiopancreatography (ERCP)	Cholangiopancreatography, Endoscopic Retrograde	Chapter 9
Fecal Analysis	Fecal Analysis	Chapter 10
Lipase	Lipase	Chapter 1
Magnesium	Magnesium, Blood	Chapter 1
Oxygen Saturation (Pulse Oximetry)	Pulse Oximetry	Chapter 14
Ultrasound	Ultrasound, Abdomen	Chapter 21
	Ultrasound, Pancreas	Chapter 21
WBC Count and Differential	Complete Blood Count, WBC Count and Differential	Chapter 2

STEP 1: DATA COLLECTION

Pathophysiology

The pancreas has two primary functions. The first is to act as an exocrine gland producing enzymes that empty through ducts into the duodenum. The second is to act as an endocrine gland producing hormones that enter directly into the bloodstream. The overall function of the pancreas is to aid in the digestion of protein, fats, and starches while secreting hormones to aid in regulation of blood glucose.

As a function of an endocrine gland, the islets of Langerhans within the pancreas secrete insulin and glucagon. Insulin and glucagon are hormones that balance blood glucose and play a vital role in lipid and carbohydrate metabolism. As a function of an exocrine gland, acinar cells produce the pancreatic juices trypsinogen and chymotrypsinogen, which convert to trypsin and chymotrypsin in the duodenum and are used to digest protein. Additional enzymatic functions include pancreatic lipase being released to digest triglycerides and the release of amylase to digest starch.

The tricky part about diagnosing pancreatitis is making sure the symptoms are not caused by something else. Pancreatitis begins at the cellular level with the inflammation of acinar cells. One type of pancreatitis is interstitial or edematous, a result of fluid accumulation and swelling. About 80% of all pancreatic cases fall into this category with a 5%–10% mortality rate. Hospitalization for treatment is between 3 and 5 days. Positive prognosis is minimal organ dysfunction, no necrotic injury, and a recovery without complication.

Pancreatitis can also be classified as necrotizing, a severe form of the disease causing cell death, tissue damage, and systemic complications. Necrotizing pancreatitis usually requires intensive support for multiple life-threatening problems, including sepsis, necrosis, infection, and multisystem disease. About 20% of all pancreatic cases fall into this category, with 50% of those ending in death. Prognosis is poor.

Risk Factors

Pancreatitis is also viewed as being an acute or chronic inflammatory process. Normally the digestive enzymes used to break down protein and fat are not activated until they enter the duodenum. Pancreatitis disrupts this process.

Acute Inflammatory Pancreatitis

Acute inflammatory pancreatitis is usually the result of ductal obstruction from gallstones or stenosis of the sphincter of Oddi. Of these two, gallstones are the most common reason that pancreatic ducts fail to drain into the duodenum. The sphincter of Oddi normally assists the flow of pancreatic juices forward into the duodenum; stenosis interferes with this process, causing reflux. When pancreatic juices are blocked from entering the duodenum, they activate prematurely inside the pancreas, causing autodigestion and destruction of the acinar cells and islet cell tissue. This is followed by leakage of enzymes into the surrounding tissues. Simply stated, the pancreas turns its digestive enzymes on itself, initiating inflammation and causing pancreatitis. Other causes of acute pancreatitis are tumors, trauma, radiation therapy, ulcer disease, and inflammation.

Chronic Inflammatory Pancreatitis

Chronic inflammatory pancreatitis is the result of acute alcoholism 90% of the time. Alcohol abuse promotes a vicious cycle of decreased pancreatic blood flow, followed by ischemic episodes and cellular damage with circular episodes of increasingly frequent and severe attacks. Alcohol irritates the pancreas and stimulates production of protein precipitates, which block acinar ducts and trap enzymes within the pancreas. Other metabolic causes of chronic pancreatitis include diabetic ketoacidosis, hypercalcemia, hyperlipidemia, and drugs such as acetaminophen and estrogen.

Trauma-Associated Pancreatitis

Trauma-associated pancreatitis has multiple causes. Contrast injections, high-pressure injections, contrast shot directly into an acinar cell, or poor operator performance during an endoscopic retrograde cholangiopancreatography (ERCP) can all trigger an episode. Patients who have undergone cardiac, renal, or abdominal surgery may have some pancreatic trauma or temporary blockage of the pancreas. Any event that causes prolonged pancreatic ischemia could result in pancreatitis.

Infection-Triggered Pancreatitis

Infection is another trigger for pancreatitis. Immunosuppressant drugs such as azathioprine can leave the patient open to infection, causing pancreatitis. Bacterial or viral organisms and parasites are thought to precipitate pancreatitis. Causal viral organisms may be mumps, measles, rubella, Coxsackie virus, Epstein-Barr virus, or hepatitis B. Bacterial organisms include *Legionella, Mycobacterium tuberculosis*, and *campylobacter*. The more common causal parasites include *Ascaris* and *Clonorchis*. It is believed that infection precipitates pancreatitis by triggering trypsinogen and chymotrypsinogen to activate and begin to digest the pancreas.

Failure to discover the cause of pancreatitis after a good diagnostic evaluation and careful history is considered to be *idiopathic*. A diagnosis of idiopathic pancreatitis means that the cause is unknown. Some health-care providers (HCPs) believe idiopathic pancreatitis is associated with inflammation and fibrosis. Diagnosis of idiopathic pancreatitis occurs in about 25% of all cases.

Other Causes of Pancreatitis

Genetic predisposition toward pancreatitis is a causal possibility. Genetic mutation can cause trypsinogen to convert to trypsin inside of the pancreas instead of waiting until it enters the duodenum.

Causes of pancreatitis vary by age and gender. Men tend to have pancreatitis associated with alcohol abuse and dependence. Women tend to have pancreatitis associated with gallstones and the biliary tract. Cystic fibrosis is usually the cause of pancreatitis in children, whereas in older adults it is associated with a high-fat diet.

A definitive diagnosis of pancreatitis can be made if the serum amylase and lipase levels are elevated. The pancreas releases these enzymes on the first day of illness. Serum amylase may decrease within 24 hr of the event, but the serum lipase remains elevated for up to 14 days. Laboratory results can be skewed by advanced chronic pancreatitis with a large amount of organ damage. Cells that have been destroyed over time with repeated pancreatic episodes no longer secrete enzymes. This cellular destruction will be reflected in the laboratory results. Generally, a diagnosis can be made when the amylase is elevated to four times the highest reference point.

In summary, mild acute pancreatitis, or interstitial edematous pancreatitis, results in a pancreas that is inflamed and edematous. This form of pancreatitis usually resolves over time with a complete recovery. Severe, chronic, or necrotizing pancreatitis are aggressive inflammatory responses. Severe pancreatitis causes the pancreatic tissue to bleed and become necrotic with the potential of infection and abscess formation. This form of pancreatitis is slow to resolve, and the outcome can be life threatening. Acute pancreatitis can become chronic if treatment is not successful.

Signs and Symptoms

Pancreatitis usually has a rapid onset associated with the recent ingestion of alcohol, a fatty meal, or obstruction. The classic symptom is the sudden onset of acute pain caused by an increase in the release of pancreatic enzymes. Individuals usually describe the pain as a severe, boring, knife-like pain in the epigastric and abdominal area, with some radiation to the back. Pain worsens with walking or lying flat, while sitting up and leaning forward can relieve some of the pain. Assess the abdomen for bowel sounds, which would be hypoactive, and abdominal tenderness, which would be present, with guarding or rigidity. Remember to listen to the bowel prior to palpation for assessment accuracy.

Skin should be carefully assessed. Check for any bluish discoloration around the flanks (Grey Turner sign), or the umbilicus (Cullen sign), indicating that blood is pooling under the skin. Respirations may be shallow from an increase in the size of the abdomen, causing diminished breath sounds in the lower lobes. Ask about family history of pancreatitis, medication use, alcohol consumption, diet history, and intensity and character of the pain. Observe for nonverbal cues of pain such as restlessness, facial grimace, clenched fists, tachycardia, diaphoresis, or rapid shallow breathing. Ask if stools have been foul smelling or fatty. Report this information to the HCP, who may request that a stool sample be sent for fecal analysis. Find out if there has been any nausea, vomiting, or previous attack. There should be a discussion about alcohol use, both frequency and amount.

Acute pancreatitis presents with nausea, vomiting, epigastric or abdominal pain, abdominal distention, decreased bowel sounds, low-grade fever, tachycardia, hypotension, and cool, clammy skin.

Chronic pancreatitis presents as persistent periodic episodes of epigastric, abdominal or back pain, anorexia, vomiting, nausea, weight loss, gas, constipation, and steatorrhea (fatty, foul-smelling stool). Unlike the severe pain experienced during acute pancreatitis, those with chronic disease may actually have less pain or no pain as with every episode of pancreatitis more tissue is destroyed or damaged. With less tissue to attack there is less pain. That is why the severity of chronic pancreatitis cannot be based solely upon pain intensity but must be evaluated in other ways.

Complications

Acute pancreatitis has the potential of multiple complications. Hypovolemic shock can occur as fluid shifts into the small bowel. There may be bleeding into the retroperitoneal space. Turner and Cullen signs can provide evidence of bleeding. A pancreatic pseudocyst can develop as cells damaged from autodigestion create a wall around a collection of blood, fluids, and necrotic debris within the abdominal cavity. Ruptured pseudocysts can cause infection, abscess, fistulae, and peritonitis. Abscesses caused by collecting secretions and necrotic products pose a mortality risk. Pancreatic islet cells can be damaged or destroyed, resulting in diabetes. Other complications include pancreatic hemorrhage, shock, acute respiratory distress syndrome (ARDS), atelectasis, pleural effusion, pneumonia, paralytic ileus, chronic kidney disease, and multiorgan dysfunction syndrome.

Chronic pancreatitis is irreversible with damage to the small ducts of the pancreas from calcified proteins with scar tissue formation. Edema and distention cause an irreversible loss of acinar cells as they become fibrotic and necrotic. Structural changes within the pancreas permanently alter the organ's functionality. Symptoms of this alteration are evidenced by weight loss from malabsorption, malnutrition, and digestive dysfunction, and the development of type 2 diabetes. Additional complications include peptic ulcer disease, portal hypertension, opioid addiction, and risk of pancreatic cancer.

Laboratory Studies

Laboratory studies guide the HCP in distinguishing between acute and chronic disease as well as severity of that disease. Evaluation for infection and inflammation along with enzyme changes will be important. Results may show an elevated WBC, serum amylase greater than 110 units/L, lipase greater than 60 units/L, and elevated blood sugar greater than 105 mg/dL. Low laboratory values would include low serum calcium less than 8.2 mg/dL and low serum magnesium less than 1.6 mg/dL. Fecal analysis may be requested by the physician to evaluate malabsorption or pancreatic insufficiency.

Diagnostic Studies

Diagnostic studies will be looking for signs of blockage and inflammation. Requested studies may include abdominal x-rays or ultrasound of the abdomen and pancreas, which would show inflammatory changes to the pancreas, including inflammation and gallstones. Computerized tomography (CT) can differentiate between acute and chronic pancreatitis and visualize an abscess, pseudocyst, and enlarged pancreas with fluid collection. Endoscopic retrograde cholangiopancreatography (ERCP), can diagnose chronic pancreatitis and visualize bile ducts. However, caution should be used as ERCP can precipitate an event of acute pancreatitis in some patients. Computed tomography–guided percutaneous fine-needle aspiration can check for cancer versus chronic disease.

General/Medical Management

Treatment for pancreatitis encompasses a medical management and/or surgical approach. The approach taken is dependent on the severity of the disease. The general focus is on minimizing pancreatic damage. The treatment of chronic pancreatitis focuses on pain management, the replacement of deficient enzymes and hormones, and nutritional support. Suppressing pancreatic enzyme secretion with use of a synthetic hormone such as octreotide can decrease pain.

Resting the Pancreas

Pancreatic damage can be minimized by resting the pancreas. This can be achieved by making the patient NPO (nothing by mouth), without ice chips or sips of water until the acute phase has passed. Nasogastric intubation (NGT) placed to intermittent suction may also be used to prevent the release of gastric secretions into the duodenum, decreasing the release of pancreatic secretions.

Fluid Management

Appropriate fluid management is a necessary standard of care in managing pancreatitis. Adequate hydration is important to prevent hypotension, maintain electrolyte balance, and prevent hypervolemia, which may precipitate renal and cardiac complications. Urinary output should be monitored as a marker of adequate hydration and perfusion. Output should exceed 0.5 mL/kg/hr, as less than that can indicate hypoperfusion concerns. Fluids should be titrated to meet this goal. The type of fluid used for hydration may be normal saline or lactated Ringer solution as per physician preference. Besides improved urine output, the effect of adequate fluid replacement will be seen in improved vital signs, decreased hemoconcentration, and an improvement in the patient's blood urea nitrogen. If unsuccessful, consideration should be given to the efficacy of adding a medication such as dopamine to support renal function.

Fluid imbalances can cause other problems. Hydration and electrolyte replacement will be needed to replace fluids lost by inflammation. Magnesium can be lost with the calcium, and potassium can be lost through vomiting. Ventricular dysrhythmia can occur if the process is not reversed. Those patients who do not improve may need to be transported to critical care.

Oxygenation

Oxygenation can be a concern. Pulse oximetry should be used to monitor saturation with a maintenance goal of greater than 95%. Oxygen appliances may vary depending on the situation, ranging from nasal cannula to mechanical ventilation. Hypoxia may occur from pleural effusion, atelectasis, pulmonary emboli, and ARDS. Arterial blood gas evaluation should be considered for those with an oxygen saturation of less than 95%. Pancreatic fluid leaking into the pleural space can cause an effusion, placing the patient at risk for pneumonia.

Nutrition

Once the pancreas has had a chance to recover, the diet should be slowly resumed. Oral feedings can begin when the pain has improved, there is no ileus, and the nausea and vomiting have resolved. The physician may order a clear liquid diet initially. Ongoing dietary recommendations include adhering to a low-fat diet of small, frequent meals. Dietary tolerance should be evaluated and adjustments made as needed. Spicy foods and caffeinated drinks should be avoided, and alcohol should be forbidden, as it will exacerbate the disease and may precipitate an attack. Chemical dependency support may be necessary to assist the patient to quit drinking. Social services may be needed to assist the patient in recognizing and adapting to abstinence from alcohol.

For those patients who are unable to eat, alternative methods of nutritional support will be necessary. Total parental nutrition (TPN) can support caloric needs until the patient is able to eat again and may begin as early as within 5 days of diagnosis. Lipids will be withheld because they can increase triglyceride levels and exacerbate the situation. Total parenteral nutrition (TPN) should be used for those patients who do not tolerate enteral feedings. Gemfibrozil may be ordered to reduce the liver's ability to produce triglycerides through fatty acid uptake.

Enteral feedings are another option to provide nutrition. Enteral nutrition may be a better choice than TPN in some circumstances to avoid the catheter-related concerns of sepsis, pneumothorax, embolism, and thrombophlebitis. The goal of enteral feedings is to provide nutrition while preventing pancreatic enzyme release. Enteral feedings may begin within 72 hr of pancreatitis onset if oral feedings are not recommended or tolerated. One benefit of using enteral nutrition as compared with using TPN is that the cost is much less while still providing adequate nutrition, maintaining bowel integrity, and supporting the immune system.

Pain Management

The narcotic use for pain management may be limited due to the risk of addiction over time. Patient-controlled analgesia (PCA) seems to be the best choice for acute pain management. The choices of drugs for PCA administration include hydromorphone and fentanyl. The evaluation should be made to determine if the patient needs a PCA basal infusion along with a bolus selection for adequate pain management. Pain management for chronic pancreatitis will be dependent on what works best for the patient. One nonpharmacological intervention for pain management is to use bed rest to decrease basal metabolism, thereby decreasing pain.

Other Medications

Blood glucose can be altered from damage to pancreatic islet cells. Blood glucose elevations can occur from TPN administration, decreased insulin release, or decreased glucose use. The patient's blood sugar should be monitored closely, and insulin should be given to address hyperglycemic events.

Infection concerns can be addressed with the use of broad-spectrum prophylactic antibiotics. Suggested drugs to address infection prophylactically are imipenem and meropenem.

Other drugs that may be helpful are histamine antagonists to decrease acid production and antacids to neutralize gastric secretions. Other medications useful in decreasing gastric acidity are omeprazole or ranitidine. Oral enzymes may be given to aid digestion and absorption of nutrients.

Surgical/Interventional Management

Surgical or interventional procedures may be used in combination with medical management to resolve the pancreatitis. Percutaneous computed tomography (CT)–guided aspiration can be used to remove fluid and debris. For patients with gallstone pancreatitis, stones may be removed by surgical intervention or through ERCP with papillotomy. Stent placement may be used to facilitate drainage and decrease the risk of post-ERCP pancreatitis. The recommended time frame for this procedure is within the first 72 hr of onset. If surgical intervention is needed for stone removal, cholecystectomy may be performed when the patient is medically cleared.

Débridement (necrosectomy) may be necessary to remove necrotic tissue from the pancreas. This may be accomplished using a surgical or less invasive endoscopic approach. Peritoneal lavage and repeated débridement may be necessary.

Social Services

Patients experiencing pancreatitis may have feelings of hopelessness and apathy because of the debilitating nature of the disease. Assistance may be required to help the patient and family to cope.

Patient Education

The prevention of a repeat episode is the focus of patient education. Having a clear understanding of medication, diet, what to expect when an attack occurs, and when to seek medical attention is very important. There are times when a patient will be diagnosed with pancreatitis and the physician will not be able to identify the cause. The diagnosis will be idiopathic. Prevention is a large part of disease management. How do you provide education to a patient regarding a diagnosis where the physician cannot identify the cause? One approach found to be effective is to discover the risk factors that are readily identifiable and educate to those in addition to general information. The management of pain and nutrition will probably be high on the patient's priority list.

STEP 2: POTENTIAL PROBLEMS/ DIAGNOSES

It is important that nurses understand and consider the science of the disease process and consider the possibilities prior to applying that knowledge to a patient situation. We begin that process with questioning.

Question: Based upon your review of the content presented what possible *potential problems* would you expect for a patient with these diagnoses?

Answer: Pain, nutrition, deficient fluid, gas exchange, and infection

STEP 3: POTENTIAL INTERVENTIONS AND EXPECTED OUTCOME

💬 **Question:** Based upon your identification of patient problems, what possible interventions would you recommend for these diagnoses, and what would you expect to happen? This would be considered your "grocery list" of the possible actions you could use to assist your patient.

💬 **Answer:** See the following problems, interventions, and expected outcomes:

Problem	Interventions	Expected Outcomes
Pain	Assess intensity with a 0/10 scale. Monitor the effects of opioid use, manage PCA use, and monitor medication effectiveness. Maintain nothing by mouth (NPO) status. Position the patient for comfort and limit movement.	Self-report of satisfactory pain relief
Nutrition	Maintain NPO status with small meals when eating again. Monitor diet tolerance, weigh daily, provide low-fat foods, and use TPN as needed. Avoid caffeine, spicy foods, and alcohol. Self-monitor for steatorrhea.	Baseline body weight will be maintained, nutritional status will be supported.
Deficient Fluid	Monitor intake and output, blood pressure, heart rate, and breath sounds. Administer IV fluids and volume expanders. Replace electrolytes. Record daily weight.	Normovolemic, balanced electrolytes, and stable weight
Gas Exchange	Monitor respiratory rate and oxygenation. Assess for changes in mental status. Assess breath sounds.	Adequate gas exchange, normal mental status, respiratory rate 12–20 per minute
Infection	Check temperature every 4 hr. Obtain blood culture, for temperature spikes. Administer antibiotics. Use good hand hygiene. Monitor mental status.	Patient remains afebrile and free of infection

PUTTING IT ALL TOGETHER: APPLICATION OF THE NURSING PROCESS

Putting it all together is where the art and science of nursing meet to provide the best patient outcomes. We take the possibilities and place them into the context of the patient situation. To accomplish this we use nursing diagnosis, nursing interventions, nursing outcomes, and nursing theory to provide the palate for nursing care.

STEP 4: ASSESSMENT

PATIENT INFORMATION: John Adams is a 53-year-old Caucasian male and an unemployed construction worker.

CHIEF COMPLAINT: Acute unrelieved abdominal pain, nausea, vomiting, and abdominal tenderness

HISTORY OF THE PRESENT ILLNESS: Was at his buddy's house having beer and burgers last night. Woke up this morning with severe pain, nausea, and vomiting, had one emesis (vomiting) prior to coming to the emergency department (ED).

PAST MEDICAL HISTORY: None; never sees a doctor.

FAMILY HISTORY: Single, no children. Parents deceased, history unknown.

CHART REVIEW AND REPORT: John was admitted through the ED 4 hours ago. Vital signs on admission were BP of 156/94 mm Hg, pulse 126 beats per minute, respirations 26 breaths per minute, temperature 99.6°F. A hydromorphone PCA with a lockout of 10 minutes was started after a bolus for pain management. Pain was rated at greater than a 10/10 prior to hydromorphone administration, and afterward pain was rated 5/10. Pain is described as stabbing and persistent. Abdomen is tender and slightly distended, with hypoactive bowel sounds and mild nausea. John says he is most comfortable when sitting up in bed. A nasogastric tube (NGT) has been placed to intermittent low suction with a return of 225 mL green gastric drainage. John is currently NPO and an IV of normal saline is infusing at 100 mL/hr.

Repeat vital signs are BP of 138/86 mm Hg, a pulse of 102 beats per minute, respirations of 20 breaths per minute, and a temperature of 99°F.

SUBJECTIVE ASSESSMENT: You enter the room and say, *"Good morning! My name is Arvin James (AJ) and I will be your nurse today. How are you feeling this morning, Mr. Adams?"* "Call me John," says Mr. Adams. *"OK. How you are feeling, John?"* John replies, "I feel wretched! My belly is killing me and I have this stupid tube down my nose. What the heck happened to me?" Concerned, AJ asks, *"Has your doctor talked to you about why you are in here?"* "Yes, but the guy ran in, said a bunch of stuff I couldn't understand, and then ran out like his tail was on fire. I don't trust him as far as I could throw him." Understanding John's concern, AJ continues, *"What did he say?"* "He said I have pancrea...something, who the heck knows, it didn't make a lick of sense to me. He just said I had to keep this tube in my nose for a couple of days, that I couldn't have anything to eat, and that I needed to stop drinking beer, as if *that's* gonna happen. Drinking with my buddies is the only thing I really enjoy in this life." AJ asks, *"Did the doctor explain why you have the tube down your nose, or can't eat, or should stop drinking?"* John bitterly replies, "He didn't explain nothing—just ran out of here like the fool he is." Politely, AJ asks, *"Would you like me to explain it to you?"* John shakes his head and says, "No. Maybe later, but I am too fed up with this place to listen right now." "OK," AJ replies placatingly, *"We will talk about it later. How is the pain in your belly right now? Is it better or worse?"* John grimaces and says, "Better than it was. When I came in it was over the top, then after the medicine it got better. Right now it is a 4/10, which is OK for me—I can take it." AJ asks, *"Would you like me to call the doctor and adjust your dose?"* John laughs, "No, I'm good. I'll let you know if I need something more." *"Are you still nauseated?"* AJ asks. John replies, "Not much; this nose sucker tube takes everything out of my stomach so I don't feel too barfy. I'm still tender around my belly button but the bloating is gone, and I am peeing a river so I guess I am going in the right direction. I do feel a little better this morning, and I want to go home as soon as I can."

OBJECTIVE ASSESSMENT: John appears slightly pale, is not restless, and is alert and oriented. Although cooperative, it is obvious that John is upset with his physician and is not interested in being educated about his disease. Current vital signs are BP of 132/84 mm Hg, pulse 98 beats per minute, respirations 20 breaths per minute, temperature 99°F. John's NGT is set to low intermittent suction with a continued output of green gastric secretions. John remains NPO with IV as ordered. John's abdomen is nondistended and tender at the umbilicus with pain rated at a 4/10. John reports that the pain is less stabbing but more achy. There is no discoloration at umbilicus or flank. Bowel sounds are hypoactive. Breath sounds are clear. The head of the bed is in high Fowler position with John confirming that this is his position of comfort.

- *Laboratory Studies:*
  - Amylase, 640 units/L
  - Lipase, 586 units/L
  - Serum calcium, 9.6 mg/dL
  - Blood glucose of 98 mg/dL
  - K^+ of 3.9 mEq/L
  - Cl^- of 103 mEq/L
  - NA^+ 140 mEq/L
- *Diagnostic Study:*
  - CT scan shows pancreatic enlargement and inflammation
- *Medications:*
  - Zantac, 50 mg IVPB (IV piggyback) every 6 hr
  - IV imipenem and cilastatin 500 mg IVPB every 6 hr
  - PCA morphine for pain management

STEP 5: REALITY CHECK: DETOUR AHEAD

Reality Check occurs when the nurse takes a moment to think about individualized patient information that needs to be considered in framing diagnoses and interventions. This information is retrievable from any legitimate source (e.g., family, case management, other nurses, any ancillary, a physician, etc.). These are the "wrenches" that create challenging situations, such as culture, religion, socioeconomic status, level of education, developmental level, marital status, employment, age, and gender.

Psychosocial History

John Adams is a 53-year-old unemployed construction worker. He dropped out of high school at the age of 15. His father was in jail and his mother was on drugs, and John ran away from home to escape an abusive situation. Having never married and without children or any close family, John spends all of his free time with his buddies eating a high-fat diet of burgers and buffalo wings and drinking beer. It is estimated that he drinks 2 six-packs of beer a day.

Critical Thinking Moment

You have just completed the assessment of John Adams and need to make a decision about the patient's *actual* problems and nursing diagnoses based on the data you have collected and the potential problems you identified. Outcomes must be realistic and measurable.

STEP 6: ACTUAL PROBLEMS/DIAGNOSES

The *first step* in problem identification is to revisit the list of *potential diagnoses* and choose *actual diagnoses* based upon the learner's evaluation of the case study information provided. A problem statement must be completed for each identified problem/diagnosis. The actual problems/diagnoses for this case study are pain, nutrition, and deficient fluid risk.

STEP 7: PLANNING: ACTUAL INTERVENTIONS

After actual diagnoses have been chosen, it is necessary to evaluate the list of *potential interventions* and choose *actual interventions* that will fit within the patient's reality and meet expected outcomes. Each intervention requires a rationale. Interventions are identified in three categories: (1) assessment, (2) therapeutic, and (3) education.

Diagnostic Statement

Pain related to pancreatic inflammation is evidenced by elevated amylase and a report of pain at 4/10 with facial grimace.

Assessment

- Assess pain using a 0/10 scale. *Rationale: This assists with an ongoing evaluation of disease progress and pain management effectiveness.*
- Assess response to Dilaudid PCA. *Rationale: This allows you to evaluate the effectiveness of management and the need for alterations in dosage.*
- Monitor respiratory status. *Rationale: Respiratory depression is associated with narcotic use.*

Therapeutic Interventions

- Adequate pain management with the use of PCA morphine. *Rationale: Unrelieved pain can stimulate the secretion of pancreatic enzymes.*
- Maintain NPO status and NGT patency. *Rationale: Gastric and pancreatic secretions aggravate pain, and alleviate nausea and vomiting.*
- Position in high Fowler. *Rationale: This promotes self-reports of comfort.*

Education

- Limit activities. *Rationale: Limiting activities will decrease basal metabolism and rest the pancreas.*
- Use pain medication early. *Rationale: This disease is very painful. The proactive use of medications can prevent pain from getting out of control.*
- Abstain from alcohol use. *Rationale: Alcohol use can precipitate pancreatitis.*

Expected Outcome

- Pain will be at a level acceptable to John.

Diagnostic Statement

Nutritional imbalance related to NPO status, NGT to suction, and pancreatic dysfunction is evidenced by nausea and hypoactive bowel sounds.

Assessment

- Monitor stool color, odor, consistency. *Rationale: Fat in the stool can indicate worsening pancreatitis.*
- Assess bowel sounds. *Rationale: Evaluate the return of bowel motility so the patient's diet can be resumed.*
- Monitor the amount of diet eaten once ordered. *Rationale: This allows you to assess diet tolerance.*

Therapeutic Interventions

- Daily weight. *Rationale: Ongoing evaluation of nutritional status is based upon weight.*
- Maintain NPO status until able to eat. *Rationale: Doing so rests the pancreas and decreases pain.*
- Discuss with the physician the necessity of starting enteral feedings or TPN for nutrition support. *Rationale: This is needed if there is a significant delay in restarting oral feedings.*

Education

- Once diet is resumed, eat frequent, small, low-fat meals. *Rationale: This makes the lifestyle change from a high-fat to a low-fat diet to promote digestion.*
- Avoid caffeine, spicy foods, and alcohol. *Rationale: This prevents a pancreatitis reoccurrence.*
- Self-monitoring of stool. *Rationale: Observe for steatorrhea.*

Expected Outcome

- Baseline body weight will be maintained, and nutritional status will be supported.

Diagnostic Statement

Deficient fluids related to the loss of gastric secretions as evidenced by NGT suctioning and NPO status

Assessment

- Monitor intake and output. *Rationale: Evaluate fluid balance.*
- Monitor blood pressure and heart rate. *Rationale: Falling blood pressure and increasing heart rate can indicate fluid loss.*
- Monitor breath sounds. *Rationale: Adventitious breath sounds can indicate a too aggressive fluid replacement strategy.*

Therapeutic Interventions

- Administer IV normal saline at 100/mL per hour as ordered. *Rationale: This supports homeostasis.*

- Ask health-care provider about adding KCL to IVF. *Rationale: This maintains the patient's potassium level.*
- Weigh daily, and note trends. *Rationale: Doing so can monitor fluid increase or decrease.*

Education

- Report shortness of breath. *Rationale: This allows you to monitor for excessive fluids with overload.*
- Report dizziness. *Rationale: This allows for an assessment of orthostatic hypotension.*
- Report muscle twitching. *Rationale: This symptom is associated with calcium loss.*

Expected Outcome

- Maintain adequate fluid status with balanced electrolytes, and maintain stable weight.

STEP 8: IMPLEMENTATION

Nursing Theory

Imogene King, who development the Theory of Goal Attainment, looks at how to frame health-care goals while considering the reality of the patient's situation. Mr. Adams is an unemployed construction worker who is single and has no other family. Through your interaction with him, you realize that his support group is his drinking buddies. It may be difficult to convince him to stop drinking beer with his social group. It will be necessary to assess for John's receptiveness and see what mutual goals can be set.

Rosemarie Rizzo Parse, the creator of the Human Becoming Theory of Nursing, reminds us that it is the nurse's role to guide the patient to make good choices and to respect the patient's decisions. Ultimately, John is responsible for the choices made and will have to live with the consequences. However, the nurse needs to make sure that John has all the pertinent information so that informed choices can be made. John is going to need a lot of supportive education to understand how his drinking is causing his disease. John will also need a "reality check" of what may happen in the future if he continues down this path.

Ancillary Support

The clinical dietician may be a valuable tool for assisting John in understanding how to incorporate dietary restriction into his lifestyle. A chemical dependency consult may be assistive in starting the process of alcohol abstinence. The case manager or social services can provide referral information for alcohol support groups.

STEP 9: PLAN OF CARE

The plan of care is a road map for patient care and should be used as a communication tool between disciplines. Expected entries on the plan of care would be each identified problem (e.g., pain, nutrition, fluid deficit risk) with corresponding interventions and expected outcomes, including any information from ancillaries. In John's case, other information that should be included on the plan is his long-standing alcohol use and lack of supportive family. There should be some notation that he considers his drinking buddies to be his primary support group and source of social interaction. This is especially important because alcohol use is a primary factor in this pancreatic episode, and unless John's alcohol consumption gets under control, it is likely that episodes like this will continue to occur. Social services should have some discussion with John about chemical dependency support as an outpatient, and that information should be noted.

STEP 10: EVALUATION

Evaluation is an active process in which the nurse "connects the dots" to decide if the expected outcomes (goals) that were established have been met, partially met, or not met. If the goals are met, we continue with the plan as outlined. If the goal was partially met, we revise the parts of the plan that did not work. If the goals were not met, we start all over with a new plan.

In the case of John, pain, nutrition, and deficient fluid risk were identified as the primary problems. Have we achieved our expected outcomes (goals), and have they been met? What is John's overall status at the end of the shift? Is he improving, is there no change, or is he declining? If our goals were not met, how will we modify the plan(s) to achieve the stated goal(s)?

End-of-Shift Narrative

AJ enters the room at the end of his shift to check on John. *"I just wanted to check in on you before I leave."* "Thanks," John replies. *"How is the pain?"* AJ asks. *"Is it any better?"* "I think so," John replies, and says, "The pain had been running at a 5/10 but this pain medication seems to keep me pretty comfortable, maybe a 3–4/10, but I have no complaints." AJ responds, *"I'm glad you are comfortable,"* and John smiles, "So am I." AJ asks, *"Are you still nauseated?"* "Not really," John responds. "This tube in my nose is irritating but I would rather have that than keep throwing up. I noticed that there is not as much green stuff coming out." AJ says, *"Yes, you had only about 100 mL out this shift. And your hydration is good, your urine and NGT output are in balance* with the IV fluid you are taking in." John asks, "Is it ok that I'm not eating anything?" AJ continues, *"The doctor and I did talk about starting you on TPN, but we are hoping you will start eating soon. We are going to see how you are doing tomorrow and decide then. Your bowels are still a little hypoactive but they seem better."* "Good," John slowly smiles. "I trust you to take care of me, and make sure the doc is on board." AJ nods toward the standing scale in the corner of the room, *"We are going to check your weight every morning so we can keep track of your fluid and nutritional status."* John remarks, "Yeah, I weighed myself again a while ago and it's pretty much the same." AJ says, *"Did the social worker speak with you about attending an alcohol support group?"* John looks very serious and replies, "Yes, but I am not sure I can do that. I'll have to think about it a little more."

Problem Evaluation

PROBLEM 1: **Pain.** The expected outcome is that pain will be at a level acceptable to John. The goal is met: John's last report of pain was 3–4/10, he stated that he is comfortable and satisfied with his pain management. He is considering joining an alcohol support group.

PROBLEM 2: **Nutrition.** The expected outcome is that John's baseline body weight will be maintained, and his nutritional status will be supported. The goal is met: John's nutritional status is presently supported with IV fluids of normal saline, and a discussion has occurred to evaluate the need for TPN in the near future. Bowel sounds remain hypoactive but are less so. Although John has weighed himself and is confident that he is okay, his first official daily weight post-baseline will be in the morning; if needed, the plan will be revised.

PROBLEM 3: **Deficient Fluid Risk.** The expected outcome is that there is no risk at this time. The goal is met: Intake and output are balanced, and electrolytes are within normal limits.

Overall Evaluation

Based on the comparison of John's assessment at the beginning and at the end of the shift, it is evident that John is improving.

REFERENCES

Amerine, E. (2007). Get optimum outcomes for acute pancreatitis. Nursing2007 Critical Care, 2(2), 54–61.

Beers, M., Porter, R., Jones, T., Kaplan, J., & Berkwits, M. (Eds.). (2006). Pancreatitis. The MERCK Manual (18th ed., pp. 128–132). Whitehouse Station; NJ: Merck Research Laboratories.

Cole, L. (2002, May/June). Unraveling the mystery of acute pancreatitis. Dimension of Critical Care Nursing, 21(3), 86–89.

Giamouzis, G., Butler, J., Starling, R.C., et al. (2010). Impact of dopamine infusion on renal function in hospitalized heart failure patients: results of the Dopamine in Acute Decompensated Heart Failure (DAD-HF) Trial. Journal of Cardiac Failure, 16(12), 922–930. Retrieved from http://www.ncbi.nlm.nih.gov/pubmed/21111980

Gulanick, M., & Meyers J. (2013). Nursing care plans nursing diagnosis and intervention (8th ed.). St Louis, MO: Mosby.

Histology Laboratory Manual. Endocrine Pancreas—Islets of Langerhans. Retrieved from http://histologylab.ccnmtl.columbia.edu/lab17/pancreas_-_islets_of_langerhans.html

Holloway, N. (2004). Asthma. In Medical-Surgical Nursing Care Planning (4th ed., pp. 259–266). Philadelphia, PA: Lippincott Williams & Wilkins.

LeMone, P., & Bauldof, G. (2010). Medical surgical nursing: Critical thinking in client care (5th ed.). Menlo Park, CA: Benjamin Cummings.

Phillips, R. (2006, September/October). Inflammation gone wild, acute pancreatitis. Nursing Made Incredibly Easy, 4(5), 18–28.

Rodgers, S. (2008). Medical surgical nursing care plans. Clifton Park, NY: Thomson Delmar.

Sargent, S. (2006). Pathophysiology, diagnosis and management. British Journal of Nursing, 15(18), 999–1005.

Sommers, M., Johnson, S., & Beery, T. (2007). Diseases and disorders: a nursing therapeutics manual (3rd ed.). Philadelphia, PA: F.A. Davis.

Swearingen, P. (2008). All in one care planning resource (2nd ed.). St Louis, MO: Mosby.

Twedell, D. (2008, August). Clinical updates. Journal of Continuing Education in Nursing, 29(8), 10.

Up to date: Renal actions of dopamine. Retrieved from http://www.uptodate.com/contents/renal-actions-of-dopamine

Up to date: Treatment of acute pancreatitis. Retrieved from http://www.uptodate.com/contents/treatment-of-acute-pancreatitis

Van Leeuwen, A., & Bladh, M. (2015). Davis's comprehensive handbook of laboratory and diagnostic testing with nursing implications (6th ed.). Philadelphia, PA: F.A. Davis Company.

Venes, D., Fenton, B., Patwell, J., & Enright, A. (2009). Tabers cyclopedic medical dictionary (21st ed.). Philadelphia, PA: F.A. Davis.

Wilkinson, J., & Ahern, N. (2009). Nursing Diagnosis Handbook (9th ed.). Upper Saddle River, NJ: Prentice Hall.

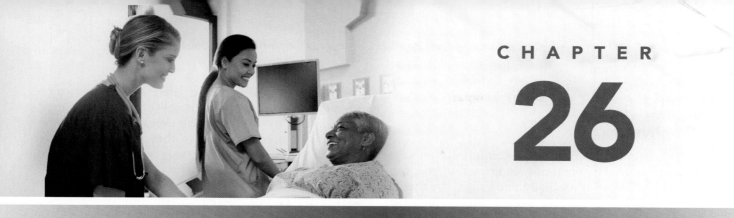

Female Genitourinary System and Breasts

Case Study: Endometriosis

Common Nursing Study Name	Section 1 Study	Section 1, Chapter Number
Biopsy	Laparoscopy, Gynecologic	Chapter 9
Cancer Antigen 125 (CA-125)	Cancer Antigens: CA 15-3, CA 19-9, CA 125, and Carcinoembryonic	Chapter 5
Complete Blood Count (CBC)	Complete Blood Count, Hematocrit	Chapter 2
	Complete Blood Count, Hemoglobin	Chapter 2
	Complete Blood Count, Platelet Count	Chapter 3
	Complete Blood Count, RBC Count	Chapter 2
	Complete Blood Count, RBC Indices	Chapter 2
	Complete Blood Count, RBC Morphology and Inclusions	Chapter 2
	Complete Blood Count, WBC Count and Differential	Chapter 2
Cultures (to rule out gonorrhea and chlamydia)	Culture, Bacterial, Anal/Genital, Ear, Eye, Skin, and Wound	Chapter 19
	Chlamydia Group Antibody, IgG and IgM	Chapter 5
HCG (Human Chorionic Gonadotropin)	Human Chorionic Gonadotropin	Chapter 1
Laparoscopy	Laparoscopy, Gynecologic	Chapter 9
Papanicolaou (PAP)	Papanicolaou Smear	Chapter 20
Pelvic Ultrasound	Ultrasound, Pelvis (Gynecologic, Nonobstetric)	Chapter 21
Prothrombin Time (PT) with International Normalized Ratio (INR)	Prothrombin Time and International Normalized Ratio	Chapter 3

STEP 1: DATA COLLECTION

Pathophysiology

Endometriosis is a hormonal and immune system disease characterized by an abnormal growth of endometrial tissue in places other than the lining of the uterus. Estimates indicate that this disease occurs in up to 15% of women of reproductive age between 30 and 40 years. Endometriosis can occur anywhere in the body but is typically found on or around the ovaries, cul-de-sac, cervix, rectovaginal septum, sigmoid colon, uterosacral ligaments, round ligaments, and pelvic peritoneum.

Endometriosis Severity

Endometriosis is a cyclic disease that responds to estrogen production with associated tissue swelling and inflammation. The severity of endometriosis is individualized. The disease can worsen with each successive menstrual cycle, with effects that range from being asymptomatic to experiencing crippling pain and infertility. The size of endometrial lesions varies from microscopic to large, with a dark reddish brown appearance. In general, endometriosis is considered to be a progressive disease that stops after menopause.

Causes of Endometriosis

The cause of endometriosis is unknown. What we do know is that by some mechanism, endometrial tissue ends up where it is not supposed to be. During a woman's reproductive years endometrial tissue that has planted itself where it does not belong responds to the same hormonal stimulation as does normal endometrial tissue within the uterus. The process of tissue growth followed by bleeding is a normal occurrence. For women with endometriosis the tissue implanted within the pelvic cavity also bleeds, draining into the peritoneal cavity. This causes pressure, inflammation, fibrosis, and adhesions that can lead to blockage or distortion of surrounding organs. Various thoughts on how endometrial tissue ends up inside the pelvic cavity include the following: (1) endometrial tissue spreads through the vascular and lymphatic system; (2) immature cells spread during a woman's embryonic phase while in the womb, showing up as metaplasma during adulthood; (3) by some unknown process, cells lining the peritoneum transform into metaplastic cells; and (4) due to a genetic family link.

A commonly accepted theory of how endometriosis occurs is by *retrograde menstruation*. Retrograde menstruation is a backflow of endometrial tissue from the uterus, through the fallopian tubes, and into the pelvic cavity. If this theory is true, then women with more frequent menstrual cycles or those with longer menstrual cycles are at greater risk. Many believe endometriosis to be a combination of these events. Whatever you believe the cause to be, the result is the same: pain, infertility, and dysmenorrhea.

Signs and Symptoms

Symptoms of endometriosis vary with the location of the implanted tissue. As stated earlier, the three classic symptoms associated with endometriosis are dysmenorrhea, dyspareunia, and infertility. These symptoms can vary in severity over time and may be constant or cyclical.

Pain

Dysmenorrhea is defined as pain associated with menstruation and is different from normal cramping. Pain is probably the most common symptom of endometriosis. Endometrial pain is thought to be associated with stimulation of tissue growth from estrogen and progesterone. The pain is described as a deep, aching, pressing, grinding pain located in the lower abdomen, low back, vagina, or posterior pelvis. There are also reports of painful bowel movements and heaviness or pressure in the pelvic area, which can increase in the presence of large masses.

Pain typically occurs a day or two prior to menstruation and can last up to 2–3 days, repeating each month during the menstrual cycle until after menopause. It is believed that the severity of the pain is associated with the location and depth of the infiltrating tissue. Deep implants in highly innervated areas are usually the most painful.

Dyspareunia is painful intercourse. The degree of pain can vary but is often worse with deep penetration. This can be very disruptive and embarrassing to those in an intimate relationship.

Infertility

Infertility is a serious concern for women with endometriosis. Even moderate endometriosis can contribute to pelvic adhesions, distorting pelvic anatomy and interfering with normal tubal and ovarian function. Endometriosis can destroy ovarian and tubular tissue, making conception difficult. Infertility is usually expected in women with significant damage to the reproductive organs. What is interesting is that women with minimal and mild endometriosis who present with normal pelvic anatomy except for a few lesions also have infertility problems—and no one knows why. One theory is that excessive peritoneal fluid secondary to the endometriosis interferes with the process of ovulation, ovum pick-up, and tubal function. Regardless of the cause, women diagnosed with this disease should have children as soon as possible. Up to 40% of women with fertility problems are diagnosed with endometriosis.

Other Physical Findings

Physical examination is an important step in the diagnosis of endometriosis. Completing the physical examination during the menstrual cycle can provide evidence of tender nodules associated with endometriosis. Examination may also show a cervix that is displaced to the right or left of midline. Palpation may disclose nodules in the uterosacral ligament, tenderness in the posterior fornix, restricted and/or painful movement of the uterus, a fixed and retroverted uterus, or ovarian enlargement. Caution should be used when completing a direct physical examination during acute flare-ups of endometriosis, because it can cause acute abdominal or suprapubic pain. Tissue implants may be seen during visual inspection located in incisions from episiotomy, or cesarean sections. A definitive diagnosis of endometriosis should not be made on visual inspection alone, because some patients have no abnormal physical findings.

A thorough history is another piece in the diagnosis of endometriosis. It is important to differentiate this disease from other likely options such as pelvic inflammatory disease, tumor, or ovarian cancer. The presentation of endometriosis can vary from patient to patient. Questions should be asked regarding menstruation as well as sexual and contraceptive practices. A detailed description of symptoms will assist in making a definitive diagnosis. Endometriosis can be strongly suspected with a solid history of infertility, dysmenorrhea, and dyspareunia. Endometriosis should always be suspected in women of productive years who present with complaints of pelvic pain and infertility.

Other reported symptoms include spotting, nausea, diarrhea, and bloody urine or stool. It cannot be emphasized enough that patient presentations vary from no symptoms to infertility only to devastating symptoms. There is little correlation between the degree of symptoms and the severity of the disease.

Laboratory Studies

There are no laboratory studies that definitively diagnose endometriosis. However, there are studies that can point in that direction and rule out other possibilities. Cancer antigen 125 is a small molecule that appears on the surface of abnormal cells. A normal finding is 0–35 units/mL. Because elevated levels are associated with various gynecological and nongynecological conditions, CA-125 is not considered to be a useful tool in diagnosing endometriosis. However, elevated levels of this antigen are directly correlated with the severity of the disease and can be useful in assessing the effectiveness of treatment and in the diagnosis of ovarian cancer. Cultures can be done to rule out gonorrhea and chlamydia. A pregnancy test for hCG (human chorionic gonadotropin) levels should be completed to check for pregnancy prior to beginning treatment. Completion of a complete blood count (CBC) with WBC count and differential to evaluate for infection and hemoglobin (Hgb)/hematocrit (Hct) to check for anemia is valuable information.

Diagnostic Studies

Diagnostic studies are more useful tools to identify endometriosis than are laboratory studies. Laparoscopy or laparotomy provides evidence of the presence or absence of ectopic tissue by direct visualization. Normal results show no visualization of ectopic tissue. Abnormal results show visualization of endometrial tissue and confirm a diagnosis of endometriosis. This procedure can be accompanied by biopsy. Biopsy is used to evaluate malignancy of the endometrial tissue. A normal finding would be benign tissue, which confirms the diagnosis of endometriosis. Malignancy would be cancer. Biopsy may be necessary to confirm suspicions. Papanicolaou (PAP) smear may be taken to rule out other medical problems, and a pelvic ultrasound may be done to rule out fibroids and reveal the extent of the disease.

General/Medical Management

Because the discussion of the effects of endometriosis will include reproduction and sexual relations, it is important to be aware of the cultural and ethnic influences associated with each patient situation. Careful education of the cause of the disease and treatment options is important. Factors that will give direction to the plan of care are the severity of symptoms, desire for fertility, and degree of disease. A combination of interventions can be chosen to meet each patient's therapeutic goals. Management is usually completed on an outpatient basis unless there is some reason for admission, such as surgery.

Generally, treatment can be placed into two categories. Women who want to have children and those who do not. Because infertility is a concern, those who wish to have children should be instructed to begin their family as soon as possible. There are two benefits from this, first the women have the children that are desired. Second, pregnancy and lactation suppress the menstrual cycle, which in turn can shrink implanted endometrial tissue. This has been known to provide relief for symptoms for years after the pregnancy.

Women with endometriosis who are not having children or are nearing menopause are usually treated as symptoms arise. If there are no symptoms, no treatment will be provided other than monitoring the progression of the disease to start treatment, if necessary.

Endometriosis can cause significant pain with sexual intercourse. Encouragement should be provided for the couple to discuss the disease and its effect on their relationship as well as collaborate on acceptable interventions.

Surgical Interventions

The goal of surgery is to seek and destroy all endometrial tissue and remove all adhesions while maintaining reproductive function. Surgery should be offered as an option in women with adnexal masses, symptoms which are unresponsive to treatment, or if fertility is to be maintained. If surgery becomes necessary, there are two types of surgical options available—conservative and definitive.

A conservative surgical approach is used for women who wish to maintain reproductive function. Conservative surgery is performed by laser during a laparoscopy or laparotomy. Carbon dioxide laparoscopy is used to vaporize endometrial tissue and is useful for women with minimal to moderate endometriosis. Laparoscopic surgery is used most often for women with multiple implants and adhesions. Laser ablation or electrocautery of adhesions may be an option. Assisted reproduction is a viable option for women with endometriosis who wish to have children.

Definitive surgery is used for women who no longer wish to have children, the symptoms are severe and unmanageable by medical means, or the disease has seriously affected bowel and bladder function. Definitive surgery, the only real cure for endometriosis, is a hysterectomy with bilateral salpingo-oopherectomy and removal of all endometrial lesions. All other interventions provide relief only, not a cure. A presacral neurectomy can be performed in women with severe debilitating pain that does not respond to other therapeutic treatments.

Pharmacological Interventions

One of the best ways to treat endometriosis is to interrupt and/or decrease the swelling and bleeding of implanted endometrial tissue. This can be achieved through pharmacologic means by interrupting the cyclic process of tissue stimulation and bleeding associated with monthly menstrual cycles. Medications can be used to create a state of pseudopregnancy, pseudomenopause, or chronic anovulation. However, recurrence of endometriosis after completion of pharmacologic management occurs in up to 50% of women. Table 26.1 provides information about specific medications.

Nonpharmacological Interventions

Nonpharmacologic interventions that have shown some success are lying on the side with knees bent to relieve cramping, warm baths, a heating pad (or other warming device) to the lower abdomen (be careful of burning), herbal teas, yoga, and biofeedback.

Psychosocial Interventions

There are no preventative strategies for endometriosis. Psychosocial interventions may be necessary due to emotional effects of this disease. Women should be assessed for depression associated with chronic pain. Hormonal changes can contribute to mood swings and loss of libido. Continued pain during intercourse can have a detrimental effect on sexual relations.

Complications

There are very few true complications for endometriosis. The most common complication is infertility associated with scarring and adhesions due to bleeding from atypical endometrial tissue. Adhesions in the pelvic cavity can fix the uterus in a retroverted position and block fallopian tubes, thus preventing conception. Endometriosis can also contribute to anemia and spontaneous abortion. Renal function may be impaired if ureters become obstructed. Ovarian torsion or rupture can occur, contributing to peritonitis.

Depression is another complication of concern due to the long-term chronic nature of the disease. Pain, interference in activities of daily living, impaired sexual function, and fertility concerns can contribute to depression.

Patient Education

Sexuality and intimacy are very personal and private topics for many people. Some cultures do not discuss this with others. The big educational issues are pain management and medical and surgical interventions. Consideration should be given to the emotional impact of this disease and ways to provide education that will encourage collaboration with social services and support groups for chronic conditions.

TABLE 26.1 *Medications to Treat Endometriosis*

Medication	Dose	Action	Rationale
Hormonal Therapy: Goal is to interrupt the cycle of endometrial tissue stimulation and bleeding			
Progestins			
Medroxyprogesterone acetate (Provera)	10–30 mg daily for 6–9 months	Shrinkage and resorption of endometrial implants	Suppresses cyclic hormonal fluctuations
(Depo-Provera)	100 mg IM every 2 weeks for four doses, followed by 200 mg IM monthly for 4 months	Creates a hypoestrogenic environment	Used for women who have mild to moderate endometriosis
Norethindrone	5 mg daily		
Megestrol acetate	40 mg daily		
Danazol (Danocrine)	400–800 mg per day in two divided doses for about 6–9 months	Synthetic androgenic steroid similar to testosterone Resorption of endometrial implants Suppresses endometrial growth	Induces amenorrhea Creates a hypo-estrogen environment preventing the growth of endometrial tissue Used for women with mild to moderate endometriosis Return to fertility Relieves pain
Nafarelin (Synarel)	Metered nasal spray twice daily 400–800 mg for 6 months	Gonadotropin-releasing hormone (GnRH) agonist Decreases secretion of FSH and LH Creates a hypoestrogenic environment	Restricts hormone production, suppresses endometrial implants
Gonadotropin-releasing hormone	Administered for 3–6 months	Creates a pseudomenopause	Relief of pain Resorption of endometrial implants Return to fertility
Ethylnorgestrienone (Gestrinone)	2.5 mg two to three times a week	Suppression of and resorption of endometrial tissue Amenorrhea	Pain relief Return to fertility
Leuprolide (Lupron)	3.75 mg IM monthly, or 11.25 mg every 3 months	Gonadotropin-releasing hormone (GnRH) agonist	Restricts hormone production, suppresses endometrial implants
Goserelin (Zoladex)	3.6 mg SQ monthly for 6 months	Gonadotropin-releasing hormone (GnRH) agonist	Restricts hormone production, suppresses endometrial implants
Aromatase (Anastrozole)	1 mg or 2.5 mg daily	Interferes with the conversion of androgen to estrogen	Interferes with growth of endometrial tissue
Oral contraceptives			
Ethinyl estradiol	35 mcg	Suppresses cyclic hormonal response of endometrial implants	Pain relief
Norethindrone	0.35–0.5 mg		Suppression and resorption of endometrial tissue
Conjugated estrogens	1.25 mg daily for 2 weeks or 2.5 mg daily for 1 week	Creates an androgen effect by using small amounts of estrogen and large amounts of progestin	Return to fertility
Analgesic therapy: Goal is to relive pain and decrease inflammation			
Acetaminophen	650–1000 mg		Pain relief, preferable to NSAIDS to decrease bleeding risk
NSAIDS			
Ibuprofen	200–800 mg qid	Anti-inflammatory	Relief of dysmenorrhea
Naproxen	550 mg tid		

STEP 2: POTENTIAL PROBLEMS/ DIAGNOSES

It is important that nurses understand and consider the science of the disease process and consider the possibilities prior to applying that knowledge to a patient situation. We begin that process with questioning.

💬 *Question:* Based upon your review of the content presented, what possible *potential problems* would you expect for a patient with these diagnoses?

💬 *Answer:* Pain, anxiety, disputed sexuality, reduced self-esteem, and depression

STEP 3: POTENTIAL INTERVENTION AND EXPECTED OUTCOME

💬 *Question:* Based upon your identification of patient problems, what possible interventions would you recommend for these diagnoses, and what would you expect to happen? This would be considered your "grocery list" of the possible actions you could use to assist your patient.

💬 *Answer:* See the following problems, interventions, and expected outcomes:

Problem	Interventions	Expected Outcome
Pain	• Administer medication to decrease pain and medication to decrease hormone secretion, thereby also decreasing pain. • Use nonpharmacologic measures to decrease pain, such as a heating pad, positioning, imagery, and relaxation techniques. • Provide education on the cause of the pain.	Pain level acceptable to the patient
Anxiety	• Encourage the patient's expression of feelings. • Answer all questions about treatment and fertility concerns honestly. • Discuss the benefit of having children sooner rather than later. • Provide education about monitoring fertility, such as basal body temperature.	Patient experiences decreased anxiety to a manageable level
Disrupted Sexuality	• Suggest alternate positions for intercourse. • Encourage the discussion of intimacy concerns. • Recommend counseling/referral as appropriate. • Educate the patient about the relationship from painful intercourse to disease pathology. • Allow for a release of grief as a result of a potential loss of intimacy. • Assess the patient's feelings and coping strategies. • Discuss the efficacy of medications relative to decreasing the pain associated with intercourse.	Psychological healing, with a collaborative effort in a plan of action to decrease painful intercourse
Self-Esteem	• Include the patient in treatment planning. • Provide clear answers regarding medications and the disease process. • Assist the patient in making informed choices. • Encourage rest and nutrition. • Provide emotional support. • Encourage a discussion regarding fertility concerns. • Prepare for potential surgery.	Patient has increased involvement in care and decisions, and verbalizes increased self-esteem
Depression	• Assist the patient to adapt to stressors. • Facilitate the use of analgesics to manage pain. Monitor the effectiveness of pain management. • Assess nutritional intake. • Consider recommending psychiatric evaluation. Recommend the support of social services. • Provide positive reinforcement. • Support the identification and use of coping strategies. • Monitor sleep patterns.	Patient shows improved melancholy and adaptation

PUTTING IT ALL TOGETHER: APPLICATION OF THE NURSING PROCESS

Putting it all together is where the art and science of nursing meet to provide the best patient outcomes. We take the possibilities and place them into the context of the patient situation. To accomplish this, we use nursing diagnosis, nursing interventions, nursing outcomes, and nursing theory to provide the palate for nursing care.

STEP 4: ASSESSMENT

PATIENT INFORMATION: Lucy Nguyen, a 35-year-old female, married

CHIEF COMPLAINT: Painful intercourse, persistent infertility

HISTORY OF THE PRESENT ILLNESS: Painful intercourse which has worsened progressively, unable to conceive after 2 years without birth control

PAST MEDICAL HISTORY: None

FAMILY HISTORY: Mother is a breast cancer survivor, father is deceased

CHART REVIEW AND REPORT: Lucy was admitted for a laparoscopy with possible laser ablation and resection. The physician suspects that Lucy has endometriosis based upon physical examination and a history of painful menstruation, painful intercourse, and infertility. Conservative treatment in the form of oral contraceptives has been offered by the physician but rejected by the family. The previous nurse reports that Lucy's surgery has been delayed at her husband Jason's request. Jason is on the way into the hospital to speak with his wife. On the phone Jason seemed to be upset and was curt with the nurse who took the message. Lucy is NPO except for ibuprofen with a sip of water. You are told that she barely slept last night and has been uncommunicative, refusing pain medication when offered. Lucy's appetite has been poor, eating less than 25% of each meal.

SUBJECTIVE ASSESSMENT: As you enter the room you see Lucy sitting on a chair looking out of the window with a grimace on her face and a protective hand over her abdomen. *"Good morning, my name is Arvin James and I will be your nurse today, how are you feeling?"* "I am fine," replies Lucy without looking up. AJ continues, *"You look worried, is there anything you want to discuss?"* "No, nothing, my husband is on the way in, did you know that?" *"Yes,"* replies AJ, *"your last nurse told me. Are you worried about your husband coming?"* AJ asks. Lucy just shrugs and does not answer. AJ decides to change the subject, asking, *"Are you in any pain?"* "No," Lucy replies. AJ continues, *"You do have pain medication ordered if you need it."* "I know," Lucy responds without making eye contact. *"You do have that heating pad that you can use if you don't want to take any pain medication,"* Lucy just shrugs without responding. AJ asks, *"Are you aware that your husband called in and requested your surgery be postponed?"* "No," Lucy responds. AJ continues, *"Until we know more, I would like you to continue to abstain from eating or drinking."* "OK," Lucy responds, "I'm not hungry anyway."

OBJECTIVE ASSESSMENT: Lucy is alert, oriented, and withdrawn; efforts to draw her out into conversation are unsuccessful. It is obvious that she is concerned about something. Physical assessment is normal except for some abdominal tenderness. Lucy denies pain, but you observed some facial grimace during palpation. You also notice that Lucy places her hand protectively over her abdomen. Vital signs are BP of 110/60 mm Hg, an apical pulse of 82 beats per minute, respirations of 16 breaths per minute, and a temperature of 98.4°F.

- *Laboratory Studies:*
  - Hgb: 9.8 g/dL
  - Hct: 29.6%
  - WBC: 7.8×10^3/microL
  - Pregnancy test negative
  - INR: 1.5
- *Diagnostic Studies:*
  - Preoperative pelvic ultrasound shows possible endometrial tissue with small submucous fibroids
- *Medications:*
  - Ibuprofen 800 mg PO every 8 hr prn has been ordered for moderate abdominal pain

STEP 5: REALITY CHECK: DETOUR AHEAD

Reality Check occurs when the nurse takes a moment to think about individualized patient information that needs to be considered in framing diagnoses and interventions. This information is retrievable from any legitimate source (family, case management, other nurses, any ancillary, physician, etc.). These are the "wrenches" that create challenging situations (culture, religion, socioeconomic status, level of education, developmental level, marital status, employment, age, and gender).

Psychosocial History

Lucy Nguyen and her husband, Jason, met through a social network. After corresponding for more than a year, Jason went to Vietnam to meet Lucy. Following their marriage in Vietnam 3 years ago, Lucy immigrated to the United States. Jason's view of family is very traditional. He believes that the husband is the head of the home and makes all major decisions. Lucy cares for the home, and Jason supports the family. Jason fully expects his wife to agree with all of his decisions. Both Lucy and Jason are Catholic. Lucy believes that her illness and inability to conceive are punishment for being prideful. Lucy has recently refused to have intimate relations with her husband due to painful intercourse, which put a strain on their relationship. She feels these things make her a failure as a woman and a wife.

Critical Thinking Moment

You have just completed the assessment of Lucy Nguyen and need to make a decision about the patient's *actual* problems and nursing diagnoses based on the data you have collected and the potential problems you identified. Outcomes must be realistic and measurable.

STEP 6: ACTUAL PROBLEMS/DIAGNOSES

The *first step* in problem identification is to revisit the list of *potential diagnoses* and choose *actual diagnoses* based upon the learner's evaluation of the case study information provided. A problem statement must be completed for each identified problem/diagnosis. The actual problems for this case study are pain, depression, and self-esteem.

STEP 7: PLANNING: ACTUAL INTERVENTIONS

After actual diagnoses have been chosen, it is necessary to evaluate the list of *potential interventions* and choose *actual interventions* that will fit within the patient's reality and meet expected outcomes. Each intervention requires a rationale. Interventions are identified in three categories: (1) assessment, (2) therapeutic, and (3) education.

Diagnostic Statement

Pain related to swelling and inflammation during the menstrual cycle secondary to hormonal stimulation of the implantation of ectopic tissue as evidenced by visual facial grimace and abdominal guarding.

Assessment

- Assess pain using a pain scale. *Rationale: This allows you to assess the intensity of pain.*

- Assess the physical signs of pain. *Rationale: Lucy may not verbalize pain due to a culture of stoicism.*
- Assess for abdominal tenderness and guarding. *Rationale: These symptoms are associated with disease progression.*

Therapeutic Interventions

- Administer ibuprofen 800 mg as ordered. *Rationale: This decreases inflammation and relieves pain.*
- Encourage use of a heating pad to the abdomen. *Rationale: Heat can decrease abdominal pain.*
- Encourage a position of comfort. *Rationale: Moving to a new position may decrease pain.*

Education

- Teach relaxation techniques. *Rationale: Relaxation may assist in managing pain.*
- Explain the purpose of analgesic use. *Rationale: This addresses addiction concerns, if any exist.*
- Explain the causes of pain. *Rationale: This enhances Lucy's understanding of the disease process.*

Expected Outcome

- The reduced pain level will be acceptable to Lucy.

Diagnostic Statement

Depression related to a sense of hopelessness secondary to chronic pain and failure to conceive as evidenced by withdrawal and melancholy

Assessment

- Assess for the presence of coping strategies. *Rationale: This allows you to evaluate areas of needed support and the types of strategies used.*
- Assess for the effectiveness of coping strategies. *Rationale: This allows you to assess the need for a change in approach to meet coping challenges.*
- Assess affect and effort at communication. *Rationale: This allows you to evaluate Lucy's emotional status.*

Therapeutic Interventions

- Record accurate intake and output. *Rationale: Depression may lead to anorexia.*
- Request a psychiatric consult. *Rationale: Doing so provides a supportive intervention for hopelessness and depression.*
- Request a social service visit. *Rationale: Explore the efficacy of support groups in meeting Lucy's emotional needs.*

Education

- Importance of pain management. *Rationale: This helps to improve Lucy's understanding of how pain management can assist in meeting health management goals.*

- Overall plan of care with expected outcome. *Rationale: Collaboration with the plan of care can improve patient satisfaction and promote positive outcomes.*
- Benefits of support groups. *Rationale: The support of those with similar medical conditions can assist in meeting emotional needs.*

Expected Outcome

- Lucy will exhibit a reduction of melancholy with increased participation in the plan of care.

Diagnostic Statement

Altered self-esteem related to failure to conceive and perceived altered sexuality as evidenced by stated feelings of failure, and self-blame

Assessment

- Assess Lucy's understanding of the treatment plan. *Rationale: Collaboration with Lucy increases the chance of success.*
- Assess Lucy's understanding of the cause of infertility. *Rationale: Evaluate Lucy's understanding of her disease to establish a baseline for education and areas of support.*
- Assess personal strengths and emotional lability. *Rationale: This allows you to evaluate the appropriateness of openly addressing fertility concerns and a sense of blame.*

Therapeutic Interventions

- Encourage discussion regarding fertility concerns. *Rationale: This allows for the evaluation of self-blame and to assist in making informed choices.*
- Provide emotional support. *Rationale: This step assists in coping during emotional stressful times.*
- Prepare for surgery, with information on expected outcome related to improved fertility. *Rationale: This ensures that Lucy understands the risk and benefits of surgery as explained by the physician prior to surgery.*

Education

- Reinforce surgery benefits and risks as outlined by the physician. *Rationale: Lucy may not have understood all of the information presented by the physician.*
- Educate Lucy about the importance of rest and adequate nutrition. *Rationale: Understanding may improve compliance with activity and nutrition requirements.*
- Educate Lucy about medications and the disease process. *Rationale: Understanding the purpose of the prescribed medication in relation to the disease process may improve compliance with health management.*

Expected Outcome

- Diminished self-blame and improving self-esteem

STEP 8: IMPLEMENTATION

Nursing Theory

Ernestine Wiedenbach believes the role of the nurse is to help the patient. Therefore, it is necessary to be aware of the realities of care situations such as culture, age, and view of health. Care should be compassionate with emotional support for both Jason and Lucy while dealing with this sensitive health issue. It will be important to identify expected outcomes and use them as a measure of success while collaborating with the family. Nursing care should be professional regardless of personal views.

Ancillary Support

Ancillary support will be tricky. Lucy and Jason may not want to discuss such a private and personal subject with outsiders. The best approach may be to provide information and let them decide what to do with it. Proactive action from social services will be necessary, and more than one attempt may be necessary. Cultural considerations will be required for any measure of success.

STEP 9: PLAN OF CARE

The plan of care is a road map for patient care and should be used as a communication tool among disciplines. Expected entries on the plan of care would be each identified problem: pain, depression, and altered self-esteem. There is a definitive cultural aspect to Lucy's care that must be addressed. It is evident that Jason is the decision maker, and Lucy will follow her husband's lead. It is possible that Jason will become upset if health-care decisions are discussed with his wife before he is approached as head of the household. This must be noted in the plan of care. It is also evident that Lucy is in pain but is not going to ask for medication. Pain management may be better addressed by around-the-clock administration of ibuprofen. A comment can be made on the plan of care to suggest this approach.

STEP 10: EVALUATION

Evaluation is an active process in which the nurse "connects the dots" to decide if the expected outcomes (goals) that were established have been met, partially met, or not met. If the goals are met, we continue with the plan as outlined. If the goal was partially met, we revise the parts of the plan that did not work. If the goals were not met, we start all over with a new plan.

End-of-Shift Narrative

As you are going down the hall, you hear what sounds like glass breaking from Lucy's room. You enter the room and see a white-faced Lucy dressed in her street clothes, sitting in a chair, facing her husband who is standing beside the bed. There is broken glass on the floor; it appears to have been a religious icon of some kind. You recognize it as the one that Lucy's friend brought in earlier during your shift. You ask, *"Is everything alright, Lucy?"* Lucy does not answer you but continues to stare at her husband. Finally, her husband looks at you and says, "She is fine. Call the doctor and let him know we are going home." You ask, *"Can you tell me what the problem is? Maybe I can help."* Lucy finally looks at you and says, "No one can help me; this is my fault." Jason continues with irritation, "We don't need any help…we can solve this on our own. Just call the doctor so we can get out of here." You ask, *"Have you changed your mind about having the surgery?"* Lucy will not meet your eyes. "Yes, we have changed our minds," Jason says in a tight voice. You ask, *"Lucy is there anything I can do?"* "No," she whispers brokenly. "Just call the doctor so we can go." Impatiently, Jason turns to Lucy, saying, "Just get your things; we are leaving now." You look at Jason and ask, *"Can I get the doctor on the phone? Maybe you would like to talk to him about your concerns."* "We have already spoken. He knows my mind, and I know his. We are leaving," Jason returns bitingly. "Look," Jason continues, "It doesn't matter anymore… we are leaving. He can call me at home if he wants to." Jason holds a hand out to Lucy saying, "Come on Lucy, let's go." You interrupt him, saying, *"Sir, if you leave without being discharged, you are leaving against medical advice [AMA]. I need to inform the doctor and have you sign yourself out."* Jason bristles, "Okay—get the papers. I will sign them, and then we are leaving." As you are leaving the room you notice that Lucy is holding a hand over her abdomen and grimacing as if in pain. While you go to get the AMA forms, you ask the charge nurse to contact Lucy's physician, but he is unreachable. Lucy and her husband leave, Lucy softly crying on the way out. The surgery is canceled, and when the physician calls in, he is briefed on what occurred.

Problem Evaluation

Because of Jason's insistence that they must leave, none of Lucy's goals were met. Lucy would not accept the offered pain medication or use the heating pad. It was very apparent that she was despondent, and Jason was angry. Unfortunately for AJ, he is unable to prevent the departure of the patient, and without speaking to the physician, has no understanding of why Jason reacted this way.

Overall Evaluation

Based on the comparison of Lucy's assessment at the beginning and at the end of the shift, it is evident that Lucy is declining. There was something we missed, and the patient left AMA.

REFERENCES

American College of Obstetricians and Gynecologists (ACOG). (2010, July). Practice bulletin, no. 114: Management of endometriosis. Obstetrics and Gynecology, 116(1), 223–234.

Applebaum, H. (2010, August). Membranous dysmenorrhea: A complication of treatment for endometriosis. *Obstetrics and Gynecology*, 116(2), 488–490.

Berek, J. S. (Ed.). (2002). In: Novak's gynecology (13th ed., pp. 935–957). Philadelphia, PA: Lippincott Williams & Wilkins.

DeCherney, A., Nathan, L., Goodwin, M., & Laufer, N. (2007). In: Current diagnosis and treatment obstetrics and gynecology (10th ed., pp. 712–719). New York, NY: McGraw-Hill.

George, J. (2010). Nursing theories: the base for professional nursing practice (6th ed.). Upper Saddle River, NJ: Pearson.

Gulanick, M., & Meyers J. (2013). Nursing care plans: nursing diagnosis and intervention (8th ed.). St Louis, MO: Mosby.

Guarnaccia, M., Silverberg, K., & Olive, D. (2007). Endometriosis and adenomyosis. In: Copeland, L. J., Jarrel, J. F., and McGregor, J. A. (Eds.), Textbook of gynecology (2nd ed., pp. 687–710). Philadelphia, PA: W. B. Saunders.

Holloway, N. (2004). Medical-surgical nursing care planning (4th ed.). Philadelphia , PA: Lippincott Williams & Wilkins.

LeMone, P., Burke, K., & Baldoff, G. (2011). Medical surgical nursing. Critical thinking in patient care (5th ed.). Upper Saddle River, NJ: Pearson.

Rodgers, S. (2008). Medical surgical nursing care plans. Clifton Park, NY: Thomson Delmar.

Van Leeuwen, A., & Bladh, M. (2015). Davis's comprehensive handbook of laboratory and diagnostic testing with nursing implications (6th ed.). Philadelphia, PA: F.A. Davis Company.

Wilkinson, J., & Ahern, N. (2009). In: Nursing diagnosis handbook (9th ed.). Saddle River, NJ: Prentice Hall.

Wilson, B., Shannon, M., & Stang, C. (2006). Nurses drug guide. Upper Saddle River, NJ: Prentice Hall.

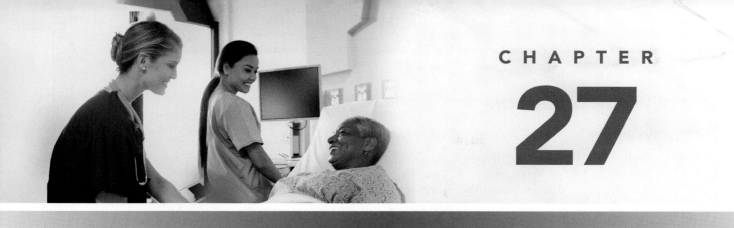

27

Genitourinary System: Male

Case Study: Benign Prostatic Hyperplasia

Common Nursing Study Name	Section 1 Study	Section 1 Chapter Number
Abdominal Ultrasound	Ultrasound, Abdomen	Chapter 21
Abdominal X-Rays, Plain (KUB)	Kidney, Ureter, and Bladder Study	Chapter 16
Blood Sugar	Glucose	Chapter 1
Creatinine (Serum)	Creatinine, Blood	Chapter 1
Cystoscopy	Cystoscopy	Chapter 9
DRE (Digital Rectal Examination)	Ultrasound, Prostate (Transrectal)	Chapter 21
Electrolytes	Carbon Dioxide Chloride, Blood Potassium, Blood Sodium, Blood	Chapter 1 Chapter 1 Chapter 1 Chapter 1
Hematocrit (Hct) and Hemoglobin (Hgb)	Complete Blood Count, Hematocrit Complete Blood Count, Hemoglobin	Chapter 2 Chapter 2
Intravenous Pyelogram (IVP)	Intravenous Pyelography	Chapter 15
Pelvic Ultrasonography	Ultrasound, Abdomen Ultrasound, Bladder	Chapter 21 Chapter 21
Postvoid Residual	Cystometry	Chapter 11
Prostate-Specific Antigen (PSA)	Prostate-Specific Antigen	Chapter 5
Oxygen Saturation (Pulse Oximetry)	Pulse Oximetry	Chapter 14
Transrectal Ultrasound (TRUS)	Ultrasound, Prostate (Transrectal)	Chapter 21
Urinalysis	Urinalysis	Chapter 22
Urine Flow Study	Cystometry	Chapter 11

STEP 1: DATA COLLECTION

Pathophysiology

The truth about benign prostatic hyperplasia (BPH) is that no one really knows what causes it. The three most popular theories that explore the whys and wherefores of BPH involve hormones, age, and genetics. Many consider BPH to be a normal part of a man's aging process. Estimates are that 50% of men at age 50 and 80% of men at age 80 have some degree of BPH. As a young boy, the prostate gland is about the size of a pea. As boys grow up, the prostate grows to the size of a walnut. About age 25, the prostate has a growing spurt with the normal healthy prostate weighing about 20 g. This remains 20 g unless and until BPH develops.

Normal prostate growth is linked to the release of the hormone dihydrotestosterone (DHT), which occurs as boys mature into adulthood. The *hormone theory* for BHP is that as men age, the ongoing production of DHT encourages cell growth, resulting in an enlarged prostate. Others suggest that DHT levels in prostate tissue are no different in men with or without BPH.

The *aging theory* focuses on the production of testosterone and estrogen. Men normally produce both. The belief is that as men age, the level of testosterone decreases and the level of estrogen increases, resulting in prostate growth.

The *genetic theory* is that a cellular glitch reboots prostate growth in middle age, mimicking the initial prostate growth of their youth. There is some evidence that BPH runs in families, so if a father has been diagnosed, a son's risk increases fourfold. Of these three suggested causes of BPH, the aging theory is the most popular choice. However, no one really knows for sure; it could be a combination of factors. Whatever reason, the outcome is essentially the same. The prostate grows and presses on the urethra, causing uncomfortable urinary symptoms. Diagnosis is made based on the patient's history and evaluation of the urinary tract. Men will complain of the bladder not emptying completely, a weak urinary stream, nocturia, hesitancy, frequency, and urgency. BPH is a growth of hyperplastic tissue which compresses the urethra, causing urinary flow problems of varying degrees.

Laboratory Studies

Prostate-specific antigen (PSA) is considered to be a screening tool for cancer in men with BPH. There has been a lot of discussion regarding the efficacy of PSA screening. The general consensus is that when there is a concern, the patient and physician should have a discussion regarding the benefits versus risks based on the patient's individual circumstances. When to screen is dependent on at-risk status. Consideration of PSA screening for those at average risk is recommended at age 50. Higher-risk patients with a first-degree family history of cancer prior to the age of 65, or of African American descent should consider PSA screening beginning at age 45. Those at highest risk who have more than one first-degree relative with prostate cancer younger than the age of 65 should consider screenings beginning at age 40. Re-screening every 2 to 4 years or sooner may be considered based on individual circumstances and patient physician collaboration. Serum creatinine level and urinalysis are used to rule out infection, kidney problems, or urinary insufficiency as the cause. If the lab results are positive, it may be necessary to complete an abdominal ultrasound to distinguish between obstructive urinary causes, infection, and kidney problems. Urinalysis is also used to evaluate for hematuria. If more than five red blood cells are seen on visual examination of the urine sample, the patient should be evaluated for cancer.

Diagnostic Studies

There are several diagnostic studies that help to diagnose BHP, some are simple and some are more complex. In all cases, the possibility of prostate cancer should be considered.

Digital Rectal Exam

The simplest form of prostate evaluation is the digital rectal exam (DRE), which should be completed on all men over the age of 50. Rectal exams provide the physician with information regarding prostate size and presence of large lesions. Rectal exams are not useful for identification of lesions smaller than 1.5 cm.

Urine Flow Study

Urine flow study is another simple test that evaluates the speed of urination. The patient simply urinates into a device that measures how fast the urine comes out. The average rate of flow is age dependent. Men ages 46 to 65 have an average flow rate of 12 mL/sec, those age 66 to 80 have an average flow rate of 9 mL/sec. The slower the speed, the higher is the chance of urinary problems.

Transrectal Ultrasound

More complex evaluative tools are a little more invasive. Transrectal ultrasound (TRUS) is performed when prostate cancer is expected. An ultrasound probe is placed inside the rectum and sound waves create a screen image of the size and shape of the prostate. Rectal ultrasound can be completed if the cause of BPH is not clear and cancer is suspected.

Intravenous Pyelogram (IVP)

Intravenous pyelogram (IVP) is an invasive procedure wherein intravenously injected contrast provides visual images about the urinary tract such as obstruction or narrowing. Multiple images are taken to record any abnormal information.

Postvoid Residual

To evaluate bladder emptying, a postvoid residual can be done to measure how much urine is left in the bladder after the patient voids. Completion of this test requires catheterization of the patient directly after voiding. The amount remaining is measured and reported as the postvoid or residual urine. Bladder scanning is a noninvasive evaluation of residual urine. Normal postvoid residual is less than 30 to 50 mL of urine.

Cystoscopy

When direct visual examination is needed, a cystoscopy should be completed. A cystoscopy allows the physician to visually examine the prostate for size and/or obstruction by inserting a tiny lighted lens into the urethra. Pelvic ultrasonography of the abdomen and bladder and plain abdominal x-rays are useful to evaluate for bladder calculus, or obstruction of kidneys or ureters.

General/Medical Management

There are three primary approaches to managing BPH: (1) watchful waiting, (2) administering medications to decrease prostate size, and (3) performing invasive procedures.

Watchful Waiting

"Watchful waiting" is a phrase commonly associated with BPH when discussing disease management, and this means that before we use drugs or invasive procedures, let's wait and see what happens. Sometimes patients will find that the symptoms improve without any intervention. A way to evaluate the severity of symptoms is by using a questionnaire called the American Urological Association Symptom Index (AUSI) (also known as the IPSS, the International Prostate Symptom Score). The AUSI questionnaire is designed to help make decisions about the severity of symptoms and provide direction to appropriate treatment. AUSI uses a series of seven questions that look at individual symptoms over a 30-day period. The questions focus on frequency, nocturia, urgency, hesitancy, intermittence, speed of urinary stream, and complete bladder emptying. The results of the AUSI scoring system are as follows: 0 to 7 indicates mild BPH; 8 to 19 indicates moderate BPH; and 20 to 35 indicates severe BPH. Watchful waiting is recommended for patients with a score of 0 to 7. A voiding diary is useful in keeping a record of urinary frequency and severity of complaints, and may assist the physician in determining the best course of treatment.

Pharmacological Management

Pharmacological management focuses on decreasing the size of the prostate and improving urinary flow. Medications are used before invasive therapies are considered. Alpha-adrenergic antagonists are more effective for short-term treatment of BPH; 5-alpha-reductase inhibitors are more effective for long-term therapy. Both reduce the need for surgery. It has been suggested that the use of medication from both classes is more beneficial to the patient than exclusive use of one or the other.

ANTIANDROGENS AND ALPHA-1 ADRENERGIC BLOCKERS: Hyperplasic tissue is androgen dependent. Antiandrogens (5-alpha-reductase) convert testosterone to DHT, which shrinks the prostate and the tissue around the prostate. The two approved drugs of this class are finasteride and dutasteride. Finasteride is frequently prescribed as 5 mg daily for BPH. It is estimated that use of finasteride may decrease the need for surgery by 55%. Dutasteride is administered as 0.5 mg daily and should not be handled by pregnant women. Alpha-1 adrenergic blockers act by releasing the smooth muscle of the bladder and prostate, which improves urine flow. Prescribed medications are terazosin, alfuzosin, doxazosin mesylate, and tamsulosin. This class of medications has been found to improve mild BPH symptoms in about 70% of patients. Side effects of these medications include dizziness, hypotension, headache, and fatigue.

TERAZOSIN: Terazosin lowers blood pressure and should be taken at bedtime. The recommended dosage of terazosin is 1 to 10 mg/day. Side effects include postural hypotension, drowsiness, headache, dizziness, impotence, and weight gain. Dosage will be advanced based on effectiveness.

DOXAZOSIN: Doxazosin mesylate should also be given at bedtime. The initial dose is 1 mg which is then titrated up to a maximum dose of 8 mg a day. Side effects include postural hypotension, edema, drowsiness, and dizziness.

TAMSULOSIN: Tamsulosin is considered to be more urinary specific than the other alpha-1-adrenergic blockers. The recommended dosage of Tamsulosin is 0.4 to 0.8 mg taken 30 minutes after the same meal daily. Side effects include postural hypotension, dizziness, headache, drowsiness, and impotence.

HERBAL REMEDIES: Herbal remedies for BPH include saw palmetto, pygeum africanum, and stinging nettles. The most commonly used herbal remedies are saw palmetto and pygeum africanum because of the amount of beta-sitosterol they contain. The favorite herbal choice is saw palmetto at a dose of 60 mg twice a day. Some evidence supports the premise that saw palmetto may decrease urinary frequency, urgency, dysuria, impaired flow, and nocturia.

OTC MEDICATIONS: Medications such as over-the-counter decongestants and sinus medication can worsen BPH symptoms and should be avoided. When medications fail to become effective, invasive measures may be recommended.

Invasive Procedures

Invasive procedures are used after medication therapy has been tried and failed. Potential therapies consist of minimally invasive or surgical procedures using a variety of methods including microwaves, radio waves, and electricity. The goal of all of these therapies is to increase urinary flow and decrease BPH symptoms.

Minimally invasive procedures will usually be tried first. Transurethral microwave therapy (TUMT) is a procedure that takes one or two hours and is used to decrease frequency, straining, urgency, and intermittent urine flow. This is done by putting a catheter into the bladder, then threading a microwave antenna through the catheter and into the prostate tissue. Heat produced from the microwave applied over 30 to 60 seconds destroys excess prostate tissue.

Transurethral needle ablation (TUNA) uses low-level radio waves at 456 kHz instead of microwaves to destroy excessive prostate tissue. This procedure is completed under local anesthesia with the goal of improving urinary flow. The radio waves heat the tissue to 160 to 200 degrees, removing excess prostate tissue.

Surgical Interventions

When minimally invasive procedures fail, surgery needs to be considered. A transurethral resection of the prostate (TURP) is the second most common surgical procedure performed in the older adult age group. A TURP is performed by inserting a resectoscope into the urethra, then using a wire loop to cut away strips of excess tissue, manually cutting away the prostate. TURP is the preferred surgical procedure when other interventions have failed and is considered to be the gold standard for BHP treatment. The surgery itself takes about 60 to 90 minutes and requires a 24-hour hospital stay. The result is a sizable increase in urinary flow rate. A prophylactic antibiotic may be ordered to prevent infection. Early complications associated with TURP are perforation, infection, need for recatheterization, and hemorrhage. Late complications include stricture requiring dilatation, obstruction requiring a second TURP, or persistent incontinence. If a TURP is not feasible or desirable, an optional solution is laser surgery. Laser surgery is performed by using an Nd:YAG laser in 30- to 60-second bursts to vaporize excess prostate tissue, shrinking the prostate in size. This procedure improves urinary flow rate almost as much as TURP with the benefits of less blood loss and a quicker recovery time. Electrovaporization (TVP) is another option. TVP works by removing prostate tissue by vaporization using electrical energy. This procedure will increase urinary flow with less tissue sloughing or bleeding than is found with a TURP. If the prostate is larger than can be managed by either a TURP or laser surgery, an open prostatectomy may be the best option for a prostate greater than 50 g. This surgery is considered by some to be a radical procedure with complications of bleeding and infection. The benefits are increased flow rate and decreased postvoid residual.

If the situation occurs in which pharmacological therapy is not beneficial and surgery or other invasive procedures are not options, patients may undergo either a urethral stent or balloon urethroplasty. A urethral stent is a piece of flexible tube-shaped mesh which is placed inside the narrowed section of the urethra to keep it open for urinary flow. However, due to tissue regrowth around and through the stent, this procedure has been abandoned by some urologists. A balloon urethroplasty is when a balloon attached to a catheter inflates inside the narrowed section of the urethra to widen the narrow section to improve urinary flow.

Patient Education

Patients need to understand their options from watchful waiting to surgical intervention. Patients should be given a simple explanation of the pathophysiology involved in prostate disease progression. Understanding the signs and symptoms that can occur will help them to know when to contact the physician. Any laboratory studies or diagnostic studies should be discussed at length with the patient so the patient has a clear understanding of their importance. As in all cases, the information provided will allow the patient to make informed decisions that will fit his specific needs.

STEP 2: POTENTIAL PROBLEMS/ DIAGNOSES

It is important that nurses understand and consider the science of the disease process and consider the possibilities prior to applying that knowledge to a patient situation. We begin that process with questioning.

💬 *Question:* Based upon your review of the content presented, what possible *potential problems* would you expect for a patient with these diagnoses?

💬 *Answer:* Bleeding/fluid volume, pain, infection, sexual dysfunction, urinary elimination, and confusion risk

STEP 3: POTENTIAL INTERVENTIONS AND EXPECTED OUTCOME

💬 *Question:* Based on your identification of patient problems, what possible interventions would you recommend for these diagnoses, and what would you expect to happen? This would be considered your "grocery list" of the possible actions you could use to assist your patient.

💬 *Answer:* See the following problems, interventions, and expected outcomes:

Problem	Interventions	Expected Outcome
Fluid Deficit/Bleeding	Monitor blood pressure and heart rate. Monitor catheter drainage and intake and output. Maintain catheter traction. Administer stool softeners. Administer bladder irrigation.	Patient will have stable vital signs, normal fluid volume, and an absence of gross hematuria
Infection	Monitor labs. Monitor temperature. Monitor the color and odor of urine. Maintain closed sterile drainage system. Encourage an adequate, high-protein diet. Administer antibiotics and antipyretics.	Patient will be free of infection
Pain	Assess pain quality and intensity. Administer pain medication and an antispasmodic. Maintain catheter traction.	Pain decreased to an acceptable level to the patient
Sexuality	Assess the patient's understanding of surgery side effects. Assess the patient's understanding of the effects of surgery on sexual function. Provide education about possible sexual dysfunction, such as retrograde ejaculation. Educate the patient about urinary incontinence (dribbling). Refer for sexual counseling.	The patient becomes comfortable in discussing the potential effects of surgery on sexual function
Urination	Assess the patient's pattern of elimination. Assess for hematuria. Encourage fluids. Administer antibiotics. Document accurate input and output (I&O). Provide catheter management.	Unobstructed urine flow
Confusion	Assess a baseline level of consciousness. Assess the patient's hydration status. Monitor pulse oximetry. Check the patient's blood sugar (fingerstick). Complete and monitor labs, including electrolytes. Monitor I&O and blood loss.	Baseline normal mental status will be restored

PUTTING IT ALL TOGETHER, APPLICATION OF NURSING PROCESS

Putting it all together is where the art and science of nursing meet to provide the best patient outcomes. We take the possibilities and place them into the context of the patient situation. To accomplish this, we use nursing diagnosis, nursing interventions, nursing outcomes, and nursing theory to provide the palate for nursing care.

STEP 4: ASSESSMENT

PATIENT INFORMATION: Joshua Holmes is a 56-year-old Black male.

CHIEF COMPLAINT: Symptoms of urinary urgency, frequency, not emptying bladder

HISTORY OF THE PRESENT ILLNESS: Diagnosed with BHP 6 years ago, which has worsened over the past 3 months.

Urinary urgency and frequency are interfering with his job and social activities.

PAST MEDICAL HISTORY: Hypertension, BHP

FAMILY HISTORY: Parents deceased, father of prostate cancer, mother of acute myocardial infarction (MI)

CHART REVIEW AND REPORT: Admitted for a TURP. The admission screening was completed yesterday, and the patient is being admitted at 0400 for surgery at 0900.

SUBJECTIVE ASSESSMENT: Arvin James (AJ) enters the room and introduces himself by saying, *"Good morning! My name is Arvin James and I will be your nurse today."* Joshua smiles, "I am so glad to be here. This prostate problem has been miserable—I need to have it fixed." AJ asks, *"Has your physician explained your surgery to you?"* "Yes," Joshua responds. "He told me that he is going to cut away the extra tissue around my prostate so that I won't have to go to the bathroom so often. This is ruining my life. I am an airplane pilot and can't be getting up to the bathroom every 5 minutes. I can't be up all night going to the bathroom either—I need my sleep."

OBJECTIVE ASSESSMENT: General appearance calm, and cooperative, steady gait, alert and oriented ×4. Physical assessment vital signs BP of 138/88 mm Hg, pulse 98 beats per minute, respirations 20 breaths per minute, temperature 98.4°F. Postoperative report shows that Joshua returned to his room accompanied by the recovery room nurse. Joshua is sleepy but arouses easily. Joshua is well hydrated and his IV site is clear and was converted to saline lock. Catheter traction is in place; the physician will come in the evening to assess if traction can be discontinued. Continuous bladder irrigation is infusing with normal saline to be titrated until the urine is clear. Foley catheter drainage (a mix of urine and irrigation) is reddish with several small clots noted. Postoperative orders a regular diet as tolerated and the medications listed below. Current vital signs are BP of 122/78 mm Hg, pulse 90 beats per minute, respiratory rate 18 breaths per minute, temperature 98°F. Joshua had moderate blood loss during surgery. He currently rates his pain at a 5/10 and is requesting acetaminophen/hydrocodone 5 mg be administered. A belladonna and opium suppository was given for bladder spasms in recovery.

- *Preoperative Laboratory Studies:*
  - Hgb: 17.3 g/dL
  - Hct: 51.9%
  - Cr: 0.9 mg/dL
- *Postoperative Laboratory Studies:*
  - Hgb: 15.1 g/dL
  - Hct: 45.3%
- *Diagnostic Studies:*
  - Urinary flow study: 11 mL/sec
  - Postvoid residual: 95 mL

- *Preoperative Medications:*
  - Lisinopril 10 mg daily
  - Tamsulosin hydrochloride 0.8 mg daily
- *Postoperative Medications:*
  - Cefazolin 1 g IV piggyback (IVPB) every 8 hours for three doses
  - Acetaminophen 1,000 mg every 4 hours prn mild pain rated 0 to 3/10
  - Acetaminophen/hydrocodone 5 mg every 4 hours prn moderate pain rated 4 to 6/10
  - Morphine sulfate 2 mg IVPB every 6 hours for severe pain rated 7/10
  - Docusate sodium 100 mg daily
  - Lisinopril 10 mg daily
  - B&O suppository daily prn

STEP 5: REALITY CHECK: DETOUR AHEAD

Reality Check occurs when the nurse takes a moment to think about individualized patient information that needs to be considered in framing diagnoses and interventions. This information is retrievable from any legitimate source (e.g., family, case management, other nurses, any ancillary, a doctor, etc.). These are the "wrenches" that create challenging situations, such as culture, religion, socioeconomic status, level of education, developmental level, marital status, employment, age, and gender.

Psychosocial History

Joshua is single, Christian but not religious, and works as an airline pilot. He is an only child with deceased parents. He considers his job and social life to be the most important aspects of his life. He states he is "very sexually active" and describes himself as being a "ladies' man." Joshua declines to give specifics of his sexual activity.

Critical Thinking Moment

You have just completed the assessment of Joshua and need to make a decision about the patient's *actual* problems and nursing diagnoses based on the data you have collected and the potential problems you identified. Outcomes must be realistic and measurable.

STEP 6: ACTUAL PROBLEMS/ DIAGNOSES

The *first step* in problem identification is to revisit the list of *potential diagnoses* and choose *actual diagnoses* based on the learner's evaluation of the case study information provided. A problem statement must be completed for each identified problem/diagnosis.

The actual problems for this case study are fluid deficit, pain, and sexual dysfunction risk.

STEP 7: PLANNING: ACTUAL INTERVENTIONS

After actual diagnoses have been chosen, it is necessary to evaluate the list of *potential interventions* and choose *actual interventions* that will fit within the patient's reality and meet expected outcomes. Each intervention requires a rationale. Interventions are identified in three categories: (1) assessment, (2) therapeutic, and (3) education.

Diagnostic Statement

Fluid deficit related to postsurgical bleeding as evidenced by report of moderate blood loss, reddish drainage, Hgb results 15.1 g/dL, and Hct results 45.3%.

Assessment

- Monitor Joshua's blood pressure and heart rate. *Rationale: This allows you to trend recovery progress alterations in blood pressure and heart rate, which can indicate hemodynamic instability.*
- Monitor catheter drainage closely for the first 24 hours. *Rationale: This allows you to assess for bleeding and check for clots.*
- Monitor intake and output. *Rationale: This allows the assessment of the difference between the amount of irrigation and urine.*

Therapeutic Interventions

- Maintain catheter traction until the physician visit. *Rationale: Doing so decreases bleeding risk by the application of pressure.*
- Administer Colace as ordered. *Rationale: This prevents constipation, straining, and hemorrhage.*
- Titrate normal saline continuous bladder irrigation. *Rationale: This allows you to monitor clots and bleeding, and help prevents obstruction.*

Education

- Do not remove penile traction. *Rationale: Early removal may result in hemorrhage.*
- Use pain medication. *Rationale: Good pain management promotes healing.*
- Call if bright red blood is noted in the catheter tubing. *Rationale: Bright red blood could indicate arterial bleeding.*

Expected Outcome

- Stable vital signs, normal fluid volume, and an absence of gross hematuria

Diagnostic Statement

Pain related to bladder spasms as evidenced by Joshua's complaint of moderate spasms with pain rated 5/10.

Assessment

- Assess pain every 4 hours. *Rationale: Check for changes after establishing a baseline.*
- Assess the quality of pain. *Rationale: The treatment approach may change based on incisional pain versus bladder spasm.*
- Assess the occurrence of pain. *Rationale: This helps you determine if there is an association with bladder irrigation.*

Therapeutic Interventions

- Anticipate the need for pain medication and administer as needed. *Rationale: This prevents peaking pain and promotes healing.*
- Administer a B&O suppository as needed. *Rationale: This provides pain relief with bladder spasm.*
- Maintain penile traction. *Rationale: Doing so decreases bladder spasms.*

Education

- Know how to accurately rate pain. *Rationale: Collaborate with the patient to ensure that pain management is appropriate.*
- Be aware of types of pain medication available. *Rationale: This empowers Joshua in care selections.*
- Encourage minimal movement. *Rationale: This helps Joshua understand that this can decrease the incidence of spasms.*

Expected Outcome

- Pain is at a level acceptable to Joshua.

Diagnostic Statement

Sexual dysfunction risk related to operative perineal nerve damage.

Assessment

- Assess Joshua's understanding of the potential effects of surgery on sexual function. *Rationale: This establishes a baseline for conversation.*
- Assess if Joshua wants information before or after discharge. *Rationale: Identify his willingness to learn.*
- Assess Joshua's expectation of postoperative sexual function. *Rationale: Evaluate Joshua's knowledge of potential alterations in sexuality.*

Therapeutic Interventions

- Discuss with Joshua that retrograde ejaculation may occur. *Rationale: This provides the patient with information that ejaculate goes into the bladder instead of the urethra.*
- Discuss the possibility of urinary incontinence (dribbling) postoperatively. *Rationale: Prepare Joshua for a lifestyle change issue related to management.*

- Refer for sexual counseling if requested. *Rationale: This addresses the patient's educational needs due to a change in sexuality.*

Education

- Identify retrograde ejaculation. *Rationale: This allows Joshua to understand that if this occurs, the urine will be cloudy.*
- Inform that urinary dribbling does not impede sexual activity. *Rationale: This addresses sexual function concerns.*
- Teach Kegel exercises (i.e., exercises to strengthen the pelvic floor). *Rationale: This is a proactive action that Joshua can take to strengthen the pelvic floor, decrease dribbling, and improve his quality of life.*

Expected Outcome

- Joshua is comfortable discussing the potential effects of surgery on sexual function.

STEP 8: IMPLEMENTATION

Nursing Theory

Callista Roy's theory (the Adaptation Model of Nursing) encourages nurses to assess a patient's coping mechanisms and check on how Joshua is adapting to his health-care situation. A TURP is painful surgery that can leave concerns about sexual function postoperatively. Since Joshua is very social, sexual dysfunction may be devastating to him. Nurses should assess Joshua's response to education and evaluate the level of coping and adaptation. Florence Nightingale would be an influence in maintaining a clean environment for postoperative healing. Joshua needs to understand good hand hygiene and the signs of symptoms of infection to collaborate with the physician in reporting infection concerns.

Ancillary Support

Social services could be contacted to provide information for support groups postoperatively. Since Joshua is an airline pilot, the resources would need to be more global than local, possibly an Internet chat group. A list of available resources or websites should be provided to him to meet this goal. If sexual dysfunction should occur, Joshua will need assistance to adapt to his altered physical status. Those who are experiencing the same thing will most helpful.

STEP 9: PLAN OF CARE

The plan of care is a road map for patient care and should be used as a communication tool between disciplines. Expected entries on the plan of care would be

each identified problem; bleeding/fluid deficit, pain, and sexual dysfunction with interventions; and expected outcomes, including any information from ancillaries. To individualize Joshua's care, there should be information regarding the challenges he will have because of his job on being connected with support groups. Available groups should be noted either by nursing or social services. Joshua seems to be alone in the world. A discussion with him regarding whom to contact in the case of emergency would be important, as no surgery or postoperative course is without risk. Coordinating the follow-up visits with the physician will be a challenge again because of his work schedule. Discharge planning may need to be included to assist and the outcomes documented on the plan of care. It should also be noted that Joshua prefers to take the acetaminophen/hydrocodone for pain on a schedule of every 4 hours without having to call the nurse.

STEP 10: EVALUATION

Evaluation is an active process in which the nurse "connects the dots" to decide if the expected outcomes (goals) that were established have been met, partially met, or not met. If the goals are met, we continue with the plan as outlined. If the goal was partially met, we revise the parts of the plan that did not work. If the goals were not met, we start all over with a new plan.

End-of-Shift Narrative

AJ enters the room at the end of the shift to evaluate Joshua's progress. *"Good evening, Joshua. I just wanted to check on you before I go. How are you feeling?"* Joshua responds, "The pain medication worked pretty well. If I don't move around too much I don't get those horrible bladder spasms. Most of the time the pain is a 4/10 with the acetaminophen/hydrocodone. Taking it every 4 hours around the clock works perfectly for me. Otherwise I think the pain would be much worse." AJ asks, *"Do you need something stronger?"* Joshua smiles, "No the acetaminophen/hydrocodone works fine and a 4/10 is OK. I have a pretty high pain tolerance, and the spasms are much better." Joshua continues, "I have been thinking about the discussion we had about how this surgery might change my sexual life. The doctor had told me it was a possibility, but I didn't give it much thought at the time. I think I would like to be able to get in touch with some kind of support group for a while when I go home. Is there some kind of chat group or something? I can't go to a meeting since I fly all over the place." AJ asks, *"Did the social worker see you yet?"* "No, but she should be in tomorrow." AJ smiles. *"I will call and remind him to come and see you. I think he will be able to answer all of your questions."* Joshua folds his arms over his chest and says, "Good, I will look forward to it." AJ sits next to Joshua, *"I think you are doing well. Your urine is pink instead of red. The doctor told me he would be in later this evening and if your urine keeps getting lighter he plans to take off the traction."* Joshua gives a sigh of relief, "Great news. Is my blood pressure OK?" *"Yes,"* AJ responds, *"your last blood pressure was 126/78 mm Hg, and your pulse was 88 beats per minute."* Joshua grins, "That's more my normal. I check my blood pressure all of the time at home." AJ comments, *"Well, it looks like we are going in the right direction."*

Problem Evaluation

PROBLEM 1: Fluid Deficit/Bleeding. The expected outcome is that Joshua should show stable vital signs, normal fluid volume, and an absence of gross hematuria. The goal is met: Vital signs are BP of 126/88 mm Hg, a pulse of 88 beats per minute, and catheter drainage has moved from red to pink.

PROBLEM 2: Pain. The expected outcome is a pain level acceptable to the patient. The goal is met: Even though the pain level is reported as a 4/10, Joshua states this is acceptable to him and also verbalizes that the bladder spasms are much improved.

PROBLEM 3: Risk of Sexual Dysfunction. The expected outcome is that Joshua is comfortable discussing the potential effects of surgery on sexual function. The goal is met: Joshua verbalizes that he appreciates their earlier conversation and is looking forward to a social service visit to get information about a support group.

Overall Evaluation

Based on the comparison of Joshua's assessment at the beginning and at the end of the shift, it is evident that Joshua is improving.

REFERENCES

American Cancer Society. How is prostate cancer treated? Retrieved from http://www.cancer.org/cancer/prostatecancer/detailedguide/prostate-cancer-treating-general-info

American Urological Association. AUA releases new clinical guideline on prostate cancer screening. Retrieved from www.auanet.org/advnews/press_releases/article.cfm?articleNo=290

Beers, M., Porter, R., Jones, T., Kaplan, J., & Berkwits, M. (Eds.). (2006). Prostate disease: The MERCK Manual (18th ed., pp. 2042–2045). Whitehouse Station; NJ: Merck Research Laboratories.

Drugs.com. Doxazosin dosage, last updated 9/1/13, 9/2/13, 9/16/13. Retrieved from http://www.drugs.com/dosage/doxazosin.html#Usual_Adult_Dose_for_Benign_Prostatic_Hyperplasia

Drugs.com. Flomax dosage, last updated September 1, 2, and 16, 2013. Retrieved from http://www.drugs.com/dosage/flomax.html

George, J. (2010). Nursing theories: The base for professional nursing practice (6th ed.). Upper Saddle River, NJ: Pearson.

Gilchrist, K. (2004). Benign prostatic hyperplasia: Is it a precursor to cancer. The Nurse Practitioner 29(6), 30–39.

Gilchrist, K. (2005, November/December). Twin perils of health benign prostatic hypertrophy prostate cancer. Nursing Made Incredibly Easy, 3(6), 30–43.

Gulanick, M., & Meyers, J. (2013). Nursing care plans nursing diagnosis and intervention (8th ed.). St Louis, MO: Mosby.

Holloway, N. (2004). Medical-surgical nursing care planning (4th ed.). Philadelphia, PA: Lippincott Williams & Wilkins.

International Prostate Symptom Score (IPSS). Appendix H. Retrieved from http://www.ncbi.nlm.nih.gov/pubmedhealth/PMH0033859/

King, D. (2003). Benign prostatic hyperplasia. Nursing 2003, 33(5), 44–45.

LeMone, P., Burke, K., & Baldoff, G. (2011). Medical surgical nursing. Critical thinking in patient care (5th ed.). Upper Saddle River, NJ: Pearson.

Matsukawa, Y., Goth, M., Komatsu, T., Funahashi, Y., Sassa, N., & Halton, R. (2009, December). Benign prostatic hyperplasia. Journal of Urology, 182(6), 2831–2835.

Mayo Clinic. PSA Test. Retrieved from http://www.mayoclinic.com/health/psa-test/MY00180/DSECTION=results

Medline Plus. Uroflometry. Retrieved from http://www.nlm.nih.gov/medlineplus/ency/article/003325.htm

Parker, M. (2006). Nursing theories and nursing practice (2nd ed.). Philadelphia, PA: FA Davis.

Rodgers, S. (2008). Medical surgical nursing care plans. Clifton Park, NY: Thomson Delmar.

Swearingen, P. (2008). All in one care planning resource (2nd ed.). St Louis, MO: Mosby.

Urine Flow Study. Retrieved from http://www.nlm.nih.gov/medlineplus/ency/article/003325.htm

Van Leeuwen, A., & Bladh, M. (2015). Davis's comprehensive handbook of laboratory and diagnostic testing with nursing implications (6th ed.). Philadelphia, PA: F.A. Davis Company.

Wilkinson, J., & Ahern, N. (2009). Nursing Diagnosis Handbook (9th ed.). Upper Saddle River, NJ: Prentice Hall.

Wilson, B., Shannon, M., & Stang, C. (2006). Nurses drug guide. Upper Saddle River, NJ: Prentice Hall.

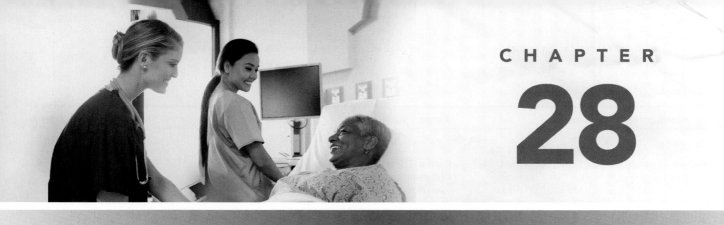

Hematopoietic System

Case Study: Sickle Cell Anemia

Common Nursing Study Name	Section 1 Study	Section 1 Chapter Number
Arterial Blood Gas (ABG)	Blood Gases	Chapter 14
Blood and Wound Cultures	Culture, Bacterial, Anal/Genital, Ear, Eye, Skin, and Wound	Chapter 19
	Culture, Bacterial, Blood	Chapter 5
Bone Scan	Bone Scan	Chapter 13
Chest X-Ray	Chest X-Ray	Chapter 16
Complete Blood Count (CBC)	Complete Blood Count, Hematocrit	Chapter 2
	Complete Blood Count, Hemoglobin	Chapter 2
	Complete Blood Count, Platelet Count	Chapter 3
	Complete Blood Count, RBC Count	Chapter 2
	Complete Blood Count, RBC Indices	Chapter 2
	Complete Blood Count, RBC Morphology and Inclusions	Chapter 2
	Complete Blood Count, WBC Count and Differential	Chapter 2
Computed Tomography (CT) of the Abdomen	Computed Tomography, Abdomen	Chapter 7
Computed Tomography (CT) of the Head	Computed Tomography, Brain	Chapter 7
DNA Testing	Amniotic Fluid Analysis and Lecithin/ Sphingomyelin Ratio	Chapter 6
	Biopsy, Chorionic Villus	Chapter 20
Electrolytes	Carbon Dioxide	Chapter 1
	Chloride, Blood	Chapter 1
	Potassium, Blood	Chapter 1
	Sodium, Blood	Chapter 1
Hemoglobin Electrophoresis	Hemoglobin Electrophoresis	Chapter 2
Hepatic Panel	Alanine Aminotransferase	Chapter 1
	Albumin and Albumin/Globulin Ratio	Chapter 1
	Alkaline Phosphatase and Isoenzymes	Chapter 1
	Aspartate Aminotransferase	Chapter 1
	Bilirubin and Bilirubin Fractions	Chapter 1
	Protein, Blood, Total and Fractions	Chapter 1
Magnetic Resonance Imaging (MRI), Brain	Magnetic Resonance Imaging, Brain	Chapter 12
Oxygen Saturation (Pulse Oximetry)	Pulse Oximetry	Chapter 14

Continued

Table Continued

Common Nursing Study Name	Section 1 Study	Section 1 Chapter Number
Newborn Screening	Newborn Screening	Chapter 1
Partial Thromboplastin Time, Activated (aPTT) and Prothrombin Time and International Normalized Ratio (INR)	Partial Thromboplastin Time, Activated Prothrombin Time, and International Normalized Ratio	Chapter 3 Chapter 3
Reticulocyte Count	Reticulocyte Count	Chapter 2
Sickle Turbidity Testing	Sickle Cell Screen	Chapter 2
Transfusions	Blood Groups and Antibodies (ABO, Rh and Antibody Screen)	Chapter 4
Urinalysis	Urinalysis	Chapter 22

STEP 1: DATA COLLECTION

Pathophysiology

Sickle cell anemia (SCA) is one of the more common genetic disorders that occurs from an autosomal recessive genetic mutation in hemoglobin synthesis that is inherited from both parents (homozygous). When the SCA gene is inherited from only one parent, the individual is a "carrier" and has the ability to pass the disease trait but not get the disease her- or himself (heterozygous). Carriers can have sickle cell symptoms that appear from physical stress, dehydration, infection, temperature extremes, or drastic pressure changes.

One in 600 people of African American descent have SCA, and about 8% are carriers. Sickle cell disease is also found in 1 of every 1,000 Hispanic American births. Other at-risk groups are those from the Mediterranean, Asia Minor, India, Central America, South America, Turkey, Greece, Italy, and the Middle East. Genetic counseling is recommended for carriers, because those who marry have a much greater risk of passing on the disease.

Sickle cell anemia is one of a group of diseases classified as *hemoglobinopathies* in which normal hemoglobin (Hgb A) is replaced by abnormal hemoglobin (Hgb S). The most common trio of these diseases is SCA, sickle cell C disease, and sickle cell thalassemia. Each version is characterized by the substitution of Hgb S for Hgb A through amino acid alteration in the beta chain.

Half of SCA patients fail to survive beyond age 20, and the rest beyond age 50. Infants born with SCA have a lag time between birth and symptom development because fetal hemoglobin (Hgb F) protects them until 3 to 6 months of age. Symptoms occur as Hgb F is replaced with increasing amounts of Hgb S.

Sickle cell mutation is most evident in the altered shape of the red blood cell from the normal flexible biconcave disc shape to an altered crescent half-moon shape. The difference between the normal Hgb A cell and the altered Hgb S cell is the substitution of the amino acid valine for glutamine in the hemoglobin molecule of both beta chains. The sickle shape is the result of the Hgb S gene changing the structure of the beta chain within the hemoglobin molecule.

Normal red cell function is to partner with hemoglobin to transport oxygen and nutrients to the body's tissues by way of the circulatory system. During oxygen pickup, both the normal Hgb A cells and the altered Hgb S cells retain the normal biconcave disc shape. The difference occurs when oxygen is off-loaded. Normal Hgb A cells retain their normal disc shape. Altered Hgb S cells form rod-shaped structures from a crystallized insoluble fluid which cluster together and create a chain, bending the cell into a crescent sickle shape. Carriers of SCA have up to 40% of Hgb S cells in their system. Those with active SCA have up to 70% or more of Hgb S cells. Altered Hgb S cells have a lower oxygen-carrying capacity, a lower hemoglobin content, and a life span shortened from 120 to 20 days from constant sickling and unsickling.

The premature destruction of the Hgb S cell increases the demand for more cells by the bone marrow. These cells are immature and fragile, contributing to the shortened life span. Altered Hgb S cells change into their sickle shape and stick to capillary walls and each other, which increases blood viscosity and plugs capillaries during a crisis. Cyclic repetition causes tissue hypoxia, metabolic acidosis, and cellular damage, slowly destroying organs and tissues. Platelet activation has been found to be increased during sickling events.

Signs and Symptoms

Sickle cell anemia is marked by episodes of wellness and deterioration. The degree of symptoms experienced is dependent on the amount of altered Hgb S present in the blood. Any event that changes the condition of the blood can trigger a crisis. Strenuous exercise, infection, high altitudes, any high-oxygen demand event, decreased plasma volume, decreased blood pH, or increased plasma osmolality from dehydration can precipitate a crisis.

The severity of symptoms varies from person to person. Severe pain is the number one primary defining symptom of sickle cell anemia. The cause of pain is thought to be from muscle necrosis, tissue ischemia, or tissue infarct due to a disrupted oxygen supply. The intensity of the pain will vary with the severity of the attack. Acute attacks of pain may last minutes, days, or weeks at a time, ranging in intensity from transient or mild to debilitating. Acute pain may require hospitalization for adequate management. The frequency of acute painful episodes depends on the individual's hemoglobin phenotype and physical condition.

Chronic pain comes from the inflammatory response to bone marrow changes, or from cumulative ischemic tissue damage and fibrosis. Concurrent medical conditions, mental health issues, and societal variables are also factors. Chronic hypoperfusion from sickling events can damage the brain, lungs, liver, spleen, kidneys, bones, and eyes. Extensive sickling can impair circulation with sequestration of large amounts of blood in the spleen and liver. Blood pooling may cause intense pain in the back, chest, or abdomen. Bone pain may be associated with an infection such as osteomyelitis.

Common sickling symptoms are hemolytic anemia, pallor, fatigue, jaundice, and irritability. Children may present as small for their age with narrow shoulders, hips, long extremities, and a curved spine. Heart rates may be faster with noticeable murmurs. Children start to fall off the growth chart around 7 years of age from insufficient nutrients at the cellular level. Puberty may be delayed.

The effects of this disease on body organs or systems can be devastating. Patients may experience an enlarged spleen due to cell congestion. Repeated sickling events can cause splenic infarction, cause functional asplenia, or increase infection risk due to the spleen's altered ability to filter bacteria and release phagocytic cells. The liver may fail or become necrotic, with anemia, impaired hepatic blood flow, hepatomegaly, and abdominal pain or swelling. The kidneys can become ischemic, with scaring, necrosis, hematuria, enuresis, progressive renal failure, and altered urine concentration.

The musculoskeletal system can present with changes such as lumbar and thoracic skeletal deformities (e.g., lordosis, kyphosis) from a weakened bone structure. Osteomyelitis can occur from chronic hypoxia and osteoporosis from bone marrow congestion. Femoral and humeral head aseptic necrosis can occur

from chronic ischemia. Patients may have bone pain and swollen hands and feet (hand-foot syndrome) from infarction of the short tubular bones along with chronic arthroplasty and bone infarctions.

Central nervous system (CNS) changes are related to vascular interruption from cyclic occlusion, ischemia, and infarct at the cellular level. The effects of this can be stroke, transient ischemic attack, headache, paralysis, aphasia, weakness, convulsions, progressive or complete blindness, retinopathy or retinal detachment, or hemorrhage and cognitive impairment. Cardiac stress can occur from chronic anemia associated with decompensation and failure. The patient may experience cardiomegaly, murmur, or septal hypertrophy. The respiratory system can be affected by chest pain, cough, dyspnea, chills, fever, and pulmonary embolism. The peripheral vascular system can experience venous stasis ulcers from vaso-occlusion, tissue ischemia, and extremity pain. In addition to effecting body systems, sickle cell anemia can retard growth with altered height and weight, can delay sexual maturity, and can decrease fertility. Please visit the U.S. Department of Health and Human Services at www.nhlbi.nih.gov/health/dci/Diseases/Sca/SCA_SignsAndSymptoms.html for a further review of disease symptoms.

Crises

Crises or flares occur during periods of disease exacerbation. The severity depends on the extent of cellular damage over time. There are four common types of crises that place an individual at serious risk: vaso-occlusive, hematologic, aplastic, and infectious.

VASO-OCCLUSIVE CRISIS: A *vaso-occlusive crisis* is a common painful episode that can be caused by stress, surgery, blood loss, dehydration, hypoxia, or infection. During this crisis, blood cells clump together, causing vasospasms that obstruct blood flow and interfere with microcirculation. Ischemic pain can be located anywhere in the body where the abnormal Hgb S cells clog up "the works" with variations of tissue ischemia, tissue infarction, and structural damage. The first vaso-occlusive event can occur as early as 6 months of age. Pain is migratory, localized, or generalized; can be found in the back, chest, abdomen, and extremities; and can last from hours to days. Abdominal pain may indicate organ infarction, bone pain may indicate aseptic necrosis, stroke can occur from the occlusion of a cerebral vessel, and stasis ulcers can result from the disruption of blood to the skin. Small vessel infarction can cause swelling of the hands, feet, and large joints. Repetitive sickling events can exacerbate these injuries.

HEMATOLOGIC CRISIS: A *hematologic crisis* occurs when sickled cells become trapped inside the spleen. Splenic sequestration is characterized by rapidly worsening anemia and rapidly falling hemoglobin. The spleen grows progressively larger as blood pools with trapped cells. This is a life-threatening event that requires immediate transfusion and/or spleen removal. Death can occur in acute sequestration from decreased blood volume, profound anemia, and cardiovascular collapse. Chronic sequestration is called *hypersplenia*. Hepatic sequestration can also occur with sickle cells trapped inside the liver, which requires aggressive transfusions.

APLASTIC CRISIS: An *aplastic crisis* occurs when red cell production from the bone marrow alters or is stopped. Profound anemia occurs when decreased cell production is coupled with rapid cell destruction. Laboratory studies will show decreased hemoglobin and hematocrit levels, and a decreased reticulocyte count. Patients will present with dizziness, pallor, weakness, and dyspnea. Treatment for an aplastic event is hospitalization with blood transfusions.

INFECTIOUS CRISIS: An *infectious crisis* is common among those with SCA due to the damaged spleen's inability to support the body's immune system. A compromised spleen leaves SCA sufferers open to bacterial infection and possible death, sometimes within 12 hours of fever onset. Infected individuals usually present with fever and pain. Serious infections include sepsis, pneumonia, meningitis, chest syndrome, and osteomyelitis. Aggressive antibiotic therapy can help to prevent death. The prophylactic administration of penicillin can prevent infection from the time of birth to 5 years of age. The most serious infections occur as a result of *Streptococcus pneumoniae*, *Neisseria meningitis*, *Salmonella species*, *Mycoplasma pneumoniae*, and *Staphylococcus aureus*.

Laboratory Studies

The method of diagnosing SCA depends on the age of the individual. Prior to birth, DNA testing can be completed on amniotic fluid or chorionic villus tissue to identify hemoglobin variants. After birth, blood samples can be obtained by heel stick or from cord blood. The blood is then tested using electrophoresis, high-performance liquid chromatography, and/or thin-layer isoelectric focusing to distinguish among the types of hemoglobin in the infant's blood in order to identify Hgb S. Newborn screening for SCA is mandated in all 50 states.

Older children or adults diagnosed with SCA can be screened using a combination of tests focused on distinguishing between hemoglobin variants and Hgb S identification. Positive identification of Hgb S by two or more tests is considered to be a confirmation of the disease. Stained blood smear can provide visual confirmation of sickled cells. Sickle turbidity testing uses anticoagulated blood mixed with a special solution that becomes cloudy (turbid) when mixed with Hgb S. Complete blood count can check for an aplastic crisis; bleeding, transfusion-related hyperhemolysis; chronic anemia; or a distorted cell shape. Infection risk can be assessed by monitoring the white blood count; chronic neutrophilia (an increased number of neutrophils over other white blood cell [WBC] types, expressed as a percentage of greater than 80% the total WBC count) is often present. Blood and wound cultures can isolate an infecting organism. Urinalysis can assess for kidney infection. Electrolytes can provide hydration information. Coagulation studies (PT, PTT) are used to check coagulation function. Jaundice can be assessed with hepatic panel. Bilirubin can be elevated from the degradation of old, damaged, and abnormal RBCs. Arterial blood gas analysis can help to manage oxygenation and assess oxygen demand. Hemoglobin electrophoresis can diagnose SCA by identifying the types and percentages of Hgb present in the blood.

Diagnostic Studies

There are no diagnostic studies that can diagnose SCA. However, diagnostic studies can be used to measure the damage caused by SCA on an individualized basis. Diagnostic studies focus on identifying the cause of observed symptoms. Chest x-ray can assess for a compromised lung from infection. A computed tomography (CT) scan of the abdomen may provide information about splenic or hepatic sequestration. CT of the head may be used to assess for headache causes, such as stroke, aneurysm, or meningitis. Magnetic resonance imaging can also help in identifying the cause of severe headache, changes in mental status, or changes in speech pattern. Bone scan may be completed in the presence of bone pain.

General/Medical Management

There are two main goals for management of SCA: (1) to prevent sickling and (2) to treat crises. Management is usually event based. As each flare-up occurs, treatment is provided based on precipitating factors and presenting symptoms. The plan of care includes minimizing activity and increasing oxygen utilization, hydration using oral and IV fluids, electrolyte replacement to keep metabolic acidosis from stimulating sickling, analgesics for pain, transfusion for anemia and combating increased blood viscosity, and antibiotics for infection.

Oxygen Therapy

Oxygen therapy can be useful for short durations but does not reverse sickling because the clogged capillary system prevents oxygen from reaching ischemic areas. Over-oxygenation can adversely affect bone marrow activity, which worsens anemia. Oxygen should be administered to treat or prevent hypoxia for a saturation below 90%. Caution is necessary because routine oxygen use may place the patient at risk for erythropoiesis.

Hydration

Adequate hydration can prevent sludging (hyperviscosity) of the circulatory system and tissue hypoxia. Because sickling impairs the kidneys' ability to concentrate urine, dilute urine is an inadequate indicator of hydration. The recommended oral intake may be 150 mL/kg/day, and hypotonic fluids such as 5% dextrose and 0.45% normal saline.

Transfusion

Transfusions can replace depleted red cell stores and help to decrease the percentage of circulating altered Hgb S. Complications can be prevented by screening for comorbidities associated with sickle cell disease prior to transfusion. Possible complications are stroke, myocardial infarction, multiple organ system failure, or RBC sequestration. If any of these concerns are noted, a leukocyte-depleted transfusion may be preferred. Blood hyperviscosity is a concern, so a post-transfusion hematocrit of 36% or less is recommended, with an Hgb level between 9 and 10 g/dL. Transfusions can support failing organs, improve generalized weakness, and treat lethargy. Fluid overload and iron overload are risks with multiple transfusions. Partial exchange transfusion may be beneficial as a treatment modality when multiple transfusions are necessary and iron overload is a concern.

Pain Management

Pain management is a key component of sickle cell treatment. Standardized pain scales appropriate for a pediatric population are a necessary component of care. The Wong-Baker FACES pain scale is an appropriate example. Medication should provide rapid and steady pain relief over a period of time with the least amount of risk. The route of administration may be oral or IV. Successful management may require trying several different medications before discovering what works. Doses can be titrated to patient response and an adequate therapeutic level. Suggested drugs include sustained-release morphine, oxycodone, hydromorphone, and methadone. Ketoprofen is a nonsteroidal anti-inflammatory drug used for pain management. Patient-controlled analgesia (PCA) is recommended for around-the-clock pain management. Monitoring for adverse reactions such as itching, respiratory depression, nausea, vomiting, hypotension, constipation, and alterations in bladder tone is necessary. Hydroxyurea can decrease painful sickle cell episodes by 50% and can increase red cell survival. Alternative pain management techniques include behavior modification, relaxation, and music therapy.

Infection

Infection should be treated with broad-spectrum antibiotics until culture results provide direction for more narrowed antibiotic management. Vigilant hand washing, adequate nutrition, frequent medical checks, and isolation from known sources of infection can prevent infection.

Other Medications

Due to the variety of presentations and symptoms, a selection of other medications may be useful for disease management. Clotrimazole is an antifungal drug that can help retain RBC hydration and reduce sickling by preventing potassium loss. Nitric oxide acts as a vasodilator and may slow or reverse RBC sickling, and decrease cell "stickiness." Folate can reduce RBC production demands and assist in treating an aplastic crisis. Vaccination against common pathogens may protect against opportunistic hosts.

Emotional Support

Sickle cell disease is emotionally devastating for the entire family. Psychological distress can occur from altered self-esteem and body image changes. Cognitive memory may be challenged from damage to the frontal lobe of the brain. Parental guilt is present from passing a potentially fatal genetic disorder to a beloved child. Social Services can provide emotional support for the family. Protocols that can help prevent disease complications are receipt of all immunizations, including pneumococcal conjugated vaccine, flu vaccine, and meningococcal vaccine. Routine prophylactic antibiotic therapy, from age 2 months to 5 years, to prevent infection is recommended. Penicillin is the antibiotic of choice unless there is an allergy, in which case erythromycin may be used. There is no known viable cure for sickle cell disease. Bone marrow transplants and stem cell research are under debate, neither with great success.

Patient Education

Can you imagine a loved one with a disease that may be fatal? How do you assist a parent and a child to cope with a disease such as this? The best way is to give them all of the information that you have available to you. However, there is so much information available that you must make sure you provide it in manageable chunks. Be cautious in completing a good literacy and cultural evaluation so that you can most effectively provide that education. Remember also that experience is sometimes the best form of education. Counsel your SCA families to attend support groups, which can give them good commonsense suggestions for care. Also, make sure you consider both the emotional and physical impact of SCA in your educational approach.

STEP 2: POTENTIAL PROBLEMS/ DIAGNOSES

It is important that nurses understand and consider the science of the disease process and the possibilities prior to applying that knowledge to a patient situation. We begin that process with questioning.

💬 *Question:* Based on your review of the content presented, what possible *potential problems* would you expect for a patient with these diagnoses?

💬 *Answer:* Pain, infection, tissue perfusion, hydration, family process, and gas exchange

STEP 3: POTENTIAL INTERVENTIONS AND EXPECTED OUTCOMES

💬 *Question:* Based on your identification of patient problems, what possible interventions would you recommend for these diagnoses, and what would you expect to happen (expected outcomes)? This would be considered your "grocery list" of the possible actions you could use to assist your patient.

💬 *Answer:* See the following problems, interventions, and expected outcomes:

Problem	Interventions	Expected Outcome
Pain	• Assess pain location, as well as the intensity, quality, and duration. • Administer narcotics and an anti-inflammatory medication and hydroxyurea. • Apply warm, moist heat. • Explain and encourage the use of a PCA. • Discuss the importance of adequate hydration, and how activity conservation may decrease pain. • Schedule pain medication around the clock rather than prn. • Educate the patient regarding addiction risks. • Carefully position and support painful areas; use distraction to support pain management.	Pain controlled at a level acceptable to the patient
Infection	• Educate the patient about the importance of adequate nutrition and the importance of routine immunizations. • Discuss the need to report any signs of infection. • Ensure the patient understands the importance of complying with antibiotic treatment, giving meticulous care to any open sores, and participating in vigilant handwashing.	Patient remains infection free, no postoperative infection.
Tissue Perfusion	• Assess capillary refill, skin temperature, skin color, peripheral pulses, edema, and stasis ulcers. • Monitor labs, including Hgb electrophoresis, bilirubin, CBC, and arterial blood gas. • Administer humidified oxygen and monitor oxygenation. • Administer IV fluids and encourage oral fluid intake. • Apply moist heat to affected joints and elevate the head of the bed. • Administer a transfusion as ordered.	Peripheral pulses will be strong with a capillary refill of less than 3 seconds
Hydration	• Identify the recommended daily fluid intake. • Increase the fluid intake during high-stress periods. • Educate the family about the importance of adequate fluid intake • Encourage fluid intake and offer alternate forms of fluid to increase intake. • Educate about the signs and symptoms of dehydration, and the ways fluid is lost, such as overheating. • Administer IV fluids as ordered and strictly monitor intake and output.	Maintain adequate hydration with no signs of dehydration

Family Process	• Educate the patient and the patient's family about the cause and effect of disease, the importance of consistent physician visits, and the importance of notifying the physician about any flare symptoms.	Family will demonstrate understanding of disease process and treatments
	• Educate them about crisis symptoms (fever, pallor, respiratory distress, pain), genetic counseling, and the importance of teacher notification regarding flare symptoms.	
	• Support agency referrals.	
Gas Exchange	• Administer oxygen, monitor oxygen saturation, assess respiratory rate and effort, and assess the use of accessory muscles.	Saturation greater than 90%
	• Administer a bronchodilator and antibiotics as ordered.	
	• Elevate the head of the bed.	
	• Administer blood as ordered.	

PUTTING IT ALL TOGETHER: APPLICATION OF THE NURSING PROCESS

Putting it all together is where the art and science of nursing meet to provide the best patient outcomes. We take the possibilities and place them into the context of the patient situation. To accomplish this, we use nursing diagnosis, nursing interventions, nursing outcomes, and nursing theory to provide the palate for nursing care.

STEP 4: ASSESSMENT

PATIENT INFORMATION: 13-year-old male of mixed Hispanic/African American descent

CHIEF COMPLAINT: Acute severe pain in bilateral knees

HISTORY OF THE PRESENT ILLNESS: Started having knee pain while playing touch football

PAST MEDICAL HISTORY: Diagnosed with SCA at 6 months of age with swelling of the hands and feet. Good control until age 12 years, when he ignored restrictions in order to "fit in" with friends

FAMILY HISTORY: Mother is Hispanic and father is African American. Genetic testing shows both are SCA carriers. A brother, age 14, and a sister, age 16, are carriers. There are no other known cases of active SCA in their family circle. Subsequent genetic testing has identified multiple carriers.

CHART REVIEW AND REPORT: Jeremiah Jones was admitted 2 days ago for acute pain of both knees from a combination of strenuous activity and dehydration. Initial pain was severe at a 10/10 and is now rated at a 6/10. Pain is localized and grinding with generalized achiness. Jeremiah weighs 187 pounds. Pain management is basal rate morphine PCA at 2 mg/hour, and 1 mg on demand every 15 minutes for breakthrough pain. Current vital signs are a temperature of 100.4°F,

a pulse of 96 beats/minute, respirations of 22 breaths/minute, and a BP reading of 106/70 mm Hg. An electrolyte panel on admission K$^+$4.3 mEq/L, Na$^+$ 148 mEq/L, Cl$^-$ 109 mEq/L indicated dehydration. Intravenous fluids of D5/0.45 NS are running at 80 mL/hour until oral intake can support hydration needs. Oral intake over the past 4 hours is 200 mL. Jeremiah is receiving cefuroxime 250 mg IVPB for his temperature, his CXR is negative for infiltrates, and pulse oximetry is 93% on room air. The off-going nurse tells you Jeremiah has been fidgety and uncommunicative, staring off into space. He has two units of packed RBCs on hold for an Hgb level that is less than 8 g/dL. He refuses to use warm, moist heat to his knees to decrease the pain.

SUBJECTIVE ASSESSMENT: As you enter the room you see Jeremiah watching TV. *"Good morning, how are you feeling?"* Jeremiah is pale and thin and is staring off into space with a flat affect. "How is the pain? It feels like someone is squeezing my knees to see if they will pop. It's like a horrible toothache. This stuff," he gestures to the PCA, "is helping, as much as it usually does." *"What does that mean?"* AJ asks. "Nothing," Jeremiah replies heatedly, "I'm just tired of this." *"How bad is the pain?"* "It's an 8," Jeremiah responds. *"You know that you can give yourself some extra pain medicine just by pushing the button on the machine,"* AJ explains. "I know, but my friends said I'll become a drug addict," Jeremiah returns sullenly. *"That's not true, you will just suffer needlessly. Use the medicine when you need it to help the pain. You said the pain is an 8/10 right now, and that's a little worse than last night, isn't it?"* "Yes," Jeremiah replies, "but it always gets worse after I go to the bathroom." *"Do you want a urinal?"* "No, way, can I get rid of this bag of fluid?" *"Yes, if you start drinking more we can take out the IV."* "Whatever," Jeremiah replies dismissively, "why don't you go away and leave me alone, I'm just a freak, why me."

OBJECTIVE ASSESSMENT: Jeremiah's movements in bed appear slow and painful, with a facial grimace and a slight moan noted. He is emotionally withdrawn, and fatigued. Bilateral knees are moderately swollen, tender, and warm to the touch; tactile stimulation seems to make the pain worse. Current temperature is 100.2°F, otherwise vital signs are unchanged. All other assessments are within normal limits.

- *Laboratory Studies:* Jeremiah's morning laboratory results are:
  - WBC 12×10^3/microL
  - Hgb/Hct 7.8 g/dL and 23%
  - Platelets 145×10^3/microL
  - Hemoglobin electrophoresis indicates significant current sickling.
- *Diagnostic Studies:*
  - A repeat chest x-ray shows the lungs to be clear of infiltrates.
- *Medications:*
  - Folic acid 1 mg daily
  - Cefuroxime 250 mg IVPB every 6 hours
  - Hydroxyurea at 15 mg/kg/day increasing by 5 mg/kg/day until peak effectiveness is reached
  - PCA morphine 2 mg/hour as a basal rate with 1 mg every 15 minutes for breakthrough pain
  - Two units of packed RBCs are on hold for transfusion.

STEP 5: REALITY CHECK: DETOUR AHEAD

Reality Check occurs when the nurse takes a moment to think about individualized patient information that needs to be considered in framing diagnoses and interventions. This information is retrievable from any legitimate source (e.g., family, case management, other nurses, any ancillary, a doctor, etc.). These are the "wrenches" that create challenging situations, such as culture, religion, socioeconomic status, level of education, developmental level, marital status, employment, age, and gender.

Psychosocial History

Jeremiah is the only child with active SCA. Jeremiah first had symptoms of the disease at age 6 months. Crawling was painful, and his parents noticed his hands and feet seemed swollen. Jeremiahs' diagnosis with SCA came as a shock. There has been a lot of guilt on the part of the parents who have provided the best of care possible to help him have a "normal life." Jeremiah has been cooperative with his restrictions, but lately he has been angry and resentful, making choices that place his health at risk. Jeremiah's parents are at a loss as to where to go from here.

Critical Thinking Moment

You have just completed the assessment of Jeremiah and need to make a decision about the patient's *actual* problems and nursing diagnoses based upon the data you have collected and the potential problems you identified. Outcomes must be realistic and measurable.

STEP 6: ACTUAL PROBLEMS/DIAGNOSES

The *first step* in problem identification is to revisit the list of *potential diagnoses* and choose *actual diagnoses* based on the learner's evaluation of the case study information provided. A problem statement must be completed for each identified problem/diagnosis. The actual problems for this case study are pain, dehydration (hydration), and family process.

STEP 7: PLANNING: ACTUAL INTERVENTIONS

After actual diagnoses have been chosen, it is necessary to evaluate the list of *potential interventions* and choose *actual interventions* that will fit within the patient's reality and meet expected outcomes. Each intervention requires a rationale. Interventions are identified in three categories: (1) assessment, (2) therapeutic, and (3) education.

Diagnostic Statement

Pain related to clumped sickled cells and vascular occlusion as evidenced by knee pain of 6 to 8/10, as well as facial grimace and moan with movement.

Assessment

- Assess pain characteristics (location, intensity, quality, and duration). *Rationale: This allows for a baseline assessment to be obtained as well as direction for appropriate pain management.*
- Assess the effectiveness of basal PCA morphine on the patient's pain intensity. *Rationale: This allows for alterations to be made, if needed.*
- Assess coping. *Rationale: Pain can cause stress that may require assistance with coping.*

Therapeutic Interventions

- Administer basal PCA morphine at 2 mg/hour for pain relief. *Rationale: This allows for Jeremiah's pain management needs to be met.*
- Apply warm, moist heat to Jeremiah's knees. *Rationale: Vasodilatation improves cellular oxygenation, which decreases pain.*

- Administer hydroxyurea per pharmacist direction. *Rationale: This increases the amount of Hgb F, which decreases sickling and thereby decreases pain.*

Education

- Explain using a PCA to manage pain effectively. *Rationale: This assists Jeremiah in having control over his pain.*
- Explain the importance of drinking fluids. *Rationale: This assists Jeremiah in understanding that decreased viscosity will decrease sickling.*
- Provide Jeremiah with education about addiction risks. *Rationale: This helps to prevent undermedication and poor pain management.*

Expected Outcome

- Pain will be at a level acceptable to Jeremiah.

Diagnostic Statement

Dehydration related to increased physical exertion, insensible fluid loss, and inadequate fluid intake oral intake as evidenced by altered electrolytes K$^+$ 4.3 mEq/L, Na$^+$ 148 mEq/L, Cl$^-$ 109 mEq/L.

Assessment

- Assess Jeremiah's current fluid intake. *Rationale: This assures that Jeremiah is taking in a sufficient amount of fluid.*
- Assess Jeremiah's awareness of oral fluid choices. *Rationale: This helps to improve Jeremiah's compliance (not everyone likes water).*
- Monitor electrolytes. *Rationale: This allows you to assess Jeremiah's hydration status.*

Therapeutic Interventions

- Strictly monitor the patient's intake and output. *Rationale: This allows you to monitor Jeremiah's hydration status.*
- Administer D5/ ½ NS at 80 mL/hour. *Rationale: This allows for enhanced hydration.*
- Offer optional forms of fluids or oral fluids. *Rationale: This helps to increase Jeremiah's overall fluid intake.*

Education

- Explain the signs and symptoms of dehydration. *Rationale: Jeremiah's understanding will improve his compliance.*
- Discuss the ways that fluid is lost, such as overheating. *Rationale: This allows Jeremiah to make positive health choices.*
- Review appropriate fluid choices and daily intake. *Rationale: This helps to ensure that Jeremiah consumes adequate fluids.*

Expected Outcome

- Jeremiah's oral intake will increase to 800 mL this shift to improve hydration.

Diagnostic Statement

Altered family process related to the disease process (SCA) as evidenced by Jeremiah's denial of lifestyle restrictions, as evidenced by anger, resentment, and acting out.

Assessment

- Assess Jeremiah's understanding of the disease process. *Rationale: This allows you to establish a baseline for conversation.*
- Assess Jeremiah's willingness to comply with lifestyle restrictions. *Rationale: This allows you to better identify needed resources.*
- Assess Jeremiah's willingness to report any flare. *Rationale: This allows you to facilitate prompt medical treatment.*

Therapeutic Interventions

- Connect Jeremiah and his family with an SCA support group, especially one that focuses on teenage challenges. *Rationale: This allows for the provision of real-life support from those experiencing the same challenges.*
- Make a recommendation for a psychotherapy consult. *Rationale: This allows for a safe environment in which Jeremiah can discuss issues.*
- Discuss teacher notification, education, and support at school and with Jeremiah's peer group. *Rationale: This assists Jeremiah in making positive health choices.*

Education

- Educate Jeremiah about the disease pathophysiology. *Rationale: Understanding the cause and effect may improve Jeremiah's compliance.*
- Stress the importance of Jeremiah's monitoring for crisis symptoms. *Rationale: This allows Jeremiah to get early medical treatment.*
- Discuss with Jeremiah the potential impact of the disease on his life. *Rationale: Understanding may improve Jeremiah's compliance to lifestyle restrictions.*

Expected Outcome

- Jeremiah will verbalize an understanding of disease and an acceptance of lifestyle limitations.

STEP 8: IMPLEMENTATION

Nursing Theory

Jeremiah has a disease that makes it difficult for him to interact socially with his peers. He wants to be just like everyone else and is not complying with his health restrictions. The theory of Myra Levine focuses on individualized patient care. Sickle cell anemia symptoms can vary over time based on precipitating events. By necessity, Jeremiah will be dependent on the care provider, which requires adaptation to the immediate situation. During a crisis, he will need to conserve energy and manage his pain. Nurses help Jeremiah to focus on "keeping it together" during sickle cell flares. Nursing should partner with Jeremiah and his parents to achieve care goals while at the same time maintaining individual integrity. Special attention should be given to supporting his self-worth and societal identification. Consideration needs to be given to Jeremiah's community connections that can be used to provide support after discharge.

Ancillary Support

Jeremiah is striking out over his frustration with the limitations SCA has placed on his life. His teenage angst places him at risk for life-threatening crises. Support is needed to convince him to cooperate with his care and prevent placing his life at risk. Parental influence is no longer effective. Social Services should collaborate with the family in selecting a support group that complements his age-related needs. Family counseling may be beneficial in solving some issues and may provide Jeremiah with a safe haven to explore his own feelings.

STEP 9: PLAN OF CARE

The plan of care is a road map for patient care and should be used as a communication tool between disciplines. Expected entries on the plan of care would be each identified problem, intervention, and expected outcome, including any information from ancillaries. Nursing-sensitive concerns should be addressed. How are we going to get buy-in from Jeremiah to make choices that decrease the risk of another flare when he is determined to do otherwise?

STEP 10: EVALUATION

Evaluation is an active process in which the nurse "connects the dots" to decide if the expected outcomes (goals) that were established have been met, partially met, or not met. If the goals are met, we continue with the plan as outlined; if the goal was partially met, we revise the parts of the plan that did not work; and if the goals were not met, we start all over with a new plan.

End-of-Shift Narrative

It has been a difficult day. Jeremiah's parents had a terrible argument with their son. Jeremiah insists he is going to continue to do whatever he wants, including playing football with his friends. His parents are terrified and have requested help. Social Services has contacted some teenagers with SCA to talk to Jeremiah, who became belligerent and refused. AJ enters the room while Jeremiah is eating dinner. *"I received a call from a girl your age with SCA, she would like to visit you."* "Forget it. It was nice of her to call but I probably won't call back." AJ continues, *"Can you think about it?"* "OK, just get off my back." *"You're drinking more, almost a whole liter since this morning, so maybe we can get rid of the IV on the next shift."* Jeremiah smiles, "You were right about drinking more, I do feel better." *"Your blood work looks better too, the fluids help your blood to be less concentrated. How is the pain level now?"* AJ asks. Jeremiah smiles, "Better. The pain medicine is working and the moist heat makes the achiness better." *"How would you rate the pain?"* AJ asks. "Probably at a 4. It still bothers me but it's much better. I think my knees are less swollen. Maybe I can go home soon." *"I heard you had a fight with your parents. Is there anything I can do?"* "Yeah, stay out of my business."

Problem Evaluation

PROBLEM 1: **Pain.** The expected outcome is that pain will be at a level acceptable to Jeremiah. The goal is met: The pain level has decreased to a 4/10 with successful use of the PCA. The moist heat to the knees has added to the pain relief.

PROBLEM 2: **Dehydration.** The expected outcome is that oral intake will increase to 800 mL this shift to improve hydration. The goal is met: AJ's suggestion of having other fluids besides water has been successful. IV fluids may be discontinued on the following shift if Jeremiah's oral intake remains consistent, and electrolytes demonstrate less hemoconcentration.

PROBLEM 3: **Patient Understanding.** Jeremiah verbalizes understanding of the disease process and acceptance of lifestyle limitations. The goal is not met: Jeremiah remains angry about his disease and states he is not going to conform to suggested limitations, saying he is going to do whatever he wants. He will not listen or follow his parents' or anyone else's advice. A revised plan would be to further pursue interaction with a peer from an SCA support group. Both Jeremiah and his parents should receive individual and family counseling.

Overall Evaluation

Based on the end-of-shift assessment and the comparison of Jeremiah's progress during this shift, Jeremiah is found to be improving.

REFERENCES

Camp-Sorrell, D., & Hawkins, R. (2006). Clinical manual for oncology: Advance practice nurse edition (2nd ed.). Pittsburgh, PA: ONS Publishing.

George, J. (2011). Nursing theories: The base for professional nursing practice (6th ed.). Upper Saddle River, NJ: Pearson Education.

Gill, V., Lavin, J., & Sim, M. (2010, November/December). Managing sickle cell disease. Nursing Made Incredibly Easy, 27–31.

Gulanick, M., & Meyers, J. (2013). Nursing care plans: Nursing diagnosis and intervention (8th ed.). St Louis, MO: Mosby.

Holloway, N. (2004). Medical surgical nursing care planning (4th ed.). Springhouse, PA: Lippincott Williams & Wilkins.

How is sickle cell anemia diagnosed? Retrieved from www.nhlbi.nih.gov/health/health-topics/topics/sca/diagnosis.html

Jaeckel, R., Thieme, M., Czeslick, E., and Sablotzki, A. (2010). The use of partial exchange blood transfusion and anaesthesia in the management of sickle cell disease in a perioperative setting: Two case reports. Journal of Medical Case Reports, 4, 82. Retrieved from www.ncbi.nlm.nih.gov/pmc/articles/PMC2838918/

LeMone, P., & Burke, K. (1996). Medical surgical nursing: Critical thinking in client care. Menlo Park, CA: Benjamin Cummings.

Luxor, K. (2005). Delmar's pediatric care plans (3rd ed.). Clifton, NY: Delmar.

Mone, P., & Burke, K. (2008). Medical surgical nursing (4th ed.). Upper Saddle River, NJ: Prentice Hall.

Parker, M. (2006). Nursing theories and nursing practice (2nd ed.). Philadelphia, PA: FA Davis.

Platt, A. (2007). How much do you know about sickle cell disease. LPN2007, 3(4), 32–37.

Potts, N., & Mandleco, B. (2007). Pediatric nursing (2nd ed.). Clifton, NY: Delmar.

Rodgers, S. (2008). Medical surgical nursing care plans. Clifton Park, NY: Thomson Delmar

Sickle cell anemia. Retrieved from http://www.mayoclinic.com/health/sickle-cell-anemia/DS00324/METHOD=print

Sickle cell anemia. Also called: Hemoglobin SS disease. Retrieved from www.nlm.nih.gov/medlineplus/sicklecellanemia.html

Sickle cell disease (SCD). Retrieved from www.cdc.gov/ncbddd/sicklecell/treatments.html

Van Leeuwen, A., & Bladh, M. (2015). Davis's comprehensive handbook of laboratory and diagnostic testing with nursing implications (6th ed.). Philadelphia, PA: F.A. Davis Company.

Wagner, K., Johnson, K., & Hardin-Pierce, M. (2005). *High Acuity Nursing* (5th ed.). Boston, MA: Pearson Education.

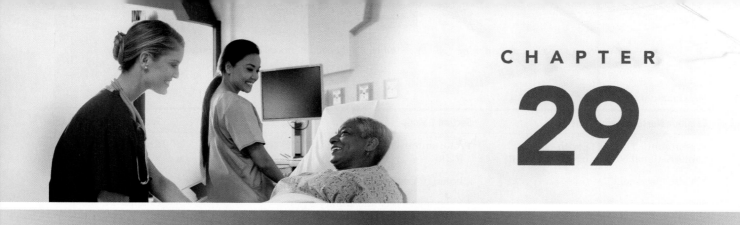

Hepatobiliary System

Case Study: Cholecystitis

Common Nursing Study Name	Section 1 Study	Section 1 Chapter Number
Abdominal X-Rays, Plain (KUB)	Kidney, Ureter, and Bladder Study	Chapter 16
Alanine Aminotransferase	Alanine Aminotransferase	Chapter 1
Alkaline Phosphatase	Alkaline Phosphatase and Isoenzymes	Chapter 1
Amylase	Amylase	Chapter 1
Aspartate Aminotransferase	Aspartate Aminotransferase	Chapter 1
Bilirubin	Bilirubin and Bilirubin Fractions	Chapter 1
Complete Blood Count (CBC)	Complete Blood Count, Hematocrit	Chapter 2
	Complete Blood Count, Hemoglobin	Chapter 2
	Complete Blood Count, Platelet Count	Chapter 3
	Complete Blood Count, RBC Count	Chapter 2
	Complete Blood Count, RBC Indices	Chapter 2
	Complete Blood Count, RBC Morphology and Inclusions	Chapter 2
	Complete Blood Count, WBC Count and Differential	Chapter 2
Computed Tomography (CT), Biliary Tract and Liver	Computed Tomography, Biliary Tract and Liver	Chapter 7
C-Reactive Protein (CRP)	C-Reactive Protein	Chapter 1
Culture and Sensitivity (C&S), Sterile Fluid	Culture, Bacterial, Anal/Genital, Ear, Eye, Skin, and Wound	Chapter 19
Endoscopic Retrograde Cholangiopancreatography (ERCP)	Cholangiopancreatography, Endoscopic Retrograde	Chapter 9
Hepatobiliary Iminodiacetic Acid (HIDA)	Hepatobiliary Scan	Chapter 13
Magnetic Resonance Cholangiopancreatography (MRCP)	Magnetic Resonance Imaging, Abdomen	Chapter 12
Magnetic Resonance Imaging (MRI), Abdomen	Magnetic Resonance Imaging, Abdomen	Chapter 12
Percutaneous Transhepatic Cholangiography (PTHC)	Cholangiography, Percutaneous Transhepatic	Chapter 15

Continued

Table Continued

Common Nursing Study Name	Section 1 Study	Section 1 Chapter Number
Prothrombin Time (PT) with International Normalized Ratio (INR)	Prothrombin Time and International Normalized Ratio	Chapter 3
T-Tube Placement	Cholangiography, Postoperative	Chapter 15
Ultrasonography, Biliary Tract	Ultrasound, Liver and Biliary System	Chapter 21
Vancomycin	Antimicrobial Drugs—Aminoglycosides: Amikacin, Gentamicin, Tobramycin; Tricyclic Glycopeptide: Vancomycin	Chapter 1

STEP 1: DATA COLLECTION

Pathophysiology

Cholecystitis is a common gallbladder disease that affects more than 20 million Americans annually. The gallbladder is a small pear-shaped organ located between the right and left lobes of the liver. The function of the gallbladder is to store bile, the by-product of the liver. Bile is a combination of cholesterol, phospholipids, water, electrolytes, bilirubin, bile salts, and other waste products. About one quart of bile is produced each day. The gallbladder gets larger or smaller based on the amount of bile it contains. Bile production is stimulated by food that enters the small intestine. Bile is mostly used to break down and metabolize fats. Bile is also used to help remove toxins, drugs, bacteria, viruses, and other foreign substances from the liver. These substances are transported to the intestines for removal from the body through the common bile duct. Gallbladder disease is associated with the abnormal flow of bile through the common bile duct, resulting in inflammation and infection. Problems begin when the flow of bile is blocked or slows down, which usually results from stone formation.

Stone formation, known as *cholelithiasis*, is the most common cause of gallbladder disease. Stones are made of a combination of bile products, cholesterol, and calcium salt. Infection and inflammation can occur, and stones can form either in the gallbladder itself or in the ducts that transport the bile. However, most stones form in the gallbladder rather than in a duct. Stones that are small and remain in the gallbladder do not usually cause any symptoms.

Acute cholecystitis is associated with inflammation and infection. Inflammation occurs from a combination of obstructing stones, increased pressure, ischemia, and chemical irritation from retained bile. Inflammation can also be caused from trauma or crystals trapped in the gallbladder walls. Ongoing inflammation creates a cycle of increasing edema, ischemia caused by obstruction, and possible infection with necrosis or perforation.

Types of Gallbladder Stones

There are three types of gallbladder stones. Cholesterol stones are the most common and are found in patients who live in industrialized countries like the United States. Cholesterol stones can grow in excess of 2.5 cm in size. Slow gallbladder motility is commonly associated with the development of cholesterol stones, which allows the stones to form. Black stones are found more often in those who have a chronic hemolytic disorder such as sickle cell anemia or cirrhosis of the liver. Black stones have also been found in older adults. In the United States, black stones are found in patients about 30% of the time. Brown stones are found in patients in whom the biliary tract or gallbladder is impacted.

Risk Factors

There are several risk factors associated with development of cholecystitis. Some risk factors are modifiable, and some are not. Modifiable risk factors are primarily weight and diet. Cholecystitis can be precipitated by excess weight or rapid weight loss. A very low-calorie diet, or a diet high in refined carbohydrates or fasting can also place an individual at risk.

Nonmodifiable risk factors are age, gender, and ethnicity. Women, people over the age of 60, or those of Native American, Northern European, or Hispanic ethnicity are more at risk. Other contributing factors are medical conditions such as pregnancy, diabetes, cystic fibrosis, pancreatic insufficiency, small intestine disease, and cancer treatment. Medications such as birth control pills, total parental nutrition, and some cholesterol-lowering medications can also place one at risk. The classic cholecystitis patient is a middle-aged woman who has gained weight over time from pregnancy and aging.

Signs and Symptoms

Severe symptoms occur in patients up to 30% of the time. Yet more than half of the time there are no symptoms. Individuals with early symptoms of cholecystitis most often describe feeling colicky, gassy, or just really full after eating a large fatty meal. These first mild symptoms can worsen progressively over time. Frank abdominal pain is the hallmark of cholecystitis. Pain may vary from moderate to severe or from intermittent to continuous. The pain location can also vary. Pain often starts in the right upper quadrant of the abdomen with guarding and tenderness radiating between the back and shoulder on the right side. Pain is aggravated by movement such as sitting or standing and deep breathing. Acute pain occurs from spastic contractions of the bile ducts lasting up to 18 hours. After the acute pain has passed, the patient may experience soreness for another 24 hours.

Severe epigastric pain is occasionally mistaken for heart attack. Additional symptoms of cholecystitis that occur in tandem with the pain are nausea, vomiting, and fever with chills. Jaundice and liver damage can occur if there is significant backflow of bile into the liver. Symptoms of cholecystitis can be acute or chronic. Chronic cholecystitis can alternate from mild symptoms to no symptoms at all and is characterized by recurrent acute episodes from the persistent presence of stones. The pain experienced is usually less severe and is often perceived as gastric upset with mild right upper quadrant abdominal discomfort after eating.

Physical assessment findings can point toward a diagnosis of gallbladder disease. *Murphy sign* is a classic symptom of cholecystitis and is positive when the patient has tenderness under the right costal margin with deep palpation. *Boas sign* is tenderness to the right of the 10th to 12th thoracic vertebrae. *Courvoisier sign* is positive when there is a distended palpable nontender gallbladder, which suggests obstruction due to tumor. If abdominal rigidity is present, there may be peritoneal inflammation. Dark urine or light-colored stools may be noted in conjunction with jaundice.

Complications

The complications of cholecystitis include empyema (pus inside of the gallbladder), gangrene, perforation, peritonitis, and abscess. In some cases, a fistula can form with nearby organs.

Laboratory Studies

Laboratory studies will focus on the differentiation of gallbladder disease from other possible causes of pain, as well as from inflammation, infection, and jaundice. A complete blood count (CBC) can be ordered to check for inflammation, which can be assessed by evaluating the leukocyte count. Leukocytosis is indicated if the leukocyte count is greater than 11×10^3/microL. Inflammation and infection are considered if the results range from 12×10^3/microL to 15×10^3/microL. A result greater than 20×10^3/microL may be suspect for perforation or gangrene.

Bilirubin (total, direct, indirect) will all be elevated in the presence of cholecystitis that results from obstructed bile flow. Patients may have jaundice with values greater than 2.5 mg/dL. An evaluation of the serum amylase level may be done in combination with bilirubin to check for the presence of any pancreatitis associated with gallbladder disease.

Culture and sensitivity of a body fluid specimen can be used to identify the infectious organism and to provide direction for the selection of the antibiotic to treat it. Other laboratory studies that may be elevated in the presence of gallbladder disease are alanine aminotransferase, aspartate aminotransferase, and alkaline phosphatase.

Diagnostic Studies

The purpose of diagnostic studies is to differentiate gallbladder disease from other abdominal disorders. Ultrasonography is a fairly inexpensive noninvasive procedure that can be used to check for the presence of stones and to evaluate the ability of the gallbladder to empty. Ultrasound works by deflecting sound waves to look for stones in the gallbladder or common bile duct. Ultrasound is often the diagnostic study of choice, because it is 95% accurate and can be used for most patients, including those with jaundice and liver disease. Ultrasound can also help to differentiate between acute cholecystitis (inflammation and infection) or cholelithiasis (just stones).

Computed Tomography (CT)

Computed tomography (CT) is more expensive and is considered a less sensitive indicator than ultrasound to identify gallstones. However, CT is thought to be better at identifying biliary dilatation and stones in the common bile duct. Endoscopic ultrasonography (EUS) is a noninvasive diagnostic tool that can be used to detect stones smaller than 3 cm in size. This type of ultrasonography is also useful in assessing for the presence of cholesterol microcrystals or bilirubin granules. Oral cholecystogram is an older test that is used to assess the motility of the gallbladder. Motility is assessed by having the patient take an oral dye and then monitoring the ability of the gallbladder to excrete bile.

Hepatobiliary Iminodiacetic Acid (HIDA) Scanning

Hepatobiliary iminodiacetic acid (HIDA) scanning is a nuclear medicine study used to show that the gallbladder is not filling, which confirms obstruction. This scan is used most often in the diagnosis of cholecystitis.

Endoscopic Retrograde Cholangiopancreatography (ERCP)

Endoscopic retrograde cholangiopancreatography (ERCP) is an invasive procedure used to measure the resting pressure of the sphincter of Oddi. If the pressure is greater than 40 mm Hg, pain may be experienced due to interference with bile flow. During an ERCP, stones can be located, and those larger than 1.5 cm can be broken and removed. Stones that require ERCP for diagnosis may be treated with broad-spectrum antibiotics to prevent sepsis.

Percutaneous Transhepatic Cholangiography (PTHC)

Percutaneous transhepatic cholangiography (PTHC) is an invasive procedure in which the patient is injected with a contrast that allows visualization of the bile ducts inside and outside of the liver. This is useful in identifying the location, extent, and cause of the obstruction.

Magnetic Resonance Cholangiopancreatography (MRCP)

Magnetic resonance cholangiopancreatography (MRCP) is a fast, noninvasive way to visualize the pancreatobiliary tree. An MRCP does not have the same therapeutic capability as an ERCP. However, it does allow assessment of the liver and pancreas for masses, fluid, abscesses, and pseudocysts, whereas an ERCP does not. MRCP imaging helps to find difficult to visualize impacted gallstones that are located in the neck of the duct, and biliary dilation both inside and outside of the liver. The procedure is also useful for those with contraindications for ERCP, such as children and the elderly.

Other Diagnostic Studies

Other diagnostic studies that may be considered are magnetic resonance imaging (MRI) of the abdomen to locate small areas of perforation that may not be visible with other diagnostic tools such as ultrasound and CT. Abdominal flat-plate x-ray can be useful in picking up calcium deposits in the stones.

General/Medical Management

Treatment choices can be noninvasive or invasive. Noninvasive management of cholecystitis is useful for patients too frail for surgery or for those who refuse surgery.

Medication Administration

A common noninvasive treatment is the administration of oral bile acids to dissolve stones. Small cholesterol stones can be dissolved by lowering the stone cholesterol content. Suggested medications are ursodiol or chenodiol. These drugs act to reduce cholesterol production within the liver, which reduces the cholesterol content of the bile. Possible side effects are altered liver enzymes and diarrhea. Cholestyramine is another drug that can inhibit gallbladder disease by binding bile salts and promoting excretion, and is useful for patients with jaundice.

Antibiotics are used to treat infection or are used prophylactically prior to surgery. Drug choices may include second-, third-, or fourth-generation cephalosporins or a combination of aminoglycoside and metronidazole. Suggested drugs include ceftriaxone, cefepime, ofloxacin, or ciprofloxacin. Patients who have their gallbladder removed or who have uncomplicated cholecystitis may not need antibiotic therapy. Vancomycin may be used if enterococcus is suspected. An anticholinergic agent, such as dicyclomine, can be used during gallbladder "attacks" to relax smooth muscle, which prevents contraction and pain.

Dietary Changes

Dietary changes will be necessary because ingested fat can stimulate a gallbladder contraction. Patients are usually placed on a low-fat diet and are asked to avoid foods such as whole milk products; deep-fried foods and pastries; avocados; meats such as hot dogs, sausage, and bacon; cream-based gravy; chips; nuts; peanut butter; and chocolate.

Shock Wave Lithotripsy

Extracorporeal shock wave lithotripsy (ESWL) is a noninvasive procedure that is an option in breaking up small stones. The negative in using this treatment is that the diseased gallbladder remains in place and can continue to form stones, resulting in future episodes. Patients may receive a mild sedative and prophylactic antibiotics prior to the procedure. Patients may need to be NPO for a specific period, and may receive a bowel preparation. General anesthesia may or may not be used. Explain to the patient that the procedure is done under fluoroscopy and may take up to an hour to complete. The goal is to use the shock waves to pulverize the stone so that it may be excreted with the urine. Some patients may have a tube inserted to help drain urine until all the pieces of stone are passed. Postprocedure nurses will be asked to monitor for bleeding by assessing the color of the urine. Accurate intake and output will be required.

Endoscopy and Surgery

Invasive procedures include endoscopy and surgery. Endoscopy is preferred for those who need decompression of the biliary tree. Pressure within the common bile duct can be relieved by placing a T-tube, which allows for bile drainage. The color consistency and amount of drainage needs to be recorded. The amount of drainage should decrease daily. Management of the T-tube includes placing the patient in the Fowler position to promote drainage, monitoring output, protecting the skin, and ensuring the patient does not pull on the tube.

The surgical intervention is to remove the gallbladder. Removal can be accomplished either by an open cholecystectomy or laparoscopic cholecystectomy. Open cholecystectomy involves the physician making one large incision to remove the gallbladder. Laparoscopic cholecystectomy involves the physician making four small incisions to insert a scope, a video camera, and other instruments to remove the gallbladder.

Ideally, a cholecystectomy should be completed within 72 hours of admission in the absence of patient deterioration. Exceptions would be if emergency surgery is needed or if the patient has a history of previous cholecystitis, diabetes, or is older than 70 years of age.

Laparoscopic cholecystectomy is the most common invasive surgery for gallbladder disease. The procedure is often completed within 48 to 72 hours of admission and is considered to be the gold standard for treatment. During the procedure, carbon dioxide is used to raise the abdominal musculature away from the organs so that the surgeon can see the organs and perform the surgery. This laparoscopic approach has generally replaced the traditional open cholecystectomy.

An open cholecystectomy is more likely to be used when the patient has large stones or other abnormalities that require investigation. Surgical intervention can be delayed in order to allow the patient to recover from an acute episode.

Patient Education

Patients can assist in managing their gall bladder disease by altering their diet, losing weight, and avoiding high-cholesterol and high-fat foods. The inclusion of fresh fruits and vegetables with whole grains is beneficial. When assessing pain, ask about timing and frequency in relation to meals. See if there has been any nausea or vomiting associated with these events.

STEP 2: POTENTIAL PROBLEM/ DIAGNOSES

It is important that nurses understand and consider the science of the disease process and consider the possibilities prior to applying that knowledge to a patient situation. We begin that process with questioning.

💬 *Question:* Based upon your review of the content presented, what possible *potential problems* would you expect for a patient with these diagnoses?

💬 *Answer:* Pain, conflicted decision making, and infection

STEP 3: POTENTIAL INTERVENTIONS

💬 *Question:* Based on your identification of patient problems, what possible interventions would you recommend for these diagnoses, and what would you expect to happen? This would be considered your "grocery list" of the possible actions you could use to assist your patient.

💬 *Answer:* See the following problems, interventions, and expected outcomes:

Problem	Interventions	Expected Outcome
Pain	• Place in a position of comfort. • Administer an analgesic. • Assess opiate tolerance. • Identify pain intensity and characteristics. • Consider culture and religion in pain management strategies. • In discussing pain, use words understandable by the patient based on age and developmental level. • Identify what makes the pain better or worse, assess for nonverbal pain cues, and use nonpharmacological interventions such as imagery, relaxation, and hot or cold application. • Correct the patient's misconceptions about addiction.	Pain will be managed at a level acceptable to the patient.
Conflicted Decision	• Assess understanding of health-care choices. • Assess the patient's stress level relative to decision making. • Identify the discrepancy between the patient's view of a decision and the health-care provider's view. • Provide clear information to facilitate decision making and utilize available resources to assist with decision making (i.e., family, chaplain, special services). • Assist the patient in expressing feelings or concerns over the decision and assess the patient's decision-making ability. • Act as a liaison between the patient and others on the health-care team, and assist the patient in articulating health-care goals.	Positive health-care decisions

Continued

Table Continued

Problem	Interventions	Expected Outcome
Infection Risk	• Monitor for signs of infection, including vital signs. • Observe the wound for redness, swelling, or drainage. • Monitor laboratory values that could indicate infection (i.e., WBC, CRP). • Encourage good personal hygiene and hand washing. • Explain why there is an infection risk, and instruct the patient about proper hand washing and about the signs and symptoms of infection.	No postoperative infection

PUTTING IT ALL TOGETHER: APPLICATION OF THE NURSING PROCESS

Putting it all together is where the art and science of nursing meet to provide the best patient outcomes. We take the possibilities and place them into the context of the patient situation. To accomplish this, we use nursing diagnosis, nursing interventions, nursing outcomes, and nursing theory to provide the palate for nursing care.

STEP 4: ASSESSMENT

PATIENT INFORMATION: Ruby Baker, a 54-year-old elementary school bus driver

CHIEF COMPLAINT: Chest and right upper quadrant abdominal pain rated 10/10

HISTORY OF THE PRESENT ILLNESS: While driving the bus this morning, Ruby experienced severe chest and right upper quadrant abdominal pain and was brought to the emergency department for treatment.

PAST MEDICAL HISTORY: Moderately overweight, delivery of three healthy children

FAMILY HISTORY: Mother died of a heart attack at the age of 42; father is alive and in good health.

CHART REVIEW AND REPORT: Ruby was admitted through the emergency department (ED) for chest and upper abdominal pain. Ruby thought she was having a heart attack, stopped the school bus she was driving so no children would be injured, and called 911. Another driver took the children home from school. Ruby reported the pain to be a 10/10 on the pain scale. The pain was described as sharp and stabbing in the right side of her abdomen and chest. While in the ED, Ruby was medicated with morphine sulfate 2 mg IVP with good relief at 2/10 on the pain scale. Vital signs on admission were a BP of 128/72 mm Hg, a pulse of 88 beats per minute, a temperature of 100.9°F, and respirations of 18 breaths per minute. On physical assessment there is pain in the right upper subcostal area of the abdomen with deep palpation, a positive Murphy sign. EKG and cardiac enzyme studies were normal. The remainder of the physical examination is unremarkable. Ruby has been transported to the surgical unit for suspected gallbladder disease. A surgical consult has been ordered. Ultrasound is tied up with an emergency and Ruby will have an ultrasound to confirm gallbladder disease later in the day. Ruby is currently NPO with IV fluids of D5/ ½ NS running at 100 mL/hr. Ruby has had one dose of cefazolin, 1 mg.

SUBJECTIVE ASSESSMENT: As you enter the room, you see Ruby staring out of the window. You introduce yourself saying, *"Good morning, my name is Arvin James and I will be your nurse today. How are you feeling?"* Ruby looks at you with tearful eyes. "I thought I was going to die. Today when I was driving the bus and the pain started, it was so awful, I thought I was going to die. All I could think about is that I had to stop so the kids didn't get hurt and then call for help. I have never been so scared in my entire life." *"Are you having any pain now?"* "No, that's what's so crazy, the pain was so awful and now it is gone, how is that possible?" *"What did the doctor say?"* "He said it isn't my heart, that he thinks it's my gallbladder. He says I might need surgery." *"Sometimes the gallbladder acts like that—it can be really painful and then just stop."* "Will the pain start up again?" *"It is possible that is why he was thinking of doing surgery."* You inform Ruby that she is scheduled for an ultrasound of her gallbladder in about an hour to see if that is the cause of her pain. Ruby appears worried and tearful, saying "The doctor told me I may need to have surgery today." *"Does that worry you?"* "Yes, I have insurance through the school so I'm not worried about the bill, but I don't have any sick leave time. Money is so tight with my three boys. I can't lose time or money—we are barely making it now."

OBJECTIVE ASSESSMENT: Current vital signs are a temperature of 101.1°F, a pulse of 88 beats per minute, BP of 118/76 mm Hg, and respirations of 20 breaths per minute. The right upper quadrant of the abdomen is tender to gentle palpation. You see that there is dark-colored urine in the bedside commode. All other assessment findings are within normal limits. IV fluids continue to infuse as ordered. Ruby is to remain NPO until after her ultrasound as she may be scheduled for surgery later this afternoon.

- *Laboratory Studies:*
  - White blood count is 12.3 × 10³/microL.
  - Prothrombin time (PT) is 20 seconds, and international normalized ratio (INR) is 1.7.
- *Diagnostic Studies:*
  - Ultrasound was positive for gallbladder disease with stones located in the gallbladder and common bile duct.
- *Medications:*
  - Morphine sulfate 2 mg IV push every 2 hours as needed for pain.
  - Cefazolin 1 gram every 6 hours by IV piggyback

STEP 5: REALITY CHECK: DETOUR AHEAD

Reality Check occurs when the nurse takes a moment to think about individualized patient information that needs to be considered in framing diagnoses and interventions. This information is retrievable from any legitimate source (e.g., family, case management, other nurses, any ancillary, a doctor, etc.). These are the "wrenches" that create challenging situations, such as culture, religion, socioeconomic status, level of education, developmental level, marital status, employment, age, and gender.

Psychosocial History

Ruby is a hard-working single mom of three teenage boys. Ruby was a stay-at-home mom until 3 years ago, when her husband Robert died during a trucking accident. Since that time, Ruby attended driving school to learn how to drive a bus. This career was chosen so that she would only be working while her boys were at school. Ruby is the sole financial support as there is no family in the state. Recently Ruby's mother died of a heart attack, causing her to take off 2 weeks, using up all of her vacation days. Each day that Ruby is in the hospital she is losing income. Losing their father was very difficult for the boys, and they are just now beginning to act like their old selves. Ruby is terrified of what would happen to her boys if something should happen to her. Ruby's mother's death was devastating for her. It was not until she was sitting in the bus afraid for her life that she recognized her very real fear of dying and leaving her children alone. Because she is

not having a heart attack and the pain is gone, Ruby is thinking she should just go home so she can get back to work and take care of this health problem later. After Ruby voices her plan, you contact the surgeon who agrees that if the surgery is uncomplicated, he may allow Ruby to return to work on Tuesday next week with light duty, resuming full duty the following week so that she does not lose income. Ruby is considering his proposal.

Critical Thinking Moment

You have just completed the assessment of Ruby and need to make a decision about the patient's actual problems and nursing diagnoses based on the data you have collected and the potential problems you identified. Outcomes must be realistic and measurable.

STEP 6: ACTUAL PROBLEMS/DIAGNOSES

The *first step* in problem identification is to revisit the list of *potential diagnoses* and choose *actual diagnoses* based upon the learner's evaluation of the case study information provided. A problem statement must be completed for each identified problem/diagnosis. The actual problems for this case study are pain, conflicted decision making, and infection.

STEP 7: PLANNING: ACTUAL INTERVENTIONS

After actual diagnoses have been chosen, it is necessary to evaluate the list of *potential interventions* and choose *actual interventions* that will fit within the patient's reality and meet expected outcomes. Each intervention requires a rationale. Interventions are identified in three categories: (1) assessment, (2) therapeutic, and (3) education.

Diagnostic Statement

Pain related to inflammation of the gallbladder secondary to obstruction of the common bile duct as evidenced by pain rated at a 10/10 on admission.

Assessment

- Assess what makes pain better or worse. *Rationale: Assessing this assists with pain management interventions.*
- Assess the patient's pain intensity and characteristics. *Rationale: This establishes a baseline for comparison.*
- Assess the patient's understanding of pain interventions. *Rationale: This helps to identify areas of needed education.*

Therapeutic Interventions

- Administer morphine IVP every 2 hours for pain. *Rationale: This allows the goal of having a pain level acceptable to Ruby and follow-up within 1 hour to gauge the medication's effectiveness.*
- Keep the patient NPO. *Rationale: This allows Ruby to rest her gut and prepare for possible surgery.*
- Place the patient in the Fowler position. *Rationale: This position decreases pressure on the gut and decreases inflammation, thereby decreasing pain.*

Education

- Discuss the purpose for the patient's remaining NPO. *Rationale: This assists in resting the abdomen until bowel sounds are heard and the digestion of foods can be resumed.*
- Discuss potential common side effects of morphine, and instruct the patient to notify the nurse of any occurrence. *Rationale: Collaboration with pain management will improve its effectiveness.*
- Discuss how positioning may reduce the patient's pain. *Rationale: This assists Ruby in managing her pain.*

Expected Outcome

- Pain at a level acceptable to the patient

Diagnostic Statement

Conflicted decision related to the need for surgery as evidenced by the desire to improve health versus the need to prevent loss of income for family support.

Assessment

- Assess Ruby's demeanor. *Rationale: This allows you to evaluate whether or not she is capable of making an informed decision.*
- Assess Ruby's willingness to listen to options. *Rationale: This establishes a baseline for conversation.*
- Assess Ruby's ability to make decisions. *Rationale: This allows you to evaluate if she is emotionally labile.*

Therapeutic Interventions

- Discuss options and potential outcomes. *Rationale: This facilitates Ruby's making informed decisions.*
- Speak to the surgeon about patient concerns and inform the health-care team of Ruby's decisional conflict. *Rationale: Clear communication and collaboration are part of the nursing role.*
- Keep Ruby NPO. *Rationale: This makes surgery possible, if agreed to.*

Education

- Collaborate with health-care team members. *Rationale: This facilitates the goal of early treatment and discharge.*
- Educate Ruby about the possible consequences of delayed treatment. *Rationale: Understanding will assist the decision process when the patient is conflicted about how to proceed.*
- Educate Ruby about the benefits of early treatment. *Rationale: A clear understanding of the benefits of early treatment to her overall health will increase the likelihood of agreement to the plan of care.*

Expected Outcome

- Agreement to positive health-seeking behavior
- Laparoscopic surgery

Diagnostic Statement

Infection related to gallbladder inflammation and surgical intervention as evidenced by a temperature of 101.1°F and a WBC of 12.3×10^3/microL.

Assessment

- Monitor for changes in temperature. *Rationale: Temperature is an indicator of infection.*
- Monitor the postoperative incision site for redness, swelling, drainage, and warmth. *Rationale: This allows you to check for signs of infection.*
- Monitor laboratory values such as WBC. *Rationale: Changes could indicate infection.*

Therapeutic Interventions

- Assess environmental factors that may place Ruby at risk for infection. *Rationale: A clean immediate environment will decrease the risk of exposure to opportunistic organisms.*
- Administer cefazolin 1 g every 6 hours. *Rationale: Cefazolin treats the infection.*
- Encourage good hand hygiene. *Rationale: This prevents exposure to infecting organisms.*
- Observe Ruby's performance of hygiene. *Rationale: This ensures adequate infection control measures.*

Education

- Educate Ruby about the signs and symptoms of infection. *Rationale: An understanding of infection symptoms can facilitate necessary therapeutic interventions.*
- Explain how good hygiene and hand washing can prevent infection. *Rationale: Vigilant hand washing by the patient and family will decrease the risk of germ transmission.*
- Explain how cefazolin can treat the infection and discuss possible side effects. *Rationale: Understanding increases compliance with the plan of care and improved health maintenance activities. Ensuring a patient's understanding of a medication's possible side effect is part of the nursing role.*

Expected Outcome

- Absence of postoperative infection

STEP 8: IMPLEMENTATION

Nursing Theory

Ruby was terrified when she started to have pain; she really thought she was going to die of a heart attack like her mom did. This emotional response to the physical illness and her concern over losing money seem to be more of a worry to her than the illness itself. Emotional support will be a necessary part of helping Ruby through the decisional process related to agreeing to surgery. Anne Boykin's and Savina Schoenhofer's theory of caring encourages the nurse to make a personal connection with Ruby. This caring connection sets the stage for understanding the best way of helping and nurturing Ruby. Although nursing tasks are important, the focus of this theory is the artistic application of nursing as a social contract between Ruby and the nurse. The discussion would be, "How are *we* going to deal with this situation?" This is a dynamic process of understanding and acceptance within the immediate circumstances of Ruby's situation.

Emotional concerns have to be tempered by physical realities. Ruby will need to recognize that her physical health will affect her ability to care for her family. Nursing theorist Imogene King would recognize that Ruby and the nurse meet as strangers, and they need to develop a relationship in order to enable them to set mutual goals. However, goal setting needs to be done within the context of Ruby's reality, which is that of a single mom with no sick days left to cover time lost due to this illness. Goal setting needs to be done within Ruby's reality in order to be successful. Carefully consider verbal and nonverbal cues when providing and evaluating care. Remember that reality is defined as whatever Ruby says it is. Our job is to provide Ruby with information that will allow her to make informed decisions.

Ancillary Support

Ancillary support would be minimal in this situation. Social services may be able to assist Ruby in obtaining food and other supplies so that her limited funds can be used for more expensive demands such as rent. If there should be any need for other ancillary support, it would be based on events as they occur.

STEP 9: PLAN OF CARE

The plan of care is a road map for patient care and should be used as a communication tool between disciplines. Expected entries on the plan of care would be each identified problem, intervention, and expected outcome. The problems already discussed—pain, conflicted decision making, and infection—will be part of the plan. However, Ruby's plan of care will also need to focus heavily on how to assist her to meet her family obligations within the context of her illness. Contact with social support groups, local charities, and community churches may be good resources that could be included in the plan with Ruby's approval.

STEP 10: EVALUATION

Evaluation is an active process in which the nurse "connects the dots" to decide if the expected outcomes (goals) that were established have been met, partially met, or not met. If the goals are met, we continue with the plan as outlined. If the goal was partially met, we revise the parts of the plan that did not work. If the goals were not met, we start all over with a new plan.

End-of-Shift Narrative

The ultrasound confirmed that Ruby had gallstones. Ruby was kept NPO in the hopes that she could go to surgery today. In advocating for Ruby, you spoke with the surgeon and explained her financial and home situation. There was a long discussion with Ruby about the risks and benefits of surgery now versus later. The discussion considered the cost of readmission, the reoccurrence of pain, and the distress of this reoccurring situation to her sons, with possible worsening condition that would keep her out of work longer. After much thought, Ruby agreed to have the surgery if it could be done today and she could go home tomorrow. Luckily, the surgeon had a cancellation and Ruby was picked up by the transporter an hour ago. Based on Ruby's concern about being away from home and having too much time off, the surgeon agreed that if the gallbladder extraction was unremarkable she could be discharged tomorrow morning after his visit. Because today is Thursday, the surgeon plans to have Ruby come to his office on Monday, which is a school holiday. Assuming all goes well, Ruby may be able to go back to work on Tuesday of the next week, losing only 1 day of work over the 4-day holiday weekend. Ruby understands that it will be important to prevent infection after surgery and has been receptive to all of the infection prevention information provided. Ruby verbalizes her understanding that any signs and symptoms of infection should be reported immediately to the physician. Although distressed by the events, Ruby is greatly relieved that she will not lose too many hours. Ruby has expressed her thanks at working with her and helping to get everything set up so that she could have the surgery today and go home tomorrow. As Ruby was leaving for surgery, she said, "You will never know how much this means to me and my boys. Thank you so much for your help."

Problem Evaluation

PROBLEM 1: Pain. The expected outcome is that pain will be at a level acceptable to the patient. The goal is met: The morphine ordered for Ruby kept her pain at a level between 0/10 and 2/10.

PROBLEM 2: Conflicted Decision Making. While Ruby was originally conflicted about her decision to have surgery, the expected outcome is her agreement to positive health-seeking behavior, which is laparoscopic surgery. The goal is met: Although Ruby is unwilling at first to have the surgery, she recognized the benefit of surgery versus a possible worsening situation later. The opening in the surgical schedule coupled with the long weekend convinced Ruby that she should not put off the surgery.

PROBLEM 3: Infection. The expected outcome is that there will be an absence of a postoperative infection. The goal is partially met. Ruby has agreed to have the surgery, but we do not yet have any information about whether there will be a postoperative infection. However, Ruby has agreed to follow all of the physician's recommendations and was receptive to the infection prevention information provided. The expected outcome is that the infection will be resolved.

Overall Evaluation

Based on the end-of-shift assessment and the comparison of Ruby's progress during this shift, Ruby is found to be improving.

REFERENCES

Beers, M., Porter, R., Jones, T., Kaplan, J., & Berkwits, M. (Eds.). (2006). Urinary calculi. The MERCK Manual (18th ed., pp. 1967). Whitehouse Station; NJ: Merck Research Laboratories.

Camp-Sorrell, D., & Hawkins, R. (2006). Clinical manual for the oncology advanced practice nurse (2nd ed.). Pittsburgh, PA: ONS Publishing.

George, J. (2011). Nursing theories: The base for professional nursing practice (6th ed.). Upper Saddle River, NJ: Pearson Education.

Griffin, N., Charles-Edwards, G., & Grant, L.A. (2012). Magnetic resonance cholangiopancreatography: The ABC of MRCP. Insights Imaging, 3(1), 11–21. Retrieved from http://www.ncbi.nlm.nih.gov/pmc/articles/PMC3292642/

Gulanick, M., & Meyers, J. (2013). Nursing care plans nursing diagnosis and intervention (8th ed.). St Louis, MO: Mosby.

Holloway, N. (2004). Medical surgical nursing care planning (4th ed.). Springhouse, PA: Lippincott Williams & Wilkins.

LeMone, P., Burke, K., & Baldoff, G. (2011). Medical surgical nursing, Critical thinking in patient care (5th ed.). Upper Saddle River, NJ: Pearson.

Lithotripsy. Retrieved from http://www.nlm.nih.gov/medlineplus/ency/article/007113.htm

Parker, M. (2006). Nursing theories and nursing practice (2nd ed.). Philadelphia, PA: FA Davis.

Rodgers, S. (2008). Medical surgical nursing care plans. Clifton Park, NY: Thomson Delmar.

Swearingen, P. (2008). All in one care planning resource (2nd ed.). St Louis, MO: Mosby.

Van Leeuwen, A., & Bladh, M. (2015). Davis's comprehensive handbook of laboratory and diagnostic testing with nursing implications (6th ed.). Philadelphia, PA: F.A. Davis Company.

Wilkinson, J., & Ahern, N. (2009). In Nursing Diagnosis Handbook (9th ed.). Saddle River, NJ: Prentice Hall.

Wilson, B., Shannon, M., & Stang, C. (2006). Nurses drug guide. Upper Saddle River, NJ: Prentice Hall.

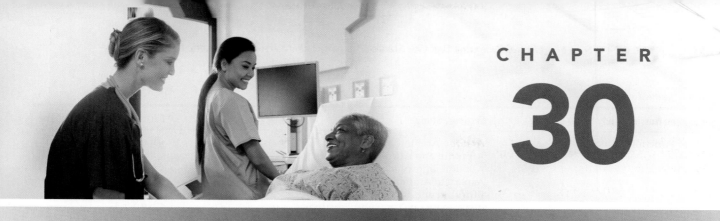

Immunologic System

Case Study: Systemic Lupus Erythematosus

Common Nursing Study Name	Section 1 Study	Section 1 Chapter Numbers
Amitriptyline	Antidepressant Drugs (Cyclic): Amitriptyline, Nortriptyline, Protriptyline, Doxepin, Imipramine	Chapter 1
Antinuclear Antibody (ANA) Panel	Antibodies, Antinuclear, Anti-DNA, Anticentromere, Antiextractable Nuclear Antigen, Anti-Jo, and Antiscleroderma	Chapter 5
Antiphospholipid (ALP)	Antibodies, Cardiolipin, Immunoglobulin A, Immunoglobulin G, and Immunoglobulin M	Chapter 5
	Lupus Anticoagulant Antibodies	Chapter 5
Blood Sugar	Glucose	Chapter 1
Blood Urea Nitrogen (BUN)	Urea Nitrogen, Blood	Chapter 1
Chest X-Ray	Chest X-Ray	Chapter 16
C3 and C4 Complement Levels	Complement C3 and Complement C4	Chapter 5
Complete Blood Count (CBC)	Complete Blood Count, Hematocrit	Chapter 2
	Complete Blood Count, Hemoglobin	Chapter 2
	Complete Blood Count, Platelet Count	Chapter 3
	Complete Blood Count, RBC Count	Chapter 2
	Complete Blood Count, RBC Indices	Chapter 2
	Complete Blood Count, RBC Morphology and Inclusions	Chapter 2
	Complete Blood Count, WBC Count and Differential	Chapter 2
C-Reactive Protein (CRP)	C-Reactive Protein	Chapter 1
Creatinine, Urine	Creatinine, Urine, and Creatinine Clearance, Urine	Chapter 22
Creatinine (Serum) (Cr)	Creatinine, Blood	Chapter 1
Echocardiogram	Echocardiography	Chapter 21
Erythrocyte Sedimentation Rate (ESR)	Erythrocyte Sedimentation Rate	Chapter 2
Knee X-Ray	Radiography, Bone	Chapter 16

Continued

Table Continued

Common Nursing Study Name	Section 1 Study	Section 1 Chapter Numbers
Liver Function Tests	Alanine Aminotransferase	Chapter 1
	Albumin and Albumin/Globulin Ratio	Chapter 1
	Alkaline Phosphatase and Isoenzymes	Chapter 1
	Aspartate Aminotransferase	Chapter 1
	Bilirubin and Bilirubin Fractions	Chapter 1
	Protein, Blood, Total and Fractions	Chapter 1
Methotrexate	Immunosuppressants: Cyclosporine, Methotrexate, Everolimus, Sirolimus, and Tacrolimus	Chapter 1
Protein Clearance	Protein, Urine: Total Quantitative and Fractions	Chapter 22
Syphilis Testing	Syphilis Serology	Chapter 5

STEP 1: DATA COLLECTION

Pathophysiology

You may be thinking to yourself, my patient has all of these weird symptoms and no one can figure out what is wrong. If that is the case, your patient might have lupus. Systemic lupus erythematosus (SLE) is a chronic inflammatory autoimmune disease of the connective tissue with no known specific cause or cure, and has the potential to affect every organ in the body.

Lupus occurs in women more often than in men. Groups most at risk are African American women followed by Hispanic, Native American, and Asian women. Those at greatest risk are between the ages of 15 and 45 during childbearing years or after menopause. For this reason, some believe sex hormones may be involved with the development of lupus. However, the truth is that no one really knows. Triggers for SLE are thought to be chemicals, environment, heredity, stress, sunlight, infection, injury, radiation exposure, vaccination, and drug-induced causes.

So what happens to the body when lupus occurs? Lupus is characterized by the production of antibodies that fight against normal tissue. This begins when T cells and B cells fail to moderate the immune response. The body's immune system becomes confused and overreacts. Antibodies designed to protect the body against attack are unable to distinguish between themselves and foreign invaders. The confused antibodies begin to attack tissues throughout the body, which results in multisystem microvascular inflammation. Antibodies combine with antigens to form immune complexes that deposit in tissues. Damage occurs to the skin, heart, kidneys, lungs, blood vessels, and central nervous system. Systemic responses can range from mild during periods of remission to severe during episodes of flare.

Lupus can be categorized into types: discoid, drug induced, and systemic lupus. Discoid lupus affects the skin and is characterized by scaly plaques found most often on the head, neck, ears, and scalp. Scalp lesions may lead to hair loss, and old lesions may lead to scarring. Hair may return once the lesions are healed. Some individuals with discoid lupus may transition to systemic lupus. Drug-induced lupus is triggered by a medication that has been prescribed for a medical problem. The most common drugs triggers are procainamide, hydralazine, isoniazid, quinidine, and phenytoin. When a drug-induced event occurs, the drug should be immediately discontinued. Symptoms of drug-induced lupus are similar to SLE. Systemic lupus erythematosus is the most damaging to the body and is presented in this case.

Signs and Symptoms

The signs and symptoms of lupus can be vague, nonspecific, and easily confused with other diseases, hence the term "the great imitator." The symptoms and severity of lupus will vary widely from person to person with episodes of exacerbation called *flares* and episodes of wellness or *remission*. This fluctuation can be devastating both physically and psychologically. To assist physicians in diagnosing lupus, the American College of Rheumatology has created a criteria-based classification system. Presenting symptoms are used to diagnose the disease. Anyone who has 4 or more of the 11 identified lupus signs and/or symptoms either simultaneously or within an observed period of time is considered to have SLE.

The following symptoms do not have to manifest at the same time:

- Malar rash—rash over the cheeks, sometimes described as a butterfly rash
- Discoid rash—red, raised patches
- Photosensitivity—exposure resulting in the development of or an increase in skin rash
- Oral ulcers
- Nonerosive arthritis involving two or more peripheral joints

- Pleuritis or pericarditis
- Renal disorder—as evidenced by excessive protein in the urine or the presence of casts in the urine
- Neurological disorder—seizures or psychosis in the absence of drugs known to cause these effects
- Hematological disorder—hemolytic anemia, leukopenia, lymphopenia, thrombocytopenia in which the leukopenia or lymphopenia occurs on more than two occasions and the thrombocytopenia occurs in the absence of drugs known to cause it
- Positive antinuclear antibody (ANA) in the absence of a drug known to induce lupus, or immunological disorder—evidenced by positive anti-double-stranded (anti-ds) DNA, positive anti-Smith (anti-Sm), positive antiphospholipid such as anticardiolipin antibody, positive lupus anticoagulant test, or a false-positive serological syphilis test, known to be positive for at least 6 months and confirmed to be falsely positive by a negative *Treponema pallidum* immobilization or FTA-ABS

The Systemic Lupus International Collaborating Clinics met and created easily identifiable clinical and immunologic criteria for diagnosing lupus. See Fig. 30.1 for the classification system of the American College of Rheumatology.

When assessing for SLE, a clear systematic head-to-toe assessment approach should be used so that nothing is missed. Skin should be inspected for any rash. Butterfly rash, a classic symptom of SLE, is found on the cheeks and nose. This is seen in about half of the patients, and can be either malar or discoid. Most patients are photosensitive. Exposure to light exacerbates skin rashes and system effects. Hair loss on the scalp or other areas of the body may be seen.

Musculoskeletal complaints of joint pain, swelling, stiffness, and muscular weakness are the most common symptoms of SLE. The way to differentiate SLE joint symptoms from other orthopedic problems is that bone and cartilage are not destroyed and symptoms are not static but move to different parts of the body. Musculoskeletal symptoms also come and go.

Kidney problems may be early presenting symptoms of SLE in the form of nephritis. Patients may not notice nephritis symptoms such as proteinuria, casts, and red cells until the disease is advanced and damage is done. Cardiovascular involvement may include pericarditis, endocarditis, and vasculitis. Myocarditis from cardiac inflammation may lead to heart failure. The assessment of cardiac valve dysfunction and ventricular or atrial gallop is recommended.

The pulmonary effects of SLE may be life-threatening and include pulmonary hemorrhage, pulmonary embolism, pulmonary hypertension, pleuritis, and interstitial lung disease. Cardiopulmonary status can be assessed by auscultation of the lungs to check for pleural friction rub, or crackles. Hematologic effects of the disease include anemia, leukopenia, thrombocytopenia, and lymphopenia. Neurologic involvement can vary from mild to severe. Symptoms may range from severe headache to seizure, from peripheral neuropathy to confusion, or from being severely altered or exhibiting psychosis. The assessment of orientation can help to evaluate cognitive function. Gastrointestinal assessment should include a careful evaluation of the abdomen for pain or distention that may indicate peritonitis, pancreatitis, intestinal vasculitis, or bowel infarction. Depression can occur as a result of changes in the quality of life from pain and from disfigurement caused by chronic skin conditions.

Laboratory Studies

The challenge in using laboratory studies used to check for SLE is that although positive results are highly suggestive of a diagnosis, some tests can be positive when the disease is not present. All laboratory findings need to be used in combination with symptom analysis and physical assessment. An ANA panel is a laboratory test used to diagnose multiple systemic autoimmune disorders, including SLE. ANA checks to see if there are antibodies that mistake normal cells for non-normal cells and attack them. Most individuals with SLE will have a positive ANA. However, this test is considered to be nonspecific because it can also be positive when an individual has scleroderma, autoimmune hepatitis, and bacterial or viral infections. Some

---

SLICC† Classification Criteria for Systemic Lupus Erythematosus

Requirements: ≥4 criteria (at least 1 clinical and 1 laboratory criteria OR biopsy-proven lupus nephritis with positive ANA or Anti-DNA)

Clinical Criteria	Immunologic Criteria
1. Acute Cutaneous Lupus* 2. Chronic Cutaneous Lupus* 3. Oral or nasal ulcers* 4. Nonscarring alopecia 5. Arthritis* 6. Serositis* 7. Renal* 8. Neurologic* 9. Hemolytic anemia 10. Leukopenia* 11. Thrombocytopenia ($<100,000/mm^3$)	1. ANA 2. Anti-DNA 3. Anti-Sm 4. Antiphospholipid Ab* 5. Low complement (C3, C4, CH50) 6. Direct Coombs' test (do not count in the presence of hemolyticanemia)

†SLICC: Systemic Lupus International Collaborating Clinics
*See notes for criteria details

FIGURE 30.1 SLICC Classification for Identifying Symptoms of Lupus. *From www.rheumtutor.com/2012-slicc-sle-criteria/. Please visit the website for a complete analysis of SLE Symptoms. Used with permission of Raj Carmona, MBBS, FRCPN; Assistant Professor of Medicine, McMaster University/St. Joseph's Healthcare.*

medications—diabetic, diuretic, and anticonvulsant—can also cause a false-positive result.

Anti-Sm testing is a laboratory test that is specific for SLE but only has a positive result in up to 30% of patients. Anti-ds DNA is positive in up to 70% of individuals with SLE because it is specific to antibodies against native DNA. Antiphospholipid (APL) antibodies, anticardiolipin and lupus anticoagulant antibodies, are found in about 50% of patients with SLE, but is also positive in individuals without SLE. Syphilis testing with repeated false-positive results may be a clue that the individual has SLE. A complete blood count (CBC) can assess for anemia caused by chronic inflammation. This laboratory study can also be used to check for leukopenia and lymphopenia. Liver function tests can be used to monitor the body's response to immunosuppressive or nonsteroidal anti-inflammatory medications.

Measures of blood urea nitrogen (BUN) and creatinine (Cr) are used to assess renal function, which can be compromised by nephritis. These laboratory tests can be used to complement the 24-hour urine test in the assessment of renal function. A 24-hour urine test can be used to assess renal function by checking the kidneys for creatinine and protein clearance.

Measuring the erythrocyte sedimentation rate (ESR) is not specific to diagnosing SLE but is useful as an early indicator of acute widespread inflammation that may occur in an autoimmune disorder. An elevated ESR result could be indicative of an SLE flare. C-reactive protein (CRP) is produced by the liver. An elevated CRP level is an indication of inflammation somewhere in the body. It is not specific to SLE but is useful in confirming the presence of an inflammatory response. The measure of serum complement can be used as an indicator of autoimmune disease, such as SLE. Two frequently measured serum complement proteins, C3 and C4, assist in the immunological and inflammatory responses associated with autoimmune diseases by destroying and removing foreign materials. Serum C3 and C4 complement levels will therefore be decreased in SLE due to their increased rate of consumption during the mechanisms involving the autoimmune process.

Diagnostic Studies

There is no diagnostic study used to diagnose SLE. Chest x-ray can check for pleural effusion, cardiomegaly, or lung infiltrates. Echocardiogram can assist in the diagnosis of pulmonary hypertension, and to assess for effusion or valvular pathology.

General/Medical Management

SLE is not curable, but it is treatable. Untreated SLE can end in death. The plan chosen to manage SLE is customized to the presenting symptoms and treatment goals. Goals are focused on preventing the exacerbation of the disease, treating occurring flares, and limiting complications.

Steroid Administration

Preventing exacerbation is mostly accomplished through the administration of medications that treat SLE by decreasing inflammation and reducing pain. Some medications are used to treat more than one symptom. Corticosteroids are the classic anti-inflammatory drug prescribed in various dosages and durations to meet treatment needs. Corticosteroids can be administered as an oral or IV medication and act to decrease inflammation. The dosage is dependent on presenting symptoms. Low doses can relive joint inflammation, and higher doses are used for organ involvement. Steroids are contraindicated if there is a history of diabetes, glaucoma, ulcers, heart failure, or liver or kidney disease.

Pain Management

Pain management can be accomplished using different types of drugs. Nonsteroidal anti-inflammatory drugs can treat joint pain and swelling, as well as fever and fatigue. Opioids such as combination hydrocodone and acetaminophen can provide relief for pain that is not managed by other medications. Contraindications related to comorbidities should be considered in pain drug selection.

Antimalarial Drugs

Antimalarial drugs may be used to treat fatigue, skin rashes, mouth sores, lung inflammation, and joint pain. Hydroxychloroquine, chloroquine, and quinacrine hydrochloride are some of the suggested drugs of choice. Antimalarial drugs can take months to reach a therapeutic drug level. Individuals will need to be reminded to be patient and take drugs as prescribed. Visual field changes can occur when antimalarial drugs are taken, therefore yearly eye exams are recommended.

Immunosuppressive Medications

Immunosuppressive medications are useful in reducing inflammation of the heart, lungs, central nervous system, and kidneys in the presence of severe SLE. Immunosuppressive drugs are considered a good alternative to steroid use but can increase the risk of nausea and vomiting. Suggested medication choices include azathioprine, cyclophosphamide, methotrexate, and ciclosporin. Patients taking these medications should be monitored for bone marrow suppression as the use of these drugs can place the patient at risk for an infection that could be life-threatening.

Emotional Support

Depression is a real concern in SLE sufferers. Antidepressants such as amitriptyline can assist in managing the depression that occurs in those with chronic illness. Other medication therapies that may be beneficial are vitamins A, B$_{12}$, D, folic acid, and St. John's Wort to assist in managing osteoporosis as well as fighting fatigue and depression.

Belimumab has been approved by the U.S. Food and Drug Administration (FDA) to treat lupus. This newer drug works by decreasing the number of abnormal B cells, and by diminishing SLE activity and symptoms such as joint pain. Belimumab seems to be most effective when used in combination with other lupus medications and is contraindicated for use in the presence of severe nephritis or central nervous system problems.

Limiting and Treating Flares

Limiting SLE complications is dependent on good patient education. An SLE patient who comprehends the risks and potential consequences of poor health management is more likely to adhere to his or her treatment plan. Being able to recognize symptoms is part of this process. A daily question should be, "how am I feeling today?" If the answer is "I am feeling bad," with increasing pain, headache, fatigue, fever, or a new-onset rash, a flare may be starting. Flares can last for days or weeks and can become dangerous if untreated, causing serious organ damage. Recognizing a flare, however subtle, is an important factor in SLE management. Suspected flares should be reported immediately to the health-care provider (HCP).

Helping patients understand what causes them to experience a flare is an important part of management. Collaboration between the patient and the physician related to identifying flare causes and successful treatments is necessary. Treating flares as they occur is very important to overall health.

Renal flares precipitate weight gain from water retention due to excessive protein loss with swelling of the feet, legs, and ankles. Foamy, frothy urine and nocturia may also occur. Cardiovascular flares are related to inflammation and may include pericarditis, myocarditis, or endocarditis. Flares that affect the central nervous system may be initially attributed to other causes. Symptoms include fatigue, headache, fever, memory loss, stroke, vision changes, confusion, altered behavior, and seizure. Flares that affect the skin are obvious as they are easily seen. Skin flares can occur from exposure to sunlight, fluorescent light, or other light sources when exposed for extended periods of time.

Infection is one of the primary causes of death in SLE sufferers and is often associated with the use of immunosuppressive medications. Recognizing the symptoms of infection and acting in ways to prevent infection is important. Good hygienic habits are important. Keeping appointments for laboratory work that may catch an infection early is important. Being aware of the symptoms of infection is key to staying healthy.

Understanding the importance of taking all prescribed medications is necessary to controlling SLE and preventing flares. Medications should never be stopped or changed without discussion with the prescribing physician. Each medication is necessary to support good health. Patients should know the medication dose, the expected action, side effects, and administration times.

Living a healthy lifestyle can assist in preventing flares. Undue stress can exacerbate SLE. Care should be taken to avoid stress, which can be supported by family and friends. Adequate rest and good nutrition are a part of healthy living. Unhealthy habits such as smoking and excessive alcohol intake should be avoided.

Patient Education

How do you tell someone that his or her entire life has just changed? The multiple challenges that accompany a diagnosis of SLE are legion. You will need to find out what is most important to your patient and design your education to meet his or her immediate needs. Some may despair what they perceive as severe restrictions on their personal choices. Compliance is necessary to prevent flares with devastating results. Help patients understand that they may be able to keep a modified version of their current lifestyle. Clear understanding of the disease and collaboration with their HCP may allow them to keep their dreams.

STEP 2: POTENTIAL PROBLEM/DIAGNOSES

It is important that nurses understand and consider the science of the disease process and consider the possibilities prior to applying that knowledge to a patient situation. We begin that process with questioning.

Question: Based upon your review of the content presented, what possible *potential problems* would you expect for a patient with these diagnoses?

Answer: Systemic lupus erythematosus can present in multiple ways. The problems chosen for this case are mobility, pain, fatigue, body image, and skin.

STEP 3: POTENTIAL INTERVENTIONS AND EXPECTED OUTCOMES

Question: Based upon your identification of patient problems, what possible interventions would you recommend for these diagnoses, and what would you expect to happen? This would be considered your "grocery list" of the possible actions you could use to assist your patient.

💬 *Answer:* See the following problems, interventions, and expected outcomes:

Problem	Interventions	Expected Outcome
Mobility	<ul><li>Assess current range of motion and evaluate mobility history.</li><li>Administer analgesic for pain.</li><li>Explain nonpharmacologic measures that can be taken to control pain, and use moist heat treatment for joint comfort.</li><li>Exercise regularly.</li><li>Learn to balance/bundle activity and rest.</li><li>Facilitate physical therapy and encourage good posture and body mechanics.</li><li>Assess the safety of the home environment, and evaluate the need for assistive devices.</li><li>Explain how the disease affects mobility.</li><li>Refer to a support group.</li></ul>	The patient can comfortably perform activities of daily living
Pain	<ul><li>Assess pain with a pain scale.</li><li>Assess the characteristics of pain, as well as the location, duration, and precipitating and relieving factors.</li><li>Apply moist or cold heat.</li><li>Administer drugs as needed: anti-inflammatory medications, NSAIDs, antimalarial drugs, cytotoxic drugs, and corticosteroids.</li><li>Monitor blood sugar if on steroids.</li><li>Facilitate physical therapy.</li><li>Educate the patient to exercise regularly, and to use relaxation techniques and imagery.</li><li>Provide diversional activities.</li></ul>	Pain relief at a level comfortable for the patient
Fatigue	<ul><li>Encourage pacing activities and periods of rest.</li><li>Assess for physical signs of fatigue and limit visitors to prevent fatigue.</li><li>Plan activities for times of high energy, such as early morning.</li><li>Increase the intake of high-energy foods such as organ meats, chicken, and whole grains.</li></ul>	Positive fatigue management
Skin	<ul><li>Assess the patient's understanding of skin changes.</li><li>Assess the nose and mouth for ulcers, assess the scalp for lesions, and assess the trunk for rashes.</li><li>Use nonperfumed lotion on skin and use nonperfumed shampoo.</li><li>Discuss clothing choices that can protect against the sun, and discuss using sunscreen SPF greater than 30 to protect against UV light.</li></ul>	The patient can state the cause of the rash and exacerbation prevention techniques
Body Image	<ul><li>Assess the patient's feelings about disease-related physical changes and provide assurance that the patient's feelings about identified changes are normal.</li><li>Provide privacy to prevent embarrassment when performing activities of daily living.</li><li>Educate the patient about skin care in order to protect skin and prevent disfigurement.</li><li>Discuss the use of wigs or other types of hairpieces for alopecia.</li><li>Arrange a visit from a support group member to discuss body image issues.</li><li>Monitor interpersonal interactions with family and friends.</li><li>Monitor for withdrawal or depression; administer an antidepressant if needed.</li><li>Consider the patient's religion in relation to body image changes.</li><li>Consider recommending psychosocial counseling and provide information on community support groups.</li></ul>	The patient verbalizes the impact of an altered body image and considers positive solutions

PUTTING IT ALL TOGETHER: APPLICATION OF THE NURSING PROCESS

Putting it all together is where the art and science of nursing meet to provide the best patient outcomes. We take the possibilities and place them into the context of the patient situation. To accomplish this we use nursing diagnosis, nursing interventions, nursing outcomes, and nursing theory to provide the palate for nursing care.

STEP 4: ASSESSMENT

PATIENT INFORMATION: Martha Jackson, an 18-year-old African American female

CHIEF COMPLAINT: Increasingly severe joint pain in her knees, a rash on her face that will not go away, fatigue, and morning stiffness

HISTORY OF THE PRESENT ILLNESS: Complaint of severe, debilitating knee pain for the past 2 weeks without relief; was seen in the emergency department last evening stating that the ibuprofen given to her by the doctor is not working and she is seeking further treatment for pain relief

PAST MEDICAL HISTORY: Unremarkable

FAMILY HISTORY: Mother has rheumatoid arthritis; father died at war and received the Purple Heart prior to her birth and was in good health at the time of his death

CHART REVIEW AND REPORT: Martha arrived as a direct admission from the emergency room. She had been seen by her family physician earlier in the day with complaints of pain at a 6/10 and stiffness in both knees. Her physician prescribed 800 mg of ibuprofen every 8 hours. Martha had no pain relief during the night so she came to the emergency room for treatment. Her current pain level is reported as a 10/10. The pain is described as being like a constant toothache in her knees. The emergency room physician in consultation with her primary care doctor decided to admit her for pain management and evaluation. Martha has a red rash across the bridge of her nose and told the nurse she thinks she has psoriasis because of the scaly patches on her scalp. Her vital signs are BP of 116/74 mm Hg, a pulse of 76 beats per minute, a temperature of 99.8°F, respirations of 16 breaths per minutes, and a WBC on the low side at 5.5×10^3/microL. Martha has been given morphine sulfate 2 mg IV push and is reported to be sleeping.

SUBJECTIVE ASSESSMENT: Arvin James (AJ) has floated to the observation unit for the day due to multiple sick calls that have left this unit short. AJ received a brief orientation to the floor and then was assigned to Martha. The report that AJ receives about Martha is incomplete and very brief since the nurse caring for her left early due to a family emergency. AJ receives an update from the charge nurse who tells him that Martha arrived on the unit 2 hours ago. She has been admitted and her last pain medication was morphine 2 mg IVP administered in the emergency department (ED). There are no pending laboratory studies, and an x-ray of the knees was negative. AJ is told that Martha's admission vital signs were normal except for a low-grade fever. A urinalysis collected in the ED was reported to have some cellular casts and red cells. AJ reviews the ED notes and sees that Martha has a rash on her face, has reported scaling on her scalp, and has a low WBC.

Upon entering the room, AJ sees that Martha is now awake, and he introduces himself as the nurse for the day. Martha appears to be restless and fidgety in bed, and asks, "Can you get me more pain medication? I just got back from the bathroom and the pain was so bad I could barely walk. What is wrong with me? I'm as stiff as an old woman. This is more than sore muscles like my doctor said." *"How severe would you rate the pain?"* AJ asks. "A 10/10," Martha returns, "Please just get me something—I can't take this pain." AJ looks concerned and continues, *"Can you tell me what makes the pain worse?"* Martha grimaces, "Any kind of walking early in the morning is painful and difficult." *"Have you done anything at home that seems to help?"* AJ asks. "Sometimes I put on hot, wet towels and that has helped some but not enough, I need the morphine." Martha sobs. AJ leaves and returns with another dose of morphine 2 mg, which he administers via an IV push. *"Martha, I am going to leave you to rest and let this medication work and then I will come back and check on you, is that alright?"* "Perfect," Martha replies, and then closes her eyes as AJ leaves the room.

OBJECTIVE ASSESSMENT: Fifteen minutes after the administration of the morphine, AJ returns to complete the morning assessment. As he enters the room, he sees that Martha is awake. *"How is the pain now?"* AJ asks. "Much better," Martha replies. "I would give it a 3/10, still a little achy but tolerable." AJ asks, *"Can I look at your knees now if that's all right?"* "Sure," Martha replies as she pulls back the covers. Martha's knees are moderately swollen, warm, and tender to the touch. AJ asks, *"Are you having pain anywhere else?"* "No," Martha replies. "But this rash on my face is getting worse, and I have these scaly patches on my scalp. My mom says it is psoriasis. I noticed when I was brushing my teeth this morning that there are some sores in my mouth. I didn't know they were there. They don't hurt but it worries me. Do you think it is herpes?" AJ steps closer, saying, *"Open your mouth and let me check."* After a quick visual assessment, AJ replies,

"They don't look inflamed. I'll let your doctor know so he can take a look when he comes in." Current vital signs are BP of 112/70 mm Hg, a pulse of 70 beats per minutes, a temperature of 99.8°F, and respirations of 16 breaths per minute. All other assessments are within normal limits.

- *Laboratory Studies:*
  - No new studies have been ordered.
- *Diagnostic Studies:*
  - Knee x-rays are negative.
- *Medications:*
  - Ibuprofen 800 mg PO every 8 hours as needed for mild pain
  - Hydrocodone 5/500 one tablet every 4 hours for moderate pain
  - Morphine 2 mg IV push every 2 hours for severe pain

STEP 5: REALITY CHECK: DETOUR AHEAD

Reality Check occurs when the nurse takes a moment to think about individualized patient information that needs to be considered in framing diagnoses and interventions. This information is retrievable from any legitimate source (e.g., family, case management, other nurses, any ancillary, a doctor, etc.). These are the "wrenches" that create challenging situations, such as culture, religion, socioeconomic status, level of education, developmental level, marital status, employment, age, and gender.

Psychosocial History

Martha wants to be a photojournalist and graduated from her high school with a GPA of 3.6. Her mother is a musician and plays the violin in the local philharmonic orchestra. Martha has applied to several colleges but is concerned that they cannot afford the college with the program she wants to attend. As a way to earn college tuition, Martha entered an essay competition and landed a summer job at a premier camp. The job is 8 weeks long and consists of taking groups of campers on nature hikes. Martha is worried that if she is unable to take the job because of the pain in her knees, she may not have money for school. Martha has been having symptoms like this for the past 3 years; sometimes it is her knees that hurt and sometimes it is other joints. She has not said anything to her mother because she is worried they cannot afford medical care, and she has been secretly sexually active since the age of 14 and wonders if she has a sexually transmitted disease. About 6 months ago Martha went to a clinic for venereal disease testing, which came back positive. Martha was very upset and with her friend's urging was retested with the same results, positive. Martha saw a physician at the clinic who examined her and told her regardless of the laboratory results she did not have a venereal disease. Martha does not want her mother to know about this incident and so has not shared her fears. After the last clinic visit, Martha decided to abstain from sexual activity and has kept that promise to herself.

Critical Thinking Moment

You have just completed the assessment and need to make a decision about the patient's *actual* problems and nursing diagnoses based upon the data you have collected and the potential problems you identified. Outcomes must be realistic and measurable.

STEP 6: ACTUAL PROBLEMS/ DIAGNOSES

The *first step* in problem identification is to revisit the list of *potential diagnoses* and choose *actual diagnoses* based on the learner's evaluation of the case study information provided. A problem statement must be completed for each identified problem/diagnosis.

The actual problems for this case study are that Martha has been seen by an immunologist who feels that there is enough evidence to support a diagnosis of SLE. She has been told and is unsure what the diagnosis means but is glad that she does not have a sexually transmitted disease. The immunologist explained to her that the false-positive venereal disease results were probably due to the SLE. Martha has been started on hydroxychloroquine 310 mg twice a day (bid), and may be started on prednisone. Based on the previous information, the problems chosen for this case study are mobility, pain, and skin.

STEP 7: PLANNING: ACTUAL INTERVENTIONS

After actual diagnoses have been chosen, it is necessary to evaluate the list of *potential interventions* and choose *actual interventions* that will fit within the patient's reality and meet expected outcomes. Each intervention requires a rationale. Interventions are identified in three categories: (1) assessment, (2) therapeutic, and (3) education.

Diagnostic Statement

Altered physical mobility related to joint inflammation as evidenced by swelling, tenderness, complaints of morning stiffness, joint pain of 10/10, and stated difficulty in getting to the bathroom.

Assessment

- Assess Martha's current range of motion. *Rationale: This helps you determine baseline functionality.*
- Assess Martha's need for any assistive devices. *Rationale: These devices may make it easier for Martha to be self-sufficient. Evaluate her fall risk.*
- Assess Martha's gait when she is out of bed. *Rationale: This helps you evaluate how severely her mobility is limited.*

Therapeutic Interventions

- Administer hydrocodone 5 mg to Martha as needed for pain. *Rationale: Pain relief increases mobility.*
- Encourage performance of range-of-motion exercises prior to getting out of bed in the morning. *Rationale: This limbers joints and facilitates mobility.*
- Administer morphine 2 mg IVP to Martha for severe pain. *Rationale: Adequate pain management is essential to healing.*

Education

- Teach Martha good body mechanics. *Rationale: This protects joints from injury and reduces joint stress.*
- Teach Martha to bundle activities. *Rationale: This decreases stress on the joints.*
- Explain to Martha how the disease can affect joints and mobility. *Rationale: This improves compliance.*

Expected Outcome

- Improved mobility tolerance with better pain management

Diagnostic Statement

Pain related to joint swelling and inflammation as evidenced by a report of pain in the knees of 10/10 and fidgety restlessness movement.

Assessment

- Assess Martha's pain using the 0/10 scale. *Rationale: This establishes a baseline for pain management.*
- Assess precipitating factors to Martha's pain, including the time of onset; aggravating factors; relieving factors; and the location, duration, and character of the pain. *Rationale: This helps to accurately understand the relationship between pain and function in order to create a pain management plan.*
- Assess pain relief with the current medication. *Rationale: This helps you determine if alterations need to be made for appropriate pain management.*

Therapeutic Interventions

- Administer hydrocodone or morphine as needed. *Rationale: This reduces pain.*

- Administer ibuprofen 800 mg every 8 hours. *Rationale: This is an anti-inflammatory that decreases pain.*
- Administer hydroxychloroquine 310 mg bid. *Rationale: This decreases the progression of the disease over time.*

Education

- Report any vision loss to the physician. *Rationale: Hydroxychloroquine can cause vision loss.*
- Take medications on a dosing schedule rather than as needed. *Rationale: This provides better pain relief.*
- Report increased pain. *Rationale: This may indicate a flare.*

Expected Outcome

- Pain at a level acceptable to Martha

Diagnostic Statement

Skin integrity alteration as related to an inappropriate autoimmune response evidenced by a butterfly rash on the face and a scaly rash on the scalp.

Assessment

- Assess the degree of rash on the face. *Rationale: This allows you to evaluate whether or not the rash is improving.*
- Assess the scalp for lesions and hair loss. *Rationale: This allows you to establish a baseline.*
- Inspect Martha's skin to see if there are any other rashes present. *Rationale: This allows you to check for malar and discoid rashes.*

Therapeutic Interventions

- Use nonperfumed skin lotion to prevent dryness. *Rationale: The alcohol content in perfumed lotion can irritate sensitive skin.*
- Take hydroxychloroquine 310 mg bid. *Rationale: Control of the disease may improve the rash.*
- Keep windows in the room closed to prevent sun exposure. *Rationale: This reduces skin irritation.*

Education

- Avoid exposure to the sun. *Rationale: Sun exposure can exacerbate the rash.*
- Discuss the use of SPF 25 or higher lotion. *Rationale: This protects the skin from ultraviolet sunlight.*
- Discuss how appropriate clothing can protect the skin from UV light. *Rationale: This can help prevent flares.*

Expected Outcome

- Martha will understand that the rash on her face and scalp may improve over time with treatment.

STEP 8: IMPLEMENTATION

Nursing Theory

Martha has been diagnosed with a disease that will fundamentally change how she approaches her life choices. The potentially debilitating nature of SLE makes it important that Martha clearly understand the consequences of choices she may make. Faye Glenn Abdellah was one of the pioneers of the concept of nursing diagnoses. The focus of Abdellah's theory is on the nurse's ability to identify and solve nursing problems, with prevention, rehabilitation, and wellness as the goal. Martha will need to understand flare triggers and how healthy choices associated with SLE will affect her life. Abdellah recognizes that obvious nursing problems such as pain and a lack of skin integrity may intermingle with more emotional problems such as altered body image. Both types of problems could be interrelated, and solving one may solve the other. Abdellah's assumption is that correctly identifying Martha's problems will guide the nurse to the correct choices of interventions and positive outcomes.

Margaret Newman is a theorist who views health and wellness as a pattern and rhythm of living that is encompassed within the movement of time and space. In this theory, Martha would be viewed as a dynamic entity capable of making choices that will move her to a higher level of consciousness. The disease of SLE is perceived as patterns that provide information to assist Martha and her nurse in setting goals. Goal setting is viewed as a collaborative effort that includes ancillaries and other HCPs. Newman emphasizes looking at the problem as a whole instead of objectifying it. In Martha's case, her nurse would not just address the disease process of SLE but would take in the whole situation, including Martha's age, culture, life goals, and overall health. Illness is considered to be a transformative event in Martha's life.

Ancillary Support

Martha is at the beginning of the illness, and the symptoms of SLE are limited to joint pain and rash. Ancillary support for the current situation would include case management and physical therapy. Case management can provide resources for Martha such as support groups as well as educational offerings. Online resources can be provided so that when Martha is at home she can begin to absorb the implications of the diagnosis and how it will affect her personal goals. The physical therapist may be able to provide Martha with some simple body mechanic ideas that will help her to prevent joint injury. Additional ancillary support may be needed in the future as the disease progresses or as flares occur. The specific ancillary used to support Martha would be dependent on the symptoms she is exhibiting.

STEP 9: PLAN OF CARE

The plan of care is a road map for patient care and should be used as a communication tool between disciplines. Expected entries on the plan of care would be each identified problem, interventions, and expected outcomes.

Pertinent information to include in the plan of care is pain management specifics. Note Martha's preferred pain medication and when to best provide medication in order to meet her mobility goals. Martha's preference for online education to get a better understanding of the disease process can also be noted. Support group contact information that has been provided to Martha should be listed here.

STEP 10: EVALUATION

Evaluation is an active process in which the nurse "connects the dots" to decide if the expected outcomes (goals) that were established have been met, partially met, or not met. If the goals are met, we continue with the plan as outlined. If the goal was partially met, we revise the parts of the plan that did not work. If the goals were not met, we start all over with a new plan.

End-of-Shift Narrative

AJ enters the room at the end of the shift to check on Martha. Earlier, Martha's physician arrived with an immunologist, and they told her that based on her symptoms and laboratory results, she has SLE. Martha did not understand what that meant. AJ gave Martha some education materials that he was able to print from the hospital online patient education system, and provided a computer with a list of websites she could review. AJ is anxious to discover what Martha thinks and if she has any questions. *"How you are feeling, Martha?"* AJ asks. "I don't know how to feel," she replies. "All of my life I had this dream of traveling all over the world as a photojournalist. Now because of the stupid disease, I don't think I can do that anymore." *"Why not?"* AJ asks. "Why? It sounds like I have to live the life of a monk. Stay out of the sun, lots of rest, no stress, a completely boring life. I am just 18 years old and my life is done, over, the end." *"Is that what the immunologist said?"* AJ continues. "Not exactly, he said that there was medicine that could help me. I have to take hydroxychloroquine and that I might have to take prednisone. My aunt took prednisone for her asthma, and she gained a ton of weight, so I told him I don't really want to take it unless I have to, and he said we could wait and see. He is thinking about starting me on belimumab soon. The doctor also told me I should go to classes and talk to some other people with SLE. I don't see how that will help." *"Can I make a suggestion?"* AJ asks. "Sure." *"I would do just what the doctor asked you to do. You may discover some wonderful ideas about how to protect your health and be a photojournalist."* "I don't know, it all seems pointless." *"What would be the harm in just checking it out? All I ask is that you just think about it some more before deciding not to go,"* AJ gently remarks. "All right," Martha says with a smile. "I'll think about it." *"How is the pain in your knees?"* AJ asks. *"It has been about 4 hours since I gave you the hydrocodone. Do you need another one?"* "Yes, that would be great." AJ continues, *"Do you think the pain is less than it was? It was a 10/10 this morning, but then you wanted to switch to the pills, and how do you rate the pain now?"* Martha smiles, "Right now it is a 4/10. If I don't move too much the pain is less. It's when I get up and walk around that it gets worse." AJ asks, *"Does the hydrocodone keep you comfortable?"* "Yes, it does, thanks. My pain drops down to a 2 to a 3 after I take it." AJ looks concerned and asks, *"Have you tried to bundle your activities so that you don't have to get up so often?"* Martha, looking grateful, remarks, "Yes, and it has helped. Thanks for the suggestion. Taking the pain medication a little before walking also helps—thanks. I have decided I will try those range-of-motion exercises in the morning. Maybe it will help with the stiffness." AJ continues, *"Are you still worried about the rash on your face?"* Shaking her head no, Martha remarks, "I know I should be but compared to the pain, it's bearable." *"Did you read the information I gave you about the rash, that it can come and go?"* "Yes," Martha replies, "and I put on the cream you gave me. I don't think it will help the rash, but it makes my skin feel better." *"What about your scalp?"* "There aren't that many patches, I just have to keep reminding myself not to pick at them." *"Do you understand why it is important to keep out of the sun?"* "Yes, and I will try." *"Do you have any other questions?"* "Not really, thanks."

Problem Evaluation

PROBLEM 1: **Mobility.** The patient should have improved mobility tolerance with better pain management. The goal is met when Martha verbalizes that if she bundles activities, it is easier for her to get around, and that taking the pain medication first really helps. She is willing to try range-of-motion exercises in the morning to decrease stiffness.

PROBLEM 2: **Pain.** Pain should be at an acceptable level for the patient. Although Martha was in severe pain at the beginning of the shift, the morphine helped, and her transition to hydrocodone was successful, as evidenced by rating her pain at a 3/10.

PROBLEM 3: **Skin Integrity.** Martha will understand that a rash on the face and scalp may improve over time with treatment. Martha verbalizes that the cream provided to her can help to keep her skin moist and has

used it. She may still have some questions regarding the rash but is willing to attend a support group.

Overall Evaluation

Based on the end-of-shift assessment and the comparison of Martha's progress during this shift, Martha is found to be improving.

REFERENCES

2012 SLICC SLE Criteria. Retrieved from www.rheumtutor.com/2012-slicc-sle-criteria/

Appendix A. American College of Rheumatology Criteria for Classification of Systemic Lupus Erythematosus. Retrieved from www.ncbi.nlm.nih.gov/pubmedhealth/PMH0041704/

Beers, M., Porter, R., Jones, T., Kaplan, J., & Berkwits, M. (Eds.). (2006). Systemic lupus erythematosus. The MERCK Manual (18th ed., pp. 266–272). Whitehouse Station, NJ: Merck Research Laboratories.

Benlysta. (2012, March). Retrieved from www.benlysta.com/?google=e_& rotation=12014&banner=89745&kw=3605&gclid=CK_16N21nbcCFcU5QgodBU4AQg

Childs, S. (2006, March/April). The pathogenesis of systemic lupus erythematosus. Orthopaedic Nursing, 25(2), 140–145.

George, J. (2011). Nursing theories: The base for professional nursing practice (6th ed.). Upper Saddle River, NJ: Pearson Education.

Gulanick, M., & Meyers J. (2013). Nursing care plans nursing diagnosis and intervention (8th ed.). St. Louis, MO: Mosby.

Holloway, N. (2004). Medical surgical nursing care planning (4th ed.). Springhouse, PA: Lippincott Williams & Wilkins.

LeMone, P., Burke, K., & Baldoff, G. (2011). Medical surgical nursing. Critical thinking in patient care (5th ed.). Upper Saddle River, NJ: Pearson.

Man, B.L., & Mok, C.C. (2005). Serositis related to systemic lupus erythematosus: Prevalence and outcome. Lupus, 14(10), 822–826. Retrieved from www.ncbi.nlm.nih.gov/pubmed/16302677

McClintock, R. (2004). What can you say about systemic lupus erythematosus. Nursing 2004, 34(8), 32–34.

Parker, M. (2006). Nursing theories and nursing practice (2nd ed.). Philadelphia, PA: FA Davis.

Petri, M., Orbai, A.M., Alarcón, G.S., et al. (2012). Revision of Classification Criteria for Systemic Lupus Erythematosus. doi:10.1002/art.34473 [Epub ahead of print]. Retrieved from www.lupus.org/research-news/entry/revision-of-classification-criteria-for-systemic-lupus-erythematosus

Pullen, R. (2008, January/February). Stay in the loop with lupus. Nursing Made Incredibly Easy, 44–51.

Rodgers, S. (2008). Medical surgical nursing care plans. Clifton Park, NY: Thomson Delmar.

Rooney, J. (2005). Systemic lupus erythematosus unmasking the great imitator. Nursing 2005, 35(11), 54–60.

Syphilis Tests. Retrieved from www.webmd.com/sexual-conditions/syphilis-tests

Systemic Lupus Erythematosus (Lupus). Retrieved from www.rheumatology.org/practice/clinical/patients/diseases_and_conditions/lupus.asp

Thompson, C. (2011, April 15). SLE. American Journal of Health-care Systems Pharmacy, 68, 646.

Van Leeuwen, A., & Bladh, M. (2015). Davis's comprehensive handbook of laboratory and diagnostic testing with nursing implications (6th ed.). Philadelphia, PA: F.A. Davis Company.

Wilson, B., Shannon, M., & Stang, C. (2006). Nurses drug guide. Upper Saddle River, NJ: Prentice Hall.

Wilkinson, J., & Ahern, N. (2009). In Nursing Diagnosis Handbook (9th ed.). Saddle River, NJ: Prentice Hall.

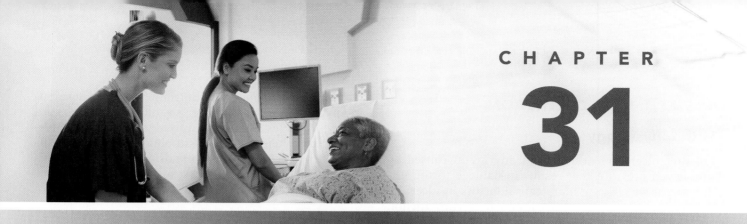

CHAPTER 31

Integumentary System

Case Study, Pressure Ulcer

Common Nursing Study Name	Section 1 Study	Section 1 Chapter Number
Abdominal X-Rays, Plain (KUB)	Kidney, Ureter, and Bladder Study	Chapter 16
Albumin	Albumin and Albumin/Globulin Ratio	Chapter 1
Bioelectric Impedance Analysis	Bioelectric Impedance Analysis (in chapter Overview: Chapter 8, Electrophysiologic Studies)	Chapter 8 Overview
C-Reactive Protein	C-Reactive Protein	Chapter 1
Gentamycin	Antimicrobial Drugs—Aminoglycosides: Amikacin, Gentamicin, Tobramycin; Tricyclic Glycopeptide: Vancomycin	Chapter 1
Prealbumin	Prealbumin	Chapter 1
Stool Culture	Culture, Bacterial, Stool	Chapter 10
Culture and Sensitivity (C&S), Wound	Culture, Bacterial, Anal/Genital, Ear, Eye, Skin, and Wound	Chapter 19
X-Ray	Radiography, Bone	Chapter 16

STEP 1: DATA COLLECTION

Pathophysiology

Pressure ulcers are described as any lesion caused by unrelieved pressure that results in damage to the underlying tissue. The primary causal factors in ulcer development are pressure in combination with friction and shear. The National Pressure Ulcer Advisory Panel (NPAUP) defines a pressure ulcer as an injury to the skin or underlying tissue that occurs as a result of a combination of these three.

Pressure is the compression of tissue between an external surface and bone, causing ischemia and necrosis. Moderate pressure over a long period of time is just as damaging as excessive pressure over a short duration. Friction and shear are partners in pressure ulcer formation. *Friction* is the force that resists the movement of the skin and is usually visible on the skin surface, such as an abrasion. *Shearing* is a force parallel to the skin surface, causing an injury beneath the surface of the skin. Think about a patient who slips down in bed: the muscle and deep fascia slip with gravity while the external skin sticks to the sheets. This combination of pressure, friction, and shear are the classic triad of pressure ulcer development.

There are two theories of how a pressure ulcer begins: from the inside out and from the outside in. The inside-out theorists believe a pressure ulcer begins from a deep tissue injury near the bone, with tissue damage moving from the bone to the skin. The outside-in theorists believe tissue damage begins at the skin and moves downward toward the bone.

Either way, over time, unrelieved pressure will occlude capillary blood flow and lymphatic circulation. When pressure is relieved, the body can compensate, blood vessels will dilate, and blood flow will return. Blanchable erythema is a sign of improved blood supply. Nonblanchable erythema can indicate deep tissue injury. Tissue malnutrition occurs from impaired blood supply from prolonged pressure. Waste products collect and leak into tissues, causing edema and hypoxia. Over time, the combination of pressure, friction, shear, malnutrition, tissue edema, and the release of waste products contribute to cellular death, and a pressure ulcer is born.

Pressure ulcers occur most often over a bony prominence. Adults develop pressure ulcers on the coccyx or sacrum, heels, and hips. Children with mobility problems develop pressure ulcers in the same areas. Children without mobility problems have pressure ulcers most often on the back of the head. Medical devices such as oxygen, casts, cervical collars, and endotracheal tubes can also cause pressure ulcers.

Medical problems that contribute to ulcer development are malnutrition, age, steroid use, spinal cord injury, diabetes, smoking, vascular disease, anemia, altered body temperature, skin abnormalities, and impaired cognitive function. Exposure to skin irritants that would cause maceration, such as urine, stool, or other moisture, is also a causal factor.

Staging

Pressure ulcers are staged according to the amount of soft tissue loss and damage observed on assessment. The NPAUP defines six stages of pressure ulcers: (1) suspected deep tissue injury, (2) stage I, (3) stage II, (4) stage III, (5) stage IV, and (6) unstageable pressure ulcers. Stage I and stage II pressure ulcers are partial-thickness wounds, stage III and stage IV are full-thickness wounds. Acquiring a stage III or stage IV pressure ulcer after being admitted to the hospital is a "never event," meaning that it should never happen and is reportable to the Department of Health. Although rare, it is recognized that some ulcers are unavoidable due to patient condition. Documentation should reflect risk assessment and chosen interventions, with reassessment and revision of interventions.

Signs and Symptoms

- *Suspected deep tissue injury* looks like a purple or maroon discolored area. Skin may still be intact or appear as a blood-filled blister from soft-tissue damage, pressure, or shear. The injured area may feel different: firmer, softer, warmer, cooler, or more painful.
- *Stage I* pressure ulcers have reddened, nonblanchable intact skin over a bony prominence, such as the coccyx or heel. Skin may look slightly red in those with light-colored skin, and discolored with a red, blue, or purple hue in those with a darker skin tone. Skin may feel too warm or too cool. The consistency may feel too boggy or too firm. The patient may complain of pain or tingling. This stage has the least amount of tissue damage and there is no open wound.
- *Stage II* pressure ulcers have an open wound with partial-thickness loss of the epidermis and/or dermis. The ulcer may look like a shallow open crater with a pink wound bed, a blister that may or may not be ruptured, or it may look like an abrasion.
- *Stage III* pressure ulcers move further into the dermis with full-thickness tissue loss. Subcutaneous fat may be visible, but not bone or tendon. The ulcer may have the appearance of a deeper crater. Undermining and/or tunneling may or may not be present, and slough may be present.

- *Stage IV* pressure ulcers involve full-thickness tissue loss with visualization of bone, tendon, or muscle. There is extensive tissue destruction. Slough and/or eschar may be present, along with undermining and tunneling with damage to the bone, muscle, or supporting structures.
- *Unstageable pressure ulcers* are covered by slough or eschar, making it impossible to see how deep the wound is, thereby making it unstageable. Staging will occur after the slough and eschar are removed so that the wound bed can be seen. In some cases, eschar can act as a natural cover for a pressure ulcer and, depending on patient circumstances, may not be removed.

The correct identification of ulcer type is used to guide treatment choices. Ask yourself, is the tissue observed slough, eschar, or granulation tissue? Both slough and eschar are devitalized necrotic tissue, and granulation tissue is healthy tissue. Slough looks like a moist fibrous gray, yellow, or tan tissue. Eschar looks like a brownish-black, leathery scab-like substance. Both slough and eschar may be seen in stage III and stage IV pressure ulcers. Wound healing can be delayed by moist necrotic tissue. Granulation tissue looks like raw hamburger.

Tunneling occurs just the way it sounds, delving down into the tissue. Undermining occurs when the ulcer extends to just under the edges of the skin parallel to the wound bed.

When the ulcer begins to heal, the tissue bed will be moist, and the amount of moisture will be determined by the size of the wound. A sudden increase in moisture or a change in odor could indicate an infection. Drainage type should be documented as serosanguineous, sanguineous, or purulent. Tissue that appears pale or dusky may have oxygenation problems.

Healing also occurs by epithelization, which is a closing of the wound by moving cells across the open wound surface. Wound edges will become pink as healing progresses. Those with a stage I or stage II pressure ulcer will heal from the wound edges inward until the wound closes. Those with a stage III or stage IV ulcer heal by a combination of secondary intention and wound epithelization. Skin edges that roll under during healing will have to be cut back to allow for continued healing. Skin around the pressure ulcer should be assessed for a change in color, temperature, induration, tenderness, or maceration. Slough and eschar impede wound healing.

Documenting ulcer stage includes location, size, tunneling or undermining, color consistency, and the amount of drainage, odor, necrotic, or granulation tissue. Colors can be described as black to indicate eschar, yellow to indicate slough, and red to indicate granulation.

Laboratory Studies

There are no laboratory studies that diagnose pressure ulcer. However there are studies that can identify the degree of risk. Protein is necessary for cell growth. Several laboratory studies can assess the risk of malnutrition and provide direction for care. Prealbumin is useful in assessing nutritional status. A normal adult prealbumin level is 12 to 42 mg/dL. A prealbumin of 10 mg/dL indicates mild nutritional depletion. Less than 7 mg/dL indicates severe depletion. Albumin may also be used to measure the patient's protein level. A normal albumin is age dependent. Adults ages 20 to 40 is 3.7 to 5.1 g/dL; ages 41 to 60, 3.4 to 4.8 g/dL; ages 61 to 90, 3.2 to 4.6 g/dL; and older than age 90, 2.9 to 4.5 g/dL. An albumin of less than 3.4 g/dL indicates hypoalbuminemia. Wound culture is a valuable tool in identifying the organism that causes the infection and the best antibiotic to kill it.

Diagnostic Studies

There are no diagnostic studies that point to pressure ulcer, but there are studies that can help identify risk. Bioelectric impedance analysis is a noninvasive analysis that evaluates the composition of body cell mass, extracellular mass, and fat to assess nutritional status. The body's cells should be functioning at 100% efficiency. A result of less than 95% indicates that cellular function is compromised, which may in turn compromise wound healing. X-ray can be used to assess for osteomyelitis that develops as a result of pressure ulcer development.

General/Medical Management

The assessment of risk is the first step in pressure ulcer management. The Braden Scale is a risk assessment tool with the categories of sensory perception, moisture, activity, mobility, nutrition, friction, and shear. Each category is assessed and assigned a number. The numbers are totaled, and the patient receives an overall risk score. A score less than 9 indicates a very high risk, 10 to 12 a high risk, 13 to 14 a moderate risk, and 15 to 18 indicates some risk. A score of 18 or less requires a skin prevention plan. Never assume that a score greater than 18 will protect against an ulcer.

Skin assessment begins on admission. Skin should be evaluated a minimum of every 24 hours or per policy, as well as with any change in condition. The best time to evaluate skin is during the bath or a head-to-toe assessment. Special attention should be given to the inspection of all bony prominences. Long-term care facilities may assess skin on admission and then weekly for the first 4 weeks, quarterly, and with change of condition. Home health agencies may assess skin on admission and with each visit. Skin assessment should be linked with appropriate interventions.

Interventions to treat pressure ulcers consist of three concepts: (1) to control and remove the causative factor, (2) to support the patient's health, and (3) to provide an environment that supports wound healing. To control or remove the cause of an ulcer requires interventions that address friction, shear, pressure, and moisture. This begins with prevention. During admission, screen ulcer risk by asking about connective tissue disorders, previous surgeries, healing issues, and mobility limitations. Ask about smoking or alcohol use and home support. Look for any existing pressure ulcers. Identified ulcers should be photographed, measured, and documented with wound location, size (length, width, and depth), any undermining or tunneling, and stage identification. Document the color and odor of any exudates, wound edge epithelialization, and integrity of the surrounding skin.

Tissue Load Management

Interventions to prevent or reduce pressure, friction, and shear are usually bundled as a group. Turn the patient every 2 hours or as needed. Move the patient completely off the pressure area if possible and if not contraindicated. Removing pressure helps to prevent capillary occlusion and ongoing ischemia. Use lifting devices to reduce friction and shear during repositioning. This involves tissue load management. Tissue load management refers to positioning the patient to prevent ulcer development by keeping pressure off areas of concern. The best positioning is to keep the head of the bed elevated no more than 30 degrees. Higher elevation places the patient at risk for increased pressure, friction, and shear by slipping and sliding in bed. Support all bony prominences using pillows or foam wedges. Heels can be supported by the use of pressure relief boots, or floated off the mattress with the use of pillows. Keep the patient's weight off the ulcer, or decrease the patient's weight on the ulcer. Once a patient has been positioned, care should be given to assure it is maintained. Hourly rounding, a turning schedule, and informed family assistance can be helpful.

Interventions to reduce friction and shear include the use of lift teams, lift sheets, or ceiling lifts, and specialty beds or a foam mattress overlay. Specialty support surfaces are useful in redistributing weight while reducing moisture, friction, and shear.

Moisture Control and Moisturization

Excess moisture contributes to maceration, making it more likely that skin will be damaged during turning and repositioning. Urine, stool, sweat, and other sources of moisture need to be contained or eliminated to minimize skin irritation that can cause breakdown. Bathing frequency should be adjusted to fit patient needs. Incontinence should be cleaned as soon as possible with a pH-appropriate mild product. Harsh rubbing during cleansing should be avoided to prevent damage and shear. Water should be a moderate temperature to prevent burning, and skin should be patted dry. Lotion can be used to keep the skin from becoming dry. A topical skin barrier is recommended to protect against frequent exposure to incontinent urine or stool. Skin should be checked for fungal infections, and a bowel or bladder program may be started, if appropriate. A moisture-absorbing pad with a quick-dry surface may be helpful if necessary.

Supporting overall health can assist with pressure ulcer prevention and wound healing. Protein is a necessary component of wound repair. During admission, complete a nutritional assessment, asking questions about involuntary weight loss and decreased appetite. Laboratory work can be used to assess nutritional status. Consult with the dietician to evaluate calorie, carbohydrate, and protein needs. Dietary supplements and vitamins A, B complex, E, C, magnesium, selenium, and zinc may be ordered.

Nutritional Support

Caloric intake needs to be calculated to ensure enough energy for wound repair. Daily protein should be increased to 1.25 to 1.5 g/kg per day, with a total calorie intake of 35 to 40 kcal/kg/day. The diet should be 55% carbohydrate with fats and other nutrient sources. Enteral or parenteral nutrition can be used if oral intake is not possible. Monitor intake and output closely.

Wound Débridement

Before healing can begin, the wound must be ready. Wound care nurses are a great resource. Wound care nurses can assess the ulcer for needed débridement and provide a course of action. Débridement removes necrotic tissue and allows for the growth of healthy granulation tissue. The type of débridement is dependent on physician preference and the amount of necrotic tissue to be removed. Necrotic tissue can be removed surgically, at the bedside using a sharp instrument, mechanically, by the application of chemicals, or by biologic means.

Surgical débridement removes large amounts of necrotic tissue followed by closure with a tissue flap. Wounds retaining necrotic tissue will require other treatment until surgically ready. Sharp débridement using a scalpel or other sharp instrument takes place at the bedside by the physician or wound care nurse. This can be painful, requiring local anesthetic prior to the procedure. Sharp débridement may need to be repeated to clear away all necrotic tissue.

Mechanical débridement uses force to clean out the wound. The types of force may include pulsed lavage, whirlpool therapy, and wet to dry dressings, although these are rarely used due to tissue damage.

Chemical enzymes can destroy necrotic tissue while leaving healthy tissue alone. The process is slower but less painful. Topical enzymes include papain/urea foam and sterile enzymatic débriding ointments. Enzymatic remedies are always changing, so check with the wound care nurse for the most recent selection. Remember to keep products off of healthy skin to prevent stinging or burning. Biologic débridement is done by placing medically approved maggots in the wound for up to 48 hours to feed on the necrotic tissue and clean the wound.

Wound Vacuuming

Wound vacuum has become a common way to treat pressure ulcers. This device is used to remove tissue, fluids, infectious materials, and wound exudates through intermittent or continuous suction while assisting in the formulation of granulation tissue. Contraindications for use depend on the characteristics of the wound and the patient. Wound vacuum may not work for patients who will not adhere to protocol, have untreated malnutrition, are pain intolerant, have an allergy to the adhesive or foam, have a wound where the vacuum cannot make a seal, or have a bleeding disorder. Wound characteristics that would contraindicate use are an inadequately prepared wound bed, a wound that is too small to create a negative pressure, or one that is freshly débrided, or is fibrotic, devitalized, or desiccated. Ulcers treated with a wound vacuum should be reevaluated every 2 weeks for wound size (length, width, and depth); a change in color; the presence of granulation tissue; a decrease in necrotic tissue, odor, and drainage; and the condition of the surrounding skin. Without improvement, this device should be discontinued in favor of other treatments. Chosen interventions are determined by the stage of the pressure ulcer. Treatment for a stage III or stage IV pressure ulcer will be more involved and may include a variety of modalities. A healing pressure ulcer should show signs of improvement in 2 to 4 weeks.

Vigilance and Education

Vigilance by *all* health-care staff is the best protection again pressure ulcer development. Extra pairs of eyes may be the best intervention of all. Education should be provided to family and all staff caring for patients. Organizational policy should be reviewed regarding the management of pressure ulcers. Home health can assist in reinforcing family education regarding ulcer care and can evaluate the quality of care provided in the home.

Patient Education

Pressure ulcers are a sensitive subject for nurses and family. No one wants the patient's skin to break down. The education to prevent pressure ulcers begins on admission. First, complete a good skin assessment to check for any current breakdown. Second, develop a plan for how to prevent breakdown from occurring or getting worse if present on admission. One classic barrier to preventing breakdown is the patient's or family's refusal to move in bed. Your challenge is to discover why they are refusing. Is there a cultural issue, a language barrier, or are they afraid of pain? Provide clear education about the benefits of pressure ulcer prevention and the risks involved if ignored. Other health-care professionals such as respiratory therapy, occupational therapy, registered dietician, clinical pharmacist, and unit educator can help reinforce patient education. It is the nurse's job to coordinate the education, communicate patient concerns, and document the goals on the plan of care.

STEP 2: POTENTIAL PROBLEM/ DIAGNOSES

It is important that nurses understand and consider the science of the disease process and consider the possibilities prior to applying that knowledge to a patient situation. We begin that process with questioning.

Question: Based upon your review of the content presented, what possible *potential problems* would you expect for a patient with these diagnoses?

Answer: Skin, issue integrity, infection, and home care management

STEP 3: POTENTIAL INTERVENTIONS

Question: Based upon your identification of patient problems, what possible interventions would you recommend for these diagnoses, and what would you expect to happen? This would be considered your "grocery list" of the possible actions you could use to assist your patient.

💬 *Answer:* See the following problems, interventions, and expected outcomes:

Problem	Interventions	Expected Outcome
Skin Integrity	• Turn the patient every 2 hours or as indicated. • Use pillows, foam, or pads to support bony prominences. • Elevate the head of the bed 30 degrees or less. • Lift when moving the patient—do not drag. • Raise the patient's heels off the bed surface. • Refrain from massage over bony prominences to prevent skin damage. • Clean the skin promptly when soiled. • Use a foam overlay on the mattress; use a specialty bed. • Use the Braden Risk Scale for skin assessment.	Skin will remain intact.
Tissue Integrity	• Consider requesting a skin care consult. • Maintain a moist physiologic environment. • Provide wound care as ordered, and provide dressing change as ordered with meticulous aseptic technique. • Bathe the patient as needed to keep skin clean and dry. • Apply heel protectors as needed. • Pad equipment that comes in contact with the patient's skin. • Keep linens clean and dry; change linens frequently if soiled or if there is excessive perspiration. • Provide education about the importance of ulcer prevention measures. • Identify the pressure ulcer stage. • Educate the patient about pressure relief measures. • Assess for pre-existing chronic conditions. • Assess the patient's nutritional status. • Assess for friction, shear, and pressure.	Signs of healing are noted, and the patient demonstrates the correct care of the pressure ulcer
Infection	• Assess the pressure ulcer for drainage color and odor. • Complete wound cultures. • Administer antibiotics. • Monitor laboratory values associated with infection. • Monitor urinary and fecal incontinence. • Administer medication for diarrhea. • Consider a request for urinary catheter insertion. • Assess the patient's dietary intake. • Monitor vital signs. • Explain the importance of wound cleanliness to prevent infection. • Complete ordered wound care. • Order a dietary consult for inadequate caloric intake. • Administer enteral or parenteral nutrition.	The infection should be free of foul-smelling exudate
Home Care Management	• Assess the family's understanding of the long-term nature of pressure ulcer care/prevention. • Assess the ability of the family to provide pressure ulcer treatment. • Assess the family's understanding of the importance of a high-calorie, high-protein diet in wound healing.	The patient's family will successfully provide care

PUTTING IT ALL TOGETHER: APPLICATION OF THE NURSING PROCESS

Putting it all together is where the art and science of nursing meet to provide the best patient outcomes. We take the possibilities and place them into the context of the patient situation. To accomplish this, we use nursing diagnosis, nursing interventions, nursing outcomes, and nursing theory to provide the palate for nursing care.

STEP 4: ASSESSMENT

PATIENT INFORMATION: 89-year-old Asian male

CHIEF COMPLAINT: Diarrhea and fever with dehydration and weight loss

HISTORY OF THE PRESENT ILLNESS: Diarrhea four to five times a day for the past week with fever, poor appetite, progressive weakness; the patient was admitted for diarrhea, etiology unknown

PAST MEDICAL HISTORY: Hypertension, benign prostatic hyperplasia

FAMILY HISTORY: Unknown; emigrated from China

CHART REVIEW AND REPORT: Joe Kim was admitted 3 days ago with fever and diarrhea. Joe had three large watery brown stools on the previous shift. Joe's daughter Lori changes his diaper leaving it for the staff to check. Joe has become increasingly weak, and his appetite remains poor eating only about 20% of each meal. Daily weight shows a loss of 4 pounds in the last 3 days. IV is infusing at D51/2NS with KCl 20 mEq at 100 mL/hr. Stool culture is in process; there are no results yet. Vital signs are BP of 146/88 mm Hg, a temperature of 99.6°F, a pulse of 102 beats per minute, and respirations of 16 breaths per minute. Joe spends most of his time on his back. He refuses to comply with his turning schedule. The off-going nurse reports that his skin is clear of any pressure ulcers.

SUBJECTIVE ASSESSMENT: Arvin James (AJ) enters the room and sees Joe lying on his back. His daughter Lori is at the bedside and reports leaving a dirty diaper in the bathroom. AJ sees that the stool in the diaper is loose and not watery as reported. After checking the diaper, AJ returns. *"Good morning, Mr. Kim. My name is AJ and I will be your nurse today."* Mr. Kim glances disdainfully then says, "Good morning." *"How are you feeling today?"* Lori interjects, "He's about the same as he was when we got here." AJ smiles at Lori and continues, *"Mr. Kim, do you feel like you are getting better?"* Again Lori answers for her father, forcefully saying,

"He is not better." *"Do you agree with that?"* AJ asks. "Yes," he replies. AJ asks, *"Besides still having diarrhea, what is not better?"* "My bottom hurts, my belly is sore, I am weak, no appetite." *"Where does your bottom hurt?"* "Right on my fanny." *"What about your belly, where does it hurt?"* "Around my belly button." *"How bad is the pain on a scale of 0 to 10?"* Mr. Kim asks his daughter something in Mandarin, she answers back and says to AJ, "the pain on his bottom is a 6 if I don't touch it, when I clean him it is a 10. The pain in his belly is a 3." *"Has anyone offered pain medication?"* Lori gives AJ a flat look, "No one has asked and I have not told them. I do not want my father shamed."

OBJECTIVE ASSESSMENT: Joe Kim is thin and frail. His a.m. weight was 105 pounds; his admission weight was 109 pounds. Lori says he usually weighs about 123 pounds. Current vital signs are BP of 138/86 mm Hg, a pulse of 98 beats per minute, a temperature of 100.6°F, and respirations of 18 breaths per minute. The IV site is clear and fluids are infusing as ordered. The abdomen is soft and tender in all quadrants, bowel sounds are a little hyperactive, and skin turgor is fair. AJ asks Joe to roll on his side so that he can check his bottom where he says he has been having pain, he refuses. AJ asks, *"Do you always wear a diaper?"* "Yes, it makes me feel better, safer, no mess. My daughter brought them from home." *"You told me that your bottom hurts, I need to check and make sure everything is OK."* Lori interrupts, "No one else has done that since we got here." AJ explains, *"Your father has been having diarrhea, and wearing diapers can keep the moisture in. I just think it is important to check his skin and make sure it looks OK."* "Alright, you can check," replies Joe. AJ is horrified by what he sees. There is a stage III ulcer on his coccyx. The wound base is covered in grayish slough, there is a pungent foul odor, and there is oozing greenish purulent drainage. The surrounding skin is macerated and looks like raw meat. AJ asks, *"When did this start?"* Lori says, "Right after we got here, and it has been getting worse. I told the nurse but she ignored me, this is her fault. No one here cares about my father; no one comes when he calls, so I stay to take care of him." AJ measures the pressure ulcer at 5 cm in length, 3 cm in width, and 2 cm in depth. The skin around the pressure ulcer is macerated, boggy, and warm to the touch. AJ takes pictures and lets Lori and her father know that he is going to contact the physician and ask to have the skin care nurse visit him. AJ tells Joe, *"I want you to turn on your side to keep the pressure off of your bottom for a while."* Joe becomes visibly upset, "No, my hip hurts from arthritis; I have to lie on my back." Lori becomes angry, insisting he be left alone to rest. An hour later the wound care nurse visits and sends cultures to the lab. The physician starts Joe on IVPB ampicillin sodium, gentamycin sulfate until culture results can confirm the infecting organism and adjustments can be made as appropriate. Oral vitamins are also started. Because of the concern that Joe will not adhere to positioning suggestions, a specialty bed has been ordered.

- *Laboratory Studies:*
  - Electrolytes: K^+ 4.1 mEq/L, Na^+ mEq/L 140, Cl^- mEq/L 103
  - Prealbumin: 9 mg/dL
  - Hemoglobin: 15.2 g/dL
  - Hematocrit: 49%
  - White blood count: 13.9×10^3/microL
  - C-reactive protein: 5.9 mg/L
- *Diagnostic Studies:*
  - Radiographic study of the kidney, ureter, and bladder (KUB) was completed to assess the abdominal pain with negative results.
- *Medications:*
  - Diphenoxylate/atropine 1 tablet every 6 hours as needed for diarrhea
  - Ampicillin sodium 2 g IVPB every 6 hours
  - Gentamycin sulfate 125 mg IVPB every 8 hours
  - Zinc 50 mg tid
  - Vitamin C 500 mg bid
  - Oxycodone/acetaminophen 1 tablet every 4 hours as needed for moderate pain rated 5 to 7

STEP 5: REALITY CHECK: DETOUR AHEAD

Reality Check occurs when the nurse takes a moment to think about individualized patient information that needs to be considered in framing diagnoses and interventions. This information is retrievable from any legitimate source (e.g., family, case management, other nurses, any ancillary, a doctor, etc.). These are the "wrenches" that create challenging situations, such as culture, religion, socioeconomic status, level of education, developmental level, marital status, employment, age, and gender.

Psychosocial History

Joe Kim is a naturalized citizen of 50 years. His wife died giving birth to Lori due to physician negligence. Lori barely survived. Joe never remarried. He sued and received a cash settlement that he used to open his own restaurant, which he ran until the age of 78 years when he lost his business to government reclamation of land. He has always felt that if he was not a Chinese immigrant that it would never have happened. His anger and distrust were passed on to his daughter. His family has rejected him for his conversion from Buddhism to Christianity.

 Critical Thinking Moment

You have just completed the assessment of Joe and need to make a decision about the patient's *actual* problems and nursing diagnoses based on the data you have collected and the potential problems you identified. Outcomes must be realistic and measurable.

STEP 6: ACTUAL PROBLEMS/DIAGNOSES

The *first step* in problem identification is to revisit the list of *potential diagnoses* and choose *actual diagnoses* based on the learner's evaluation of the case study information provided. A problem statement must be completed for each identified problem/diagnosis. The actual problems for this case study are tissue integrity, infection, and skin integrity.

STEP 7: PLANNING: ACTUAL INTERVENTIONS

After actual diagnoses have been chosen, it is necessary to evaluate the list of *potential interventions* and choose *actual interventions* that will fit within the patient's reality and meet expected outcomes. Each intervention requires a rationale. Interventions are identified in three categories: (1) assessment, (2) therapeutic, and (3) education.

Diagnostic Statement

Altered tissue integrity related to poor nutrition, immobility, and incontinence as evidenced by a refusal to turn, 20% dietary intake, and the development of a stage III ulcer

Assessment

- Assess Joe's pressure ulcer daily during the dressing change. *Rationale: This allows you to document the progress of chemical débridement and the development of granulation tissue.*
- Assess Joe's skin surrounding the pressure ulcer daily. *Rationale: This ensures that the chemical débridement is not worsening the already macerated skin and damaging healthy skin.*
- Assess Joe's tolerance to dressing changes. *Rationale: The family already feels uncared for, and good pain management is important for success.*

Therapeutic Interventions

- Application of a sterile enzymatic débriding ointment twice daily after irrigation with normal saline. *Rationale: This débrides the wound.*

- Administration of oxycodone/acetaminophen 30 minutes prior to wound care. *Rationale: This decreases patient discomfort.*
- Measure the pressure ulcer weekly with photography. *Rationale: This allows for the documentation of progress.*

Education

- Explain the purpose of applying a sterile enzymatic débriding ointment in relation to wound healing. *Rationale: Understanding can increase compliance with the proposed plan.*
- Explain that pain medication can make the process more comfortable. *Rationale: Adequate pain management increases the likelihood of positive collaboration.*
- Begin educating Lori about how to care for the pressure ulcer. *Rationale: Family involvement increases the probability of positive outcomes.*

Expected Outcome

- Decreased slough and development of granulation tissue

Diagnostic Statement

Infection of a pressure ulcer related to contamination of the wound base with stool, poor communication with the family, and a lack of skin inspection as evidenced by oozing, pungent, smelly green drainage, CRP of 5.9 mg/dL, WBC 13.9×10^3/microL, and a temperature of 100.6°F.

Assessment

- Assess the amount, color, and odor of wound drainage. *Rationale: Decreasing drainage is evidence of a resolving infection.*
- Monitor WBC and CRP. *Rationale: This allows you to monitor the progression of infection and the effect of antibiotics.*
- Monitor the results of the wound culture and sensitivity. *Rationale: This ensures that the antibiotic the patient is on will kill the germ causing the infection.*

Therapeutic Interventions

- Administer ampicillin every 6 hours as ordered. *Rationale: This antibiotic treats bacterial infections.*
- Administer gentamycin every 8 hours as ordered. *Rationale: This antibiotic treats bacterial infections.*
- Ensure that the gentamycin peak and trough are drawn in a timely manner. *Rationale: The drug levels will indicate if the dose needs to be changed in order to treat the infection.*

Education

- Explain the purpose of the wound culture. *Rationale: This helps the patient understand that the culture will identify the infecting organism.*

- Explain the purpose of the antibiotic administration. *Rationale: This is to kill the suspected infecting organism while waiting for culture confirmation.*
- Explain the purpose of the gentamycin sulfate drug level. *Rationale: The patient should understand that there is enough antibiotic in the system to kill the infection.*

Expected Outcome

- Resolving wound infection

Diagnostic Statement

Altered skin integrity related to poor appetite, refusal to turn, and incontinent diarrhea as evidenced by the development of a stage III pressure ulcer and maceration of the surrounding skin.

Assessment

- Assess Joe's skin over the bony areas. *Rationale: This will allow you to monitor for the development of additional pressure ulcers.*
- Assess Joe's ability to move himself in bed. *Rationale: This helps in developing a mobility plan.*
- Assess Joe's tolerance to the prescribed diet. *Rationale: This helps you identify needed revisions to increase Joe's protein intake.*

Therapeutic Interventions

- Pad reddened heels and float them off the bed with the use of a pillow. *Rationale: This keeps the pressure off the heels and prevents the development of a pressure ulcer.*
- Have the family bring food that he likes to eat from home. *Rationale: This increases caloric intake.*
- Place the patient on a specialty bed. *Rationale: This helps relieve pressure points and decreases further risk.*

Education

- Educate the patient about the importance of keeping his weight off his coccyx. *Rationale: This promotes Joe's understanding that weight adjustment in necessary to promote healing.*
- Educate the patient about the importance of turning every 2 hours. *Rationale: This promotes Joe's understanding of how to prevent ulcers on other bony prominences.*
- Educate the patient about the importance of containing incontinent urine and stool. *Rationale: This promotes understanding of how to prevent transition to a stage IV ulcer.*

Expected Outcome

- Agree to a turning schedule, keep off the coccyx, and increase caloric intake

STEP 8: IMPLEMENTATION

Nursing Theory

Joe and Lori are distrustful. Joe's conversion to Christianity has created a rift between himself and his family, who remain Buddhist. Joe feels betrayed by Western medicine because of the death of his wife through negligence. Helen Erickson and Mary Tomlin use the concept of modeling and role modeling to create a patient-centered approach to nursing. Modeling consists of developing an understanding of Joe's world. Role modeling is completed by facilitating Joe's health. AJ's goal should be to promote a trusting relationship toward positive orientation and perceived control, and that allows the setting of mutual goals that are self-directed. AJ will then assist Joe and Lori to provide self-care while assessing their ability to perform. The focus of care should always be on Joe as an individual and not on the disease. The plan of care and interventions should be individualized. AJ will need to talk to Joe and Lori to find out what they think is the best way to promote his health. Once that is done, AJ will then need to partner with them to get it done. During the process, acceptance of the patient is unconditional and nonjudgmental.

Ancillary Support

Several ancillary groups can be assistive in Joe's care. The most important of these is the wound care nurse who will direct the pressure ulcer care and provide family education. Case management will need to arrange home health visits to assist pressure ulcer care at home. A clinical dietician can organize a culturally appropriate diet to meet caloric needs.

STEP 9: PLAN OF CARE

The plan of care is a road map for patient care and should be used as a communication tool between disciplines. Expected entries on the plan of care would be each identified problem, intervention, and expected outcome. There should also be some information about the family's distrust of the medical community. Consistency in assignment planning should be included as a way to work with the family.

STEP 10: EVALUATION

Evaluation is an active process in which the nurse "connects the dots" to decide if the expected outcomes (goals) that were established have been met, partially met, or not met. If the goals are met, we continue with the plan as outlined. If the goal was partially met, we revise the parts of the plan that did not work. If the goals were not met, we start all over with a new plan.

End-of-Shift Narrative

Joe has been seen by the skin care nurse, placed on a specialty bed, and started on sterile enzymatic débriding ointment as chemical débridement. A wound culture was obtained. A dietary consult was ordered, Lori is bringing food from home, and Joe's intake has improved to almost 50%. Lori is aware that parenteral nutrition may be necessary but continues to refuse this alternative. Antibiotics have been started. Pressure ulcer education has been provided. Joe has agreed to stay off his coccyx. Risk management was notified of the stage III pressure ulcer. The admitting nurse confirms there was a stage II ulcer that she forgot to document. When confronted, Lori angrily denies this, saying that it is our fault and so is going to sue.

AJ has been asked to continue caring for Joe because he has some rapport with the family. Lori told the Unit Coordinator that AJ is the only nurse who treats her father like a real person, and she trusts him. Currently, Lori refuses to learn to care for the pressure ulcer. She has agreed to call the nurse when her father has diarrhea and needs to be cleaned. The family has agreed to adhere to a turning schedule. Heel pads were refused, but they did agree to keep Joe's heels off the bed with pillows. The pressure ulcer has been reported to the Department of Health.

Problem Evaluation

PROBLEM 1: **Altered Tissue Integrity:** The expected outcome is compliance with pressure ulcer treatment, decreased slough, and the development of granulation tissue. The goal is met: The family has agreed to dressing changes with sterile enzymatic débriding ointment. Oxycodone/acetaminophen administered prior to the procedure keeps him comfortable.

PROBLEM 2: **Infection:** The expected outcome is resolving wound infection evidenced by improved lab values and improved wound status. The goal is met: Joe agrees to take the antibiotics but blames the hospital for the pressure ulcer and his infection and plans to sue for poor care.

PROBLEM 3: **Altered Skin Integrity:** The expected outcome is that the family agrees to a turning schedule, to keep off coccyx, and to increase caloric intake. The goal is partially met in that a specialty bed has been ordered to prevent the development of further pressure ulcers, Joe has agreed to a turning schedule, and Joe is making an effort to eat more since Lori brought food from home, but he still refuses to consider parenteral nutrition. The revised plan is to continue to work toward increasing his caloric intake in collaboration with the clinical dietician.

Overall Evaluation

Based on the end-of-shift assessment and the comparison of Joe's progress during this shift, there is no change; the family's compliance is provisional.

REFERENCES

Avent, Y. (2010, September/October). Spotlight on prevention: Pressure ulcers. Nursing Made Incredibly Easy, 21–26.

Baldwin, K. (2006, January/February). Damage control, preventing and treating pressure ulcers. Nursing Made Incredibly Easy, 12–27.

George, J. (2011). Nursing theories. The base for professional nursing practice (6th ed.). Upper Saddle River, NJ: Pearson Education.

Gulanick, M., & Meyers J. (2013). Nursing care plans nursing diagnosis and intervention (8th ed.). St Louis, MO: Mosby.

Holloway, N. (2004). Medical surgical nursing care planning (4th ed.). Springhouse, PA: Lippincott Williams & Wilkins.

LeMone, P., Burke, K., & Baldoff, G. (2011). Medical surgical nursing, Critical thinking in patient care (5th ed.). Upper Saddle River, NJ: Pearson.

Lynch, S. (2010). Steps to reducing hospital-acquired pressure ulcers. Nursing 2010, 61–62.

Niezgoda, J., & Mendez-Eastman, S. (2006, January/February). The effective management of pressure ulcers. Advances in Skin and Wound Care, 3–15.

Nutrition Care Systems. (n.d.). Hypoalbuminemia: Malnutrition versus inflammatory response. Retrieved from www.nutrition caresystems.com/hypoalbuminemia-malnutrition-versus-inflammatory-response

Pressure ulcer stages. (2011). Retrieved from www.npaup.org

Rodgers, S. (2008). Medical surgical nursing care plans. Clifton Park, NY: Thomson Delmar.

Swearingen, P. (2008). All in one care planning resource (2nd ed.). St Louis, MO: Mosby.

Van Leeuwen, A., & Bladh, M. (2015). Davis's comprehensive handbook of laboratory and diagnostic testing with nursing implications (6th ed.). Philadelphia, PA: F.A. Davis Company.

VanRijswijk, L., & Ledger, C. (2008, November). Pressure ulcers: Were they there on admission? American Journal of Nursing, 108(11), 27.

Vincent, J., Dubois, M., Navickis, R., & Wilkes, M. (2003). Hypoalbuminemia in acute illness: Is there a rationale for intervention? Annals of Surgery, 237(3), 319–344. Retrieved from www.ncbi.nlm.nih.gov/pmc/articles/PMC1514323

Wilkinson, J., & Ahern, N. (2009). In Nursing Diagnosis Handbook (9th ed.). Saddle River, NJ: Prentice Hall.

Wilson, B., Shannon, M., & Stang, C. (2006). Nurses drug guide. Upper Saddle River, NJ: Prentice Hall.

Zulkawski, K., & Gray-Leach, K. (2009, January). Staging pressure ulcers: What's the buzz. American Journal of Nursing, 109(1).

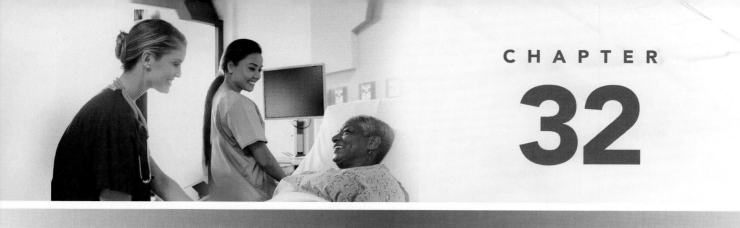

Musculoskeletal System

Case Study: Total Hip Replacement

Common Nursing Study Name	Section 1 Study	Section 1 Chapter Number
Arthroscopy	Arthroscopy	Chapter 9
Chemistry Panel	Calcium, Blood	Chapter 1
	Carbon Dioxide	Chapter 1
	Chloride, Blood	Chapter 1
	Creatinine, Blood	Chapter 1
	Glucose	Chapter 1
	Potassium, Blood	Chapter 1
	Sodium, Blood	Chapter 1
	Urea Nitrogen, Blood	Chapter 1
Chest X-Ray	Chest X-Ray	Chapter 16
Coagulation Studies (for Prothrombin Time [PT] and International Normalized Ratio [INR] and Partial Thromboplastin Time, Activated [aPTT])	Partial Thromboplastin Time, Activated	Chapter 3
	Prothrombin Time and International Normalized Ratio	Chapter 3
Complete Blood Count (CBC)	Complete Blood Count, Hematocrit	Chapter 2
	Complete Blood Count, Hemoglobin	Chapter 2
	Complete Blood Count, Platelet Count	Chapter 3
	Complete Blood Count, RBC Count	Chapter 2
	Complete Blood Count, RBC Indices	Chapter 2
	Complete Blood Count, RBC Morphology and Inclusions	Chapter 2
	Complete Blood Count, WBC Count and Differential	Chapter 2
Electrocardiogram	Electrocardiogram	Chapter 8
Magnetic Resonance Imaging (MRI), Musculoskeletal	Magnetic Resonance Imaging, Musculoskeletal	Chapter 12
Type and Screen	Blood Groups and Antibodies (ABO, Rh & Antibody Screen)	Chapter 4
Urinalysis	Urinalysis	Chapter 22
X-Ray, Hips and Pelvis	Radiography, Bone	Chapter 16

STEP 1: DATA COLLECTION

Pathophysiology

The incidence of hip fracture is related to aging baby boomers, increased life expectancy, occupational and recreational risk taking, disease, and chronic illness associated with falls. The hip is considered to be a ball-and-socket joint, consisting of the femoral head (ball) and acetabulum (socket). Ligaments stabilize the ball-and-socket joint and connect them together. Bone surface is covered by cartilage, which creates a cushion for movement. A thin tissue called the *synovial membrane* provides lubrication to prevent friction.

The causes of hip fracture revolve around bone and/ or cartilage degradation and injury. One cause is osteoarthritis, which progresses slowly over time, wearing down collagen and cartilage until both are lost. Bone on the femoral head and inside the acetabulum rub together, causing joint pain, stiffness, and loss of mobility. Aging, obesity, and the overuse of joints through physical activity also contribute to osteoarthritis. This is a common cause of hip fracture. Rheumatoid arthritis and osteonecrosis are less common causes of hip fracture. Rheumatoid arthritis is an autoimmune disease that causes an inflammatory response that destroys soft tissue, bone, and joint cartilage. Osteonecrosis occurs when the blood supply to the femoral head is destroyed or interrupted. Interruption of the blood supply can occur from trauma, dislocation, fracture, long-term corticosteroid therapy, glandular disease, or alcoholism.

Hip fractures are classified by type or site and degree.

Types of Fractures

The type or site of a fracture is designated as *intracapsular* or *extracapsular*. Intracapsular fracture is more common and occurs at the femoral head or neck. Treatment options are fixation with cannulated screws, removal and replacement of the femoral head (hemiarthroplasty), or a total hip replacement (arthroplasty).

Extracapsular fracture occurs farther down at the trochanteric or subtrochanteric region. Fractures range from simple to complex, requiring surgery or manipulation to reduce and stabilize the fracture. Extracapsular subtrochanteric fractures are the most difficult to treat because bone in this area heals more slowly. These fractures are usually treated by open reduction and internal fixation.

Degrees of Fractures

The degree of a fracture is classified as *stable* or *unstable*. A stable fracture is not displaced or deformed. X-ray verification is difficult, thereby requiring further examination using magnetic resonance imaging (MRI) for visualization. An unstable fracture occurs when the neck of the femur is displaced, becoming clearly detectable on x-ray. Both are common in the older adult.

Risk Factors

The risk factors for fracture are varied. More than 90% of fractures occur after the age of 50 and are from a fall, a motor vehicle accident, an industrial injury, or a sports accident. Those at greatest risk are women with a slight build who are of Caucasian or Asian descent, with osteoporosis, or with a family history of osteoporosis. Chronic medical conditions such as cancer, osteoarthritis, deficiency of vitamin D or calcium, and nutritional disorders such as anorexia or bulimia will also place one at risk. Alcohol use, smoking, and steroid use can cause bone loss, which contributes to fractures. Home hazards such as poor lighting and loose floor rugs can contribute to falls, resulting in fractures.

Signs and Symptoms

The diagnosis of fracture is based upon presenting symptoms, a history of injury, physical assessment, and radiological findings. Pain is the most common complaint with hip fracture. Pain may be located in the knees, thighs, back, anterior hip, groin, and buttocks. Pain may worsen with motion such as walking, and may or may not improve at rest. Sometimes the pain is described as stiffness or tightness. Physical exam may show external rotation or shortening of one leg, with swelling or bruising of the hip.

Laboratory Studies

There is no laboratory study used to diagnose hip fracture. Baseline studies are completed as a preoperative evaluation and may include a chemistry panel, coagulation studies (for prothrombin time [PT] and activated partial thromboplastin time [aPTT]), complete blood count, urinalysis, and a type and screen with crossmatch for transfusion.

Diagnostic Studies

X-ray of the hips and pelvis may be done both pre- and postoperatively. The purpose is to identify the fracture site, type, nonunion issues, and any nonalignment concerns. Preoperative x-ray may be weight-bearing anterior and posterior pelvis, and anterior and posterior lateral view to rule out deformity. Preoperatively, MRI can be used to diagnose osteonecrosis, necrosis, metastatic lesions, and soft-tissue injury, and to visualize hip and femur structure. Additional preoperative studies include chest x-ray and electrocardiogram.

Medication administration will focus on infection, prophylaxis for deep vein thrombosis (DVT), pain management, improving blood stores, and bowel elimination. An antibiotic such as cefazolin or cefuroxime may be ordered preoperatively to prevent infection. Enoxaparin sodium or warfarin may be used to prevent DVT.

Vitamins C and D may be ordered to support bone health. Erythropoietin may be ordered for patients who cannot be transfused with a Hgb between 10 and 13 g/dL. Analgesics such as acetaminophen and ibuprofen can be used for mild-to-moderate pain and to decrease inflammation. Codeine, morphine, oxycodone, and others may be used for moderate-to-severe pain. Patients may receive a stool softener, and may increase fiber in their diet to prevent constipation from narcotic use and immobility.

General/Medical Management

Medical management focuses on treating the primary symptoms of pain and impaired mobility. Surgery becomes an option when medical management is no longer effective. The most common reason for hip replacement surgery is ongoing pain from arthritis, fracture, congenital hip disease, and failed previous surgery. Weight loss can help to lessen symptoms. Assistive devices can improve mobility. Steroid injections and NSAIDS can lessen pain.

The goal of surgery is to decrease pain and restore mobility and range of motion by stabilizing the fracture. Choosing a surgical approach is dependent upon the severity and location of the fracture. Fractures from a fall associated with a medical event such as stroke may require treating the stroke before the fracture. In this case, surgery will be delayed until the patient has been medically cleared. While awaiting surgery, pain medication coupled with Buck traction may be the treatment of choice. Buck traction is used to decrease the pain and muscle spasms associated with hip fracture, and to maintain alignment and stabilize the fracture.

Hemiarthroplasty and total hip arthroplasty are the most common types of surgery for hip fracture.

Hemiarthroplasty

A hemiarthroplasty replaces the head of the femur (ball) *or* the acetabulum (socket) and is considered a repair of the hip. A total hip arthroplasty replaces both the head of the femur (ball) *and* acetabulum (socket).

Stable, nondisplaced fractures can be repaired by a hemiarthroplasty with an open reduction and internal fixation. Stabilization is achieved using pins, cannulated screws, and metal plates with a femoral head implant. This approach is used for less active patients in whom there is a decreased risk of cartilage wear. If unsuccessful, a total hip arthroplasty can be used to remove and replace the damaged femoral head and acetabulum with a prosthetic device.

Total Hip Arthroplasty

Total hip arthroplasty is used for unstable or displaced fractures, or in situations in which medical management has become ineffective, diminishing quality of life. Those with rheumatoid arthritis and osteoarthritis in whom the cartilage is worn away may require hip replacement. As long as there is no infection, any patient with unrelieved hip pain that interferes with activities and sleep is a surgical candidate. This surgery is used more often for active patients. During surgery, the acetabulum (socket) is smoothed out so that a metal cup and a polyethylene liner can fit inside. The head of the femur (ball) is removed and replaced with an implant that is then attached to the repaired socket. The prosthetic device can last for 10 to 15 years.

Other Surgeries

Alternatives are available for patients for whom surgery would not be the best choice. Hip fusion is beneficial in cases of severe arthritis or an infection in which an individual is involved in high-impact activities that a normal hip replacement could support. However, a fusion limits mobility, and the patient will walk with a limp. Osteotomy is another option in which the diseased or damaged bone is cut out and realigned and then allowed to heal over a 6- to 12-month period. The length of time needed for healing is a concern, and the surgery may need to be repeated. Arthroscopy allows the surgeon to look at the joint and decide how best to proceed.

Presurgical Evaluation

Prior to surgery, the patient's health status is evaluated. A medication history should be completed. NSAIDs should be discontinued 1 week prior to surgery to decrease bleeding risk. Anticoagulants such as warfarin should be discontinued or decreased 3 to 5 days prior to surgery for the same reason. Active infection would be a contraindication to surgery.

Presurgical Education

Before surgery, education should be provided to help the patient have a clear, realistic understanding of the surgical procedure and expected outcomes. This includes activity restrictions, exercise expectations to prevent accidental dislocation, ways to promote joint stability, and the prevention of muscle atrophy and venous stasis. Incentive spirometry with cough and deep breathing should be taught to prevent respiratory complications. Medications used for pain management, and DVT or infection prophylaxis should be reviewed and discussed.

Postsurgical Education

Postoperative hip precaution education is an important part of preoperative teaching. Dislocation risk is greatest in the first postoperative months. Hip precaution education includes not crossing the legs, not flexing the hips greater than 90 degrees, and not rotating the operative hip inward. Assistive devices such as raised toilet seats, shower benches, and abductor pillows can assist in meeting this goal.

Postsurgical Care

Social workers can complete a home visit prior to surgery to evaluate fall hazards such as loose carpets or dangling electrical wires. Nutrition can be provided by Meals on Wheels. Those needing a blood transfusion should be educated on donor options. Those having elective surgery can benefit from improving their upper body strength with exercise 3 months before surgery. Patients without support at home, or those who do not progress as expected, may need to be transferred to a lower level of care, such as a transitional care unit or an extended care facility.

Scheduled home health visits can bridge the gap between the hospital and the home to evaluate progress and catch any concerns early.

Postoperative care focuses on managing pain, preventing dislocation, monitoring for bleeding and infection, monitoring mobility, preventing complications, and preparing for discharge. Pain management should be individualized to the patient's needs. Careful monitoring of sedation and pain level is important. Patient-controlled analgesia (PCA) is commonly used. Strategies change when spinal anesthesia is used. The incision should be monitored for infection and the amount of wound drainage. The amount of drainage in the first 24 hours can range from 200 to 500 mL, but should decrease to about 30 mL 48 hours after surgery. The first dressing change may be done by the surgeon and then delegated to nursing. Inspection of the incision is an important part of wound management with documentation of the findings.

RESPIRATORY CARE: Respiratory care consists of encouraging the use of the incentive spirometer with cough and deep breathing at regular intervals to decrease pneumonia risk. Respiratory concerns should be reported immediately to the physician. Respiratory therapists are a resource for any concerns.

MOBILITY: Mobility focuses on getting the patient up and moving as well as on maintaining hip alignment during activity and rest. Weight-bearing ambulation should start as ordered by the physician and as tolerated by the patient. The degree of weight-bearing is dependent upon the type of surgical procedure and the individual patient. Physical therapy in collaboration with the nurse and physician will decide the correct amount of weight the patient can bear on the affected limb. Gait training, weight-bearing practices, stair training, and home exercises will be taught prior

to discharge. Physical therapy may be ongoing on an outpatient basis.

COMPLICATIONS: Complications are possible and include compartment syndrome, DVT, infection, dislocation, leg length discrepancy, malunion, and nonunion.

- *Compartment syndrome* is a serious complication that can lead to necrosis and amputation. Compartment syndrome occurs when pressure from bleeding or edema within the fascia of the joint causes nerve damage, impaired tissue perfusion, and necrosis. The symptoms of compartment syndrome are unrelieved pain, pallor, decreased capillary refill, numbness and tingling, pulselessness, or paralysis.

- *DVT* is a common complication that poses the highest risk of death. To decrease risk, patients may begin a low molecular weight heparin such as enoxaparin sodium with monitoring of hemoglobin and hematocrit. The use of warfarin requires monitoring of the prothrombin time (PT) and international normalized ratio (INR) for a therapeutic INR range between 2 and 3. Bleeding precautions should be adhered to when anticoagulant therapy is in use. Compression stockings or sequential compression devices may also be useful as a DVT preventative strategy.

- *Infection* can occur whenever there is a break in the skin. Antibiotics such as cefazolin or cefuroxime are often administered preoperatively and up to 24 hours postoperatively to prevent infection. Physicians have been known to order antibiotics for longer periods of time when a wound drain stays in place. Indwelling urinary catheters can contribute to urinary tract infection and should be removed as soon as possible. Patients who have an active infection preoperatively need to have completed their antibiotics for 48 hours before surgery with no evidence of residual infection. Infections occur most often in patients who touch or pick at their incisions, who have multisystem diagnoses such as diabetes, or who have intraoperative contamination. Infection may not be noticed until the patient arrives home. Symptoms of infection should be reported to the physician immediately. Severe infections may necessitate the removal of surgical hardware with wound débridement.

- *Dislocation* can occur from flexion, adduction, or internal rotation of the leg. Wear and tear on the prosthetic device can also cause dislocation. Contributors to dislocation are age, weight, poor cementing, poor implant design, and poor biologic integration between the prosthesis and the bone. A culture of joint fluid may be needed to distinguish between prosthetic loosening and joint infection.

- *Leg length discrepancy* is the number one cause of postoperative lawsuits. Inequality in leg length can necessitate the use of shoe lifts, limping, and back pain. This possible outcome should be discussed. Every effort should be made to ensure leg length accuracy.
- *Malunion* occurs when the bones are not united correctly, resulting in improper gait and obvious hip deformity. Surgical revision would be required to restore the normal union of the fracture and correct the gait.
- *Nonunion* occurs when the surgery does not take. This can occur from infection, poor compliance with weight-bearing instructions, interference of bone fragments, or poor blood supply. Alternative treatments would have to be tried and failed before repeat surgery would be considered. Surgical revision is not the first treatment of choice.

Patient Education

Independent physical function is the desire of most people. For the majority of patients, the most important point of education is the answer to the question, "how are you going to help me retain my independence?" Education should focus on getting them to where they want to go. The answer can be complex. In devising your strategy you need to know the patient's functionality prior to this event. Are there additional barriers to mobility? Are they medically compromised by diabetes or another disease? This will be your baseline starting point and will help determine your goal.

All patients want to get back all of their previous function or better. That is why they have hip surgery. The education you give needs to be specific to each person's desire, needs, and functional ability.

STEP 2: POTENTIAL PROBLEM/DIAGNOSES

It is important that nurses understand and consider the science of the disease process and consider the possibilities prior to applying that knowledge to a patient situation. We begin that process with questioning.

💬 *Question:* Based upon your review of the content presented, what possible *potential problems* would you expect for a patient with these diagnoses?

💬 *Answer:* Pain, mobility, skin, and infection

STEP 3: POTENTIAL INTERVENTIONS

💬 *Question:* Based upon your identification of patient problems, what possible interventions would you recommend for these diagnoses, and what would you expect to happen? This would be considered your "grocery list" of the possible actions you could use to assist your patient.

💬 *Answer:* See the following problems, interventions, and expected outcomes:

Problem	Interventions	Expected Outcome
Pain	• Monitor vital signs and compare to the baseline for changes in respiratory effort and blood pressure. • Assess pain intensity and the effectiveness of alternate methods of pain relief. • Provide education about the effective use of PCA and choose a pain scale appropriate for the patient. • Use Buck traction to decrease spasms. • Educate the patient about how to rate pain and explain the value of distraction to decrease the patient's focus on pain. • Educate the patient to move slowly and carefully to decrease spasm risk.	Pain relief at a level acceptable to the patient
Mobility	• Use a trapeze to assist movement. • Facilitate physical therapy. • Assess the patient's understanding of the purpose of traction and apply and maintain Buck traction as appropriate. • Assess neurovascular status, and educate the patient about the signs and symptoms of neurovascular instability. • Assess the patient's understanding, and educate him or her about the importance of range-of-motion exercises. • Maintain proper alignment, and assist with range of motion as needed.	Maintains proper alignment and peripheral neurovascular integrity

Continued

Table Continued

Problem	Interventions	Expected Outcome
Skin	• Educate the patient about how to use a trapeze to shift weight and about how repositioning can protect skin. • Teach the patient to shift weight a minimum of every 2 hours and assist in shifting weight as needed. • Assess Buck traction to ensure proper application. • Assess the patient for the ability to have independent movement and evaluate self-care deficits. • Assess skin pressure points for breakdown. • Keep linens clean, dry, and wrinkle free. Collaborate with the skin care nurse regarding the use of a specialty bed to prevent breakdown. • Explain the risk of skin breakdown associated with inactivity. • Discuss the relationship between adequate pain management, decreased mobility, and skin breakdown.	Maintenance of skin integrity
Infection	• Administer antibiotics as ordered. • Use sterile technique with dressing change, and monitor the character of the incision. • Culture the drainage if necessary. • Teach the patient to notify the health-care provider if the incision should have increased drainage or become warm and tender to the touch. • Monitor for an elevated temperature or change in respiratory rate and heart rate. • Assess for altered mental status. • Remind patients to wash their hands prior to touching the incision site. • Discuss maintaining an adequate diet to facilitate healing.	The incision will not become infected.

PUTTING IT ALL TOGETHER, APPLICATION OF NURSING PROCESS

Putting it all together is where the art and science of nursing meet to provide the best patient outcomes. We take the possibilities and place them into the context of the patient situation. To accomplish this, we use nursing diagnosis, nursing interventions, nursing outcomes, and nursing theory to provide the palate for nursing care.

STEP 4: ASSESSMENT

PATIENT INFORMATION: Melissa, a 62-year-old female, widowed

CHIEF COMPLAINT: Left hip pain after a fall from a ladder at home

HISTORY OF PRESENT ILLNESS: Melissa is a retired secretary who came to the emergency department (ED) with her daughter Lori after falling off a ladder while painting the kitchen. Lori says her mother did not fall far but is concerned and brought her to the ED for evaluation.

PAST MEDICAL HISTORY: Chronic left hip pain associated with osteoarthritis that was successfully treated with glucosamine and NSAIDS. No other history.

FAMILY HISTORY: Both parents are deceased: her mother of cancer and her father of heart disease.

CHART REVIEW AND REPORT: Melissa was admitted after being seen in the ED for a fall from a ladder at home that caused a left hip fracture. Radiographic x-ray shows an unstable displaced fracture of the femoral head. After consultation with an orthopedist by the primary physician, the decision has been made for a total hip arthroplasty. Melissa is currently NPO for surgery at 1200 today. The consent has been signed for both the surgery and possible blood transfusion. Preoperative medical screening has been completed; there is no medical history or active infection that would contraindicate surgery. The shift report received states that Melissa currently has 10 pounds of Buck traction to the left leg. Intravenous fluid of 5% dextrose and ½ normal saline is running at 100 mL/hr. Pain management consists of morphine PCA. Pain is currently rated at a 6/10. Melissa only uses the PCA minimally, stating "I can take the pain." Melissa refused acetaminophen and hydrocodone 5 mg, saying "pills never work on me." Preoperative education still needs to be completed. Melissa is refusing to move because of the pain and has been in the same position for the last 16 hours. A urinary catheter was placed after Melissa's insistence that she "needed it."

SUBJECTIVE ASSESSMENT: *"Good morning, my name is Arvin and I will be your nurse today. How are you feeling this morning?"* Melissa replies, "I feel ridiculous, all of this fuss over a little fall. I can't believe I am going to need surgery." AJ says, *"Your surgery is scheduled for 1200 and I would like to give you some information before you go so you will know what to expect."* Melissa continues, "I'm really not up to a big, long, drawn-out explanation. My leg is killing me and my rear end is numb from sitting in one position all night. Can't we just skip it till later? I told that other nurse I wasn't interested." The patient's daughter interrupts, "Mom, I think you should listen to what the nurse says," Melissa snaps saying, "Then you listen, I am fed up with all of this." The daughter addresses AJ, "I have never seen her like this. I am so frustrated she won't listen to anyone." AJ asks Melissa if he can do his morning assessment. She grumpily replies, "OK, but be quick." As he leaves the room, AJ notices that Melissa seems more relaxed when she listens to classical music.

OBJECTIVE ASSESSMENT: Melissa appears to be in moderate pain. She is fidgety and picking at the sheets. Buck traction 10 pounds is in place to the left leg, and a sequential compression device is in place to the right leg. IV fluids are infusing as ordered, and the site is clear. Morning vital signs are BP 132/90 mm Hg, a temperature of 98.8°F, a pulse of 92 beats per minutes, and a respiratory rate of 20 breaths per minute that is regular and unlabored. The left hip has a large, dark purple bruise. Melissa denies tingling or numbness in the left leg or foot, capillary refill is less than 3 seconds bilaterally, pedal pulses are equal, and feet are pink and warm bilaterally. Urinary catheter is in place and draining 300 mL light amber urine. Other assessments are normal. Melissa has been typed and crossmatched for two units of packed cells that are on hold in the blood bank.

- *Laboratory Studies:*
  - Hgb 14.7 g/dL and /Hct 44%
  - WBC 10.8×10^3/microL
  - Chemistry K$^+$ 4.1 mEq/L, Na$^+$ 142 mEq/L, Cl$^-$ 108 mEq/L , BUN 11 mg/dL, Cr 0.8 mg/dL
  - Coagulation study results: PT 11.6 seconds, INR 2.1, and aPTT 29 seconds
  - Urinalysis: normal
- *Diagnostic Studies:*
  - Chest x-ray: normal
  - Pelvis x-ray: a fracture of the femoral head of the left hip
  - EKG: normal
- *Medications:*
  - Cefazolin 1 gram IVPB on call to surgery and every 8 hours for three doses postoperatively
  - Stool softener 100 mg daily
  - Morphine sulfate 2-mg intravenous push every 2 hours as needed for pain
  - Enoxaparin sodium 30 mg twice a day subcutaneously to be started postoperatively

STEP 5: REALITY CHECK: DETOUR AHEAD

Reality Check occurs when the nurse takes a moment to think about individualized patient information that needs to be considered in framing diagnoses and interventions. This information is retrievable from any legitimate source (e.g., family, case management, other nurses, any ancillary, a doctor, etc.). These are the "wrenches" that create challenging situations, such as culture, religion, socioeconomic status, level of education, developmental level, marital status, employment, age, and gender.

Psychosocial History

Melissa is a retired elementary school teacher. Her ethnicity is Caucasian of Eastern European descent. She is recently widowed; her husband of 45 years died from pancreatic cancer. The funeral was 3 months ago, and Lori has stayed with her mom to keep her company. Lori reports her mother has been angry with the doctors since her father's death and blames them for not saving him. Her husband was her best friend, and she has no other support group. Melissa has no financial concerns and considers herself to be an atheist.

Critical Thinking Moment

You have just completed the assessment of Melissa and need to make a decision about the patient's *actual* problems and nursing diagnoses based upon the data you have collected and the potential problems you identified. Outcomes must be realistic and measurable.

STEP 6: ACTUAL PROBLEMS/ DIAGNOSES

The *first step* in problem identification is to revisit the list of *potential diagnoses* and choose *actual diagnoses* based upon the learner's evaluation of the case study information provided. A problem statement must be completed for each identified problem/diagnosis. The actual problems for this case study are pain, mobility, and skin.

STEP 7: PLANNING: ACTUAL INTERVENTIONS

After actual diagnoses have been chosen, it is necessary to evaluate the list of *potential interventions* and choose *actual interventions* that will fit within the patient's reality and meet expected outcomes. Each intervention requires a rationale. Interventions are identified in three categories: (1) assessment, (2) therapeutic, and (3) education.

Diagnostic Statement

Pain related to left hip fracture of femoral head and muscle spasms as evidenced by a self-report of pain rated at 6/10.

Assessment

- Monitor vital signs and compare to the baseline. *Rationale: Analgesics may cause changes in respiratory effort and may decrease blood pressure.*
- Assess pain intensity (0/10). *Rationale: Increasing pain may indicate complications such as compartment syndrome.*
- Assess the effectiveness of alternate methods of pain relief *to see if it works. Rationale: Melissa likes to listen to classical music.*

Therapeutic Interventions

- Assist in the appropriate use of a pain scale. *Rationale: This will allow you to evaluate the use of PCA morphine for effective pain relief.*
- Apply Buck traction 10# as ordered, and monitor its use. *Rationale: This decreases pain and muscle spasms.*
- Use the distraction of classical music to relieve pain. *Rationale: Melissa's daughter verbalized that this will help her mom.*

Patient Education

- Teach Melissa how to rate pain and use the PCA effectively. *Rationale: This better meets the patient's pain management needs.*
- Teach Melissa the value of distraction. *Rationale: This decreases Melissa's focus on pain and decreases spasms.*
- Teach Melissa to move slowly and carefully. *Rationale: This decreases the risk of spasms, which may increase pain.*

Expected Outcome

- A decrease in pain to less than 6/10 and an increased level of comfort

Diagnostic Statement

Impaired mobility related to pain, a fear of moving with fracture, and the use of Buck traction as evidenced by Melissa's refusal to move for the last 16 hours and a self-report of pain of 6/10.

Assessment

- Assess Melissa's neurovascular status. *Rationale: This provides a baseline for comparison.*
- Assess Melissa's understanding of the purpose of traction. *Rationale: This ensures the correct use of this therapy.*
- Assess Melissa's understanding of range-of-motion exercises. *Rationale: This facilitates her participation in mobility.*

Therapeutic Interventions

- Maintain proper body alignment. *Rationale: This promotes neurovascular stability.*
- Assist with range of motion to the unaffected limbs. *Rationale: This prevents atrophy and maintains joint mobility and function.*
- Maintain Buck traction and ensure weights are off the floor. *Rationale: This supports hip alignment and promotes neurovascular stability.*

Education

- Educate Melissa about the importance of range-of-motion activities. *Rationale: This prevents atrophy and maintains joint function.*
- Educate Melissa about the purpose of Buck traction. *Rationale: This traction supports joint stability.*
- Educate Melissa about the signs and symptoms of neurovascular instability. *Rationale: This promotes collaborative cooperation.*

Expected Outcome

- Maintenance of neurovascular stability and participation in prescribed range-of-motion activities

Diagnostic Statement

Skin integrity related to decreased mobility and the presence of Buck traction as evidenced by Melissa's refusal to move.

Assessment

- Assess Buck traction. *Rationale: This ensures proper application as well as the evaluation of pressure points.*
- Assess Melissa's ability to move herself. *Rationale: This allows the evaluations of self-care deficits.*
- Assess Melissa's skin pressure points. *Rationale: This allows the evaluation of skin breakdown.*

Therapeutic Interventions

- Assist Melissa in shifting her weight every 2 hours. *Rationale: Even a minimal change in position can prevent skin breakdown.*
- Keep linens clean, dry, and wrinkle free. *Rationale: This prevents pressure points and maceration.*
- Collaborate with the skin care nurse regarding the use of a specialty bed. *Rationale: This promotes skin integrity and decreases pressure on the coccyx.*

Education

- Educate Melissa about the use of a trapeze for shifting weight and repositioning. *Rationale: This prevents skin breakdown.*
- Educate Melissa about the risk for skin breakdown associated with inactivity. *Rationale: This promotes cooperation in care.*
- Educate Melissa about the relationship among adequate pain management, increased mobility, and a decreased risk of skin breakdown. *Rationale: This promotes cooperation with the plan of care.*

Expected Outcome

- Skin will remain intact, and Melissa will participate in the prevention of breakdown.
- *Preoperative Note*: Surgery scheduled for 1200 was postponed until 1400 to make room for an emergency surgery. Melissa is upset and shouts at the nurse stating, "This is the worst hospital around; if I could, I would get up and walk out of here." Her daughter apologizes for her mother's behavior, again stating, "She has never been like this. She is just angry all of the time." At 1430 Melissa is transported to surgery without further incident. AJ has communicated to the holding area concerns about the patient's emotional state, including the refusal to receive preoperative education.

STEP 8: IMPLEMENTATION

Nursing Theory

Virginia Henderson encourages the nurse to assist the patient to meet basic care needs. Nurses should use ancillaries as needed to achieve this goal. Ancillaries that may be helpful to Melissa are Case Management, Occupational Therapy, Physical Therapy, Chaplain, and Social Services. Florence Nightingale reminds us that environment matters and should be manipulated to achieve wellness. In Melissa's case, the use of a specialty bed may assist in preventing skin breakdown. Traction can assist to stabilize the fracture. Rosemarie Parse explains that the nurse's role is to guide patients to make good choices and to respect their decisions. Although Melissa is not being cooperative, AJ needs to continue to communicate the surgical information.

Ancillary Support

Occupational therapy and physical therapy may both be involved with Melissa postoperatively. Collaboration between occupational therapy and physical therapy can assist with postoperative total hip replacement education and make recommendations for assistive devices. The therapist should help to identify areas of daily living that may need to be adjusted. There should be education about how best to adapt activities of daily living to adhere to hip precautions. Typically, this includes bathing; dressing; transfers; bed mobility; getting into cars, the tub, or the shower; and using the toilet. Consideration should be given to family expectations, the layout of the house, and if Melissa has help at home. Physical therapy will work with Melissa in gait training and weight-bearing of the new hip. Outpatient physical therapy can be arranged if needed. Social services and the Chaplain may be of assistance in helping Melissa deal with her anger, and in encouraging cooperation with the plan of care. If needed, the skin care nurse can assist in helping Melissa understand the risk of breakdown by her continued refusal to move in bed. Case management can assist in coordinating home care needs.

STEP 9: PLAN OF CARE

The plan of care is a road map for patient care and should be used as a communication tool between disciplines. Expected entries on the plan of care would be each identified problem, intervention, and expected outcome. Within the plan of care there should be a notation that Melissa is a recent widow, that she is resistive to taking pain medication, and that she likes classical music. A safety notation should be made that Melissa needs to be closely monitored to prevent falling since she will not verbally agree to the current plan. Contact information for Lori should be documented for easy access.

STEP 10: EVALUATION

Evaluation is an active process in which the nurse "connects the dots" to decide if the expected outcomes (goals) that were established have been met, partially met, or not met. If the goals are met, we continue with the plan as outlined. If the goal was partially met, we revise the parts of the plan that did not work. If the goals were not met, we start all over with a new plan.

End-of-Shift Narrative

Melissa returned from surgery at 1830. AJ received the following report from the recovery room nurse: "Melissa tolerated the surgery without complication. She has a stage I pressure ulcer on her coccyx. Vital signs are stable. One unit of packed cells was transfused during surgery to replace blood loss of about 150 mL. IV fluid of 5% dextrose and ½ normal saline is infusing at 100 mL/hr. Melissa received cefazolin 1 gm IVPB at 1800 in recovery. Another dose is to be given in

8 hours and then discontinued. Postoperative pain is rated at a 6/10, and medication was refused. PCA morphine is to be continued postoperatively for pain management. Melissa is currently NPO until fully awake, and then she can start clear liquids and progress to a regular diet. The urinary catheter is draining 300 mL amber urine and is to be discontinued in 12 hours. Physical therapy is to see Melissa in the morning to begin adjusted weight-bearing activity. Hip precautions are to be strictly enforced, with an abductor pillow for use in bed.

Currently Melissa denies tingling or a sensation loss in the left foot. Pedal pulses are strong with a capillary refill of less than 3 seconds. Dressing to her left hip is dry and intact with a Jackson-Pratt drain intact with 50 mL of bloody drainage. Postoperative medications include the last dose of cefazolin 1 gm, a stool softener 100 mg daily, and enoxaparin sodium 30 mg subcutaneous twice a day. AJ attempts to speak to Melissa and explain her postoperative restrictions. She looks directly at him and says, "Just leave me alone, all I want to do is sleep." Lori, who is at the bedside, shakes her head, "I apologize for my mother's attitude." AJ persists, stating, *"Please don't try to get out of bed. The physical therapist will get you up in the morning."* Melissa closes her eyes, "Yea, whatever, I don't plan to do physical therapy." Lori assures AJ she will stay the night and make sure her mother follows everyone's instructions.

Problem Evaluation

PROBLEM 1: Pain. Melissa should have a decrease in her pain intensity to a level that is acceptable. The goal is not met because Melissa has refused both the hydrocodone and the PCA morphine. Yet her pain is a 6/10. A revised plan is to partner with daughter to educate Melissa about the positive effects of pain management to the overall healing process. Have a discussion with the physician about the possibility of setting a PCA basal rate for the next 48 hours.

PROBLEM 2: Mobility. Melissa should have neurovascular stability in preparation for postoperative physical therapy. The goal is partially met because there is no neurovascular compromise, but Melissa is reticent about following postoperative guidelines. The revised plan is to collaborate with Lori to elicit her mother's cooperation in assisting to meet physical therapy goals. Social services should be contacted for a consult, and the Chaplain for grief counseling.

PROBLEM 3: Skin. Melissa should maintain skin integrity. The goal is not met because she now has a small stage I ulcer on her coccyx from lying on her back for 16 hours and refusing to move. The revised plan is to discuss the effects of immobility with Melissa and her daughter. Arrange a visit with the skin care nurse.

Overall Evaluation

Based on the end-of-shift assessment and the comparison of Melissa's progress during this shift, her overall evaluation is declining: Her skin is breaking down, her pain is not managed, and mobility continues to be an issue.

Postscript: Melissa continued to be uncooperative with the staff and refused to listen to her daughter. Three hours after her urinary catheter was removed, she attempted to get out of bed without assistance while her daughter was briefly out of the room. As a result, she fell and fractured her right hip. Melissa has become more verbally abusive.

REFERENCES

Altizer, L. (2005, July/August). Hip fractures. Orthopaedic Nursing 24(4), 283–292.

Eby, A. (2008, May/June). Get hip to hip replacement. Nursing Made Incredibly Easy, 22–30.

George, J. (2011). Nursing theories. The base for professional nursing practice (6th ed.). Upper Saddle River, NJ: Pearson Education.

Gulanick, M., & Meyers, J. (2013). Nursing care plans nursing diagnosis and intervention (8th ed.). St Louis, MO: Mosby.

Hohler, S. (2005). Looking into minimally invasive total hip arthroplasty. Nursing 2005, 35(6), 54–57.

Holloway, N. (2004). Medical surgical nursing care planning (4th ed.). Springhouse, PA: Lippincott, Williams & Wilkins.

Honkanen, L. (2002). An overview of hip fracture prevention. Topics in Geriatric Rehabilitation, 20(4), 285–296.

Keston, V. (1998, Winter). Total hip replacement: A case history. Health Care Management, 23(1) 7–17.

LeMone, P., Burke, K., & Baldoff, G. (2011). Medical surgical nursing, Critical thinking in patient care (5th ed.). Upper Saddle River, NJ: Pearson.

Neville, D., Dvorkin, M., Chittenden, M., & Fromm, L. (2008, November/December). The new era of hip replacement. OR Nurse, 2(10) 18–25.

Neville-Smith, M., Trujillo, L., & Ammundson, R. (2000, June). Special feature: Consistency in post-operative education programs following total hip replacement. Topics in Geriatric Rehabilitation, 14(4), 68–76.

Parker, M. (2006). Nursing theories and nursing practice (2nd ed.). Philadelphia, PA: FA Davis.

Rodgers, S. (2008). Asthma. In Medical-Surgical Nursing Care Plan (pp. 140–147). Clifton Park, NY: Thomson Delmar Learning.

Swearingen, P. (2008). All in one care planning resource (2nd ed.). St Louis, MO: Mosby.

Van Leeuwen, A., & Bladh, M. (2015). Davis's comprehensive handbook of laboratory and diagnostic testing with nursing implications (6th ed.). Philadelphia, PA: F.A. Davis Company.

Wilkinson, J., & Ahern, N. (2009). In Nursing Diagnosis Handbook (9th ed). Saddle River, NJ: Prentice Hall.

Wilson, B., Shannon, M., & Stang, C. (2006). Nurses drug guide. Upper Saddle River: NJ Prentice Hall.

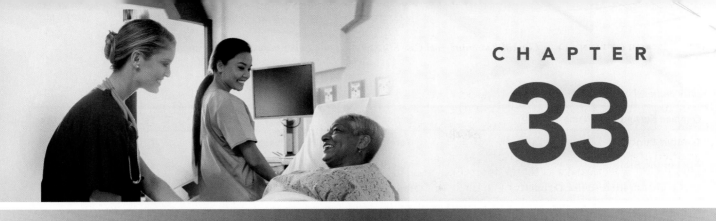

Neurologic System

Case Study: Stroke, Brain Attack

Common Nursing Study Name	Section 1 Study	Section 1 Chapter Number
Carotid Angiography	Angiography, Carotid	Chapter 15
Audiometry	Audiometry, Hearing Loss	Chapter 17
Blood Glucose	Glucose	Chapter 1
Carotid Doppler	Ultrasound, Arterial Doppler, Carotid Studies	Chapter 21
Computed Tomography (CT) (Noncontrast) and Xenon-Enhanced CT of the Head	Computed Tomography, Brain	Chapter 7
C-Reactive Protein (CRP)	C-Reactive Protein	Chapter 1
Digital Subtraction, Carotid Angiography	Angiography, Carotid	Chapter 15
Echocardiography	Echocardiography	Chapter 21
Electrocardiogram (ECG)	Electrocardiogram	Chapter 8
Electroencephalogram (EEG)	Electroencephalography	Chapter 8
Electrolytes	Chloride, Blood	Chapter 1
	Carbon Dioxide	Chapter 1
	Potassium, Blood	Chapter 1
	Sodium, Blood	Chapter 1
Evoked Response Tests	Evoked Brain Potentials	Chapter 8
Hemoglobin A_1C	Glycated Hemoglobin	Chapter 1
Hemogram and Platelet Count	Complete Blood Count, Hematocrit	Chapter 2
	Complete Blood Count, Hemoglobin	Chapter 2
	Complete Blood Count, Platelet Count	Chapter 3
	Complete Blood Count, RBC Count	Chapter 2
	Complete Blood Count, RBC Indices	Chapter 2
	Complete Blood Count, WBC Count	Chapter 2
Lipid Panel	Cholesterol, HDL and LDL	Chapter 1
	Cholesterol, Total	Chapter 1
	Triglycerides	Chapter 1

Continued

Table Continued

Common Nursing Study Name	Section 1 Study	Section 1 Chapter Number
Lumbar Puncture	Cerebrospinal Fluid Analysis	Chapter 6
MRI of the Brain	Magnetic Resonance Imaging, Brain	Chapter 12
Oxygen Saturation (Pulse Oximetry)	Pulse Oximetry	Chapter 14
Phenytoin	Anticonvulsant Drugs: Carbamazepine, Ethosuximide, Lamotrigine, Phenobarbital, Phenytoin, Primidone, Valproic Acid	Chapter 1
Partial Thromboplastin Time, Activated (aPTT)	Partial Thromboplastin Time, Activated	Chapter 3
Positron Emission Tomography (PET), Brain	Positron Emission Tomography, Brain	Chapter 13
Prothrombin Time (PT) with International Normalized Ratio (INR)	Prothrombin Time and International Normalized Ratio	Chapter 3
Swallowing Evaluation	Barium Swallow Upper Gastrointestinal and Small Bowel Series	Chapter 15 Chapter 15
Toxicology Screening	Drugs of Abuse	Chapter 22
Troponin	Troponins I and T	Chapter 1
Videofluoroscopy	Barium Swallow Upper Gastrointestinal and Small Bowel Series	Chapter 15 Chapter 15

STEP 1: DATA COLLECTION

Pathophysiology

Stroke or brain attack is the leading cause of adult disability. Strokes can be progressive, with deficits that worsen over time, or completed with the maximum deficit level reached. Stroke severity is assessed using the Glasgow Coma Scale or National Institutes of Health Stroke Scale.

Eighty percent of the blood to the brain is supplied by the internal carotid artery and the other 20% by the vertebral arteries. The brain has the highest metabolic rate within the body, receiving about 25% of the cardiac output. Because the brain does not store oxygen or nutrients, it needs a continuous blood supply to support brain function.

Types of Stroke

There are two kinds of stroke: *ischemic* and *hemorrhagic.* Ischemic stroke occurs in about 88% of reported cases, and hemorrhagic stroke occurs in about 12%. Both types disrupt blood supply to the brain, causing tissue damage and neurological deficits.

An ischemic stroke occurs when a clot deprives a part of the brain of oxygen and nutrients. The occluded vessel could be large or small. Large vessel occlusions occur when an artery narrowed from atherosclerosis becomes completely occluded by a clot. Large vessel strokes have a high mortality rate, occurring most often in the middle cerebral artery or branches. Large vessel clots are also found in the basilar, internal carotid, vertebral, anterior cerebral, or posterior cerebral arteries. Small vessel occlusions occur more often in hypertensive smokers or diabetics. Vessel involvement varies, but prognosis is better than in large vessel strokes.

Hemorrhagic stroke occurs when a ruptured artery bleeds into the brain causing cerebral pressure and cell death. Bleeding into the brain is an intracranial hemorrhage occurring at the bifurcation of the major arteries. Bleeding around the brain is a subarachnoid hemorrhage and occurs around the circle of Willis. Intracranial hemorrhage is more common than subarachnoid hemorrhage. Causes of hemorrhagic stroke are hypertension, trauma, congenital defects, or atherosclerosis. Common stroke sites are the circle of Willis, anterior and posterior cerebral and anterior communicating arteries, and the middle cerebral arteries.

Risk Factors

Stroke risk factors can be characterized as modifiable and nonmodifiable. Modifiable risk factors can be changed either by medication or lifestyle changes. These include smoking, hypertension, heart disease, diabetes, hyperlipidemia, carotid stenosis, weight, and activity.

Smoking has been shown to double stroke risk by contributing to atherosclerosis, platelet clustering, and increased blood viscosity. Hypertension is most easily modifiable through use of medications, diet changes, and daily exercise. Stroke risk is four times greater with hypertension. Weight loss and dietary changes with moderate exercise can reduce stroke risk.

Due to plaque buildup, stroke risk can be six times greater in diabetics than in nondiabetics. Risk can be adjusted using insulin, oral glycemic medications, and statins to control lipids. Atrial fibrillation, cardiomyopathy, and valvular or congenital defects can increase the risk of a cardioembolism. Stroke risk doubles with advanced atherosclerotic plaque buildup and stenosis. Elevated low-density lipoprotein (LDL) and cholesterol increase the risk of atherosclerosis.

Transient ischemic attack (TIA) is a warning sign of imminent stroke. TIA occurs from a temporary decrease in blood flow and oxygen with neurological deficits that usually clear within 24 hours. Immediate medical attention is necessary.

Nonmodifiable risk factors include age, gender, ethnicity, and genetic make-up. Increasing age doubles stroke risk every 10 years after the age of 55. More women die of stroke than men. Mexican Americans and African Americans are at greater risk of stroke than Caucasians. Mexican Americans have a higher risk of hemorrhagic stroke due to diabetes. African Americans have a higher incidence of disability and death associated with hypertensive stroke.

Signs and Symptoms

Stroke presents with a rapid onset of neurological deficits. The challenge is in differentiating stroke from other possible causes associated with the presenting symptoms.

General signs and symptoms of stroke can be defined using categories, as seen in Table 33-1. Patients can present with one, several, or none of the signs and symptoms from each of the neurological, motor, and sensory categories.

The expression of neurological deficits is dependent on the area of the brain affected. Deficits appear on the opposite side of the damaged brain with the exception of cranial nerve injury, which will appear on the same side. Symptoms can recede as cerebral edema decreases. Brain tissue damage can occur in the left, right, and deep hemisphere, brainstem, and cerebellum. Left hemisphere stroke presents with right-sided deficits. Right hemisphere stroke presents with left-sided deficits, a mirror image of the left hemisphere stroke.

Deep hemisphere stroke presents a little differently. Patients may have a pure motor stroke with hemiparesis and no change in sensation, or a pure sensory loss without visual, speech, or mental deficits. Clumsy-hand dysarthria, impaired speech from loss of muscle control, unilateral hand weakness, or loss of motor control on one side may be seen. Brainstem stroke presents with motor and sensory deficits in all extremities.

TABLE 33.1 *General Signs and Symptoms of Stroke*

Neurological	Motor	Sensory
• Irritability	• Weakness	• Visual field loss (hemianopsia)
• Memory loss	• One-sided paralysis (hemiparesis)	• Double vision (diplopia)
• Disorientation	• Partial paralysis	• Blindness
• Withdrawal	• Difficulty swallowing (dysphagia)	• Involuntary eye movement (nystagmus)
• Confusion	• Uncoordinated muscle movement (ataxia)	• Ear ringing (tinnitus)
• Stupor	• Difficulty chewing	• Numbness (paresthesia)
• Coma		• Expressive aphasia, difficulty with speaking or expression
• Dizziness (vertigo)		• Receptive aphasia, the inability to understand the written or spoken word. Verbal speech is nonsensical.
• Unequal or fixed pupils		• Broca aphasia, the loss of control over the lips, tongue, or vocal cords
• Seizure		• Altered auditory comprehension, difficulty with naming or finding correct words, sequencing phonemes
• Positive Babinski		• Global aphasia, complete breakdown in written and verbal language skills including auditory comprehension
• Spatial neglect, ignoring a side of the body as if it does not exist		• Impaired conjugate gaze; eyes do not track together when looking to the right or left
		• Hemisensory loss

The patient may also have ataxia, dysarthria, or dysphagia. Stroke of the cerebellum presents with gait ataxia, same-sided limb ataxia, hemisensory loss, nausea, vomiting, hiccups, dizziness, ringing or buzzing in the ears, and altered level of consciousness. Symptoms can vary with each individual case; bowel and bladder disturbances, nausea, vomiting, and incontinence are other commonly encountered changes.

Laboratory Studies

When a patient presents with a possible stroke, it is important that initial lab studies screen the patient's suitability to receive recombinant tissue plasminogen activator (tPA). These laboratory tests would include a hemogram and platelet count, electrolytes, activated partial thromboplastin time (aPTT), and prothrombin time (PT) with international normalized ratio (INR). Suggested follow-up laboratory tests are hemoglobin A_1C, lipid panel, C-reactive protein, and toxicology screening.

Diagnostic Studies

Diagnostic testing is used to identify the type, cause, and severity of stroke while ruling out other potential diagnoses. Electrocardiogram (ECG) can rule out a cardiac event, check for atrial fibrillation, and check for myocardial ischemia. Noncontrast computed tomography (CT) scan of the head can differentiate between ischemic and hemorrhagic stroke and can determine stroke size and location, the presence or absence of ventricular blood or cerebral spinal fluid, and any shift in brain structures. CT is the examination of choice for unstable patients; however, the extent of necrosis may not be certain until 48 to 72 hours poststroke. A xenon-enhanced CT scan can evaluate blood flow, and a carotid angiography can evaluate blood vessels. Magnetic resonance imaging (MRI) helps identify stroke size, including smaller strokes located in deep brain tissue. MRI can provide information on brain structure shift and cerebral edema. Diffusion and perfusion studies can differentiate between an acute and a chronic stroke. Positron emission tomography (PET) scans can localize damage from an ischemic stroke. Electroencephalogram can measure brain waves and check for seizure, nerve transmission, and brain wave activity.

Carotid Doppler can evaluate the patency of the carotid arteries. Transcranial Doppler ultrasound is non-invasive and can supply information about intracranial pressure and blood flow. Echocardiography assesses for clots attached to heart valves or walls. Angiography, cerebral or carotid, can differentiate between cerebral aneurysm and arteriovenous malformation, including size, location, and vessel involvement. Digital subtraction angiography can visualize blood flow and detect abnormalities. Lumbar puncture can confirm the presence of a subarachnoid hemorrhage by evaluating for increased intracranial pressure if the CT scan is negative or inconclusive.

Evoked response tests can determine the brain's ability to react to stimuli to assess for abnormal areas. Swallowing evaluation assesses the ability of the patient to swallow safely. Video fluoroscopy can be used to identify the swallowing problem and provide direction for appropriate treatment. Patients who choke on thin liquids such as saliva are at high risk for aspiration and should not have this test.

Audiometry can be used to assess patients who continue to complain of ringing in the ears and who are able to follow directions in the performance of this hearing evaluation.

General/Medical Management

Thrombolytic Therapy

The overarching goal of stroke management is to limit or reverse brain tissue damage. The gold standard to treat an ischemic stroke is thrombolytic therapy using tPA, which can be administered safely after patient screening. Inclusion criteria for tPA administration are as follows: 18 years of age, ischemic stroke, measurable deficits that are not minor and do not clear, occurrence within 3 hours, neurology consult, and informed consent. Exclusion criteria are hemorrhagic stroke; subarachnoid hemorrhage symptoms; history of seizure with postictal presentation; stroke, heart attack, or head trauma in the past 3 months; surgery or trauma in the past 3 weeks; genitourinary or gastrointestinal hemorrhage in the past 3 weeks; pregnancy; history of anticoagulant use with INR greater than 1.5; BP greater than 185/110 mm Hg at the time of tPA administration; blood sugar less than 50 mg/dL or greater than 400 mg/dL; and platelets less than 100×10^3/microL.

Once the inclusion criteria are met, tPA should be administered as soon as possible. After the administration of tPA, the patient should be closely monitored for any bleeding associated with the procedure such as puncture sites, signs, or symptoms indicative of internal bleeding, or blood in the urine. Careful observation of the level of consciousness will be necessary to monitor for intracranial bleeding. Hemorrhagic stroke patients do not receive tPA.

Oxygenation

Oxygen is necessary to prevent hypoxia. Interventions to support oxygenation are suctioning, intubation, elevating the head of the bed 30 degrees, encouraging cough and deep breathing, and frequent turning. Oxygenation saturation (pulse oximetry) should be minimally maintained at a SpO_2 of 94%.

Monitoring of Fever, Blood Glucose, and Cardiac Rhythms

Fever has been associated with an increase in mortality rate and degrading neurological status. Fever, if present, should be treated with cooling blankets and acetaminophen. Altered blood glucose can adversely affect brain health. Management may require the use of insulin to maintain blood glucose between 80 and 110 mg/dL. Rhythm disturbances in the form of atrial fibrillation are common. Patients may be placed on monitored units or have frequent ECGs. Vigilance in assessment of cardiac rate, rhythm, and chest pain is necessary.

Anticoagulant Use

The judicious use of anticoagulants may help prevent a repeat stroke and provide some benefit in reducing neurological deficits. Bleeding precautions are necessary if anticoagulants are used. Anticoagulants are contraindicated in hemorrhagic stroke. Limited mobility can contribute to a host of problems. Early activity can help keep joints mobile and prevent the development of clots in the legs or lungs. Lack of early physical therapy contributes to deconditioning, which is a failure to maintain optimal muscular tone and functionality. Assistive devices (canes, walkers, etc.) should be used to facilitate mobility. Frequent active and passive range of motion should be used if other activity is not possible.

Use of the Neglected Side

Spatial neglect is another mobility challenge. Forcing recognition of the neglected side is the best course of action. For example, approach the patient from the neglected side, place the bedside table on the neglected side, and use the neglected side in all care activities. Voluntary spastic movement may be treated with tizanidine, baclofen, or dantrolene sodium.

Prevention of Skin Breakdown and Ensurance of Nutrition

Skin breakdown and pressure ulcers are a concern for stroke patients. Two important factors affecting skin integrity are nutrition and continence. Malnutrition increases the risk of pressure ulcers, yet nutrition is a challenge because of the presence of dysphagia and altered levels of consciousness. A swallowing evaluation must be completed by a speech pathologist or trained registered nurse to assess aspiration risk before a diet can begin. Swallowing deficits that require interventions such as thickening liquids should be part of the plan of care. Enteral feedings by nasogastric or gastrostomy tube may be an option for those who cannot swallow safely. Total parenteral nutrition (TPN) is another temporary caloric alternative. Intake and output should be monitored to check for fluid deficit or overload.

Urine or stool incontinence can contribute to skin breakdown. Skin should be protected by frequent turning. Special attention should be given to the sacrum and heels. Skin should be kept clean and dry, and a consult with the skin care nurse should be considered.

Infection Control

Hospital-acquired infections can develop at any invasive procedure site such as blood draws. Pressure ulcers, pneumonia, and uncontrolled diabetes can also contribute to infections. Timely changing of lines, removal of urinary catheters, and correct aseptic technique with vigorous hand hygiene can act as barriers to infection.

Antiseizure Measures

Seizure activity is a possible complication that can occur as the result of cerebral irritation poststroke. If embolism was the cause of the stroke, it is likely that a seizure will occur within 30 days. Suggested antiseizure medications are fosphenytoin and phenytoin. Seizure precautions should be instituted.

Fall Precautions

Safety is a concern when there are neurological deficits from a stroke. Denial of physical limitations can precipitate an injury when attempting to get out of bed without assistance. Fall precautions should be put into place, such as use of a bed alarm. Short-term memory loss can interfere with the patient's ability to remember the provided instructions. If impulsive behavior continues, a sitter may be needed to prevent injury.

Communication Alterations

Communication is a challenge for stroke patients. Aphasia can manifest itself in different ways such as in the inability to name objects, express thoughts, and comprehend written or spoken language, and it can alter the ability to understand and follow commands. Speak slowly and clearly to the aphasic patient; the use of yes-or-no questions may be helpful. Culturally appropriate hand gestures may be used to enhance communication.

Non-Health-Care Services

Stroke patients can be emotionally fragile owing to their drastic change in health status. Feelings of frustration, fear, anxiety, anger, sadness, grief, and depression are common after a stroke. Patients and their families should be closely observed for emotional issues. When the patient is the primary source of income, there may also be financial concerns. The assistance of social services, case management, or pastoral care may be helpful.

Special Intervention for Hemorrhagic Stroke

Hemorrhagic stroke requires some special interventions. The goal is to stop the bleeding. Initial treatment will be to focus on diminishing cerebral irritation to prevent an increase in intracranial pressure. Interventions include placing the patient on bedrest, using sedation to prevent agitation, minimizing external stimuli, providing pain medication, and treating hypertension and vasospasm if present. Anti-epileptics may be used for seizures or antipyretics for fever. Elevating the head of the bed, administering diuretics, and adequately managing blood glucose can decrease cerebral pressure. Surgery in the form of craniotomy may be needed for decompression if there is no improvement. If an aneurysm is detected before it ruptures, a clip or wrap can be used to cut the aneurysm off from the blood supply and prevent rupture.

Endarterectomy and stent placement can be used to increase the size of the carotid artery lumen to prevent stroke. Antiplatelet medications such as clopidogrel, dipyridamole, or ticlopidine are also helpful.

Patient Education

Education begins as soon as the patient arrives in crisis. Initially the education may be provided to the family while awaiting a decision on the severity and type of stroke. Remember that this is a life-changing event for all of them. All of the information discussed thus far should be considered within the context of the clinical situation. You must choose the moment to begin the process of education, and assist them in adapting to their new reality.

STEP 2: POTENTIAL PROBLEMS/DIAGNOSES

It is important that nurses understand and consider the science of the disease process and consider the possibilities prior to applying that knowledge to a patient situation. We begin that process with questioning.

💬 *Question:* Based on your review of the content presented, what possible *potential problems* would you expect for a patient with these diagnoses?

💬 *Answer:* Mobility, communication, nutrition, skin integrity, coping, and self-care

STEP 3: POTENTIAL INTERVENTIONS AND EXPECTED OUTCOMES

💬 *Question:* Based on your identification of patient problems, what possible interventions would you recommend for these diagnoses and what would you expect to happen? This would be considered your "grocery list" of the possible actions you could use to assist your patient.

💬 *Answer:* See the following problems, interventions, and expected outcomes:

Problem	Interventions	Expected Outcome
Mobility	• Assess for joint pain or tenderness. • Assess for range of motion. • Assess for the ability to move and change position. • Assess fine and gross motor movement. • Assess the degree of weakness. • Place the patient in the correct body alignment with the head of the bed elevated 30 degrees. • Maintain bedrest for the first 24 hours poststroke. • Encourage wearing well-fitting shoes to prevent foot drop, wearing a sling on the affected arm when out of bed for support, moving from small to larger tasks, and consulting with a physical therapist. • Teach the correct technique for turning or moving. • Teach the family not to pull on the affected arm to correct its position and how to transfer toward the unaffected side.	The patient can demonstrate an increased ability to manage mobility within functional limits.
Communication	• Assess the ability to speak, to follow directions, and to read, write, and name common objects. • Suggest a speech therapist referral, use communication technique that works, decrease distraction during communication, and praise patient efforts to communicate. • Teach the family to speak directly and slowly to the patient, to give the patient plenty of time to respond, and to recommend alternative modes of communication to the family.	The patient can demonstrate improved communication of basic needs.

Problem	Interventions	Expected Outcome
Nutrition	• Assess the patient's ability to swallow the diet ordered, to identify food preferences, and to assess an understanding of how to safely swallow. • Use thickening agents, have the family bring in desired foods, plan meals for when the patient is rested, provide good oral care, and feed slowly. • Encourage the use of provided assistive devices, eating small frequent meals, using good oral hygiene, and reducing environmental distractions.	The patient's dietary intake will increase.
Skin Integrity	• Assess general condition of the skin, including turgor, injury, and capillary refill. Assess for breakdown on bony prominences. • Assess for the ability to move. • Start a turning schedule, place on a pressure relief mattress, maintain functional alignment, and pad bony areas. • Teach that an adequate diet and turning a minimum of every 2 hours decreases the risk for skin breakdown. • Emphasize reporting any suspected skin problems immediately.	The patient's skin integrity will be maintained.
Coping	• Assess the patient's current emotional status, available support mechanisms, and understanding of changes related to stroke. • Establish a caring relationship with the patient to assist with coping, encourage focusing on the positive, and facilitate the setting of realistic goals. • Provide education about stroke causes, encourage the sharing of feelings, emphasize patience with progress, recognize some level of depression may occur, discuss support groups, and discuss the benefit of stress management techniques.	The patient can make a positive effort to recognize and cope with current health reality.
Self-Care	• Assess the patient's ability to perform activities of daily living (ADLs), his or her willingness to assist, and the need for assistive devices. • Encourage the patient to provide self-care, collaborate to identify a time to perform ADLs, and assist in setting realistic goals. • Move all ADL items to the unaffected side if spatial neglect is present, and provide any necessary assistive devices. • Teach the patient to follow instructions given by the occupational therapist and to begin self-care when well rested. • Teach the family that being overly attentive can be a deterrent in regaining functionality. • Teach the patient and family that clothes that are one size larger or have Velcro closure will facilitate success.	The patient will make an effort to participate in self-care.

PUTTING IT ALL TOGETHER: APPLICATION OF THE NURSING PROCESS

Putting it all together is where the art and science of nursing meet to provide the best patient outcomes. We take the possibilities and place them in the context of the patient situation. To accomplish this, we use nursing diagnosis, nursing interventions, nursing outcomes, and nursing theory to provide the palate for nursing care.

STEP 4: ASSESSMENT

PATIENT INFORMATION: Joy Lewis, a 65-year-old female admitted for recurring syncope, etiology unknown

CHIEF COMPLAINT: Recurrent dizziness with loss of balance

HISTORY OF THE PRESENT ILLNESS: Brought to the emergency department (ED) by her husband, who stated that after eating dinner, his wife became very dizzy and was unable to stand without the risk of falling

PAST MEDICAL HISTORY: Hypertension, obesity

FAMILY HISTORY: Parents deceased in a car accident when the patient was 8 years old

CHART REVIEW AND REPORT: Joy Lewis was admitted from the ED with the diagnosis of syncope. The electrocardiogram (EKG) completed in ED was normal, and initial computed tomography (CT) scan was negative.

Her vital signs are BP of 126/82 mm Hg, an apical pulse of 98 beats per minute, respirations of 18 breaths per minute, and a temperature of 98.8°F. Admission laboratory results are as follows: PT 10.8 seconds; INR 0.9; aPTT 36 seconds; platelets 230 × 10^3/microL; glucose 106 mg/dL; red blood cell count (RBC) 4.5 × 10^6/microL; hemoglobin (HgB) 14.2 g/dL; hematocrit (Hct) 38.7%; white blood cell count (WBC) 8.6 × 10^3/microL; K$^+$ 4.1 mEq/L; CL$^-$ 103 mEq/L; NA$^+$ 138.6 mEq/L; and troponin 0.1 ng/mL. Joy's admitting orders are saline lock and Tylenol 650 mg as needed (prn) orally for mild pain. Joy told the physician that she will not take any other medications until after she has seen her tribal healer. Her husband supports this decision. The off-going nurse reports that Joy slept all night. Although told to call for assistance before going to the bathroom, she was seen an hour ago by the certified nurse assistant (CNA) while getting back into bed. When asked what she had been doing, Joy admitted that she had been up to the bathroom, but said she was not dizzy. Joy was reminded again of her fall risk and has agreed to call for help from now on. The assessment of all body systems was within normal limits.

SUBJECTIVE ASSESSMENT: You enter the room saying, *"Good morning! My name is Arvin James (AJ) and I will be your nurse today. How are you feeling?"* Joy's back is partially turned toward you, but the position looks awkward. You wonder if she heard you. As you walk to the other side of the bed you see that Joy's eyes are open and she appears to be panicked. You ask, *"Can you speak?"* Joy's tears are your only response.

OBJECTIVE ASSESSMENT: A quick 30-second focused assessment reveals that Joy has right-sided weakness with garbled slurred speech. The rapid response team (RRT) is called as the physician arrives for morning rounds. Current vital signs are BP of 156/98 mm Hg, a pulse of 106 beats per minute, respirations of 20 breaths per minute, and a temperature of 98.4°F. The RRT team arrives during the physician's examination and he calls a Code Stroke. In response, a stat (immediate) noncontrast CT of the head is ordered, and Joy is ordered to be transferred to critical care. Unfortunately, one of the critical care units is closed because of a biohazard spill. A bed will not be available until after that situation is resolved. A critical care nurse who is a member of the stroke team will stay to assist in caring for Joy during this emergent period.

Joy's last known normal neurological status was 1 hour ago when she was assisted to the bathroom. Neurologic deficits after examination include moderate right-sided weakness of arm and leg and garbled speech. Informed consent for administration has been obtained from Joy's husband.

After tPA infusion, AJ enters the room and asks the critical care nurse, *"How is she doing?"* "Time will tell, it's a good thing that you saw her first thing this morning otherwise she wouldn't be getting any tPA." *"Do you think it will work?"* AJ asks. "I hope so; I think we got to her in time so her chances are good." *"How soon will we see some reversal if it does work?"* "Sometimes we see changes pretty fast, other times it takes several hours; it just depends on the extent of the damage and size of the clot. Right now we will just have to wait and see." AJ moves closer to Joy and takes her hand; she clings to him, crying again. AJ attempts to comfort her saying, *"You are in good hands. I'll come in and check on you from time to time."* Joy responds with a lopsided smile, and AJ notes a right facial droop.

- *Laboratory Studies:*
  - PT: 10.5 seconds
  - INR: 0.8
  - aPTT: 35 seconds
  - Platelets: 220 × 10^3/microL
  - No significant change in hemogram, troponin, electrolytes, or blood glucose
- *Diagnostic Studies:*
  - Noncontrast CT scan of the brain reveals an ischemic large vessel stroke located in the right hemisphere
- *Medications:*
  - Physician orders immediate tPA screening with tPa infusion per clinical pharmacist recommendation at 0.9 mg/kg

STEP 5: REALITY CHECK: DETOUR AHEAD

Reality Check occurs when the nurse takes a moment to think about individualized patient information that needs to be considered in framing diagnoses and interventions. This information is retrievable from any legitimate source (e.g., family, case management, other nurses, any ancillary, a doctor, etc.). These are the "wrenches" that create challenging situations, such as culture, religion, socioeconomic status, level of education, developmental level, marital status, employment, age, and gender.

Psychosocial History

Joy Lewis is a Native American of the Navajo Tribe; she grew up on the reservation and speaks both Navajo and English. Joy was educated through the eighth grade, at which time she went to work in a local market to help support a family of five brothers and two sisters. Joy met her husband Eric at the market where she worked. Joy and Eric are the same age. Eric is a Native American of the Sioux tribe; they were married at the age of 18 and are childless. Both Joy and Eric have dedicated their lives to improving the education of the children who live on the reservation. Although Eric respects "Western" medicine, he wants the tribal healer to visit his wife. He has also asked that his wife's health not be discussed with her until after the healer has visited and given his opinion. They have no health-care insurance and live on a meager salary.

Critical Thinking Moment

You have just completed the assessment of Joy Lewis and need to make a decision about the patient's *actual* problems and nursing diagnoses based upon the data you have collected and the potential problems you identified. Outcomes must be realistic and measurable.

STEP 6: ACTUAL PROBLEMS/ DIAGNOSES

The *first step* in problem identification is to revisit the list of *potential diagnoses* and choose *actual diagnoses* based on the learner's evaluation of the case study information provided. A problem statement must be completed for each identified problem/diagnosis. The actual problems for this case study are mobility, communication, and coping.

STEP 7: PLANNING: ACTUAL INTERVENTIONS

After actual diagnoses have been chosen, it is necessary to evaluate the list of *potential interventions* and choose *actual interventions* that will fit within the patient's reality and meet expected outcomes. Each intervention requires a rationale. Interventions are identified in three categories: (1) assessment, (2) therapeutic, and (3) education.

Diagnostic Statement

Mobility related to neuromuscular impairment secondary to left hemisphere stroke as evidenced by moderate right-sided weakness of the arm and leg

Assessment

- Assess Joy's ability to move and change position. *Rationale: This provides a baseline evaluation.*
- Assess her fine and gross motor movement. *Rationale: This is the baseline evaluation of motor function change.*
- Assess her degree of weakness. *Rationale: This is the assessment of her self-care deficit.*

Therapeutic Interventions

- Her correct body alignment should be supported with pillows. *Rationale: This is done so that the patient does not lean to her weak side; make sure she is placed in safe positioning.*

- Ensure bed rest for the first 24 hours poststroke. *Rationale: This is a safety measure that puts less stress on the body system.*
- Elevate the head of her bed 30 degrees. *Rationale: This decreases cerebral edema and improves function.*

Education

- Teach Joy the technique for turning or moving using her stronger extremity. *Rationale: This is so Joy can safely move with activity and prevent injury.* Do not pull on the patient's arm to correct her position. *Rationale: Doing so could cause a potential injury to her shoulder.*
- Encourage Joy to do as much as possible for herself. *Rationale: This increases her control over movement.*

Expected Outcome

- Demonstrate an increased ability to manage mobility within functional limits

Diagnostic Statement

Communication related to aphasia secondary to ischemic stroke of left hemisphere as evidenced by garbled, slurred speech

Assessment

- Assess Joy's ability to speak without slurring her words. *Rationale: This assesses for the presence and degree of any communication deficits.*
- Assess Joy's ability to follow directions. *Rationale: This provides a baseline evaluation of cognitive function.*
- Assess Joy's ability to read, write, and name common objects. *Rationale: This provides a baseline evaluation of the presence of types of aphasic communication deficits.*

Therapeutic Interventions

- Use what works (yes, no, hand gestures, etc.). *Rationale: This facilitates communicative interaction.*
- Decrease distraction during communication. *Rationale: This better focuses Joy's efforts.*
- Praise her efforts to communicate. *Rationale: This helps prevent Joy from giving up.*

Education

- Have Joy's husband speak directly and slowly to her. *Rationale: This facilitates communication.*
- Have her husband give Joy plenty of time to respond. *Rationale: This supports her efforts and helps prevent her giving up.*
- Recommended alternative modes of communication to the family. *Rationale: This decreases frustration.*

Expected Outcome

- Joy will demonstrate improved communication.

Diagnostic Statement

Coping related to a sudden change in health status secondary to neurological deficits as associated with stroke and as evidenced by crying

Assessment

- Assess Joy's current emotional status. *Rationale: This provides a baseline to develop a plan of care.*
- Assess Joy's available support mechanisms. *Rationale: This helps to identify support and potential areas of need.*
- Assess Joy's and her family's understanding of changes related to stroke. *Rationale: Understanding may assist with coping.*

Therapeutic Interventions

- Establish a relationship with the patient. *Rationale: An ongoing relationship can establish trust, which may assist in coping.*
- Encourage Joy to focus on the positive, building on strengths and successes rather than negatives. *Rationale: This can assist in coping.*
- Facilitate the patient's setting of realistic goals. *Rationale: This can help Joy move in a positive direction and decrease feelings of helplessness.*

Education

- Provide education about stroke causes. *Rationale: Understanding may increase coping.*
- Allow Joy to convey her feelings. *Rationale: Verbalization may assist emotional stability.*
- Patience will be necessary in the rehabilitation period. *Rationale: This will allow the prevention of frustration and depression with the understanding that recovery will take time.*

Expected Outcome

- The patient will make a positive effort to recognize and cope with her current health reality.

STEP 8: IMPLEMENTATION

Nursing Theory

Dorothea Orem's theory focuses on the assessment of self-care and self-care deficits. Self-care is described as what the patient can do for herself or himself. Orem assumes that patients want to care for themselves if they are able to. A self-care deficit occurs when the patient is not able to meet his or her own needs and nursing intervention is required. In the case of Joy Lewis, the nurse will need to ask what kind of help is required. Does Joy require total assistance, partial assistance, or is she independent? Then the nurse will develop a plan based on the assessment findings.

Because Joy and Eric come from an American Indian cultural base with which they completely identify,

the approach to care will need to be a blend of their cultural perspective with the identified plan to achieve the expected outcomes. If Joy does not agree to the plan because it is not culturally congruent, it will not be successful. Imposing a cultural view on Joy and her husband will cause frustration. In this case, it will be necessary to accommodate Eric's desire to have their tribal healer see his wife.

Ancillary Support

Dietary consult may be needed to ensure that Joy is receiving foods that she will eat or to make recommendations for nutritional support if she is at risk for aspiration. Social services may be assistive in helping Joy cope with her altered health status as well as act as an advocate for addressing financial concerns in collaboration with case management. Pastoral care can provide spiritual support during a stressful time, and a chaplain or pastoral nurse can act as a conduit in facilitating a visit from the tribal healer and spiritual guide. The physical therapist can assist in providing an evaluation of Joy's current mobility status and develop a plan for activity when it is appropriate to do so. Occupational and speech therapy can help Joy identify her strengths and weaknesses by evaluating her ability to perform fine and gross motor skills and assessing her ability to swallow.

STEP 9: PLAN OF CARE

The plan of care is a road map for patient care and should be used as a communication tool between disciplines. Expected entries on the plan of care would be each identified problem (e.g., mobility, communication, and coping) with corresponding interventions and expected outcomes. Additionally, there should be some information regarding the cultural aspects of Joy's care with contact information for the tribal healer.

STEP 10: EVALUATION

Evaluation is an active process in which the nurse "connects the dots" to decide if the expected outcomes (goals) that were established have been met, partially met, or not met. If the goals are met, we continue with the plan as outlined. If the goal was partially met, we revise the parts of the plan that did not work. If the goals were not met, we start all over with a new plan.

End-of-Shift Narrative

Toward the end of the shift, AJ returns to Joy's room to see how she is doing and get an update from the critical care nurse. AJ asks, *"Is the tPA working?"* The critical care nurse replies, "Yes; her speech has cleared some, and she is beginning to move her right side. Joy is still very upset and asking for her healer, and the social worker is making special arrangements for the healer to visit. Her husband Eric said the healer will leave the reservation and visit later today; he is bringing her a medicine bag. Both she and her husband believe that this visit may cure her. They are a little late but should be here soon. She's not worried about it. "AJ looks concerned and comments to the critical care nurse, *"Joy still seems pretty upset. When I walked in she started to cry again."* "Yes," the critical care nurse replies, "she keeps doing that, I think when the healer comes she will be less tearful." AJ asks, *"Is she worried about anything else?"* The critical care nurse replies, "According to her husband she is worried about money. I think they both are. The case manager is seeing what resources are available to them." AJ asks, *"May I speak to her?"* "Of course," the critical care nurse replies. Joy's husband Eric arrives as AJ enters the room. Upon seeing AJ, Eric offers his hand in a light handshake saying, "Thank you for helping my wife. The doctor said it was because you saw Joy was in trouble that we have a chance to help her." *"You are very welcome,"* AJ responds. Joy grins with an almost symmetrical smile and with less garbled speech says, "Thank you." You also note increased mobility of the right hand and arm. After leaving the room, the critical care nurse tells AJ that the next day they will have a better idea of how far her deficits will reverse. The neurologist has ordered physical therapy, occupational therapy, speech therapy, and a swallow evaluation.

Problem Evaluation

PROBLEM 1: Mobility. The expected outcome is that Joy will demonstrate an increased ability to move her right hand and arm. The goal is met, although assessment shows some resolution mobility deficits.

PROBLEM 2: Communication. The expected outcome is that Joy will demonstrate improved communication. The goal is met, although Joy is in the emergent first 24 hours. Some of her language skills have improved, and her speech is less garbled and more understandable. There is the possibility that there will be further improvement.

PROBLEM 3: Coping. The expected outcome is that Joy will make a positive effort to cope with her current health reality. The goal is partially met: Joy's neurological status is improving; however, she is still very tearful. Revised plan: Facilitate the visit of her tribal healer and allow him to give her a medicine bag that she believes will help her to improve.

Overall Evaluation

Based on the end-of-shift assessment and comparison of Joy's progress during this shift, Joy is found to be improving.

REFERENCES

Baldwin, K. (2006, March/April). Stroke is a knockout punch. Nursing Made Incredibly Easy, 4 (2), 10–23.

George, J. (2011). Nursing theories. The base for professional nursing practice (6th ed.). Upper Saddle River, NJ: Pearson Education.

Gulanick, M., & Meyers J. (2013). Nursing care plans nursing diagnosis and intervention (8th ed.). St Louis, MO: Mosby.

Harvey, J. (2007, Fall). Countering brain attack. ED Insider. 37, 7–10.

Holloway, N. (2004). Medical surgical nursing care planning (4th ed.). Springhouse, PA: Lippincott Williams & Wilkins.

LeMone, P., & Burke, K. (1996). Medical surgical nursing: Critical thinking in client care. Menlo Park, CA: Benjamin Cummings.

Miller, J. (2005). Call a stroke code. Nursing 2005, 35(3), 58–63.

Miller, J. (2009, May). Acute ischemic stroke: Not a moment to lose. Nursing 2009. 39(5), 36–42.

Parker, M. (2006). Nursing theories and nursing practice (2nd ed.). Philadelphia, PA: FA Davis.

Quinn, C. (2006, July). Quick my patient is having an ischemic stroke. Nursing 2006. 36(7), 56cc1–56cc4.

Rodgers, S. (2008). Medical surgical nursing care plans. Clifton Park, NY: Thomson Delmar.

Swearingen, P. (2008). All in one care planning resource (2nd ed.). St Louis, MO: Mosby.

Taft, K.A. (2009, July/August). Raising awareness of hemorrhagic stroke. 7(4), 42–52.

Tinnitus, Tests and diagnosis. Retrieved from http://www.mayoclinic.org/diseases-conditions/tinnitus/basics/tests-diagnosis/con-20021487

Van Leeuwen, A., & Bladh, M. (2015). Davis's comprehensive handbook of laboratory and diagnostic testing with nursing implications (6th ed.). Philadelphia, PA: F.A. Davis Company.

Wilkinson, J., & Ahern, N. (2009). In Nursing diagnosis handbook (9th ed.). Upper Saddle River, NJ: Prentice Hall.

Wilson, B., Shannon, M., & Stang, C. (2006). Nurses drug guide. Upper Saddle River, NJ: Prentice Hall.

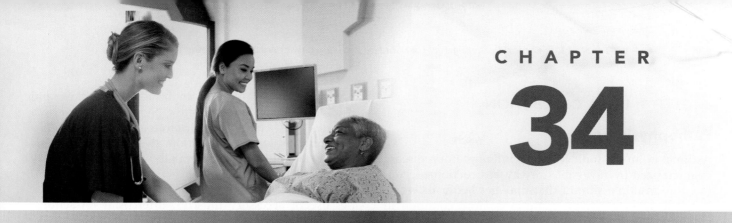

Respiratory System

Case Study: Asthma

Common Nursing Study Name	Section 1 Study	Section 1 Chapter Number
Allergen-Specific IgE	Allergen-Specific Immunoglobulin E	Chapter 5
Arterial Blood Gas (ABG)	Blood Gases	Chapter 14
Chest X-Ray	Chest X-Ray	Chapter 16
Complete Blood Count (CBC) and Differential	Complete Blood Count, Hematocrit Complete Blood Count, Hemoglobin Complete Blood Count, Platelet Count Complete Blood Count, RBC Count Complete Blood Count, RBC Indices Complete Blood Count, RBC Morphology and Inclusions Complete Blood Count, WBC Count and Differential	Chapter 2 Chapter 2 Chapter 3 Chapter 2 Chapter 2 Chapter 2 Chapter 2
Electrolytes	Chloride, Blood Carbon Dioxide Potassium, Blood Sodium, Blood	Chapter 1 Chapter 1 Chapter 1 Chapter 1
IgE Levels (Nonspecific)	Immunoglobulin E	Chapter 5
Nasal Cytology (included in Allergen-Specific IgE)	Allergen-Specific Immunoglobulin E	Chapter 5
Pulmonary Function Tests	Pulmonary Function Studies	Chapter 14
Oxygen Saturation (Pulse Oximetry)	Pulse Oximetry	Chapter 14
Radioallergosorbent (RAST) or ImmunoCAP® (part of Allergen-Specific IgE) Testing	Allergen-Specific Immunoglobulin E	Chapter 5
Sputum Culture	Culture, Bacterial, Sputum	Chapter 6

STEP 1: DATA COLLECTION

Pathophysiology

Asthma is an episodic chronic inflammatory disease characterized by reversible airway obstruction precipitated by multiple stimuli that may get better or worse but will never go away. Asthma is more common in children, with half of asthmatics under the age of 10. Asthmatics can have long periods free of symptoms until an exaggerated airway response is triggered, leading to compromised ventilation and possibly death. The degree of responsive hyperactivity is dependent on the amount of inflammation.

An asthmatic episode begins like this. Trigger(s) create a cyclical acute inflammatory response in the mast cells lining the airways. Mast cells release histamine and other inflammatory agents. Mediators cause circulating inflammatory cells to travel to the lungs. Once in the lungs bronchospasm occurs from increased airway responsiveness. Stimulation of the vagus nerve and beta-adrenergic reception airways facilitate ongoing bronchospasm. Continued mast cell stimulation and continued release of leukotrienes and bradykinins create a vicious cycle leading to further bronchospasm and inflammation. This results in impaired gas exchange as hypersecretion leads to increased mucous production narrowing and constricting the airways. If the cycle is not broken by therapeutic interventions, status asthmaticus can occur.

Status asthmaticus is a severe form of asthma characterized by increased mucous production where airways narrow from bronchial smooth muscle spasms. Ongoing spasms create a cascade event with an increase in eosinophils, neutrophils, and macrophages, ending in more inflammation, more airway obstruction, and possibly death.

Asthma can be classified as intrinsic or extrinsic. Intrinsic asthma can be triggered by cold air, emotional upset, bronchial irritant, respiratory infections, exercise, beta blockers, NSAIDs (including aspirin), sulfites used as a food preservative, and emotional stress. Extrinsic asthma is triggered by environmental allergens including pollen, animal dander, dust, tobacco smoke, irritating gases, noxious fumes, and chemicals. Asthma can be triggered by a combination of intrinsic and extrinsic factors. Diagnosis is based on evaluation of airway hyperreactivity, recurrence, and reversibility. An individual who has respiratory symptoms associated with a trigger, and has repeated episodes of this event that improve with specific treatment has asthma.

Signs and Symptoms

Asthmatic triggers can cause symptoms within minutes or hours. Frequency and severity of asthma attacks vary from one individual to another. Attacks can fluctuate from mild to continuous, with episodic life-threatening exacerbations. Symptoms can be abrupt or slow and insidious, lasting hours or days. Symptoms of asthma include chest tightness, inspiratory and expiratory wheezing, prolonged expiration, dyspnea, tachycardia, tachypnea, and cough, especially at night and early mornings.

Symptoms of worsening asthma include nasal flaring, use of accessory muscles, intercostal retractions, and audible wheezing. Some may complain about having a "tight airway" or fatigue, anxiety, and apprehension. Severe dyspnea may prevent speech of more than one or two words at a time. Prolonged asthma that does not respond to treatment can result in respiratory failure, hypoxia, hypercapnia, and acidosis. Correction may require intubation, mechanical ventilation, and aggressive pharmacological support. Respiratory failure is marked by inaudible breath sounds, reduced wheezing, and ineffective cough. A silent chest is a severe obstruction indicating very little air movement. This is an emergency situation and can result in death in a very short amount of time.

When considering a diagnosis of asthma, ask these questions: are there occasional episodes of airflow obstruction or hyper-responsiveness, is the airflow obstruction somewhat reversible, and have other potential diagnosis have been excluded? Asthmatics 5 years and older can be classified based on severity of daytime and nighttime symptoms prior to treatment. Classifications are intermittent, mild-persistent, moderate-persistent, or severe-persistent.

Intermittent asthmatics have symptoms twice a week or less, nighttime symptoms twice a month or less, and an absence of interference with normal activity. Treatment consists of using a short acting beta2-agonist inhaler twice a week or less for symptom control.

Mild Persistent Asthma

Mild persistent asthmatics have daytime symptoms more than twice a week, but less than daily. Nighttime symptoms occur three to four times a month, and there is some minor limitation of normal activities. Treatment consists of a low dose of inhaled corticosteroid. Frequency of using a short-acting beta2-agonist increases to more than twice a week. Leukotriene receptor antagonist, cromolyn, nedocromil, or theophylline may be considered. Immunotherapy should be considered if there is the presence of allergic asthma.

Moderate Persistent Asthma

Moderate persistent asthmatics have daily daytime symptoms, with nighttime symptoms occurring more than weekly, but not nightly. Limitation of daily activities is increased. A short-acting beta2-agonist is being used daily. Treatment consists of a low-to-medium inhaled corticosteroid and a daily long-acting beta2-agonist. Leukotriene receptor antagonist, cromolyn, nedocromil, or theophylline may be considered along with oral corticosteroids. Consultation with an asthma specialist is recommended. Immunotherapy should be considered if there is the presence of allergic asthma.

Severe Persistent Asthma

Severe persistent asthmatics have continual daytime symptoms and frequent nighttime symptoms. Short-acting beta2-agonist is being used several times a day. Activity is extremely limited, and symptom control is difficult. High-dose inhaled corticosteroids may be used in combination with long-acting beta2-agonist. Oral systemic corticosteroids, leukotriene receptor antagonist, and theophylline may be considered. Consultation with an asthma specialist is recommended.

Laboratory Studies

Laboratory studies focus on assessing the oxygenation status and checking for an allergen trigger and inflammation. Arterial blood gas (ABG) can evaluate blood pH, oxygenation, and carbon dioxide levels. Initial ABG results may show a low pO_2 from tachypnea, hypoxemia, and an elevated pH with respiratory alkalosis. Increasingly compromised ventilation results in significant hypoxia. Respiratory acidosis can occur with a pCO_2 greater than 42 mm Hg, and a pH of less than 7.35, indicating a need for mechanical ventilation.

Allergic triggers can be assessed using a complete blood count (CBC) and differential, allergen-specific IgE, and nonspecific IgE levels. The white blood count (WBC) may be elevated greater than 12×10^3/microL due to the inflammation. Neutrophil levels may also be elevated and correlate with the severity of the asthma. An absolute eosinophil count greater than 500 cells/mm^3 or greater than 4% of the WBC differential, and nonspecific IgE greater than 150 International Units/L is suggestive but not diagnostic of asthma related to an allergic response. To identify which allergen may be causing the allergic response, **radioallergosorbent (RAST)** or **ImmunoCAP®** testing may be necessary. These methods are used as an alternative to pinprick skin testing to discover which allergens are causing the allergic reaction that is triggering asthma. Nasal cytology assesses checks for airway hyperresponsiveness by checking increased nasal eosinophils, WBCs, and sputum mast cells. Sputum culture and sensitivity may show the presence of bacteria; bacterial infection can be an issue in cases of severe asthma.

Diagnostic Studies

Diagnostic studies can evaluate the effects of asthmatic triggers. Chest x-ray may be ordered to assess for hyperinflation found during exacerbation. Electrocardiogram may show signs of arrhythmia including tachycardia and supraventricular tachycardia.

Pulmonary function tests can evaluate the degree of airway obstruction and the effectiveness of therapies used to reverse the obstruction. Residual volume may be found to be increased and vital capacity decreased or normal in the presence of remission. Forced expiratory volume and peak expiratory flow rate are more sensitive indicators of the severity of the asthmatic event and effectiveness of interventions. Identifying a baseline peak flow provides a point for comparison that can be used in evaluating ongoing respiratory status.

Pulse oximetry is a noninvasive measurement of oxygen saturation. Normal results are greater than 95%; results for asthmatics may be less than 93%.

General/Medical Management

Management of asthma focuses on prevention and the early intervention of asthmatic events.

Prevention

Prevention is all about avoiding allergens and environmental triggers. Home modification focuses on controlling dust by removing carpets, covering mattresses and pillows, removing pets, and installing air filtration systems. Personal choices can decrease exposure to triggers such as covering the mouth and nose with a scarf to warm the air by adding humidification during breathing on cold days. Staying away from dander; not smoking; avoiding second-hand smoke, wood smoke, and strong odors such as perfume; and avoiding odors from paints may prevent an attack. Staying indoors on high pollen days, closing windows, and using air conditioning to avoid extreme heat can help.

Prevention also includes the ability to recognize worsening symptoms, as treatment will be stepped up or down based on the severity of symptoms as needed. It is important to understand the purpose and action of each medication as well as which inhaler is for daily use and which is for emergency use.

Emotional control is necessary to prevent triggering an asthmatic attack. Panic will only worsen the situation. Learning cognitive behavior techniques may assist in emotional control.

Oxygen Therapy

Asthma may require hospitalization. Once this occurs, treatment focuses on oxygen therapy, medication administration, and consideration of the necessity of intubation and mechanical ventilation. Oxygen therapy's goal is to maintain saturation between 90% and 95%. Use of a high-flow oxygen device such as a partial or complete nonrebreather mask may be necessary. Unsuccessful attempts to support oxygenation by noninvasive means may require intubation and mechanical ventilation. Indicators for ventilator use include increased pulsus paradoxus (exaggerated normal inspiratory decrease in systolic blood pressure), exhaustion, decreased mental status, worsening ABG values, lactic acidosis, and hypoxemia.

Nurses will need to be vigilant in monitoring oxygenation, cardiac status, and medication effectiveness. Feeling unable to breathe is terrifying. Asthmatics will need reassurance to stay calm. Presenting a calm, supportive exterior with the use of relaxation techniques and imagery, and inclusion of pursed lip breathing can be of assistance in controlling asthma.

Remember, the overarching goal of asthma management is to maintain normal pulmonary function, prevent or reduce exacerbation, identify and reduce exposure to triggers, maintain normal activity, relieve acute episodes, provide appropriate patient education, and improve quality of life. Treatment will be stepped up or down depending on symptoms and the effectiveness of treatment.

Medications

Pharmacological interventions emphasize preventing obstruction and treating acute episodes. Medications are used for long-term control, or for quick relief in emergency situations. Long-term medication therapy focuses on controlling persistent airway inflammation rather than intervening in acute episodes. Medications choices include inhaled steroids, inhaled cromolyn and nedocromil, oral leukotriene modifiers, oral or inhaled long-acting beta2-agonists, and oral or IV theophylline.

The treatment for each stage of asthma is step based, moving from lower dosages and few medications, to higher dosages and more medications. Moving up or down a step in treatment depends on the effectiveness of therapeutic interventions and presenting symptoms. The goal is to control the asthma and prevent exacerbation.

STEROIDS: Steroids can be administered in inhaled, oral, or IV form. Inhaled corticosteroids are considered to be most effective for long-term control of asthma by reducing bronchial hyperresponsiveness and decreasing airway swelling without the systemic absorption that can lead to side effects. Severe attacks may require oral or IV steroids to alleviate symptoms. The most commonly used inhaled long-term steroids include beclomethasone, fluticasone, budesonide, flunisolide, and triamcinolone. Long-term use of steroids can cause side effects such as growth suppression, osteoporosis, elevated cholesterol, cataracts, diabetes, muscle weakness, and thin skin. Short-term side effects of steroid use include increased appetite, fluid retention, mood alteration, and weight gain.

Steroids such as prednisone and methylprednisolone can be administered orally or intravenously to decrease airway swelling. A short course of oral steroids used in combination with short-acting beta2-agonists can be useful for those who experience moderate to severe asthma. The rule of thumb is that if an individual is using a rescue inhaler more than twice a week, the physician should be contacted to adjust the medications.

INHALED CROMOLYN: Inhaled cromolyn acts as a mast cell stabilizer to prevent airway swelling. Cromolyn can lessen the number and severity of asthma attacks but cannot prevent an attack from occurring. Leukotriene modifiers also prevent airway swelling by attacking leukotrienes and are especially helpful in preventing a flare up from exercise or cat dander.

LONG-ACTING BETA2-AGONISTS: Long-acting beta2-agonists open the airway so that more air can get out. Oral and inhaled beta2-agonists include salmeterol, albuterol, and formoterol. Side effects of beta2-agonists are nervousness, tremors, anxiety, headache, nausea, tachycardia, and dizziness. An effective treatment combination for moderate to severe asthma is use of inhaled corticosteroids with beta-agonists.

THEOPHYLLINE: Theophylline is given to inhibit the inflammatory response and relax smooth muscles around the airways but is rarely used and is considered to be more of a last-ditch choice. However, if theophylline is included as a treatment modality, drug levels should be attained to prevent overdose or inadequate therapeutic levels. Therapeutic levels would be a serum concentration between 5 and 20 mcg/mL, and toxicity occurs with levels greater than 25 mcg/mL. When theophylline is used, consideration should be given to potential interactions with other medications.

QUICK-RELIEF MEDICATIONS: Quick-relief medications are used to intervene in the event of an asthma attack. Asthmatics should keep a rescue inhaler with them at all times. Quick-relief medications work within approximately 3 minutes by stimulating smooth muscle relaxation and bronchodilation, which allows more air to get out. Suggested beta2 rescue inhalers are albuterol, pirbuterol, and levalbuterol. Inhaled anticholinergics such as ipratropium can also open the airway so that more air can get out. Ipratropium provides acts as a bronchodilator and can be used in combination with short-acting beta2-agonists to manage acute exacerbation.

Patient Education

Imagine that you are not able to breathe. There are so many variables that can feed into the asthmatic event that tailoring your education to meet each clinical situation can be a challenge. Talk to your patient, talk to their family. Try to assist them to identify the events that occurred before their asthma flare. Once those triggers have been verbalized, then you can focus your education on what is most important to them. For asthmatics, education needs to be as individualized as their therapeutic interventions for positive outcomes.

STEP 2: POTENTIAL PROBLEMS/ DIAGNOSES

It is important that nurses understand and consider the science of the disease process and consider the possibilities prior to applying that knowledge to a patient situation. We begin that process with questioning.

💬 *Question:* Based on your review of the content about asthma, what *possible problems* would you expect for a patient with this diagnosis?

💬 *Answer:* Breathing, gas exchange, airway clearance, anxiety, fatigue, and family coping

STEP 3: POTENTIAL INTERVENTIONS AND EXPECTED OUTCOMES

💬 *Question:* Based on your identification of patient problems, what possible interventions would you recommend for these diagnoses, and what would you expect to happen? This would be considered your "grocery list" of the possible actions you could use to assist your patient.

💬 *Answer:* See the following problems, interventions, and expected outcomes:

Problem	Interventions	Expected Outcomes
Airway Clearance	• Administer albuterol and corticoid steroids as ordered. • Encourage cough and deep breathing every 2 hours and position in high Fowler position. • Encourage oral fluids and consider insensible water loss.	• Decreased work of breathing • Diminished nasal flaring • Decreased retractions • Slower respiratory rate
Fatigue	• Assess work of breathing every 4 hours and as needed. • Monitor for hypoxia characterized by restlessness, fatigue, irritability, dyspnea, tachycardia, or change in level of consciousness. • Provide a calm, quiet atmosphere and calming support.	• Less fatigue, irritability, and restlessness with improved sleeping pattern • Ability to perform activities of daily living (ADLs)
Anxiety	• Explain all procedures and the purpose of equipment. • Provide a calm restful environment; the presence of family is calming. • Suggest using comforting objects from home. • Use imagery and relaxation techniques. • Consider the use of music.	Decreased anxiety
Gas Exchange	• Monitor oxygen saturation. • Assess lung sounds; assess respiratory rate, depth, work of breathing; assess sputum production. • Monitor mental status, restlessness, confusion and level of consciousness. • Monitor for cyanosis, electrolyte levels, and ABG results. • Administer medications to open airway and improve ventilation as ordered.	Improved respiratory effort
Breathing	• Assess respiratory rate, pattern, and breath sounds. • Assess for symptoms of altered breathing pattern such as shallow respirations, nasal flaring, retractions of the intercostal muscles, and diminished or absent breath sounds. • Monitor vital signs and lab reports. • Assist with ADLs and pace activities with inclusion of rest periods. • Assist in controlling breathing by use of pursed lip breathing, abdominal breathing, and relaxation techniques including visualization. • Administer medications as ordered.	Patient will have an uncompromised breathing pattern
Family Coping	• Assess emotional lability, level of interference, level of support and readiness to learn. • Facilitate chaplain and social services to visit family member(s). • Minimize the disruption of care. • Provide education. • Review the plan of care. • Listen to family.	Family/caregiver will cooperate and collaborate with staff in provision of care

PUTTING IT ALL TOGETHER: APPLICATION OF THE NURSING PROCESS

Putting it all together is where the art and science of nursing meet to provide the best patient outcomes. We take the possibilities and place them into the context of the patient situation. To accomplish this, we use nursing diagnosis, nursing interventions, nursing outcomes, and nursing theory to provide the palate for nursing care.

STEP 4: ASSESSMENT

PATIENT INFORMATION: 10-year-old Jesus Taki

CHIEF COMPLAINT: Chest tightness and difficulty breathing

HISTORY OF THE PRESENT ILLNESS: Jesus was running in the playground at school and started having trouble breathing. Budesonide and albuterol sulfate inhalers were used without relief. He was brought to the emergency department (ED) by ambulance for respiratory distress.

PAST MEDICAL HISTORY: Jesus was diagnosed with mild persistent asthma at the age of 6.

FAMILY HISTORY: Father is of Japanese descent and has mild hypertension. Mother was Hispanic and is deceased from ovarian cancer last year.

CHART REVIEW AND REPORT: Jesus arrived in the ED in asthma exacerbation. He was treated with continuous albuterol free flow for an hour followed by five additional hourly treatments, two of which were administered in the ED and the other three on the pediatric unit. While receiving the last hourly treatment, Jesus' grandmother, Petra Gonzales, became very upset and vocal, telling the respiratory therapist to leave Jesus alone so that he could sleep. Petra would not listen to any explanation regarding the necessity of the treatments. Eventually, the pediatric hospitalist had to explain why the treatments were needed. Petra has become more cooperative but continues to question everything and writes down the answers along with the individual's name. Jesus was placed on 6 L of oxygen by mask to improve his oxygenation with a saturation of 94%. ABG results were pH 7.29, pCO$_2$ 47 mm Hg, and Petra has refused any repeat ABGs. Petra keeps removing the oxygen mask when Jesus complains that it is bothering him with a resulting desaturation to 88%. The respiratory therapist has changed the oxygen to 4 L via nasal cannula to keep Jesus more comfortable, with a resulting oxygen saturation of 92%. Petra has been more cooperative in leaving the oxygen on since the delivery device was changed.

Jesus has an occasional nonproductive cough with tight diminished breath sounds and slight wheezing on the last assessment. Dexamethasone 11 mg IV push was given in the ED as a onetime dose. The last set of vital signs was pulse 128 beats per minute, respiratory rate 28 breaths per minute, temperature 99.6°F, and BP of 118/72 mm Hg. Accessory muscles are being used to support ventilation, with mild intercostal retractions and nasal flaring. Jesus has been sitting in the Fowler position, with pillows behind his back for comfort. Chest x-ray shows lung hyperinflation. CBC shows increased eosinophils at 6% of the WBC differential, with a total WBC of 17.8 × 10^3/microL, IV fluids are infusing, D5/1/2 normal saline at 80 mL/hr.

SUBJECTIVE ASSESSMENT: As you enter the room you see that Jesus is sleeping. You introduce yourself to Petra who is reading at the bedside and say, *"Good morning! My name is Arvin James (AJ). I will be his nurse today."* Petra interrupts, "Don't wake him up. Those idiots kept him up all night. He just went to sleep." You continue, *"I will do my best but it is important that I check him to make sure he is breathing all right."* Petra rolls her eyes and comments, "You all say the same thing. I told my son-in-law he should go home with me, but he wouldn't listen. The only reason we are still here is because I promised him I wouldn't take him out." You can tell by Petra's body language and tone of voice that she is defensive. You say, *"I understand the hospitalist spoke to you last night about the treatment plan."* Petra responds, "Bah! What does he know—he looks like he's 18 years old." You offer, *"I can ask the doctor to come back if you wish, but I do need to see how he is doing."* Grudgingly, Petra agrees and says, "OK, but be quick and try not to wake him up."

OBJECTIVE ASSESSMENT: Jesus appears to be slightly pale and fatigued with a slight audible wheeze; his skin is slightly cool to the touch. On auscultation breath sounds are coarse with inspiratory and expiratory wheezing, with improved air movement. An IV of D5/1/2 normal saline is infusing at 80 mL/hr. Oxygen of 4 L by nasal cannula is in place with a saturation of 92% at rest. The head of the bed remains in Fowler position, with two pillows behind his back for comfort. Jesus has no noticeable nasal flaring or use of accessory muscles but still has some mild intercostal retractions. Respiratory rate is 24 breaths per minute, pulse is 98 beats per minute, and BP is 106/70 mm Hg. Petra refuses to allow a temperature. As you complete your assessment, Jesus wakes up anxious and crying. Petra glares at you saying, "See what you've done, you woke him up! I want you to leave now and don't come back." Once awake you notice that Jesus has a weak, nonproductive, ineffective cough. It is difficult to gauge cognitive status because Petra is very upset and pushing you out of the room. You leave the room and decide to contact the chaplain and social services for assistance in meeting Petra's emotional needs, while supporting the treatment plan. The most current laboratory values are WBC 13.6×10^3/microL with decreasing eosinophils. Jesus is on albuterol free flow treatment 2.5 mg hourly adjusted per protocol, and Solu-Medrol 40 mg IV push every 6 hours. Jesus has a teddy bear given to him by his mother that provides him with comfort.

STEP 5: REALITY CHECK: DETOUR AHEAD

Reality Check occurs when the nurse takes a moment to think about individualized patient information that needs to be considered in framing diagnoses and interventions. This information is retrievable from any legitimate source (e.g., family, case management, other nurses, any ancillary, a doctor, etc.). These are the "wrenches" that create challenging situations, such as culture, religion, socioeconomic status, level of education, developmental level, marital status, employment, age, and gender.

Psychosocial History

Petra is Jesus' maternal grandmother and primary caregiver while his father is absent. Jesus' father, Mori, is currently in Japan, and Jesus' mother died last year from stage IV ovarian cancer. Since her daughter's death, Petra has assumed the mothering role and has been empowered to make health-care decisions in Mori's absence. Petra is very much into folk medicine and does not trust doctors or "modern medicine." She blames the death of her daughter on the failure of the health-care system. Mori is a highly paid executive with Sony and is frequently out of the country. Mori is Buddhist, and Petra is Catholic, which often causes conflict in the family. Jesus is being raised as a Catholic against his father's wishes.

⏺ Critical Thinking Moment

You have just completed the assessment on Jesus Taki and need to make a decision on the patient's *actual* problems and nursing diagnoses based on the data you have collected and the potential problems you identified. Outcomes must be realistic and measurable.

STEP 6: ACTUAL PROBLEMS/DIAGNOSES

The *first step* in problem identification is to revisit the list of *potential diagnoses* and choose *actual diagnoses* based on the learner's evaluation of the case study information provided. A problem statement must be

completed for each identified problem/diagnosis. The actual problems for this case study are airway, breathing, and family coping.

STEP 7: PLANNING: ACTUAL INTERVENTIONS

After actual diagnoses have been chosen, it is necessary to evaluate the list of *potential interventions* and choose *actual interventions* that will fit within the patient's reality and meet expected outcomes. Each intervention requires a rationale. Interventions are identified in three categories: (1) assessment, (2) therapeutic, and (3) education.

Diagnostic Statement

Ineffective airway clearance related to bronchospasm and bronchoconstriction as evidenced by intercostal retraction, a respiratory rate of 24 breaths per minute, diminished breath sounds, and wheezing.

Assessment

- Assess Jesus' adequacy of respirations every 1 to 2 hours; rate, depth, chest movement, and breath sounds. *Rationale: The respiratory status can change quickly, so vigilant assessment is required.*
- Assess Jesus' cough effort, sputum color, consistency, and amount. *Rationale: An ineffective cough with diminished sputum production can indicate oncoming respiratory failure.*
- Assess Jesus' skin color, temperature, and cognitive status. *Rationale: This allows you to evaluate for hypoxia.*

Therapeutic Interventions

- Position Jesus in the Fowler position. *Rationale: This promotes lung expansion and facilitates breathing.*
- Administer oxygen 4 L via nasal cannula. *Rationale: This reduces hypoxia and decreases anxiety.*
- Administer hourly nebulized albuterol. *Rationale: Doing so opens airways, loosens secretions, and promotes ventilation.*

Education

- Explain how to evaluate the work of breathing. *Rationale: Understanding may facilitate cooperation.*
- Explain oxygen use as a form of medication. *Rationale: This may elicit cooperation in maintaining oxygen therapy.*
- Explain albuterol use to help open airways and decrease work of breathing. *Rationale: This facilitates cooperation in the treatment plan.*

Expected Outcome

- Jesus will breathe more easily as evidenced by decreased respiratory rate and retractions, and improved breath sounds; Petra will be on board with therapeutic interventions.

Diagnostic Statement

Ineffective breathing related to altered lung ventilation and expansion and emptying as evidenced by a rapid respiratory rate and anxiety.

Assessment

- Assess Jesus' respiratory rate, pattern, breath sounds, shallow respirations, nasal flaring, intercostal retractions, and diminished or absent breath sounds. *Rationale: This allows for the early identification and initiation of appropriate interventions.*
- Assess Jesus' vital signs and oxygenation. *Rationale: Elevated blood pressure, an increased respiratory rate and pulse, and hypoxia are signs of compromised respiratory status.*
- Monitor Petra's attitude toward interventions. *Rationale: Petra may need the assistance of social services.*

Therapeutic Interventions

- Administer albuterol breathing treatments. *Rationale: This opens airways.*
- Administer Solu-Medrol IV push as ordered. *Rationale: This step decreases inflammation.*
- Demonstrate pursed lip breathing. *Rationale: This is a way to help keep airways open.*

Education

- Teach use of pursed lip breathing. *Rationale: This is a way to keep airways open and have some control over therapy.*
- Review the medications and their purpose. *Rationale: The patient's buy-in will improve adherence to the treatment regimen.*
- Discuss environmental changes. *Rationale: This helps to avoid allergens and prevent future flare-ups.*

Expected Outcome

- Jesus' work of breathing will be less with decreasing retractions, nasal flare, and the use of accessory muscles.

Diagnostic Statement

Ineffective family coping related to Petra's overprotectiveness and disruption of care as evidenced by interference with therapeutic interventions and negative statements.

Assessment

- Assess Petra's emotional lability. *Rationale: This establishes a baseline for appropriate conversation.*
- Assess Petra's level of interference with necessary therapeutic activities. *Rationale: This helps you determine the patient's willingness to adhere to the plan of care.*
- Assess Petra's interaction with Jesus. *Rationale: This helps to determine if she is supportive of care or not.*

Therapeutic Interventions

- Arrange a chaplain visit. *Rationale: This will allow for a discussion of concerns with a nonclinical person.*
- Arrange a social services visit. *Rationale: This will assist the patient in meeting challenges and in identifying support groups within the community that are culturally congruent.*
- Minimize the disruption of care. *Rationale: This provides the best care for the patient.*

Education

- Review the purpose of the plan of care. *Rationale: She loves her grandson and is more likely to be cooperative if she understands the plan.*
- Provide information about asthma and preventative measures. *Rationale: This helps to better prepare Petra in assisting Jesus to avoid additional asthmatic episodes.*
- Listen to concerns and provide point-by-point specific answers. *Rationale: Understanding Petra's point of view will enhance collaboration.*

Expected Outcome

- Petra will verbalize support for and participate in the plan of care.

STEP 8: IMPLEMENTATION

Nursing Theory

Jesus is a mixture of two distinct cultures: a Japanese father who embraces modern medicine and insists that his son be in the hospital, and a Hispanic grandmother who feels betrayed by modern medicine and prefers folk care. Jesus' father is supportive of the plan of care, but he is out of the country, leaving Petra to make the health-care decisions. The nursing challenge is to find a way to work with Petra while addressing her concerns and getting buy-in for the plan of care.

Madeleine Leininger, who originally developed transcultural nursing theory, reminds us that it is important to consider the culture of the individual and how it will influence both the care and the outcome. If Petra does not agree to the plan because it is not culturally congruent, it will not be successful and will result in frustration for everyone. It is clear that Petra is frustrated with the care and has become hostile to the staff, which creates a barrier to care. Ernestine Wiedenbach, who developed the *helping art of clinical nursing*, points out that it is the role of the nurse to help the patient. This includes being aware of the reality of care situations that are influenced by factors such as culture, age, and view of health. The reality for Jesus is that Petra does not trust modern medicine because it failed to prevent her daughter's death, and she is afraid of losing her grandson, too. Petra also has a strong cultural belief in folk medicine that will require careful handling. However, the discussions proceed, the nursing care should be professional regardless of personal views, and the nurse should partner with Petra to develop a plan of care, clarify problems, and set mutually acceptable goals and expected outcomes. The goal is to help the family and Jesus in health promotion activities.

Ancillary Support

Social services should be asked to visit Petra to assist in identifying specific concerns and relieve some of her fears. Petra has a strong faith and keeps her rosary with her at all times. Asking the chaplain to see her may assist her in coming to grips with her daughter's death, and thereby become more open to the plan of care for Jesus. Respiratory therapy will need to reinforce the importance of vigilance in providing timely and consistent treatments to resolve the asthma.

STEP 9: PLAN OF CARE

The plan of care is a road map for patient care and should be used as a communication tool between disciplines. Expected entries on the plan of care would be each identified problem (e.g., airway, breathing, and family coping) with corresponding interventions, and expected outcomes, including any information from ancillary health-care providers. Concerns individual to Jesus and his family should also be addressed. In this instance, note should be made of Petra's distrust of the health-care system associated with her daughter's death. The conflict between Petra and Mori regarding how to approach Jesus should be noted along with the understanding that at this time Petra is the primary caregiver. Notation should be made regarding Petra's apparent lack of understanding about how asthma is triggered and how far the education has progressed. Jesus' coping strategy of keeping his teddy bear with him to help stay calm, social services, the chaplain, and respiratory therapy approaches should also be part of the plan.

STEP 10: EVALUATION

Evaluation is an active process in which the nurse "connects the dots" to decide if the expected outcomes (goals) that were established have been met, partially met, or not met. If the goals are met, we continue with the plan as outlined. If the goal was partially met, we revise the parts of the plan that did not work. If the goals were not met, we start all over with a new plan.

End-of-Shift Narrative

At the end of the shift, AJ enters the room to check on Jesus and Petra. *"Good evening, Petra. Jesus, I'm leaving soon and I wanted to check one more time to see how you all are doing."* Jesus grins, "I'm good, I can breathe and talk and I ate almost all of my hamburger and French fries." Jesus holds up his gown pointing, "See my chest doesn't suck in anymore and I don't breathe so fast. I'm not coughing either." AJ smiles at Jesus and says to Petra, *"Jesus' vital signs are improved, his respiratory rate is 20 breaths per minute, his pulse is 90 beats per minute, his BP is 90/60 mm Hg, and his temperature is 98.6°F. His intercostal retractions are gone, his treatments are every 3 hours instead of hourly, and I don't hear any audible wheezing. I agree with Jesus—he is indeed better."* Petra looks fondly at Jesus and says to AJ, "I want to thank you for having the chaplain visit today. She helped me understand that everyone here is trying to help Jesus get better. I was just so afraid of losing him." AJ says, *"I'm glad the chaplain was able to help. We all have the same goal; we want Jesus to get better so that you can take him home."* Petra smiles, "I know that now, thanks for being so patient. Kara from social services came by and told me there is a movie I can watch about asthma. I think that will help." AJ nods, *"Yes of course, I can set that up right away."* Petra sighs in relief, "Thank you!"

Problem Evaluation

In the case of Jesus Taki, airway clearance, effective breathing, and family coping were identified as the primary problems. Have we achieved our expected outcomes (goals), and have they been met? What is our patient's overall status at the end of the shift? Is Jesus improving, is there no change, or is Jesus declining? If our goals were not met, how will we modify the plan(s) to achieve the stated goal(s)?

PROBLEM 1: Airway Clearance. The expected outcome is that Jesus will breathe more easily, as evidenced by decreased respiratory rate and retractions and improved breath sounds, and that Petra will be on board with therapeutic interventions. The goal is met: Intercostal retractions are diminished, the respiratory rate is 20 breaths per minute, and wheezing is decreased.

PROBLEM 2: Breathing. The expected outcome is that the work of breathing will be less with decreasing retractions, nasal flare, and the use of accessory muscles. The goal is met: Assessment shows a diminished use of accessory muscles, decreased fatigue, a decreased respiratory rate of 20 breaths per minute, and Jesus' ability to speak easily and eat lunch.

PROBLEM 3: Family Coping. The expected outcome is that Petra will verbalize support for and participate in the plan of care. The goal is met. Petra has apologized for her obstructive behavior, has felt supported by the chaplain and social services, and is willing to participate in education that will better allow her to care for her grandson's asthma.

Overall Evaluation

Based on the comparison of Jesus' status at the beginning and end of the shift, it is evident that he is improving.

REFERENCES

Beclomethasone Nasal Inhalation, Why is this Medication Prescribed? Retrieved from www.nlm.nih.gov/medlineplus/druginfo/meds/a681047.htm

California Asthma Public Health Initiative. Revised 02/16/2010 Summary of the NAEPP's EPR- National Asthma Education and Prevention Program: Expert Report 3. Guidelines for the diagnosis and management of asthma.. Retrieved from http://www.nhlbi.nih.gov/files/docs/guidelines/asthgdln.pdf

Carroll, C. (2005). Helping your patients manage adult onset asthma. LPN2005, 1(2), 28–31.

Fluticasone Nasal Spray. Why is this medication prescribed. Retrieved from www.nlm.nih.gov/medlineplus/druginfo/meds/a681047.html

George, J. (2011). Nursing theories. The base for professional nursing practice (6th ed.). Upper Saddle River, NJ: Pearson Education.

Gulanick, M., & Meyers, J. (2013). Nursing care plans nursing diagnosis and intervention (8th ed.). St Louis, MO: Mosby.

Holloway, N. (2004). Asthma. In Medical-surgical nursing care planning (4th ed., pp. 259–266). Philadelphia, PA: Lippincott Williams & Wilkins.

LeMone, P., Burke, K., & Baldoff, G. (2011). Medical surgical nursing. Critical thinking in patient care (5th ed.). Upper Saddle River, NJ: Pearson.

Parker, M.E. (2006). Nursing theories and nursing practice (2nd ed.). Philadelphia, PA: F.A. Davis.

Pope, B. (2005). Asthma. LPN2005, 1(2), 32–37.

Rodgers, S. (2008). Asthma. In Medical-surgical nursing care plan (pp. 140–147). Clifton Park, NY: Thomson Delmar Learning.

McCormick, M. (2009, January/February). Boost your asthma IQ. Nursing Made Incredibly Easy, 7(1), 42–52.

http://www.nhlbi.nih.gov/files/docs/guidelines/07_sec3_comp4.pdf

Sims, J. (2006). Asthma. Dimensions of Critical Care Nursing, 25(6), 264–268.

Swearingen, P. (2008). All in one care planning resource (2nd ed.). St Louis, MO: Mosby.

Van Leeuwen, A., & Bladh, M. (2015). Davis's comprehensive handbook of laboratory and diagnostic testing with nursing implications (6th ed.). Philadelphia, PA: F.A. Davis Company.

Wilkinson, J., & Ahern, N. (2009). In Nursing diagnosis handbook (9th ed.). Saddle River, NJ: Prentice Hall.

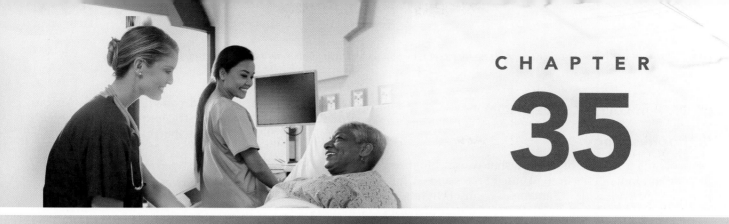

Sensory: Auditory and Ocular

Case Study: Glaucoma

Common Nursing Study Name	Section 1 Study	Section 1 Chapter Number
Complete Blood Count (CBC)	Complete Blood Count, Hematocrit	Chapter 2
	Complete Blood Count, Hemoglobin	Chapter 2
	Complete Blood Count, Platelet Count	Chapter 3
	Complete Blood Count, RBC Count	Chapter 2
	Complete Blood Count, RBC Indices	Chapter 2
	Complete Blood Count, RBC Morphology and Inclusions	Chapter 2
	Complete Blood Count, WBC Count and Differential	Chapter 2
Computed Tomography (CT) of the Head	Computed Tomography, Brain	Chapter 7
Dilated Eye Exam	Slit-Lamp Biomicroscopy	Chapter 18
Electrolytes	Carbon Dioxide	Chapter 1
	Chloride, Blood	Chapter 1
	Potassium, Blood	Chapter 1
	Sodium, Blood	Chapter 1
Fundus Photography	Fundus Photography	Chapter 18
Gonioscopy	Gonioscopy	Chapter 18
Pachymetry	Pachymetry	Chapter 18
Tonometry	Intraocular Pressure	Chapter 18
Visual Acuity Test	Refraction	Chapter 18
Visual Field Testing	Visual Fields Test	Chapter 18

STEP 1: DATA COLLECTION

Pathophysiology

Glaucoma is a disease of the eye that causes blindness in 3 million individuals in the United States and 61 million people worldwide. Glaucoma is caused by an increase of aqueous humor within the eye that increases intraocular pressure (IOP) and damages optic neurons. Glaucoma can be chronic and progressive or acute and emergent. The excess of aqueous humor is due to overproduction or a blockage that prevents aqueous humor outflow. Both result in increased IOP, which is the major cause of glaucoma. Some individuals get glaucoma without an increase in IOP, and we do not know why. Either way, IOP is the focus of treatment in glaucoma.

Aqueous humor is the clear fluid produced in the posterior chamber of the eye by the ciliary body that fills the space between the lens and the cornea. The ciliary body is the circular structure that surrounds the iris. The function of the aqueous humor is to inflate the eye globe while maintaining IOP, provide nourishment to tissues, and remove waste products. The fluid itself is composed of electrolytes, proteins, antibodies, glucose, and antioxidants designed to protect the eye's cornea and lens.

The normal flow of aqueous humor is from the posterior to the anterior chamber of the eye through the pupil and out through the trabecular meshwork (a sieve-like structure made up of tiny channels). From there the aqueous humor flows into the venous bloodstream by way of the canal of Schlemm, where it is absorbed. When this pathway is disrupted or fluid is overproduced, the pressure on the optic disc increases, damaging the optic nerve. The optic nerve is composed of about 1 million nerve fibers whose purpose is to relay visual information from the eye to the brain. When nerve fibers are damaged or die, visual acuity can be permanently altered, including a loss of peripheral vision, the occurrence of blind spots, and the potential for total blindness. Both eyes are usually affected, although the degree may differ a little from eye to eye.

A normal IOP is 10 to 20 mm Hg. The pressure is determined by a combination of resistance to aqueous fluid flow, the rate of fluid production, and the efficiency of outflow drainage. Changes in pressure can occur as a result of diet, exercise, time of day, or medication use. A sustained IOP above 21 mm Hg can contribute to visual field loss.

Risk Factors

Risk factors for development of glaucoma include the following: advancing age, diabetes, cardiovascular disease, myopia, migraines, early-onset menopause, trauma, long-term steroid use, family history, a thin cornea, an increased cup-to-disc ratio, African American or Hispanic ancestry, previous eye surgery, systemic hypertension, and hyperthyroidism.

Types of Glaucoma

There are two types of glaucoma: open angle and angle closure.

OPEN-ANGLE GLAUCOMA: Open-angle glaucoma occurs when the outflow of aqueous humor is restricted by a narrowing at the opening of the trabecular meshwork. Angle-closure or secondary glaucoma is due to an obstruction or occlusion within or on the trabecular meshwork which affects the outflow of aqueous humor. Increased pressure causes the bowing of the peripheral iris so that it blocks the trabecular meshwork. In both cases, aqueous humor fluid is trapped inside the eye, causing IOP to increase.

Open-angle glaucoma is the most common type of glaucoma and accounts for about 90% of all glaucoma cases. In this type of glaucoma, the anterior angle is structurally normal, but the outflow of aqueous humor is hampered by obstruction from degenerative changes of the trabecular meshwork or the canal of Schlemm. An increase of IOP occurs over time with subtle visual changes not noticed by the patient. The risk of optic nerve damage increases with age.

ANGLE-CLOSURE GLAUCOMA: Angle-closure glaucoma, also known as *narrow-angle* or *closed-angle glaucoma*, is less common and is more often seen in acute or subacute situations as may occur in trauma or in older adult women as a chronic condition. This type of glaucoma usually occurs from a forward displacement of the iris. The angle between the iris and cornea (the iridocorneal angle) either narrows or closes from the lens of the eye, enlarging and pushing the iris forward and displacing it. The disruption usually occurs by way of a shallow or closed anterior chamber angle and blockage of the trabecular meshwork. The blockage causes an accumulation of aqueous humor within the eye, resulting in an increased IOP with visual field loss and blindness. Angle-closure glaucoma can be corrected by opening the angle. This type of glaucoma may be seen in only one eye at a time with a risk of development in the other eye.

Signs and Symptoms

Open-angle glaucoma affects both eyes, has very few initial symptoms, and is usually found during a routine eye exam. It is often called the *silent thief of sight* due to the slow loss of peripheral vision associated with irreversible damage to the optic disc. Most people do not notice any loss of vision until the glaucoma is advanced. When looking at the optic disc, there will be an indentation in the center that is called the cup. Damage is evidenced by "cupping" of the optic disc. Cupping is measured as the ratio between the size of the optic cup and the optic disc. Normally, the cup is about one-third the size of the disc. When the cup enlarges, visual field losses can occur. Fundus photography is used to document changes in the optic disc.

Symptoms of open-angle glaucoma start with a gradual loss of peripheral vision, development of tunnel vision, a sense that the individual's eyes are "bothering" her or that she sees halos around lights. There may some complaint about vision being foggy or tired, or of having to change her lens prescription frequently. These visual field changes are a result of nerve damage and permanent vision loss. Open-angle glaucoma cannot be cured, but it may be managed.

The symptoms of acute angle-closure glaucoma are more dramatic and indicate a medical emergency that, if untreated, will result in blindness. Symptoms may be sudden and severe. Individuals may present with eye redness, eye pain, headache, nausea and vomiting, and blurred vision with multicolored, "rainbow-colored halos." The IOP can be as high as 50 mm Hg. Pain severity will increase as the IOP increases. When visualized, the pupil may be fixed or mid-dilated. Dilation of the pupil should be prevented in order to prevent a greater increase in the IOP. Laser iridotomy may be completed to lower the IOP with long-lasting results. This procedure is a revision of the iris with removal of a small portion of the outer edge to allow for the drainage of aqueous humor. Delay in treatment of sustained, elevated IOP can result in varying degrees of permanent vision loss progressing to blindness.

Laboratory Studies

There are no laboratory studies that can diagnose glaucoma.

Diagnostic Studies

The diagnosis of glaucoma is based on a combination of patient history and the results of visual eye exams. Ideally, screening for glaucoma begins before symptoms appear. Recommendations for screening divide individuals into two groups: people with risk factors for glaucoma and those without.

Anyone over the age of 40 is at risk of developing glaucoma. Screenings should be done more often on those with risk factors. Glaucoma screening should be completed for all at-risk individuals at the age of 60. African Americans who are at greater risk should have glaucoma screenings beginning at the age of 40. Repeat screenings should be completed every 1 to 2 years or sooner for those at higher risk without the disease. Those with the disease should have re-screenings based on their disease progression and health-care provider (HCP) recommendation.

Visual Eye Exams

Visual eye exams are the gold standard for examining the eye and diagnosing glaucoma. The following are eye exams that may be completed to assist in the diagnosis of glaucoma.

VISUAL ACUITY TEST: A visual acuity test is used to evaluate how well an individual can see at a distance of 20 feet. This information is compared to what an individual with normal vision would see.

TONOMETRY: Tonometry is a measurement of the IOP. This eye exam is completed by putting anesthetic drops into the eyes and measuring the IOP with a tonometer. A normal reading is 10 to 20 mm Hg. A reading of 22 to 28 mm Hg would be considered elevated, and a reading greater than 35 mm Hg would be a serious finding. Tonometry as part of an eye exam may act as an early indicator of glaucoma and can be used to assess ongoing risk.

GONIOSCOPY: Gonioscopy evaluates the angle or depth between the iris and the cornea to see if the angle is open or closed (the iridocorneal angle). This exam is completed by putting anesthetic drops in the eye and then looking at the eye through a special lens (goniolens, or gonioscope) to get a 360-degree look at the angle. With open-angle glaucoma, the angle will be open. This exam is considered to be the gold standard for diagnosis of angle-closure glaucoma.

DILATED EYE EXAM: A dilated eye exam is used to check the retina, blood vessels, and the optic disc for physical damage. This exam is completed by dilating the eye and using an ophthalmoscope to get a close-up look at the eye.

VISUAL FIELD TESTING: A visual field test evaluates and measures the loss of peripheral vision or blind spots. The test is performed by asking the individual to look at a fixed point and then measuring where vision occurs peripherally.

FUNDUS PHOTOGRAPHY: Fundus photographs can provide a baseline evaluation of the optic disc. The results can be used for later comparison in monitoring the progression of optic disc damage.

PACHYMETRY: Pachymetry is completed by using ultrasound to assess the thickness of the cornea. This test may be used to evaluate ongoing glaucoma risk. Normal corneal thickness is 535 micron to 555 micron.

General/Medical Management

The primary goal of glaucoma treatment is to slow disease progression and preserve as much of the vision as possible. Although increased IOP does not seem to be a factor in all cases of glaucoma, it is the one symptom that responds well to treatment and therefore remains the focus of therapeutic management. The overarching goal is to use medications, surgery, and laser therapy to help maintain eye health. Each approach may be used individually or in combination to decrease the production of aqueous humor, increase the outflow of aqueous humor, or both.

Medication Administration

Medication administration is used first to manage glaucoma by lowering the IOP. Medications are used to decrease the production of or improve the outflow of aqueous humor. Classifications of medications used to treat glaucoma are miotics, mydriatics, adrenergic agonists, nonselective beta blockers, alpha-adrenergic agonists, carbonic anhydrase inhibitors, and prostaglandin analogues.

Miotics such as pilocarpine hydrochloride decrease IOP and increase the outflow of aqueous humor while decreasing its production. Miotic drops are useful to open the angle during an emergent event of angle-closure glaucoma. Some HCPs may avoid the use of miotics because of the detrimental effect on night vision.

Mydriatics such as atropine sulfate decrease IOP by dilating the pupil and blocking the reaction of the iris to cholinergic stimulation. Adrenergic agonists such as epinephrine reduce the production of aqueous humor and increase outflow. Cholinergic drugs such as pilocarpine also increase aqueous humor outflow.

Nonselective beta blockers such as timolol decrease the production of aqueous humor. This class of drugs is often used as an initial treatment modality. However, there may be systemic side effects such as bradycardia, hypotension, and an exacerbation of pulmonary diseases. Therefore, administration is contraindicated in patients with asthma, chronic obstructive pulmonary disease (COPD), second- or third-degree heart block, cardiac failure, or bradycardia.

Alpha-adrenergic agonists such as brimonidine decrease the production of aqueous humor, increase aqueous humor outflow, and lower the IOP somewhat. Carbonic anhydrase inhibitors such as methazolamide can be used in combination with other drugs to decrease the production of aqueous humor. Prostaglandin analogues such as travoprost can increase the outflow of aqueous humor through the ciliary muscle to decease intraocular pressure. Mannitol can act as an emergency drug to treat narrow-angle glaucoma and decrease aqueous fluid production and IOP.

Surgical and Laser Interventions

Surgical or laser interventions consist of laser trabeculoplasty, laser iridotomy, trabeculectomy, or shunt placement.

LASER TRABECULOPLASTY: Laser trabeculoplasty is performed on the angle of the iris to open drainage channels. This is done by burning holes into the trabecular meshwork and widening the canal of Schlemm. Aqueous humor drains out and decreases the IOP. Trabeculoplasty is recommended when medications do not lower the IOP, compliance in medication use is poor, or medications are not tolerated. Trabeculoplasty cannot be used if the physician cannot see the trabecular meshwork. The success rate is about 80%, and this procedure may need to be repeated.

LASER IRIDOTOMY: Laser iridotomy removes the blockage between the iris and the pupil by making several small holes in the iris so that the aqueous humor can drain into the canal of Schlemm. The side effects of this procedure include burns to the cornea, lens, and retina, which may prohibit its use. Iridotomy should not be used if there is any corneal edema, because it would interfere with visualizing and targeting the laser site. Pilocarpine may be prescribed after this procedure to prevent closure of the iridotomy. This is a procedure that may be used to treat angle-closure glaucoma.

TRABECULECTOMY: Trabeculectomy is a surgical procedure designed to create an alternate drainage pathway for the aqueous humor. This is an option used when medications and laser trabeculoplasty have failed. An opening is made by removing part of the trabecular meshwork, allowing the aqueous humor to drain, which decreases the IOP. Prevention of scarring at the surgical site is necessary to prevent closure of the new opening. Medications such as mitomycin (an antimetabolite) may be used during the surgery for this purpose. Possible complications are hemorrhage, an IOP that is too low, inflammation, and drainage failure. Surgery can be repeated if needed.

SHUNT PLACEMENT: Sometimes a very small open tube called a shunt may be placed into the anterior chamber to keep the pathway open, allowing aqueous humor to drain. A shunt is used when repeated trabeculectomies fail.

Postsurgical Interventions

Patients should be taught to avoid activities that may increase IOP. This includes bending at the waist, lifting heavy objects, coughing, vomiting, and bowel strain. Medications should be taken as ordered, and all follow-up appointments should be kept.

Treatment for Open-Angle Glaucoma

Open-angle glaucoma is best treated by a combination of drugs that will both open the pathway for fluid drainage and decrease fluid production. Miotics can be used to increase outflow, and a beta-adrenergic blocker or carbonic anhydrase inhibitor can be used to decrease production. If drops do not work, laser trabeculoplasty can facilitate fluid drainage with more invasive choices as needed.

Treatment for Closed-Angle Glaucoma

The treatment of closed-angle glaucoma is focused on immediately lowering the IOP followed by eye surgery. The type of surgery would be dependent on the clinical presentation. Iridotomy or trabeculectomy is the best choice. The other eye may also be operated on as a preventative measure, as may be seen in chronic conditions. A miotic may be used to move the iris away from the cornea with aqueous humor draining out via lymph spaces, and a carbonic anhydrase inhibitor may be administered to decrease the production of aqueous humor.

Patient Education

Our senses keep us in touch with our world. As educators, we rely heavily on the sense of vision when teaching. Our patients rely heavily on the same sense when learning. Patients with compromised vision will require a very personal approach in discovering alternate ways in which education can be provided. An example is an educational CD that can be given to the patient and listened to when needed. Engaging the family in the learning process is recommended to support the correct use of medications and other treatment modalities. Talk to the patient to find out what kinds of alternative learning methodologies have worked for them in the past. This will provide useful information in making decisions about how to move forward.

STEP 2: POTENTIAL PROBLEM/ DIAGNOSES

It is important that nurses understand and consider the science of the disease process and consider the possibilities prior to applying that knowledge to a patient situation. We begin that process with questioning.

💬 *Question:* Based on your review of the content presented, what possible *potential problems* would you expect for a patient with these diagnoses?

💬 *Answer:* Visual perception, injury, anxiety, and knowledge

STEP 3: POTENTIAL INTERVENTIONS

💬 *Question:* Based on your identification of patient problems, what possible interventions would you recommend for these diagnoses, and what would you expect to happen? This would be considered your "grocery list" of the possible actions you could use to assist your patient.

💬 *Answer:* See the following problems, interventions, and expected outcomes:

Problem	Interventions	Expected Outcome
Visual Perception	• Assess for peripheral vision loss, halos, headache, and poor night vision. • Assess for eye pain. • Orient to the room environment. • Use bright lights and large print in teaching. • Monitor the results of diagnostic tests. • Administer eyedrops; teach the correct technique for eyedrop administration.	The patient will be able to compensate for visual deficiencies.
Injury	• Assess environmental hazards. • Orient the patient to the environment; turn the patient's head from side to side to get the full visual view. • Encourage the use of wall rails; assist with ambulation. • Teach the patient to avoid picking up heavy objects and to place frequently used items within the visual field. • Assess the patient's ability to provide self-care. • Encourage the use of bed side rails.	The patient remains injury free.
Anxiety	• Assess the patient's level of anxiety. • Encourage the patient's verbalization of concerns. • Assess the patient's coping strategies. • Provide information about the disease. • Encourage the patient to consider support groups. • Administer anti-anxiety medication. • Discuss the effects of the disease on the patient's lifestyle	The patient has manageable anxiety

Continued

Table Continued

Problem	Interventions	Expected Outcome
Knowledge	<ul><li>Assess the patient's readiness to learn and the knowledge baseline.</li><li>Create an environment conducive to learning.</li><li>Teach the patient how to instill eye drops.</li><li>Educate the patient about the disease process.</li><li>Explain the purpose of the test and procedures.</li><li>Explain the purpose of regular eye exams.</li><li>Explain the importance of adhering to the medication regime.</li><li>Teach the patient to avoid bending and lifting.</li><li>Teach the patient the symptoms to report to the physician.</li><li>Assess that the patient has the resources to follow the plan of care.</li><li>Provide written detailed instructions regarding eye care and disease process.</li></ul>	The patient verbalizes understanding of disease process and associated treatments.

PUTTING IT ALL TOGETHER: APPLICATION OF THE NURSING PROCESS

Putting it all together is where the art and science of nursing meet to provide the best patient outcomes. We take the possibilities and place them into the context of the patient situation. To accomplish this, we use nursing diagnosis, nursing interventions, nursing outcomes, and nursing theory to provide the palate for nursing care.

STEP 4: ASSESSMENT

PATIENT INFORMATION: A 64-year-old female, Toafa Chun

CHIEF COMPLAINT: Motor vehicle accident

HISTORY OF THE PRESENT ILLNESS: Rear-ended on the freeway and the vehicle rolled over, she was unconscious when paramedics arrived and was admitted for observation.

PAST MEDICAL HISTORY: Hypertension

FAMILY HISTORY: Parents deceased, both died of cardiac arrest in their mid 90s

CHART REVIEW AND REPORT: Toafa Chun was seen in the emergency department (ED) after being involved in a car accident in which she was rear-ended with enough force to cause her car to roll. The teenage driver of the car that hit her died at the scene; it is suspected that he fell asleep at the wheel. When paramedics arrived, Toafa was unconscious with a large laceration to the low forehead. Toafa regained consciousness when she got to the ED. Other than feeling sore with a headache and pain at the laceration site, she denied any other injuries. Lack of brain injury was confirmed by physical examination and a negative computed tomography (CT) scan of the head. Toafa has two black eyes with moderate swelling. Because she was unconscious for almost 30 minutes, Toafa is to be admitted for observation. The physician has requested a consultation with an ophthalmologist just to make sure there are no residual visual problems from the impact. The last set of vital signs is BP of 136/82 mm Hg, a pulse of 96 beats per minute, a temperature of 97.8°F, and respirations of 16 breaths per minute. Neurological assessment is normal. Toafa was given hydrocodone with acetaminophen for head pain rated at 6/10, with relief to a 2/10. The previous nurse reports that Toafa is to be discharged home after being seen by the ophthalmologist. CBC values and electrolytes are normal.

SUBJECTIVE ASSESSMENT: As you enter the room you see Toafa sitting in a chair looking out onto the garden patio. *"Good morning, my name is Arvin James, and I will be your nurse today, how are you feeling"* "Lucky to be alive," replies Toafa with a small smile. "Did you know that that poor boy driving the car died?" *"Yes, I had heard that."* "They told me he was only 16 years old, just got his license last week, his parents must be devastated." *"Did you know him?"* "No, but I have a nephew his age, such a loss." *"Does your head still hurt?"* "A little," admits Toafa. *"On a 0/10 scale how would you rate the intensity of your pain?"* "I think it is still a 2, just enough to know it's there but not too bad." *"What does the pain feel like?"* "Like a nagging headache, the black eyes bother me more. I look like someone hit my face with a bat. I'm glad that the eye doctor will be checking me, I don't want any problems with my eyes." AJ asks, *"Did you know you're to go home after the eye doctor sees you?"* "Yes, I told my cousin that I would give him a call and let him know when to come." *"Is there anything else I can do for you before I go."* "No, I'm fine, thanks." As AJ was leaving the room, the ophthalmologist, Dr. Gerber, arrived to examine Toafa's eyes. During the eye exam AJ notices that Dr. Gerber has a concerned look on his face. He asks her to look straight ahead and tell him when she sees his finger in her peripheral vision. Dr. Gerber's finger is almost to the front of her face before she tells him she sees it. Toafa's peripheral vision is much less than it should be. Dr. Gerber asks, "Have you had any trouble with your vision lately?" "A little," Toafa admits with a frown, "that's why I was so anxious for you to check my eyes. Over the last year I've noticed my eyes bother me. Sometimes at night I see circles around lights at night. I was thinking I might need glasses." While examining her eyes with an ophthalmoscope, it is noted that the cup-to-disc ratio is off. The cup is larger than it should be. These findings are an indication that Toafa has glaucoma. Dr. Gerber tells Toafa and asks her to see him in his office to complete a more in-depth eye exam. Toafa readily agrees, stating "I don't know anything about glaucoma, so I had best learn." When she stands to hug the doctor she trips over the small stool to her left and is saved from falling by Dr. Gerber. Toafa gives a little laugh and says, "Where did that come from?" Dr. Gerber is starting her on latanoprost eyedrops.

OBJECTIVE ASSESSMENT: Toafa is alert and oriented. When standing to move from the chair to the bed, you note that her gait is normal with no evidence of dizziness. The remainder of her neurological assessment is negative. The stitches to her forehead are dry and intact. She has moderate bruising and swelling to both eyes but denies any trouble seeing. Vital signs are a BP of 128/78 mm Hg, a pulse of 88 beats per minute, a temperature of 98.2°F, and respirations of 16 breaths per minute. The pain rating for her head pain remains at a 2/10, and no pain medication is requested.

- *Laboratory Studies:*
  - Hgb 14.8 g/dL
  - Hct 44.8%.
- *Diagnostic Studies:*
  - CT scan of the head: negative
- *Medications:*
  - Hydrocodone with acetaminophen 5 mg PO every 4 hours prn moderate pain rated 5 to 7
  - Acetaminophen 650 mg every 4 hours prn mild pain rated 2 to 4
  - Atenolol 25 mg daily
  - Latanoprost one drop both eyes every night at bedtime

STEP 5: REALITY CHECK: DETOUR AHEAD

Reality Check occurs when the nurse takes a moment to think about individualized patient information that needs to be considered in framing diagnoses and interventions. This information is retrievable from any legitimate source (e.g., family, case management, other nurses, any ancillary, a doctor, etc.). These are the "wrenches" that create challenging situations, such as culture, religion, socioeconomic status, level of education, developmental level, marital status, employment, age, and gender.

Psychosocial History

Toafa is a part of a very large Samoan family and is the Matai (leader) of her family. As such, she is given great respect by her children and grandchildren. This is an obligation she takes very seriously, sometimes to the detriment of her own health. Toafa is known to ignore her own needs in order to serve her family. Currently, she has been using all of her financial resources to assist her uninsured niece, who is in the hospital. As a result, she is at risk for losing her home. The car insurance lapsed, and the young man who caused the accident was also uninsured. Work replaced school early in life; she dropped out of school in the seventh grade. She now lives on Social Security. Toafa is Christian and was on the way to church when the accident occurred.

Critical Thinking Moment

You have just completed the assessment of Toafa and need to make a decision about the patient's *actual* problems and nursing diagnoses based on the data you have collected and the potential problems you identified. Outcomes must be realistic and measurable.

STEP 6: ACTUAL PROBLEMS/ DIAGNOSES

The *first step* in problem identification is to revisit the list of *potential diagnoses* and choose *actual diagnoses* based on the learner's evaluation of the case study information provided. A problem statement must be completed for each identified problem/diagnosis. The actual problems for this case study are visual perception, injury, and knowledge.

STEP 7: PLANNING: ACTUAL INTERVENTIONS

After actual diagnoses have been chosen, it is necessary to evaluate the list of *potential interventions* and choose *actual interventions* that will fit within the patient's reality and meet expected outcomes. Each intervention requires a rationale. Interventions are identified in three categories: (1) assessment, (2) therapeutic, and (3) education.

Diagnostic Statement

Altered visual perception related to aqueous humor buildup and associated with nerve fiber destruction as evidenced by the loss of peripheral vision, optic disc cupping, visual halos, and "seeing funny"

Assessment

- Assess visual ability. *Rationale: This establishes a baseline to guide a plan of care.*
- Assess the need for visual aids. *Rationale: This provides appropriate reading material and enhances self-care.*
- Assess mobility. *Rationale: This acts as a safety baseline assessment.*

Therapeutic Interventions

- Provide information in large print. *Rationale: The patient has stated that small print is hard to read.*
- Encourage Toafa to move her head from side to side. *Rationale: This allows accurate visual scanning of the environment.*
- Assist with mobility as needed. *Rationale: This helps to prevent injury.*

Education

- Educate Toafa about the importance of adequate lighting. *Rationale: This enhances visual acuity.*
- Educate Toafa about the importance of using visual aids. *Rationale: This enhances visual acuity.*
- Provide Toafa with referral information. *Rationale: This provides for ongoing support after discharge.*

Expected Outcome

- Toafa demonstrates the ability to compensate for visual deficiencies.

Diagnostic Statement

The **risk for injury** related to altered visual acuity is evidenced by the patient's tripping over a stool and nearly falling. The patient remarks that she did not see the stool.

Assessment

- Assess the environment for clutter that may increase the risk of injury. *Rationale: The loss of visual acuity can increase fall risk.*
- Assess Toafa's orientation to the environment. *Rationale: Poor orientation can increase injury risk.*
- Assess Toafa's self-care ability. *Rationale: This provides assistance when needed to decrease the risk of injury.*

Therapeutic Interventions

- Orient Toafa to the environment. *Rationale: This awareness can decrease the injury risk.*
- Remove items from traffic areas. *Rationale: This helps prevent falls.*
- Place meal trays and frequently used items within Toafa's reach. *Rationale: This increased accessibility decreases the potential for falls in Toafa's seeking personal items.*

Education

- Educate Toafa that the purpose for asking for assistance is to enhance safety. *Rationale: Understanding promotes collaboration and compliance.*
- Educate Toafa that the purpose for room orientation is to prevent trips and falls. *Rationale: This helps avoid injury.*
- Educate Toafa about the relationship between visual acuity loss and injury risk. *Rationale: This improves compliance with safety measures and decreases injury risk.*

Expected Outcome

- Injury prevention

Diagnostic Statement

A **knowledge deficit** related to altered visual acuity secondary to glaucoma as evidenced by the patient's statement, "I don't know anything about this disease so I had best learn"

Assessment

- Assess Toafa's understanding of latanoprost use. *Rationale: This helps you identify any necessary areas of teaching.*
- Assess Toafa's understanding of visual loss. *Rationale: This helps evaluate her injury risk.*
- Assess Toafa's understanding of the disease process related to continued vision loss and her blindness risk. *Rationale: This decreases the risk of future vision loss.*

Therapeutic Interventions

- Assist in the proper technique to instill latanoprost. *Rationale: Proper technique enhances the effects of the medication.*
- Answer questions about open-angle glaucoma and its long-term effects on vision loss. *Rationale: This emphasizes the importance of adhering to a therapeutic regime to prevent potential blindness.*
- Ask Toafa to describe the prediagnosis symptoms she experienced. *Rationale: In order to prevent increased vision loss, the patient's describing her previous symptoms underscores what may be experienced if glaucoma advances.*

Education

- Provide written material on glaucoma in large print. *Rationale: Large print makes reading with visual deficits easier.*
- Explain the importance of adhering to eye medications relative to disease progression. *Rationale: Agreeing to the therapeutic regime will help preserve visual acuity.*

- Explain the importance of keeping eye appointments. *Rationale: This allows Toafa to look for disease advancement early.*

Expected Outcome

- Verbalizes an understanding of the disease process and treatment methodologies

STEP 8: IMPLEMENTATION

Nursing Theory

Toafa has been diagnosed with a disease that leads to lost vision. Although the eyedrops may help to prevent further vision loss, she will not regain what is already lost. It is essential to discover how the amount of vision already lost affects her ability to care for herself, and identify areas of needed assistance. Dorothea Orem's nursing theory is based on the idea of *self-care* and *self-care deficits. Self-care* is described as what patients can do for themselves. Orem assumes that patients want to care for themselves if they are able to. A *self-care deficit* occurs when a patient is not able to meet her or his own needs and nursing intervention is required. Nursing assistance should be given in an organized manner by diagnosing the problem, creating a plan of care, and using support mechanisms to provide care. Toafa's ability to assist in care is evaluated at each step while deciding whether to provide total assistance, partial assistance, or educational support. Nurses are encouraged to identify needs while giving direction for tasks.

Toafa is at risk for putting responsibilities as the Matai of her family before her own health. Madeleine Leininger recognizes that culture plays a part in health-care decisions. Leininger's theory encourages us to consider how care is given within a cultural context. Nurses need to recognize that peoples of different cultures will have alternative views of health and health practices that may not be congruent with Western ideas. Culturally congruent nursing care will allow care decisions to blend with Toafa's culture, values, beliefs, and ways of living to promote positive outcomes. Because Toafa is here such a short time, this situation can be challenging.

Ancillary Support

Ancillary support should focus on providing information about glaucoma support groups. This can be done by Case Management or Social Services.

STEP 9: PLAN OF CARE

The plan of care is a road map for patient care and should be used as a communication tool between disciplines. Expected entries on the plan of care would be each identified problem (visual perception, injury, and knowledge), intervention, and expected outcome.

There needs to be some notation about Toafa's role within the family and financial status as it may impact her decision. Because she is Christian and very active in supporting her church, contact information for the pastor should be noted. Support in meeting the financial aspects of her care may be assisted by the parish members and may save her eyesight. Because time is limited, this will be a challenge.

STEP 10: EVALUATION

Evaluation is an active process in which the nurse "connects the dots" to decide if the expected outcomes (goals) that were established have been met, partially met, or not met. If the goals are met, we continue with the plan as outlined. If the goal was partially met, we revise the parts of the plan that did not work. If the goals were not met, we start all over with a new plan.

End-of-Shift Narrative

Dr. Gerber has left a prescription for latanoprost eyedrops: 1 drop HS to both eyes for Toafa's glaucoma. AJ has explained how to administer the drops, and Toafa has demonstrated how to correctly instill them. Dr. Gerber has also asked Toafa to see him in his office tomorrow to complete additional eye exams that consist of tonometry, gonioscopy, and fundus photography. AJ gave Toafa this information as part of her discharge instructions. Toafa replies, "Dr. Gerber is a very nice man and I will see him as soon as I can, but I'm not sure that I can do it tomorrow. My niece is in the hospital and needs me to be there. Her mother died last year, and we are very close. I think my eyes will be fine for another few days. I'll use the eyedrops though, that should help." AJ responds by saying, *"It's important to keep your eye appointment. Dr. Gerber needs to take a closer look at your eyes to make sure that the treatment we are giving you is the right one. Would you be able to take a break from visiting your niece in the hospital just long enough to get your eyes checked?"* Toafa pats AJ's hand, "Don't you worry about me, if she is doing OK then, maybe, we'll see how it goes." AJ continues, *"Do you remember what the doctor said about taking time to look around so that you don't fall and hurt yourself like you almost did this morning?"* "Yes, and I will be careful. My mother broke her hip later in her life and she was never able to get around the same anymore. I have too many responsibilities for that, so I will be very careful, that I can promise you." *"I know that I have given you a lot of information about glaucoma. Do you have any questions for me?"* Toafa smiles, "I don't think I have any questions yet. This is all still new to me. I did read what you gave me. If I think of any questions, I'll ask Dr. Gerber when I see him. Thanks for giving me the large print version. I didn't realize I was having so much trouble reading. It really helps, otherwise I would probably just get frustrated and quit." *"Toafa is there anything else I can do for you?"* "Yes," she replies with a laugh, "get the wheelchair so I can get out of here."

Problem Evaluation

PROBLEM 1:   **Altered Visual Perception:** The expected outcome is that Toafa will be able to demonstrate the ability to compensate for her visual deficiencies. The goal is met: Reading materials with large print have allowed Toafa to review information about her newly diagnosed glaucoma. However, Toafa does not seem to be very concerned about her eyes. This could be a problem for the future.

PROBLEM 2:   **Risk for Injury:** The expected outcome is injury prevention. The goal is met: Toafa agreed to scan open areas before walking to make sure that she did not trip over anything else. However, it is difficult to fully evaluate whether or not she will take the necessary precautions at home.

PROBLEM 3:   **Knowledge Deficit:** The expected outcome is Toafa's understanding of the disease process and the treatment methodologies. The goal is met: Toafa has verbalized her understanding of the written material, has successfully demonstrated how to instill her eyedrops, and has noted the importance of seeing Dr. Gerber for follow-up care. Whether or not she will be compliant is in question.

Overall Evaluation

Based on the end-of-shift assessment and the comparison of Toafa's progress during this shift, there is no change.

REFERENCES

Comer, S. (2005). Geriatric nursing care plans (3rd ed.). New York, NY: Delmar.

George, J. (2011). Nursing theories. The base for professional nursing practice (6th ed.). Upper Saddle River, NJ: Pearson Education.

Gulanick, M., & Meyers, J. (2013). Nursing care plans: Nursing diagnosis and intervention (8th ed.). St Louis, MO: Mosby.

Holloway, N. (2004). Medical surgical nursing care planning (4th ed.). Springhouse, PA: Lippincott Williams & Wilkins.

LeMone, P., Burke, K., & Baldoff, G. (2011). Medical surgical nursing, Critical thinking in patient care (5th ed.). Upper Saddle River, NJ: Pearson.

McCann, J. (2006). Lippincott manual of nursing practice (8th ed.). Amber, PA: Lippincott Williams & Wilkins.

McCarren, K. (2009, March/April). The blue haze of glaucoma. Nursing Made Incredibly Easy, 27–36.

Milley, C., & Sharts-Hopko, N. (2009, February). Primary open angle glaucoma catching and treating the sneak thief of sight. American Journal of Nursing, 109(2), 40–47.

Mohn-Brown, E., & Burke, K. (2007). Medical surgical nursing care plans (3rd ed.). Boston, MA: Pearson.

Monk, H. (2007, January/February). Focusing on the aging eye glaucoma and macular degeneration. LPN, 47–54.

National Eye Institute Statement on Detection of Glaucoma and Adult Vision Screening. Retrieved from www.nei.nih.gov /nehep/programs/glaucoma/detection.asp

Rodgers, S. (2008). Medical surgical nursing care plans. Clifton Park, NY: Thomson Delmar.

Sommers, M., Johnson, S., & Beery, T. (2007). Diseases and disorders: A nursing therapeutics manual. Philadelphia, PA: F.A. Davis.

Swearingen, P. (2008). All in one care planning resource (2nd ed.). St. Louis, MO: Mosby.

Tonometry. Retrieved from http://www.nlm.nih.gov/medlineplus /ency/article/003447.htm

Van Leeuwen, A., & Bladh, M. (2015). Davis's comprehensive handbook of laboratory and diagnostic testing with nursing implications (6th ed.). Philadelphia, PA: F.A. Davis Company.

Wilson, B., Shannon, M., & Stang, C. (2006). Nurse's drug guide. Upper Saddle River, NJ: Prentice Hall.

Wilkinson, J., & Ahern, N. (2009). In Nursing Diagnosis Handbook (9th ed.). Saddle River, NJ: Prentice Hall.

INDEX

Note: Page numbers followed by b indicate boxes; f, figures; t, tables/tabular material.

Table for the Practical Application of Nursing Theories

Theorist	Premise	Clinical Application
Florence Nightingale	Theory focus is on manipulation of the environment. Areas of the environment nursing should focus on are ventilation, warmth, light, noise, bed and bedding, cleanliness and nutrition. Nightingale's theory instructs nurses to evaluate the environment surrounding the patient and make any necessary adjustments based on the patient's response to said environment. Nursing should assist the patient to find balance, prevent unnecessary expenditures of energy, and allow nature to take its course to promote health.	Evaluate the patient's environment. Ask the question, "what specific environmental changes need to be made to improve patient outcomes?" An example would be using a specialty bed for a patient with pressure ulcers. Hand washing remains a key component of environmental safety.
Hildegard Peplau	Focus is on development of an interpersonal relationship between patient and nurse. The purpose of the relationship is to create a collaborative atmosphere to identify patient problems, and health-care goals. Conflict is possible when there is disagreement on how to proceed. Development of the relationship is viewed as sequential: (1) *orientation*, getting to know each other; (2) *identification*, clarification of expectations within the nurse-patient relationship; (3) *exploitation*, patient makes demands for and takes advantage of all available services; and (4) *resolution*, patient needs have been met through collaborative efforts and the relationship is terminated. Various roles can be assumed by the nurse during each phase: (1) *teacher*, imparting knowledge; (2) *resource*, providing information; (3) *counselor*, assisting in problem resolution; (4) *leader*, providing direction; (5) *technical expert*, provision of physical care; and (6) *surrogate*, taking the place of another. Personal and professional growth is a benefit of the relationship.	Talk to your patient. Partner with them to clarify problems, set mutually acceptable goals, and determine expected outcomes. Both the patient and the nurse learn and grow from the interaction.
Virginia Henderson	Focus is on activities required to maintain health, recover from illness, or have a peaceful death. Henderson was among the first to suggest the importance of explicit expected outcomes. Her original outcomes list consists of • Breathe normally, eat and drink adequately, eliminate body wastes • Move and maintain desirable postures, sleep and rest, dress and undress with suitable clothing • Maintain body temperature within normal range by adjusting clothing and environment • Keep body clean and well groomed, skin protected, and safe from environmental dangers • Communicate needs, emotions, fears, and opinions, and worship according to one's faith • Participate in forms of recreation, appropriate use of health facilities • Verbalize health promotion activities Nurses are to work with the patient to create a therapeutic relationship and do for the patients what they cannot do for themselves. The goal is to move the patient from a dependant to independent state. Consideration should be given to working with an interdisciplinary team to achieve goals while maintaining the professional nursing role.	Nurses should assist the patient in meeting their basic care needs while encouraging them to become independent. The relationship between the nurse and patient helps to facilitate this process. Nurses should use ancillaries as needed to meet nursing goals. It is important to identify expected outcomes in relation to interventions and planned care.
Lydia Hall	View of nursing is based on the concept of interlocking circles of *core, cure,* and *care* as dynamic interrelated aspects of nursing care. *Core* is focused on assisting the patient to use reflection as a means of making health-care choices and lifestyle changes to promote health. *Cure* views the nurse as the patient advocate during implementation of prescribed therapies. Hall recognizes that there are times the nurse may be a source of pain and discomfort for the patient. *Care* is considered to be specific to nursing and directs the nurse to assist the patient in meeting his or her basic needs in a nurturing environment. The overall emphasis of this theory is a total person approach to care.	Nurses are to nurture the patient and assist him or her to think about what the patient can do to improve his or her health. Nurses are to carry out physician orders. Goals can be completed independently by the nurse or with the assistance of ancillaries.

Theorist	Premise	Clinical Application
Dorothea Orem	Construct centers on the notion of *self-care* and *self-care deficits*. *Self-care* is described as what the patient can do for himself or herself. Orem assumes that patients want to care for themselves if they are able to. A *self-care deficit* occurs when the patient is not able to meet his or her own needs and nursing intervention is required. Age is a consideration as Orem views adults as independent, and children, infants, aged, and ill as requiring assistance. *Self-care agency* is the ability and willingness of the patient to perform activities independently of the nurse for his or her own benefit. *Nursing systems/agency* is viewed as tasks the nurse performs for the benefit of the patient. Assistance is provided in an organized manner: (1) diagnoses and prescription of the patient's problem, (2) design of nursing systems and plan for delivery of care, and (3) production and management of nursing systems. Methods of assisting in care include acting, doing, guiding, directing, physical and psychological support, personal development, and teaching. The patient's ability to assist in care is evaluated at each step in the process and may be identified as providing total assistance (wholly compensatory), partial assistance (partly compensatory), or support and education (supportive-educative) to achieve the nursing goal. Nurses are encouraged to identify patient needs and give direction for tasks to be performed.	Can the patient care for himself or herself, or does the patient need help? If the patient needs help, what kind of help is required? Does the patient require total assistance, partial assistance, or is he or she independent? Always consider the patient's age, gender, general health, developmental level, family, sociocultural factors, lifestyle, and availability of resources in planning care. Use a systematic approach to care such as problem identification, plan of care, implementation of plan, and evaluation. The level of the patient's ability to assist in his or her own care will indicate the amount of support required by the nurse to achieve stated goals.
Dorothy E. Johnson	The basic principle of this theory is that people develop a set of behaviors that are unique to them as individuals. An individual's behavioral pattern determines how they react to/interact with environment, stress, illness, objects, and events. Patients' behavioral interactions are categorized in designated subsystems: (1) attachment, social intimacy/bonds; (2) dependency, seeking nurturing and approval; (3) ingestive, biological intake and output; (4) eliminative, excretion of wastes; (5) sexual, procreation; (6) aggressive, protection and self-preservation; and (7) achievement, personal accomplishment. Nursing intervention is needed when there are discrepancies, insufficiencies, and incompatibilities between systems or dominance of one system over the other.	The patient is an individual with specific behavioral patterns. Identification of behavioral patterns will make it easier to successfully plan care. The nurse may need to modify the patient behavior to achieve identified goals. Patient/nurse collaboration is limited. Care is nurse driven, focusing on the nurse designing and implementing activities to meet the patient's needs.
Ida Jean Orlando	The focus of this theory is on the nurse-patient relationship and recognizing the patient as an individual. Orlando gives consideration to the thoughts and perceptions of the nurse in relation to patient care, and encourages nurses to base their practice upon critical thinking rationale and not on specified protocols. The nurse is seen as directly responsible to ensure that the patient's needs are met by their own actions or by the assistance of others. *Orlando's theory moves nursing from being the handmaiden of the physician to being the advocate for the patient.* Leadership and supervision in the health-care setting are viewed as part of the nursing role. Nurses are encouraged to evaluate patient behavior in planning effective care. Behavior may be *verbal* in the form of complaints, requests, or questions, and *nonverbal* in the form of fear, crying, yelling, or laughter. Ineffective patient behavior may hinder the nurse-patient relationship and delay appropriate interventions. Nursing perceptions in relation to patient behavior stimulate a nursing reaction which is acted upon after patient verification.	Think critically about what you are doing and why. Talk to the patient about the goals of the day, or goals of the shift. Plan with the patient how those goals will be met. Take body language into consideration with every patient interaction as well as the spoken word. If tasks are delegated, it is the nurses' responsibility to follow up on those tasks. Evaluation is ongoing, and success of a plan is based upon observable outcomes.

Continued

Theorist	Premise	Clinical Application
Faye Glenn Abdellah	The focus of this theory is on the nurse's ability to identify and solve nursing problems. Health is perceived as prevention and rehabilitation with wellness as the goal. Nursing problems could be covert, meaning difficult to perceive such as emotional issues. Problems could be overt, meaning an obviously apparent condition. Both types of problems could be interrelated, and solving one may solve the other. *The goal of this theory is to move away from medical diagnoses and into the concept of nursing diagnoses.* The approach to problem solving is systematic and similar to nursing process. The assumption is that correct identification of patient problems will guide the nurse to correct choices of interventions and positive outcomes. This theory is strongly nurse centered and nurse directed. Although Abdellah specifically identified 21 potential problems, this premise has been significantly expanded with the current definition of Nursing Diagnoses.	Identify patient problems, and create nursing diagnoses. Consider both emotional and physical problems associated with the diagnosis. Develop a plan of action based on problem identification. Evaluate and revise the problems and interventions as appropriate. Recognize that emotional and physical problems may be interrelated.
Ernestine Wiedenbach	Considers nursing to be a process of *nurture* and *care* for another in a motherly fashion. Nurses are to be sensitive to the nuances in care situations and look for inconsistencies that may indicate a problem. Emphasis is placed on the nurse as a professional person in his or her own right. Nurses are to inspire confidence, and have a practice philosophy of care, compassion, and selfless service to others. Nurses also need to recognize the reality in care situations, be aware of their own limitations, and have an expected outcome in mind as part of the overall plan. Nursing is an active deliberate process and not a passive one.	The role of the nurse is to help the patient. Be aware of the realities of care situations such as culture, age, and view of health. Care should be compassionate with emotional support when facing health issues. Identify expected outcomes and use them as a measure of success. Also be aware that nursing care should be professional regardless of personal views.
Myra Levine	Emphasis of this theory is on *individualized* patient care, and taking care of someone in need. Patients seeking assistance will become dependent on the care provider, requiring adaptation to the immediate situation. It is important for the patient to conserve energy during this process to help to regain and maintain homeostasis. Nurses can assist in energy conservation by focusing on the individual and helping the individual *"keep it together"* during the health-care experience. Nursing care will engage the patient as a partner so as to maintain individual integrity. Nursing should support the healing process, the individual's self-worth, and societal identification. Consideration needs to be given to the patient's community connections such as ethnicity, religion, vocation, education, and socioeconomic status.	Provide care when needed. Partner with the patient or family to promote healing and conserve energy in order to regain and maintain pre-illness levels of health. Ask questions like what works and what does not for problems such as pain. Care provided needs to include consideration of cultural and societal identification.
Imogene King	Focus of care is on *partnering* with the patient within the health-care environment to achieve goals. For this to be successful, nurses need to work within the patient's reality. The definition of reality is whatever the patient says it is. Within the definition of an individual's reality are the concepts of growth and development, body image, personal space, learning, and time orientation. Face-to-face communication is an essential part of providing care. Communication can be verbal or nonverbal. The relationship between patient and nurse is progressive and moves from meeting as strangers to mutual goal setting and goal attainment. The patient has the right to be involved in his or her own care decisions. Nurses have the responsibility to provide information that will allow the patient to make informed decisions.	Recognize that the nurse and patient meet as strangers and need to develop a relationship where it is possible to set mutually acceptable goals. Goal setting should be done within the patient's reality to be successful. For example, one person's reality may be as a homeless individual who is alone versus an employed individual who has a family. Each situation will require careful consideration in provision of care. Consider verbal and nonverbal cues when providing and evaluating care. Provide clear information to facilitate informed decisions and consent.

Theorist	Premise	Clinical Application
Martha Rogers	People are dynamic entities that interact with the environment and are in a constant state of change. Rogers calls this the *principles of hemodynamics*. Environment is explained as anything external to the patient, including the nurse. Interaction with the environment is an association that is mutual, continuous, and to the benefit of the individual's personal growth. The interaction of individual and environment is rhythmical and innovative with diverse and complex outcomes. The goal of the nurse is to work within the patient's environment and participate in the change process in a way that will have positive outcomes. Nurses are to partner with the patient, not do to the patient. The primary focus is to view the patient as a whole which would include the patient, and the patient's current and past environment.	Nursing care is a dynamic living process of interaction with patient and environment. Nurses partner with the patient to create a plan of care. Thought needs to be given to the whole patient, not just what the patient was admitted for. Care should be individualized. Nurses need to be aware of external forces that can affect the patient such as family, job, hospital culture, and more. An accurate patient history and evaluation of current events are important in providing care and achieving outcomes.
Callista Roy	Roy views the individual as a dynamic entity who interacts with and *adapts* to a changing environment. Learning to cope with this process is an integral part of the theory. Coping could be purposeful on the part of the patient or it could be physiological such as a response to infection, or therapeutic interventions. Some coping mechanisms are learned and some are intuitive. Roy focuses on patient responses and nurse's evaluation of those responses. Responses could be observed by the nurse, reported to the nurse by the patient, or intuitively perceived. Stressors could be internal or external in origin. Stressors are defined as focal, contextual, or residual stimulus. A focal stressor originates with the individual and is anything that has the greatest impact on the person. Contextual stimuli are additional factors that contribute to the situation with positive or negative results. Residual stimuli are anything else that may or may not have an effect on the situation. Roy also views coping mechanisms as *"regulator,"* meaning the adaptive physiologic response to an event, or *"cognator,"* individual choices made which will impact the outcome. Roy reminds us that people will learn from experience and use that information to adapt to future events.	Assess the patient's coping mechanisms and check on how they are adapting to their health-care situation. An example would be evaluating response to a new diagnosis such as diabetes. Is the patient responding to learning about the disease and is the patient coping with the required lifestyle changes? Monitor diagnostic tests to evaluate the physiological response to illness and therapeutic modalities. Subjective and objective assessment of the patient is an important part of care. Nurses should give credence to their intuitive perceptions in providing care. Patient outcomes can be affected by stressors. Nurses should try to identify the stressors and address them. The nursing goal is to promote and support adaptive responses.
Betty Neuman	Neuman's theory focuses on the individual and his or her *reaction to stress* within the environment. The basic premise of the theory is a set of barriers that protect the core of the individual. The individual is defined as a person, family, community, or any part thereof. The defending barriers are named *lines of resistance, normal line of defense,* and *flexible line of defense*. As each barrier is breached, the individual's risk of serious problems increases. This theory promotes the concept of primary, secondary, and tertiary levels of care. *Primary* prevention focuses on reducing the possibility of illness and strengthening overall health. *Secondary* prevention is early diagnosis and treatment of illness. *Tertiary* prevention assists the patient to regain and maintain stability, adapt to health changes, and provide re-education to decrease the risk of future occurrences. To promote optimal health, it is important to view the patient holistically. This requires evaluation of the patient at the psychological, psychosocial, sociocultural, developmental, and spiritual levels.	This is applicable at all levels of nursing practice. The nurse would consider how to assist the patient to return to baseline health status by accurate assessment, interventions, and evaluation. The nurse is the link between the patient and the environment. Levels of care should be used to promote the best outcome.

Continued

Theorist	Premise	Clinical Application
Josephine Paterson and Loretta Zderad	These theorists take *an existential humanistic* approach to health care and explore the *"meaning"* of the experience from the point of view of the nurse and patient. This "meaning" will be a personal lived experience to those involved colored by their own worldview. The goal of the nurse is to comfort and nurture another in time of need. Recognizing the relationship between the art and science of nursing is essential in promoting positive outcomes. The mutuality of the relationship should promote responsible choices and healing.	Nurses need to recognize that they come to the bedside with their own set of values which are separate from the patient, and will have an impact on the care given. Nurses need to find a way to create a reciprocal relationship that will nurture the patient and promote health. Artistic application of scientific principles is important to this process.
Jean Watson	The essence of this theory is the *science of caring*. The nurse and patient work within the framework of a caring relationship to promote health changes. Watson characterizes carative factors as <ul><li>Presence of a humanistic-altruistic value system</li><li>Instillation of faith-hope</li><li>Presence of a help-trust relationship</li><li>Promotion/acceptance of positive/negative feelings</li><li>Use of scientific problem solving</li><li>Promotion of interpersonal teaching-learning</li><li>Presence of a supportive environment</li><li>Assistance with the gratification of needs</li></ul> Watson allows for the existence of existential forces as the building blocks of her theory. Encourages nurses to focus on the patient using the best information available to them.	Speaks to the importance of evidence-based practice in promoting positive outcomes. The nurse should work as a partner with the patient in a caring and nurturing manner. There is recognition of the spiritual aspect of individuals in relation to care. As a result, the person, rather than the technology, is the focus of care. This relationship allows the nurse the opportunity for personal and professional growth.
Rosemarie Parse	Conceptualizes the *"Human"* experience as a process of *"Becoming."* The *"Human"* experience involves choice and accountability. Choices made may offer new opportunity while at the same time close the door on others. Humans coexist within their environment and universe in a process of give and take. Humans have untold potential that may be revealed over time. *"Becoming"* is a process of human unfolding, experiencing life, relating value priorities, and being one with the universe. Parse believes in being open to the possibilities. Clinically Parse asks nurses to be accountable for their actions, be competent, use nursing theory, embrace the new, and take pride in their job. In interpersonal relationships, Parse asks nurses to respect differences in views, value the other as a human presence, be respectful, appreciate the mystery of life and discovery, and recognize the moments of joy in the struggle of living.	The nurse's role is to guide the patient to make good choices and to respect his or her decisions. Ultimately, the patient is responsible for the choices made and will have to live with the consequences. The nurse needs to make sure the patient has all the pertinent information so that informed choices can be made. Nurses should be open to *"new ways"* of nursing. Always look at the patient as a person, never as an object.
Helen Erickson, Evelyn Tomlin, and Mary Ann Swain	*Modeling and Role-Modeling* is a patient-centered approach to nursing. Modeling is defined as developing an understanding of the patient's world; role-modeling is defined as facilitating health. The goal of nursing is to promote trust, positive orientation, perceived control, and strengths, and set mutual goals that are self-directed. Nurses are to assist the patient to provide self-care. This would include knowing and understanding his or her own personal health as well as having insight into available internal and external strengths and support in planning self-care implementations. This theorist considers attachment and separation from a significant other as a motivating factor. How well an individual copes with his or her situation will have an impact on the individual's ability for self-care.	Focus of care should always be on the individual, not on the nurse, the care, or the disease. Plan of care and interventions should be individualized to the patient. Engage the patient and find out what the patient thinks is the best way to promote his or her own health. Then partner with the patient to get it done. Acceptance of the patient is unconditional and nonjudgmental. Consideration should be given to how the patient's personal relationships affect care.